CONTENTS

Evolve®

YOU'VE JUST PURCHASED

MORE THAN A TEXTBOOK!

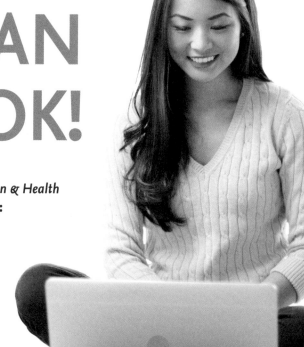

Evolve Student Resources for *Jarvis: Physical Examination & Health Assessment, Third Canadian Edition,* include the following:

- Animations
- Assessment Videos
- Bedside Assessment Summary Checklists
- Case Studies
- Complete Physical Examination Form
- Examination Review Questions
- Health Promotion Guides
- Key Points
- Review Questions
- Physical Examination Summary Checklists
- Quick Assessments for Common Conditions
- Review Questions

Activate the complete learning experience that comes with each textbook purchase by registering at

http://evolve.elsevier.com/Canada/Jarvis/examination/

REGISTER TODAY!

ELSEVIER

2018v1.0

PHYSICAL EXAMINATION
& HEALTH ASSESSMENT

JARVIS

PHYSICAL EXAMINATION & HEALTH ASSESSMENT

THIRD CANADIAN EDITION

Carolyn Jarvis, PhD, APN, CNP
Professor of Nursing
School of Nursing
Illinois Wesleyan University
Bloomington, Illinois
Family Nurse Practitioner
Bloomington, Illinois

Original Illustrations by
Pat Thomas, CMI, FAMI
East Troy, Wisconsin

Assessment Photographs by
Kevin Strandberg
Professor of Art
Illinois Wesleyan University
Bloomington, Illinois

CANADIAN EDITORS

Annette J. Browne, RN, PhD
Professor & Distinguished University Scholar
School of Nursing
University of British Columbia
Vancouver, British Columbia

June MacDonald-Jenkins, RN, BScN, MSc
Dean, School of Health, Human & Justice Studies
Loyalist College
Belleville, Ontario

Marian Luctkar-Flude, RN, PhD
Assistant Professor
School of Nursing
Queen's University
Kingston, Ontario

ELSEVIER

ELSEVIER

PHYSICAL EXAMINATION & HEALTH ASSESSMENT, THIRD CANADIAN EDITION

Copyright © 2019 Elsevier Inc. All rights reserved.

Copyright © 2014 Elsevier Canada, a division of Reed Elsevier Canada, Ltd. Copyright © 2012, 2008, 2004, 2000, 1996, 1993 by Saunders, an Imprint of Elsevier Inc.

Adapted from *Physical Examination & Health Assessment,* 7th edition, by Carolyn Jarvis. Copyright © 2016 by Elsevier, Inc. All rights reserved. ISBN: 978-1-4557-2810-7.

This adaptation of *Physical Examination & Health Assessment,* 7th edition by Carolyn Jarvis is published by arrangement with Elsevier and has been undertaken by Elsevier Inc. at its sole responsibility.

Notices

Library of Congress Control Number: 2018959772

ISBN: 978-1-77172-154-7
Ebook ISBN: 978-1-77172-155-4

VP Education Content: Kevonne Holloway
Content Strategist, Canada Acquisitions: Roberta A. Spinosa-Millman
Senior Content Development Specialist: Heather Bays
Publishing Services Manager: Julie Eddy
Project Manager: Abigail Bradberry
Copy Editor: Claudia Forgas
Design Direction: Maggie Reid

Printed in Canada

1 2 3 4 5   22 21 20 19 18

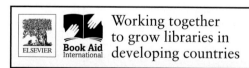

To Paul, who read every word, with love and thanks
Carolyn Jarvis

The work and ideas I have contributed are dedicated to Rachel Browne,
Don Browne and Eva Minkoff, who instilled in me values of social justice.
Annette J. Browne

My work in this edition is dedicated in memory of my brother Dan,
much loved and missed.
June MacDonald-Jenkins

My work on this book is dedicated with love to Richard,
for your patience and support and all that you do. PYZ.
Marian Luctkar-Flude

ABOUT THE AUTHOR

Carolyn Jarvis received her BSN cum laude from the University of Iowa, her MSN from Loyola University (Chicago), and her PhD from the University of Illinois at Chicago, with a research interest in the physiologic effect of alcohol on the cardiovascular system. She has taught physical assessment and critical care nursing at Rush University (Chicago), the University of Missouri (Columbia), and the University of Illinois (Urbana), and she has taught physical assessment, pharmacology, and pathophysiology at Illinois Wesleyan University (Bloomington).

Dr. Jarvis is a recipient of the University of Missouri's Superior Teaching Award; has taught physical assessment to thousands of baccalaureate students, graduate students, and nursing professionals; has held 150 continuing education seminars; and is the author of numerous articles and textbook contributions.

Dr. Jarvis has maintained a clinical practice in advanced practice roles—first as a cardiovascular clinical specialist in various critical care settings and as a certified family nurse practitioner in primary care. She is currently a Professor at Illinois Wesleyan University; is a nurse practitioner in Bloomington, Illinois; and is licensed as an advanced practice nurse in the state of Illinois. During the last 8 years, her enthusiasm has focused on using Spanish language skills to provide health care in rural Guatemala and at the Community Health Care Clinic in Bloomington. Dr. Jarvis has been instrumental in developing a synchronous teaching program for Illinois Wesleyan students both in Barcelona, Spain, and at the home campus.

ABOUT THE CANADIAN EDITORS

Annette J. Browne's career began as an outpost nurse, living and working in northern First Nations and Inuit communities in Canada. She holds a master's degree as a family nurse practitioner from the University of Rhode Island and a PhD in nursing from the University of British Columbia (UBC). Dr. Browne is a professor at the UBC School of Nursing and has taught advanced health assessment to nurse practitioners and post-RNs for many years. Dr. Browne is an active researcher who focuses on health and health care inequities, with a particular focus on fostering health equity with Indigenous peoples. She conducts research on strategies to improve care in primary health care settings and emergency departments, cultural safety, women's health, and health equity interventions to improve health outcomes. By working in partnership with policy leaders, leaders in the health care sector, and clinicians at the point of care, her work is aimed at closing the health equity gap through improvements in health care delivery and policy.

June MacDonald-Jenkins began her career as an outpost nurse working with Indigenous populations in Northern Ontario. She then went to work for over 20 years in a variety of acute care and specialty environments. June holds an undergraduate in nursing from Laurentian University and a Master from McMaster. She is a recognized expert in hybrid course delivery e-learning, having worked in this field for many years. Over 15 years' experience as a nursing professor in the Durham College/University of Ontario Institute of Technology (UOIT) BScN program, Ms. MacDonald-Jenkins brings strong education experience to the team. She has taught health assessment to thousands of students, from those enrolled in diploma to advanced practice programs. She is currently the Dean of Health, Human and Justice Studies at Loyalist College in Belleville, Ontario. Ms. MacDonald-Jenkins's research interests are primarily in the areas of assessing core competencies across curriculum, simulation, and continuous improvement in education through alternative delivery methodologies. Ms. MacDonald-Jenkins has presented across the country to numerous nursing faculties and internationally on the concept of creating engaging hybrid learning environments. She is a faculty member with SIM_One–Ontario Simulation Network focusing on the enhancement of e-Learning strategies.

Marian Luctkar-Flude received her BScN and MScN from the University of Ottawa, her critical care nursing diploma from St. Lawrence College (Kingston), and her PhD from Queen's University (Kingston). She has over 20 years' medical–surgical nursing experience, and over 15 years' experience as an educator. She is now an Assistant Professor at Queen's University School of Nursing where she has taught Nursing Health Assessment and Nursing Research, and currently teaches Medical Surgical Nursing and the Project in Evidence-Based Practice courses. She has expertise in clinical simulation and curriculum development, and was the recipient of the International Nursing Association for Clinical Simulation and Learning (INACSL) 2016 Excellence in Research Award. Her educational research interests include use of simulation in undergraduate nursing education, interprofessional education, and virtual simulation games, and her clinical research interests include breast cancer survivorship care, neurofeedback for postcancer cognitive impairment, and knowledge translation interventions for primary care providers and cancer survivors.

Dana S. Edge, RN, PhD
The co-contributor to Chapter 2: Health Promotion in the Context of Health Assessment, Dana Edge received a BSN from the University of Iowa, a MSN in primary care from the University of North Carolina at Chapel Hill, and a doctorate degree in epidemiology from the University of Toronto. Dr. Edge practised nursing in Minnesota, Colorado, Alaska, and North Carolina before moving to Newfoundland and Labrador in 1986. As a full-time faculty member, she taught health assessment between 1986-2007 to Outpost nursing students at Memorial University of Newfoundland, to undergraduate students at the University of Northern British Columbia, and to both undergraduate and graduate students at the University of Calgary. In addition to her university responsibilities, she was a relief nurse in nursing stations in Labrador and in a rural hospital in northern British Columbia. In 2007, Dr. Edge joined Queen's University, School of Nursing, in Kingston, Ontario, where she is currently an associate professor.

Dianne Groll, RN, PhD
The co-contributor for Chapter 31, Functional Assessment of the Older Adult, is an Associate Professor and Research Director in the Department of Psychiatry at Queen's University. Her research interests include factors affecting physical function and quality of life, and the impact of comorbid illness on patient outcomes.

Lynn Haslam, RN (EC), MN
The contributor for Chapter 10, pain Assessment, Lynn Haslam is Nurse Practitioner who currently works at the Sunnybrook Hospital in Toronto and is engaged in doctoral studies at Queen's University. She is one of the first graduates of the Canadian NP in Anesthesia Certificate program through the Lawrence S Bloomberg faculty of Nursing, where she is an adjunct lecturer. lecturer.

Barbara Wilson Keates, RN, PhD
The co-contributor for Chapter 17, Nose, Mouth and Throat, is an Academic Coordinator in the Faculty of Health Disciplines at Athabasca University. She has over 25 years' experience in adult medicine and cardiac and critical care nursing, and has assisted with the development and implementation of clinical simulation in undergraduate nursing programs in Ontario and Alberta.

Laraine Michalson, RN, MSN
The co-contributor for Chapter 7: Substance Use and Health Assessment, Laraine Michalson has worked as a nurse at the Sheway Program, since 1998. Sheway is a community-based, pregnancy outreach program in the Downtown Eastside of Vancouver. The interdisciplinary team provides health and social services to women with substance use issues during pregnancy and after. The care and services provided to these families are based on harm-reduction and trauma-informed practices. The focus of the program is to help women have healthy pregnancies and positive parenting experiences. Laraine is also an Adjunct Professor at the University of British Columbia School of Nursing.

Andrea Miller, RD, MHSc
Andrea Miller graduated with honours from Ryerson University's undergraduate program in human nutrition and her Master's degree in Health Sciences at the University of Ontario Institute of Technology, in Oshawa. Andrea has worked in a wide range of dietetic practice settings, including Family Health Teams, Long Term Care, Teaching and Community hospitals. Andrea was on the Board of Directors of Dietitians of Canada from 2011-2014, she has been a National Media spokesperson for Dietitians of Canada and she is Co-chair of two provincial Nutrition Networks, for the profession.

Victoria Smye, RN, PhD
The contributor to Chapter 6: Mental Health Assessment, Victoria (Vicki) Smye is faculty and the director of the Arthur Labatt School of Nursing, Faculty of Health Sciences, at Western University. Vicki began on an academic career path after over 20 years in clinical practice, primarily in mental health. Currently Vicki's program of research is focused on addressing health and social inequity (e.g., stigma and discrimination, violence, poverty and homelessness) in the area of mental health and Indigenous health. The aim of her research is to promote culturally safe, effective mental health policy and practice. Currently, Vicki is completing a study entitled, Aboriginal Men's Health Narratives: Reclaiming our Lives. In addition, she has co-led and been a co-investigator on several studies, including health equity research in primary health care. Also, at this time, Vicki is a co-investigator on a study examining an intervention for health enhancement and living (iHeal) for women who have left an abusive partner.

Christina Vaillancourt, RD, CDE, MHSc
The co-contributor for Chapter 12: Nutritional Assessment and Nursing Practice, Christina Vaillancourt is a Registered Dietitian and Certified Diabetes Educator. Christina completed her undergraduate degree in Foods and Nutrition at Ryerson University and a Masters of Health Science at the University of Ontario Institute for Technology. She has taught nutrition at Georgian College, Durham College and the University Of Ontario Institute Of Technology. Her work experience includes acute care, long-term care, ambulatory care, health care management and health policy.

Colleen Varcoe, RN, PhD
The contributor to Chapter 3: Cultural and Social Considerations in Health Assessment and Chapter 8: Interpersonal Violence Assessment, and the co-contributor to Chapter 7: Substance Use and Health Assessment, Colleen Varcoe teaches at undergraduate and graduate levels with a focus on culture, ethics, inequity, and policy at the University of British Columbia. Her research focuses on violence and inequity, with an emphasis on the intersections between interpersonal violence (including intimate partner violence) and structural forms of violence (such as systemic racism, poverty and multiple types of stigma, including stigma related to gender, mental health problems and substance use). Her program of research is aimed at promoting ethical practice and policy in the context of violence and inequity. She recently completed a study of a health care intervention for Indigenous women who have experienced violence and is now co-leading a randomized control trial of the intervention for Indigenous and non-Indigenous women. She recently co-led an intervention study to promote equity in primary health care and is currently leading a test of the same intervention in Emergency settings.

Ellen Vogel, RD, FDC, PhD
The co-contributor for Chapter 12: Nutritional Assessment and Nursing Practice, Ellen Vogel is an associate professor in the faculty of Health Sciences at the University of Ontario institute of Technology. Dr. Ellen Vogel completed an undergraduate degree in Foods and Nutrition from the University of Manitoba in Winnipeg in 1975; a Master of Health Education degree from the University of Manitoba in 1985; and a PhD in Nutrition and Metabolism from the University of Alberta 2001. She is a fellow with Dietitians of Canada; a past chair of the Dietitians of Canada's Board of Directors; and the recipient of numerous awards for leadership and innovation in dietetic practice.

Nancy Watts, RN, MN, PNC (C)
The co-contributor for Chapter 30, Pregnancy, is a Clinical Nurse Specialist, Women's and Infant's Program at Sinai Health Care in Toronto, Ontario, with a focus on family-centered care around labour, birth and postpartum. She is a past President of the Canadian Association of Perinatal and Women's Health Nurses, and has authored several chapters on pregnancy and high risk labour and birth.

Erin Wilson, NP(F), MSN, PhD
The contributor for Chapter 18: Breasts and Regional Lymphatics, Erin Wilson is a family nurse practitioner and assistant professor at the University of Northern British Columbia. Her undergraduate degree is from the University of Manitoba, her MSN from the University of British Columbia, and completed her doctorate in Interdisciplinary Health Sciences at the University of Northern British Columbia. Her clinical practice is in primary care and she has worked in rural, remote, and urban locations in Manitoba, British Columbia, and the Yukon. She teaches health assessment to undergraduate nursing students, registered nurses, and first and second year medical students. Her research informs her teaching and practice and is centred on areas of rural health, interprofessional teams, and primary health care.

Judy A.K. Bornais, RN, BA, BScN, MSc, PhD(c)
Experiential Learning Specialist
Teaching Leadership Chair
Faculty of Nursing
University of Windsor
Windsor, Ontario

Vickie Bruce, RN
Program Coordinator
Health and Wellness
Georgian College of Applied Arts and Technology
Owen Sound, Ontario

Andrea Carver, LPN
PN Instructor
Staff Nurse
ER, Acute, Med Surg, Day Surgery
St. Paul Health Centre
Portage College
St. Paul, Alberta

Catherine Moore Coburn, RN, BScN, MSN
Professor of Nursing
Health, Wellness and Sciences
Georgian College
Owen Sound, Ontario

Sara Craig, RN, BA, BScN, MN
Professor
Health Sciences
St. Lawrence College
Brockville, Ontario

Deirdre Duncan RN, BSN, Med
Nurse Educator
School of Health Sciences
Vancouver Community College
Vancouver, British Columbia

Louise Ethier, RN, BScN
Nursing instructor
Nursing program coordinator
Faculty of Nursing
Champlain College Lennoxville
Sherbrooke, Quebec

Bonnie Hessler, RN, BScN, MN
Nursing Faculty
Nursing Education and Health Studies
Grande Prairie Regional College
Grande Prairie, Alberta

Lauren Irving, MN, NP(F)
Adjunct Professor
Nursing Program
University of Northern British Columbia
Prince George, British Columbia

Paul Jeffrey, RN(EC), MN/ACNP, NP-Adult, DNP (student)
Professor, Nursing
School of Health Sciences
Humber Institute of Technology and Advanced Learning
Toronto, Ontario

Melanie Neumeier, RN, MN
Assistant Professor
Department of Nursing Science
Faculty of Nursing MacEwan University
Edmonton, Alberta

Rebecca Pauls, BScN, RN
Registered Nurse
Cardiology
Royal Victoria Regional Health Center
Hamilton Health Sciences
McMaster University
Barrie Ontario, Hamilton Ontario

Kara Sealock, RN, BN, MEd., CNCC(C)
Instructor
Faculty of Nursing
University of Calgary
Calgary, Alberta

PREFACE

It is important that students develop, practise, and then learn to trust their health history and physical examination skills. In this book we give you the tools to do that. Learn to listen to the patient—most often they will tell you what is wrong (and right) and what you can do to meet his or her health care needs. Then learn to inspect, examine, and listen to the person's body. The data are all there and are accessible to you by using just a few extra tools. High-technological machinery is a smart and sophisticated adjunct, but it cannot replace your own bedside assessment of your patient.

Whether you are a beginning examiner or an advanced-practice student, this book holds the content you need to develop and refine your clinical skills. The **Third Canadian Edition** of *Physical Examination & Health Assessment* is a comprehensive textbook of health history-taking methods, physical examination skills, health promotion techniques, and clinical assessment tools.

Thank you for your enthusiastic anticipation of this third Canadian edition. We are excited to be able to bring you an established, successful text with a focus on Canadian issues and content to further meet the needs of both novice and advanced practitioners in Canada.

DUAL FOCUS AS TEXT AND REFERENCE

Physical Examination & Health Assessment is both a **text for beginning students** of physical examination and also a **text and reference for advanced practitioners such as nurse practitioners and clinical nurse specialists.** The chapter progression and format permit this scope without sacrificing one use for the other.

Chapters 1 through 8 focus on **health assessment of individuals and families,** including preventive health care recommendations and other health promotion recommendations across the lifespan; the importance of **relational practice** in health assessment; **cultural and social considerations in assessment;** interviewing and complete health history gathering; and approaches to use for **mental health assessment, substance use assessment,** and **interpersonal violence assessment.**

Chapters 9 through 12 begin the approach to the **clinical care setting,** describing physical data-gathering techniques, how to set up the examination site, body measurement and vital signs, pain assessment, and nutritional assessment.

Chapters 13 through 27 focus on the **physical examination and related health history** in a body-systems approach. This is the most efficient method of performing the examination and is the most systematic and logical method for student learning and retrieval of data. **Each chapter has five major sections:** Structure and Function, Subjective Data (history), Objective Data (examination skills and findings), Documentation and Critical Thinking, and Abnormal Findings, An additional section Special Considerations for Advanced Practice is included in selected relevant chapters. The novice practitioner can review anatomy and physiology and learn the skills, expected findings, and common variations for generally healthy people and selected abnormal findings in the Objective Data sections. The sections on Special Considerations for Advanced Practice were created to address assessment approaches that are particularly relevant for **advanced practice nurses,** for example clinical nurse specialists or nurse practitioners. These sections also help to delineate the boundaries between basic assessments and more advanced assessments that may be conducted by advanced practice nurses.

Chapters 28 through 31 **integrate the complete health assessment.** Chapters 28 and 29 present the choreography of the head-to-toe examination for a complete screening examination in various age groups and for the focused examination of a hospitalized adult. Special populations are addressed in Chapters 30 and 31—the health assessment of the pregnant woman and the functional assessment of the older adult.

Students continue to use this text in subsequent courses throughout their education, and experienced clinicians will use this text as part of their advanced nursing practice. Given that each course demands more advanced skills and techniques, students can review the detailed presentation and the additional techniques in the Objective Data sections as well as variations for different age levels. Students can also study the extensive pathology illustrations and detailed text in the Abnormal Findings sections.

This text is valuable to both advanced practice students and experienced clinicians because of its comprehensive approach. *Physical Examination & Health Assessment* can help clinicians learn the skills for advanced practice, refresh their memory, review a specific examination technique when confronted with an unfamiliar clinical situation, and compare and label a diagnostic finding.

NEW TO THE THIRD CANADIAN EDITION

All chapters are **revised and updated** to include Canadian concepts, terminology, statistics, standards and guidelines, and assessment tools commonly used in Canadian health care settings. Six revised **Promoting Health** boxes are presented. These boxes describe an important health promotion topic related to the system discussed in each chapter—a topic you can use to enhance preventive recommendations and other types of patient education initiatives.

Special Considerations for Advanced Practice sections provided in selected chapters identify assessment approaches that are particularly relevant for advanced practice nurses. **Critical Findings** textboxes are placed strategically throughout the chapters to alert practitioners to assessment findings that require immediate attention, action, and decision-making. The New **Social Determinants of Health Considerations** sections have been newly written in each chapter to reflect content relevant to Canada. The social and economic factors that influence health, illness, and access to health care are discussed, and implications requiring consideration in the context of health assessment are identified. Highlights of Canadian content in each chapter are outlined below.

Chapter 1, **Critical Thinking and Evidence-Informed Assessment,** includes new perspectives on critical thinking and diagnostic reasoning as integral to health assessment. The relevance of conducting assessments based on evidence-informed decisions is emphasized. Relational approaches to nursing practice are discussed to foster nurses' capacities to convey respect, and as a means to avoid objectifying people in the process of health assessment.

Chapter 2, **Health Promotion in the Context of Health Assessment,** is newly written and integrates the latest Canadian guidelines for health promotion, illness prevention, screening, immunizations, and health education across the lifespan. Emphasis is placed on health promotion opportunities and actions that can be taken in the process of conducting health assessments.

Chapter 3, **Cultural and Social Considerations in Health Assessment,** is newly written to reflect the increasingly diverse populations in Canada. Examples of current trends in health, socioeconomic, and gender inequities are reviewed and discussed in terms of the implications for health assessment. New content relevant to Indigenous peoples is provided included an overview of the recently released Truth and Reconciliation Commission of Canada Calls to Action. Guidelines are provided for conducting assessments that respectfully take into account the social and economic contexts shaping people's lives.

Chapter 6, **Mental Health Assessment,** is newly written to provide content reflecting Canadian perspectives on the personal and social factors that shape people's mental health. New content relevant to Indigenous populations is provided, including strategies for conducting relevant, respectful assessments. The chapter provides strategies for conducting mental health assessments, including mental status examinations and risk assessments for suicide. The developmental adaptations that are required to conduct meaningful assessments across the lifespan are also discussed.

Chapter 7, **Substance Use in the Context of Health Assessment,** is a cutting-edge, new chapter—one of the first of its kind in a nursing health assessment textbook. It provides clinicians with the knowledge and skills to integrate assessments regarding substance use across a range of practice settings and with patients of all ages. Factors influencing the use of substances and the health effects of substance use are discussed. An entirely new section on harm reduction, including the principles of harm reduction and the relevance to health assessment, is provided. Emphasis is placed on the non-judgmental, non-stigmatizing approaches for assessing substance use.

Chapter 8, **Interpersonal Violence Assessment,** has also been heavily revised to include guidelines for assessing intimate partner violence, sexual assault, child abuse, and elder abuse as important problems for health care professionals to recognize and respond to. The chapter discusses the long-term effects of violence on health and the implications in the context of health assessment. Mandatory reporting requirements are also discussed, and practical strategies for assessing violence in a nonjudgmental and supportive manner are emphasized.

Chapter 9, **Assessment Techniques and the Clinical Setting,** focuses on assessment techniques and includes the Canadian Hypertensive Education Program guidelines for diagnosis. The chapter will help both novice and advanced practitioners make clinical decisions based on accurate assessment techniques.

Chapter 11, **Pain Assessment,** has been updated to include assessment tools for both conscious and unconscious patients. These additions reflect a growing trend toward caring for palliative patients in the community setting and the increased complexity of caring for the patient found outside the intensive care environment.

Chapter 12, **Nutritional Assessment and Nursing Practice,** has been updated to reflect growing concerns around food safety and security and assessment tools to better address nutrition, determinants of health, and reinforce the latest information concerning dietary reference intakes and nutrition labeling in Canada.

Chapter 14 has focused content related to head injuries and the Return to Play requirements for post-concussion assessment and recommendations.

Chapter 17, **Nose, Mouth, and Throat,** has included new health promotion content related to E-cigarettes.

Chapter 26, **Male Genitourinary System**, and Chapter 27, **Female Genitourinary System** both have new content related to assessment of the genitalia for transgender persons, and the latest Canadian recommendations for HPV vaccines for males and females.

Chapter 29, **Bedside Assessment and Electronic Health Recording,** includes an expanded section describing electronic health recording and patient safety.

APPROACHES USED IN THIS EDITION

The Third Canadian Edition of *Physical Examination & Health Assessment* builds on the strengths of the U.S. Seventh Edition and is designed to engage students and enhance learning:

1. **Method of examination** (Objective Data section) is clear, orderly, and easy to follow. Hundreds of original examination illustrations are placed directly with the text to demonstrate the physical examination in a step-by-step format.
2. **Two-column format** begins in the Subjective Data section, where the running column highlights the rationales for asking various history questions. In the Objective Data section, the running column highlights

selected abnormal findings to show a clear relationship between normal and abnormal findings.

3. **Abnormal Findings tables** organize and expand on material in the examination section. These have been revised and updated with many new clinical photos. The atlas format of these extensive collections of pathology and original illustrations helps students recognize, sort, and describe abnormal findings. When applicable, the text under a table entry is presented in a Subjective Data–Objective Data format.

4. **Developmental approach** in each chapter presents prototypical content on the adult, then age-specific content for the infant, child, adolescent, pregnant woman, and older adult so that students can learn common variations for all age groups.

5. **Social Determinants of Health Considerations** are discussed throughout as factors that shape health, illness, and access to health care. In addition to Chapter 3, where these issues are discussed in depth, social and economic considerations are included throughout the chapters to orient readers to relevant issues in the Canadian context.

6. **Stunning full-colour art** shows detailed human anatomy, physiology, examination techniques, and abnormal findings.

7. **Health history** (Subjective Data) appears in two places: Chapter 4, The Interview, has the most complete discussion available on the process of communication and on interviewing skills, techniques, and potential traps to avoid. This chapter includes guidelines for communicating with people whose primary language differs from yours and for working with interpreters to conduct sensitive and accurate health assessments. In Chapter 5, The Complete Health History, and in pertinent history questions that are repeated and expanded in each chapter, history questions are included that highlight health promotion opportunities and activities. This approach to emphasizing history questions helps students to understand the relationship between subjective and objective data. Because the history and examination data are considered together, as they would be in the clinical setting, each chapter can stand on its own if a person has a specific problem related to that body system.

8. **Summary checklists** toward the end of each chapter provide a quick review of examination steps to help you develop a mental checklist.

9. **Sample recordings** of normal findings show the written language you should use to ensure that charting is complete yet succinct.

10. **Focused assessment and clinical case studies** of frequently encountered situations demonstrate the application of assessment techniques to patients of different ages in differing clinical situations. These case histories, in subjective-objective-assessment-plan (SOAP) format, ending in diagnosis, are presented in the language actually used during recording.

11. **Integration of the complete health assessment** for the adult, infant, and child is presented as an illustrated essay in Chapter 28. This approach integrates all the steps into a choreographed whole. Included is a complete write-up of a health history and physical examination.

12. **User-friendly design** makes the book easy to use. Frequent subheadings and instructional headings help readers to easily retrieve content.

13. Bedside Assessment of the Hospitalized Adult, in Chapter 29, provides a unique photo sequence that **illustrates a head-to-toe assessment** suitable for each daily shift of care. It would be neither possible nor pertinent to perform a complete head-to-toe examination on every patient during every 24-hour stay in the hospital; therefore, this sequence shows a consistent specialized examination for each 8-hour shift that focuses on certain parameters pertinent to areas of medical, surgical, and cardiac step-down care.

The Canadian content that appears in the book—particularly the content about dealing with hospitalized patients, older adults, and pain assessment; relating to substance use and interpersonal violence; and cultural and social considerations—form part of the standard repertoire of knowledge from which Canadian examiners can draw.

CONCEPTUAL APPROACH

The Third Canadian Edition of *Physical Examination & Health Assessment* reflects a commitment to the following approaches:

- **Relational practice** in clinical practice recognizes that health, illness, and the meanings they hold for people are shaped by one's gender, age, ability, and social, cultural, familial, historical, and geographical contexts. These contexts influence how nurses and other health care professionals view, relate, and work with patients and families. By practising relationally, health care professionals will be optimally prepared to conduct accurate health assessments and to respond meaningfully to the patient's health, illness, and health promotion needs.

- **Health promotion** is discussed in depth in Chapter 2, with an emphasis on how to integrate health promotion into the process of health assessment. Health promotion textboxes are also provided in most chapters outlining the latest health promoting practices.

- Engaging with the patient as an **active participant in health care** involves encouraging discussion of what the person is currently doing to promote his or her health and supporting people to participate in health promoting practices given the social contexts of their lives.

- **Social determinants of health considerations** take into account our global society and the shifting landscape of Canada's populations. Strategies are provided for integrating attention to the wide range of social, economic and ethnocultural diversity within Canada in health assessment.

- Assessing individuals **across the lifespan** reflects the understanding that a person's state of health must be considered in light of their developmental stage.

Developmental anatomy; modifications of examination techniques; and expected findings for infants and children, adolescents, pregnant women, and older adults are provided. **Developmental Considerations** are provided in each relevant chapter, along with strategies for adapting health assessment approaches and techniques across the lifespan.

ANCILLARIES

- The *Pocket Companion for Physical Examination & Health Assessment* continues to be a handy and current clinical reference that provides pertinent material in full colour, with over 150 illustrations from the textbook.
- The *Student Laboratory Manual* with physical examination forms is a workbook that includes a student study guide, glossary of key terms, clinical objectives, regional write-up forms, and review questions for each chapter. The pages are perforated so that students can use the regional write-up forms in the skills laboratory or in the clinical setting and turn them in to the instructor.
- The revised *Health Assessment Online* is an innovative and dynamic teaching and learning tool with more than **8000 electronic assets**, including video clips, anatomic overlays, animations, audio clips, interactive exercises, laboratory/diagnostic tests, review questions, and **electronic charting activities**. Comprehensive **Self-Paced Learning Modules** offer increased flexibility to faculty who wish to provide students with tutorial learning modules and in-depth capstone case studies for each body system chapter in the text. The **Capstone Case Studies** now include **Quality and Safety Challenge** activities. Additional **Advance Practice Case Studies** put the student in the exam room and test history taking and documentation skills. The comprehensive **video clip library** shows exam procedures across the life span, including clips on the pregnant woman. Animations, sounds, images, interactive activities, and video clips are embedded in the learning modules and cases to provide a dynamic, multimodal learning environment for today's learners.
- *Physical Examination & Health Assessment Video Series* is an 18-video package developed in conjunction with this text. There are 12 body system videos and 6 head-to-toe videos, with the latter containing complete examinations of the neonate, child, adult, older adult, pregnant woman, and the bedside examination of a hospitalized adult. This series is available in DVD or streaming online formats. There are over 5 hours of video footage with highlighted Cross-Cultural Care Considerations, Developmental Considerations, and Health Promotion Tips, as well as Instructor Booklets with video overviews, outlines, learning objectives, discussion topics, and questions with answers.

- The companion *EVOLVE Website* (http://evolve.elsevier.com/Canada/Jarvis/examination/) contains learning objectives, more than 300 multiple-choice and alternate-format review questions, system-by-system exam summaries, bedside exam summaries, printable key points from the chapter, and a comprehensive physical exam form for the adult. **Case studies**—including a variety of developmental and cultural variables—help students apply health assessment skills and knowledge. These include 25 in-depth case studies with critical thinking questions and answer guidelines, as well as printable health promotion handouts. Also included is a complete Head-to-Toe Video Examination of the Adult that can be viewed in its entirety or by systems, as well as a new printable section on Quick Assessments for Common Conditions.
- *Simulation Learning System.* The new *Simulation Learning System* (SLS) is an online toolkit that incorporates medium- to high-fidelity simulation with scenarios that enhance the clinical decision-making skills of students. The SLS offers a comprehensive package of resources, including leveled patient scenarios, detailed instructions for preparation and implementation of the simulation experience, debriefing questions that encourage critical thinking, and learning resources to reinforce student comprehension.
- For instructors, the Evolve website presents TEACH for Nursing, PowerPoint slides with Audience Response Questions for iClicker and Case Studies, a comprehensive Image Collection, and a Test Bank. **TEACH for Nurses** provides annotated learning objectives, key terms, teaching strategies for the classroom in a revised section with strategies for both clinical and simulation lab use and critical thinking exercises, websites, and performance checklists. The **PowerPoint** slides include 2000 slides with integrated images. **Audience Response Questions** provide 90 questions for in-class student participation. A separate 1200-illustration **Image Collection** is featured and, finally, the ExamView **Test Bank** has over 1000 multiple-choice and alternate-format questions with coded answers and rationales.

IN CONCLUSION

Throughout all stages of manuscript preparation and production, every effort has been made to develop a book that is readable, informative, instructive, and vital. Your comments and suggestions have been important to this task and continue to be welcome for this new Canadian edition.

Carolyn Jarvis
Annette J. Browne
June MacDonald-Jenkins
Marian Luctkar-Flude

ACKNOWLEDGEMENTS FOR THE U.S. SEVENTH EDITION

I am grateful for the many talented and dedicated colleagues who helped make the revision of the 7th edition of this textbook possible.

Thank you to the bright, hardworking professional team at Elsevier. I am fortunate to have the support of Laurie Gower, Content Development Manager. Laurie is positive and skilled in directing the big picture of the books, as well as the endless details. She has a calm and forthright manner that is so welcome. Also, I am grateful to work daily with Heather Bays, Senior Content Development Specialist. Heather juggled all the deadlines, readied all the manuscript for production, searched out endless photos for abnormal examination findings, kept current with the permissions, and so many other daily details. Her work is pivotal to our success. I feel lucky she joined our team.

I had a wonderful production team and I am most grateful to them. Debbie Vogel, Publishing Services Manager, supervised the schedule for book production. I am especially grateful to Jodi Willard, Senior Project Manager, who has been in daily contact to keep the production organized and moving. She works in so many extra ways to keep production on schedule. I am pleased with the striking colors of the interior design of the 7th edition and the beautiful cover; both are the work of Julia Dummitt, Book Designer. The individual page layout is the wonderful work of Leslie Foster, Illustrator/Designer. Leslie hand-crafted every page, always planning how the page can be made better. Because of her work, I added 45 new case studies and scores of new art and tables, and we still came out with comparable page length for the 7th edition.

I have gifted artistic colleagues, who made this book such a vibrant teaching display. Pat Thomas, Medical Illustrator, is so talented and contributes format ideas as well as brilliant drawings. Kevin Strandberg patiently sets up equipment for all our photo shoots and then captures lovely exam photos of children and adults. Julia Jarvis also photographed our infant photos with patience and clarity.

I am fortunate to have dedicated research assistants. Molly Gray Guenette searched and retrieved countless articles and sources. She was always prompt and accurate. Karolina Sierzputowska just joined as a research assistant and has helped in many ways. I am most grateful to Paul Jarvis, who read and reread endless copies of galley and page proof, finding any errors and making helpful suggestions.

Thank you to the faculty and students who took the time to write letters of suggestions and encouragement—your comments are gratefully received and are very helpful. I am fortunate to have the skilled reviewers who spend time reading the chapter manuscript and making valuable suggestions.

Most important are the members of my wonderful family, growing in number and in support. Their constant encouragement has kept me going throughout this process.

Carolyn Jarvis

ACKNOWLEDGEMENTS FOR THE THIRD CANADIAN EDITION

Carolyn Jarvis's text has been a constant companion throughout my clinical and teaching career. The opportunity to adapt this classic textbook to reflect Canadian perspectives, content, and guidelines is a major honour. I have thoroughly enjoyed thinking critically about the range of content to include, especially given the diverse range of students, clinicians, and faculty who may use this text. I want to thank Dr. Sally Thorne, a professor at the University of British Columbia School of Nursing, for encouraging me to take on this project. I am also grateful to June MacDonald-Jenkins and Marian Luctkar-Flude for adapting this text in significant ways to reflect the unique context of nursing practice in Canada. I am fortunate to be able to draw on the expertise of Dr. Dana Edge, Dr. Vicki Smye, Dr. Colleen Varcoe, Laraine Michalson, and Dr. Erin Wilson as chapter authors and contributors, and I thank them for providing highly pertinent and cutting-edge content. Finally, thank you to John, whose loving support makes this work possible.

Annette J. Browne

What a pleasure to have been given the opportunity to potentially influence the learning of students across the country. My thanks to every student who risked taking a stance of inquiry, looked for more, and sought the answers; you are the reason that editing this text was such a pleasure. I, too, would like to thank the editorial team at Elsevier Canada; they have been gracious and supportive while ensuring that we met timelines for publication of the Third Canadian Edition. I would like to thank my colleagues Dr. Ellen Vogel, Christina Vaillancourt, and Andrea Miller for contributing to Chapter 12, Nutritional Assessment and Nursing Practice, and to Lynn Haslam for her work on Chapter 11, Pain Assessment. I extend my thanks to these four professionals for hours of collaboration and consultation to ensure the inclusion of a truly national perspective. Many thanks, as well, to my co-editors Annette and Marian; your knowledge and insight have truly shaped the perspective of this text. I would like to thank my family for their endless support and indulgence of my "adventures:" my husband, Dean, and my three daughters, Sarah, Emily, and Mackenzie.

June MacDonald-Jenkins

I am truly grateful for having had the opportunity to participate in the development of the Third Canadian Edition of Jarvis's *Physical Examination & Health Assessment*. The support of the Elsevier Canada staff throughout this process has been invaluable. In particular, I would like to thank Heather Bays and Claudia Forgas for their guidance. I would also like to thank my colleagues Barbara Wilson-Keates and Dianne Groll for their contributions to the Nose, Mouth, and Throat, and Functional Assessment of the Older Adult chapters; and Nancy Watts for contributing to the Pregnancy chapter, as these are not my areas of expertise. I would like to thank my Canadian coeditors, Annette J. Browne and June MacDonald-Jenkins, for their long-distance collaboration. It has been a pleasure and a great learning experience to work with each of you. And, finally, I would like to acknowledge the support of those dearest to me, my wonderful family, Richard, Curtis and Sarena, Cameron and Katurah, Corey, and Brianna, and my colleague and friend Jane.

Marian Luctkar-Flude

CHAPTER 1

Critical Thinking and Evidence-Informed Assessment

Written by Carolyn Jarvis, PhD, APN, CNP
Adapted by Annette J. Browne, PhD, RN

ⓔ http://evolve.elsevier.com/Canada/Jarvis/examination/

The ability to conduct a high-quality health assessment and physical examination is foundational to nursing practice. Similarly, to provide relevant, timely, and appropriate nursing and health care, nurses must be able to accurately describe assessment findings to patients, families, and other members of the interprofessional team. Assessments must be conducted in ways that convey respect for the whole person, to avoid objectifying people. Learning to conduct systematic assessments is integral to developing confidence in clinical abilities and capacity to respond effectively to patients' needs.

You work in a primary health care clinic in a Canadian city. Ellen K. is a 23-year-old woman whom you have seen several times over the past 2 months (Fig. 1.1). She has been admitted for observation at the emergency department because of sudden onset of shortness of breath.

The health care provider in the emergency department documented a health history and performed a complete physical examination. Examples of the preliminary list of significant findings recorded in her health record are as follows:

- *Appearance: Sitting quietly alone in the examination room. Facial expression appears sad. Eyes fill with tears when she discusses her partner.*
- *Elevated BP [blood pressure]; 142/100 at end of examination today.*
- *Diminished breath sounds, with moderate expiratory wheeze and scattered rhonchi at both bases.*
- *Grade II/VI systolic heart murmur, left lower sternal border.*
- *Resolving hematoma, 2 to 3 cm, R [right] infraorbital ridge.*
- *Missing R lower first molar, gums receding on lower incisors, multiple dark spots on front upper teeth.*
- *Well-healed scar, 28 cm long × 2 cm wide, R lower leg, with R leg 3 cm shorter than L [left], sequelae of auto accident at age 12.*
- *Altered nutrition: omits breakfast; daily intake has no fruits, no vegetables; meals at fast food restaurants most days.*

- *Oral contraceptives for birth control × 3 years, last pelvic examination 1 year ago.*
- *Smokes a half PPD [pack of cigarettes per day] × 2 years, prior use one PPD × 4 years.*
- *Started using alcohol at age 16. For past 2 years, has equivalent of 3 to 4 drinks per day × 4 to 5 days a week. Last intake of alcohol was yesterday.*
- *Currently is unemployed × 6 months. Receives employment insurance (≈$680/month). Previous work as cashier in large department store.*
- *History of emotional and physical abuse related to current relationship with partner. Today has orbital hematoma as a result of being struck by partner. States, "We had a big fight."*
- *Relationships: Over past 12 months, has not been in communication with her parents, who live in another city. Has one close woman friend who lives nearby. Significant relationship is with partner of 2 years, with whom she resides in a rented small basement suite.*

The examiner analyzed and interpreted all the data; clustered the information, sorting out which data to refer and which to treat; and identified the diagnoses. Of interest is how many significant findings are derived from data the examiner collected. Not only physical data but also cognitive, psychosocial, and behavioural data are significant for an analysis of Ellen's health state. Also, the findings are interesting when considered from a life cycle perspective; that is, Ellen is a young adult who normally should be concerned with the developmental tasks of emancipation from parents, building an economically stable life, and developing caring relationships.

A body of clinical evidence has validated the importance of using assessment techniques in Ellen's case. For example, measuring blood pressure is a way to screen for hypertension, and early intervention can prevent heart attack and stroke. Listening to breath sounds is a way to screen (in Ellen's case) for asthma, which is compounded by the use of tobacco. Listening to heart sounds reveals Ellen's heart murmur, which could be innocent or functional, or a sign of a structural abnormality in a heart valve; further examination will yield further data.

1.1

ASSESSMENT: POINT OF ENTRY IN AN ONGOING PROCESS

Assessment is the collection of data about an individual's health state. Throughout this text, you will study the techniques of collecting and analyzing **subjective data** (i.e., what the person *says* about himself or herself during history taking) and **objective data** (i.e., what you as the health care provider *observe* by inspecting, percussing, palpating, and auscultating during the physical examination). Together with the patient's record, laboratory studies, and other diagnostic tests, these elements form the **database**. For example, in the preceding case of Ellen, an example of subjective data is "History of emotional and physical abuse related to current relationship with partner." An example of objective data is "Resolving hematoma, 2 to 3 cm, R infraorbital ridge."

From the database, you make a clinical judgement or diagnosis about the individual's health state or response to actual health problems or risk factors and life processes, as well as diagnoses about overall levels of wellness. Thus, the purpose of assessment is to make a judgement or diagnosis on the basis of data from various sources.

An organized assessment is the starting point of diagnostic reasoning. Because all health care diagnoses, decisions, and treatments are based on the data you gather during assessment, it is paramount that your assessment be factual and complete.

Diagnostic Reasoning

The step from data collection to diagnosis can be a difficult one. Most beginning examiners perform well in gathering the data, with adequate practice, but then treat all the data as being equally important. This makes decision making slow and laboured.

Diagnostic reasoning is the process of analyzing health data and drawing conclusions to identify diagnoses. It has four major components: (a) attending to initially available cues; (b) formulating diagnostic hypotheses; (c) gathering data relative to the tentative hypotheses; and (d) evaluating each hypothesis with the new data collected, thus arriving

at a final diagnosis. A *cue* is a piece of information, a sign or symptom, or a piece of laboratory data. A *hypothesis* is a tentative explanation for a cue or a set of cues that can be used as a basis for further investigation.

For example, Ellen K., the patient described at the beginning of this chapter, presents with a number of initial cues, one of which is the resolving hematoma under her eye. (a) You can recognize this cue even before history documentation begins. Is it significant? (b) If Ellen were to say she ran into a door, mumbles as she speaks, and avoids eye contact, you formulate a hypothesis of trauma. (c) During the history documentation and physical examination, you gather data to support or reject the tentative hypothesis. (d) You synthesize the new data collected, which support the hypothesis of trauma but eliminate the accidental cause. The final diagnoses are "resolving right orbital contusion" and "risk for trauma."

Diagnostic hypotheses are activated very early in the reasoning process. Consider a hunch that Ellen has suffered physical trauma. A hunch helps diagnosticians adapt to large amounts of information because it clusters cues into meaningful groups and directs subsequent data collection. Later, you can accept your hunch or rule it out.

Once you complete data collection, you can develop a preliminary list of significant signs and symptoms and all patient health needs. This list is less formal in structure than your final list of diagnoses will be and is in no particular order. (Such a list for Ellen is found on p. 1 of the opening vignette.) Cluster or group together the assessment data that appear to be causal or associated. For example, for a person in acute pain, associated data may include rapid heart rate and anxiety. Organizing the data into meaningful clusters is slow at first; experienced examiners cluster data more rapidly.[1]

Validate the data you collect to make sure they are accurate. As you validate your information, look for gaps in data collection. Be sure to find the missing information because identifying missing information is an essential critical thinking skill. How you validate your data depends on experience. If you are unsure of the blood pressure, validate it by repeating the measurement yourself. Eliminate any extraneous variables that could influence blood pressure results, such as recent activity or anxiety over admission. If you have less experience analyzing breath sounds or heart murmurs, ask an expert to listen. Even for nurses with years of clinical experience, some signs always require validation (e.g., a breast lump).

Critical Thinking and the Diagnostic Process

The **nursing process** is a systematic method of planning and providing patient care organized around series of phrases that integrate evidence-informed practice and critical thinking.[2] The nursing process typically includes five phases: (a) assessment, (b) nursing diagnosis, (c) planning, (d) implementation, and (e) evaluation. As shown in Fig. 1.2, the nursing process is a dynamic, interactive process requiring clinicians to move back and forth within the phases.

The method of moving from novice to becoming an expert practitioner is through the use of critical thinking.[1]

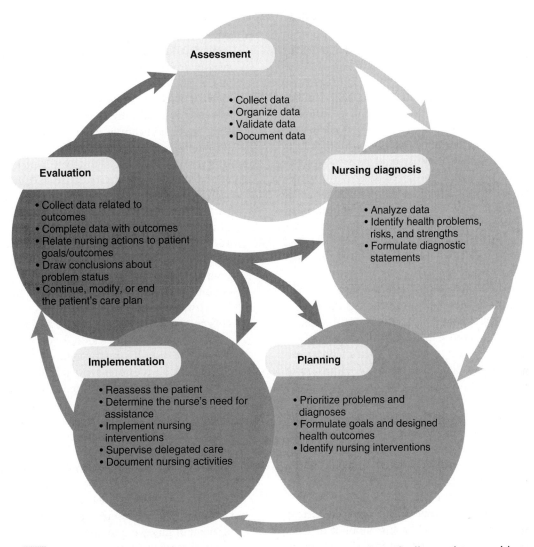

1.2   The clockwise arrow indicates how the nursing process is typically used to provide patient care. While not depicted, counterclockwise arrows are "at play" and help us to understand how information acquired in on step of the nursing process informs the previous step. Note that evaluation relates to nursing diagnosis, planning, and implementation. (Cullen, M. L., & Wagner, S. (2015). The nursing process in the 21st century. In D. M. Gregory, C. Raymond-Seniuk, L. Patrick, et al. (Eds.), *Fundamentals: Perspectives on the art and science of Canadian nursing* (pp. 164–191). Philadelphia: Wolters Kluwer Health.)

All nurses start as novices, when clear-cut rules are needed to guide actions. Critical thinking is the means by which nurses learn to assess and modify, if indicated, before acting.

The following critical thinking skills are organized in a logical progression according to how these skills might be used in the nursing process.[3] Although the skills are described sequentially here, they are not used that way in the clinical area. Rather than a step-by-step linear process, critical thinking is a multidimensional thinking process. With experience, you will be able to apply these skills in a rapid, dynamic, and interactive way. You will also be able to conduct health assessments and physical examinations in ways that convey genuine positive regard for and acceptance of the person, and that show you are not viewing people with regard merely to their bodily parts. For now, follow Ellen's case study through these steps:

1. *Identify assumptions.* That is, recognize that you could take information for granted or see it as fact when actually there is no evidence for it. Ask yourself what you may be taking for granted here. For example, in Ellen's situation, you might have assumptions of a "typical profile" of a person who uses alcohol or who experiences physical violence on the basis of your past experience or exposure to media coverage. However, the facts of Ellen's situation are unique.

2. *Identify an organized and comprehensive approach to assessment.* This approach depends on the patient's priority needs and your personal or institutional preference. Ellen has many physical and psychosocial issues, but at her time of admission, she is not acutely physically ill. Thus you may use any organized format for assessment that is feasible for you: a head-to-toe approach, a body

systems approach (e.g., cardiovascular, gastro-intestinal), a regional area approach (e.g., pelvic examination), or the use of a preprinted assessment form developed by the hospital or clinic.

3. *Validate or check the accuracy and reliability of data.* For example, in addiction treatment, a clinician corroborates data with a family member or friend to verify the accuracy of Ellen's history. In Ellen's particular case, her significant others are absent or nonsupportive, and the corroborative interview may need to be with a social worker.

4. *Distinguish normal from abnormal when signs and symptoms are identified.* This is the first step in problem identification, and your ease will grow with study, practice, and experience. Increased blood pressure, wheezing, and heart murmur are among the many abnormal findings in Ellen's case.

5. *Make inferences or hypotheses.* This skill involves interpreting the data and deriving a correct conclusion about the health status. It is a challenge for the beginning examiner because both a baseline amount of knowledge and experience are needed. Is Ellen's blood pressure increased as a result of the stress of admission or as a result of a chronic condition? Is the heart murmur "innocent" or a sign of heart valve disease?

6. *Cluster related cues, which helps you see relationships among the data.* For example, heavy alcohol use, social and interpersonal consequences of alcohol use, academic consequences, and occupational consequences are a clustering of cues that suggest a pattern of alcohol use that results in significant harms.

7. *Distinguish relevant from irrelevant.* A complete history and physical examination yield a vast amount of data. Look at the clusters of data, and consider which data are important for a health problem or a health promotion need. This skill is also a challenge for beginning examiners and one area in which the expertise of a clinical mentor can be invaluable.

8. *Recognize inconsistencies.* Ellen explains that she ran into a door (subjective data), which is at odds with the location of the infraorbital hematoma (objective data). With this kind of conflicting information, you can investigate and further clarify the situation.

9. *Identify patterns.* Awareness of patterns helps you fill in the whole picture and discover missing pieces of information. To decide whether the systolic murmur is a problem for Ellen, you need to know the usual function of the heart, characteristics of innocent murmurs, and risk factors for abnormal or pathological murmurs.

10. *Identify missing information, gaps in data, or a need for more data to make a diagnosis.* Ellen will likely require further diagnostic tests to determine whether her respiratory issues are asthma-related to specify a diagnosis.

11. *Promote health by identifying priorities with the patient, assessing risk factors, and considering a patient's social context.* This skill applies to generally healthy people and concerns disease prevention and health promotion.

To accomplish this skill, you need to identify and work with each patient to manage known risk factors for the individual's age group and social context. Managing risk factors drives the health promotion goals and priorities. For example, safety planning is an important intervention for Ellen, inasmuch as she identified interpersonal violence as an immediate concern. Following Ellen's lead, you would convey acceptance of her and a willingness to listen, and you would tell Ellen that the abuse she experiences is not her fault (see Chapter 8). You would ask Ellen whether she is interested in developing a safety plan to ensure that she has a safe place to go to if her partner becomes abusive, or whether she is interested in discussing other issues that she identifies as priorities. You might ask her whether she would like to talk to a social worker who could help her address her social, economic, or housing needs. Depending on her priorities, you might also refer Ellen to a dental clinic that provides low-cost or no-cost dental care.

12. *Diagnose actual and potential (risk) problems from the assessment data.* These include, for example, potential for alcohol use disorder; right orbital contusion (resolving); elevated blood pressure; systolic heart murmur; diminished respiratory function related to wheezes and rhonchi; interpersonal violence and trauma. Medical and nursing diagnoses should not be considered isolated from each other; interprofessional perspectives and assessment data are needed to fully understand a person's health status. **Nurse practitioners**, for example, have expanded scopes of practice. Nurse practitioners are registered nurses who typically have master's degrees and have advanced education in health assessment and the diagnosis and management of illnesses and injuries, including the ability to order diagnostic texts and prescribe medications. Nurse practitioners provide a direct point of entry to the health care system for case management, diagnosis, treatment, prevention, and promotion, and, in some cases, palliative care.[4] For example, it makes sense that the medical diagnosis of asthma be reflected in the nursing diagnoses, in view of the nurse's knowledge of the signs of asthma. In this book, common nursing diagnoses are presented along with medical diagnoses to illustrate common abnormalities. It is important to observe how these two types of diagnoses are interrelated.

With regard to Ellen's case, for example, the medical diagnosis is used to evaluate the cause of disease. The nursing diagnosis is used to evaluate the response of the whole person to actual or potential health problems. Note that the admitting nurse and later the physician auscultate Ellen's lung sounds and determine that they are diminished and that wheezing is present. Diminished breath sounds, with moderate expiratory wheeze and scattered rhonchi at both bases, represent both medical problems and nursing clinical problems. The physician or nurse practitioner listens to diagnose the cause of the abnormal sounds (in this case, asthma) and to order specific diagnostic tests or medication

TABLE 1.1   Identifying Immediate Priorities

Principles of Setting Priorities

1. **Make a complete list of current medications, medical problems, allergies, and reasons for seeking care.** Refer to them frequently because they may affect how you set priorities.

2. **Determine the *relationships* among the problems:** If problem Y causes problem Z, problem Y takes priority over problem Z. **Example:** If pain is causing immobility, *pain management* is a high priority.

    Setting priorities is a dynamic, changing process: at times, the order of priority changes, depending on the seriousness and relationship of the problems.

    Example: If abnormal laboratory values are at life-threatening levels, they become a higher priority; if the patient is having trouble breathing because of acute rib pain, managing the pain may be a higher priority than dealing with a rapid pulse (first-level priority, listed in the following section of this table).

Steps to Setting Priorities

1. Assign high priority to *first-level* priority problems (immediate priorities): Remember the "ABCs plus V":
    - **A**irway problems
    - **B**reathing problems
    - **C**ardiac/circulation problems
    - **V**ital sign concerns (e.g., high fever)

    Exception: With cardiopulmonary resuscitation (CPR) for cardiac arrest, begin chest compressions immediately. Go online to https://resuscitation.heartandstroke.ca/guidelines/position/CPR for the most current CPR guidelines.

2. Next, attend to *second-level* priority problems:
    - Mental status change (e.g., confusion, decreased alertness)
    - Untreated medical problems that necessitate immediate attention (e.g., for a diabetic patient who has not had insulin)
    - Acute pain
    - Acute urinary elimination problems
    - Abnormal laboratory values
    - Risks of infection, to safety, or to security (for the patient or for others)

3. Address *third-level* priority problems (later priorities):
    - Health problems that do not fit into the previous categories (e.g., problems with lack of knowledge, activity, rest, family coping)

Source: Adapted from Alfaro-LeFevre, R. (2017). *Critical thinking and clinical judgment: A practical approach* (6th ed.). Philadelphia: W.B. Saunders.

treatment. The nurse listens to detect abnormal sounds early, to monitor Ellen's response to treatment, and to initiate supportive measures and health education.

13. *Set priorities when a patient has more than one health or illness issue occurring concurrently (which is often the case).* In the acute care hospital setting, the initial problems are usually related to the reason for admission. However, the acuity of illness, as well as the person's social and family context, often determines the order of priorities of the person's problems (Table 1.1).

For example, **first-level priority problems** are those that are emergencies, life-threatening, and immediate, such as establishing an airway or supporting breathing. **Second-level priority problems** are those that are next in urgency: those necessitating your prompt intervention to forestall further deterioration, such as mental status change, acute pain, acute urinary elimination problems, untreated medical problems, abnormal laboratory values, risks of infection, or risk to safety or security. Ellen has abnormal physical signs that fit in the category of untreated medical problems. For example, Ellen's adventitious breath sounds are a cue to further assess respiratory status to determine the final diagnosis. Ellen's mildly elevated blood pressure also needs monitoring.

Third-level priority problems are those that are important to the patient's health but can be addressed after more urgent health problems are addressed. In Ellen's case, the data indicating diagnoses of knowledge deficit, social isolation, risk for other-directed violence, and risk for situational low self-esteem fit in this category. Interventions to treat these problems are lengthier, and the response to treatment is expected to take more time.

Collaborative problems are those in which the approach to treatment involves multiple disciplines, and nurses often have the primary responsibility to diagnose the onset and monitor the changes in status. For example, the data regarding alcohol use represent a collaborative problem. With this problem, the sudden withdrawal of alcohol has profound implications on the central nervous and cardiovascular systems. Ellen's response to the rebound effects of these systems is managed.

14. *Identify patient-centred expected outcomes.* What specific, measurable results that will show an improvement in the person's problem after treatment will you expect? The outcome statement should include a specific time frame. For example, before discharge from the emergency department, and nurses will talk with Ellen to help her consider a safety plan for dealing with interpersonal violence that fits with her life context (see Chapter 8).

15. *Determine specific interventions that will achieve positive outcomes.* These interventions aim to prevent, manage, or resolve health problems. They constitute the health care plan. For specific interventions, state who should perform the intervention, when and how often, and the method used.

16. *Evaluate and revise your thinking.* Observe the actual outcomes, and evaluate them in relation to the expected outcomes (do the stated outcomes match the individual's actual progress?). Then, analyze whether your interventions were successful or not. Continually think about what you could be doing differently or better.

17. *Determine a comprehensive plan or evaluate and update the plan.* Record the revised plan of care and keep it up to date. The use of electronic health records is widespread in Canada; nurses play an important role in

influencing the flow, use, and management of information. Communicate the plan to the multidisciplinary team. Be aware that the plan of care is a legal document, and accurate recording is important for accountability purposes, billing purposes, quality assurance and evaluation, and research.

EVIDENCE-INFORMED ASSESSMENT

All patients must be provided with the most current best-practice techniques. The term **evidence-informed practice (EIP)** is increasingly used in the literature to encompass a more inclusive view of what "counts" as evidence than is conventionally implied when using the term *evidence-based practice*.[5] Many forms of evidence inform clinical decision making and the delivery of nursing care, including evidence generated through intervention studies, clinical trials, ethnographic research, systemic reviews, policy analyses, and evaluation studies, among others—hence the relevance of the term *evidence-informed practice*. EIP is more than the use of best-practice techniques to treat patients; it can be defined as "a paradigm and life-long problem solving approach to clinical decision-making that involves the conscientious use of the best available evidence (including a systematic search for and critical appraisal of the most relevant evidence to answer a clinical question) with one's own clinical expertise and patient values and preferences to improve outcomes for individuals, groups, communities, and systems."[6] Many EIP guidelines, including those developed by the RNAO (see http://rnao.ca/bpg), are applicable in a number of jurisdictions in Canada. As shown in Fig. 1.3, note how clinical decision making depends on all four factors: the best and most appropriate evidence from a critical review of research

literature; the patient's own context and preferences; the clinician's experience and expertise; and finally, physical examination and assessment. Assessment skills must be practised with hands-on experience and refined to a high level.

Although assessment skills are foundational to EIP, it is important to question tradition when no compelling research evidence exists to support it. Some time-honoured assessment techniques have been omitted from the examination repertoire because clinical evidence has shown them to be less than useful. For example, the traditional practice of auscultating bowel sounds was found not to be the best indicator of returning gastro-intestinal motility in patients who have had abdominal surgery.[7] Madsen and colleagues[7] first reviewed earlier studies suggesting that early postoperative bowel sounds probably do not represent the return of normal gastro-intestinal motility and that listening to the abdomen is therefore not useful in this situation. Research did show the primary markers for returning gastro-intestinal motility after abdominal surgery to be the return of flatus and the first postoperative bowel movement. Madsen and colleagues instituted a new practice protocol and monitored patient outcomes to check whether discontinuing the auscultation of bowel sounds was detrimental to patients who had undergone abdominal surgery. Detrimental outcomes did not occur; the new practice guideline was shown to be safe for patients' recovery and a better allocation of staff time.

EXPANDING THE CONCEPT OF HEALTH

Assessment is the collection of data about an individual's health state. A clear idea of an individual patient's health status is important because it determines which assessment data should be collected. In general, the list of data that must be collected has lengthened as the concept of health has broadened.

According to the **biomedical model**, which is the predominant model of the Canadian health care system, health is the absence of disease (Fig. 1.4). Health and disease are viewed as two ends of a continuum. Disease is assumed to be caused by specific agents or pathogens. Thus the biomedical focus is the diagnosis and treatment of those pathogens and the curing of disease. Assessment factors are a list of biophysical symptoms and signs. A person is certified as healthy

Evidence from research and evidence-informed theories

Patient preferences and values

Evidence-informed clinical decision making

Physical examination and assessment of patient

Clinical expertise

1.3

1.4

when these symptoms and signs have been eliminated. When disease does exist, the medical diagnosis is worded to identify and explain the cause of disease.

Accurate diagnosis and treatment of illness are important parts of health care. However, the medical model has limiting boundaries. According to the **behavioural model**, health care extends beyond treating disease to include secondary and primary preventions, with emphasis on changing behaviours and lifestyles (e.g., quitting smoking or eating nutritiously).[8] The **socioenvironmental model** incorporates sociological and environmental aspects in addition to the biomedical and behavioural ones. The socioenvironmental perspective parallels the definition provided by the World Health Organization,[9] which defines *health* as a resource for living and as the abilities to realize goals or aspirations, meet personal needs, and change or cope with everyday life. Building on these ideas, the *Ottawa Charter for Health Promotion*[9] identified the prerequisites to health as peace, shelter, education, food, income, a stable ecosystem, sustainable resources, social justice, and equity. Although the *Ottawa Charter* was written in 1986, many people in Canada still lack these basic prerequisites, and their health is profoundly compromised as a result.

By developing the *Ottawa Charter for Health Promotion*, Canada has taken a leading international role in emphasizing the importance of the **social determinants of health**. Social determinants are the social, economic, and political conditions that shape the health of individuals, families, and communities.[10] For example, some of the best predictors of adult-onset diabetes, mental illness, heart attack, and stroke are low income, inability to afford nutritious foods, and crowded housing or lack of affordable housing. These are issues that also affect patients' and families' abilities to engage in health-promoting practices.

As discussed in Chapter 2, Canada has also been a major international leader in the area of **health promotion**. *Health promotion* can be defined as a comprehensive social and political process of enabling people to increase control over the determinants of health and thereby improve their health.[10] Health-promoting actions focus on strengthening the skills and capabilities of individuals and families and are directed toward changing social, economic, and environmental conditions to improve health.

A RELATIONAL APPROACH TO NURSING PRACTICE

The concept of "relational" is increasingly used to describe the complex, interrelated nature of health, people, society, and nursing practice.[8] *Relational* is not the same as *relationships*: Although relationships between people are important, relational practice refers to more than interpersonal relationships. A **relational approach in nursing practice** accounts for the fact that health, illness, and the meanings they hold for a person are shaped by the person's social, cultural, family, historical, and geographical contexts, as well as the person's gender, age, ability, and other individual contexts. Relational approaches focus nurses' attention on what is significant to people in the context of their everyday lives and how capacities and socioenvironmental limitations shape people's choices. One of the central skills of relational practice is *reflectivity*, a process of continually examining how you view and respond to patients on the basis of your own assumptions, cultural and social orientation, past experiences, and so on. Approaching nursing practice relationally promotes (a) understanding across differences rather than defensiveness and (b) responsiveness rather than a sense of frustration or powerlessness. The application of relational approaches in clinical practice are discussed further in Chapters 3, 4, and 6–8.

Nurses need to draw on a variety of perspectives. For example, if you were working with Ellen, the young woman in the chapter opening case study, you would use a biomedical perspective to assess and treat her underlying respiratory infection. From a behavioural perspective, you might focus on providing information and teaching Ellen about how to eat more nutritious foods. The socioenvironmental model would attune you to assessing Ellen's risks for violence and supporting her to develop a safety plan in case she needs to remove herself quickly from a violent situation at home. Considering the social determinants of health, you would focus attention on whether Ellen could afford fresh fruits or vegetables or pay for the prescription necessary to treat her respiratory infection. A relational stance would prompt you to consider what biases or assumptions might be influencing you in relation to Ellen and would involve your exploring with her the issues she thought were most important at this point in her life. For example, the health assessment process might indicate that the most important health-promoting intervention would be a referral to a women's social support agency in the community.

COLLECTING FOUR TYPES OF DATA

Every examiner needs to collect four different kinds of data, depending on the clinical situation: (a) complete, (b) episodic or problem-centred, (c) follow-up, and (d) emergency.

Complete (Total Health) Database

The complete database includes a complete health history and results of a full physical examination. It describes the current and past health states and forms a baseline against which all future changes can be measured. It yields the first diagnoses.

In primary care, the complete database is compiled in a primary care setting, such as a pediatric or family practice clinic, independent or group private practice, college health service, women's health care agency, visiting nurse agency, or community health care agency. When you work in these settings, you are the first health care provider to see the patient, and you have primary responsibility for monitoring the patient's health care. For the well person, this database must describe the person's health state, perception of health, strengths or assets such as the ability to engage in health maintenance or health-promoting practices, support systems, current developmental tasks, and any risk factors or social issues. For the ill person, the database also includes a description of the person's health problems, perception of illness, and response to the problems.

In acute hospital care, the complete database also is compiled after the patient's admission to the hospital. In the hospital, data related specifically to disease may be collected by the admitting physician. You collect additional information about the patient's perception of illness, functional ability or patterns of living, activities of daily living (ADLs), health maintenance behaviours, response to health problems, coping patterns, interaction patterns, and health goals.

Episodic or Problem-Centred Database

The episodic database is for a limited or short-term problem. It is a "mini-database," smaller in scope and more focused than the complete database. It concerns mainly one problem, one cue complex, or one body system. It is used in all settings: hospital, primary care, or long-term care. For example, 2 days after surgery, a hospitalized person suddenly has a congested cough, shortness of breath, and fatigue. The history and examination focus primarily on the respiratory and cardiovascular systems. In another example, a person presents with a rash in an outpatient clinic. The history and examination follow the direction of this presenting concern, such as whether the rash had an acute or chronic onset, was associated with a fever, and was localized or generalized. Documentation of the history and examination must include a clear description of the rash.

Follow-Up Database

The status of any identified problems should be evaluated at regular and appropriate intervals. What change has occurred? Is the problem getting better or worse? What coping strategies are used? The follow-up database is used in all settings to monitor short-term or chronic health problems.

Emergency Database

The emergency database calls for a rapid collection of the data, often compiled while life-saving measures are occurring. Diagnosis must be swift and sure. For example, in a hospital emergency department, a person is brought in with suspected substance overdose. The first history questions are "What did you take?", "How much did you take?", and "When did you take it?" The person is questioned simultaneously while their airway, breathing, circulation, level of consciousness, and disability are being assessed. Clearly, the emergency database requires more rapid collection of data than does the episodic database.

FREQUENCY OF ASSESSMENT

The frequency of assessment varies with the person's age, sex, gender, ability, social context, and illness and wellness needs. Most ill people seek care because of pain or some abnormal signs and symptoms they have noticed. Their visit

to a health care facility prompts an assessment: the gathering of a complete, an episodic, or an emergency database.

For the well person, however, opinions are changing about assessment intervals. The term *annual checkup* is vague. What does it constitute? Is it necessary or cost effective? Does it sometimes give an implicit promise of health and thus provide false security? What about the classic situation in which a person suffers a heart attack 2 weeks after a routine checkup that includes normal findings on an electrocardiogram? The timing of some formerly accepted recommendations have now changed; for example, the Papanicolaou (Pap) test for cervical cancer in females is no longer required annually depending on past test results and the female's health history.[11] Screening guidelines for the use of mammography, breast self-examination, and clinical breast examination to screen for breast cancer have also recently changed, and recommendations vary significantly in different provinces and territories.[11] The same annual routine physical examination cannot be recommended for all persons because health priorities vary among individuals, different age groups, and risk categories.

In Canada, there are various guidelines for disease prevention and health promotion. New national and provincial guidelines are developed regularly for particular populations; an example is the 2017 updated recommendations on human papillomavirus (HPV) vaccine guidelines for girls, women, boys, and men.[12]

National standards for **immunizations** are contained in the *Canadian Immunization Guide*, and updates to information are published as a Table of Updates several times a year.[13] Each province and territory adapts these standards slightly according to its population's needs. It is important to check the provincial or territorial guidelines where you practice. **Periodic health examinations** are designed to prevent morbidity and mortality by identifying modifiable risk factors, social determinants of health, early signs of treatable conditions, and counsel on lifestyle issues (e.g., diet and exercise).[14] In 1980, the Canadian Task Force on the Periodic Health Examination produced its first evidence-informed clinical practice guidelines. The task force was renamed the *Canadian Task Force on Preventive Health Care* in 1984, and many of the guidelines were updated in 2006, again in 2013, and new guidelines and appraisals continue to be added online.[15]

Since 2006, the Public Health Agency of Canada[16] has taken the lead in developing and distributing health promotion, disease prevention, and other guidelines for children, adults, pregnant women, and older adults. The Canadian Medical Association's[17] *Clinical Practice Guidelines* are also updated regularly and include prevention, promotion, and treatment guidelines for use by nurses, nurse practitioners, and physicians.

For infants and children, clinical practice guidelines developed at the provincial and territorial level are accessible; these guidelines include the following:
- Developmental screening tools
- Schedules for periodic well-child assessments

- Health promotion, injury prevention, and disease prevention strategies for various age groups
- Depression screening tools for adolescents
- Strategies to promote healthy parenting
- Strategies to support psychosocial and emotional development in children

For example, the *Rourke Baby Record*[18] is an evidence-informed health maintenance and prevention guide that can be used by community health nurses, nurse practitioners, and physicians caring for children during the first 5 years of life. The Canadian Paediatric Society[19] and the World Health Organization[20] also have evidence-informed developmental and preventive screening guidelines.

Tables 1.2, 1.3, 1.4, and 1.5 contain examples of clinical preventive health care recommendations per age group, beginning with birth to 9 years of age. These recommendations are periodically updated, and they vary from one province or territory to another, as noted previously; however, these tables provide a good overview of preventive guidelines over the lifespan. Addressing health promotion in the context of health assessment is discussed in depth in Chapter 2.

ASSESSMENT THROUGHOUT THE LIFE CYCLE

It makes good sense to consider health assessment from a life cycle approach. First, you must be familiar with the usual and expected developmental tasks for each age group. This knowledge alerts you to which physical, psychosocial, cognitive, and behavioural tasks are currently important for each person. Next, once assessment skills are learned, they are more meaningful when considered from a developmental perspective. Your knowledge of communication skills and health history content is enhanced as you consider how they apply to individuals throughout the life cycle. The physical examination also is more relevant when you consider age-specific data about anatomy, the method of examination, normal findings, and abnormal findings (see Fig. 10.5 pm p. 168). For example, an average normal blood pressure for a female Ellen K.'s age is 116/70 mm Hg.

For each age group, the approach to health assessment arises from an orientation toward wellness, quality of life, and health maintenance. The nurse learns to capitalize on the patient's strengths. What is the patient already doing that promotes health? What other areas are amenable to health teaching so that the patient can further build the potential for health?

 ## SOCIAL DETERMINANTS OF HEALTH CONSIDERATIONS

Considerations with respect to the social determinants of health are critical in health and physical assessments. An introduction to key concepts related to the social determinants of health is provided in Chapter 3. These concepts are threaded throughout the text as they relate to specific chapters, and a relational stance in your clinical practice will help you to attend to the varying contexts that shape people's health and well-being.

As you will read in more depth in Chapter 3, Canada's population, estimated at 35 151 728, has increased 5.0% since 2011.[21,22] Although the majority of the population is Canadian born, the Canadian population is increasingly diverse, primarily as a result of international migration. According to the 2016 census, 4.9% of the total population reported "Aboriginal identity".[23] As discussed in Chapter 3, the term *Aboriginal* is commonly used, for example, by Statistics Canada, to refer to Indigenous peoples, and in Canada, Indigenous peoples includes First Nations, Métis, and Inuit.

In Canada, health and social inequities are widening, which has had a negative influence on the health of Canadians.[10,24] At least 15% of Canadians live in impoverished circumstances, and these rates are dramatically higher for women who are raising children on their own (51%).[10] Evidence continues to demonstrate that poverty is the primary cause of poor health among Canadians.[10] For example, living in inadequate or overcrowded living conditions increases people's risk for respiratory illness, mental health problems, and injuries.[24] Nurses and other health care providers therefore require the skills and knowledge to effectively—and respectfully—explore these interrelated social, economic, and cultural factors affecting peoples' physical and mental health.

TABLE 1.2 **Clinical Preventive Health Care Recommendations: Birth to Age 9 Years**
Leading Causes of Death (2008)[a]
Conditions originating in perinatal period (<1 year)
Congenital anomalies (<1 year)
Sudden unexpected infant death (SUID) (<1 year)
Unintentional injuries
Cancer
Nervous system diseases

[a]Data from Public Health Agency of Canada. (2016). *Leading causes of death, Canada, 2008 males and females combined, counts*. Retrieved from http://www.phac-aspc.gc.ca/publicat/lcd-pcd97/table1-eng.php.

Continued

TABLE 1.2   Clinical Preventive Health Care Recommendations: Birth to Age 9 Years—cont'd

Interventions for the Pediatric Population[b]

Screening

Hip examination, serial
Eye examination, serial
Hearing and ear examination, serial
Visual acuity screen, serial
Skin and scalp, serial
Nose and mouth, serial
Chest and abdomen, serial
Serial height, weight, head circumference measurements, serial
Developmental milestones: language, social, and emotional issues, serial
Sleep and eating habits, serial
Blood test to screen for 15+ treatable disorders depending on province or territory at time of birth (most common: congenital hypothyroidism [CH], cystic fibrosis [CF], medium-chain acyl-CoA dehydrogenase deficiency [MCAD], and phenylketonuria [PKU] [at birth]).

Counselling

Injury Prevention:

Child safety car seats and boosters (<5 years)
Seatbelts (<5 years)
Violence and firearms safety
Helmet safety
Trampoline safety
Water safety (e.g., swimming and boating)
Smoke detector, flame-retardant sleepwear
Set hot water heater temperature below 48.9°C (120°F)
Window and stair guards, pool fence
Poison control phone number (see website of the Canadian Association of Poison Control Centres: http://www.capcc.ca)

Diet and Exercise:[c]

Infant Diet (0–12 Months):

- Recommend exclusive breastfeeding for the first 6 months and sustained up to 2 years (individually counsel those families who have made a fully informed choice not to breastfeed on the use of breast milk substitutes).
- Recommend that all exclusively breastfed, healthy, term infants in Canada receive 10 μg/day (400 IU/day) of vitamin D, and that this dosage should continue until the infant diet includes at least 10 μg/day (400 IU/day) from other sources.[d]
- Recommend meat, meat alternatives, and iron-fortified cereal as an infant's first complementary foods.
- Advise parents and caregivers not to give honey to a child under 1 year of age to prevent infant botulism.

Toddler and Older Children Diet (12 Months+):

- Recommend a regular schedule of meals and snacks, offering a variety of whole, nonprocessed foods from the four food groups.
- Recommend foods prepared with little or no added salt or sugar.
- Explain to parents and caregivers that nutritious, higher-fat foods are an important source of energy for young children.
- Encourage continued breastfeeding, or offering 500 mL per day of homogenized (3.25% M.F.) cow milk.
- Recommend limiting fruit juice and sweetened beverages. Encourage offering water to satisfy thirst.
- Encourage parents and caregivers to be role models and instill lifelong healthy eating habits.
- Encourage adequate vitamin D intake.

[b]Andreatta, D. (2013, August 25). Canada has no national standard for newborn screening: Here's why it should. *The Globe and Mail.* Retrieved from http://www.theglobeandmail.com/life/health-and-fitness/health/canada-has-no-national-standard-for-newborn-screening-heres-why-it-should/article13940675/; Canadian Paediatric Society. (2013). *Schedule of well-child visits.* Retrieved from http://www. caringforkids.cps.ca/handouts/schedule_of_well_child_visits; Perinatal Services BC. (2017). *Disorders screened.* Retrieved from http://www. perinatalservicesbc.ca/health-professionals/professional-resources/screening/newborn/disorders-screened.
[c]Data from Canadian Paediatric Society (2012). *Healthy active living: physical activity guidelines for children and adolescents.* Retrieved from http://www.cps.ca/en/documents/position/physical-activity-guidelines; Health Canada. (2015). *Nutrition for health term infants: recommendations from six to 24 months.* Retrieved from http://www.hc-sc.gc.ca/fn-an/nutrition/infant-nourisson/recom/recom-6-24-months-6-24-mois-eng.php.
[d]Canadian Paediatric Society. (2017). *Vitamin D supplementation: Recommendations for Canadian mothers and infants.* Retrieved from https://www.cps.ca/en/documents/position/vitamin-d.

TABLE 1.2 Clinical Preventive Health Care Recommendations: Birth to Age 9 Years—cont'd

Exercise (Infant to 9 Years Old):

- Infants (<1 year) should be physically active several times daily—particularly through interactive floor-based play.
- Toddlers (1–2 years) and preschoolers (3–4 years) should accumulate at least 180 min of physical activity at any intensity spread throughout the day. Exercise includes a variety of activities in different environments and activities that develop movement skills. There should be progression toward at least 60 min per day of energetic play by 5 years of age.
- Children (5–11 years) should accumulate at least 60 min of moderate-to-vigorous-intensity physical activity daily. Exercise includes vigorous-intensity activities at least 3 days per week and activities that strengthen muscle and bone at least 3 days per week.

Anticipatory Guidance:

Inquiries about developmental milestones

Night-time crying

Skin cancer:
- Sun exposure and protective clothing

Electronic media[e]
- TV/tablet/smartphone screen time (<2 years, not recommended; 2+ years, 0–2 hr/day maximum)
- Hearing protection

Substance use:
- Effects of second-hand smoke
- Antismoking message

Dental health:
- Regular visits to dental care provider
- Flossing once daily, brushing with fluoride toothpaste twice daily

Social support:
- Abuse and violence
- Mental health
- Body image and dieting
- Peer relationships and bullying

Immunizations (Examples)[f]

Diphtheria–tetanus–acellular pertussis–inactivated poliovirus (DTaP-IPV)[g]

Haemophilus influenzae type b (Hib) conjugate[h]

Measles-mumps-rubella (MMR)[i]

Varicella (chicken pox) (Var)[j]

Hepatitis B (HB)[k]

Pneumococcal conjugate (Pneu-C-13)[l]

Meningococcal C conjugate (Men-C)[m]

Influenza (Inf)[n]

Rotavirus (Rot)[o]

[e]Data from Screen Smart. (2010). *Screens and health.* Retrieved from http://www.screensmart.ca/screens_health.

[f]Data from Public Health Agency of Canada. (2017). *Canada's provincial and territorial routine (and catch-up) vaccination programs for infants and children.* Retrieved from https://www.canada.ca/content/dam/phac-aspc/documents/services/provincial-territorial-immunization-information/childhood_schedule.pdf.

[g]At ages 2, 4, 6, and 18 months and 4–6 years.

[h]At ages 2, 4, 6, and 18 months.

[i]At ages 12 months and 4–6 years.

[j]At age 12 months and 4-6 years.

[k]Three doses in infancy or two or three doses in preteen or teen years, depending on province.

[l]At ages 2, 4, and 12 months.

[m]Infancy: 12 months. At least one dose in primary infant series should be given after age 5 months. Earlier doses may be recommended depending on province or territory.

[n]One dose at age 6–23 months.

[o]At ages 2 and 4 months.

Continued

TABLE 1.2   Clinical Preventive Health Care Recommendations: Birth to Age 9 Years—cont'd

Chemoprophylaxis[p]

Ocular prophylaxis (birth) is no longer routinely recommended. More effective means of preventing ophthalmia neonatorum include screening all pregnant women for gonorrhea and chlamydia infection, and treatment and follow-up of those found to be infected. Mothers who were not screened should be tested at delivery. Infants of mothers with untreated gonococcal infection at delivery should receive ceftriaxone. Infants exposed to chlamydia at delivery should be followed closely for signs of infection.

Interventions for Populations at High Risk

POPULATION	POTENTIAL INTERVENTIONS
First-time mothers of low socioeconomic status (SES); lone caregivers or teenage mothers at risk for child maltreatment	Home visitation by nurses during perinatal period through infancy
Children at high risk for dental caries	Fissure sealants
Infants at high risk for iron deficiency anemia	Routine hemoglobin testing
Children at high risk for exposure to lead	Blood lead screening
Indigenous children born in Canada; parental history of intravenous drug use, HIV-positive status, or alcohol abuse	Tuberculin (TB) skin test
Recent immigrant and refugee children[q]	TB skin test, blood test, infectious disease tests, thyroid and other biochemical function tests

[p]Recommendations from Canadian Paediatric Society. (2015). Preventing ophthalmia neonatorum. Retrieved from http://www.cps.ca/en/documents/position/ophthalmia-neonatorum.

[q]Recommendations from Canadian Paediatric Society. (2016). Caring for kids new to Canada. Retrieved from http://www.kidsnewtocanada.ca/care/assessment.

TABLE 1.3   Clinical Preventive Health Care Recommendations: Ages 10 to 17 Years

Leading Causes of Death (2008)[a]
Unintentional injuries
Suicide
Cancer
Homicide
Nervous system diseases

Interventions for the Preadolescent and Adolescent Population
Screening[b]
Height, weight measurements
Physical assessment of head, neck, chest, back, abdomen, gastro-intestinal tract, skin
Visual acuity screen
Blood pressure
Pelvic examination and sexually transmitted infection (STI) testing (females; can include cis-gendered young women, trans young men, and others)[c]
Sexual maturity rating
Menstrual issues
Assessment for eating disorders
Assessment for depression and other mental health concerns
Assessment for problem drinking and other substance use

[a]Data from Public Health Agency of Canada. (2016). *Leading causes of death, Canada, 2008 males and females combined, counts.* Retrieved from http://www.phac-aspc.gc.ca/publicat/lcd-pcd97/table1-eng.php.

[b]Canadian Paediatric Society. (2016). *An update to the Greig health record: Preventative health care visits for children and adolescents aged 6 to 17 years—Technical report.* Retrieved from http://www.cps.ca/documents/position/greig-health-record-technical-report.

[c]Screening for cervical cancer under the age of 21 is not recommended. STI testing is recommended in all sexually active women, at least annually. There is insufficient evidence to recommend screening in males, unless they have specific risk factors (Canadian Paediatric Society. [2016]. *An update to the Greig health record: Preventative health care visits for children and adolescents aged 6 to 17 years—Technical report.* Retrieved from http://www.cps.ca/documents/position/greig-health-record-technical-report).

TABLE 1.3	Clinical Preventive Health Care Recommendations: Ages 10 to 17 Years—cont'd

Counselling

Injury Prevention:

Seatbelts

Violence and firearms safety

Helmet safety

Trampoline safety

Water safety (e.g., swimming and boating)

Smoke detector, flame-retardant sleepwear

Poison control phone number (see website of the Canadian Association of Poison Control Centres: http://www.capcc.ca/index.html)

Avoidance of the combination of underage alcohol and drug use with activities such as driving, swimming, and boating

Diet and Exercise:[d]

Limiting bad fats and cholesterol (e.g., processed foods); maintaining caloric balance; emphasizing whole grains, fruits, vegetables, and proteins

Adequate calcium intake

Adequate vitamin D intake

Regular exercise: children (5–11 years) and youth (12–17 years) should accumulate at least 60 min of moderate-to-vigorous-intensity physical activity daily. Exercise includes vigorous-intensity activities at least 3 days/week, and activities that strengthen muscle and bone at least 3 days/week

Anticipatory Guidance:

Electronic media[e]
  • TV/Tablet/smartphone screen time (10+ years, 0–2 hours/day maximum)
  • Hearing protection

Skin cancer:
  • Limiting sun exposure and wearing protective clothing

Substance use:
  • Antismoking message
  • Avoidance of underage drinking, underage marijuana consumption, and other illegal drugs

Sexual behaviour:
  • STI prevention: avoiding high-risk behaviour; using male or female condoms; abstinence; and barrier with spermicide
  • Prevention of unintended pregnancy: using contraception

Dental health:
  • Regular visits to dental care provider
  • Flossing once daily and brushing with fluoride toothpaste twice daily

Social support:
  • Abuse and violence
  • Mental health
  • Body image and dieting
  • Peer relationships and bullying

Immunizations (Examples—For Full List, See Source in Note f)

Diphtheria–tetanus–acellular pertussis (DTap) vaccine[f]

Hepatitis B

Human papillomavirus (HPV) vaccine

Interventions for Populations at High Risk

POPULATION	POTENTIAL INTERVENTIONS
Indigenous children born in Canada; parental history of intravenous drug use, HIV-positive status, or alcohol abuse	Tuberculin (TB) skin test
Recent immigrant and refugee children[g]	TB skin test, blood test, infectious disease tests, thyroid and other biochemical function tests

[d]Canadian Paediatric Society. (2012). *Healthy active living: physical activity guidelines for children and adolescents.* Retrieved from http://www.cps.ca/en/documents/position/physical-activity-guidelines.

[e]Screen Smart. (2010). *Screens and health.* Retrieved from http://www.screensmart.ca/screens_health.

[f]Caring for Kids. (2017). *Diphtheria-tetanus-acellular pertussis (dTap) vaccine.* Retrieved from https://www.caringforkids.cps.ca/handouts/diphtheria_tetanus_acellular_pertussis_vaccine.

[g]Canadian Paediatric Society. (2016). *Caring for kids new to Canada.* Retrieved from http://www.kidsnewtocanada.ca/care/assessment.

TABLE 1.4   Clinical Preventive Health Care Recommendations: Ages 18 to 64 Years

Leading Causes of Death (2008)[a]

Ages 18–44:	**Ages 45–64:**
Unintentional injuries	Cancer
Suicide	Circulatory system diseases
Cancer	Digestive system diseases

Interventions for the Adult Population[b]

Screening

Height, weight measurements

Blood pressure

Pelvic examination, sexually transmitted infection (STI) testing, and cervical testing (females; can include cis-gendered women, trans men, and others)[c]

Fecal occult blood test for colorectal cancer[d] (≤50 years)

Mammography ± clinical breast examination[e]

Screening for depression[f]

Clinical and risk factor screening for osteoporosis (≤50 years)[g]

Assessment for problem drinking and other substance use

[a]Data from Public Health Agency of Canada. (2016). *Leading causes of death, Canada, 2008 males and females combined, counts.* Retrieved from http://www.phac-aspc.gc.ca/publicat/lcd-pcd97/table1-eng.php.

[b]Data from Canadian Task Force on Preventive Health Care. (2013). *Guidelines.* Retrieved from http://canadiantaskforce.ca.

[c]Cervical screening recommendations are presented for screening asymptomatic females who are or have been sexually active. They do not apply to females with symptoms of cervical cancer, previous abnormal screening results (until they have been cleared to resume normal screening), those who do not have a cervix (due to hysterectomy), or who are immunosuppressed (Canadian Task Force on Preventive Health Care. [2013]. Screening for cervical cancer. *Canadian Medical Association Journal, 185*(1), 35–45). Screening for cervical cancer under the age of 21 is not recommended. STI testing is recommended in all sexually active females, at least annually. There is insufficient evidence to recommend screening in males, unless they have specific risk factors (Canadian Paediatric Society. [2016]. *An update to the Greig health record: Preventative health care visits for children and adolescents aged 6 to 17 years—Technical report.* Retrieved from http://www.cps.ca/documents/position/greig-health-record-technical-report).

- For females aged 20 to 24, we recommend not routinely screening for cervical cancer (weak recommendation; moderate-quality evidence).
- For females aged 25 to 29, we recommend routine screening for cervical cancer every 3 years (weak recommendation; moderate-quality evidence).
- For females aged 30 to 69, we recommend routine screening for cervical cancer every 3 years (strong recommendation; high-quality evidence).

[d]At least once every 2 years.

[e]Recommendations vary in different provinces: be sure to check your local guidelines. The following recommendations are presented for the use of mammography and clinical breast examination to screen for breast cancer (Canadian Task Force on Preventive Health Care. [2011]. Recommendations on screening for breast cancer in average-risk women aged 40–74. *Canadian Medical Association Journal, 183*(17), 1991–2001. Retrieved from http://www.cmaj.ca/content/183/17/1991.full#sec-3). These recommendations apply only to females at average risk for breast cancer aged 40 to 74 years. They do not apply to females at higher risk due to personal history of breast cancer, history of breast cancer in a first-degree relative, known *BRCA1/BRCA2* mutation, or prior chest wall radiation. No recommendations are made for females aged 75 and older, given the lack of data. The Canadian Task Force on Preventive Health Care recommends the following:

- For females aged 40–49, we recommend not routinely screening with mammography (weak recommendation; moderate-quality evidence).
- For females aged 50–69, we recommend routinely screening with mammography every 2 to 3 years (weak recommendation; moderate-quality evidence).
- For females aged 70–74, we recommend routinely screening with mammography every 2 to 3 years (weak recommendation; low-quality evidence).
- We recommend not routinely performing clinical breast examinations alone or in conjunction with mammography to screen for breast cancer (weak recommendation; low-quality evidence).

[f]These recommendations on screening for depression are provided for adults 18 years of age or older who present at a primary care setting with no apparent symptoms of depression (Canadian Task Force on Preventive Health Care. [2013]. *Screening for depression in primary care.* Retrieved from http://canadiantaskforce.ca/guidelines/all-guidelines/2005-screening-for-depression-in-primary-care/). These recommendations do not apply to people with known depression, with a history of depression, or who are receiving treatment for depression.

- For adults at average risk for depression, we recommend not routinely screening for depression (weak recommendation; very-low-quality evidence).
- For adults in subgroups of the population who may be at increased risk for depression, we recommend not routinely screening for depression (weak recommendation; very-low-quality evidence).

[g]The key predictors of fracture related to osteoporosis are low bone mineral density (BMD), prolonged use of glucocorticoids, use of other high-risk medications, prior fragility fracture, age, and family history. A detailed history and a focused physical examination are recommended to identify risk factors for low BMD, falls, and fractures, as well as undiagnosed vertebral fractures. In selected individuals, BMD should be measured with dual-energy X-ray absorptiometry (Papaioannou, A., Morin, S., Cheung, A. M., et al. [2010]. 2010 clinical practice guidelines for the diagnosis and management of osteoporosis in Canada: Summary. *Canadian Medical Association Journal, 182*[17], 1864–1873).

- Measure height annually, and assess for the presence of vertebral fractures.
- Assess history of falls in the past year. If there has been such a fall, a multifactorial risk assessment should be conducted, including the ability to get out of a chair without using arms.

TABLE 1.4 Clinical Preventive Health Care Recommendations: Ages 18 to 64 Years—cont'd

Counselling

Injury Prevention:[h]

Seatbelts and car seats

Avoidance of the combination of alcohol and drug use with activities such as driving, swimming, and boating

Smoke detector

Workplace safety

Diet and Exercise:

Limiting bad fats and cholesterol (e.g., processed foods); maintaining caloric balance; emphasizing whole grains, fruits, vegetables, and proteins

Adequate calcium intake

Adequate vitamin D intake

Regular physical activity that fits with health regime (e.g., low impact on joints)—at least 30 min of moderate-to-vigorous-intensity physical activity daily

Sexual Behaviour:

STI prevention: avoidance of high-risk behaviour; use of male or female condoms; and barrier with spermicide

Prevention of unintended pregnancy: contraception

Skin Cancer:

Limiting sun exposure and wearing protective clothing

Substance Use:

Smoking cessation

Responsible alcohol consumption

Harm reduction

Dental Health:

Regular visits to dental care provider

Flossing once daily and brushing with fluoride toothpaste twice daily

Immunizations (Example)

Diphtheria-tetanus (Td)[i]

Chemoprophylaxis

Multivitamin with folic acid (women planning or capable of pregnancy)

Calcium (≥50 years)

Vitamin D supplements (all adults)

Interventions for High-Risk Populations[b]

POPULATION	POTENTIAL INTERVENTIONS
• Recent immigrants and refugees from endemic areas; Indigenous people born in Canada; parental history of intravenous drug use, HIV-positive status, or high alcohol and substance use	Tuberculin (TB) skin test
• Individuals at high risk for type 2 diabetes (e.g., hypertension, dyslipidemia)	Fasting plasma glucose test

[h]More information available at Parachute Canada. (2017). *Resources*. Retrieved from http://www.parachutecanada.org/resources.
[i]Td booster every 10 years. Based on Public Health Agency of Canada. (2018). *Canadian immunization guide*. Retrieved from https://www.canada.ca/en/public-health/services/canadian-immunization-guide.html. Be sure to consult more specific provincial and territorial guidelines in your local area.

TABLE 1.5 Clinical Preventive Health Care Recommendations: Ages 65 Years and Older

Leading Causes of Death (2008)[a]

Circulatory system diseases

Cancer

Respiratory system diseases

Mental health disorders

Nervous system diseases

[a]Data from Public Health Agency of Canada. (2016). *Leading causes of death, Canada, 2008 males and females combined, counts*. Retrieved from http://www.phac-aspc.gc.ca/publicat/lcd-pcd97/table1-eng.php.

Continued

TABLE 1.5 **Clinical Preventive Health Care Recommendations: Ages 65 Years and Older—cont'd**

Interventions for the Older Adult Population[b]
Screening

Height, weight measurements

Blood pressure

Cholesterol

Diabetes

Pelvic examination, sexually transmitted infection (STI) testing, and cervical testing (females; can include cis-gendered women, trans men, and others)[c]

Fecal occult blood test[d]

Mammography ± clinical breast examination[e]

Screening for depression[f]

Visual screening (Snellen eye chart)

Hearing screening

Fall prevention (postfall multidisciplinary team assessment)

Bone mineral density (BMD)[g]

Assessment for problem drinking and substance use

---

[b]Data from Canadian Task Force on Preventive Health Care. (2013). *Guidelines.* Retrieved from http://canadiantaskforce.ca.

[c]Cervical screening recommendations are presented for screening asymptomatic females who are or have been sexually active. They do not apply to females with symptoms of cervical cancer, previous abnormal screening results (until they have been cleared to resume normal screening), those who do not have a cervix (due to hysterectomy), or who are immunosuppressed (Canadian Task Force on Preventive Health Care. [2013]. Screening for cervical cancer. *Canadian Medical Association Journal, 185*[1], 35–45). For women aged ≥70 who have been adequately screened (i.e., three successive negative Pap tests in the last 10 years), we recommend that routine screening may cease. For females aged 70 or over who have not been adequately screened, we recommend continued screening until 3 negative test results have been obtained (weak recommendation; low-quality evidence).

[d]Recommendations from the Canadian Task Force on Preventive Health Care suggest:
- Screening adults aged 60–74 for colorectal cancer (CRC) with fecal occult blood test (FOBT) (either guaiac FOBT [gFOBT] or fecal immunochemical test [FIT]) every two years OR flexible sigmoidoscopy every 10 years (strong recommendation; moderate-quality evidence)
- Screening adults aged 50 –59 for CRC with FOBT (either gFOBT or FIT) every two years OR flexible sigmoidoscopy every 10 years (weak recommendation; moderate-quality evidence)
- Not screening adults aged 75 and over for CRC (weak recommendation; low-quality evidence)
- Not using colonoscopy as a screening test for CRC (weak recommendation; low-quality evidence) (Canadian Task Force on Preventive Health Care. [2013]. *Colorectal cancer.* Retrieved from http://canadiantaskforce.ca/guidelines/published-guidelines/colorectal-cancer/)

[e]Recommendations vary in different provinces: be sure to check your local guidelines. The following recommendations are presented for the use of mammography and clinical breast examination by the Canadian Task Force on Preventive Health Care (Canadian Task Force on Preventive Health Care. [2011]. Recommendaitons on screening for breast cancer in average-risk women aged 40–74. *Canadian Medical Association Journal, 183*(17), 1991–2001. Retrieved from http://www.cmaj.ca/content/183/17/1991.full#sec-3). These recommendations apply only to females at average risk for breast cancer aged 40 to 74 years. They do not apply to females at higher risk due to personal history of breast cancer, history of breast cancer in first-degree relative, known *BRCA1/BRCA2* mutation, or prior chest wall radiation. No recommendations are made for women aged 75 and older, given the lack of data. The Canadian Task Force on Preventive Health Care recommends the following:
- For females aged 50–69, we recommend routinely screening with mammography every 2 to 3 years (weak recommendation; moderate-quality evidence).
- For females aged 70–74, we recommend routinely screening with mammography every 2 to 3 years (weak recommendation; low-quality evidence).

[f]These recommendations on screening for depression are provided for adults 18 years of age or older who present at a primary care setting with no apparent symptoms of depression. These recommendations do not apply to people with known depression, with a history of depression or who are receiving treatment for depression.
- For adults at average risk for depression, we recommend not routinely screening for depression (weak recommendation; very-low-quality evidence).
- For adults in subgroups of the population who may be at increased risk for depression, we recommend not routinely screening for depression (weak recommendation; very-low-quality evidence) (Canadian Task Force on Preventive Health Care. [2013]. *Screening for depression in primary care.* Retrieved from http://canadiantaskforce.ca/guidelines/all-guidelines/2005-screening-for-depression-in-primary-care/).

[g]The key predictors of fracture related to osteoporosis are low bone mineral density (BMD), prolonged use of glucocorticoids, use of other high-risk medications, prior fragility fracture, age, and family history. A detailed history and a focused physical examination are recommended to identify risk factors for low BMD, falls and fractures, as well as undiagnosed vertebral fractures. In selected individuals, BMD should be measured with dual-energy X-ray absorptiometry (Papaioannou, A., Morin, S., Cheung, A. M., et al. [2010]. 2010 clinical practice guidelines for the diagnosis and management of osteoporosis in Canada: Summary. *Canadian Medical Association Journal, 182*[17], 1864–1873). Best practices for an older population include measuring height annually, assessing for presence of vertebral fractures, and history of falls in past year. If there has been such a fall, conduct a multifactorial risk assessment, which includes the ability to get out of a chair without using arms (Canadian Task Force on Preventive Health Care. [2013]. *Prevention of osteoporosis and osteoporotic fractures in postmenopausal women.* Retrieved from http://canadiantaskforce.ca/guidelines/all-guidelines/2002-prevention-of-osteoporosis-and-osteoporotic-fractures-in-postmenopausal-women/).

TABLE 1.5 Clinical Preventive Health Care Recommendations: Ages 65 Years and Older—cont'd

Counselling
Injury Prevention:[h]
Nonslip surfaces in place of residence
Using grab bars and other safety aids
Using medication wisely
Seatbelts
Moving slowly out of bed and chair
Avoidance of the combination of alcohol and drug use with activities such as driving, swimming, and boating
Smoke detector
Workplace safety

Diet and Exercise:
Limiting bad fats and cholesterol (e.g., processed foods); maintaining caloric balance; emphasizing whole grains, fruits, vegetables, and proteins
Adequate calcium intake
Adequate vitamin D intake
Regular physical activity that fits with health regime (e.g., low impact on joints)—at least 30 min of moderate-to-vigorous-intensity physical activity daily

Sexual Behaviour:
STI prevention: avoidance of high-risk behaviour; use of male or female condoms

Skin Cancer:
Limiting sun exposure and wearing protective clothing

Substance Use:
Smoking cessation
Responsible alcohol consumption
Harm reduction

Dental Health:
Regular visits to dental care provider
Flossing once daily and brushing with fluoride toothpaste twice daily

Immunizations (Examples)
Diphtheria-tetanus (primary series for previously unimmunized adults or booster dose every 10 years)[i]
Influenza[j]
Pneumococcal vaccine[k]
Shingles vaccine[l]

Chemoprophylaxis
Calcium and vitamin D supplements[m]

Interventions for High-Risk Populations[b]

POPULATION	POTENTIAL INTERVENTIONS
Individuals who experience cognitive decline or a memory complaint; this information may be self-reported or come from caregivers or others close to the person	Cognitive assessment and careful follow-up required
Individuals with vascular risk factors for dementia (elevated systolic blood pressure, dyslipidemia)	Management of hypertension; physical exercise
Individuals at high risk for type 2 diabetes (e.g., hypertension, dyslipidemia)	Fasting plasma glucose test
Recent immigrants and refugees from endemic areas; parental history of intravenous drug use, HIV-positive status, or alcohol abuse	Tuberculin (TB) skin test

[h]Public Health Agency of Canada. (2016). *You can prevent falls*. Retrieved from http://www.phac-aspc.gc.ca/seniors-aines/publications/public/injury-blessure/prevent-eviter/index-eng.php.
[i]Td booster every 10 years. Based on Public Health Agency of Canada. (2018). *Canadian immunization guide: Part 4—Active vaccines*. Retrieved from https://www.canada.ca/en/public-health/services/canadian-immunization-guide.html. Be sure to consult more specific provincial and territorial guidelines in your local area.
[j]Annually.
[k]Given once after age 65.
[l]HealthLinkBC. (2017). *Shingles vaccine*. Retrieved from https://www.healthlinkbc.ca/healthlinkbc-files/shingles-vaccine.
[m]For people without documented osteoporosis, there is fair evidence that calcium and vitamin D supplementation alone prevents osteoporotic fractures (grade B recommendation) (Canadian Task Force on Preventive Health Care. [2013]. *Prevention of osteoporosis and osteoporotic fractures in postmenopausal women*. Retrieved from http://canadiantaskforce.ca/guidelines/all-guidelines/2002-prevention-of-osteoporosis-and-osteoporotic-fractures-in-postmenopausal-women/).

REFERENCES

1. Benner, P. (2001). *From novice to expert: Excellence and power in clinical nursing practice.* Upper Saddle River, NJ: Prentice Hall.
2. Cullen, M. L., & Wagner, S. (2015). The nursing process in the 21st century. In D. M. Gregory, C. Raymond-Seniuk, L. Patrick, et al. (Eds.), *Fundamentals: Perspectives on the art and science of Canadian nursing* (pp. 164–191). Philadelphia: Wolters Kluwer Health.
3. Alfaro-LeFevre, R. (2017). *Critical thinking and clinical judgment: A practical approach* (6th ed.). Philadelphia: Elsevier.
4. Canadian Nurses Association (2017). *Nurse practitioners.* Ottawa: Author. Retrieved from https://cna-aiic.ca/en/professional-development/advanced-nursing-practice/nurse-practitioners.
5. Ciliska, D. K., & Patrick, L. (2015). Nursing research and evidence-informed practice. In D. M. Gregory, C. Raymond-Seniuk, L. Patrick, et al. (Eds.), *Fundamentals: Perspectives on the art and science of Canadian nursing* (pp. 205–215). Philadelphia: Wolters Kluwer Health.
6. Registered Nurses Association of Ontario. (2014). *Promoting evidence-based practice and healthy work environments* (p. 2). Retrieved from http://rnao.ca/sites/rnao-ca/files/vision-docs/RNAO-Vision-Nurturing-Evidenced-Based-Practice-and-HWE.pdf.
7. Madsen, D., Sebolt, T., Cullen, L., et al. (2005). Listening to bowel sounds: An evidence-based practice project: Nurses find that a traditional practice isn't the best indicator of returning gastrointestinal motility in patients who've undergone abdominal surgery. *American Journal of Nursing, 105*(12), 40–50.
8. Doane, G. A., & Varcoe, C. (2015). *How to nurse: Relational inquiry with individuals and families in changing health and health care contexts.* Baltimore: Lippincott Williams & Wilkins.
9. World Health Organization. (1986). *Ottawa charter for health promotion.* Retrieved from http://www.who.int/healthpromotion/conferences/previous/ottawa/en/.
10. Raphael, D. (Ed.), (2016). *Social determinants of health: Canadian perspectives* (3rd ed.). Toronto: Canadian Scholars' Press.
11. Canadian Task Force on Preventive Health Care. (2013). *Screening for cervical cancer: Recommendations 2013.* Retrieved from https://canadiantaskforce.ca/wp-content/uploads/2016/06/2013-cervical-cancer-guideline-presentation-en.pdf.
12. Public Health Agency of Canada. (2017). *An Advisory Committee Statement (ACS) National Advisory Committee on Immunization (NACI) updated recommendations on human papillomavirus (HPV) vaccines: 9-valent HPV vaccine 2-dose immunization schedule and the use of HPV vaccines in immunocompromised populations.* Retrieved from https://www.canada.ca/content/dam/phac-aspc/documents/services/publications/healthy-living/updated-recommendations-human-papillomavirus-immunization-schedule-immunocompromised-populations/updated-recommendations-human-papillomavirus-immunization-schedule-immunocompromised-populationsv3-eng.pdf.
13. Public Health Agency of Canada. (2018). *Canadian immunization guide.* Retrieved from https://www.canada.ca/en/public-health/services/canadian-immunization-guide.html.
14. Ponka, D. (2014). The periodic health examination in adults. *CMAJ, 186*(16), 1245.
15. Canadian Paediatric Society. (2016). *Caring for kids new to Canada.* Retrieved from http://www.kidsnewtocanada.ca/care/assessment.
16. Public Health Agency of Canada. (2017). *Canada's provincial and territorial routine (and catch-up) vaccination programs for infants and children.* Retrieved from https://www.canada.ca/content/dam/phac-aspc/documents/services/provincial-territorial-immunization-information/childhood_schedule.pdf.
17. Canadian Medical Association. (2017). *Clinical practice guidelines.* Retrieved from http://www.cma.ca/cpgs.
18. Rourke Baby Record. (2017). *Rourke baby record: 2017 edition.* Retrieved from http://www.rourkebabyrecord.ca/default.asp.
19. Canadian Paediatric Society. (2017). *Clinical tools and resources.* Retrieved from https://www.cps.ca/en/tools-outils.
20. World Health Organization. (2017). *The WHO child growth standards.* Retrieved from http://www.who.int/childgrowth/en/.
21. Statistics Canada. (2017). *Population growth: Migratory increase overtakes natural increase.* Retrieved from http://www.statcan.gc.ca/pub/11-630-x/11-630-x2014001-eng.htm.
22. Statistics Canada (2017). *Population size and growth in Canada: Key results from the 2016 census.* Retrieved from http://www.statcan.gc.ca/daily-quotidien/170208/dq170208a-eng.htm.
23. "Aboriginal identity" definition from Statistics Canada. (2017). *Dictionary, census of population, 2016.* Retrieved from http://www12.statcan.gc.ca/census-recensement/2016/ref/dict/pop001-eng.cfm.
24. Canadian Institute for Health Information (2016). *Trends in income-related health inequalities in Canada.* Ottawa: Author. Retrieved from https://secure.cihi.ca/free_products/trends_in_income_related_inequalities_in_canada_2015_en.pdf.

CHAPTER 2

Health Promotion in the Context of Health Assessment

Written by Dana S. Edge, PhD, RN

http://evolve.elsevier.com/Canada/Jarvis/examination/

Changes in the conceptualization about the meaning of health began with the World Health Organization's 1946 declaration that health is "not merely the absence of disease."[1] Since that time, the definition of health has transformed from being a two-dimensional concept to one that accounts for the importance of the environment, both physical and social, in defining health. It is not enough simply to have access to good health care services. In this chapter, you are introduced to the role that Canada has played in health promotion, the foundational concepts of disease prevention and health promotion, and how nurses assess health-promoting behaviours in clinical settings.

HEALTH PROMOTION: DEVELOPMENT AND CONCEPTS

Prevalent patterns of disease and mortality in North America changed from infectious diseases in the early 1900s to chronic conditions by the late 1950s. Sanitation improvements and the discovery of penicillin played a role in this shift. Many individuals were spared contracting potentially fatal cases of polio, diphtheria, and pertussis with the development of vaccines in the 1940s and early 1950s.

The three levels of disease prevention are (a) primary, (b) secondary, and (c) tertiary prevention, which represent the biomedical approach to health promotion (Fig. 2.1). Sanitation and immunization are examples of **primary prevention**, whereby people and populations are prevented from becoming ill, sick, or injured in the first place. The definition of *primary prevention* continues to evolve, but currently it refers to the promotion of health and the prevention of illness by assisting individuals, families, and communities to prevent known health problems, protect existing states of health, and promote psychosocial wellness.[2] Often, primary prevention entails the dissemination of health information so that individuals, families, and communities have the necessary tools to keep themselves healthy and prevent disease. Primary prevention strategies, however, need to be tailored to peoples' needs and social contexts to be relevant, feasible, and effective.

Primary prevention was first discussed by American academics Hugh R. Leavell and Edwin G. Clark in the 1940s; they further described **secondary prevention** as early detection of disease, before symptoms emerge, and **tertiary prevention** as the prevention of complications when a condition or disease is present or has progressed.[3] Screening tests, such as mammography, lipid profiles, and the Papanicolaou (Pap) test, are examples of secondary prevention. As you teach a patient with newly diagnosed diabetes how to care for their feet, you are engaging in tertiary prevention activities designed to help the patient avoid complications of diabetes, such as a diabetic ulcer or infection. Box 2.1 illustrates the levels of prevention for tobacco-related illnesses.

Nurses' ability to understand the natural history of a particular disease, to know the patterns of disease occurrence, and to detect a condition early all factor into how they intervene to prevent disease. Prevention strategies are not static; as the understanding about a condition evolves, so do the prevention and treatment approaches. For example, before 1982, peptic ulcer disease was attributed to oversecretion of gastric acid, and stress was considered to be a major contributor to the excess acid. Treatment with antacids and, in severe cases, surgery, were the norms. The discovery that a bacterium, *Helicobacter pylori*, is a major risk factor in the development of gastric and duodenal ulcers[4,5] totally shifted the management and prevention of the condition, including nurses' approach to health teaching.[6]

Despite medical breakthroughs and advances in technology, curative approaches to health have limits.[7] Canada has been a leader since the 1970s in the development of health promotion frameworks. The 1974 *Lalonde Report* highlighted the limitations of the health care system to Canadians and to the international community. The traditional approach to health shifted from biomedical responses to the influences of lifestyle, human biology, and the social environment with this development.[8,9] The report laid the foundation for future health promotion initiatives in Canada. The *Declaration of Alma-Ata* reinforced health promotion principles in 1978, which heralded a shift in power from health care providers to consumers of health care and their communities.[7] Moreover, in 1986, the *Ottawa Charter for Health Promotion* was released with five action strategies to improve the health of populations.[10] **Health promotion**, as defined by the World Health Organization, is "the process of enabling people to increase control over, and to improve their health. It moves beyond a focus on individual behaviour towards a wide

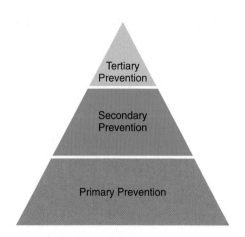

2.1 Levels of health prevention.

BOX 2.1 **Prevention of the Damaging Effects of Tobacco**

Primary: Teaching a group of Grade 3 students about the harmful effects of tobacco use.
Secondary: Providing tobacco cessation or reduction strategies to a current smoker who has expressed an interest in attempting to quit or cut down.
Tertiary: Limiting second-hand smoke exposure to a patient with chronic obstructive lung disease.

---

range of social and environmental interventions."[11] In 1984, the World Health Organization set out five principles of health promotion, which continue to guide practice today:

1. Health promotion involves the population as a whole in the context of their everyday lives.
2. Health promotion is directed toward action on the social determinants of health.
3. Health promotion combines diverse but complementary methods.
4. Health promotion seeks to achieve effective and concrete public participation.
5. Health promotion is nurtured and enabled by health care providers, particularly those in primary health care.[12]

How much do environmental, social, and biological factors influence health? We now know that 50% of all health outcomes can be attributed to social and economic factors, 25% to health care services, 15% to biology and genetics, and 10% to the built and natural environment.[13] The **social determinants of health** as outlined by the Public Health Agency of Canada (PHAC) include the following elements: income and social status; social support networks; education and literacy; employment/working conditions; social environments; physical environments; personal health practices and coping skills; healthy child development; biology and genetic endowment; health services; gender; and culture.[14] The socioeconomic environment, in particular, has a profound influence on individuals' health. Income, social status, social support networks, education, employment, and social environments are components of the socioeconomic

environment. **Disparities in health** occur when the combination and interaction of the social determinants of health result in differences in health status between segments of the population. When disparities are avoidable, but outside the control of individuals, **health inequities** result.[15]

Certain populations in Canada are at increased risk for disease and disability as a result of growing social and health inequities.[16] For example, First Nations and Inuit peoples have shorter life expectancy and higher rates of morbidity from infectious diseases, such as tuberculosis, than do the rest of Canadians.[17] Temporary foreign workers, whose numbers have doubled in Canada between 2004 and 2013, also experience health inequities. They are employed predominantly in the agricultural sector, and concerns have been raised about their working conditions.[18] Questionable working conditions, inadequate housing, and vulnerability affect temporary workers' ability to work and, ultimately, their health.[19] Undocumented immigrants and refugee claimants face similar challenges in terms of their ability to access health care.[20] Poor health indicators can be linked directly to social and economic conditions such as overcrowding, low income, and lack of access to nutritious foods, particularly for those living on-reserve or in remote locations.

THE POPULATION HEALTH PROMOTION MODEL AS A GUIDE TO NURSING ASSESSMENT

Nursing assessment occurs at the individual, family, community, and population levels. The Population Health Promotion Model provides a multifaceted approach to considering the social determinants of health in our nursing health assessment, whether one is working in a tertiary hospital, an outpatient clinic, long-term care, home care, a public health agency, or working as a policy analyst. The Population Health Promotion Model was developed in 1996 by Hamilton and Bhatti (Fig. 2.2). A three-dimensional cube rests on a base foundation of the values and assumptions of a society upon which evidence-informed decision making occurs. Three faces of the 3-D cube are visible. On the top, a continuum from the individual to society is depicted, representing with *who or whom* health care providers are to engage with. On one side, the five action strategies of the Ottawa Charter provide guidance as to *how* we can take health promotion action. Finally, the original nine social determinants of health are listed on the opposite side of the cube, indicating on *what* we can take action to promote health (today, Canada also recognizes social environments, gender, and culture as social determinants of health). The model illustrates the larger context and societal influences that affect individuals, families, communities, and populations.

Health promotion forces nurses to focus upstream* to the root causes of health conditions that afflict individuals.

---

*Taking action to avoid a problem before it occurs is referred to as "moving upstream" and is the hallmark of primary prevention.[8]

WHO: With whom can we act?
(The levels within society
where action can be taken)

WHAT: On what can we
take action?
(The determination of
health care areas where
action could improve
health)

HOW: How can we take
action to improve health?
(The Ottawa Charter
action strategies)

WHY: Why take action to improve health?
(Using the best available information to make
decisions that are consistent with community
needs, values, and resources)

2.2 The Population Health Promotion Model.

Health care providers alone cannot tackle many of the barriers to adequate health in populations. Instead, public policy, by nurses and others, must promote sustainable employment, sound education, food security, environmental protection, political stability, and affordable health care. Enacting such policies necessitates that multiple players, including the public, understand the importance of the social determinants of health and act to improve them.

In addition to influencing health policy, health care providers play a pivotal role in promoting health at individual, family, and community levels through health education and counselling, immunization, and screening activities. Inquiry into the social determinants of health is completed during health history encounters with patients and families (Table 2.1). Health education is one specific intervention strategy that is employed by all nurses to promote patients' health. The Population Health Promotion Model can be used to consider social determinants of health during health encounters with patients, and to guide health promotion strategies when working with individuals, families, and communities. At a higher societal level, the Population Health Promotion Model serves to influence change in health, social, and environmental policies.

SPECIFIC HEALTH PROMOTION INTERVENTIONS

Consider Randy, a 45-year-old single man who seeks health care for recurrent early morning insomnia. During your interview with him, Randy reports that he falls asleep easily at night but awakens around 3:00 A.M. and spends hours unable to fall back asleep, sitting in front of the television in his armchair. As the interview proceeds, Randy indicates that he was a chief engineer at a major automotive assembly plant but was "let go" 4 weeks ago; he is not sure how he will be able to pay his bills or his mortgage. His aging

TABLE 2.1   Social Determinants of Health and the Health History

Social Determinants of Health[b]	Corresponding Components of the Health History[a]
Socioeconomic environment: • Income and social status • Social support networks • Education and literacy • Employment/working conditions • Social environments	Biographical data; functional assessment (interpersonal relationships; social and economic contexts; spiritual resources; occupational health)
Physical environments	Functional assessment (environmental hazards)
Healthy child development	Developmental history
Personal health practices and coping skills	• Health promotion and harm reduction approaches • Functional assessment (self-concept; coping and stress management)
Biology and genetic endowment	Family history
Health services	Most recent examination (medical, dental, immunizations)
Gender	Biographical data
Culture	Biographical data; cultural perception of health

[a]See Chapter 5 in this book.
[b]From Public Health Agency of Canada. (2017). *What determines health?* Retrieved from http://www.phac-aspc.gc.ca/ph-sp/determinants/index-eng.php#determinants.

parents, who live in another province, are not aware of his situation. Randy reveals that he has lost 5 kg during the past month and is not interested much in eating. At this point in the encounter, you have information about his presenting concern, socioeconomic status, and his coping skills. At this visit, more detail about his social supports and how he can manage financially is required. Future visits could explore his physical environment, personal health practices, family history, social and cultural contexts, and use of preventive health care services.

Your assessment and interventions in relation to Randy's presenting symptom of insomnia are affected by the knowledge that the suicide rate among Canadians is highest for men between ages 40 and 59 (32.5 per 100 000).[21] Randy is experiencing the loss of a valued occupational role and social isolation, which increase the risk for self-harm. Your interventions today focus on identifying any deviations from health in your physical examination that could explain the insomnia, screening for depression and suicidal ideation (see Chapter 6), and working with Randy on a plan to support him during this period of upheaval in his life. The approach used with Randy is illustrative of a counselling intervention to support healthy practices and behaviours, given the context of his life, and to promote overall health. Depending on Randy's responses, screening for suicidal ideation may be required (see Chapter 6). From the previous description, several social determinants of health have been assessed in this one encounter between you and Randy.

HEALTH EDUCATION AND COUNSELLING ACTIVITIES IN HEALTH PROMOTION

Focusing on patients' strengths, capacities, and resources, nurses can inquire about patients' injury prevention, diet, exercise, sexual health, substance use, dental health, anticipatory guidance, and primary prevention of specific cancers during health encounters.[22] Any health education intervention should be informed by the developmental level and the cultural, social, and economic context of the individual (and the family); the readiness of the person to engage in discussions related to health information; the availability of local resources; and the prevalent health conditions for which the individual may be at risk. For example, Canadian men younger than 20 are at risk for injuries during recreational and organized sports activities.[23] During a health care visit by a young man, you are provided with the opportunity to learn about the man's interests, his health-protective behaviours (e.g., protective gear), and his beliefs about vulnerability, and you can tailor your health education messages accordingly.

Health education and counselling can be utilized at all three levels of prevention. As exhibited in in Box 2.1, the primary and secondary tobacco prevention examples are health education strategies; an example of tobacco-related health education at the tertiary prevention level is the proper instruction of inhaler use for a hospitalized patient with smoking-related chronic obstructive pulmonary disease (COPD). With tertiary prevention, the goal is to assist patients in preventing complications of disease and illness. It is important to recognize that health education is one strategy of health promotion. Furthermore, health education is not synonymous with health promotion, as health education is a limited approach when the resources to implement recommended health promotion strategies or influence economic and social change are unavailable.[24]

IMMUNIZATIONS

Active immunization through the use of either vaccines or toxoid preparations elicits immunological self-response within the host body that provides protection at a later exposure date. The measles-mumps-rubella (MMR) immunization is an example of a vaccine, whereas protection against diphtheria and tetanus is provided through the administration of a toxoid.[25,26] In some instances, antibodies are administered in the form of immune globulin to people who have already been exposed to a disease; this action is known as *passive immunization*, and the effects are short-lived. As mentioned previously, immunization is a primary prevention activity. Inadequate coverage or lack of booster vaccinations can result in re-emergence of infectious disease in susceptible hosts, such as mumps outbreaks in 2014 and 2017 among National Hockey League (NHL) players.[27] Opportunities to check immunization status with patients, including booster status, occur with nearly every health encounter, and yet it is an opportunity frequently missed in many health care settings due to a variety of factors.[28]

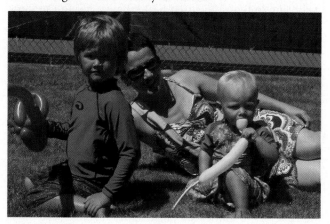

SCREENING

Early detection of a condition or disease is possible when a sensitive and effective tool for detection is available; when the natural history of the condition has a long latency period before symptoms appear; and when an acceptable treatment method is available.[29] Some malignancies are amenable to early detection, including cervical, breast, colon, skin, and prostate tumours. Nurses can also screen to identify individuals at risk for falls, depression, visual acuity loss, problematic alcohol or substance use, and hearing loss. Screening is based on the prevalence of the disease in the population; therefore, routine screening is reasonable when the prevalence is relatively high in a specific age group, gender, or ethnic population. The natural history of disease, the pattern of the disease in the population, and other epidemiological indicators, in addition to the individual's risk profile, provide the evidence to support the decision of whether to screen.

SCREENING TOOLS FOR DEVELOPMENTAL TASKS

Before its revision in 1989, public health nurses in Canada used the Denver Developmental Screening Test (DDST), a professionally administered test, extensively. By the early 1990s, however, the Canadian Task Force on Preventive Health Care had reported insufficient evidence for the routine developmental screening of children.[30] Because of the lack of evidence of effectiveness, as well as funding cuts in public health, the routine use of the DDST ceased. In its place, several provincial programs now use the Nipissing District Developmental Screen (NDDS), a parent-report screening tool (Fig. 2.3 shows the screening tool for 2-year-olds).

The NDDS originated in 1993 from the work of a multidisciplinary committee of health professionals within the Nipissing District of Ontario; by 1997, the screen was being used across Canada, and since that time, the tool has been revised and analyzed for cultural sensitivity, Grade 5 literacy level, and reliability. Currently, Ontario, New Brunswick, and the Nunavut have endorsed the NDDS as the screening tool of choice in provincial programs, and the forms are free of charge to Ontario residents.[31] Translated versions in French, Spanish, and Vietnamese are available, and the tool can be accessed electronically, with interactive screens. The NDDS elicits a "yes" or "no" response from parents for a set of developmental milestones appropriate to the age of the child; a "no" response highlights a potential developmental delay. Other available parent-report developmental screening tools that were developed in North America include the Ages and Stages Questionnaires (ASQ), the Child Development Inventory (CDI), and the Parents' Evaluation of Developmental Status (PEDS). Weighing the evolving discoveries in neuroscience and the effects of environment on early childhood development, the Canadian Paediatric Society endorsed the systematic use of a developmental screening tool (e.g., NDDS, ASQ, PEDS) at each 18-month well-baby visit.[32] An overview of developmental tasks for each age group can be found on the Evolve website.

CASE EXAMPLE: INCORPORATING HEALTH PROMOTION STRATEGIES

Mary is a 72-year-old Cree woman who is living with five members of her extended family in a three-bedroom bungalow on-reserve. For the past 10 years, Mary has been living with type 2 diabetes and has been seen by health care providers on a regular basis. Over the past 6 months, her glucose levels have not been at target, despite the adjustment of her oral hypoglycemic agent. She has come today to clinic because she just does not feel "right." You check her glucose level and find that it is moderately elevated. What

information do you need to gather to properly care for Mary? What are potential factors that may have contributed to Mary's diabetes? What else might be happening in her environment that might be contributing to her not feeling "right"? How will you determine the focus of your health assessment? What are relevant cultural and social considerations that should inform your health messages and health promotion strategies? Let's consider how an appreciation of health promotion concepts, including the social determinants of health, can assist in your assessment.

As you begin to gather Mary's story about not feeling "right," be mindful of living conditions and circumstances within the community. A larger appreciation of the cultural and historical influences in Mary's community provides context for potential health inequities that may have contributed to Mary's ill health.[33,34]

You need to begin by reviewing with Mary what her typical day has been like over the past 6 months, particularly with regard to her diet, medication, and exercise patterns. Mary's understanding of the disease process, her social support, factors potentially impeding her ability to walk in the community (as her form of exercise), plus your understanding of local food availability and affordability all contribute to a better understanding of the situational influences affecting Mary.[33,34] You can ask Mary several questions: "You told me that you don't feel 'right.' Can you describe what you mean by 'not right'?" "You've been told you have diabetes, Mary. Tell me what diabetes means to you." "How do the diabetes pills make you feel? Any problems with taking them?" "Mary, tell me about what you ate yesterday. Today?" "How often are you able to eat traditional food?" "Mary, who prepares the meals in your home?" "How often are you able to purchase fresh fruits or vegetables?" "What do you think may be wrong, Mary?" Inquiry into Mary's daily activities and any recent departures from her routines, along with her beliefs about what might be causing her to feel "not right," can provide immeasurable insights into her beliefs and behaviours. These assessment data are critical for beginning a plan with Mary to develop health promotion strategies that are acceptable to her. Such an approach leads to safer, more appropriate care.[35] Exploration of Mary's experience may also lead to identification of community-level health issues such as the need for more affordable access to fruits and vegetables that can be addressed locally or advocated for at a regional, provincial, or federal level for change.

SUMMARY

Individuals and their families reside in communities that are part of a much larger sociopolitical environment. As you focus on caring for an individual, you must remain mindful of the larger context and engage in upstream thinking to more fully understand the person's particular situation. Health care providers frequently undervalue the influence of a well-placed question or comment to a patient. Even short health assessment encounters offer the opportunity to inquire about health-promoting behaviours within the

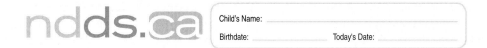

Child's Name: _____

Birthdate: _____ Today's Date: _____

The ndds checklist is designed to
help monitor your child's development.

Y N   BY **TWO YEARS** OF AGE, DOES YOUR CHILD:

○ ○ 1 Understand one and two step directions? *("close the door", "go find your book and show it to grandma")**

○ ○ 2 Ask for help using words?

○ ○ 3 Learn and use one or more new words a week? *(may only be understood by family)*

○ ○ 4 Join two words together? *("want cookie", "car go", "my hat")**

○ ○ 5 Eat most foods without coughing and choking?

○ ○ 6 Eat with a utensil with little spilling?**

○ ○ 7 Take off own shoes, socks, or hat?**

○ ○ 8 Try to run?

○ ○ 9 Play in a squat position? *A*

○ ○ 10 Walk backwards or sideways pulling a toy?

○ ○ 11 Make scribbles and dots on paper or in sand?

○ ○ 12 Put objects into a small container? *B*

○ ○ 13 Like to watch and play near other children?

○ ○ 14 Say "no", and like to do some things without help?**

○ ○ 15 Use toys for pretend play? *(give doll a drink)**

○ ○ 16 Use skills already learned and develop new ones? *(no loss of skills)*

○ ○ 17 Copy your actions? *(you clap your hands and he/she claps hands)**

2
YEARS
English

* Examples provided are only suggestions.
 You may use similar examples from your family experience.

** Item may not be common to all cultures.

Always talk to your healthcare or childcare professional if you have any questions about your child's development or well being.
See reverse for instructions, limitation of liability, and product license. NDDS © 2011 NDDS Intellectual Property Association. All rights reserved.

2.3 Nipissing District Developmental Screen.

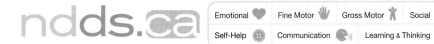

The following **activities for your child** will help you play your part in your child's development.

I am learning about my feelings. Give me words for my feelings and show that you understand.

Let me open and close plastic containers by twisting and turning the lids. Help me find the right lid to put on each container.

I love to pour water from containers during my bath.

I enjoy stringing beads or buttons on a shoelace, string, or pipe cleaner. Talk to me about the colour and count the beads as I lace them. Remember, I may still put things in my mouth, so watch me.

Provide me with toys that allow me to push or pedal with my feet. This will help me learn to climb on and off and to pedal. Make sure I have lots of room. Praise my efforts.

Let's practise climbing and jumping. I love to get in and out of a box or jump from a bottom step. We can have fun together.

Let's sing *Old MacDonald* and move our bodies like the animals: hop like a frog or bunny, squat or waddle like a duck, or jump up and down like a kangaroo.

I love sharing storybooks with you. Cuddle me while we read together.

Let's play a game. Use two shoeboxes and two toys. We each get a box and a toy. Let's take turns putting our toy in, over, under, behind, and on the box. Talk to me about what we are doing.

I want to become independent. Encourage me to get dressed and undressed, do household tasks, turn lights on and off, and open and close doors.

Sing songs with me throughout the day and repeat them often. This helps me learn to sing them on my own. Leave out parts of the song or rhyme for me to finish.

Help me learn new words. Talk to me during bathing, feeding, dressing, and doing daily chores. Name my clothing and body parts. Let me help set the table, sort the laundry, and put groceries away.

I like to play sorting games with you. We can sort objects by shape, touch, colour, and size. Use spoons, blocks, toys, and clothing.

I am learning to make decisions; offer me choices throughout the day.

I may get ear infections. Talk to my doctor about signs and symptoms.

Always talk to your healthcare or childcare professional if you have any questions about your child's development or well being
See reverse for instructions, limitation of liability, and product license. NDDS © 2011 NDDS Intellectual Property Association. All rights reserved.

2.3, cont'd

context of the visit (e.g., asking about bicycle helmet use during an assessment of a minor sports-related injury). The key is to attend to what is being said and not said, to appreciate the environmental context, and to demonstrate genuine respect. The effect of the social determinants of health on an individual's health status cannot be underestimated, and the opportunities to promote health are endless.

REFERENCES

1. World Health Organization. (1946). *Preamble to the Constitution of the World Health Organization as adopted by the International Health Conference*, New York, 19–22 June, 1946; signed on 22 July 1946 by the representatives of 61 States (Official Records of the World Health Organization, no. 2, p.

100) and entered into force on 7 April 1948. Retrieved from http://www.who.int/kobe_centre/about/faq/en/.

2. Bloom, M., & Gullotta, T. P. (2014). Definitions of primary care. In T. P. Gullotta & M. Bloom (Eds.), *Encyclopedia of primary prevention and health promotion* (pp. 3–12). New York: Springer U.S.

3. McPherson, N. C., Belton, K. L., & Watson-Creed, G. (2017). Population health action: Prevention and harm reduction. In A. R. Vollman, E. T. Anderson, & J. McFarlane (Eds.), *Canadian community as partners: Theory & multidisciplinary practice* (4th ed., pp. 157–170). Philadelphia: Wolters Kluwer.

4. Lanas, A., & Chan, F. K. L. (2017). Peptic ulcer disease. *Lancet, 390*(10094), 613–624. doi: https://doi.org/10.1016/S0140-6736(16)32404-7.

5. Lynch, N. A. (2000). *Helicobacter pylori* and ulcers: A paradigm revised. *FASEB Breakthroughs in Bioscience*. Retrieved from http://www.faseb.org/Portals/2/PDFs/opa/pylori.pdf.

6. Barba, K., Fitzgerald, P., & Wood, S. (2007). Managing peptic ulcer disease. *Nursing, 37*(7), 56hn1–56hn4.

7. Catford, J. (2014). Turn, turn, turn: Time to reorient health services. *Health Promotion International, 29*(1), 1–3.

8. Kirk, M., Tomm-Bonde, L., & Schreiber, R. (2014). Public health reform and health promotion in Canada. *Global Health Promotion, 21*(2), 15–22.

9. Lalonde, M. (1974). *A new perspective on the health of Canadians*. Ottawa: Minister of Supply and Services Canada.

10. World Health Organization (1986). *Ottawa Charter for Health Promotion: First international conference on health promotion, Ottawa, 21 November 1986*. Geneva: Author. Retrieved from http://www.who.int/healthpromotion/conferences/previous/ottawa/en/.

11. World Health Organization (2017). *Health promotion*. Geneva: Author, para. 1. Retrieved from http://www.who.int/topics/health_promotion/en/.

12. Catford, J. (2004). Health promotion's record card: How principled are we 20 years on? *Health Promotion International, 19*(1), 1–4.

13. The Standing Senate Committee on Social Affairs, Science and Technology; the Honourable Wilbert Joseph Keon, Chair, and the Honourable Lucie Pepin, Deputy Chair. (2009). *A healthy productive Canada: A determinant of health approach. Final report of the Senate Subcommittee on Population Health*. Retrieved from https://sencanada.ca/content/sen/Committee/402/popu/rep/rephealthjun09-e.pdf.

14. Public Health Agency of Canada. (2017). *What determines health?* Retrieved from http://www.phac-aspc.gc.ca/ph-sp/determinants/index-eng.php#determinants.

15. Pan-Canadian Health Inequalities Data Tool. (2017). *A joint initiative of the Public Health Agency of Canada, the Pan-Canadian Public Health Network, Statistics Canada and the Canadian Institute of Health Information*. Retrieved from http://infobase.phac-aspc.gc.ca/health-inequalities/.

16. Canadian Institute for Health Information (2016). *Trends in income-related health inequalities in Canada*. Ottawa: Author. Retrieved from https://www.cihi.ca/sites/default/files/trendshealthinequalities_inddefs_sept2016_combined_en_web_0.pdf.

17. Public Health Agency of Canada (2016). *Health status of Canadians 2016: A report of the chief public health officer*. Ottawa: Author. Retrieved from http://www.healthycanadians.gc.ca/publications/department-ministere/state-public-health-status-2016-etat-sante-publique-statut/index-eng.php.

18. United Food and Commercial Workers Union. (2015). *Report on the status of migrant workers in Canada, 2015*. Retrieved from http://www.ufcw.ca/index.php?option=com_content&view=article&id=59&Itemid=2&lang=en.

19. Preibisch, K., & Hennebry, J. (2011). Temporary migration, chronic effects: The health of international migrant workers in Canada. *Canadian Medical Association Journal, 183*(9), 1033–1038. doi:10.1503/cmaj.090736.

20. Campbell, R. M., Klei, A. G., Hodges, B. D., et al. (2014). A comparison of health access between permanent residents, undocumented immigrants and refugee claimants in Toronto, Canada. *Journal of Immigrant and Minority Health, 16*, 165–176.

21. Navaneelan, T. (2015). *Suicide rates: An overview* (Catalogue no. 82-624-X). Retrieved from http://www.statcan.gc.ca/pub/82-624-x/2012001/article/11696-eng.htm.

22. Zenzano, T., Allan, J. D., Bigley, M. B., et al. (2011). The roles of healthcare professionals in implementing clinical prevention and population health. *American Journal of Preventive Medicine, 40*(2), 261–267.

23. Billette, J.-M., & Janz, T. (2015). *Injuries in Canada: Insights from the Canadian Community Health Survey* (Catalogue no. 82-624-X). Retrieved from http://www.statcan.gc.ca/pub/82-624-x/2011001/article/11506-eng.htm.

24. Whitehead, D. (2006). Health promotion in the practice setting: Findings form a review of clinical issues. *Worldviews on Evidence-based Nursing, 3*(4), 165–184.

25. Public Health Agency of Canada. (2018). *Canadian immunization guide*. Retrieved from https://www.canada.ca/en/public-health/services/canadian-immunization-guide.html.

26. Sanford, C. A., & Jong, E. C. (2016). Immunizations. *Medical Clinics of North America, 100*, 247–259.

27. Osbourn, E. (2014). NHL mumps outbreak: 7 big questions answered. *CBC News*. Retrieved from http://www.cbc.ca/news/health/nhl-mumps-outbreak-7-big-questions-answered-1.2873761. and Wawrow, J. (2017). NHL players hope league can contain latest mumps outbreak. *CTV News*. Retrieved from http://www.ctvnews.ca/sports/nhl-players-hope-league-can-contain-latest-mumps-outbreak-1.3305508.

28. Gingold, J. A., Bricetti, C., Zook, K., et al. (2016). Context matters: Practitioner perspectives on immunization delivery quality improvement efforts. *Clinical Pediatrics, 55*(9), 825–837.

29. Association of Faculties of Medicine of Canada. (2013). *AFMC primer on population health*. Mountain View, CA: Author, Chapter 4. Retrieved from https://afmc.ca/sites/default/files/documents/en/Medical-Education/Public-Health/AFMC-Primer-on-Population-Health-2013-08-14.pdf.

30. Canadian Task Force on Preventive Health Care. (2016). Recommendations on screening for developmental delay. *Canadian Medical Association Journal, 188*(8), 579–587.

31. Nipissing District Developmental Screen. (2017). *About NDDS*. Retrieved from http://www.ndds.ca/about.html.

32. Williams, R., Clinton, J., & Canadian Paediatric Society, Early Years Task Force. (2011). Getting it right at 18 months: In support of an enhanced well-baby visit. *Paediatrics & Child Health, 16*(10), 647–650.

33. Hackett, C., Feeny, D., & Tompa, E. (2016). Canada's residential school system: Measuring the intergenerational impact of familial attendance on health and mental health outcomes. *Journal of Epidemiology and Community Health, 70*, 1096–1105.

34. Turin, T. C., Saad, N., Jun, M., et al. (2016). Lifetime risk of diabetes among First Nations and non-First Nations people. *Canadian Medical Association Journal, 188*(16), 1147–1153.

35. Rhodes, P., Campbell, S., & Sanders, C. (2015). Trust, temporality and systems: How do patients understand patient safety in primary care? A qualitative study. *Health Expectations, 19*, 253–263.

3 CHAPTER

Cultural and Social Considerations in Health Assessment

Written by Annette J. Browne, PhD, RN, and Colleen Varcoe, PhD, RN

http://evolve.elsevier.com/Canada/Jarvis/examination/

Who is the person you are meeting for the first time? Where does the person come from? How does the person identify in relation to his, her, or their cultural, social, or family background? What is the person's heritage, gender, ethnicity, and religious orientation? What language(s) does the person understand, speak, and read? What are the person's health and illness beliefs and practices? As discussed in Chapter 1, operating from a **relational** standpoint,* you should ask yourself: "Who am I? Where do I come from? What is my social, cultural, and family background? How would I identify in terms of my heritage, ethnicity, gender, and religion? What is my primary language? Do I understand, speak, and read a language other than English? What are my health and illness beliefs and practices?" A **relational approach** to health assessment prompts you to ask: "How do my social, cultural, and professional backgrounds shape my ability to relate to, and my assumptions about, the various people I encounter in my practice?" Approaching cultural and social considerations in health assessment from a relational stance helps you understand and attend to the contexts that shape patterns of health and illness. These contexts include people's past experiences, culture, and heritage; how they identify in terms of gender, their socioeconomic status, and history; and their understanding of health, illness, and strategies for maintaining health. By recognizing and attending to these contexts, you will be optimally prepared to conduct accurate health assessments and respond meaningfully to people's health, illness, and health promotion needs.

Over the course of your professional education, you will study the developmental tasks and the principles of health promotion across the lifespan and learn to conduct numerous assessments, such as: documentation of a complete health history, a mental health assessment, an assessment of risks for violence, a nutritional assessment, a pain assessment, and a physical examination of a patient. As a health care provider, you will continually experience similarities and differences between you and the patients (and patients' families) with whom you come in contact. These differences are based on a wide range of factors including life experiences, opportunities, circumstances, and linguistic, social, familial, and cultural traditions. A relational approach is aimed at making similarities and differences more transparent, so that we can be as responsive as possible to people's diverse needs.

The purposes of this chapter are as follows:
1. To describe concepts that are central to understanding cultural and social considerations in health assessment
2. To distinguish between cultural sensitivity, cultural competence, and cultural safety, and their implications for practice
3. To review the shifting demographic trends within the Canadian population
4. To provide examples of ethnocultural diversity within the Canadian population

---

*In this chapter, the term *relational* refers to "the complex interplay of human life, the world, and nursing practice" and is "grounded in the assumption that people are relational beings who are situated in and constituted through social, cultural, political and historical processes and communities."[1] Therefore, a relational approach to nursing practice extends beyond nurse–patient relationships to consider the contexts, structures, and forces that influence patients, nurses, the health care system, our communities, and societies.

5. To review trends in health, social, and gender inequities in Canada

6. To identify guidelines for assessing the social, cultural, and economic contexts that shape people's health

As you encounter the various questions we pose in this chapter, take a few minutes to reflect on the thoughts and reactions that may arise, and how they could impact your practice as a nurse.

CULTURAL AND SOCIAL CONSIDERATIONS: CENTRAL CONCEPTS

Culture, Ethnicity, and Culturalism: What Do Nurses Need to Know for Accurate Health Assessments?

No single definition of **culture** exists. All too often, definitions tend to be so general that they lack any real meaning or are so specific that they erase the complexity and shifting nature of culture. In disciplines such as anthropology, culture is understood as an inherently complex dimension of people's lives. That is because culture is a "dynamic relational process of selectively responding to and integrating particular historical social, political and economic, physical and linguistic" factors, and is "relationally determined and contextual."[1] Anderson and Reimer-Kirkham explain further that culture is "not therefore reduced to an easily identifiable set of characteristics, nor is it a politically neutral concept."[2]

Despite these complexities, in health care, culture tends to be viewed in a very limited and narrow way as the values, beliefs, customs, practices, and characteristics of particular ethnocultural group members (Figs. 3.1 and 3.2). These assumed "cultural traits" are typically those identified as different from "ours," the unspoken comparison being made with the assumed dominant norm. From this narrow viewpoint, nurses and other health care providers often operate on the basis of erroneous assumptions about people who are assumed to be members of particular ethnocultural groups. Operating in this manner can cause nurses and others to overlook the most salient factors that are influencing people's health.

Ethnicity is also not synonymous with *culture*. **Ethnicity** is a complex concept that can encompass multiple different aspects such as one's country of origin or ancestry, identity, and family history, languages spoken, and, in some cases, religious identity.[3,4] However, how individuals identify their ethnicity often changes as a result of new immigration flows and the changing nature of identity politics and nationalism. Some people may identify as part of an **ethnic group**, referring to a population or group who identify with each other based on a shared heritage, culture, language, or religious affiliation, but many do not.[5] These trends are complex: in Canada, the definition of *ethnicity* continues to shift and evolve. For example, in 2009, Statistics Canada began using the term *population group* in place of *ethnicity* to refer to "the population group or groups to which the person belongs."[6]

3.1 What aspects of culture do you see in this picture? Most people think of the carvings as "cultural" but how many of us see the house's architecture, the logging slash behind the house, and the various items (ladder, chimney) as also reflecting culture?

3.2 What definition of *culture* comes to your mind when looking at this picture?

In health care, because Canada and the United States have drawn so heavily on narrowly defined ideas about culture, there has been a proliferation of textbooks in nursing and medicine that provide systematized descriptions or lists of cultural characteristics for various groups. This is problematic for a number of reasons. How individuals relate to their cultural orientation develops in distinctive ways depending on where they live, their family background, socioeconomic circumstances, educational attainment, language(s) spoken, spiritual orientation, ancestry, and history as both individuals and as members of specific groups. Therefore, although culturally based characteristics are applicable to some people, within any given group, individuals will have varying health practices, differing levels of knowledge about health-related issues, and diverse points of view and family norms. For example, Chinese communities in Canada are extremely diverse. There is no predefined approach to follow in interacting with people who have recently emigrated from China. Furthermore, there are often significant differences between generations, including differences after migration. The dangers of applying presumed lists of cultural traits to patients whom you encounter lies in drawing on stereotypes and making assumptions about particular people, which, in turn, lead to unsafe health assessment practices. Nurses and other health care providers must therefore find ways of learning about all their patients, and their contexts, to understand how best to address their health needs.[1]

The process of conceptualizing culture in fairly narrow terms, or assuming that people act in particular ways because of their culture, is known as **culturalism**. From a culturalist perspective, culture is often given as the primary explanation for why certain people or populations experience various health, social, or economic problems. Research shows that health care providers frequently attribute people's social problems to their cultural characteristics.[4,7,8] Doing so would lead them to wrongly assume that violence toward women may be acceptable in particular cultural groups or that some people are more prone to using drugs or alcohol because of their "culture." Similarly, you cannot make accurate assumptions about people's health beliefs on the basis of their ethnicity. For example, it would be wrong to assume that people from China necessarily embrace the hot–cold theory of health and illness (an explanatory model in which the treatment of illness requires cold, heat, dryness, or wetness to restore balance). Such assumptions are culturalist because they are based on (a) popularized (and often stereotypical) ideas about culture as something fixed and inherent to particular groups defined by language, country of origin, or physical characteristics, and (b) the notion that culture is the primary explanation for people's health-related practices or decisions. These assumptions are problematic because they do not lead to useful information and can be erroneous in relation to providing high-quality care.

To counter this tendency toward culturalism in health care, it can be useful to define culture from a **critical cultural perspective**.[7] According to a critical cultural perspective, *culture* is a relational aspect of individuals that shifts and changes over time, depending on an individual's history, social context, past experiences, gender identity, professional identity, and so on. Viewing culture in this way does not imply that health care providers should not pay attention to patients' values, beliefs, and practices. From a critical perspective of culture, these factors are viewed as highly significant: not as determining factors in people's lives but as intersecting with broader social determinants of health. For example, rather than viewing people's diet (or other health-related practices) as determined by their "culture," a critical cultural perspective prompts you to consider the fact that people's dietary intake is equally influenced by their income, access to food resources, ability to afford fresh fruits and vegetables, geographical location, and educational levels. In many rural or remote communities, high-carbohydrate fast foods or drinks are often less expensive than milk, fresh fruits, and vegetables. This explains why people in these communities can have difficulties purchasing fresh foods that are beneficial to them. It also explains, in part, why rates of type 2 diabetes may be high in some Indigenous communities, where access to traditional foods (e.g., berries, fish, game) has been denied by government policies (e.g., the reserve system and land appropriation) and environmental damage (e.g., collapse of fisheries). Similarly, people who immigrate to Canada may have difficulty accessing familiar ingredients and therefore turn to less healthy, prepackaged foods. Thus, when a nurse documents a health history, understanding whether a person or family has the resources to purchase a healthy range of foods is as important as understanding their culturally based preferences for particular foods.

Just as each individual has a particular cultural orientation, health care has a particular culture. The Canadian health care system has particular features, sometimes referred to as the **dominant health care culture**. For example, health care providers working in the dominant health care culture often judge people negatively depending on their health practices (for example, for their failure to exercise or to stop smoking tobacco). They may also tend to value adherence or "compliance" with medical recommendations, such as technical diagnostic procedures, medications, and surgeries. However, the extent to which patients and their family members ascribe to the values of the dominant health care culture varies greatly. For some patients, the Western-style approach to history-taking (asking questions in quick succession) is not part of their pattern of communication. For some, taking a prescribed medication requires consultations with other family members. If you are alert to, and respectful of, the wide variety of health care practices and understandings about health, you will more easily find a mutually acceptable way to address people's concerns. This requires you to remain critically reflective about how you may be conveying features of the dominant health care culture in ways that can make patients feel uncomfortable or hesitant to share their perspectives.

These issues also have implications for how people will respond when asked on standard health history forms to identify their ethnicity. In the United States, people are regularly asked to identify their "race," but in Canada, this question is asked less often because "race" is understood as a social construct, not a fixed biological category. Some health history forms include categorical responses that people are asked to select from, while others include open-ended questions such as, "How would you identify your culture or ethnicity?" In some cases, people may choose to self-identify as, for example, Ukrainian, Greek, Sri Lankan, or Jewish. Increasingly, however, people who live in Canada are self-identifying as "Canadian," regardless of whether they were born in Canada or not. Others may not wish to report an ethnocultural identity other than Canadian because they are concerned that they might be treated differently because of how they identify.[3,4]

"Race" and Ethnicity: Why Is It Important to Distinguish Between These Terms?

In health care and other sectors of Canadian society, the concept of ethnicity is often used as a substitute for the idea of "race." It is essential for nurses and other health care providers to understand that although discussions about "race" are politically charged and often pervasive, **"race"** is a social construct that has no biological legitimacy. In 1951, in the aftermath of World War II, the United Nations Educational, Scientific and Cultural Organization (UNESCO) dismissed "race" as a biological category, stating that "biological differences between human beings within a single 'race' may be as great as, or greater than, the same biological differences between races."[9] As a social construct, however, the idea of "race" is powerful and continues to be used in a variety national contexts to classify humankind according to common ancestry and differentiation by physical characteristics such as skin colour, hair texture, stature, and facial characteristics.[5] This tendency occurs within the discipline of nursing and medicine as "race" becomes conflated with the fact that people have genetic characteristics. The reality is that all people, regardless of the colour of their skin or other physical appearances, are a mixture of populations. Skin colour, eye shape, and hair texture are genetically determined—and reflect heredity and ancestry—but those features do not signify any meaningful biological groupings or "races."

The idea of ethnicity operates in a similar way: it is used in various national and international contexts to categorize people, and is a social construct. For example, in Canada, **visible minorities** are defined by Statistics Canada as "persons, other than Aboriginal peoples, who are non-Caucasian in race or non-white in colour," and as consisting "mainly of the following groups: Chinese, South Asian, Black, Arab, West Asian, Filipino, Southeast Asian, Latin American, Japanese, and Korean."[10] Using the term *visible minority* to classify people by skin colour or other physical characteristics is a racializing process. Health care providers should be aware that some people view the term *visible minority* as demeaning because it does not account for people's various histories and social contexts.

Unlike in Canada, in the United States, the terms "race" and *ethnicity* are often used interchangeably to categorize people as, for example, "Black," "White," "Hispanic," or "Asian." As noted earlier, these categories signal social classifications rather than genetically linked groups of people.

Importantly, although "race" is not a biological entity, the social dynamics that occur in societies because of racialization (e.g., discrimination against people based on the colour of their skin or presumed ethnocultural characteristics) can have profound effects on patterns of health and illness. Nurses and other health care providers need to be aware of these effects and the terms used by researchers to study them.

Racialization is a process of attributing social, economic, or presumed cultural differences to "race."[11] Racialization may be conscious and deliberate (an act of **racism** in which discrimination is overt) or unconscious and unintended. Racism is founded on the view that there are supposedly biologically real divisions that involve "a hierarchy of value." Racialization exerts power through everyday actions and attitudes and from institutionalized policies and practices that disadvantage individuals and groups on the basis of presumed biological, physical, or genetic differences. For example, in our research, we have observed situations in which health care providers have erroneously assumed that alcoholism is "genetic" among Indigenous peoples, which leads them to presume that an Indigenous patient who has an unsteady gait is inebriated when, in fact, the patient may be experiencing cerebral bleeding, severe dehydration, a seizure disorder, or ataxia as a side effect of prescription medication.[12–15]

Racialization is closely linked to culturalism, because people whose behavior, practices, health or life circumstances are most likely to be explained by others as due to "culture" are those who are most likely to be racialized. For example, in Canada, people seen as Euro-Canadian (or Caucasian) are often thought not to "have a culture", because they are so fully aligned with the dominant culture, whereas non-Caucasians are often racialized and their differences explained as "cultural."

Racialization is also closely linked to discrimination. **Discrimination** is the systemic inequitable treatment of individuals or groups based on stratified classifications.[11] It refers to unfair, or morally wrong, social arrangements or acts, or the perception thereof, that have the potential for disadvantage or denial. Like other inequities, discrimination arises from social arrangements that are potentially remedial. The prevalence of certain diseases, such as hypertension, diabetes, and circulatory disease, can be higher in particular population groups and can vary according to genetic, biological, and family history. However, those factors intersect in significant ways with social factors, such as socioeconomic characteristics, gender roles and identities, and exposure to stressful experiences, including discrimination. For example, research in the United States has demonstrated that the increased incidence of high blood pressure among people of African descent, when socioeconomic and other factors are controlled, is attributable to experiences of discrimination.[16] In Canada, Nova Scotians who have African ancestry have been shown to have a higher incidence of circulatory disease, diabetes, and mental health issues that cannot be explained by socioeconomic characteristics or distance to a hospital,[17] which suggests that psychosocial stress and discrimination may explain the differences.

As a health care provider, you need to think critically about these processes and examine the categories and assumptions that you may be using (sometimes unconsciously) in relation to particular patients and families.[3,4] In health assessments, it is usually not necessary to ask people to identify their ethnicity. Instead, focusing on an individual's particular understandings, explanations, values, and practices related to health and illness will help you obtain information relevant to health and avoid making assumptions—in other words, provide culturally safe care.

CULTURAL SENSITIVITY, CULTURAL COMPETENCE, AND CULTURAL SAFETY: WHAT DO NURSES NEED TO KNOW?

Depending on the setting in which you work, you will be called on to provide culturally sensitive, culturally competent, or culturally safe care. **Cultural sensitivity** reflects the idea that people have culturally based understandings, practices, and customs, and that health care providers should be aware of and accommodate those understandings. Being culturally sensitive can be useful if it is done in a way that does not stereotype people for the ways in which they may be different from the dominant cultural norm. However, a critical cultural perspective emphasizes that health care providers must go further by recognizing that people's understandings, practices, and customs shift and change over time and context, and intersect with broader social determinants and power relations operating in society and in health care (Fig. 3.3). The Canadian Nurses Association (CNA) "believes that cultural competence is an entry-to-practice level competence for registered nurses" and defines **cultural competence** as "the application of knowledge, skills, attitudes or personal attributes required by nurses to maximize respectful relationships with diverse populations of clients and co-workers."[18] The CNA also recognizes "that cultural issues are intertwined with socioeconomic and political issues" and "is committed to social justice as central to the social mandate of nursing."[18] Regardless of the terminology used or the school of thought, it is not possible to develop knowledge about cultural and social considerations through brief

cross-cultural training programs alone. Rather, you must develop knowledge in several areas, such as the following:
1. Your own personal ethnocultural and social background
2. The culture of nursing and related professions
3. The culture of the health care system
4. The significance of social, economic, and cultural contexts
5. Your ability to critically examine your assumptions about each of these areas

The idea of *cultural safety* can assist you in gaining knowledge in these areas.

Cultural Safety

The concept of cultural safety emerged in the nursing literature in the 1990s in New Zealand, developed by Maori nurse leaders and educators who were concerned about the persistent health and health care inequities affecting Maori people (the Indigenous people of New Zealand).[19–21] The CNA recognizes **cultural safety** "as both a process and an outcome whose goal is to promote greater equity" by focusing on the root causes of "power imbalances and inequitable social relationships in health care."[13] Cultural safety is increasingly being incorporated in nursing, medicine, and other health care disciplines to provide care that takes into account the social, economic, political, and historical contexts of people's lives and how those contexts affect their health and health care experiences.[22–24] Nurses and health care providers who practice in culturally safe ways acknowledge that culturally based meanings and practices are to be respected. However, they are also directed to change the culture of health care, especially the practices and policies that perpetuate culturalism, racialization, and inequities.

Some of the main principles of cultural safety are as follows:
- Individual and institutional racism and discrimination, and culturalism create risks for patients, particularly when people from a particular group perceive they are "demeaned, diminished or disempowered" within the health care system.[25]
- Attention is shifted away from cultural differences as the source of the "problem" and onto the culture of health care as the site for transformation.[13]
- It is more important to consider how people are perceived and treated within the health care system than to determine or catalogue culturally specific beliefs or practices.[26]

Because relational approaches are concerned with relationships among providers and patients within particular historical, economic, social, and cultural contexts, relational approaches are integral to cultural safety (Box 3.1).

DEMOGRAPHIC PROFILE OF CANADA: TRENDS AND THEIR RELEVANCE TO HEALTH ASSESSMENT

Tensions and inequities often arise along the lines of perceived differences across populations and groups. For example, they can arise for people who are not fluent in either of Canada's official languages or for people who are

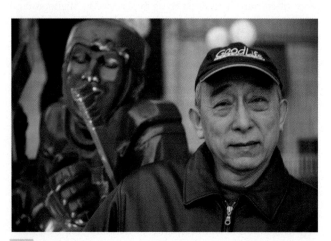

3.3   How can you counteract your own assumptions?

BOX 3.1 Using Culturally Safe Approaches

As you approach a new patient who is different from you in terms of appearance, age, skin colour, clothing, socioeconomic status, accent, or primary language spoken, take the time to ask yourself the following questions:
- What biases, assumptions, or stereotypes are influencing my verbal and nonverbal behaviours and decisions?
- What am I paying attention to, and how is that causing me to overlook certain things?
- How does the work environment (e.g., norms, colleagues, workload) contribute to, or challenge, the formation of these stereotypes and assumptions?

3.4 How does our geography shape health?

3.5 How does our geography shape health care access?

most at risk of experiencing the negative impacts of racism. Nurses need to be knowledgeable about how these dynamics can manifest in health care so that they can provide care that is consistent with the CNA's *Code of Ethics for Registered Nurses*[27] and foster health equity. For these reasons, it is important for nurses to keep up to date with Canada's changing demographic trends.

The 2016 census estimated that Canada's population is 35 151 728, an increase of 5.0% since 2011.[28] Although the majority of the population is Canadian born (around 79.4% of the total population in 2011), the Canadian population is increasing primarily as a result of international migration—which accounts for about two-thirds of Canada's population growth between 2011 and 2016.[29,30] Canada's population is diverse in terms of languages spoken, where people live, age distribution, and ethnocultural identities.

Canada's two official languages, English and French, are entrenched in the country's history. As a result of this history, rights and institutional support for English and French are entrenched in Canadian society. Notably, much less support is provided for the preservation and revitalization of Indigenous languages, despite the fact that Indigenous peoples are the original inhabitants. In 2011, nearly 58% of the Canadian population reported English as their mother tongue,* and nearly 22% reported French as their mother tongue.[31] Canada is diversifying linguistically; of significance is the fact that just over 70% of people who immigrated to Canada in 2011 reported a mother tongue other than English or French.[32,33] Many distinct Indigenous language families and dialects also exist. Strategies for communicating effectively with people whose primary language is different from yours are discussed in-depth in Chapter 4.

In 2016, 83.2% of the population lived in an urban area;[34] 70.4% of Canadians were living in one of Canada's 35 large

census metropolitan areas (CMAs)[†,35] (Figs. 3.4 and 3.5). Based on 2016 census data, the population of six CMAs exceeds 1 million: Toronto, Montreal, Vancouver, Calgary, Ottawa-Gatineau, and Edmonton.[28] Together, these cities are home to 47% of Canada's total population.

Canada's population is aging as a result of low fertility and increasing life expectancy.[35] The proportion of the population aged 65 and over has increased from 13.7% in 2006 to 16.5% in 2016. Since 2015, Canada's population of people aged 65 and older is greater than children aged 0 to 14 (the proportion of the population under 14 years of age was 16.1% in 2016).[35]

In the 2016 census, over 250 ethnic origins or ancestries were reported by the Canadian population, and 4 in 10 people reported more than one origin.[36] Ethnic origin responses are a reflection of each respondent's perception of their ethnic ancestry. An "ancestor" is usually more distant than a grandparent. As noted in the 2016 census guide:

---

*Mother tongue is defined by Statistics Canada as the first language learned at home in childhood and still understood by the individual. If the person no longer understands the first language learned, the mother tongue is the second language learned. For a person who learned two languages at the same time in early childhood, the mother tongue is the language this person spoke most often at home before starting school.

†A CMA is an area consisting of one or more neighbouring municipalities situated around a major urban core. A CMA must have a total population of at least 100 000, of which 50 000 or more live in the urban core.

BOX 3.2 Principles of Culturally Competent Care

- **Resist the practice of "othering."** This is the tendency to classify people or groups in a way that separates them from the whole. An "us" and "them" mentality supports a social hierarchy and power imbalances.
- **Everyone has a unique cultural identity.** Identities also intersect as people often identify with more than one cultural group.
- **There is as much diversity within cultures as across them.** Sex and gender, life stage, social status and other factors mean that no single cultural identity defines a cultural group. Everyone has a unique personality, aspects of shared cultural identity and a common humanity.
- **There is a difference between self-identity and being identified.** No one benefits from having their identity described and prescribed by others. People need to be able to self-identify with cultural groups. They also must choose if general information about a group applies to them. Unfortunately, people's health is partly determined by the identity imposed upon them by others.
- **Beware the dangers of stereotyping.** A stereotype is a belief or an attitude about a person or group that may not be based in reality. Stereotyping leads to the end of dialogue and understanding. For all of the above reasons, use the information provided here to inform your work but don't use it to stereotype an individual or a group.

From Nova Scotia Health Authority. (2016). *Diversity lens tool kit* (p. 6). Retrieved from https://www.cdha.nshealth.ca/diversity-inclusion.

Ethnic origin refers to a person's 'roots' and should not be confused with citizenship, nationality, language or place of birth. For example, a person who has Canadian citizenship, speaks Punjabi (Panjabi) and was born in the United States may report Guyanese ethnic origin. … In the 2016 Census, the terms 'ethnic origin,' 'ethnic group' and 'ethnic ancestry' are used interchangeably.[37]

The following were among the top 20 ethnic origins reported by the Canadian population: English (6.3 million people), Scottish (4.8 million people), French (4.7 million people), Irish (4.6 million people), Chinese (1.8 million people), East Indian (1.4 million people), and Filipino (837 130 people).[36]

The increasing ethnocultural, linguistic, and social diversity in Canadian society necessitates health care policies and practices that support providers so that they can work with a wide range of people and populations. Box 3.2 lists principles of culturally competent care recommended by the Nova Scotia Health Authority;[38] each province and territory will have standards and policies tailored to its local context. Many hospitals and health care agencies in Canada have similar standards and policies.

ETHNOCULTURAL DIVERSITY WITHIN THE CANADIAN POPULATION

Ethnocultural diversity is part of Canada's national identity. As the demographics indicate, the majority of Canadians associate themselves with the dominant linguistic groups (English and French) and with the dominant European ancestry. These patterns create the potential for "othering"* in health care, as well as the potential for modelling culturally safe, actively respectful ways of working across differences in health care. Differences are most evident when members of dominant groups provide care to people who are from racialized groups or visible minorities, such as Indigenous peoples or people who have immigrated to Canada, particularly if those persons are not fluent in one of the official languages. Therefore, to provide culturally safe care, health care providers require particular knowledge pertaining to Indigenous peoples and immigrants.

Indigenous Populations in Canada

The term *Indigenous peoples* refers to the original inhabitants of the land.[13] In Canada, Indigenous peoples includes First Nations, Métis (people of mixed European and Indigenous ancestry), and Inuit. The term *Aboriginal* is also commonly used (e.g., by Statistics Canada), and the colonial term *Indian* is still used in federal policy documents (e.g., the *Indian Act*), though the term *First Nations* is viewed as more respectful. In the 2016 census, 2.1 million people, or 6.2% of the total Canadian population, reported "Aboriginal ancestry"† (single or multiple response).[39] The 2016 census also indicated that 1 673 785 Aboriginal people in Canada reported "Aboriginal identity,"‡ accounting for 4.9% of the total population.[40] Of the three main Aboriginal groups, First Nations (North American Indians) was the largest, with 1.5 million people. Within this group, Cree (356 660), Mi'kmaq (168 480), and Ojibway (125 725) were the most common ancestries. Métis ancestry was reported by 600 000 people, and Inuit ancestry was reported by 79 125 people.[36] It is important to recognize that there is diversity within First Nations, Métis, and Inuit populations. This diversity is reflected, in part, by the more than 70 Indigenous languages currently spoken and the more than 600 unique First Nations/Indian Bands in Canada (Fig. 3.6).[41] *Registered Indians* are persons who are registered under the *Indian Act*. *Treaty Indians* are persons who belong to a First Nation or Indian band that signed a treaty with the Crown. Registered or treaty Indians are sometimes also

---

Othering is a term that refers to the projection of assumed cultural or social characteristics, differences, or identities onto members of particular groups. These projections are not based on actual differences; rather, they are based on stereotypes.

†According to Statistic Canada, *Aboriginal ancestry* refers to a person's ancestry associated with the Aboriginal peoples of Canada; that is, First Nations (North American Indian), Métis, and Inuit. "Ancestry" refers to the ethnic or cultural origins of the person's ancestors, an ancestor being usually more distant than a grandparent. A person can have more than one ethnic or cultural origin.

‡According to Statistics Canada, *Aboriginal identity* refers to a person's identification with the Aboriginal peoples of Canada; that is, First Nations (North American Indian), Métis, or Inuk (Inuit) and/or registered or treaty Indians (i.e., registered under the *Indian Act*), and/or those who have membership in a First Nation or Indian band.

3.6   What are your initial assumptions about this woman? She is the granddaughter of a renowned traditional medicine woman, Mrs. Sophie Thomas, from Saik'uz First Nation, British Columbia.

called *status Indians*.[42] In 2016, First Nations people with registered or treaty Indian status accounted for just over three-quarters (76.2%) of the First Nations population.[41]

As has been the trend in recent years, many people are moving from rural and northern communities to urban areas, often to seek employment that is not available in other regions. According to the 2016 census, among the First Nations people with registered or treaty Indian status, 44.2% lived on-reserve and the rest lived off-reserve.[41] The cities with the largest Indigenous populations in 2016 were Winnipeg, Edmonton, Vancouver, and Toronto.[43] In 2016, 72.8% of the Inuit population lived in Inuit Nunangat (the area from the western-most Arctic to the eastern shores of Newfoundland and Labrador).[41]

Policies Affecting Indigenous Peoples in Canada

In Canada, the complex history of colonialism, and current policies and practices within governments, organizations and institutions have resulted in profound social disruption within many Indigenous communities. They have contributed to a lack of employment opportunities, limited access to educational programs, inadequate and often crowded housing, and high levels of poverty.[44,45] The regulation of First Nations people's lives through the policies of the **Indian Act** and the ongoing restrictions placed on self-government, land claims, and economic development in Indigenous communities continue to shape life opportunities, economic conditions, and the overall health and social status of individuals and families.

The *Indian Act*, originally developed in 1876, was founded on the paternalistic motivation to assimilate and govern "Indians" (i.e., First Nations people). The original *Indian Act* has been amended several times, but it remains an actively applied legislation and contains all the federal policies and regulations pertaining to "registered status Indians." The *Indian Act* classifies First Nations people into registered status Indians and non-status Indians to distinguish people who receive legal recognition as First Nations citizens in

Canada from those who do not.[46] The process of obtaining registered status is complex and requires a series of applications submitted to the federal department responsible for meeting the government's constitutional, treaty, political, and legal responsibilities to First Nations people.

Until very recently, non-status First Nations people were not recognized by the federal government under the *Indian Act*, either because they were unable to prove their status or because they had lost their status rights. For example, many First Nations women and their children in Canada lost their status when they married non-status men. Although the *Indian Act* was changed in 1985 and 2011 to repeal these discriminatory policies, it is still possible for the grandchildren of status First Nations women to lose their status designation. The issue of who has status and who does not is relevant to health care providers because people who are "non-status Indians" are not entitled to the limited benefits available to people who are "status Indians." These inclusions and exclusions are also shifting: in 2016, the Supreme Court of Canada declared that Métis and non-status Indians are "Indians" for the purpose of federal Parliament's law-making jurisdiction under subsection 91(24) of the *Constitution Act, 1867*. However, the ruling does not affect Métis and non-status Indian eligibility for programs and services currently targeted to status Indians.[47,48]

Currently, First Nations people who are status Indians and Inuit receive limited health care benefits (called Non-Insured Health Benefits [NIHBs]) not covered by provincial health insurance plans.[49] NIHBs are administered by Health Canada and include selected prescription medications, limited medical supplies and equipment, short-term crisis counselling, limited coverage for glasses and vision care, medical transportation, and dental care (although many dentists do not provide services to people who have status because the dentist must wait to be reimbursed by the federal government, as opposed to receiving payment directly from the patient). Unfortunately, many members of the public, including health care providers, are unaware that the services provided through NIHBs are very limited and that these benefits do not apply to non-status people or Métis.

Another prevalent misconception is that Indigenous peoples in Canada do not pay taxes. This misconception can be a source of resentment for some Canadians. In general, Indigenous peoples are required to pay taxes on the same basis as other people in Canada, except where limited exemptions are defined by the *Indian Act* for people with status.[50] Status First Nations people are not required to pay provincial or federal taxes for goods, services, income, and property on-reserve. However, this exemption does not apply to the majority of First Nations people in Canada, who live off-reserve. Non-status people and Inuit are subject to taxation, like all other Canadians.

Inequities in Health Status

In the past in Canada, discriminatory practices and policies were aimed at assimilating Indigenous peoples into the dominant Canadian society. First Nations lands were appropriated and **reserves** were created, often of insufficient size and resources to support the reserve population and in regions with no potential for economic development. Cultural and spiritual practices were outlawed, including the work of traditional healers. Although it is not commonly known among the Canadian public, status First Nations people were not permitted to vote in federal elections until 1960, despite historically being among the most intensively governed members of Canadian society.[51] Indoctrination into the dominant culture was attempted through church- or state-run **residential schools**. Residential schools included industrial schools, boarding schools, student residences, and hostels, and they were located in every province and territory except Newfoundland, New Brunswick, and Prince Edward Island. The last residential school, located in Saskatchewan, closed in 1996. Many individuals and their family members have since come forward with emotionally painful stories of physical and sexual abuse at residential schools. In response, in 2006, the federal government approved the Indian Residential Schools Settlement Agreement (IRSSA).[52] As part of the IRRSA, the Truth and Reconciliation Commission of Canada (TRC) was launched in 2008 to create a historical record of the residential school system.[53] The TRC final report was published in December 2015, and its calls to action for Indigenous health are presented in Box 3.3.[54,55]

The inequities of the past continue to influence people's health status in the present. Despite improvements over the past three decades, the health of Indigenous populations continues to lag behind that of the overall Canadian population on virtually every measure.[13,56,57] The average projected life expectancy at birth for Indigenous peoples in 2017 was estimated to be 70.4 years for men and 77.0 years for women—8.3 and 6.3 years less, respectively, than the total Canadian population.[58] The poverty rate (based on the low-income measure after tax) among Indigenous children is more than double the national average. However, notable differences exist between populations; the poverty rate among status First Nations children is 51%, which increases to 60% for status First Nations children living on-reserve.[59] These health and social status indicators cannot be understood outside of their social, historical, and economic contexts, or viewed as "cultural" problems (Fig. 3.7). Rather, they are manifestations of the complex interplay of historical, social, political, and economic determinants influencing health status and access to equitable health care.

People Who Immigrate to Canada

A distinctive feature of Canada's history is the continuous arrival of immigrants from different regions of the world. Since the 1990s, Canada has welcomed around 235 000 immigrants per year.[29] Therefore, you have the opportunity to work with increasingly diverse groups of patients, particularly if you work in urban areas.

Since the 1970s, patterns of immigration have shifted significantly. In the past, Western European nations (such as the United Kingdom, Italy, Germany, and The Netherlands) and the United States were the primary sources of immigrants to

---

The Truth and Reconciliation Commission of Canada (TRC) detailed the effects of the residential school system on the health and well-being of survivors and their families. Effects range from the spread of infectious diseases as a result of inadequate housing and poor sanitary conditions to poor mental health as a consequence of being isolated from families, and sexual and physical abuse. The residential system has resulted in lasting trauma, the repercussions of which are apparent down the generations. TRC documented the persistent disparities in health outcomes between Aboriginal and non-Aboriginal Canadians. Its final report discussed the importance for Aboriginal people of having access to traditional practices and medicines alongside mainstream health care. To this end, 7 out of the 94 TRC's calls to action specifically relate to health:

1. It calls on Canadian governments to acknowledge that the current state of Aboriginal health is a direct result of previous Canadian government policies, and recognize and implement the health care rights of Aboriginal people as identified in international law and constitutional law, and under the Treaties.

2. It calls on the federal government to establish measurable goals to identify and close the gaps in health outcomes between Aboriginal and non-Aboriginal communities.

3. To address the jurisdictional disputes concerning Aboriginal people who do not reside on reserves, it calls on the federal government to recognize, respect, and address the distinct health needs of the Métis, Inuit, and off-reserve Aboriginal peoples.

4. It calls on the federal government to provide sustainable funding for existing and new Aboriginal healing centres.

5. It calls on the health care system to recognize the value of Aboriginal healing practices and use them in the treatment of Aboriginal patients in collaboration with Aboriginal healers and Elders where requested by Aboriginal patients.

6. It calls on all levels of government to (a) increase the number of Aboriginal health care providers; (b) ensure the retention of Aboriginal health care providers in Aboriginal communities; and (c) provide cultural competency training for all health care providers.

7. It calls on Canadian medical and nursing schools to require all students to take a course dealing with Aboriginal health issues.

Adapted from Truth and Reconciliation Commission of Canada. (2015). *Honouring the truth, reconciling for the future: Summary report of the Truth and Reconciliation Commission of Canada.* Winnipeg: Author (pp. 158–164). Retrieved from http://nctr.ca/assets/reports/Final%20Reports/Executive_Summary_English_Web.pdf.

Canada.[29] Between 2006 and 2011, people emigrating from Asia and the Middle East made up the largest proportion (56.9%) of newcomers to Canada; followed by people born in Europe (13.7%), Africa (12.5%), and Central and South America and the Caribbean (12.3%).[60]

It is important to be aware of the terms used to refer to the diverse groups of people who move to Canada. The

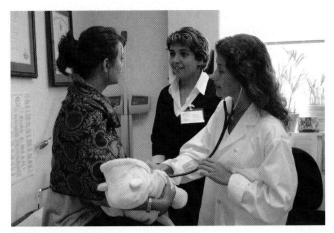

3.7 What situations challenge you most when you try to shift from the stance of "expert" to that of inquirer?

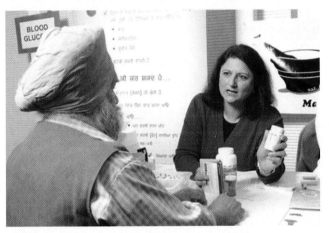

3.8 What social determinants of health do you overlook when you make assumptions/judgments based on appearances?

term **immigrant** refers to "a person who is or has ever been a landed immigrant. A landed immigrant or permanent resident is a person who has been granted the right to live in Canada permanently by immigration authorities. Immigrants are either Canadian citizens by naturalization (the citizenship process) or permanent residents (landed immigrants) under Canadian legislation. Some immigrants have resided in Canada for a number of years, while others have arrived recently. Most immigrants are born outside Canada, but a small number are born in Canada."[61] The term *visible minority* is sometimes confused with the term *immigrant*. Many people in Canada who fulfill the definition of *visible minority* are not immigrants but are from families who have resided in Canada for many generations. Nurses and other clinicians cannot assume that a person's appearance or accent has anything to do with a person's country of birth or citizenship. Rather, they need to remain amenable to learning about people's unique and multifaceted contexts, including their ethnocultural backgrounds, family origins, and social circumstances (Fig. 3.8).

People's decisions to migrate can be voluntary, involuntary, or a blend of both.[62] The "push–pull" factors in

immigration are often the need to explore new economic opportunities, family reunification, or forced relocation as a result of persecution or ecological disasters. Refugees often come from countries where conflict and war are ongoing, and they seek safer conditions in Canada (Box 3.4). The decision and ability to migrate is never easy. Immigration involves complex applications, classification, and landing procedures. Immigration applications can take many years to process. With changing eligibility requirements, those who immigrate generally must come with significant economic resources. On the other hand, people who are refugees may come with few or no resources. After immigration, the processes of integration and adaptation into a new society are often lengthy and may take an entire lifetime or many generations. The development of a healthy and vibrant society requires the ongoing commitment of both recent immigrants and Canadians already residing in Canada.

In 2011, 94.8% of Canadian immigrants lived in Ontario, British Columbia, Quebec, and Alberta; immigrants were more likely to live in a CMA than people born in Canada (91% compared with 63.3%).[60] Among these population groups, 63.4% reside in Canada's three largest CMAs: Toronto, Montreal, and Vancouver. People who were born in countries other than Canada accounted for 46% of Toronto's population, 40% of Vancouver's, and 22.6% of Montreal's.[60] In these three cities, immigration continues to be the major contributor to population growth. The most common reasons for settling in Toronto, Montreal, or Vancouver were to join social support networks of family and friends or because of the employment prospects. Most recently, an increasing number of new immigrants are settling in CMAs other than the three largest, including Calgary, Ottawa-Gatineau, Edmonton, Winnipeg, Hamilton, and London.

The Process of Immigration and Effects on Health

As a clinician, you need to recognize how the processes of migration and resettlement to another country can affect people's health and social status. Although many people are healthy when they first arrive in Canada, research shows that the health of immigrants, particularly non-Europeans, deteriorates over time in comparison with that of Canadian-born residents and immigrants from Europe.[63] This pattern of declining health status has a number of causes. Some health problems are linked to the stress of immigration itself, which involves finding suitable employment and establishing a new social support network.[63] The likelihood of a deterioration in health is also related to socioeconomic status, specifically low education and low household income. Vissandjée and colleagues showed that immigrant women, in particular, are often vulnerable to the stress that comes from trying to meet the basic needs of their families in a new country, learning a new language, and the social isolation that results from leaving family and friends behind.[64]

People who immigrate to Canada often experience difficulties getting the help they need from health care providers, hospitals, and other health care agencies.[65] Immigrants can face challenges accessing health and social services because

BOX 3.4 Resettlement of Refugees in Canada

Canada has a long history of resettling refugees. For example, Indochinese refugees immigrated to Canada following conflict in Vietnam, Laos, and Cambodia; Kosovar refugees immigrated in the late 1990s; and, more recently, Afghan, Iraqi, and Syrian refugees immigrated as a result of conflict in the Middle East.* Refugees are people fleeing conflict or persecution. They are defined in and protected by international law, which specifies that refugees must not be expelled or returned to situations where their life and freedom are at risk.† According to the UN Refugee Agency in 2015, there were nearly 21.3 million refugees worldwide. Over half come from just three countries: Syria (4.9 million), Afghanistan (2.7 million), and Somalia (1.1 million).

The Canadian government's Syrian refugee resettlement program aimed to resettle 25000 refugees by the end of February 2016. Since November 4, 2015, Canada has welcomed 40081 Syrian refugees.‡ Government-assisted refugees are provided with up to 12 months of financial support upon arrival in Canada to help with the cost of essential needs such as food, furniture, clothing, and basic household items, as well as a monthly allowance for food and shelter.§ Refugees are entitled to health care through the Interim Federal Health Program (IFHP).‖ The IFHP provides limited, temporary coverage of health care costs for people including resettled refugees, refugee claimants, rejected refugee claimants, and certain persons detained under the *Immigration and Refugee Protection Act* during their period of ineligibility for provincial or territorial health insurance. While basic coverage is similar to health care coverage provided by provincial and territorial health insurance plans and supplemental coverage is similar to supplemental coverage provided to social assistance recipients in provinces and territories, the benefits are not the same. The benefits reflect the temporary nature of the program and may vary based on the province or territory of residence.#

The Medavie Blue Cross handbook for health care providers explains the IFHP and outlines the administrative procedures for requesting reimbursement of services rendered.**

*Citizenship and Immigration Canada. (2016). *Canada: A history of refuge*. Retrieved from http://www.cic.gc.ca/english/games/teachers-corner/refugee/refuge.asp.

†UN Refugee Agency. (2015). *Figures at a glance*. Retrieved from http://www.unhcr.org/figures-at-a-glance.html.

‡Citizenship and Immigration Canada. (2017). *#WelcomeRefugees: Key figures*. Retrieved from http://www.cic.gc.ca/english/refugees/welcome/milestones.asp#popup1.

§Citizenship and Immigration Canada. (2014). *Government-assisted refugee resettlement in Canada*. Ottawa: Author. Retrieved from http://www.cic.gc.ca/english/pdf/pub/GAR_eng.pdf.

‖Citizenship and Immigration Canada. (2016). *Interim Federal Health Program policy*. Retrieved from http://www.cic.gc.ca/english/department/laws-policy/ifhp.asp.

#Citizenship and Immigration Canada. (2017). *Interim Federal Health Program: Summary of coverage*. Retrieved from http://www.cic.gc.ca/english/refugees/outside/summary-ifhp.asp.

**Medavie Blue Cross. (2016). *Information handbook for healthcare professionals*. Ottawa: Citizenship and Immigration Canada. Retrieved from http://providerifhpen.medavie.bluecross.ca/wp-content/uploads/sites/5/2016/09/IFHP-Information-Handbook-for-Health-care-Professionals-April-1-2016.pdf.

they have limited proficiency in English or French; they can feel frustrated because few health care providers can communicate in the family's language and few interpreter services are available. Immigrants may also lack a basic understanding of how the Canadian health care system works. Some people experience discrimination or prejudice in hospitals and clinics, which can lead to situations of mistrust. Clinicians, in turn, may believe that families are not following their instructions or are not abiding by hospital policies in terms of the numbers of visitors. Despite these frustrations, most people who immigrate to Canada are very appreciative of the health care they receive, particularly if services were scarce or limited in their countries of origin.

Waiting periods to qualify for provincial health care coverage can extend to several years, compromising access to health care services for children and families.[66] Studies of immigrants' economic integration in Canada have shown that those with non-European origins are more likely than those with European origins to have low-paying jobs that require little education. It has been shown that despite higher levels of education, immigrants have greater difficulties finding meaningful employment and are often forced to take low-paying jobs. These factors—in combination with experiences of racism, discrimination, and lower levels of social support—contribute to declining health status. Together, these social and economic trends have a profound effect on health status and can limit access to the resources and services necessary to maintain health in Canada.

It is important to remember that people who come from the same country may nevertheless be very diverse. They may have varying levels of education, proficiency in Canada's two official languages, socioeconomic backgrounds, and understandings of Western health care services. Applying relational approaches in clinical practice will help you assess the unique contexts, histories, and experiences that shape an individual's or a family's overall health and well-being.

HEALTH, SOCIAL, AND GENDER INEQUITIES

To understand how inequities affect health, it is useful to distinguish between concepts such as health inequality and inequity. **Health inequality** is a generic term used to designate differences, variations, and disparities in the health status of individuals and groups. An example of health inequality is the higher incidence of deaths in the prime of life among women in Canada than among men, largely because of breast and other cancers.[67–69] **Health inequity** refers to the inequalities in health that are unnecessary and avoidable, and differences that are considered unfair and unjust.[70] In Canada, and elsewhere, many of the health care services are inequitable because they reflect an unfair distribution of the underlying social determinants of health; for example, access to educational opportunities and meaningful employment, adequate income for people with physical or intellectual disabilities, access to needed health care, or the ability to afford nutritious foods. Health inequities also reflect forms of structural and individual discrimination and prejudice. For instance, people who are trans, gender nonconforming,

3.9 How do dominant ideas about families shape your assessments?

or both experience higher rates of stigma in accessing health care and other public systems (Fig. 3.9 and Box 3.5).

As indicated in Fig. 3.10, the economic, social, and political conditions in which people live are the major determinants of whether they are healthy or not. Rates of ill health are especially high among particular populations because of social, economic, and historical conditions. For example, people living in poverty, women in low-income brackets who are raising children, older women, people who experience discrimination or racism, significant numbers of the Indigenous population, women experiencing abuse, people with mental illnesses or substance use issues, refugees, and some immigrant groups are more likely than others to become ill and are less likely to receive appropriate health care services.[5,62,71–73] Assessing risk factors and promoting health therefore require consideration of the intersecting social and economic factors that go far beyond the immediately identifiable behavioural or biological risk factors (e.g., smoking, a diet high in processed foods, high blood pressure, or high cholesterol levels).

Evidence continues to show that at both the population and individual levels, poverty is the primary cause of poor health among Canadians.[73] For example, living in inadequate or overcrowded living conditions has been shown to increase people's risk for respiratory illness and psychological distress (Fig. 3.11).[71] Of major concern is the ongoing evidence indicating that inequities in health and social status are continuing to grow, despite Canada's official commitment to equity and access.[67,71,73]

Individuals who live in **relative poverty** lack the income to carry out or participate in the activities associated with the average standard of living in a country. In Canada, this kind of poverty manifests itself in a variety of ways, including limited access to the food, clothing, health care, and other amenities typically available to most Canadians; limited involvement in occupational and leisure activities; and limited participation in decision making and in civil, social, and cultural life.[73] In 2013, the national poverty rate was 13%, based on the low-income measure after tax.[74] Poverty rates differ by identity and other factors, as Canadian child poverty rates broken down by identity indicate (Fig. 3.12).

Poverty rates are highest for people living with disabilities, single mothers, and Indigenous peoples. For example, the proportion of female lone-parent families on a low income after tax in 2014 was 41.4%, considerably higher than the proportion of male lone-parent families (21.0%) and women nationally (13.5%).[75] Living in poverty is an especially significant threat to the health of children inasmuch as it has both immediate and long-lasting effects. For women, major causes of poverty include wage disparities, raising children as lone parents, lack of affordable child care, and low minimum wage rates.[73] These are important factors to consider in the context of health assessment. Recognizing how health and social inequities intersect to differentially affect people will help you to recognize and be more responsive to the range of factors that influence health and well-being.

COMPLEMENTARY AND ALTERNATIVE HEALTH CARE PRACTICES

Today, Canadians of all backgrounds draw upon a range of traditions as part of their health care (Fig. 3.13). Some wholeheartedly ascribe to the full range of *allopathic medicine* (referring to the dominant Western practice of medicine). Many also draw on other approaches, such as the use of chiropractic medicine, massage therapy, vitamins, or herbs (e.g., echinacea). **Complementary and alternative health care** "is an umbrella term used to describe numerous therapies including acupuncture, chiropractic, naturopathy, massage, herbal medicine, yoga and healing touch."[76] The term *natural health products* describes a variety of products, such as herbal medicines, homeopathic remedies, nutritional supplements, vitamins, and minerals.[77,78]

When conducting a health assessment, remember that people may draw on a combination of approaches. However, the ability to access and engage in complementary and alternative approaches varies greatly, depending on people's economic and social resources and their geographical location. For example, acupuncture, chiropractic treatments, massage, and natural health products can be prohibitively expensive. In general, most of these approaches are not covered by provincial or territorial health care plans.

Spirituality and Health

The significance of **spirituality** in people's health and healing has long been recognized. Although spirituality commonly tends to be perceived as an offshoot of religion, it is important to distinguish between religion and spirituality.[79] Spirituality has always been more central to the human experience than religion. Religions are often established by formal institutional structures, rituals, and beliefs, whereas spirituality may refer more generally to the search for meaning. Both religion and spirituality can play a significant role in the ways people deal with health and illness (Fig. 3.14).[80] As a health care provider, you do not need to know the specifics of various religious and spiritual traditions. However, it is important to convey openness, interest, and acceptance. First, you must check your own assumptions and biases. If you call places of worship "churches" in your work

BOX 3.5   The Impact of Stigma on Gender-Diverse People's Health, Well-Being, and Access to Care

Sex is a multidimensional biological construct that encompasses a person's reproductive and sexual anatomy, physiology, chromosomes, gene expression, and hormones, which together affect how we are labelled and treated in the world. In comparison, *gender* is a multidimensional social construct that is culturally and historically specific, constantly changing, and used in reference to the socially prescribed and experienced dimensions of being a woman, man, and/or gender-diverse person in society.* *Gender identity* is "an individual's experience of gender ... A person's gender identity may be the same as or different from their birth-assigned sex. Gender identity is fundamentally different from a person's sexual orientation. Gender expression is how a person publicly presents their gender. This can include behaviour and outward appearance such as dress, hair, make-up, body language and voice. A person's chosen name and pronoun are also common ways of expressing gender."[†]

In the Western world, these social and physical characteristics often operate on a binary system (e.g., male/female and woman/man); however, there are many diverse, multifaceted ways that people self-define their sex and gender. Indeed, sex and gender both exist on a spectrum.[‡] For example, gender identities include woman, man, trans, genderqueer, nonbinary, femme of centre, and two-spirit. *Two-spirit* is "a term used within some Indigenous communities, encompassing sexual, gender, cultural, and/or spiritual identity."[§] *Trans* is an "umbrella term used to describe a wide range of people whose gender identity and/or gender expression differ from their assigned sex and/or the societal and cultural expectation of their assigned sex."[||] Trans people face substantial health inequities.[#] For example, they experience a high prevalence of human immunodeficiency virus (HIV) and other sexually transmitted infections, mental health distress, and substance use and abuse.[**]

Stigma attached to gender nonconformity can lead to prejudice, discrimination, harassment, hatred, and even violence. As with racialization, discrimination can lead to "minority stress." "Minority stress is unique (additive to general stressors experienced by all people), socially based, and chronic, and may make transsexual, transgender, and gender nonconforming individuals more vulnerable to developing mental health concerns such as anxiety and depression."[††] Rates of attempted suicide among trans individuals is high; survey data from the Trans PULSE Project estimated that 10% of trans Ontarians had attempted suicide in the last year, far in excess of the average for all Canadians. Fear of discrimination also affects access to care. The Trans PULSE Project found that 21% of people surveyed avoided emergency department (ED) care for fear that their trans status would negatively affect the care they received, while 52% reported that they had had a negative ED encounter as a direct consequence of presenting in their felt gender. As well, 58% of respondents reported having had to educate their provider about trans issues. The World Professional Association for Transgender Health has published standards of care for the health of trans and gender nonconforming people.[††] As health care providers, nurses are expected and encouraged to ask *all* patients about their preferred names (which may be different than their birth name) and pronouns (*she, he, they*), rather than assuming their name and pronoun on the basis of physical appearance, gender expression, bodies, or other factors.[§]

*Canadian Institutes of Health Research. (2016). *Definitions of sex and gender.* Retrieved from http://www.cihr-irsc.gc.ca/e/47830.html.
[†]Ontario Human Rights Commission. (2014). *Policy on preventing discrimination because of gender identity and gender expression.* Toronto: Author. Retrieved from http://www.ohrc.on.ca/en/policy-preventing-discrimination-because-gender-identity-and-gender-expression.
[‡]Winter, S., Diamond, M., Green, J., et al. (2016). Transgender people: Health at the margins of society. *Lancet, 388*(10042), 390–400. doi:10.1016/S0140-6736(16)00683-8
[§]Lowik, A. J., Taylor, E., Sung, J., et al. (2016). *Promoting trans literacies: Supplementary resource.* Vancouver: Social Justice Institute. Retrieved from http://grsj.arts.ubc.ca/get-involved/promoting-trans-literacies/promoting-trans-literacies-supplementary-resource/.
[||]Transgender Health Information Program. (2017). *Trans 101.* Retrieved from http://transhealth.phsa.ca/trans-101.
[#]United Nations. (2011). *Report of the United Nations High Commissioner for Human Rights, discriminatory laws and practices and acts of violence against individuals based on their sexual orientation and gender identity, A/HRC/19/41/.* Geneva, Switzerland: Author.
**Reisner, S. L., Poteat, T., Keatley, J., et al. (2016). Global health burden and needs of transgender populations: A review. *Lancet, 388*(10042), 412–436. doi:10.1016/S0140-6736(16)00684-X
[††]Coleman, E., Bockting, W., Botzer, M., et al. (2012). Standards of care for the health of transsexual, transgender, and gender-nonconforming people, version 7. *International Journal of Transgenderism, 13*(4), 165–232. doi:10.1080/15532739.2011.700873

with patients, you are conveying a Christian bias that may discourage communication by patients who call their places of worship by other names (e.g., "temples," "mosques," or "synagogues"). Second, you need to avoid making assumptions about particular people. A person may be part of an ethnocultural group but not part of an associated religion. During the health assessment, conveying openness and inviting patients to identify what is important to them is most effective in eliciting data. For example, you might ask, "Do you have any religious beliefs or practices that you would like me to know about in relation to your health?"

GUIDELINES FOR CLINICAL PRACTICE

Assess Culturally Based Understandings and Practices

A health assessment can be completed incrementally over time. Regardless of whether you are completing a health assessment rapidly in the context of a single encounter or as part of a long-term professional relationship, building trust, engaging through listening, conveying respect for differences, and paying attention to the context of people's lives are key to culturally safe health assessments.

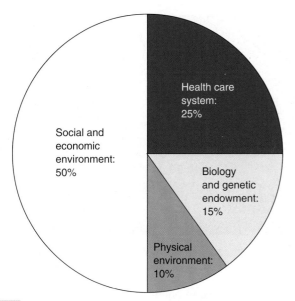

Social and economic environment: 50%

Health care system: 25%

Biology and genetic endowment: 15%

Physical environment: 10%

3.10 Estimated effect of determinants of health on the health status of the population.

3.13 How does a "critical cultural" lens shape your view differently from a "culturalist" lens?

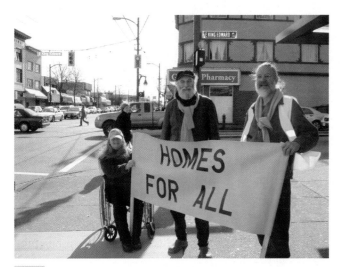

3.11 How do gender, disability, and poverty intersect to affect health?

3.14 How does your understanding of religion and spirituality influence your health assessments?

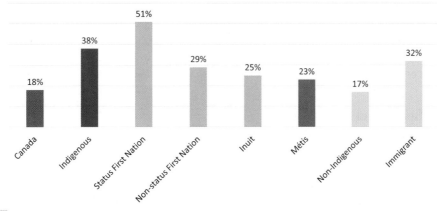

Canada 18%
Indigenous 38%
Status First Nation 51%
Non-status First Nation 29%
Inuit 25%
Métis 23%
Non-Indigenous 17%
Immigrant 32%

3.12 Breakdown of child poverty rates in Canada by identity, based on low-income measure after tax (LIM-AT) (2011).

Work to Build Trust

Although certain data must be collected in the initial interview to address the patient's presenting health issues, patients should not be expected to share sensitive information until trust has been established. Patients may be reluctant to reveal ethnocultural identity or their understandings about health and illness for fear of being dismissed as providing information that is less than legitimate. Clinicians can find out more by asking questions phrased in a nonjudgemental way, such as "What do you think may be happening to you?" or "What kinds of things have you found helpful?"

In some situations, it may be appropriate to build trust by conveying an interest in the person's life context. For example, if a person identifies as Indigenous (i.e., First Nations, Métis, Inuit, or Aboriginal) and you were interested in knowing more about the person's social and cultural context, you might ask, "What Nation or community are you from?" For people who identify themselves as new to Canada, you might ask, "In what country were you born?" or "How many years have you been in Canada?" For people who do not speak English as their primary language, you might ask, "What language(s) are you most comfortable speaking?"

Convey Respect for Differences

As this chapter discusses, you will engage with a wide range of people from diverse backgrounds. Conveying respect for differences helps build trust and welcomes patients to share their understandings. Research continues to show that patients are very quick to sense when health care providers are judging them negatively, particularly through verbal and nonverbal communication. Questions that convey respect while people's varying health practices are explored can focus on what the patients themselves have done to address their health or illness concerns. For example:

- Have you found any treatments or medications that have worked for you in the past?
- How did they help you?
- Are you using them now? If so, are they helping?
- (For people who have recently immigrated to Canada) Did you use any special treatments or medicines in other countries you have lived in that seemed to work for you?

Questions that convey an interest in hearing about traditional or complementary healing practices include the following:

- Have you used any traditional medicines or healing methods that you found helpful?
- Are you able to access those medicines or healing methods?

Pay Attention to the Social and Economic Contexts of Patients' and Families' Lives

For all patients and families, it is important to consider how people are managing with jobs, housing, child care, financial resources, care of older parents or relatives, transportation, and access to health care services. These considerations are relevant whether you are working in a community health care setting or an acute care or long-term care facility. Conveying

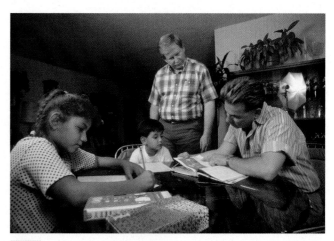

3.15 How can health care providers participate in social change?

interest in the circumstances of people's lives with a simple question such as "How have things been going for you?" is not "small talk," but rather an opportunity for you to assess a person's overall health in a nonjudgemental way (Fig. 3.15).

Assessing a patient's social and economic circumstances requires tact and effective listening and interviewing skills (as discussed in Chapter 4). Depending on the context, it may or may not be appropriate to explore this topic during your first meeting with a patient or the patient's family members. Asking direct questions about a person's finances may be seen as intrusive, and many people are embarrassed by such questions. However, inquiring about the person's ability to deal with the health, illness, or health promotion issues may be a good way to start the discussion. Anderson and associates have suggested the following questions as helpful for assessing people's social and economic circumstances:[81]

- What is particularly challenging or difficult about your health or illness, or what is needed to manage your health or illness?
- Are you working currently? Can you tell me a bit about the job you have?
- What do you need help with at home to manage (with your health or illness issues)?
- Whom do you rely on to help you at home? Do you live alone?
- Do you have family or friends nearby who can help you if needed?
- What kinds of things do you need help with?
- Are you able to afford the things you need to stay healthy, such as medications, glasses, dental work, and assistive devices such as a cane or wheelchair?
- Are you able to travel as necessary to access services or support?

Nurses must remember that many families in Canada are required to take on the extra work of caring for family members in their homes because of shortened hospital stays for acutely ill patients; the lack of affordable, high-quality long-term care facilities; and, in some cases, families' personal commitments to care for older parents in the home (Fig. 3.16). The financial circumstances of the family

3.16 What stereotypes about women, aging, and caregiving does this photo of a 101-year-old woman and her daughter challenge?

influence whether and how they are able to take on these caregiving responsibilities. These are important aspects to consider in the process of health assessment.

ADDITIONAL RESOURCES

Access Alliance—Multicultural Health and Community Services: http://www.accessalliance.ca

Assembly of First Nations: http://www.afn.ca

Canadian Centre for Policy Alternatives: https://www.policyalternatives.ca

Canadian Indigenous Nurses Association: http://www.indigenousnurses.ca

Canadian Institute for Health Information: https://www.cihi.ca/en

Canadian Nurses Association: https://www.cna-aiic.ca/en

Canadian Women's Health Network: http://www.cwhn.ca

Centre of Excellence for Women's Health: http://www.bccewh.bc.ca

Congress of Aboriginal Peoples: http://www.abo-peoples.org

Fraser, S. (201, April 30). 13 things you always wanted to know about being transgender but were afraid to ask. *CBC News*. Retrieved from http://www.cbc.ca/1.4088934

Government of Canada—Immigration and Citizenship: https://www.canada.ca/en/services/immigration-citizenship.html

Inuit Tapiriit Kanatami: https://www.itk.ca

Métis National Council: http://www.metisnation.ca

Native Women's Association of Canada: https://www.nwac.ca

Ontario Human Rights Commission—Racial Discrimination, Race and Racism (Fact Sheet): http://www.ohrc.on.ca/en/racial-discrimination-race-and-racism-fact-sheet

Public Health Agency of Canada: https://www.canada.ca/en/public-health.html

Sanctuary City Vancouver: http://www.sanctuarycityvan.com

Social Determinants of Health: The Canadian Facts: http://thecanadianfacts.org

Statistics Canada: http://statcan.gc.ca/eng/start

Status of Women Canada: http://www.swc-cfc.gc.ca

Trans Care BC: http://transhealth.phsa.ca

World Health Organization: http://www.who.int/en/

REFERENCES

1. Doane, G. A., & Varcoe, C. (2015). *How to nurse: Relational inquiry with individuals and families in changing health and health care contexts* (pp. 3–4; 139). Baltimore: Lippincott Williams & Wilkins.
2. Anderson, J. M., & Reimer-Kirkham, S. (1999). Discourses on health: A critical perspective. In H. Coward & P. Ratanakul (Eds.), *A cross-cultural dialogue on health care ethics* (pp. 47–67). Waterloo: Wilfrid Laurier University Press.
3. Varcoe, C., Browne, A. J., Wong, S. T., et al. (2009). Harms and benefits: Collecting ethnicity data in a clinical context. *Social Science and Medicine, 68*(9), 1659–1666.
4. Browne, A. J., Varcoe, C., Wong, S. T., et al. (2014). Can ethnicity data collected at an organizational level be useful in addressing health and healthcare inequities? *Ethnicity and Health, 19*(2), 240–254.
5. Henry, F., Rees, T., & Tator, C. (2010). *The colour of democracy: Racism in Canadian society* (4th ed.). Toronto: Thomas Nelson.
6. Statistics Canada. (2015). *Population group of a person.* Retrieved from http://www.statcan.gc.ca/eng/concepts/definitions/ethnicity.
7. Varcoe, C., & Browne, A. J. (2014). Culture and cultural safety: Beyond cultural inventories. In D. Gregory, C. Raymond-Seniuk, L. Patrick, et al. (Eds.), *Fundamentals: Perspectives on the art & science of Canadian nursing.* Philadelphia: Lippincott Williams & Wilkins.
8. Wyatt, R., Laderman, M., Botwinick, L., et al. (2016). *Achieving health equity: A guide for health care organizations. IHI white paper.* Cambridge, MA: Institute for Healthcare Improvement.
9. United Nations Educational Scientific and Cultural Organization. (1951). *Statement on the nature of race and race differences.* Retrieved from http://www.honestthinking.org/en/unesco/UNESCO.1951.Statement_on_Race.htm.
10. Statistics Canada. (2015). *Visible minority of person.* Retrieved from http://www23.statcan.gc.ca/imdb/p3Var.pl?Function=DECI&Id=62026.
11. Varcoe, C., Browne, A. J., & Ponic, P. (2013). *Promising theoretical contributions to the measurement of racial discrimination: Critical literature review.* Ottawa: Public Health Agency of Canada.
12. Browne, A. J., Smye, V. L., Rodney, P., et al. (2011). Access to primary care from the perspective of Aboriginal patients at an urban emergency department. *Qualitative Health Research, 21*(3), 333–348.
13. Browne, A. J., Varcoe, C., Lavoie, J. G., et al. (2016). Enhancing health care equity with Indigenous populations:

Evidence-based strategies from an ethnographic study. *BMC Health Services Research, 16*(544), 1–17.

14. Health Council of Canada. (2012). *Empathy, dignity, and respect: Creating cultural safety for Aboriginal people in urban health care.* Toronto: Author. Retrieved from https://healthcouncilcanada.ca/files/Aboriginal_Report_EN_web_final.pdf.

15. Tang, S., Browne, A. J., Mussell, B., et al. (2015). "Underclassism" and access to healthcare in urban centres. *Sociology of Health and Illness, 37*(5), 698–714.

16. Krieger, N. (2014). Discrimination and health inequities. *International Journal of Health Services, 44*(4), 643–710.

17. Etowa, J. B., Beagan, B. L., Eghan, F., et al. (2017). "You feel you have to be made of steel": The strong Black woman, health, and well-being in Nova Scotia. *Health Care for Women International, 38*(4), 379–393.

18. Canadian Nurses Association (2010). *Promoting cultural competence in nursing* (p. 1). Ottawa: Author. Retrieved from https://www.cna-aiic.ca/~/media/cna/page-content/pdf-en/ps114_cultural_competence_2010_e.pdf?la=en.

19. Papps, E., & Ramsden, I. (1996). Cultural safety in nursing: The New Zealand experience. *International Journal for Quality in Health Care, 8*(5), 491–497.

20. Ramsden, I. (1993). Kawa Whakaruruhau: Cultural safety in nursing education in Aotearoa (New Zealand). *Nursing Praxis in New Zealand, 8*(3), 4–10.

21. Ramsden, I. (2002). *Cultural safety and nursing education in Aotearoa and Te Waipounamu.* Wellington, New Zealand: University of Wellington.

22. Aboriginal Nurses Association of Canada (2010). *Cultural competence and cultural safety in nursing education introduction* [Information sheet]. Ottawa: Author.

23. Indigenous Physicians Association of Canada, & The Royal College of Physicians and Surgeons of Canada. (2009). *Cultural safety in practice: A curriculum for family medicine residents and physicians.* Winnipeg: IPAC-RCPSC Family Medicine Curriculum Development Working Group.

24. Pauly, B., McCall, J., Browne, A. J., et al. (2015). Towards cultural safety: Nurse and patient constructions of illicit substance use in hospitalized settings. *Advances in Nursing Science, 38*(2), 121–135.

25. Ramsden, I., & Spoonley, P. (1994). The cultural safety debate in nursing education in Aotearoa. *New Zealand Annual Review of Education, 3*, 161–174.

26. Polaschek, N. R. (1998). Cultural safety: A new concept in nursing people of different ethnicities. *Journal of Advanced Nursing, 27*(3), 452–457.

27. Canadian Nurses Association. (2017). *CNA Code of Ethics for registered nurses.* Retrieved from https://www.cna-aiic.ca/html/en/Code-of-Ethics-2017-Edition/files/assets/basic-html/page-1.html#.

28. Statistics Canada. (2017). *Population size and growth in Canada: Key results from the 2016 census.* Retrieved from http://www.statcan.gc.ca/daily-quotidien/170208/dq170208a-eng.htm.

29. Statistics Canada. (2016). *150 years of immigration in Canada.* Retrieved from http://www.statcan.gc.ca/pub/11-630-x/11-630-x2016006-eng.htm.

30. Statistics Canada. (2017). *Population growth: Migratory increase overtakes natural increase.* Retrieved from http://www.statcan.gc.ca/pub/11-630-x/11-630-x2014001-eng.htm.

31. Statistics Canada (2015). *Linguistic characteristics of Canadians* (Catalogue no. 98-314-X2011001). Ottawa: Author. Retrieved from http://www12.statcan.gc.ca/census-recensement/2011/as-sa/98-314-x/98-314-x2011001-eng.cfm.

32. Statistics Canada (2012). *2011 Census of population: Linguistic characteristics of Canadians.* Ottawa: Author. Retrieved from http://www.statcan.gc.ca/daily-quotidien/121024/dq121024a-eng.htm.

33. Statistics Canada (2017). *Focus on geography series, 2016 census* (Catalogue no. 98-404-X2016001). Ottawa: Author. Retrieved from http://www12.statcan.gc.ca/census-recensement/2016/as-sa/fogs-spg/Facts-can-eng.cfm?Lang=Eng&GK=CAN&GC=01.

34. Statistics Canada. (2017). *Annual demographic estimates: Subprovincial areas.* Retrieved from http://www.statcan.gc.ca/pub/91-214-x/2017000/section01-eng.htm.

35. Statistics Canada. (2016). *Population by age and sex.* Retrieved from http://www.statcan.gc.ca/pub/91-215-x/2016000/part-partie2-eng.htm.

36. Statistics Canada. (2017). *Ethnic and cultural origins of Canadians: Portrait of a rich heritage.* Census of population, 2016. Retrieved from http://www12.statcan.gc.ca/census-recensement/2016/as-sa/98-200-x/2016016/98-200-x2016016-eng.pdf.

37. Statistics Canada. (2017). *Ethnic origin reference guide, census of population, 2016.* Retrieved from http://www12.statcan.gc.ca/census-recensement/2016/ref/guides/008/98-500-x2016008-eng.cfm.

38. Nova Scotia Health Authority. (2016). *Diversity lens tool kit.* Retrieved from https://www.cdha.nshealth.ca/diversity-inclusion.

39. "Aboriginal ancestry" definition from Statistics Canada. (2017). *Dictionary, census of population, 2016.* Retrieved from http://www12.statcan.gc.ca/census-recensement/2016/ref/dict/pop145-eng.cfm.

40. "Aboriginal identity" definition from Statistics Canada. (2017). *Dictionary, census of population, 2016.* Retrieved from http://www12.statcan.gc.ca/census-recensement/2016/ref/dict/pop001-eng.cfm.

41. Statistics Canada. (2017). *Aboriginal peoples in Canada: Key results from the 2016 census.* Retrieved from http://www.statcan.gc.ca/daily-quotidien/171025/dq171025a-eng.pdf.

42. Statistics Canada. (2017). *Dictionary, census of population, 2016: Registered or treaty Indian status.* Retrieved from http://www12.statcan.gc.ca/census-recensement/2016/ref/dict/pop116-eng.cfm.

43. Statistics Canada. (2017). *Aboriginal peoples highlight tables, 2016 census.* Retrieved from http://www12.statcan.gc.ca/census-recensement/2016/dp-pd/hlt-fst/abo-aut/Table.cfm?Lang=Eng&T=102&S=88&O=A&RPP=9999.

44. Anaya, J. (2014). *Report of the special rapporteur on the rights of Indigenous peoples: The situation of Indigenous peoples in Canada.* Geneva, Switzerland: United Nations Human Rights Council. Retrieved from http://unsr.jamesanaya.org/country-reports/the-situation-of-indigenous-peoples-in-canada.

45. Greenwood, M., Leeuw, S. D., Lindsay, N. M. (Eds.), (2015). *Determinants of Indigenous peoples' health in Canada: Beyond the social.* Toronto: Canadian Scholars' Press.

46. Indigenous and Northern Affairs Canada. (2016). *Indian status.* Retrieved from https://www.aadnc-aandc.gc.ca/eng/1100100032374/1100100032378.

47. Health Canada. (2016). *Benefits information.* Retrieved from http://www.hc-sc.gc.ca/fniah-spnia/nihb-ssna/benefit-prestation/index-eng.php.

48. Indigenous and Northern Affairs Canada. (2016). *The CAP/Daniels decision—Frequently asked questions.* Retrieved

from https://www.aadnc-aandc.gc.ca/eng/1460635873455/1460635946946.

49. Government of Canada. (2016). *Non-insured health benefits for First Nations and Inuit.* Retrieved from https://www.canada.ca/en/health-canada/services/non-insured-health-benefits-first-nations-inuit.html.

50. Canada Revenue Agency. (2015). *GST/HST and Indigenous peoples.* Retrieved from http://www.cra-arc.gc.ca/tx/bsnss/tpcs/gst-tps/frstntns/menu-eng.html.

51. Furniss, E. (1999). *The burden of history: Colonialism and the frontier myth in a rural Canadian community.* Vancouver: UBC Press.

52. Indian Residential Schools Resolution Canada. (2008). *Frequently asked questions.* Retrieved from http://www.irsrrqpi.gc.ca/english/truth_reconciliation_commission.html.

53. Truth and Reconciliation Commission of Canada. (2018). *About the Commission.* Retrieved from http://www.trc.ca/websites/trcinstitution/index.php?p=39.

54. Truth and Reconciliation Commission of Canada. (2015). *Final report of the Truth and Reconciliation Commission of Canada.* Winnipeg: Author. Retrieved from http://www.trc.ca/websites/trcinstitution/index.php?p=890.

55. Truth and Reconciliation Commission of Canada. (2015). *Truth and Reconciliation Commission of Canada: Calls to action.* Winnipeg: Author. Retrieved from http://www.trc.ca/websites/trcinstitution/File/2015/Findings/Calls_to_Action_English2.pdf.

56. Allan, B., & Smylie, J. (2015). *First peoples, second class treatment: The role of racism in the health and well-being of Indigenous peoples in Canada.* Toronto: The Wellesley Institute. Retrieved from http://www.wellesleyinstitute.com/wp-content/uploads/2015/02/Report-First-Peoples-Second-Class-Treatment-Final.pdf.

57. Canadian Institute for Health Information. (2016). *Trends in income-related health inequalities in Canada: Technical report.* Ottawa: Author. Retrieved from https://www.cihi.ca/en/factors-influencing-health/health-inequalities/trends-in-income-related-health-inequalities-in.

58. Statistics Canada. (2015). *Projected life expectancy at birth by sex, by Aboriginal identity, 2017.* Retrieved from http://www.statcan.gc.ca/pub/89-645-x/2010001/c-g/c-g013-eng.htm.

59. Macdonald, D., & Wilson, D. (2016). *Shameful neglect: Indigenous child poverty in Canada.* Ottawa: Canadian Centre for Policy Alternatives.

60. Statistics Canada (2011). *Immigration and ethnocultural diversity in Canada.* Ottawa: Author. Retrieved from https://www12.statcan.gc.ca/nhs-enm/2011/as-sa/99-010-x/99-010-x2011001-eng.cfm.

61. Statistics Canada. (2015). *Definition of immigrant.* Retrieved from http://www.statcan.gc.ca/eng/concepts/definitions/immigrant.

62. Raphael, D. (Ed.), (2017). *Immigration, public policy, and health: Newcomer experiences in developed nations.* Toronto: Canadian Scholars.

63. Vang, Z. M., Sigouin, J., Flenon, A., et al. (2017). Are immigrants healthier than native-born Canadians? A systematic review of the healthy immigrant effect in Canada. *Ethnicity and Health, 22*(3), 209–241.

64. Vissandjée, B., Thurston, W., Apale, A., et al. (2007). Women's health at the intersection of gender and the experience of international migration. In M. Morrow, O. Hankivsky, & C. Varcoe (Eds.), *Women's health in Canada: Critical theory, policy and practice* (pp. 221–243). Toronto: University of Toronto Press.

65. Clarke, J. (2016). *Difficulty accessing health care services in Canada.* Retrieved from http://www.statcan.gc.ca/pub/82-624-x/2016001/article/14683-eng.htm.

66. Goel, R., Bloch, G., & Caulford, P. (2013). Waiting for care: Effects of Ontario's 3-month waiting period for OHIP on landed immigrants. *Canadian Family Physician, 59*(6), e269–e275.

67. Canadian Institute for Health Information. (2017). *Health inequalities.* Retrieved from https://www.cihi.ca/en/health-inequalities.

68. Public Health Agency of Canada. (2011). *What determines health?* Retrieved from http://www.phac-aspc.gc.ca/ph-sp/determinants/.

69. Raphael, D. (2014). Social determinants of children's health in Canada: Analysis and implications. *International Journal of Child, Youth and Family Studies, 5*(2), 220–239.

70. World Health Organization. (2017). *Health impact assessment: Glossary of terms used.* Retrieved from http://www.who.int/hia/about/glos/en/index1.html.

71. Canadian Institutes of Health Research. (2016). *Definitions of sex and gender.* Retrieved from http://www.cihr-irsc.gc.ca/e/47830.html.

72. Krieger, N. (2011). *Epidemiology and the people's health: Theory and context.* New York: Oxford University Press.

73. Raphael, D. (Ed.), (2016). *Social determinants of health: Canadian perspectives* (3rd ed.). Toronto: Canadian Scholars' Press.

74. Lammam, C., & MacIntyre, H. (2016). *An introduction to the state of poverty in Canada.* Vancouver: Fraser Institute. Retrieved from https://www.fraserinstitute.org/sites/default/files/an-introduction-to-the-state-of-poverty-in-canada.pdf.

75. Statistics Canada. (2016). *Low income statistics by economic family type, Canada, provinces and selected census metropolitan areas.* Retrieved from http://www5.statcan.gc.ca/cansim/a26?lang=eng&id=2060042.

76. Public Health Agency of Canada. (2008). *Complementary and alternative health.* Retrieved from http://www.phac-aspc.gc.ca/chn-rcs/cah-acps-eng.php.

77. College of Registered Nurses of Nova Scotia. (2017). *Complementary and alternative health care: A guideline for registered nurses and nurse practitioners.* Halifax: Author. Retrieved from https://crnns.ca/wp-content/uploads/2015/02/Complementary-and-Alternative-Health-Care.pdf.

78. Health Canada. (2016). *About natural health products.* Retrieved from http://www.hc-sc.gc.ca/dhp-mps/prodnatur/about-apropos/cons-eng.php.

79. Fowler, M. D. (2011). Religion and nursing. In M. Fowler, S. Reimer-Kirkham, R. Sawatzky, et al. (Eds.), *Religion, religious ethics, and nursing* (pp. 1–26). New York: Springer.

80. Reimer-Kirkham, S. (2014). Nursing research on religion and spirituality through a social justice lens. *Advances in Nursing Science, 37*(3), 249–257.

81. Anderson, J. M., Reimer-Kirkham, S., Waxler-Morrison, N., et al. (2005). Conclusion. In N. Waxler-Morrison, J. M. Anderson, E. Richardson, et al. (Eds.), *Cross-cultural caring: A handbook for health providers* (2nd ed., pp. 323–352). Vancouver: UBC Press.

4 CHAPTER

The Interview

Written by Carolyn Jarvis, PhD, APN, CNP
Adapted by Annette J. Browne, PhD, RN*

℮ http://evolve.elsevier.com/Canada/Jarvis/examination/

The interview is a meeting between you and your patient. The goal of this meeting is to record a complete health history. The health history helps you begin to identify the patient's health strengths and problems and contextual influences, and it functions as a bridge to the next step in data collection: the physical examination.

The interview is the first, and really the most important, part of data collection. It entails the collection of **subjective data**: what the patient says about himself, herself, or themselves. The interview is the optimal way to learn about the patient's perceptions of, understandings of, and reactions to their health state, which includes physical, mental, spiritual, and emotional health. Once people enter the health care system, power relations may change, and opportunities for relational practice may shift. The initial interview, however, is the ideal opportunity to build trust, establish rapport, and engage in relational practice. Your skill in interviewing, your nonverbal behaviours, and the attitude you convey will affect the kinds of information you elicit. If the interview is well-planned and implemented, you will be able to glean most of the necessary information needed to plan the next steps in the assessment process. The interview therefore forms the basis of a successful working relationship. To accomplish a successful interview, you must perform the following tasks:

1. Gather complete, accurate data about the patient's health state, including the description and chronology of any symptoms of illness. Listen carefully to what the patient has to say.
2. Establish rapport and trust, and convey respect, so that the patient feels accepted (versus judged by you) and thus free to share all relevant data.
3. Share information with the patient about the patient's health state so that the patient can participate in identifying problems.
4. Build rapport for a continuing therapeutic relationship; this rapport facilitates future opportunities for assessment, diagnoses, planning, and treatment.
5. Look for opportunities to engage in teaching for health promotion and illness prevention.

---

*Thank you to Taq Bhandal for her careful work on researching and integrating the revisions and updates reflected in this chapter.

THE PROCESS OF COMMUNICATION

It is challenging to teach the skill of interviewing because initially, most students think little needs to be learned. They assume that if they can talk and hear, they can communicate. However, much more than talking and hearing is necessary. Communication includes physical, mental, and emotional dimensions, and verbal and nonverbal communication. Communication can be conveyed through tone of voice, facial expressions, gestures, eye contact, body posture, and stance.

The contexts in which nurses practise can also profoundly shape how they engage in the interview process. To more mindfully and consciously choose how you will practise requires that you develop the skill of reflexivity. Critical reflection and reflexivity are the central skills of relational practice, as discussed in Chapters 1, 3, and 6–8. It involves "a combination of observation, critical scrutiny, and conscious participation ... and paying attention to whom, how, and what you are being/doing/feeling/thinking in the moment ... how you are relating to and with other people, and how they are relating to you."[1] By paying attention to how you are acting and what you are feeling in any particular situation, you can begin to see how your behaviours and responses affect other people. You will more consciously choose how to act and respond by being aware of (a) how your social and professional positioning affect how you are perceived by patients; (b) how you communicate; and (b) how your thoughts, judgements, emotions, and physical presence influence the health assessment process.

Sending

You are probably most aware of *verbal* communication: the words you speak, vocalizations, the tone of voice. *Nonverbal* communication also occurs. This is your body language: posture, gestures, facial expression, eye contact, foot tapping, touch, what you do with your hands, even where you place your chair. Because nonverbal communication is under less conscious control than verbal communication, nonverbal communication is probably more reflective of what you are feeling, thinking, or reacting to during an interaction. A high degree of critical reflection is necessary to remain attuned to your nonverbal communication during the interview and physical examination.

Receiving

Being aware of the messages you send is only part of the process. Your words and gestures must be interpreted in a *specific context* to have meaning. You have a specific context in mind when you send your words. The receiver has their own interpretation of them. The receiver attaches meaning determined by past experiences, social and family contexts, and self-concept, as well as current physical and emotional states. Sometimes these contexts do not coincide. Remember how frustrating it may have been to try to communicate something to a friend, only to have your message totally misunderstood? Your message can be misinterpreted by the listener. Mutual understanding by the sender and receiver is necessary for communication to be successful.

An even greater risk of misunderstanding exists in the health care setting than in a social setting. In the health care setting, most patients have a health problem, and this factor emotionally charges your professional relationship. It *intensifies* the communication because the patient feels dependent on you for information or support.

Attending to Power Differentials

Nurses and other health care providers are usually in a position of power in relation to patients and families.[1] They usually have more knowledge about the health care system and have influence over patients' access to health care. At the same time, nurses and health care providers are also diverse in terms of their social contexts, life experiences, knowledge, and so on. As discussed in Chapter 3, it is important to be aware of how your power and privilege in relation to patients, families, and colleagues are reflected in the way you communicate, both verbally and nonverbally, on an ongoing basis. Building awareness involves considering the effects of gender, sexual orientation, socioeconomic status, and other factors on patients' health care experiences. It also involves considering the effects of structural forces—such as reforms to the health care system, the history of colonialism in Canada, and gender inequities—on patients' health care experiences. You must continually assess how you may be using your power in relation to patients as you facilitate their access to the health care system.

Communication Skills

Cultivating the skills of relational practice during the interview involves particular communication skills. These skills include unconditional positive regard, empathy, and active listening.

Unconditional Positive Regard

One essential feature of effective communication is the ability to meet patients, individuals, and families with "unconditional positive regard."[1] Although it may be challenging, you need to develop the skills and capacity to convey unconditional positive regard to engage therapeutically with

people. Doing so means having a generally optimistic view of people: an assumption of their strengths and an acceptance of their limitations. An atmosphere of warmth and caring is necessary. The patient must feel accepted unconditionally, even if you think the patient may be engaging in behaviours or making choices that seem to be unhealthy.[2,3] Monitoring your own judgements while simultaneously conveying unconditional positive regard requires a high degree of self-reflectivity, particularly when patients or families seem to be making choices that have negative health effects.

The respect for other people extends to respect for their personal contexts and the way our society shapes people's health status. Your goal is not to make your patients dependent on you but to facilitate their capacity to manage their health. You are working toward promoting their growth. Pay attention to the cues you pick up from patients and families, and follow their lead. Be prepared to think critically about the various contexts that influence people's situations and decisions related to their health.

Empathy

Empathy means viewing the world from another person's inner frame of reference while remaining yourself. Empathy means recognizing and accepting the other person's feelings, actions, perspectives, or world views without criticism; to do this, you must be aware of your own assumptions about the person. Empathy is described as "feeling *with* the person rather than feeling *like* the person." It does not mean you become lost in the other person at the expense of your own self. If this occurred, you would cease to be helpful.

Active Listening

Listening is not a passive role in the communication process; it is active, demanding, and requires your complete attention. You cannot be preoccupied with your own thoughts, judgements, concerns, needs, or the needs of other patients, or you will miss something important. For the duration of an interview, no one is more important than the patient. To communicate you are actively listening to a patient, you can engage in positive, encouraging verbal cues (e.g., saying "Mmm-hmm" or "Go on") and convey interest through nonverbal cues (e.g., leaning toward the patient, making eye contact).

Active listening is the route to understanding. You cannot be thinking of what you are going to say as soon as the patient stops for breath. A vast difference exists between listening and simply waiting to speak.[1] Listen to *what* the patient says. The story may not be provided in the order you would expect or in the order that you will document later. Let the patient talk from their own perspective, stance, or world view; nearly everything that is said will be relevant. Listen to *the way* a patient tells the story, such as difficulty with language, impaired memory, the tone of the patient's voice, and even to what the patient is leaving out.

Attending to the Physical Setting

Prepare the physical setting. The setting may be a community health clinic, an outpatient department, a laneway or street, a hospital room, an examination room, an office, or the patient's home. In any location, optimal conditions are important for the completion of a smooth interview.

Ensuring Privacy

Aim for geographical privacy: ideally, a private space. Achieving privacy may involve asking other people who are in that space to step out for a while or finding an alternative unoccupied space. If geographical privacy is not available, "psychological privacy" by curtained partitions may suffice as long as the patient feels sure that no one can overhear the conversation or interrupt.

Refusing Interruptions

Most people resent interruptions except in cases of an emergency. Inform any support staff of your interview, and ask that they not interrupt you during this time. Discourage other health care providers from interrupting you with *their* need for access to the patient. Also be sure to turn off the ringer or other distracting noises on cellphones or other technologies. You need to concentrate and to establish rapport.

Physical Environment

- Make the distance between you and the patient about 1.5 m (twice arm's length). If you place the patient any closer, you may invade the patient's private space, which may create anxiety. If you place the patient farther away, you seem distant and aloof.
- Arrange the space (the desk and patient seating) so that the patient's back does not face the door. Patients who are seated with their back facing the door may feel "blocked in"—especially patients who may have experienced trauma and violence.
- Arrange equal-status seating. Both you and the patient should be comfortably seated, at eye level with each other (Fig. 4.1). Avoid facing a patient across a desk or table because that feels like a barrier. Placing the chairs at a 90-degree angle allows the patient either to face you or to look straight ahead from time to time. Of most

importance, avoid standing over the patient. Standing creates two negative effects: (a) it communicates your haste, and (b) it communicates your superiority. Standing makes you loom over the patient as an authority figure. When you are sitting, the opportunity to decrease the power differentials becomes more possible and facilitates the patient's sense of comfort and control in the setting.

- Arrange a face-to-face position when you interview a hospitalized, bedridden patient. The patient should not have to stare at the ceiling because doing so causes them to lose the visual message of your communication.

Taking Notes

Some use of history forms and note taking may be unavoidable. When you sit down later to record the interview, you cannot rely completely on memory to furnish details of previous hospitalizations or of the review of body systems, for example. Be sure to tell the patient in advance that you will probably take a few notes so that you can better keep track of and remember the information that the patient conveys. However, be aware that taking notes during the interview has disadvantages:

- It breaks eye contact too often. It can prevent you from conveying that you are actively listening to the patient.
- It shifts your attention away from the patient, diminishing the patient's sense of importance.
- It can interrupt the patient's narrative flow. You may say "Please slow down; I'm not getting it all." The patient's natural mode of expression is lost.
- It impedes your observation of the patient's nonverbal behaviour.
- It is threatening to the patient during the discussion of sensitive issues (e.g., amount of alcohol and drug use, number of sexual partners, or incidence of emotional or physical abuse).

Thus, keep note taking to a minimum, and try to focus your attention on the patient. Any recording you do should be secondary to the dialogue and should not interfere with the patient's spontaneity. With experience, you will not rely on taking notes as much.

Electronic Clinical Documentation

Technologies such as the electronic health record (EHR) are increasingly being used to record health histories and physical examination findings. EHRs and computer-assisted clinical documentation practices can influence interviewing practice in positive ways if used appropriately. For example, data can be shared more easily among the health care team, which would minimize redundancy (patients being asked the same questions by several members of the health care team). As with handwritten note taking, stay focused on the patient and convey that you are actively listening and interested in the patient's history.

Interviewing in a Telehealth Environment

The rapid pacing of technological advancement provides a promising form of health care communication between

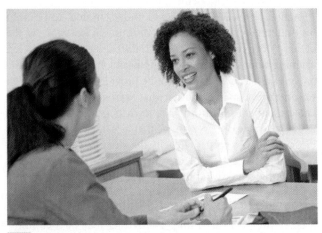

4.1   Equal-status seating.

providers and patients. Telehealth programs involve the use of synchronous (real-time) communication (e.g., instant messaging, videoconferencing on Skype, Facetime, or Google Hangouts) or asynchronous communication (e.g., text messaging) over secure channels to provide clinical consultations, continuing education, and opportunities for collaboration. Telehealth is a particularly important tool to reach rural, remote, and underserviced areas in Canada.[4]

Telehealth programs have been implemented across the country. For example, the BC First Nations Health Authority has been rolling out the Telehealth Expansion Project since 2006.[5] The Ontario Telemedicine Network's expanded its Telehomecare project to 3 500 patients with chronic disease throughout Ontario.[6] Although there is still uncertainty about how a virtual environment can affect the patient–health care provider relationship, studies continue to show that telehealth is a time-effective, accessible form of health care.[7] Similar to an in-person physical setting, nurses who use telehealth practices must attend to their verbal and non-verbal communication such as strong eye contact, awareness of voice intonation, and appropriate use of space.

TECHNIQUES OF COMMUNICATION

Introducing the Interview

If you are nervous about how to begin, remember to keep the beginning short. The patient is probably nervous, too, and is anxious to start. Address the patient using the patient's surname, and shake hands if that seems appropriate to the context and the patient, and if it feels comfortable. Introduce yourself, and state your role in the agency (if you are a student, say so). If you are gathering a complete history, give the reason for this interview:

> *"Mrs. Nagra, I would like to talk about the illness that led you to come to the hospital."*
> *"Mr. Yuan, I would like to ask you some questions about your health and your usual daily activities so that we can plan your care here in the hospital."*

If the patient is in the hospital, more than one health care team member may be documenting the history. Patients are apt to feel exasperated because they believe they are repeating the same thing unless you give a reason for this interview. You can also warn hospitalized patients that others will probably seek information from them on a frequent basis, so that they are not surprised by numerous requests for information or multiple attempts to document their history.

The Working Phase

The working phase is the data-gathering phase. Verbal skills for this phase include your questions to the patient and your responses to what the patient has said. Two general types of questions exist: open-ended and closed. Each type has a different place and function in the interview.

Open-Ended Questions

The **open-ended question** asks for narrative information. The topic to be discussed is stated, but only in general terms. Use it to begin the interview, to introduce a new section of questions, and whenever the patient introduces a new topic.

> *"What brings you to the clinic (or hospital)?"*
> *"Tell me why you have come here today."*
> *"How have you been getting along?"*
> *"You mentioned shortness of breath. Tell me more about that."*
> *"How have you been feeling since your last appointment?"*
> *"What has been most challenging?"*
> *"What would you like to be able to do, change, or address?"*
> *"Tell me how I can best help you."*
> *"What stands out for you as really important for me to know about your situation?"*

The open-ended question leaves patients free to answer in any way. This type of question encourages patients to respond in paragraphs and to give a spontaneous account in any order chosen. It lets patients express themselves fully.

As the patient answers, concentrate on how to *actively listen*. This will involve "listening to" and "listening for" particular things.[1] Also listen for things that patients may not be saying but seem relevant with regard to the other issues that have been raised or that you have observed.

What usually happens is that the patient answers with a short phrase or sentence, pauses, and then looks at you, expecting to receive some direction of how to go on. What you do next is the key to the interview. If you pose new questions on other topics, you may lose much of the initial story. Instead, respond to the first statement with "Tell me about it" or "Anything else?" or merely look acutely interested. The patient will then elaborate. Often, if you remain silent for several seconds before you respond with subsequent questions or comments, patients will continue to explain their situation. Remaining silent is challenging, inasmuch as most health care providers are socialized to rush to fill whatever silences that naturally occur in conversations. As discussed below, you will need to practise remaining silent: it is a skill that you can actively cultivate.

Closed or Direct Questions

Closed or **direct questions** ask for specific information. They elicit a short one- or two-word answer, a "yes" or "no," or a forced choice. Whereas the open-ended question allows patients to answer in a way that is more appropriate for them, the direct question limits the answer (Table 4.1).

Use direct questions after the patient's opening narrative to fill in any details that the patient left out. In addition, use direct questions when you need many specific facts, such as when asking about past health problems or during the review of systems. Direct questions are also needed when you must complete the interview in a brief time. Asking all open-ended questions can yield unwieldy amounts of data.

TABLE 4.1   Comparison of Open-Ended and Closed Questions

OPEN-ENDED	DIRECT, CLOSED
Used for narrative information	Used for specific information
Calls for longer answers	Calls for short (one- to two-word) answers
Elicits feelings, experiences, understandings, opinions, ideas	Elicits facts
Builds and enhances rapport	Limits rapport and leaves interaction neutral

Be careful, however, not to overuse closed questions. Follow these guidelines:

• Ask only one direct question at a time.
• Avoid opening the interview with closed-ended questions or bombarding the patient with long lists: "Have you ever had pain, double vision, watering, or redness in the eyes?"
• Avoid double-barrelled questions, such as "Do you exercise and follow a well-balanced diet?" The patient will not know which question to answer, and if the patient answers "yes," you will not know which question the patient has answered.

Responses: Assisting the Narrative

Some people seek health care for short-term or relatively simple needs. Their history is direct and uncomplicated; for these people, two responses (facilitation and silence) may be all you need to get a complete understanding of their situation. Other people have a complex story, a long history of interrelated chronic conditions, complex emotional responses, and may have various perceptions about the health care system in Canada. Additional responses help you gather data without cutting them off.

There are eight types of verbal responses in all. The first five responses (facilitation, silence, reflection, empathy, clarification) involve your *reactions* to the facts or feelings the patient has communicated. Your response focuses on the patient's frame of reference. Your own frame of reference does not enter into the response. In the last three responses (interpretation, explanation, summary), you start to express your *own* thoughts and feelings. The frame of reference shifts from the patient's perspective to yours. In the first five responses, the patient leads; in the last three responses, you lead.

Facilitation. These responses encourage the patient to say more, to continue with the story. Also called *general leads*, these responses show that you are interested and will listen further. Examples of verbal facilitation are "Mmm-hmm," "Go on," "Please continue," and "Uh-huh." However, simply maintaining eye contact, shifting forward in your seat with increased attention, nodding affirmatively, or using your hand to gesture "Yes, go on, I'm with you" also encourages the patient to continue talking.

Silence. Silence is a highly effective communication technique, particularly after open-ended questions. Your silent attentiveness communicates to patients that they have time to think, to organize what they wish to say without interruption. Health care providers very often disrupt this opportunity for "thinking silence," which has the effect of interrupting the patient's train of thought. The patient is often interrupted because silence is uncomfortable to novice examiners. They feel responsible for keeping the dialogue going and believe they are at fault if it stops. Silence, however, has advantages. One advantage is that it lets patients collect their thoughts. Also, silence gives you a chance to observe patients unobtrusively and to note nonverbal cues. Finally, silence gives you time to plan your next approach.

Reflection. This response echoes the patient's words. Reflection is repeating part of what the patient has just said. In this example, it focuses further attention on a specific phrase and helps the patient feel free to continue to answer:

> Patient: *"I'm here because of my water. It was cutting off."*
> Response: *"It was cutting off?"*
> Patient: *"Yes, yesterday it took me 30 minutes to pass my water. Finally I got a tiny stream, but then it just closed off."*

Reflection also can help express feeling behind a patient's words. The feeling is already in the statement. You focus on it and encourage the patient to elaborate:

> Patient: *"It's so hard having to stay on bed rest with this pregnancy. I have two more little ones at home. I'm so worried they are not getting the care or attention they need."*
> Response: *"That's understandable—you may feel that you're not 'there' for your other children?"*

Think of yourself as a mirror reflecting the patient's words or feelings. This encourages the patient to elaborate on the problem.

Empathy. A patient's physical symptom, condition, or illness is often accompanied or can even be triggered by specific emotional or mental states. Many people have trouble expressing these feelings, perhaps because of confusion or embarrassment. In the preceding reflecting example, the patient already had stated a feeling, and you echoed it. In the following example, the patient has not said it yet. An empathic response relays recognition of a feeling, puts it into words, and allows the expression of it. When the empathic response is used, the patient feels accepted and can deal with the feeling openly:

> Patient [sarcastically]: *"This is just great. I have my own business, I direct 20 employees every day and now here in hospital, I am having to call you for every little thing."*
> Response: *"It must be hard—one day having so much control, and now feeling dependent on someone else."*

4.2

Your response does not cut off further communication, as would false reassurance ("Oh, you'll be back to work in no time"). Also, it does not deny the feeling and indicate that it is not justified ("Now I don't do *everything* for you. You are feeding yourself"). An empathic response recognizes the feeling, accepts it, and allows the patient to express it without embarrassment. It strengthens rapport. The patient feels understood, which by itself is therapeutic, because it eases the feelings of isolation brought on by illness. Other empathic responses are "This must be very hard for you," "I understand," and just placing your hand on the patient's arm (Fig. 4.2).

Clarification. Seek clarification when the patient's word choice is ambiguous or confusing (e.g., "Tell me what you mean by 'tired blood'"). Clarification also is used to summarize the patient's words, to make them clearer by simplifying them, and then to ensure that you are on the right track. You are asking for agreement, and the patient can confirm or deny your understanding.

> Response: *"Now as I understand you, this heaviness in your chest comes when you shovel snow or climb stairs, and it goes away when you stop doing those things. Is that correct?"*
> Patient: *"Yes, that's pretty much it."*

Clarification may also focus on a discrepancy ("You say it doesn't hurt, but when I touch you here, you grimace"), or it may focus on the patient's affect ("You *look* sad" or "You *sound* angry").

Interpretation. Recall that in the last three types of responses (interpretation, explanation, and summary), the frame of reference shifts from the patient's perspective to yours. These responses now include your own thoughts and feelings. Use the last three responses only when merited by the situation. If you use them too often, you take over at the patient's expense. For example, interpretation is based on your inference or conclusions. It links events, makes associations, or implies cause: "It seems that every time you feel the stomach pain, you have had some kind of stress in your life." Interpretation also ascribes feelings and helps patients understand their own feelings in relation to the verbal message.

> Patient: *"I have decided I don't want to take any more treatments. But I can't seem to tell my doctor that. Every time she comes in, I tighten up and can't say anything."*
> Response: *"Could it be that you're afraid of her reaction?"*

You do run a risk of making the wrong inference. If this is the case, the patient will correct it. Even if the inference is corrected, however, interpretation helps prompt further discussion of the topic.

Explanation. With these statements, you give the patient information. You share factual and objective data. This information may be for orientation to the health care setting ("Your dinner comes at 5:30 P.M."), or it may be to explain cause ("The reason you cannot eat or drink before your blood test is that the food will affect the test results, and we would like to get as accurate a result as possible").

Summary. This is a final review of your understanding of what the patient has said. In summarizing, you condense the facts and present a survey of how you perceive the health problem or need. It is a type of validation in that the patient can agree with it or correct it. Both you and the patient should participate. When the summary occurs at the end of the interview, it signals that termination of the interview is imminent.

Ten Traps of Interviewing

The verbal skills just discussed are productive and enhance the interview. Now take time to consider nonproductive, defeating verbal messages, or *traps*. It is easy to fall into these traps because you are anxious to help. The danger is that they restrict the patient's response. The following traps are obstacles to obtaining accurate, complete data and to establishing rapport.

1. Providing False Assurance or Reassurance

A patient says, "Oh, I just know this lump is going to turn out to be cancer." How do you react? The automatic response of many clinicians is to say, "Now don't worry; I'm sure you will be all right." This "courage builder" relieves *your* anxiety and gives you the false sense of having provided comfort. For patients, however, it actually closes off communication. It trivializes their anxiety and effectively denies any further talk of it. (Also, it promises something that may not happen: that is, they may *not* be "all right"). Consider instead these responses:

> *"You are really worried about the lump, aren't you?"*
> *"It must be hard to wait for the biopsy results."*

These responses acknowledge the emotion and encourage more communication.

A genuine, valid form of reassurance does exist. You *can* reassure patients that you are listening to them, that you understand them, that you have hope for them, and that you will take care of them.

> Patient: "I feel so lost here since they transferred me to the medical centre. No one comes to see me. No one here cares what happens to me."
>
> Response: "I care what happens to you. I am here today, and I want you to know that I'll be here all week."

This type of reassurance makes a commitment to the patient, and it can have a powerful effect.

2. Giving Unwanted Advice

Know when to give advice or avoid giving it. Often, people seek health care because they want your professional advice and information on the management of a health problem: "My child has chicken pox; how should I take care of him?" This is a straightforward request for information from you that the caregiver needs. You respond by giving health information, a therapeutic plan that is based on your knowledge and experience.

In other situations, advice is different; it is based on a hunch or feeling. It is your personal opinion. Consider the woman who has just left a meeting with her consultant physician: "Dr. Msabaha just told me my only chance of getting pregnant is to have an operation. I just don't know. What would you do?" Does the woman really want your advice? An answer such as "If I were you, I would …" is a mistake. You are not that woman. If you give this answer, you have shifted the accountability for decision making from her to you instead of supporting her to consider her options or learn something about herself. Instead, a better response is reflection:

> Response: "He said you should have an operation?"
> Woman: "Yes, and I'm terrified of being put to sleep. What if I don't wake up?"

Now you know her *real* concern and can help her deal with it. She has expressed herself in the process and may be better equipped to meet her next decision.

When asked for advice, other preferred responses are as follows:

> "What are the pros and cons of [this choice] for you?"
> "What concerns do you have?"
> "What is holding you back?"

Although it is quicker just to give advice, take the time to involve patients in a problem-solving process. By participating in problem solving, patients are more likely to make decisions that fit their particular context and situation.

3. Using Authority

"Your doctor/nurse knows best" is a response that promotes dependency and inferiority. In this approach, you are talking "down," and little from the patient is going back "up." A better approach is to avoid using authority completely.

Although you and the patient may not have equality of professional skill and experience, you do have equally worthy roles in the health process, each respecting the other.

4. Using Avoidance Language

People use euphemisms such as "passed on" to avoid reality or to hide their feelings. They think if they just say the word "died," it might really happen. Thus to "protect" themselves, they may evade the issue. Although it seems that using avoidance language will make potentially fearful topics comfortable, it does not. Not talking about the fear does not make it go away; it just suppresses the fear and often makes it worse. Using direct language is the best way to deal with frightening topics. Guidelines are available for very experienced clinicians who are at a stage in their career in which they engage in discussions about serious illness care in outpatient, non-emergent settings (e.g., the Serious Illness Care Program Reference Guide for Clinicians [see the Additional Resources at the end of this chapter]).[8] Initiating these discussions is not appropriate for nurses or health care providers who are novices or still at the beginning of their career.

5. Engaging in Distancing

Distancing is the use of impersonal speech to put space between a threat and the self: "My friend has a problem; she is afraid she …," or "There is a blockage in the artery." By using "the" instead of "my," the patient may be denying any association with the health condition—as a way of coping. Health care providers use distancing, too, to soften reality. This does not work because it communicates to the patient that you also are afraid of the procedure. The use of seemingly blunt-sounding specific terms actually is preferable for defusing anxiety.

6. Overusing Professional Jargon or Casual Language

What is called a *myocardial infarction* in the health care profession is called a *heart attack* by most laypeople. What is called a *major depressive disorder* in the health care profession is called *sadness*, *the blues*, or *feeling down* by most laypeople. Use of jargon sounds exclusionary and paternalistic. You need to adjust your vocabulary to the patient, but avoid sounding condescending or too medicalized.

7. Using Leading or Biased Questions

Asking a person "You don't smoke, do you?" implies that one answer is "better" than another. If patients want to please you, either they are forced to answer in a way corresponding to your values or they feel guilty when they must admit the other answer. It is imperative to convey unconditional positive regard, regardless of your judgements or personal opinions about a patient's health status, or the behaviours or practices that may impact the patient's health.

8. Talking Too Much

Some examiners positively associate helpfulness with verbal productivity. If the air has been thick with their oratory and advice, these examiners leave thinking they have met the patient's needs. Just the opposite is true. Anxious to please, some patients let examiners talk at the expense of the need to express themselves. A good rule for every interviewer is to *listen more than talk.*

9. Interrupting

Often, when you think you know what the patient will say, you interrupt and cut the patient off. This signals that you are impatient or bored with the interview. A related trap is preoccupation with yourself by thinking of your next remark while the patient is talking. By thinking about your next step while the patient is talking, you cannot fully actively listen or understand what the patient says. Aim for a second of silence between the patient's statement and your next response.

10. Using "Why" Questions

Be careful when using "why" questions. Asking someone "Why were you so late for your appointment?" implies blame and condemnation; it puts the patient on the defensive. Instead, consider reframing your query in a more open-ended manner, such as "I noticed that you were delayed getting here, and I'm wondering how things are going for you?" The latter conveys your intention to inquire about the circumstances of the person's life, which will provide important contextual information (such as access to resources like safe, reliable transportation) pertinent to the health assessment.

Consider your use of "why" questions in the health care setting; for example, "Why did you take so much medication?" or "Why did you wait so long before coming to the hospital?" The only possible answer to a "why" question is "Because …," and the patient may not know the answer; the patient may not have reasoned it through. You will likely sound accusatory and judgemental. The patient now must produce an excuse to rationalize their own behaviour. To avoid this trap, say: "I see you started to have chest pains early in the day. What was happening between the time the pains started and the time you came to the emergency department?"

Nonverbal Skills

Learn to observe with your eyes, as well as with your ears. Nonverbal modes of communication include physical appearance, posture, gestures, facial expression, eye contact, voice, and touch. Communication patterns vary widely across families, ethnocultural groups, and social groups, even for such everyday social behaviours such as smiling and handshaking.

Physical Appearance

Your own appearance sends a message to the patient. Professional dress varies among agencies and settings. Depending on the setting, the use of a professional uniform may create a positive stereotype (comfort, expertise, or ease of identification) or a negative stereotype (distance, authority, or formality). Whatever your personal choice in clothing or grooming, the aim should be to convey a competent, professional image.

Posture

Note the patient's position. An open position with extension of large muscle groups shows relaxation, physical comfort, and a willingness to share information. A closed position with arms and legs crossed looks defensive and anxious. Note any change in posture. If a patient in a relaxed position suddenly tenses, it suggests discomfort with the new topic.

Your own calm, relaxed posture creates a feeling of warmth and trust and conveys an interest in the patient. Standing and hastily filling out a history form with periodic peeks at your watch communicates that you are busy with many things more important than interviewing the patient. Even when your time is limited, appear calm and unhurried. Sit down, even if it is only for a few minutes, and look as if nothing else matters except the patient.

Gestures

Gestures send messages. For example, nodding or an open turning out of the hand shows acceptance, attention, or agreement. Hand gestures can reinforce a patient's description of pain. When a crushing substernal chest pain is described, the patient often holds the hand twisted into a fist in front of the sternum; pain that is intense and sharply localized may be indicated by one finger pointing to the exact spot: "It hurts right here."

Facial Expression

The face reflects a wide variety of relevant emotions and conditions. The expression may look alert, relaxed, and interested, or it may look anxious, angry, and suspicious. Physical conditions such as pain or shortness of breath also show in the expression.

Your own expression should reflect a professional who is attentive, sincere, and interested in the patient. Any expression of boredom, distraction, disgust, criticism, or disbelief is picked up by the patient, and rapport dissolves.

Eye Contact

Lack of eye contact in some situations or contexts suggests that the patient is anxious, shy, withdrawn, confused, bored, intimidated, apathetic, or depressed. The same can be said of examiners who avoid eye contact, too. You should aim to maintain eye contact, but do not "stare down" the patient. Eye contact is perhaps among the most culturally variable nonverbal behaviours. Although you probably have been taught to maintain eye contact when speaking with others, people from some ethnocultural backgrounds may use eye contact in other ways. For example, some people may avert their eyes when talking with you in an effort to convey respect to people in positions of authority. Some people may look downward during conversations to indicate that the listener is paying close attention to the speaker. In some communities, people raise their eyebrows as a way to signal an affirmative response to a question, or to signal agreement, rather than nodding.

Voice

Besides the spoken words, meaning is expressed through the tone of voice, the intensity and rate of speech, the pitch, and any pauses. These factors are just as important as words in conveying meaning. For example, the tone of a patient's voice may indicate sarcasm, disbelief, judgement, sympathy, or hostility. An anxious patient often speaks in a loud, fast voice. A soft voice may indicate shyness, fear, or lack of confidence in one's self. A hearing-impaired patient may use a loud voice.

Silence

Wide variation exists in interpreting silence. Some individuals find silence extremely uncomfortable and make every effort to fill conversational lags with words. Others consider silence essential to understanding and respecting the other person. A pause after a question can signify that what has been asked is important enough to be given thoughtful consideration before responding. Silence may also be used to convey respect for another's privacy or to demonstrate respect for older adults.

Bodily Exposure and Touch

For some people, modesty in relation to bodily exposure (e.g., removing clothing for physical examinations) is particularly important in showing respect. For instance, because of past negative experiences, family norms, or culturally specific norms, a female patient or the patient's family may consider it entirely inappropriate for a male health care provider to examine the patient unless she is fully clothed; the same may be said for a female health care provider in relation to a male patient. You need to ask patients for their preferences before proceeding, be responsive to their requests, and remain attuned to the verbal and nonverbal cues conveyed by patients or their families as you proceed. In all cases, provide a clear explanation of why you are asking someone to remove part of their clothing for the purpose of examination, and be prepared to make adaptations or forgo bodily exposure of the patient in some cases.

Touching a patient is a necessary component of a comprehensive assessment. The meaning of physical touch is influenced by the patient's age, gender, ethnocultural background, other social and personal factors, their past experience, and the current setting. The meaning of touch is easily misinterpreted. Although there can be benefits in establishing rapport with patients through touch, physical contact with patients can be interpreted by patients in various ways, and have various meanings. You should be aware that the patient's significant other or family may have opinions on who is able to physically examine the patient. Touching children also may have associated meanings. Whenever possible, you should explore alternative ways to obtain information necessary for assessment of the child's condition (e.g., hold the child on the lap, observe for other manifestations of increased intracranial pressure or signs of premature fontanelle closure, or place one's hand over the caregiver's

TABLE 4.2 **Nonverbal Behaviours of the Interviewer**	
POSITIVE	**NEGATIVE**
Professional appearance is appropriate to the context	Appearance objectionable to patient
Equal-status seating	Standing
Close proximity to patient	Sitting behind desk, far away, turned away
Relaxed, open posture	Tense posture
Leaning slightly toward patient	Slouched back
Occasional facilitating gestures	Critical or distracting gestures: pointing finger, clenching fist, finger tapping, foot swinging, looking at watch
Facial animation, interest	Bland expression, yawning, tight mouth
Appropriate smiling	Frowning, lip biting
Appropriate eye contact	Shifty, avoiding eye contact, focusing on notes/computer screen/iPad, etc.
Moderate tone of voice	Strident, high-pitched tone
Moderate rate of speech	Rate too slow or too fast
Appropriate use of, and consent to touch, depending on the context	Too frequent or inappropriate touch, or touch without consent of patient and/or patient's caregiver

while asking for a description of what they feel). Overall, it is *always* necessary to ask for consent to touch. Moreover, do not use touch during the interview unless you know the patient well and are sure how the patient will interpret it.

In sum, an examiner's nonverbal messages that are productive and enhancing to the relationship are those that show attentiveness and unconditional acceptance. Defeating, nonproductive nonverbal behaviours are those of inattentiveness, authority, and superiority (Table 4.2).

Closing the Interview

The session should end gracefully. An abrupt or awkward closing can destroy rapport and leave the patient with a negative impression of the whole interview. To ease into the closing, ask the patient questions such as the following:

"Is there anything else you would like to mention?"
"Are there any questions you would like to ask?"
"Are there any other areas I should have asked about?"

Such questions give the patient the final opportunity for self-expression. Then, to indicate that closing is imminent, say something like "Our interview is just about over." No new topic should be introduced now. This is a good time to give your summary or a recapitulation of what you have learned during the interview. The summary provides a brief overview of what you and the patient have discussed. It should include positive health aspects, any health issues or priorities that have been identified, any plans for action, or an explanation of the subsequent physical examination. As you part from patients, thank them for the time spent and for their participation.

◈ DEVELOPMENTAL CONSIDERATIONS

Interviewing Caregivers

When your patient is a child, you must build rapport with two people: the child and the accompanying caregiver (which may be the child's parent or another person designated as the child's caregiver—e.g., a grandparent or guardian). Greet both by name, but with a younger child (1 to 6 years old), focus more on the caregiver. By ignoring the child temporarily, you allow the child to size you up from a safe distance. The child can observe your interaction with the caregiver, see that the caregiver accepts and likes you, and relax (Fig. 4.3).

Begin by interviewing the caregiver and child together. If any sensitive topics arise (e.g., the caregivers' troubled relationship or the child's problems at school or with peers), explore them with the caregiver later, one on one. Provide books or toys to occupy the child as you and the caregiver talk. This frees the caregiver to concentrate on the history. Also, the child's play can reveal the level of attention span or independent play. Through the interview, be alert to ways the caregiver and child interact. The history provides an ideal time to integrate discussion points related to health promotion and prevention, as noted in Chapter 2.

For younger children, the caregiver will provide all or most of the history. Thus you are collecting the child's health data from the caregiver's frame of reference. This viewpoint is usually reliable because most caregivers have the child's well-being as a priority and view cooperation with you as a way to enhance this well-being.

When you collect developmental data, avoid being judgemental about the age at achievement of certain milestones. This discussion can be an opportune time to pose

4.3

open-ended questions to caregivers about health promotion and prevention issues, such as "How does Iman like wearing her bike helmet?" Caregivers are understandably proud of their child's achievements and are sensitive to inferences that these milestones may occur late. Refer to the child by name, not as "the baby." Refer to the caregiver by name and not the label "Mother," "Dad," "Grandma," etc. Also, be clear when identifying the caregivers. In Canada and elsewhere, people may have different kinship relationships for various reasons, which influence the child's social support and health. For example, a mother's current partner may not necessarily be the child's biological father. Instead of asking about "your husband's" health, ask, "Is Joan's father in good health?"

Although most of your communication is with the caregiver, do not ignore the child completely. You need to make contact to ease into the physical examination later. Begin by asking about the books or toys the child is playing with or about a special doll or teddy bear brought from home: "Does your doll have a name?" or "What can your truck do?" Stoop down so that you are at the child's eye level. Adult size can be threatening to young children and can emphasize their smallness.

Nonverbal communication is even more important to children than it is to adults. Children are quick to pick up feelings, anxiety, or comfort from nonverbal cues. Do not try to maintain constant eye contact with a small child; it can make the child feel threatened. Use a quiet, measured voice, and choose simple words in your speech. Considering the child's level of language development is valuable in planning your communication.

Infants

Most infants look calm and relaxed when all their needs are met, and they cry when they are frightened, hungry, tired, or uncomfortable. They respond best to firm, gentle handling and a quiet, calm voice. Your calm voice is comforting, even though they do not understand the words. Older infants have anxiety toward strangers. They are more comfortable when the caregiver is kept in view.

Preschoolers

Children 2 to 6 years old are egocentric, which is a normal developmental stage. They see the world mostly from their own point of view. Only the child's own experience is relevant. Citing an example of another child's behaviour as a strategy to encourage cooperation may not work well, because it will have no meaning. Preschoolers' communication is direct, concrete, literal, and set in the present. Avoid figurative expressions such as "climbing the walls" because they are easily misinterpreted by young children. Use short, simple sentences with a concrete explanation. Take time to give a short, simple explanation for any unfamiliar equipment that will be used to examine the child. Preschoolers can have *animistic* thinking about unfamiliar objects. They may imagine that unfamiliar inanimate objects can come alive and have human characteristics (e.g., that a blood pressure cuff can wake up and bite or pinch).

School-Age Children

Children 7 to 12 years old can understand others' viewpoints. Such children are more objective and realistic. They want to know functional aspects: how things work and why things are done.

Children of this age group have the verbal ability to add important data to the history. Interview the caregiver and child together, but when the child has a presenting symptom or sign, ask the child about it first and then gather data from the caregiver. For the well child seeking a checkup, pose questions about school, friends, or activities directly to the child.

Adolescents

Adolescents want to be adults, but they do not yet have the cognitive ability to achieve their goal. They are between two stages. Sometimes they are capable of mature actions, and other times they revert to childhood response patterns, especially in times of stress. You cannot treat adolescents as children, but you cannot overcompensate and assume that their communication style, learning ability, and motivation are consistently at an adult level.

Adolescents value their peers. They crave acceptance and sameness with their peers. Most adolescents think no adult can understand them. Because of this, some act with aloof contempt, answering only in monosyllables. Some others make eye contact and tell you what they think you want to hear, but inside they are thinking, "You'll never know the full story about me." These are helpful guidelines to use when communicating with adolescents:

- Be respectful. Respect is the most important thing you can communicate to an adolescent. Adolescents need to feel validated as human beings, accepted, and worthy.
- Communicate honestly. An adolescent's intuition is highly tuned and can detect phoniness or when information is withheld. Always give adolescents the truth, or you will lose their trust. They will cooperate if they understand your rationale.
- Avoid using language or colloquialisms that are not part of your usual way of interacting. It is helpful to understand some of the jargon used by adolescents, but you cannot use those words yourself simply to try to bond with adolescent patients. Do not try to be a peer. You are not, and they will not accept you as such.
- Use conversational icebreakers. Focus first on the adolescent, not on the problem. Although adults often want to talk about their health concern immediately, adolescents respond best when the focus is on them as people. Show an interest in the adolescent. Ask open-ended, friendly questions about school, activities, hobbies, and friends. Refrain from asking questions about caregivers and family for now; these issues can be emotionally charged during adolescence.
- Explain every step about a health interview or a physical examination, and give the rationale for each step. They will feel most comfortable when they know the reason for your questions or actions. Encourage their questions. Adolescents are afraid they will sound "dumb" if they ask a question to which they assume everybody else knows the answer.
- Keep your questions short and simple. "Tell me why are you here?" sounds brazen to you, but it can be effective with adolescents. Be prepared for adolescents who do *not* know why they are there. Some adolescents are pushed into coming to the examination by a caregiver.
- Be aware of your responses. The communication responses described for adults must be reconsidered in talking with adolescents. Silent periods usually are best avoided. Giving adolescents a little time to collect their thoughts is acceptable, but a silence for other reasons is threatening. Adolescents are more sensitive to nonverbal communication than are adults. Be aware of your expressions and gestures. Adolescents are also more sensitive to any comment that can be interpreted as criticism from you and will withdraw.
- Wait until later in the interview or in a follow-up visit (after you have developed rapport with the adolescent) to address topics that are emotionally charged, including for example, sexual behaviour, multiple sexualities, alcohol and drug use, suicidal thoughts, and depression. Adolescents assume that health care providers have similar values and standards of behaviour as most of the other authority figures in their lives, and they may be reluctant to share this information. You can assure them that your questions are not intended to be curious or intrusive but cover topics that are important for most teenagers and on which you have relevant health information to share.
- If confidential material is uncovered during the interview, consider what can remain confidential and what you feel you must share for the well-being of the adolescent. Provincial and territorial laws vary with regard to confidentiality requirements with minors; several provinces (but not all) observe the "mature minors rule," and health care providers are not required to notify caregivers about, for example, birth control or treatment for sexually transmitted infections. However, if the adolescent talks about an abusive home situation, state that you must share this information with other health care providers for the adolescent's own protection. Ask the adolescent, "Do you have a problem with that?" and then discuss it. Tell the adolescent, "You will need to trust that I will handle this information professionally and in your best interest."*

---

*As discussed in more detail in Chapter 8, in Canada, all provinces have mandatory requirements for reporting suspected child abuse or other forms of abuse. If you suspect that a child is being maltreated or is at risk of maltreating others, you should involve other members of the health care team. You should be familiar with your legal obligations in the jurisdiction in which you work.

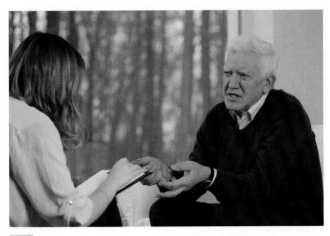

4.4

• Take every opportunity to provide positive reinforcement. Praise every action regarding the health-promoting activities in which the adolescent is engaged: "That's great that you aren't smoking cigarettes [or that you've cut down on the number of cigarettes you are smoking]. I realize that's not easy, but it's going to have a good impact on your health. And it may save you money as well."

Older Adults

Always address the patient by the last name (e.g., "Hello, Mr. Choi"; "Good morning, Ms. Tall Bear"). Some older adults resent being called by their first name by younger persons. The interview usually takes longer with older adults because they have a longer story to tell. You may need to break up the interview into more than one visit, collecting the most important historical data first. It is important to adjust the pace of the interview to older patients. Older patients have a great amount of background material to sort through, and this takes some time. Also, some older patients need a greater amount of response time to interpret questions and process their answers. Avoid trying to hurry them along. (Fig. 4.4).

Consider physical limitations when you plan the interview. Older patients may fatigue earlier and may require that the interview be broken up into shorter segments. For patients with impaired hearing, face them directly so that your mouth and face are fully visible. Do not shout; it does not help and actually distorts speech.

INTERVIEWING IN CHALLENGING SITUATIONS

Patients With Disabilities

Interviewing patients with visible and invisible disabilities requires that nurses deeply consider the process of informed consent and the appropriate tools for communication. For example, although many patients tell you in advance that they have a hearing impairment, others may not and you must recognize the impairment from clues, such as staring at your mouth and face, not responding unless looking at

you, or speaking in a voice unusually loud or with guttural or garbled sounds. Ask patients with a hearing impairment about their preferred way to communicate: by signing, lip-reading, or writing. The use of assistive devices such as Pocketalker may be useful in some situations. The Pocketalker is frequently used in Canadian hospitals to foster communication with individuals who have a hearing impairment.

There are many other spectra of disability that influence people's access to and experience of health care. For instance, you may work with patients who have intellectual disabilities. In such cases, nurses may need to be creative in their use of sign language, films, pictures, and drawings as communication tools to develop trust and rapport with patients.[9] Moreover, while there may be a caregiver in the room with you, nurses should direct their comments and questions to the patient.[10]

Acutely Ill Patients

An emergency necessitates your prompt action. You must combine interviewing with physical examination skills to determine life-saving actions. Although life support measures may be paramount, try to interview the patient as much as possible nonetheless. Subjective data are crucial for determining the cause and course of the emergency. Abbreviate your questioning. Identify the main area of distress and pose a question about that. Family or friends often can provide important data. Begin to use closed, direct questions earlier. Finally, ensure that your statements are clear. When a patient is very sick, even the simplest sentence can be misconstrued. The patient will react according to preconceived ideas about what a serious illness means, so anything you say should be direct and precise.

Patients Under the Influence of Alcohol or Drugs

As discussed in Chapter 7, people may use different kinds of substances, such as alcohol or marijuana, and they may use multiple kinds of substances. A wide range of patient behaviours may be influenced by these substances. Alcohol and the opioids (heroin, fentanyl, meperidine, oxycodone, hydromorphone, dextropropoxyphene) are central nervous system depressants. Stimulants of the central nervous system (cocaine, methamphetamine, amphetamine) can cause an intense high, agitation, and paranoid behaviour. Hallucinogens (marijuana, mushrooms, lysergic acid diethylamide [LSD]) can cause irrational, erratic, and inappropriate behaviour.

When interviewing a patient currently under the influence of alcohol or drugs or other substances, ask simple, direct questions, and convey a nonjudgemental stance (see Chapter 7). Take care to make your manner and questions nonthreatening, and convey a nonjudgemental attitude. Avoid any display of scolding or negative judgement, such as disappointment or disgust. Instead, remember that people use substances because of their life contexts, and you may not have a complete picture of the patient's life context. Conveying negative judgements will probably cause the patient to avoid subsequent contact with the health care system.

It is a priority to find out what time the patient last drank alcohol and how much was drank at that episode, as well as the name and amount of any other substances taken. Tell the patient why you are asking these questions, namely, that this information helps you assess any withdrawal patterns and needs for support. To ensure safety for your patient, seek assistance from your colleagues as needed to address the patient's issues.

Once the effects of the substances have worn off, a follow-up assessment should be performed to evaluate the extent of the problem and the meaning of the problem for the patient and family. Special interview techniques will probably be needed, which are also discussed in Chapter 7.

Personal Questions

On occasion, patients ask you questions about your personal life or opinions, such as "Are you married?"; "Do you have children?"; or "Do you smoke?" You do not need to answer every question. You may supply brief information when you feel it is appropriate, but be sensitive to the possibility that there may be a motive behind the personal questions such as loneliness or anxiety. Try directing your response back to the patient's frame of reference. Some people place a high value on developing interpersonal relationships and getting to know about a patient's family, personal concerns, and interests before they allow you to interact therapeutically.

Recognizing that time constraints frequently affect the social interchange expected by some individuals, you should strive to incorporate the patient's interactional style into the process of conducting the health history. For example, using a conversational tone of voice, you might begin the health history by inquiring about the patient's family members and their health.

You may want to consider in advance which categories of personal questions you are willing to discuss and which ones you will politely decline to discuss. The manner in which you reply to personal inquiries should be carefully worded, sensitive to the needs of the patient, and congruent with your own needs and comfort level.

Dealing With Sexual Advances

On some occasions, personal questions extend to flirtatious compliments, seductive innuendo, or advances, in part due to the prevalence of gender-based power relations in our society. Your response must make it clear that you are a health care provider who can best care for the patient by maintaining a professional relationship. Doing so may be difficult, considering that the patient's words or gestures may have left you surprised, embarrassed, and/or angry. Your feelings are normal. You need to set appropriate verbal boundaries by saying, "I am uncomfortable when you talk to me that way; please don't." A further response that would open communication is "I wonder if the way you're feeling now relates to your illness or to being in the hospital?" Each workplace will have its own procedures and policies for supporting staff members and volunteers in the case of unwanted advances or assault.

Crying

A novice examiner usually feels very concerned when a patient starts crying. Crying, however, is often a big relief to a patient. Health problems come with powerful emotions. Keeping worries about illness, death, or loss bottled up inside takes a great amount of energy. When you say something that "makes the patient cry," do not presume that you have hurt the patient. You have likely addressed a topic that is important. Do not go on to a new topic. Just let the patient cry and express their feelings fully. You can offer a tissue and wait until the crying subsides to talk. Sometimes your patient looks to be on the verge of tears but is trying hard to suppress them. Again, instead of moving on to something new, acknowledge the expression by saying, "You look sad." Do not worry that you will open an uncontrollable floodgate. The patient may cry but will be relieved, and you will have gained insight to a serious concern.

Anger

On occasion, you will try to interview a patient who is already angry. Try not to personalize this anger; usually it does not relate to you. The patient is typically showing aggression as a response to personal feelings of anxiety or helplessness. Do convey a nonjudgmental stance, ask about the anger, hear the patient out, and deal with the angry feelings before you ask anything else. This may help to diffuse the anger so that the patient can participate effectively in the health interview.

Threat of Violence

The health care setting is not immune to violent behaviour. An individual may act with such angry gestures that you feel a threat to your personal safety. Other troubling behaviours of a potentially disruptive patient include fist clenching, pacing back and forth, a vacant stare, confusion, statements indicating that the patient is out of touch with reality, statements that do not make sense, a history of recent substance use (e.g., alcohol, hallucinogen, cocaine), or perhaps even a recent history of intense bereavement (e.g., loss of spouse, loss of job). Trust your instincts. If you sense any suspect or threatening behaviour, act immediately to defuse the situation. Leave the examining room door open and position yourself between the patient and the door. Many departments have a prearranged sign or signal so that a co-worker can call 911 and the security department to send help to the setting. Do not raise your own voice or try to argue with a threatening patient. Act quite calm, and talk to the patient in a soft voice. Convey respect for the patient, even if the patient is agitated or expressing frustration toward you. Act interested in what the patient is saying, and behave in an unhurried way. Your most important goal is safety; avoid taking any risks.

Anxiety

Finally, take it for granted that nearly all sick people have some anxiety. This is a normal response to being ill. It can make some people aggressive and others dependent.

Remember that the patient is not reacting as typically as when they are healthy. When people are anxious, whether because of a health concern or not, it is important for you to convey acceptance, understanding, and patience.

 SOCIAL DETERMINANTS OF HEALTH CONSIDERATIONS

Communicating Across Cultures and Social Positions

A number of important cultural and social considerations were discussed in Chapter 3. In relation to communication, when people attempting to communicate have differing ethnocultural and sociohistorical backgrounds, the probability of miscommunication can increase. Verbal and nonverbal communication are influenced by the social position of both the health care provider and the patient, which means that both must attempt to understand the other's point of view.

Relational practice requires that you connect across differences by relating with people as they are and where they are, no matter what their context, decisions, or life history.[1] Nonetheless, you may sometimes find it challenging to relate to or communicate with patients or family members for a variety of reasons. In all situations, you need to be highly reflective about your reactions, assumptions, biases, and judgements so that you can be conscious of how you are relating to people, rather than reacting on the basis of habit.

It is particularly important to establish effective communication with people whose primary language is different from yours. Unfortunately, the current patchwork of interpreter services in Canada and different levels of understanding about the importance of effective communication in health care have led to inconsistencies in how language barriers are addressed in health care settings.[11] Studies have repeatedly shown that access to health care and the quality of health care services are seriously compromised without interpretation services for patients who need them. For example, nursing and medical errors such as misdiagnosis and inappropriate treatment, inadequate patient comprehension, and higher rates of readmission and emergency department visits can result from poor communication.[12,13]

As discussed in Chapter 3, people whose proficiency in English and French is limited and who therefore speak one or more languages other than English or French should, ideally, be offered an interpreter who is *not* a family member or friend. In some contexts and urgent situations, an interpreter may not be available, and family or friends or members of the health care team may need to translate. In either case, it is essential to determine and document whether the patient (and the family) fully understand what is happening; what the diagnosis and the implications of this diagnosis are; what procedures (diagnostic and therapeutic) are going to be performed, how the procedures will be performed, and what they mean; how medications are to be taken and when; and the prognosis derived from the given problems. Strategies

for working effectively with (and without) an interpreter are discussed later in this chapter.

Considerations Related to Gender and Sexual Orientation

As described in Box 3.5 in Chapter 3, gender and sexual identity and expression are important considerations when you communicate with patients. During the interview process, it is important to allow people to self-identify their own sex and gender identity. For example, you can say "Ryder, which gender pronouns do you prefer to use? She/her, he/him, or they/them?" Allowing people to identify their preferred first and last name and their preferred pronoun is a necessary step toward establishing trust with all patients, but particularly those that identify as trans, two-spirit, or gender nonbinary. Ethnocultural or family norms can also dictate the boundaries of appropriate professional and personal relationships between women, men, and other genders. This point is socioculturally very significant; failure to respect norms of behaviour can be viewed as a serious transgression. The best way to ensure that particular norms have been considered is to ask the patient about relevant aspects of gendered relationships, preferably at the beginning of the interview. When you have determined that gender differences are important to the patient, you might try strategies such as offering to have a third person present when this is feasible.

In interviewing people who identify as lesbian, gay, bisexual, asexual, pansexual, queer, and other diverse sexual orientations, you should be aware of heterosexist biases and the communication of these biases during the interview and physical examination. *Heterosexism* is the institutionalized belief that heterosexuality is the only natural choice of sexuality and that it is the norm. For example, most health histories include a question concerning marital status. Although many same-gender couples are married or in committed, long-term, monogamous relationships, seldom is there a category on the standard form that acknowledges this type of relationship. Although technically and legally certain patients may be "single," this designation trivializes the relationship with their significant other. This designation may also have family and decision-making implications related to caregiving roles. To mitigate heterosexist bias in your practice, you can ask patients if they have a partner or significant other and allow them to self-identify their partner's designation (e.g., girlfriend, wife, partner, boyfriend).

OVERCOMING COMMUNICATION BARRIERS

Interviewing a Patient With an Interpreter

After English and French, the most common mother tongues spoken in Canada in 2011 were Punjabi, the Chinese languages (e.g., Cantonese, Mandarin), Spanish, Italian, German, Tagalog (the national language of the Philippines), and Arabic.[14] One of the greatest challenges in cross-cultural

4.5

communication arises when you and the patient speak different languages (Fig. 4.5).

Interviewing a patient who speaks neither English nor French requires a bilingual interpreter for full communication. Even the patient from another country who has a basic command of English or French (those for whom English or French is a second language) may need an interpreter when faced with the anxiety-provoking situation of entering a hospital, describing a strange symptom, or discussing sensitive topics such as those related to reproductive or urological concerns.

Interpreters are employed in many health care agencies and hospitals in Canada; however, research demonstrates that nurses and physicians tend not to use interpreter services adequately.[15] Although Canada has a universal health care system, no legislative provisions or court precedents effectively require the availability of interpretation services for patients who need them. Only the deaf and hearing-impaired community in Canada has had success in the courts in obtaining the right to access interpreter services in health care settings.

Whenever possible, work with an interpreter who is trained in interpreting in health care settings. Trained interpreters typically know interpreting techniques, have a health care background, and understand patients' rights. The trained interpreter also is knowledgeable about culturally specific meanings and practices about health, healing, and illness. Such people can help you bridge the cultural communication gap that may exist and can advise you concerning the cultural appropriateness of your recommendations. Learn whether your institution offers training in how to work with interpreters; enhancing your skills will improve the quality of communication.

Being bilingual, however, does not necessarily mean an interpreter is able to communicate with the patient. Indigenous languages, for example, are so diverse that an Indigenous interpreter from one region of a province or territory may not necessarily understand the language or cultural practices of an Indigenous patient from another region of the same province or territory. The same can be said of South Asian languages. For example, someone who can speak and understand Hindi

may not be proficient in Punjabi, Telugu, or Bengali. Even when an interpreter and patient are from similar ethnocultural backgrounds, trained interpreters may live in urban areas and in an entirely different social context and may be unaware of particular meanings, practices, or beliefs that are important to the patient for whom they interpret.

As mentioned earlier, in some institutions, access to trained interpreters is not available. As a first preference, language services should include the availability of a bilingual staff member who can communicate directly with patients in their preferred language and dialect. If necessary, enlist the aid of a bilingual staff member at your place of employment who can interpret. For convenience, it is tempting to ask the patient's relative, friend, or even another patient to interpret because such people are readily available and probably would like to help. However, asking people who are not trained interpreters to interpret is disadvantageous because their involvement violates confidentiality for the patient, who may not want personal information shared with others. Furthermore, although they may be fluent in ordinary language usage, people who are not trained interpreters are likely to be unfamiliar with medical terminology, hospital or clinic procedures, consent, and health care ethics.

When it is not possible for a staff member to interpret, or in an immediate emergency situation, a patient's family member or friend may need to interpret. This is not desirable, and errors made in translation can be harmful. In all cases, it is your responsibility to ensure that your patients (and, in some situations, their family members) are fully informed of what you are telling them, particularly in relation to informed consent for procedures, treatments, and discharge or follow-up plans.

Working With a Trained Interpreter

When working with a trained interpreter, you are in charge of the focus and flow of the interview, and you should view yourself and the interpreter as a team. Ask the interpreter to meet the patient beforehand to establish rapport and to garner information about the patient's social, cultural, educational, and family contexts. This information enables the interpreter to communicate on the patient's level. Allow more time for interviews that require interpreters. Because the third person is repeating everything, the interview can take considerably longer than interviews with English-speaking patients. You need to focus on priority data.

There are two styles of interpreting: line by line and summarizing. Translating line by line takes more time, but it ensures accuracy. Use this style for most of the interview. Both you and the patient should speak only a sentence or two and then allow the interpreter some time. Use simple language yourself, not medical jargon that the interpreter must simplify before it can be translated. Summary translation progresses faster and is useful for teaching relatively simple health care techniques with which the interpreter is already familiar. Be alert for nonverbal cues as the patient talks. These cues can give valuable data. A good interpreter also notes nonverbal messages and passes them on to you.

Although use of an interpreter is the ideal, you may find yourself in a situation with a patient who speaks no English or French but no interpreter is available. Communicating with these patients may require that you combine verbal and nonverbal communication.

ADDITIONAL RESOURCES

Canada Health Infoway—Telehealth. https://www.infoway-inforoute.ca/en/solutions/telehealth

Canadian Association of the Deaf. http://www.cad.ca

Community Networks of Specialized Care—Health Care. http://www.community-networks.ca/health-care/

Cultural Information—Canada. https://www.international.gc.ca/cil-cai/country_insights-apercus_pays/ci-ic_ca.aspx?lang=eng

Ontario Council on Community Interpreting—Healthcare Division. http://www.occi.ca/hinredirect

Serious Illness Care Program: Reference Guide for Clinicians. http://medstaff.providencehealthcare.org/media/SICGuide-Clinician%20Reference%20Guide.pdf

Statistics Canada—CANSIM. http://www5.statcan.gc.ca/cansim/home-accueil?lang=eng

Trans Care BC—Trans 101. http://transhealth.phsa.ca/trans-101

REFERENCES

1. Doane, G. H., & Varcoe, C. (2015). *How to nurse: Relational inquiry with individuals and families in changing health and health care contexts* (p. 83). Baltimore: Lippincott Williams & Wilkins.

2. Browne, A. J., Doane, G. H., Reimer, J., et al. (2010). Public health nursing practice with "high priority" families: The significance of contextualizing "risk". *Nursing Inquiry, 17*(1), 27–38.

3. Rizvi, S. (2016). The essential aspects of building a therapeutic relationship. *Indian Journal of Positive Psychology, 7*(3), 359–361.

4. Provincial Health Services Authority. (2017). *What is telehealth?* Retrieved from http://www.phsa.ca/health-professionals/professional-resources/telehealth/what-is-telehealth.

5. First Nations Health Authority. (2018). *Together in wellness: A report on the progress of the integration and important of health services for First Nations in British Columbia.* Retrieved from https://www2.gov.bc.ca/assets/gov/government/ministries-organizations/ministries/health/office-of-indigenous-health/together-in-wellness-2016-17.pdf.

6. Canada Health Infoway. (2016). *Ontario Telemedicine Network telehomecare deployment project: Phase 2-report patient monitoring.* Retrieved from https://www.infoway-inforoute.ca/en/component/edocman/resources/reports/benefits-evaluation/3176-ontario-telemedicine-network-telehomecare-deployment-project-phase-2-remote-patient-monitoring.

7. Toh, N., Pawlovich, J., & Grzybowski, S. (2016). Telehealth and patient-doctor relationships in rural and remote communities. *Canadian Family Physician, 62*(12), 961–963.

8. Ariadne Labs: A Joint Center for Health Systems Innovation and Dana-Farber Cancer Institute. (2016). *Serious illness care program: Reference guide for clinicians.* Retrieved from http://medstaff.providencehealthcare.org/media/SICGuide-Clinician%20Reference%20Guide.pdf.

9. Thomas, B., Courtenay, K., Hassiotis, A., et al. (2014). Standardised patients with intellectual disabilities in training tomorrow's doctors. *The Psychiatric Bulletin, 38*(3), 132–136.

10. Perry, J., Felce, D., Kerr, M., et al. (2014). Contact with primary care: The experience of people with intellectual disabilities. *Journal of Applied Research in Intellectual Disabilities, 27*(3), 200–211. doi:10.1111/jar.12072.

11. Farley, R., Guillemette, R., & Rivest, F. (2015). *Canadian federal government response to language rights in health care.* Ottawa: Health Canada. Retrieved from http://www.capitaldocumentation.ca/documents/CMDLenRivest.pdf.

12. Anderson, J., Perry, J., Blue, C., et al. (2003). "Rewriting" cultural safety within the postcolonial and postnational feminist project. *ANS. Advances in Nursing Science, 26,* 196–214.

13. Segalowitz, N., & Kehayia, E. (2011). Exploring the determinants of language barriers in health care (LBHC): Toward a research agenda for the language sciences. *The Canadian Modern Language Review, 67*(4), 480–507.

14. Statistics Canada. (2015). *Linguistic characteristics of Canadians* (Catalogue no. 98-314-X2011001). Ottawa: Author. http://www12.statcan.gc.ca/census-recensement/2011/as-sa/98-314-x/98-314-x2011001-eng.cfm.

15. Gabriel, P., & Preston, E. (2016). A pilot study of telephone-based interpretation in family physician offices in British Columbia. *BC Medical Journal, 58*(8), 442–447.

5 CHAPTER

The Complete Health History

Written by Carolyn Jarvis, PhD, APN, CNP
Adapted by Annette J. Browne, PhD, RN

ⓔ http://evolve.elsevier.com/Canada/Jarvis/examination/

The purpose of the health history is to collect **subjective data**: what the patient says about himself, herself, or themselves. The history is combined with the **objective data** from the physical examination and with laboratory studies to form the database. The database is used to make a judgement or a diagnosis about the health status of the individual. As noted in Chapter 1, the use of electronic health records is widespread in Canada. Nurses can expect to use such records in documenting and managing information collected for the complete health history.

The following health history provides a complete picture of the patient's past and current health. It describes the patient as a whole and how the patient interacts with the environment. It is a record of health strengths and coping skills. In documenting the history, the nurse should recognize and affirm the patient's strengths; that is, what the patient is doing to help stay well. For the well patient, the history is used to assess overall health status, health maintenance goals, and health-promoting practices, such as exercise pattern, diet, risk and harm reduction, and preventive behaviours such as immunization status, age-appropriate health screening, limiting screen and sedentary time, or helmet use during sports activities.

For the ill patient, the health history includes a detailed and chronological record of the health problem. For all patients, the health history is a screening tool for abnormal symptoms, health problems, and concerns, and it records ways of responding to the health problems. In many settings, the patient fills out a printed history form or checklist. This allows the patient ample time to recall and consider such items as dates of health landmarks and relevant family history. The interview is then used to validate the written data and to collect more data on lifestyle management and current health problems.

Although history forms vary, most contain information on the following categories, in this sequence:

1. Biographical data
2. Reason for seeking care
3. Current health or history of current illness
4. Past health history
5. Family health history
6. Review of systems
7. Functional assessment (including activities of daily living [ADLs])

The health history outlined in the following section follows this format and constitutes a generic database for all practitioners. Nurses in clinical settings may use all of it, whereas those in a hospital may focus primarily on the history of current illness and the functional, or patterns of living, data.

HEALTH HISTORY: ADULTS

Biographical Data

By asking the patient to self-identify these characteristics (do not assume that you know), record the patient's name, age and birthdate, birthplace, other recent countries of residence, sex, gender, relationship status, and usual and current occupation or daily activity pattern (an illness or disability may have prompted a change in occupation or usual patterns of activity). Note that in some health care agencies and institutions, the primary language spoken by the patient is recorded. Therefore, the patient's primary and preferred language and authorized representative, if any, should be recorded here. This request is in response to research showing that differences in language and culture have an effect on the quality and safety of care.[1] Acquiring geographical and language information is important when undertaking the history because Canadian research shows that asking people to define their ethnocultural background during the point of care can be harmful, particularly for people who are often racialized or stigmatized.[2]

Source of History

1. Record who provides the information: the source is usually the patient, but it may be a parent or caregiver or, in some cases, a relative or friend.
2. Judge how reliable the informant seems and how willing or able the person is to communicate. Patients typically provide the same answers, even when questions are rephrased or are repeated later in the interview.

3. Note any special circumstances, such as the use of an interpreter. Sample statements are as follows:

"Patient herself, who seems reliable."
"Patient's son, John Ramirez, who seems reliable."
"Mrs. R. Fuentes, interpreter for Theresa Castillo, who does not speak English."

Reason for Seeking Care*

The reason for seeking care is a brief, spontaneous statement in the patient's own words that describes the reason for the visit. Think of it as the "title" for the story to follow. It states one (possibly two) symptoms or signs and their duration. A **symptom** is a subjective sensation that the patient feels from the disorder. A **sign** is an objective abnormality that you as the examiner could detect on physical examination or in laboratory reports. Whatever the patient says is the reason for seeking care is recorded and enclosed in quotation marks to indicate the patient's exact words:

"Chest pain" for 2 hours.
"My child has an earache and was fussy all night."
"I need a yearly physical examination for work."
"I want to start jogging, and I need a checkup."
"I would like to cut down the amount of cigarettes I smoke."

The patient's reason for seeking care should not be used for diagnosis. Avoid translating the patient's statement into the terms of a medical diagnosis. For example, a man enters with shortness of breath, and you ponder writing "emphysema." Even if he is known to have emphysema from previous visits, it is not the chronic emphysema that prompted *this* visit, but rather the "increasing shortness of breath" for 4 hours.

Some people attempt to self-diagnose on the basis of certain information: that obtained from the Internet, which may or may not be accurate; similar signs and symptoms in their relatives or friends; or conditions they know they have. For example, rather than record a woman's statement that she has "strep throat," ask her what symptoms she has that make her think strep throat is present, and record those symptoms.

On occasion, a patient may list *many* reasons for seeking care. The most important reason to the patient may not necessarily be the one stated first. Try to focus on the patient's most pressing concern by asking which one prompted the patient to seek help *now*.

Current Health or History of Current Illness

For the well patient, current health is a short statement about the general state of health. For the ill patient, this section is a chronological record of the reason for seeking care, from the time the symptom first started until now. Isolate each reason for care identified by the patient and say, for example, "Please tell me all about your headache, from the time it started until the time you came to the hospital." If the concern started months or years ago, record what occurred during that time and find out why the patient is seeking care *now*.

As the patient talks, do not jump to conclusions and bias the story by adding your opinion. Collect all the data first. Although you want the patient to respond in a narrative format without interruption from you, your final summary of any symptom the patient has should include the following eight critical characteristics:

1. *Location.* Be specific; ask the patient to point to the location. If the problem is pain, note the precise site. "Head pain" is vague, whereas descriptions such as "pain behind the eyes," "jaw pain," and "occipital pain" are more precise and are diagnostically significant. Is the pain localized to this site or radiating? Is the pain superficial or deep?

2. *Character or quality.* Ask for specific descriptive terms such as *burning, sharp, dull, aching, gnawing, throbbing, shooting,* and *viselike.* Use similes: Does blood in the stool look like sticky tar? Does blood in vomitus look like coffee grounds?

3. *Quantity or severity.* Attempt to quantify the sign or symptom, such as "profuse menstrual flow, soaking five pads per hour." The symptom of pain can be challenging to quantify because of individual interpretations. In many health care settings, patients are routinely asked to rate the intensity of their pain in this way: "How would you rate your pain on a 0 to 10 scale at the present time; that is, where 0 is 'no pain' and 10 is 'pain as bad as it could be'?" With pain, avoid adjectives and instead ask how it affects daily activities. Then the patient might say, "I was so sick I was doubled up and couldn't move" or "I was able to go to work, but then I came home and went to bed."

4. *Timing (onset, duration, frequency).* When did the symptom first appear? Give the specific date and time, or state specifically how long ago the symptom started "prior to arrival" (PTA).† "The pain started yesterday" will not mean much when you return to read the record in the future. The report must include such information as how long the symptom lasted (duration); whether it was steady (constant) or whether it would come and go during that time (intermittent); and whether it resolved completely and reappeared days or weeks later (cycle of remission and exacerbation).

5. *Setting.* Where was the patient or what was the patient doing when the symptom started? What triggers the

---

*In the past, this statement was called the "chief complaint" (CC). This description is avoided now because it implies that the patient "complains" and, of more importance, it does not include health maintenance, health promotion, or wellness needs.

---

†"Prior to arrival" (PTA) is frequently used in primary care and in emergency department settings, when it is clear that the patient arrived for health care at a particular time. For example, for a patient being assessed in an emergency department for abdominal pain, the documentation might read "gradual onset of left lower quadrant abdominal pain that started 4 hours PTA."

symptom? For example, you can ask, "Did you notice the chest pain after shovelling snow, or did the pain start by itself?"

6. *Aggravating or relieving factors.* What makes the pain worse? Is it aggravated by weather, activity, food, medication, bending over, fatigue, time of day, or season? What relieves it (e.g., rest, medication, or ice pack)? What is the effect of any treatment? Ask, "What have you tried?" or "What seems to help?"

7. *Associated factors.* Is the primary symptom associated with any others (e.g., urinary frequency and burning sensation in association with fever and chills)? Review the body system related to this symptom now rather than wait for the review of systems.

8. *Patient's perception.* Find out the meaning of the symptom by asking how it affects daily activities. "How has it affected you? Is there anything you cannot do now that you could do before?" Also ask directly, "What do you think it means?" This question is crucial because it alerts you to potential anxiety if the patient thinks the symptom may be ominous. You may find it helpful to organize this question sequence into the mnemonic **PQRSTU** to help remember all the points. Note that you still need to address the patient's perception of the problem:

P (**provocative** or **palliative**): "What brings it on? What were you doing when you first noticed it? What makes it better? Worse?"

Q (**quality** or **quantity**): "How does it look, feel, sound? How intense or severe is it?"

R (**region** or **radiation**): "Where is it? Does it spread anywhere?"

S (**severity**): "How bad is it (on a scale of 1 to 10)? Is it getting better, getting worse, or staying the same?"

T (**timing**): "Exactly when did it first occur?" (onset); "How long did it last?" (duration); "How often does it occur?" (frequency).

U (**understand** patient's perception of the problem): "What do you think it means?"

Past Health History

Past health events may have residual effects on the current health state. Also, patients' previous experience with illness may give clues as to how they respond to illness and to the significance of illness for them.

Childhood illnesses. Document a history of measles, mumps, rubella, chicken pox, pertussis, and streptococcal infection ("strep throat"). Avoid the wording "usual childhood illnesses" because an illness common in the patient's childhood (e.g., measles) may be unusual today. Ask about serious illnesses that may have sequelae for the patient in later years (e.g., rheumatic fever, scarlet fever, and poliomyelitis).

Accidents or injuries. Document a history of auto accidents, fractures, penetrating wounds, head injuries (especially if associated with unconsciousness), and burns.

Serious or chronic illnesses. Document whether the patient has diabetes, hypertension, heart disease, sickle cell disease, cancer, and seizure disorder.

Hospitalizations. Record cause, name of the hospital, how the condition was treated, how long the patient was hospitalized, and name of the treating physician.

Operations. Document type of surgery, date of surgery, name of the surgeon, name of the hospital, and how the patient recovered.

Obstetrical history. Record the number of pregnancies (gravidity, or *grav*), number of deliveries in which the fetus reached full term (*term*), number of preterm deliveries (*preterm*), number of incomplete pregnancies (therapeutic abortions, or *TA*), and number of children living (*living*). This information is recorded thus: "Grav _____ Term _____ Preterm _____ Ab _____ Living _____." For each complete pregnancy, note the course of pregnancy; the course of labour and delivery; sex, weight, and condition of each infant; and postpartum course. For any incomplete pregnancies, record the duration and whether the pregnancy resulted in spontaneous (*S*) or induced (*I*) abortion.

Immunizations. Depending on the patient's age group, ask whether the patient has received, for example, measles-mumps-rubella, polio, diphtheria-pertussis-tetanus, hepatitis B, human papillomavirus, *Haemophilus influenzae* type b, and pneumococcal vaccine. Note the dates of the most recent tetanus immunization, most recent tuberculosis skin test, and most recent influenza shot. Consult the latest immunization guidelines used in your province or territory (for an overview of current guidelines, see Chapter 1).

Most recent examination date. Document the dates of the most recent physical, dental, vision, hearing, electrocardiographic, and chest radiographic examinations.

Allergies. Note both the allergen (medication, food, or contact agent, such as fabric or environmental agent) and the reaction (rash, itching, runny nose, watery eyes, difficulty breathing). When a medication is involved, determine whether the symptom is a true allergic reaction, rather than an adverse effect.

Current medications. Note all prescription and over-the-counter medications. Ask specifically about vitamins and other supplements, birth control pills, Aspirin, and antacids, because many people do not consider them medications. For each medication, note the name, dose, and schedule, and ask, "How often do you take it each day?", "What is it for?", and "How long have you been taking it?" Finally, note use of complementary therapies, such as homeopathic or herbal remedies.

Family Health History

Ask about the ages and health, or the ages at and cause of death, of blood relatives, such as parents or other primary caregivers, grandparents, and siblings. These data may have genetic significance for the patient. Also ask about close family members, such as spouse and children. You need to know about the patient's prolonged contact with any communicable disease or the effect of a family member's illness on the patient.

Specifically ask for any family history of heart disease, high blood pressure, stroke, diabetes, blood disorders, cancer, sickle cell disease, arthritis, allergies, obesity, alcoholism, mental health issues or illness, seizure disorder, kidney disease, and tuberculosis. Construct an accurate family tree, or genogram, to show this information clearly and concisely (Fig. 5.1; Box 5.1).

🌐 SOCIAL DETERMINANTS OF HEALTH CONSIDERATIONS

Add several questions to the complete health history for people who are new immigrants:

- *Biographical data*—When did the patient come to Canada and from what country? If the patient is a refugee, what were the conditions under which they came here? Did they undergo particularly challenging experiences?

Some patients will be survivors of intergenerational or intragenerational trauma. For example, recent refugees may have come from places of resource-based and politically based conflict such as Syria, Yemen, or Iran. People who identify as Indigenous may have been residential school survivors or may be family members of people who attended residential schools. Questions regarding family and past history may evoke painful memories or may trigger past negative experiences. Such questions must be asked carefully.

- *Spiritual resources and religion*—Assess whether certain procedures need to be considered in view of the patient's spirituality or religion. For example, people who are Jehovah's Witnesses may refuse blood transfusions and may need additional decision-making supports.
- *Past health*—What immunizations were given in the patient's country of origin? For example, was the patient given *bacille Calmette-Guérin* (BCG)? This vaccine is used in many countries to prevent tuberculosis. If the patient has had BCG, the result of the tuberculin test will be positive, and further diagnostic procedures must be performed, including a sputum test and chest radiography.
- *Health perception*—How does the patient describe health and illness, and what does the patient view as the health problem?
- *Nutrition*—What foods and food combinations are taboo?

Review of Systems

The purposes of this section are (a) to evaluate the past and current health state of each body system, (b) to double-check in case any significant data were omitted in the Current Illness section, and (c) to evaluate health promotion practices. The order of the examination of body systems is approximately head to toe. The items within each system are not inclusive, and only the most common symptoms are listed. If the Current Illness section covered one body system, you do not need to repeat all the data in this section. For example, if the reason for seeking care is earache, the Current Illness section contains data about most of the symptoms listed for the auditory system. Just ask now what was not asked in that section.

Medical terms are listed in this section, but they need to be translated for the patient. (Note that symptoms and health promotion activities are merely listed here. These terms are repeated and expanded in each related physical examination chapter, along with suggested ways to pose questions and a rationale for each question.)

When recording information, avoid writing "negative" after the system heading. You need to record the *presence* or *absence* of all symptoms; otherwise the reader does not know about which factors you asked.

A common mistake made by novice practitioners is to record some physical finding or objective data here, such as "skin warm and dry." Remember that the history should be limited to the patient's statements or to subjective data: factors that the patient *says* were or were not present.

General overall health state. Ask how the patient feels overall in terms of physical, mental, emotional, and spiritual health (i.e., "How do you feel overall? Have you experienced any recent changes to your overall health status?"). Document current weight (gain or loss, period of time, by diet or other factors). Note any fatigue, weakness or malaise, fever, chills, sweats, or night sweats.

Skin, hair, and nails. Record any history of skin disease (eczema, psoriasis, hives), pigment or colour change, change in mole, excessive dryness or moisture, pruritus, excessive bruising, rash, or lesion. Document recent loss and change in texture. For nails, note change in shape, colour, or brittleness.

Health promotion. Ask what the patient is doing to stay healthy and for prevention. Depending on the patient's age, geographical location, and financial and social circumstances, ask, for example, about the amount of sun exposure and use of sunscreen, and use of appropriate footwear to prevent foot sores (for a patient with diabetes).

Head. Ask whether the patient has had any unusually frequent or severe headache, any head injury, dizziness (syncope), or vertigo.

Health promotion. Depending on the patient's age, geographical location, and social–personal circumstances, ask, for example, about use of protective gear during sports activities.

Eyes. Document any difficulty with vision (decreased acuity, blurring, blind spots), eye pain, diplopia (double vision), redness or swelling, watering or discharge, glaucoma, or cataracts.

Health promotion. Ask about the most recent eye examination. As discussed in Chapter 15, Canadians between the ages of 19 and 64 must rely on private (third-party) insurance or out-of-pocket payment to see an eye specialist for routine vision screening.[3] Many adults cannot afford the cost of vision tests or corrective lenses. You need to know which community agencies provide such services free of charge or at a reduced cost so that you can refer patients accordingly.

Document whether the patient wears glasses or contact lenses; the most recent vision check or glaucoma test; and how the patient copes with loss of vision, if any.

Ears. Record the presence of earaches, infections, discharge and its characteristics, tinnitus, or vertigo.

Drawing Your Family Tree
- Make a list of all of your family members.
- Use this sample family tree as a guide to draw your own family tree.
- Write your name at the top of your paper and the date you drew your family tree.
- In place of the words *father, mother* etc., write the names of your family members.
- When possible, draw your brothers and sisters and your parents' brothers and sisters starting from oldest to youngest, going from left to right across the paper.
- If dates of birth or ages are not known, then estimate or guess ("50s," "late 60s").

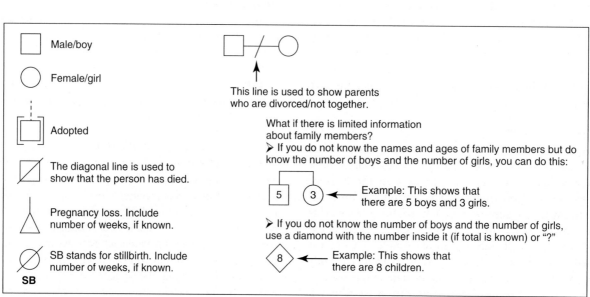

5.1 Genogram or family tree.

Health promotion. Note any hearing loss, hearing aid use, how loss affects daily life, any exposure to environmental noise, use of earplugs or other noise-reducing devices, and method of cleaning ears.

Nose and sinuses. Record discharge and its characteristics, any unusually frequent or severe colds, sinus pain, nasal obstruction, nosebleeds, allergies or hay fever, or change in sense of smell.

Mouth and throat. Document mouth pain, frequent sore throat, bleeding gums, toothache, lesion in mouth or on tongue, dysphagia, hoarseness or voice change, tonsillectomy, or altered taste.

Health promotion. Ask about the patient's pattern of daily dental care, use of prostheses (dentures, bridge), and most recent dental checkup. Be aware that dental examinations and care may require out-of-pocket payments, which many patients and families cannot afford. You need to know which community health agencies offer dental care for a reduced cost or, in some cases, free of charge, and refer patients accordingly.

Neck. Note pain, limitation of motion, lumps or swelling, enlarged or tender nodes, and goitre.

Breast. Document any pain, lump, nipple discharge, rash, history of breast disease, and any surgery on the breasts.

Health promotion. Ask about the date of most recent mammogram. Inquire as to whether the patient performs breast self-examination (see Chapter 18 for revised recommendations regarding breast self-examination).

Axilla. Note tenderness, lump or swelling, and rash.

Respiratory system. Document history of lung diseases (asthma, emphysema, bronchitis, pneumonia, tuberculosis), chest pain with breathing, wheezing or noisy breathing, shortness of breath, how much activity produces shortness of breath, cough, sputum (colour, amount), hemoptysis, and toxin or pollution exposure.

Health promotion. Ask the date of the most recent chest X-ray study.

Cardiovascular system. Note precordial or retrosternal pain, palpitation, cyanosis, dyspnea on exertion (specify amount of exertion that triggers dyspnea, such as walking one flight of stairs, walking from chair to bath, or just talking), orthopnea, paroxysmal nocturnal dyspnea, nocturia, edema, history of heart murmur, hypertension, coronary artery disease, and anemia.

Health promotion. Ask the patient about the date of the most recent electrocardiogram or other tests of heart function.

Peripheral vascular system. Document coldness, numbness and tingling, swelling of legs (time of day, activity), discoloration in hands or feet (bluish red, pallor, mottling, associated with position, especially around feet and ankles), varicose veins or complications, intermittent claudication, thrombophlebitis, and ulcers.

Health promotion. Does the patient's work involve long-term sitting or standing? Patients with vascular system issues should be advised to avoid crossing legs at the knees and to wear support hose.

Gastro-intestinal system. Note appetite, food intolerance, dysphagia, heartburn, indigestion, pain (associated with eating), other abdominal pain, pyrosis (esophageal and stomach burning sensation with sour eructation), nausea and vomiting (character), vomiting blood, history of abdominal disease (ulcer, liver or gallbladder, jaundice, appendicitis, colitis), flatulence, frequency of bowel movement (and any recent change), stool characteristics, constipation or diarrhea, black stools, rectal bleeding, and rectal conditions (hemorrhoids, fistula).

Health promotion. Document the patient's use of antacids or laxatives. (Alternatively, diet history can be described in this section.)

Urinary system. Record frequency, urgency, nocturia (the number of times the patient awakens at night to urinate; recent change), dysuria, polyuria or oliguria, hesitancy or straining, narrowed stream, urine colour (cloudy or presence of hematuria), incontinence, history of urinary disease (kidney disease, kidney stones, urinary tract infections, prostate), and pain in flank, groin, suprapubic region, or lower back.

Health promotion. Advise the patient about measures to avoid or treat urinary tract infections and the use of Kegel exercises after childbirth.

Male genital system. Note penis or testicular pain, sores or lesions, penile discharge, lumps, and hernia.

Health promotion. Ask whether the patient performs testicular self-examination and how frequently.

Female genital system. Document menstrual history (age at menarche, most recent menstrual period, cycle and duration, any amenorrhea or menorrhagia, premenstrual pain or dysmenorrhea, intermenstrual spotting), vaginal itching, discharge and its characteristics, age at menopause, menopausal signs or symptoms, and postmenopausal bleeding.

Health promotion. Ask for the date of the most recent gynecological checkup and most recent Papanicolaou (Pap) test.

Sexual health. Depending on the rapport established with the patient, and the purpose of the history, these are examples of questions that might be asked, depending on the context: Ask whether the patient is currently in a relationship involving intercourse. Are the aspects of sex satisfactory to the patient and partner? Note any dyspareunia (for a female patient), any changes in erection or ejaculation (for a male patient), and use of contraceptive. Is the contraceptive method satisfactory? Is the patient aware of contact with a partner who has any sexually transmitted infection (STI; e.g., gonorrhea, herpes, chlamydia, venereal warts, human immunodeficiency virus [HIV] infection or acquired immune deficiency syndrome [AIDS], or syphilis)?

Musculo-skeletal system. Document any history of arthritis or gout. In the joints, note pain, stiffness, swelling (location, migratory nature), deformity, limitation of motion, and noise with joint motion. In the muscles, note any pain, cramps, weakness, gait problems, or problems with coordinated activities. In the back, note any pain (location and radiation to extremities), stiffness, limitation of motion, or history of back pain or disc disease.

Health promotion. How much walking does the patient do per day? What is the effect of limited range of motion on daily activities, such as on grooming, eating, toileting, dressing? Are any mobility aids used? For older adults, ask about fall prevention strategies, such as not using throw rugs on floors but using rubberized bath mats.

Neurological system. Document any history of seizure disorder, stroke, fainting, and blackouts. In motor function, note weakness, tic or tremor, paralysis, or coordination problems. In sensory function, note numbness and tingling (paraesthesia). In cognitive function, note memory disorder (recent or distant, disorientation). In mental status, note any nervousness, mood change, depression, or any history of mental health dysfunction or hallucinations. See Chapter 6 for mental health assessment guidelines.

Health promotion. Data about interpersonal relationships and coping patterns can be placed in this section.

Hematological system. Document any bleeding tendency of skin or mucous membranes, excessive bruising, lymph node swelling, exposure to toxic agents or radiation, blood transfusion, and reactions.

Endocrine system. Record any history of diabetes or diabetic symptoms (polyuria, polydipsia, polyphagia), history of thyroid disease, intolerance to heat and cold, change in skin pigmentation or texture, excessive sweating, relationship between appetite and weight, abnormal hair distribution, nervousness, tremors, and need for hormone therapy.

Health promotion. Depending on a diabetic patient's health history, ask about use of appropriate footwear to prevent foot sores or ulcers.

Functional Assessment (Including Activities of Daily Living)

In a functional assessment, you measure a patient's self-care ability in the areas of general physical health or absence of illness; activities of daily living (ADLs), such as bathing, dressing, toileting, eating, and walking; instrumental activities of daily living (IADLs), which are activities needed for independent living, such as housekeeping, shopping, cooking, doing laundry, using the telephone, and managing finances; nutrition; social relationships and resources; self-concept and coping; and home environment.

Functional assessment may mean organizing the entire assessment around "functional health pattern areas."[4] Instruments that emphasize functional categories may help in establishing a nursing diagnosis.

Functional assessment may also mean that the health history is supplemented by a standardized instrument on functional assessment. Instruments such as the Katz Index of Activities of Daily Living (see Fig. 31.2) and the Lawton Instrumental Activities of Daily Living Scale (see Fig. 31.3) are used to objectively measure a patient's current functional status and to monitor any changes over time.[5–7]

Regardless of whether you use any of these formalized instruments, functional assessment questions such as those listed in the following sections should be included in the standard health history. These questions provide data on the lifestyle and type of living environment to which the patient is accustomed. Because some of the data may be judged private by the individual, the questions are best asked at a later point in the interview, after you have had time to establish rapport.

Self-concept, self-esteem. Ask about the patient's education level (last grade completed, other significant training), financial status (income adequate and health or social concerns), and value–belief system (religious practices and perception of personal strengths).

Activity and mobility. Obtain a daily profile that reflects usual daily activities. Ask, "Tell me how you spend a typical day." Note ability to perform ADLs: whether the patient is independent or needs assistance with feeding, bathing, hygiene, dressing, toileting, bed-to-chair transfer, walking, standing, or climbing stairs. Document any use of wheelchair, prostheses, or mobility aids. Record leisure activities enjoyed and the exercise pattern (type, amount per day or week, method of warm-up session, method of monitoring the body's response to exercise).

Sleep and rest. Record sleep patterns, daytime naps, any sleep aids used.

Nutrition and elimination. Record the diet by a recall of all food and beverages taken over the last 24 hours (see Chapter 12 for suggested method of inquiry). Ask the patient, "Is that menu typical of most days?" Describe eating habits and current appetite. Ask, "Who buys food and prepares food?", "Are your finances adequate for food?", and "Who is present at mealtimes?" Indicate any food allergy or intolerance. Record daily intake of caffeine (coffee, tea, cola drinks). Ask about usual pattern of bowel elimination and urinating, including problems with mobility or transfer in toileting, continence, and use of laxatives.

Interpersonal relationships and resources. Ask about social roles: "How would you describe your role in the family?" and "How would you say you get along with family, friends, and co-workers?" Ask about support systems composed of family and significant others: "To whom could you go for support with a problem at work, a health problem, or a personal problem?" Include contact with spouse, siblings, parents, children, chosen family, friends, organizations, and the workplace: "Is time spent alone pleasurable and relaxing, or is it isolating?"

Spiritual resources. Many people believe in a relationship between spirituality and health, and they may wish to have spiritual matters addressed in the traditional health care setting.[8] One approach to assess the role of spirituality in a patient's life is to use the faith, influence, community, and address (FICA) questions to incorporate the patient's spiritual values into the health history.[9] For *faith*: "Does religious faith or spirituality play an important part in your life? Do you consider yourself to be a religious or spiritual person?" For *influence*: "How does your religious faith or spirituality influence the way you think about your health or the way you care for yourself?" For *community*: "Are you a part of any religious or spiritual community or congregation?" For *address*: "Would you like me to address any religious or spiritual issues or concerns with you?"

Coping and stress management. Document kinds of stresses in life, especially in the past year; any change in living situation or any current stress; and methods for dealing with stress and whether these have been helpful. For children and adolescents, ask about peer relationships, as discussed in Chapter 1.

Tobacco use history. Strategies for asking about tobacco use patterns in a nonjudgemental way are included in Chapter 7. The tone with which you ask these questions is important to pre-empt people from feeling judged or stigmatized because of their smoking patterns: "We ask everyone these questions to provide the best care possible. Can you tell me if you currently smoke cigarettes or a pipe, or do you use tobacco in a vaporizer? Do you use chewing tobacco?"; "At what age did you start?"; "How many cigarettes do you tend to smoke per day?"; and "How many years have you smoked?" Often, health care providers quantify the number of cigarettes or packages of cigarettes smoked per day (based on 20 cigarettes per package) and duration. For example, 10 cigarettes per day × 5 years, or 1 pack per day (20 cigarettes/pack) × 5 years. Then ask, "People often consider ways of cutting down on smoking. Have you ever considered cutting down, and if so, how did it go?" If the person indicates interest, you can introduce plans about smoking reduction or cessation.

Alcohol. Health care providers often fail to question about alcohol or substance use despite the effect of these activities on health, quality of life, and social relationships. Asking about alcohol use can begin with asking whether the patient drinks alcohol. If the patient replies in the affirmative, you can explain that you would like to follow up with additional questions to better assess the patient's health status. Chapter 7 contains in-depth guidelines about how to discuss alcohol and substance use and how to assess the effects on health and well-being. In some cases, and in some agencies, it may be appropriate to use a screening questionnaire to identify when alcohol or other substance use is

presenting problems in relation to the patient's functional status, relationships, employment, economic status, and other areas in life. Common screening tools are discussed in Chapter 7. As explained in Chapter 7, it is imperative to convey acceptance and a nonjudgemental attitude when you discuss alcohol or substance use patterns. To do otherwise can have detrimental effects. For example, patients who feel negatively judged may not return for follow-up or may avoid seeking care altogether.

Substance use. Chapter 7 provides an overview of how to ask about substance use in a nonjudgemental and respectful manner. Depending on the patient's personal context, and the extent to which you have established rapport with the patient, you may ask specifically about marijuana, cocaine, crack cocaine, amphetamines, heroin, methadone, benzodiazepines, barbiturates, crystal methamphetamine, 3,4-methylenedioxymethamphetamine (Ecstasy), phencyclidine hydrochloride (PCP), and other drugs. Indicate frequency of use and how usage has affected the patient's work, relationships, family, or economic circumstances. In Canada, the legalization of marijuana will have implications for how people interact with this particular substance.

Environmental hazards. Ask about the patient's housing and neighbourhood (whether the patient lives alone, knows neighbours), the safety of the area, the adequacy of heat and utilities, access to transportation, and involvement in community services. Note environmental health, including hazards in the workplace, hazards at home, excessive screen use, use of seatbelts and helmets, geographical or occupational exposures, and travel to or residence in other countries, including time spent abroad during military service.

Intimate partner violence. Begin with open-ended questions. Convey openness and acceptance, and listen in a nonjudgemental manner: "How are things going at home (or at school or work)?"; "How are things at home affecting your health?"; "Is your home (or work or school) environment safe?" These are valuable questions for all patients. Specifically, in relation to intimate partner violence, patients may not recognize their situation as abusive, or they may be reluctant to discuss their situation because of guilt, fear, or shame. Follow each patient's lead to inquire more specifically. If you sense that violence is an issue, use the strategies discussed in Chapter 8.

Occupational health. Ask the patient to describe their employment situation; the patient may or may not have a clearly identifiable job. Ask whether the patient has ever worked with any health hazard, such as asbestos, inhalants, chemicals, and repetitive motion. Did the patient wear any protective equipment? Are any work programs in place in which exposure is monitored? Is the patient aware of any health problems now that may be related to work exposure?

Note the timing of the reason for seeking care and whether it may be related to work or home activities, job titles, or exposure history. Carefully document a smoking history, which may contribute to occupational hazards. Finally, ask the patient what they like or dislike about the job.

Perception of Health

Ask the patient questions such as "What does it mean to you to be healthy? How do you define health?"; "How do you view your situation now?"; "What are your concerns?"; "What do you think will happen in the future?"; "What are your health goals?"; and "What do you expect from us as [nurses, nurse practitioners, physicians, or other health care providers]?"

 DEVELOPMENTAL CONSIDERATIONS

Health History: Children

The health history is adapted to include information specific for the age and developmental stage of the child (e.g., the mother's health during pregnancy, the course of labour and delivery, and the perinatal period; Fig. 5.2). Note that the developmental history and nutritional data are listed in separate sections because of their importance for current health.

Depending on where you are working, developmental assessment tools such as the Nipissing District Developmental Screen (NDDS), the Rourke Baby Record, or the Ages and Stages Questionnaires (ASQ) are routinely used in documenting the health history. These and other assessment tools provide an excellent way to frame discussions about the importance of health promotion and disease prevention activities (see Chapters 1 and 2).

Biographical Data

Include the child's name, nickname, address, and phone number; parent or caregivers' names and work numbers; child's age and birthdate, birthplace, sex, gender, ethnocultural background; and information about other children and family members at home.

5.2

Source of History

Document the sources of historical information:
1. Person providing information and relation to child
2. Your impression of reliability of information
3. Any special circumstances, such as the use of an interpreter

Reason for Seeking Care

Record the caregiver's spontaneous statement. The reason for seeking care may be identified or initiated by the child, caregiver, or by a third party such as a classroom teacher.

Sometimes the reason stated may not be the real reason for the visit. A caregiver may have a "hidden agenda," such as the mother who brought her 4-year-old child in because "she looked pale." Further questioning revealed that the mother had heard recently from a former college friend whose own 4-year-old child had just received a diagnosis of leukemia.

Current Health or History of Current Illness

If the caregiver or child seeks routine health care, include a statement about the usual health of the child and any common health problems or major health concerns. Using the same format as for the adult, describe any presenting symptom or sign. Some additional considerations are as follows:

- Severity of pain: "How do you know the child is in pain?" (e.g., pulling at ears alerts parent to ear pain). Note effect of pain on usual behaviour (e.g., whether it stops the child from playing).
- Associated factors, such as relation to activity, eating, and body position.
- The caregiver's intuitive sense of a problem, which is often very accurate. Even if findings prove otherwise, this sense gives you an idea of the caregiver's area of concern.
- Caregiver's coping ability and the reaction of other family members to the child's symptoms or illness.

Past Health History

Prenatal status. Ask the biological mother how this pregnancy was spaced in relation to other children. Was it planned? What was the biological mother's attitude toward the pregnancy? What were other caregivers' attitudes (e.g., partner, father's, grandparent's, chosen family)? Was the biological mother under medical supervision? At what month was the supervision started? What was the biological mother's health during pregnancy? Were there any complications, such as bleeding, excessive nausea and vomiting, unusual weight gain, high blood pressure, swelling of hands and feet, infections (rubella or STIs), or falls? During which month was a diet prescribed during pregnancy? During what month were medications prescribed or taken during pregnancy (dose and duration)? Using sensitivity in posing questions, ask about the biological mother's use of alcohol, drugs, or cigarettes and any radiographs taken during pregnancy. Chapter 7 describes strategies for asking about substance use during pregnancy in ways that convey acceptance and will minimize the risk that the person will feel negatively judged and avoid care. For gender-diverse people who go through pregnancy, there may be other relevant questions to be asked.[10]

Start with an open-ended question: "Tell me about your pregnancy." If the patient questions the relevancy of the questions, mention that the question is important for obtaining a complete overview of the child's health.

Labour and delivery. Record parity of the biological mother, duration of the pregnancy, name of the hospital, course and duration of labour, use of anaesthetics, type of delivery (vertex, breech, Caesarean section), birth weight, Apgar scores, onset of breathing, any cyanosis, need for resuscitation, and use of special equipment or procedures.

Postnatal status. Note any problems in the neonatal nursery, length of hospital stay, neonatal jaundice, whether the baby was discharged with the biological mother, whether the baby was breastfed or formula-fed, weight gain, any feeding problems, "blue spells," colic, diarrhea, patterns of crying and sleeping, the biological mother's postpartum health, and the biological mother's reaction to the baby.

Childhood illnesses. Document age at onset and any complications of measles, mumps, rubella, chicken pox, whooping cough, streptococcal infection ("strep throat"), and frequent ear infections. Also note any recent exposure to illness.

Serious accidents or injuries. Record age at occurrence, extent of injury, how the child was medically treated, and complications of auto accidents, falls, head injuries, fractures, burns, and poisonings.

Serious or chronic illnesses. Document age at onset, how the child was medically treated, and complications of meningitis or encephalitis; seizure disorders; asthma, pneumonia, and other chronic lung conditions; rheumatic fever; scarlet fever; diabetes; kidney problems; sickle cell disease; high blood pressure; and allergies.

Operations or hospitalizations. Note reason for care, age at admission, name of surgeon or health care provider, name of hospital, duration of stay, how the child reacted to hospitalization, and any complications. (If the child reacted poorly, the child may be now be afraid and need special preparation for the examination that is to follow.)

Immunizations. Document age when immunizations were administered, date administered, and any reactions after immunizations. National standards for immunizations are contained in the Canadian Immunization Guide (https://www.canada.ca/en/public-health/services/canadian-immunization-guide.html), and updates to information are published as tables each year.[11] Each province and territory adapts these standards slightly according to its population's needs. It is important to check the provincial or territorial guidelines where you practise.

Allergies. Record any medications, foods, contact agents, and environmental agents to which the child is allergic and the reaction to allergens. Note allergic reactions particularly common in childhood, such as allergic rhinitis, insect hypersensitivity, eczema, and urticaria.

Medications. Document any prescription and over-the-counter medications (or vitamins and other supplements) the child takes, including the dose, daily schedule, why the medication is given, and any problems.

Developmental History

Growth. Record the height and weight at birth and at 1, 2, 5, and 10 years of age; any periods of rapid growth or weight loss; and process of dentition (age at tooth eruption and pattern of loss).

Milestones. Document the age when the child first held the head erect, rolled over, sat alone, walked alone, developed the first tooth, first said words with meaning, spoke in sentences, was toilet trained, tied shoes, and dressed without help. Does the caregiver believe this development has been normal? How does this child's development compare with that of siblings or peers?

Current development.

Children aged 1 month through preschool age. Record current gross motor skills (rolling over, sitting alone, walking alone, skipping, climbing), fine motor skills (inspecting hands, bringing hands to mouth, pincer grasp, stacking blocks, feeding self, using crayon to draw, using scissors), language skills (vocalizing, first words with meaning, sentences, persistence of baby talk, speech problems), and personal–social skills (smiling, tracking movement with eyes to midline and past midline, attending to sound by turning head, recognizing own name). If the child is undergoing toilet training, indicate the method used, age of bladder and bowel control, parents' attitude toward toilet training, and terms used for toileting.

School-age children. Document current gross motor skills (running, jumping, climbing, riding bicycle, general coordination), fine motor skills (tying shoelaces, using scissors, writing name and numbers, drawing pictures), and language skills (vocabulary, verbal ability, ability to tell time, reading level).

Nutritional History

The amount of nutritional information needed depends on the child's age; the younger the child is, the more detailed and specific the data should be. For infants, record whether breast milk or formula is used. If the child is breastfed, record nursing frequency and duration, any supplements (vitamin, iron, fluoride, formula), family support for nursing, and age at and method of weaning. If the child is formula-fed, record type of formula used, frequency and amount, any problems with feeding (spitting up, colic, diarrhea), supplements used, and any bottle propping. Record introduction of solid foods (age when the child began eating solids, which foods, whether foods are home or commercially made, amount given, child's reaction to new food, parent's reaction to feeding).

For preschool- and school-age children and adolescents, record the child's appetite, 24-hour diet recall (meals, snacks, amounts), vitamins taken, how much junk food is eaten, who eats with the child, food likes and dislikes, and parent's perception of child's nutrition. A week-long diary of food intake may be more accurate than a spot 24-hour recall.

Also, consider cultural differences in cooking and ingredients in assessing child's diet.

Family Health History

As with the adult, diagram a family tree for the child, including chosen family, caregivers, siblings, parents, and grandparents. For each, record the age and health or the age at and cause of death. Ask specifically for the family history of heart disease, high blood pressure, diabetes, blood disorders, cancer, sickle cell disease, arthritis, allergies, obesity, cystic fibrosis, alcoholism, mental health problems or illness, seizure disorder, kidney disease, intellectual disability, learning disabilities, birth defects, and sudden unexpected infant death (SUID). When interviewing caregivers individually, ask about the child's biological father and/or mother.

Review of Systems

General. Document significant gain or loss of weight, failure to gain weight appropriate for age, frequent colds, ear infections, illnesses, energy level, fatigue, overactivity, and behavioural change (irritability, increased crying, nervousness).

Skin. Note birthmarks, skin disease, pigment or colour change, mottling, change in mole, pruritus, rash, lesion, acne, easy bruising or petechiae, easy bleeding, and changes in hair or nails.

Head. Ask whether the patient suffers from headache or dizziness and whether the patient has had a head injury.

Eyes. Note strabismus, diplopia, pain, redness, discharge, cataracts, vision changes, and reading problems. Is the child able to see the board at school? Does the child sit too close to the television?

Health promotion. Document use of eyeglasses and the date of the most recent vision screening.

Ears. Note earaches, frequency of ear infections, the presence of myringotomy tubes in the ears, discharge (characteristics), cerumen, sensation of ringing or crackling, and whether the parent perceives any hearing problems.

Health promotion. Note how the child cleans their ears.

Nose and sinuses. Record discharge and its characteristics, frequency of colds, nasal stuffiness, nosebleeds, and allergies.

Mouth and throat. Document any history of cleft lip or palate, frequency of sore throats, toothache, caries, sores in the mouth or tongue, presence of tonsils, mouth breathing, difficulty chewing, difficulty swallowing, and hoarseness or voice change.

Health promotion. Record the child's pattern of brushing teeth and the date of the most recent dental checkup.

Neck. Note swollen or tender glands, limitation of movement, or stiffness.

Breast. For preadolescent and adolescent young females, ask when they noticed that their breasts were changing. What is the young female's self-perception of development? Does the older adolescent female perform breast self-examination? (See Chapter 18 for suggested phrasing of questions.)

Respiratory system. Document croup or asthma, wheezing or noisy breathing, shortness of breath, and chronic cough.

Cardiovascular system. Document congenital heart problems, history of murmur, and cyanosis (what prompts this condition). Is activity limited, or can the child keep up with peers? Does the child have any dyspnea on exertion, palpitations, high blood pressure, or coldness in the extremities?

Gastro-intestinal system. Note abdominal pain, nausea and vomiting, history of ulcer, frequency of bowel movements, stool colour and characteristics, diarrhea, constipation or stool-holding, rectal bleeding, anal itching, history of pinworms, and use of laxatives.

Urinary system. Note painful urination, polyuria or oliguria, narrowed stream, urine colour (cloudy, dark), history of urinary tract infection, whether the child is toilet trained, when toilet training was planned, any toilet training problems, and bedwetting (when the child started, frequency, association with stress, how the child feels about it).

Male genital system. Record penis or testicular pain, whether the parent was told that testes are descended, any sores or lesions, discharge, hernia or hydrocele, or swelling in scrotum during crying. Has the preadolescent or adolescent male noticed any change in the penis and scrotum? Is the male familiar with normal growth patterns, nocturnal emissions, and sex education? Screening for sexual abuse is not normally part of the routine review of systems. (See Chapter 8 for rationale.)

Female genital system. Has the female noted any genital itching, rash, or vaginal discharge? For the preadolescent and adolescent female, document when menstruation started. How did they feel, and did they feel prepared? Screening for sexual abuse is not normally part of the routine review of systems. (See Chapter 8 for rationale.)

Intersex genital system. It should be noted that a small percentage of the population identifies as intersex.

Sexual health. Depending on the rapport and trust established with the person you are interviewing, you may ask about the child's attitude toward the opposite or same sex. Who provides sex education, and does it include the diversity of possible relationships and orientations? As discussed in Chapter 3, does it recognize that gender identity (e.g., woman, man, trans, genderqueer, nonbinary, femme of centre, and two-spirit) is different from sexual orientation (e.g., heterosexual, homosexual, bisexual, pansexual, asexual)? How does the family deal with sex education and dating patterns?

Is the adolescent patient in a relationship involving sexual activity that includes intercourse? Does the patient have information on birth control and STIs? (See Chapters 26 and 27 for suggested phrasing of questions.)

Musculo-skeletal system. For bones and joints, document arthritis, joint pain, stiffness, swelling, limitation of movement, gait strength, and coordination. For muscles, document pain, cramps, and weakness. For the back, document pain, posture, spinal curvature, and any treatment.

Neurological system. Note numbness and tingling sensation. (Behavioural and cognitive issues are covered in the section Developmental Considerations and the section Interpersonal Relationships.)

Hematological systems. Record excessive bruising, lymph node swelling, and exposure to toxic agents or radiation.

Endocrine system. Record a history of diabetes or thyroid disease; excessive hunger, thirst, or urinating; abnormal hair distribution; and precocious or delayed puberty.

Functional Assessment (Including Activities of Daily Living)

Interpersonal relationships. Record the child's position within the family constellation; whether the child is adopted; who lives with the child; who is the primary caregiver; who is the caregiver if primary parents or caregivers work outside the home; and any support from relatives, neighbours, or friends.

Indicate family cohesion. Does the family enjoy activities as a unit? Has there been a recent family change or crisis (death, divorce, move)? Record information about the child's self-image and level of independence. Does the child use a security blanket or toy? Is there any repetitive behaviour (bed rocking, head banging), pica, thumb-sucking, or nail-biting? Note method(s) of discipline used. Indicate method(s) used at home. How effective is it? Who disciplines the child? Is there any occurrence of negativism, temper tantrums, withdrawal, or aggressive behaviour?

Provide information on the child's friends. Does the child make friends easily? How does the child get along with friends? Does the child play with same-age, older, or younger children?

Activity and rest. Record the child's play activities. Indicate the amount of active and quiet play, outdoor play, time watching television, and special hobbies or activities. Record information on sleep and rest. Indicate pattern and number of hours at night and during the day and the child's routine at bedtime. Is the child a sound sleeper or is the child wakeful? Does the child have nightmares, night terrors, or somnambulation? How does the caregiver respond? Does the child have naps during the day?

Record school attendance. Has the child had any experience with day care or nursery school? In what grade is the child in school? Has the child ever skipped a grade or been held back? Does the child seem to like school? What is the child's school performance? Are the caregivers and child satisfied with the performance? Were days missed at school? If yes, what was the reason for the child's absence? (Answers to these questions provide an important index to the child's functioning outside the home.)

Economic status. It may or may not be appropriate to ask about caregivers' occupations or everyday activities. However, you may respectfully want to ask if caregivers perceive their income as adequate in terms of supporting their family's health and well-being. If a child is ill, the illness may have an effect on financial status.

Home environment. Where does the family live (house, apartment)? Is the size of the home adequate? Is an outdoor play area accessible? Does the child share a room, have their own bed, and have age-appropriate toys?

Environmental hazards. Inquire about home safety (precautions for poisons, medications, household products, presence of gates for stairways, and safe yard equipment). Record information on the child's residence (adequate heating, ventilation, bathroom facilities), neighbourhood (residential or industrial, age of neighbours, safety of play areas, availability of playmates, distance to school, amount of traffic, whether the area is remote or congested and overcrowded, whether crime is widespread, the presence of air or water pollution), and the caregiver's automobile (child safety seat, seatbelts).

Coping and stress management. Does the child have the ability to adapt to new situations? Record recent stressful experiences (death, divorce, move, loss of special friend). How does the child cope with stress? Has there been any recent change in behaviour or mood? Has counselling ever been sought?

Alcohol and substance use. Has the child ever tried cigarette smoking? How much did the child smoke? Has the child ever tried alcohol? How much alcohol did the child drink weekly or daily? Has the child ever tried other drugs or substances (e.g., marijuana, cocaine, amphetamines, barbiturates)?

Health promotion. Ask the caregiver to identify whether the child has a primary health care provider, such as a physician or nurse practitioner. If no, you could ask the caregiver if they are interested in connecting with one. When was the child's most recent checkup? Who is the dental care provider, and when was the most recent dental checkup? Record the dates and results of screening for vision, hearing, urinalysis, phenylketonuria, hematocrit, tuberculosis skin test, sickle cell trait, blood lead, and other tests specific to high-risk populations.

Health History: Adolescents

Chapter 6 discusses approaches to psychosocial and mental health assessment among adolescents and young adults. This section presents a psychosocial review of symptoms intended to maximize communication with youth. The **HEEADSSS** method of interviewing focuses on assessment of the *h*ome environment, *e*ducation and employment, *e*ating, peer-related *a*ctivities, *d*rug use (substance use), *s*exuality, *s*uicide or depression, and *s*afety from injury and violence (Fig. 5.3). The tool minimizes adolescent stress because it moves from expected and less threatening questions to those that are more personal. It presents questions in three colours: green questions are considered essential to explore with every adolescent; blue questions are important to ask if time permits; and red questions delve more deeply and are asked if they are appropriate to the context or situation.[12] Interview the youth alone, while the caregiver waits outside and fills out questionnaires about past health.

It is important to review Chapters 6, 7, and 8 before asking about mental health, substance use, and interpersonal violence issues, so that those areas are explored respectfully and in ways that convey openness and acceptance. It

The HEEADSSS psychosocial interview for adolescents

Home

Who lives with you? Where do you live? Do you have your own room?
What are relationships like at home?
To whom are you closest at home?
To whom can you talk to at home?
Is there anyone new at home? Has someone left recently?
Have you moved recently?
Have you ever had to live away from home? (Why?)
Have you ever run away? (Why?)
Is there any physical violence at home?

Education and employment

What are your favourite subjects at school? Your least favourite subjects?
How are your grades? Any recent changes? Any dramatic changes in the past?
Have you changed schools in the past few years?
What are your future education and employment plans and goals?
Are you working? Where? How much?
Tell me about your friends at school.
Is your school a safe place? (Why?)
Have you ever had to repeat a class? Have you ever had to repeat a grade?
Have you ever been suspended? Expelled? Have you ever considered dropping out?
How well do you get along with the people at school? Work?
Have your responsibilities at work increased?
Do you feel connected to your school? Do you feel as if you belong?
Are there adults at school you feel you could talk to about something important? (Who?)

Eating

What do you like and not like about your body?
Have there been any recent changes in your weight?
Have you dieted in the last year? How? How often?
Have you done anything else to try to manage your weight?
How much exercise do you get in an average day? Week?
What do you think would be a healthy diet? How does that compare to your current eating patterns?
Do you worry about your weight? How often?
Do you eat in front of the TV? Computer?
Does it ever seem as though your eating is out of control?
Have you ever made yourself throw up on purpose to control your weight?
Have you ever taken diet pills?
What would it be like if you gained (lost) 10 pounds*?

Activities

What do you and your *friends* do for fun? (With whom, where, and when?)
What do you and your *family* do for fun? (With whom, where, and when?)
Do you participate in any sports or other activities?
Do you regularly attend a church group, club, or other organized activity?
Do you have any hobbies?
Do you read for fun? (What?)
How much TV do you watch in a week? How about video games?
What music do you like to listen to?

Drug Use (Substance Use)[†]

Do any of your friends use tobacco? Alcohol? Other drugs?
Does anyone in your family use tobacco? Alcohol? Other drugs?
Do you use tobacco? Alcohol? Other drugs?
Is there any history of alcohol or drug problems in your family?
Do you ever drink or use drugs when you're alone?
(Assess frequency, intensity, patterns of use or abuse, and how youth obtains or pays for drugs, alcohol, or tobacco.)

Sexuality

Have you ever been in a romantic relationship?
Tell me about the people that you've dated. *OR* Tell me about your sex life.
Have any of your relationships ever been sexual relationships?
Are your sexual activities enjoyable?
What does the term "safer sex" mean to you?
Are you interested in boys? Girls? Both?
Have you ever been forced or pressured into doing something sexual that you didn't want to do?
Have you ever been touched sexually in a way that you didn't want?
Have you ever been raped[‡], on a date or any other time?
How many sexual partners have you had altogether?
Have you ever been pregnant or worried that you might be pregnant? (females)
Have you ever impregnated someone or worried that that might have happened? (males)
What are you using for birth control? Are you satisfied with your method?
Do you use condoms every time you have intercourse?
Does anything ever get in the way of always using a condom?
Have you ever had an STI or worried that you had an STI?

Suicide and depression

Do you feel sad or down more than usual? Do you find yourself crying more than usual?
Are you "bored" all the time?
Are you having trouble getting to sleep?
Have you thought a lot about hurting yourself or someone else?
Does it seem that you've lost interest in things that you used to really enjoy?
Do you find yourself spending less and less time with friends?
Would you rather just be by yourself most of the time?
Have you ever tried to kill yourself?
Have you ever had to hurt yourself (by cutting yourself, for example) to calm down or feel better?
Have you started using alcohol or drugs to help you relax, calm down, or feel better?

Safety

Have you ever been seriously injured? (How?) How about anyone else you know?
Do you always wear a seatbelt in the car?
Have you ever ridden with a driver who was drunk or high? When? How often?
Do you use safety equipment for sports and other physical activities (e.g., helmets for biking or skateboarding)?
Is there any violence in your home? Does the violence ever get physical?
Is there a lot of violence at your school? In your neighbourhood? Among your friends?
Have you ever been physically or sexually abused? Have you ever been raped, on a date or at any other time? (If not asked previously)
Have you ever been in a car or motorcycle accident? (What happened?)
Have you ever been picked on or bullied? Is that still a problem?
Have you participated in physical fights in school or your neighbourhood? Are you still getting into fights?
Have you ever felt that you had to carry a knife, gun, or other weapon to protect yourself? Do you still feel that way?

Green represents essential questions.
Blue represents those to be asked as time permits.
Red represents optional questions or those to be asked when situation requires.

*5 kg.
[†]See Chapter 7 for the correct terms used to describe substance use (including alcohol, drug, and other substance use).
[‡]The more commonly accepted term in Canada is *sexually assaulted*.

5.3 The HEEADSSS psychosocial interview for adolescents. *STI*, sexually transmitted infection.

is imperative that you follow the adolescent's lead when exploring these areas.

Health History: Older Adults

The health history for an older adult follows the same format as that described for a younger adult and includes some additional questions. These questions address ways in which the ADLs may have been affected by normal aging processes or by the effects of chronic illness or disability. There is no specific age at which to ask these additional questions. Use them when it seems appropriate to the patient's life context. Please review Chapter 31 for complete guidelines on assessing older adults.

It is important for you to recognize positive health measures: those activities that patients may be doing to help support their health and quality of life. Many older people have spent a lifetime obtaining care from conventional health care systems that focus on pathological processes, medical problems, and what is wrong with their health. It may be a pleasant and welcome surprise to have a health care provider affirm the things that they are "doing well" and to note health strengths, social supports, and capabilities. As you read this section, keep in mind the format for younger adults. Only *additional* questions or those with a different focus are presented in this section.

Reason for Seeking Care

It may take time to figure out the reason why an older patient has come in for an examination. An older patient may shrug off a symptom as evidence of growing old and may be unsure whether it is "worth mentioning." Also, some older people have a conservative philosophy toward their health status: "If it isn't broken, don't fix it." These people come for care only when something is blatantly wrong.

An older patient may have many chronic problems, such as diabetes, hypertension, or constipation. It is challenging to filter out what brought the patient in this time. The final statement should be the *patient's* reason for seeking care, not your assumption of what the problem is.

Past Health History

General health. Document the health state over the past 5 years.

Accidents or injuries, serious or chronic illnesses, hospitalizations, operations. These areas may produce lengthy responses, and the patient may not relate them in chronological order. Let the patient talk freely; you can reorder the events later when you prepare the write-up. The amount of data included here can indicate the amount of stress the patient has faced over the lifespan. This section of the history can be filled out at home or before the interview if the patient's vision and writing ability are adequate. Then you can concentrate the remaining time of the interview on reviewing pertinent data and on the current health of the patient.

Most recent examination. Document the results of the most recent mammography, colonoscopy, and tonometry.

Obstetrical status. It is *not* necessary to collect a detailed account of each pregnancy and delivery if the person who identifies as female has passed menopause and has no gynecological symptoms. Merely record the number of pregnancies and the health of each newborn.

Current Medications

For each medication, record the name, purpose, and daily schedule. Does the patient have a system in place to remember to take the medicine? Does the medicine seem to work? Are there any adverse effects? If so, does the patient feel like skipping the medicine because of them? Also consider the following issues:

- Some older patients take a large number of medications, prescribed by different physicians.
- The patient may not know a medication name or purpose. When this is the case, ask the patient to bring in the medication (in the prescription container) to be identified.
- Is cost a problem? When a patient is unable to afford a medication, the patient may decrease the dosage, take one pill instead of two, or not refill the empty bottle immediately. Many patients cannot afford the costs of medications; be prepared to obtain input from a social worker or other team member to connect patients to agencies or services that can provide assistance with the cost of prescription and over-the-counter medications.
- Is travelling to the pharmacy to refill a prescription a problem?
- Is the patient taking any over-the-counter medications? Some people take advice from a local pharmacist or recommendations from family or friends for self-treatment.
- Has the patient ever shared medications with neighbours or friends? Some people establish "lay referral" networks by comparing symptoms and thus medications.

Family Health History

Family history is not as useful in predicting which familial diseases the patient may contract because most of those occur at an earlier age. These data, however, are useful to assess which diseases have occurred or to assess the causes of the death of relatives. These data also describe the patient's existing social network.

Review of Systems

Remember that these are *additional* items to question for the older adult. Refer to the format for younger adults for the basic list.

General. Note current weight and what the patient would like to weigh (gives idea of body image).

Skin. Document change in sensation of pain, heat, or cold.

Eyes. Record use of bifocal glasses and any trouble adjusting to far vision (e.g., problems with climbing stairs).

Ears. Document increased sensitivity to background noise and whether conversation sounds garbled or distorted.

Mouth. Note use of dentures, when the patient wears them (always, all day, only at meals, only at social occasions, or never), method of cleaning, any difficulty wearing the dentures (looseness, pain, making whistling or clicking noise), and cracks at the corners of the mouth.

Respiratory system. Document shortness of breath and level of activity that produces it. Shortness of breath is often an early sign of cardiac dysfunction, but many older people dismiss it as "a cold" or getting "winded" because of old age.

Cardiovascular system. If chest pain occurs, an older adult may not feel it as intensely as a younger person. Instead, the patient may feel dyspnea on exertion.

Peripheral vascular system. Record whether the patient wears constrictive clothing or garters, or whether stockings are rolled at the knees. Also record any colour change at the feet or ankles.

Urinary system. Document urinary retention, incomplete emptying, straining to urinate, and change in force of stream. If the stream becomes weaker, men may note the need to stand closer to the toilet. Women may note incontinence when coughing, laughing, or sneezing.

Sexual health. Consider whether there is a reason to ask about any changes in the sexual relationship the patient has experienced. It is important that you not assume that everyone is in a heterosexual relationship. There are many ways that people can assume sexual orientations, which can be fluid and change over time. From a physical standpoint, note that for older males, it is normal for an erection to develop more slowly (see Chapter 26). For older females, note any comments about vaginal dryness or pain with intercourse. In some situations where older adults are residing in residential care homes, you may need to ask whether privacy for a sexual relationship is adequate.

Musculo-skeletal system. Record gait change (balance, weakness, difficulty with stairs, fear of falling) and use of any assistive device (cane, walker). Does the patient have any joint stiffness? During what part of the day does the stiffness occur? Does pain or stiffness occur with activity or rest?

Neurological system. Does the patient have any problem with memory (recent or remote) or disorientation (time of day, in what settings)?

Functional Assessment (Including Activities of Daily Living)

In functional assessment, you measure how a patient manages day-to-day activities. For older patients, the meaning of health refers to the activities that they can or cannot perform. The *effect* of an illness on their daily activities and overall quality of life (called the *disease burden*) is more important to older people than the actual illness diagnosis or pathological features. Thus the functional assessment—because it emphasizes function—is very important in the evaluation of older patients (see Chapter 31).

Many functional assessment instruments are available for objectively measuring a patient's current functional status and monitoring any changes over time. Most instruments are used to measure the performance of specific tasks such as the ADLs and IADLs (for examples, see Figs. 31.2 and 31.3). The Comprehensive Older Adult's Evaluation (see Table 31.2) is particularly useful because it contains the basic ADL and IADL functional assessment and addresses physical, social, psychological, demographic, financial, and legal issues.

Regardless of whether a standardized instrument is used, the following functional assessment questions are important additions to an older adult's health history.

Self-concept, self-esteem. Be aware that when the older patient was an adolescent, educational opportunities may not have been as available as they are today, nor were they equally available for women, racialized people, or people who were living on low incomes in Canada. As with all patients, older patients may not be comfortable identifying the level of education they have obtained.

Occupation. Document past positions, volunteer activities, and community activities. Many people continue to work past the age of 65; they grew up with a strong work ethic and are proud to continue. If retired, how has the patient adjusted to the change in role? It may mean loss of social role or social status, loss of personal relationships formed at work, and reduced income.

Activity and mobility. How does the patient spend a typical day in work, hobbies, and leisure activities? Is there any day this routine changes (e.g., Sunday because of visits from family)? Note that the patient suffering from chronic illness or disability may have a self-care deficit, musculo-skeletal changes such as arthritis, and mental confusion.

List significant leisure activities, hobbies, sports, and community activities. Is a community centre available to older adults for nutrition, social networking, and screening of health status? What are the type, amount, and frequency of exercise? Is a warm-up included? How does the patient's body respond?

Sleep and rest. Note the usual sleep pattern: Does the patient feel rested during the day? Is energy sufficient to carry out daily activities? Does the patient need naps? Is there a problem with night awakenings, such as nocturia, shortness of breath, light sleep, or insomnia (difficulty falling asleep, awakening during the night, early morning awakening)? If the patient has no routine, does the patient tend to nap all afternoon? Does insomnia worsen with lack of a daily schedule?

Nutrition and elimination. Record a 24-hour recall of the diet. Is this diet typical of most days? (Nutrition may vary greatly. Ask the patient to keep a weekly log to bring in.) What are the meal patterns? Are there three full meals or five to six smaller meals per day? How many convenience foods and soft foods are eaten? Who prepares meals? Does the patient eat alone? Who shops for food? How are groceries transported home? Is the income adequate for groceries? Does the patient have a problem preparing meals (adequate vision, motor deficit, adequate energy)? Are the appliances, water, and utilities adequate for meal preparation? Does the patient have any difficulty chewing or swallowing? What are the food preferences? (Older adults often eat high amounts of carbohydrates because these foods are cheaper, easier to make, and easier to chew.)

Interpersonal relationships and resources. Who else is at home with the patient? Does the patient live alone? Is this living arrangement satisfactory? Does the patient have a pet? How close are chosen family or friends? How often does the patient see chosen family or friends? If visits are infrequent, is this experienced as a loss?

Does the patient live with family, such as a spouse, children, or a sibling? Is this arrangement satisfactory? What is the role in the family for preparation of meals, housework, and other activities? Are there any conflicts? Is the family caregiver experiencing any financial, physical, or social strain (see Fig. 31.4)?

Does the patient rely on any formal support programs such as social welfare or home health care? Does the patient use any semiformal supports such as church societies or older adult centres?

On whom does the patient depend for emotional support? For help with problems? Who meets affection needs?

Coping and stress management. Has the patient experienced a recent change in living conditions or social circumstances, such as loss of occupation, spouse, or friends; a move from home; illness of self or family member; or decrease in income? How does the patient deal with stress? If a loved one has died, how is the patient responding to the loss? Ask, "How do you feel about being 'alone' and having to take on unfamiliar responsibilities now?"

Environmental hazards. Record home safety: Does the home have one floor or are there stairs? What is the state of repair? Is money adequate to maintain the home? Are there exits for fire? Are heating and utilities adequate? How long has the patient lived in the current home?

Note transportation: Does the patient own a vehicle? Is income adequate for maintenance? When was the most recent driver's test? Does the patient consider themselves be a safe driver? Is public transportation accessible? Does the patient receive drives from community resources or friends?

Document aspects of the neighbourhood: Does the patient feel secure in personal safety at day or night? Is there danger of loss of possessions? What is the amount of noise and pollution? Does the patient have access to family and friends, a grocery store, a drugstore, laundry, religious communities (church, temple, mosque), and health care facilities?

REFERENCES

1. Bowen, S. (2015). *The impact of language barriers on patient safety and quality of care.* Ottawa: Société Santé en français. Retrieved from https://santefrancais.ca/wp-content/uploads/SSF-Bowen-S.-Language-Barriers-Study.pdf.

2. Browne, A. J., Varcoe, C., Wong, S. T., et al. (2014). Can ethnicity data collected at an organizational level be useful in addressing health and healthcare inequities? *Ethnicity and Health, 19*(2), 240–254.

3. Clinical Practice Guideline Expert Committee. (2007). Canadian Ophthalmological Society evidence-based clinical practice guidelines for the periodic eye examination in adults in Canada. *Canadian Journal of Ophthalmology. Journal Canadien d'Ophtalmologie, 42,* 39–45.

4. Gordon, M. (2012). *Manual of nursing diagnosis* (12th ed.). Sudbury, MA: Jones & Bartlett.

5. Granger, C. V., Ottenbacher, K. J., Baker, J. G., et al. (1995). Reliability of a brief outpatient functional outcome assessment measure. *American Journal of Physical Medicine, 74,* 469–475.

6. Mahoney, F. I., & Barthel, D. W. (1965). Functional evaluation: The Barthel Index. *Maryland State Medical Journal, 14,* 61–65.

7. Pearlman, R. (1987). Development of a functional assessment questionnaire for geriatric patients: The Comprehensive Older Person's Evaluation (COPE). *Journal of Chronic Disease, 40,* 85S–94S.

8. Reimer-Kirkham, S., & Cochrane, M. (2016). Resistant, reluctant or responsible? The negotiation of religious and cultural plurality in Canadian healthcare. In S. Sharma & D. Llewellyn (Eds.), *Religion, equality, and inequalities* (pp. 65–76). Surrey, UK: Ashgate.

9. Borneman, T., Ferrell, B., & Puchalski, C. M. (2010). Evaluation of the FICA tool for spiritual assessment. *Journal of Pain and Symptom Management, 40*(2), 163–173.

10. Obedin-Maliver, J., & Makadon, H. J. (2016). Transgender men and pregnancy. *Obstetric Medicine, 9*(1), 4–8.

11. Public Health Agency of Canada. (2018). *Canadian immunization guide.* Retrieved from https://www.canada.ca/en/public-health/services/canadian-immunization-guide.html.

12. Goldenring, J. M., & Rosen, D. S. (2004). Getting into adolescent heads: An essential update. *Contemporary Pediatrics, 21*(1), 64–75.

6 CHAPTER

Mental Health Assessment

Written by Victoria Smye, PhD, RN*

(e) http://evolve.elsevier.com/Canada/Jarvis/examination/

SIGNIFICANCE OF MENTAL HEALTH ASSESSMENT FOR CANADIANS

Depression is now the leading cause of disability worldwide, and is a major contributor to the overall global burden of disease.[1,2] "Mental, neurological and substance use disorders account for nine out of the 20 leading causes of years lived with disability worldwide (more than a quarter of all measured disability) and 10% of the global burden of disease" (which includes deaths as well as disability).[3] In terms of prevalence, one in five Canadians are affected by a mental illness† in any given year.[4] Moreover, one in three Canadians are expected to experience a mental health problem at some point in their lives.[5]

Mental illnesses account for a large percentage of hospital stays: in 2009–10, people hospitalized with a mental diagnosis represented less than 1% of the population, but they used 25% of acute care hospital days. Two-thirds of these days involved a comorbid condition.[6] Mental illness causes as many lost days of work as physical problems such as cancer, heart attack, or back pain. The economic burden of mental illness in Canada is estimated at $51 billion per year. This estimate includes health care costs, lost productivity, and reductions in health-related quality of life.[4] Thus, mental illness is not only a global health issue but also a major public health concern for this country.

In addition, Canada's population includes many diverse groups, including immigrant and refugee groups, as well as a large number of Indigenous peoples (First Nations, Métis, and Inuit) whose mental health needs often are not adequately met. People who are members of these groups often face unique challenges in maintaining cultural, social,

and economic integrity; their beliefs, "ways of knowing," and healing and medical practices historically have been excluded and are not necessarily reflected in current health policies and practices. Without adequate social resources or access to needed and appropriate services (e.g., culturally appropriate assessments), the stressors experienced by some ethnocultural and social groups in Canada can lead to an increase in mental illnesses and suicide. For example, although there are great variations in suicide rates across communities, bands, and nations, the suicide rate among First Nations communities is at least twice as high as that of the general population, and the rate among Inuit is 6 to 11 times higher than that of the general population.[7,8] These disturbingly high rates of suicide stem from the complex interplay of social determinants of health (SDOH), intergenerational and historical traumas, and ongoing racism and stigma and discrimination not adequately addressed in our current systems of care. For example, little attention has been paid to the need for trauma- and violence-informed services. See Chapter 7 for further discussion on the importance of trauma- and violence-informed care. See also Box 6.1.

Defining Mental Health and Mental Illness

Mental health is a crucial dimension of overall health and an essential resource for everyday living. Broadly defined, positive **mental health** is the capacity to feel, think, express emotions, and behave in ways that enhance personal capacity to manage challenges, adapt successfully to a range of demands, and enjoy life.[5] "It is a sense of emotional and spiritual well-being" that reflects the importance of "culture, equity, social justice, interconnections and personal dignity."[9] The World Health Organization (WHO) describes mental health as a relative and ongoing state of well-being in which individuals realize their abilities, cope with the normal stresses of life, work productively, and contribute meaningfully to the community.[2,10] Characteristics indicative of mental health include finding balance in all aspects of life—social,

---

*Thank you to Kathryn Weaver, PhD, RN, for her work on the previous edition of this chapter.

†In this chapter, the terms *mental illness* and *mental health disorder* are used interchangeably.

BOX 6.1 Trauma, Violence, and Post-Traumatic Stress Disorder

The DSM-5 defines *post-traumatic stress disorder* (PTSD) as a trauma or stressor-related disorder in which symptoms began or worsened after the experience of one or more traumatic events.[*] Evidence suggests that individual responses to trauma depend both on the nature of the trauma and on characteristics of the individual and the environment.[*†‡§] For example, in Canada, it is estimated that up to 10% of war-zone veterans, including war-service veterans and peacekeeping forces (e.g., those deployed to Afghanistan) will go on to experience PTSD, while others may experience at least some of the symptoms associated with this condition.[‖] Of note, many veterans are not covered under their medical plan if they are diagnosed with PTSD, but they are covered if diagnosed with operational stress injury (OSI)[***] or post-traumatic stress injury (PTSI) (which has the potential risk of limiting access to mental health services).

Currently, research indicates that there also are wide variations of PTSD prevalence among Indigenous communities, with some communities showing very high rates of PTSD and others demonstrating low rates.[†] In addition, according to a meta-analysis conducted by Golding, the mean prevalence of PTSD in women with a history of intimate partner violence is 63.8%.[#] Also, a high prevalence of PTSD has been found in war-affected refugees such as the Sudanese, with prevalence estimates ranging from 32%[**] to 46%[††] in this population. Refugees and immigrants often have experienced multiple losses (e.g., family, friends and home) and dislocations (e.g., culture and place); factors that can significantly impact trauma/violence experiences. Symptoms of PTSD include, but are not limited to, flashbacks, disturbing dreams (nightmares), insomnia, persistent frightening thoughts and memories, anger, irritability, concentration difficulties and substance use. See also Chapter 7 for more information on the relationship between lifetime violence, persistent pain, mental health, and substance use.

The Primary Care PTSD Screen for DSM-5 (PC-PTSD-5) was designed to identify respondents with probable PTSD; it is a five-item screen designed for use in primary care settings. The screen begins with a question on whether the respondent has had any exposure to traumatic events. If a respondent denies exposure, the PC-PTSD-5 results in a score of 0. However, if a respondent indicates having experienced a traumatic event, that respondent is asked to answer five yes/no questions about the effects of the trauma exposure during the past month. Those who screen positive (having answered "yes" to at least three of the questions) require further assessment, preferably with a structured interview such as the Clinician-Administered PTSD Scale for DSM-5 (CAPS-5), if time permits. If time is limited, it is recommended that additional assessment be conducted using the PTSD Checklist for DSM-5 (PCL-5), a psychometrically sound self-report questionnaire.[‡‡§§]

[*]American Psychiatric Association. (2013). *Desk reference to the diagnostic criteria from DSM-5.* Arlington, VA: Author.

[†]Bellamy, S., & Hardy, C. (2015). *Post-traumatic stress disorder in Aboriginal people in Canada: Review of risk factors, the current state of knowledge and directions for further research.* Prince George, BC: National Collaborating Centre for Aboriginal Health. Retrieved from https://centredoc.cssspnql.com/cgi-bin/koha/opac-detail.pl?biblionumber=1349.

[‡]Sherin, J. E., & Nemeroff, C. B. (2011). Post-traumatic stress disorder: The neurobiological impact of psychological trauma. *Dialogues in Clinical Neuroscience, 13*(3), 263–278.

[§]Yehuda, R., & LeDoux, J. (2007). Response variation following trauma: A translational neuroscience approach to understanding PTSD. *Neuron, 56*(1), 19–32.

[‖]Health Canada. (2017). *Post-traumatic stress disorder (PTSD) and war-related stress.* Ottawa: Author. Retrieved from http://www.veterans.gc.ca/eng/services/health/mental-health/publications/ptsd-warstress#Item3-1.

[#]Golding, J. (1999). Intimate partner violence as a risk factor for mental disorders: A meta-analysis. *Journal of Family Violence, 14,* 99–132.

[**]Pelzer, K. (1999). Trauma and mental health problems of Sudanese refugees in Uganda. *Central African Journal of Medicine, 45*(5), 110–114.

[††]Karunakara, U. K., Neuner, F., Schauer, M., et al. (2004). Traumatic events and symptoms of post-traumatic stress disorder amongst Sudanese nationals, refugees and Ugandans in the West Nile. *African Health Sciences, 4*(2), 83–93.

[‡‡]Prins, A., Bovin, M. J., Kimerling, R., et al. (2015). *The Primary Care PTSD Screen for DSM-5 (PC-PTSD-5).* [Measurement instrument]. Retrieved from https://www.ptsd.va.gov/professional/assessment/screens/pc-ptsd.asp.

[§§]Prins, A., Bovin, M. J., Smolenski, D. J., et al. (2016). The Primary Care PTSD Screen for DSM-5 (PC-PTSD-5): Development and evaluation within a veteran primary care sample. *Journal of General Internal Medicine, 31,* 1206–1211. doi:10.1007/s11606-016-3703-5

[***]Note: According to Public Safety Canada, an operational stress injury (OSI) is "a nonmedical term" that is generally defined as "persistent, psychological difficulties resulting from operational duties." Within the broad category of OSIs related to public safety officers and other operational personnel, a number of mental health issues can be described as post-traumatic stress injuries (PTSI), including depression, substance use, and clinically diagnosed post-traumatic stress disorder (PTSD). Operational and Trauma Stress Support Centres (OTSSC) are specialized programs within Canadian Forces Mental Health Services that ensure comprehensive and consistent assessment and treatment of patients with operational stress injuries; they provide assessment, and individual and group treatment for members of the Canadian Forces experiencing difficulties that result from operational duties. See Government of Canada (2015). *Canadian Armed Forces Mental Health Services.* Retrieved from http://www.forces.gc.ca/en/caf-community-health-services-mental/index.page?#otssc; and Public Safety Canada (2017). *Post-traumatic stress injuries and support for public safety officers.* Retrieved from https://www.publicsafety.gc.ca/cnt/mrgnc-mngmnt/mrgnc-prprdnss/ptsi-en.as.

physical, spiritual, economic, and mental—and developing resilience,[‡] flexibility, and self-actualization.[§10,12–14]

Protective factors can help shield people against mental health problems. Consider the case of First Nations communities in British Columbia, where suicide rates vary across communities (i.e., they range from no suicide, to low rates, to high rates). Researchers have found that a number of protective factors contribute to lower suicide rates. For example, communities that had sought to secure title to traditional lands and had reached some level of self-government had lower suicide rates.[15,16] Also, the greater extent to which a community governed its own health and social services, the lower the community's suicide rate. Indigenous and non-Indigenous researchers have deemed "cultural continuity" (i.e., the extent of cultural connectedness) to be a moderator of risk for suicide[15,16] and an important determinant of health and well-being.[17–19] In addition, intergenerational knowledge transmission has been found to be a central component of renewing and maintaining cultural continuity for Indigenous peoples.[17,19] In a similar, but slightly different vein, a study conducted with First Nations and Inuit community health representatives (CHRs) found that the poor health experienced by rural and remote Indigenous communities was fundamentally connected to compromised cultural connections between land and identity, the cumulative effects of environmental dispossession.[20] As the researchers noted, "In a physical sense, the effect of environmental dispossession has led to increasingly sedentary lifestyles and limited food choices, of which study participants described as pivotal determinants of obesity, diabetes and many other chronic diseases that plague their fellow community members at near-epidemic rates."[20]

Mental health means "health of the *mind* ... The brain is the physical organ of the body that produces mental activity; the mind is a set of functions and experiences resulting from a combination of brain activity and the environment in which it operates."[21] There has been a long-standing debate over which elements influence a person's mental health. Some tend to favour a biological perspective, which emphasizes the influence of biological systems (e.g., genetic and neurophysiological characteristics) on brain functioning. Others tend to favour an environmental perspective, which emphasizes the influence of family and childhood (e.g., education), culture, politics, and economy (e.g., employment, income, and housing).[21] All of these factors—both biological and environmental—are referred to as "determinants of health." Ultimately, no single factor or circumstance influences people's mental health; rather, people are affected by a complex series of intersecting factors (biological and environmental) that also include the influences of poverty, colonialism and neocolonialism, racism, and other forms of discrimination. For example, determinants of Indigenous peoples' health also include factors such as language, land (geography), culture, and "race."[22]

To add to the complexity of our understanding of mental health, many people do not hold Western notions of mental health (and illness). For some, mental health is not neatly separated from the other dimensions of health but is instead an integral part of overall health—which includes physical, mental, emotional, and spiritual health—making the discussion of mental health and the identification of mental illness sometimes challenging. For example, in a small qualitative study with Sudanese refugee women, Bhaloo found that participants had no specific term for "mental health"; the participants cautioned against the use of "mental health" because of its conflation with "insanity" and the associated stigma.[23] In addition, similar to many Indigenous peoples in Canada and worldwide, Sudanese people have historically engaged with Indigenous systems of healing and medical practice to address physical and mental illness;[24] these practices are not fully supplanted by Western biomedical systems.

For First Nations communities, **mental wellness** is supported by factors such as "culture, language, Elders, families, and creation"[25]—this concept is linked to inherent strengths, and positive well-being and functioning. Moreover, it is believed to be "necessary for healthy individual, family, and community life."[25] Physical, mental, emotional, spiritual, social, and economic well-being (whole health and balance) is achieved "through a coordinated, comprehensive approach that respects, values, and utilizes First Nations cultural knowledge, approaches, languages, and ways of knowing."[25] Purpose, hope, belonging, and meaning are key wellness outcomes; they enrich whole health, balance, and interconnectedness.[25] This notion of mental wellness also reminds us that people can live "well" with a mental disorder or illness.

Mental disorder is the medical term for mental illness and is defined and diagnosed in Canada according to criteria specified in the *Diagnostic and Statistical Manual of Mental Disorders*, Fifth Edition (DSM-5) by the American Psychiatric Association.[26] Mental disorders are depicted as constellations of co-occurring symptoms that may involve alterations in thought, experience, and emotion that are serious enough to cause distress and impair functioning, cause difficulties in sustaining interpersonal relationships and performing jobs, and sometimes lead to self-destructive behaviour and suicide.[5,27] Multiple, often intersecting factors—including the physical environment, genetics, biology, personality, culture, socioeconomic status, and life events—may contribute to the development of a mental disorder. Men and women, young

---

[‡]"Resilience is the capacity of people to confront and cope with life's challenges; to maintain their wellbeing in the face of adversity."[11] Literature and research conducted through the Mind, Mental Health Foundation suggests that three key factors support resilience: (a) engaging in activities to promote well-being, (b) building social capital (social connections), and (c) developing psychological coping strategies.

[§]According to Carl Rogers, people naturally strive to self-actualize; that is, they seek to fulfill their potential—where the "ideal self" is a fit with the "actual self"—and become a fully functioning person. Abraham Maslow considered self-actualization as the highest order need (a growth need). It appeared at the top of his hierarchy of needs, followed by esteem needs, belongingness and love needs, safety needs, and physiological needs.

and old, and people of all ethnocultural and social groups and economic brackets may be affected.

Mental Illness and Comorbid Conditions

Current evidence suggests significant comorbidity between chronic physical conditions (in particular, cardiovascular disease, hypertension, respiratory disease, diabetes mellitus, and other metabolic disorders) and mental illness.[28–31] The reason that these health challenges are connected is not fully understood. However, we do know that mental illness complicates help-seeking, diagnosis and treatment; and it influences prognosis. In addition, we know that health care services are not provided equitably for people with mental illness and that the quality of care for people with mental illness and comorbid conditions could be improved. The challenge is creating a health care system in which people with coexisting mental illness and/or problematic substance use as well as physical illness find "no wrong door" when they seek help.[31]

There is a need for strong linkages between mental health and primary health care providers to ensure continuity and appropriateness of care and knowledge exchange; for example, awareness among primary health care providers that many medications prescribed for serious mental conditions have significant metabolic and cardiovascular adverse effects is important.[32] As Kiraly, Gunning, and Leiser suggest, patients treated with second-generation antipsychotics should receive preventive counselling and treatment for cardiovascular disease.[32] Medication interactions also can lead to increased adverse effects, increased or decreased medication levels, toxicity, or treatment failure.[31] In addition, some people with mental illness will use substances (licit or illicit) to manage their symptoms, and others will use substances for a variety of other reasons, including those tied to personal and environmental factors (e.g., trauma and violence).

Concurrent Disorders: Mental Health Disorders and Problematic Substance Use

The co-occurrence of a mental health disorder and problematic substance use/substance use disorder is referred to as a "concurrent disorder."[33] Concurrent disorders also include problem/pathological gambling and problematic substance use and/or mental health disorders.[34] The DSM-5 recognizes concurrent disorders in the diagnostic criteria section of each disorder category, acknowledging that many symptoms of one disorder are often present in others.[26] According to the 2002 *Canadian Community Health Survey: Mental Health and Well-Being*, between 40 to 60% of individuals with severe mental illness will develop a substance use disorder at some point during their lives,[35] and almost 2% of Canadians (or 435 000 adults) have both a mental health disorder and a substance use disorder.[36] Rush and colleagues reported that the Canadian Community Health Survey's rate was grossly underestimated because some comorbidities, such as personality disorder and post-traumatic stress disorder (PTSD), were not included in the survey.[36] Other reports indicate that more than 50% of those engaged in treatment for substance use are also struggling with mental illness, and 15 to 20% of those engaged in treatment for mental illness are struggling with substance use.[33]

In terms of prevalence, Rush (2015)[37] found the following:

- 10 to 25% of all individuals will have an anxiety disorder at some point in their lives; among them, 24% will also have a substance use disorder
- 15 to 20% of all individuals will have a major depression at some point in their lives; among them, 27% will also have a substance use disorder
- 1 to 2% of all individuals will have bipolar disorder at some point in their lives; among them, 56% will also have a substance use disorder
- 1% of all individuals will have schizophrenia at some point in their lives; among them, 47% will also have a substance use disorder[37]

A Canadian Institute for Health Information (CIHI) study determined that the prevalence for concurrent disorders among those hospitalized for psychiatric concerns in 2010–11 was 35.6%.[38]

Because mental illnesses and problematic substance use are so closely linked, mental health and substance use services also must be integrated. Treatment of individuals with concurrent disorders can be complex; the experience of crisis, relapse, and readmission to hospital are common for those living with concurrent disorders.[33] Moreover, it is important to note that people living with concurrent disorders often have difficulty accessing appropriate services, resulting in unmet needs[39] and poor outcomes.[33,40] These facts underline the importance of collaborative care for persons living with concurrent disorders.[37,38] However, regardless of the challenges people with concurrent disorders face, it is important to remember that people with mental health disorders and problematic substance use can and do recover (Box 6.2).[41]

Lastly, mental health and substance use problems have been consistently shown to be related, and all forms of interpersonal violence have been shown to be related to mental health and substance use problems. See Chapter 7 for further details.

Mental Health, Mental Illness, and Stigma

A major disadvantage for individuals with a mental illness is stigma and its associated cycle of alienation and discrimination. In 1963, Goffman defined *stigma* is "an attribute associated with 'difference' that is deemed to be a less desirable difference by one person (the stigmatizer) in relation to another person (the stigmatized)—a difference, which at its extreme, might deem the person as bad, dangerous or weak (stereotyping)."[42] Later, Link and Phelan expanded on Goffman's definition.[43,44] They viewed stigma, in the context if mental health, as created through five interrelated and converging social processes: (a) labelling of the person with a mental illness as "crazy" or "mad"; (b) negative stereotyping by linking "difference" with undesirable characteristics and fears, such as labelling a person with a mental illness as "dangerous"; (c) "othering" by creating "us" and "them" (the labelled person) categories; (d) status loss, blame, and

BOX 6.2 Recovery-Oriented Services and Supports

Recovery Is Person-First and Holistic

Recovery-oriented mental health practice supports people to define their goals, exercise their capacities and use their strengths to attain their potential. Recovery-oriented practice acknowledges that each person's journey is both unique and complex, and assists people in maximizing their ability to direct and manage it themselves.

Core Principles

- Each person is a unique individual with the right to determine their own path toward mental health and well-being.
- Recovery is an individual process—care and services are tailored to people's preferences, life circumstances and aspirations and are integrated with their community of supports.
- Everyone's mental health and well-being is affected by multiple intersecting factors—biological, psychological, social and economic, as well as family context and cultural background, personal values and spiritual beliefs.

Six Dimensions of Recovery-Oriented Practice

1. *Creating a culture and language of hope.* Recovery is fundamentally about nurturing and generating hope.
2. *Recovery is personal.* Each person's road to mental health and well-being is unique; each person brings their own strengths and capabilities.
3. *Recovery occurs in the context of one's life.* Assisting a person to connect with those aspects of their life that support mental health and well-being is fundamental to a recovery-oriented approach (family, friends, culture, spirituality etc.).
4. *Responding to the diverse needs of everyone in Canada.* Recovery-oriented practice is grounded in principles that encourage and enable respect for diversity and that are consistent with culturally responsive, safe and competent practices.
5. *Working with First Nations, Inuit, and Métis.* Recognition of the distinct cultures, rights and circumstances of First Nations, Inuit and Métis, and understanding how recovery for Indigenous peoples is uniquely shaped by Canada's history of colonization is key for recovery-oriented practitioners.
6. *Recovery is about transforming services and systems.* Recovery needs to be reflected in everything an organization does regardless of the type of service, service location, population served or professional roles (e.g., ensuring professional development to support the delivery of recovery-oriented practice.

Source: Adapted from Mental Health Commission of Canada. (2015). *Guidelines for recovery-oriented practice: Hope. Dignity. Inclusion.* Ottawa: Author (pp. 15–17).

discrimination of the labelled person; and (e) power dynamics that create stigmatization, which hinder the labelled person's ability to access key resources such as education, employment, housing, social networks, and institutions. In addition, stigma often is exacerbated by the media when they sensationalize the rare cases of violence associated with mental illness.[45] Misperceptions (and fear) about the relationship between mental illness and violence contribute significantly to stigma. Discrimination and social exclusion are associated with mental illness regardless of the fact that studies have shown people living with mental health conditions are no more likely to engage in violent behaviour than the general population.[46] Thus, mental illness as a category of "difference" often leads to stigmatization based on the beliefs that underpin its perceived origins (e.g., that people with mental illness are violent or unable to manage their own affairs). A significant problem is that people with mental illness often internalize these societal prejudices, and the ability of labelled people to resist stigma (or not) is dependent on their own beliefs, social location, and perceived power. The adverse effects of stigma and discrimination include a delay in seeking medical treatment, early treatment discontinuation, difficulties in obtaining housing, and other negative economic effects,[47–51] sometimes with dire consequences for health and well-being.

Unfortunately, some health care providers in the mental health field (including nurses) stigmatize patients who have mental illness.[52–54] The anticipation of experiencing stigma has been identified as a significant factor in people's reluctance to seek help for a mental illness.[54,55] Reducing stigma is a responsibility shared by health care providers, communities, and people with mental illness.[51] As a nurse working within this population, it is imperative for you to self-reflect, self-monitor, and address your own stigmatizing beliefs and behaviours. It is recommended that you complete the "De-stigmatizing Practices and Mental Illness" learning module through the Mdcme.ca website: https://www.mdcme.ca/courseinfo.asp?id=167.

A key element of antistigma practice is to engage in a recovery-oriented approach to mental illness or mental disorder. Recovery-oriented approaches, although widely taken up in Canada, have not been an easy sell. Stigma remains entrenched. For example, many health care providers hold the stereotypical view that people with a mental illness can never be well enough to make responsible decisions about their lives or that people with a mental illness are dangerous to society. As well, some mental health nurses hold pessimistic beliefs about the possibility and applicability of recovery for people with complex and serious mental illness.[56] These beliefs pose ongoing social and structural challenges for making recovery a reality in many mental health care settings.[41,57–59] Demonstrating that "recovery is both possible and real" and debunking the myths associated with recovery have thus been found to be a key program element for planning and delivering effective programs[57] (see Boxes 6.2 and 6.3).

Mental Health, Mental Illness, Housing, and Homelessness

The relationship between mental illness and housing/homelessness is complex. Many studies show that people who are homeless are more likely to experience compromised mental health or mental illness than the general population.[8] For some, these issues can precede the onset

Reflect on your own values and beliefs and ask yourself the following questions.

Recovery-Oriented Practice

- What are your values and attitudes regarding mental health/wellness, mental illness, and "recovery" for persons living with mental health and/or substance use problems?
- How has your practice been responsive to individuals' expectations, recovery goals, and unique needs?
- How have you sought to understand what helps with recovery and learn from those you serve?
- Have you considered what possible alternative service offerings might be appropriate?
- Does the treatment/service plan create opportunities for attention to physical health, exercise, recreation, nutrition, expressions of spirituality, sexuality and creative outlets, in addition to stress and symptom management?
- What positive connections with referring agencies and service partnerships do you consider to offer people? Do you provide a range of options? What practices may disadvantage those you serve? For example, Do you consider access issues (transportation, child care) and the ease of access dependent on the individual's personal and social circumstances?

Recovery-Oriented Leadership

- To what extent do the systems and processes in your setting (e.g., intake, documentation, family/community involvement, the involvement of Elders) offer flexible and individualized approaches? In what ways may they disadvantage those you serve?
- Have you critically reviewed the assessment and care planning processes in use in your agency? Are these plans inclusive of contextual information (e.g., housing stability, living arrangements, personal goals, priorities, relationships, or natural supports)?
- How do you help people obtain access to a broad range of treatment approaches, services, and support options?
- In clinical governance, policies, and professional development, do leaders reinforce that the patient is central to practice? Do they provide patients with lived experience the opportunity to determine their own path of recovery and participate in decision making about their health?

Adapted from the Mental Health Commission of Canada. (2015). *Guidelines for Recovery-Oriented Practice: Hope. Dignity. Inclusion.* Ottawa: Author.

of homelessness or, through their intersection with other health determinants such as income and employment influences, contribute to homelessness. Persons living with mental illness are more vulnerable to living in poverty than persons without a mental illness.[60,61] Poverty is the one consistent factor that hovers in the background of discussions of the risks for "mental, emotional, and behavioural disorders and antisocial behaviour."[60]

Mental health also may be more compromised with continued homelessness or contribute to the duration of homelessness.[61,62] A lack of safe, stable housing renders those living with or without mental illness vulnerable and those with mental illness at greater risk for poor outcomes. Research indicates that a stable and supportive living environment is essential to maintaining the health and well-being of people with serious mental illness, and it is integral to their recovery.[60,63] Housing with support can generate positive outcomes, including enhanced life skills, improved health status, an increased sense of empowerment, and greater involvement in the community.[60,63] In her book *Dying for a Home*, Cathy Crowe—recent Order of Canada recipient, street nurse, and social justice advocate working in Toronto, Ontario—provides compelling first-hand accounts of homelessness and practical steps for making a change for the better.[64] Crowe cofounded the Toronto Relief Committee, a group that declared homelessness a national disaster in 1998. Research shows that maintaining and improving the housing of individuals with serious mental illness can contribute to a reduction in psychiatric symptoms and therefore decrease the need for emergency and treatment services.[60]

MENTAL HEALTH NURSING ASSESSMENT

When conducting a mental health nursing assessment, it is essential for the nurse to establish rapport with the patient. Relational practice is inquiry-based practice and core to nursing.[65] From a relational perspective, the nurse–patient relationship is influenced by personal, socioeconomic, and political factors in the lives of the nurse and the patient. These contextual factors include gender, age, sexual orientation, and ability; and economic, cultural, historical, and geographical elements (e.g., income [poverty], education, employment, housing, and neocolonial policies and practices). (See Chapter 3 for details on Indigenous populations in Canada and inequities in health status.) They also include issues related to living in urban, rural, remote, and reserve communities. All of these factors influence the nurse, the patient, the patient's family, and the community and, thus, the nurse–patient relationship.[65]

Before engaging in the nurse–patient relationship, nurses need to critically reflect on how personal, socioeconomic, and political factors influence the nurse–patient relationship, health care decision making, and management of health care. For example, when working with people living with mental illness, nurses need to understand their own views on mental health and wellness, mental illness, and "recovery." Nurses also need to integrate patient, family, and community perspectives in the planning and delivery of care. Inquiry-based nursing practice involves bringing nursing knowledge into the relational space and being curious about and interested in what one does not know; for example, how features of patients' and their family's lives influence their experience of living with a mental illness. Nurses need to be interested in the interrelatedness of these pieces.[65] For example, they must understand the effects of a change in income or employment opportunities (e.g., on housing) and the vulnerabilities these kinds of life changes create for patients, families, and the community.

Relational practice is respectful, nonjudgemental, and reflexive. Connecting in this way is not easy; it requires a hard look at oneself and the social and structural factors (e.g., health and social systems of care and associated policies) that advantage some and disadvantage others. It involves the ongoing quest for knowledge and understanding. Begin by asking yourself the key questions in Box 6.3. The nurse–patient relationship is directed toward advancing the best interests and best health outcome of the patient.[66] To this end, the purpose of the mental health nursing assessment is to understand the patient's mental health or wellness, illness beliefs and experiences, challenges in daily living, and strengths and resources in relation to mental health or wellness. Accordingly, the nurse partners with the patient to assess the full scope of the patient's mental health or wellness, patient interactions with health care providers and other professionals, the patient's needs, risk factors (e.g., housing stability, food security) and needed intervention. The nurse's assessment skills are often developed in settings in which mental illness has already been identified by the psychiatrist and heavily influenced by medical judgement, which may focus on "the 'cure' of patients … potentially discount[ing] their [other] experiences."[67]

Methods and Components

To provide a comprehensive mental health nursing assessment, you will integrate close observations and routine social interactions into the collection of information about the patient's circumstances. You will combine (a) observation, (b) interview, (c) examination, (d) physical assessment, and (e) collaboration with others (referred to as *collateral information*). Observing the patient at different times of the day and in different situations provides information about hygiene, grooming, attire, facial expressions, gestures, and interactions with others. You will identify disturbances in perception and thought and any inconsistencies between what the patient states and what you notice and, in addition, analyze findings from physical, mental, cognitive, and diagnostic examinations to reveal symptoms and potential problems in self-care. Through interviewing, you will build rapport with the patient, clarify the patient's perceptions and meanings, and gather factual knowledge. You also will develop and evaluate treatment plans and risk for harm through collaboration with the patient's family and with other members of the health care team. The development of trust within the therapeutic relationship is crucial;[68,69] trust builds through making yourself available, expressing interest in the patient as a person, and being accountable. Mental health nursing assessment may include the methods and components described in the following sections (Table 6.1).

Sources of Information

Patient information can be *subjective* (symptoms reported that are not directly observable or measurable) and *objective* (signs directly observed and measured, such as diagnostic test results). Although the patient is ideally the primary provider of information, collaboration with secondary sources (including family, other health care providers, and patient

TABLE 6.1 **Elements of a Mental Health History**	
ASSESSMENT METHOD	**COMPONENTS**
Interview	Complete health history
	• Source of information
	• Identification/biographical information
	• Reason for seeking care (verbatim, psychiatric diagnoses [DSM-5])
	• Past health (past illness, injury, hospitalization; chronic illnesses)
	• Family health history
	• Developmental considerations
	• Present health (allergies, immunization/HIV/hepatitis status; current medications)
Observation (may include examination)	The mental status examination is an essential part of the mental health assessment. Most of this information can be obtained indirectly while conducting a general health assessment. For example, mood can be assessed as you meet the patient.
	• Appearance
	• Behaviour (mood and affect, speech)
	• Cognitive function (level of consciousness; orientation to time, place, person, self; memory; attention and concentration; comprehension and abstract reasoning)
	• Thought (perception, content, process, judgement, insight)
Examination	Supplemental Mental Status Examination (if warranted)
Interview (with added physical assessment)	Functional assessment of activities of daily living (ADLs): nutrition patterns; sleep/rest changes; activity/mobility; elimination; interpersonal relationships and resources; self-esteem/self-concept; ethnicity/culture; spirituality; coping and stress management; smoking, alcohol and drug use, and problem gambling; home environmental hazards
Collaboration with health care team	Risk assessment (suicide, assaultive or homicidal ideation, elopement)
	Treatment plan (Global Assessment of Functioning)

HIV, human immunodeficiency virus.

records) is needed for children and when the patient is at risk for harm to self or others.

Indication for Comprehensive Mental Health Nursing Assessment

The full comprehensive mental health examination with its accompanying components for mental status assessment, as outlined previously, rarely needs to be performed in its entirety. Usually, you can assess mental health through the context of the health history interview; hence, the mental health nursing assessment follows the major subjects of the complete health history (see Chapter 5); this approach is recommended for most situations. You will collect ample data to be able to assess mental health strengths and coping skills and to screen for any dysfunction.

A distinguishing component of the mental health assessment is the **mental status examination**. (Box 6.4). The mental status examination should always be included in

the overall physical assessment of all patients. It may be an initial assessment or part of an ongoing assessment.

The mental status examination is a vital aspect of clinical care used to assess emotional and cognitive functioning; a structured way of observing and describing a person's current state of mind, under the domains of appearance, behaviour, cognition, and thought processes. The Mini-Mental State Examination (MMSE) can be used instead of the full mental status examination when time is limited.[*70–75] It is beneficial to assess mental status when you sense that something is "not quite right." If, for instance, you see a person whose speech is slow and unclear, whose eyes do not focus, whose clothes are soiled and dishevelled, and whose thoughts are confused, you suspect that something is wrong. As additional symptoms are identified, it is possible to more fully understand the impairment and subsequently design support or intervention.

It is necessary to perform the mental health assessment when you discover any abnormality in mood or behaviour and in the following situations:

- Family members are concerned about a person's behavioural changes, such as memory loss or inappropriate social interaction.
- Brain lesions (trauma, tumour, stroke): A mental health assessment documents any emotional, cognitive, or behavioural change associated with the lesion. Not recognizing these changes hinders care planning and creates problems with social readjustment.
- Aphasia (the impairment of language ability secondary to brain damage): A mental health assessment documents language function, as well as any associated emotional problems such as depression or agitation.
- Symptoms (e.g., extreme worrying and avoidance) of psychiatric mental illness, especially with acute onset, are evident.

In every mental health assessment, note the following factors that could affect your interpretation:

- Any known illnesses or health problems, such as problematic alcohol use or chronic renal disease.
- Current medications, the adverse effects of which may cause confusion or depression.
- The usual educational and behavioural level; note that factor as the normal baseline, and do not expect

---

*The Folstein Mini-Mental State Examination (MMSE) is frequently used to evaluate a person's cognitive and mental function and initially was designed as a screening test for dementia. The MMSE is also a tool that can be used to systematically and thoroughly assess mental status. It is an 11-question measure that tests five areas of cognitive function: orientation, registration, attention and calculation, recall, and language. The maximum score is 30. A score of 23 or lower is indicative of cognitive impairment. The MMSE takes 5 to 10 minutes to administer and is therefore practical to use repeatedly and routinely. In some institutions, the Montreal Cognitive Assessment (MoCA) tool is used, and was developed to enable earlier detection of mild cognitive impairment (MCI). Scores on the MoCA range from 0 to 30, with a score of 26 and higher generally considered normal.

BOX 6.4   Mental Status Examination

I. Appearance
General presentation to others.

II. Behaviour
Mood and affect: Expressing the prevailing feelings through mood (a sustained emotion that the patient is experiencing) and affect (a display of feelings or state of mind).
Speech: Using language and the voice to communicate one's thoughts and feelings. Because this is a basic tool of humans, its loss has a devastating social effect on the individual.

III. Cognition
Consciousness: Being aware of one's feelings, thoughts, and environment. This is the most elementary of mental health functions.
Orientation: Awareness of the objective world in relation to the self.
Memory: The ability to set down and store experiences and perceptions for later recall; *immediate* memory involves on-the-spot recall, *recent* memory evokes day-to-day events, and *remote* memory includes years' worth of experiences.
Attention and concentration: The power to direct thinking toward an object or topic with the ability to focus on one specific thing without being distracted by other competing stimuli.
Comprehension and abstract reasoning: Pondering a deeper meaning beyond the concrete and literal.

IV. Thinking
Perception: An awareness of objects through the five senses.
Content: What the person thinks: specific ideas, beliefs, and the use of words.
Process: The *way* a person thinks; the logical train of thought.
Insight: Awareness of the reality of the situation.
Judgement: Ability to choose a logical course of action.

performance on the mental health assessment to exceed it.

- Responses to personal history questions, indicating current stress, social interaction patterns, sleep habits, substance use (see Chapter 7 for details on incorporating knowledge of substance use in the health assessment).

 DEVELOPMENTAL CONSIDERATIONS

Children and Adolescents

All aspects of emotional and cognitive functioning are interdependent. For example, the concept of language as a social tool of communication occurs around 3 to 5 years of age, coincident with the child's readiness to play cooperatively with other children. School readiness coincides with the development of the thought process; around age 7, thinking becomes more logical and systematic, and the child is able to reason and understand. Progression through developmental stages toward independence and the full range of health determinants affects the experience of adolescence.[76,77] Abstract thinking—the ability to consider a hypothetical situation—usually develops between ages 12 and 15, although a few adolescents never achieve it.

Given the interdependence of emotional and cognitive functioning, it is important during an assessment to inquire about the achievement of educational and developmentally appropriate tasks and milestones that provide important information regarding the emotional and cognitive well-being of the child or adolescent; that is, as a means of identifying areas of strength, as well as those that may indicate attention, interpersonal, or behavioural problems. The Adverse Childhood Experiences (ACE) study, one of the largest scientific research studies of its kind (over 17 000 predominately middle-income American participants), demonstrated a relationship between health risk behaviour and disease in adulthood to the breadth of exposure to childhood emotional, physical, or sexual abuse, and household dysfunction during childhood.[78] In addition, parental death or separation at an early age often is associated with attachment difficulties in later relationships.

Consider the long-term effects of the Canadian residential school system on Indigenous people. The residential school experience perpetuated social and psychological trauma among First Nations people beyond the generation of children who attended the schools (often referred to as *intergenerational trauma*).[79] A study by Menzies demonstrated that intergenerational trauma can be linked to an array of mental health and social issues faced by Indigenous people in Canada.[79] He warned that mental health providers who focus their interventions solely on the individual will not adequately address the needs of Indigenous patients. Menzies recommended that health care providers acknowledge the role public policy has had and still has (e.g., Child Welfare) in severing the physical, mental, emotional, and spiritual ties between Indigenous peoples, and consider the implications of intergenerational trauma on individuals, families, communities, and nations.[79] When conducting an assessment, it is important to be aware that the Indigenous patient or the patient's family may have experienced trauma in relation to the residential school system.

Seventy percent of mental health disorders have their onset during childhood or adolescence.[8] The most common mental health disorders among adolescents include depression, anxiety disorders, eating disorders, attention-deficit/hyperactivity disorder (ADHD), and substance use disorder; half of diagnosable mental health disorders over the lifetime begin by age 14.[5,80] Related to eating disorders, according to the Public Health Agency of Canada (PHAC), 34% of adolescent girls in Grades 6 to 10 described themselves as too fat, whereas only 15% of those Grade 10 girls were actually overweight, based on their self-reported heights and weights.[81] The leading cause of mortality among youth in Canada is unintentional injuries, at a rate of 21.3 per 100 000 population.[82] For adolescents aged 15 to 19 years, suicide (intentional self-harm) is the second leading cause of death.

Youth who are Indigenous, immigrant, homeless, and within a sexual minority (those who identified as lesbian, gay, bisexual, transgender, or questioning) in Canada were more likely to experience discrimination, stigmatization, harassment, bullying, less sense of belonging to their school community, and a lack of appropriate education, services, and protective measures and policies—all of which increase their risk for compromised mental health.[83–86]

Young Adults

Young people aged 15 to 24 are more likely to experience mental illness and/or substance use disorders than any other age group;[87] mental health problems often are associated with academic and financial stressors,[88] and for some, adjusting to disabilities.[89] For example, 34% of Ontario high-school students indicate a moderate-to-serious level of psychological distress (symptoms of depression and anxiety), and 14% indicate a serious level of psychological distress.[88] In addition, depression and anxiety have been reported to be increasing at alarmingly high rates in the postsecondary population. The proportion of Canadian university students who experienced at least one episode of disabling depression grew from 37.5% in 2013 to 44.4% in 2016, and the proportion of Canadian university students who experienced overwhelming anxiety at least once in the past year increased from 56.5% in 2013 to 64.5% in 2016*.[90,91] Even more alarming, in 2016, 13% of university students reported having considered suicide (9.3% in 2013); 8.7% engaged in self-harm behaviours (6.5% in 2013), and 2.1% reported to have attempted suicide (1.3% in 2013).[90,91]

The transition from high school to university and/or the work environment is a time of adjustment requiring new coping skills. It also is a time when young adults tend to experience disruptions in sleep, diet, and exercise patterns, with possible implications for mental health.[92] In addition,

---

*Forty-one schools from across Canada participated in the National College Health Assessment (NCHA), a US-based research survey that provides an overview of students' health habits, behaviours and perceptions.

many young adults begin their working lives in debt from their years in postsecondary education.[93,94] To compound this issue, unemployment rates for young adults have increased since the recession in the late 2000s; the unemployment rate for young adults is 14.3%, which is twice the national average (7.2%).[95] Moreover, young adults with poor mental health have an increased risk for future unemployment and disability pension.[96]

Middle-Aged Adults

People in their 40s, 50s, and early 60s commonly process information more slowly and are more vulnerable to distraction than in their youth. They use experience to compensate for age-related deficiencies in memory and reaction time. There is evidence that the brain can remain strong and even improve its performance well through the middle-age years, a period of maximum performance for some of the more complex, higher-order mental abilities such as inductive reasoning, spatial orientation, and vocabulary.[97] Moreover, middle age may also bring more confidence, more skill at quick assessment, and adaptability. Men reach their peak performance in these abilities in their 50s and women in their early 60s. Challenges during middle age require skills in organizing, problem solving, and multitasking. For example, family obligations peak for middle-aged adults who have good health and numerous older adult relatives and whose children are just moving out and establishing their own families. The effect of being "caught in the middle," albeit not a typical experience for most Canadian adults, may be severe.[98]

High demands and low social support within the workforce can cause the development of depressive symptoms among middle-aged workers. Job losses caused by firings or layoffs reduce health, self-esteem, and the sense of control.[99] Concurrently, daily stressors directly affect emotional and physical functioning, and the accumulation of persistent irritations and overloads may result in more serious stress reactions such as anxiety and depression. Middle-aged adults with high mastery (e.g., successful problem-solving skills) reported less emotional reactivity to stressors.[100]

Biological changes related to menopause or late onset male hypogonadism may influence cognition and well-being. Middle-aged people tend to reassess their achievements in terms of ideals and may subsequently make significant changes in day-to-day life or situations, such as career, work–life balance, marriage, romantic relationships, large expenditures, or physical appearance.[101]

Older Adults

The aging process leaves the parameters of mental health mostly intact. There is no decrease in general knowledge and little or no loss in vocabulary. Because it takes a bit longer for the brain to process information and react to it, performance on timed intelligence tests may be poorer for older adults. The slower response time affects new learning; older adults have difficulty responding to a rapidly paced new presentation.[102] Recent memory, which requires some processing (e.g., medication instructions, 24-hour diet recall), decreases

somewhat with aging. Intelligence and remote memory are not affected.

Age-related changes in sensory perception can affect mental functioning. For example, vision loss (as detailed in Chapter 15) may result in apathy, social isolation, and depression. Hearing changes are common (see the discussion of presbycusis in Chapter 16). Age-related hearing loss involves sounds of high frequencies. Consonants are high-frequency sounds, and so older adults who have difficulty hearing them have problems with normal conversation. This problem produces frustration, suspicion, and social withdrawal, and it makes the person look confused. Data analyzed from a large Canadian study suggested that older adults with overall functional impairment (e.g., inability to perform housework) exhibited more cognitive impairment 5 years later than did those without functional impairment.[103]

Meanwhile, the era of older adulthood contains much potential for loss of loved ones, job status and prestige income, energy, and resilience of the body. The grief and despair surrounding these losses can affect mental health and result in disorientation, disability, or depression.

SCREENING

In 2013, the Canadian Task Force on Preventive Health Care recommended that routine screening for depression is unnecessary in those adults (18 and over) in primary care settings who do not have apparent symptoms of depression and are at average risk for depression (weak recommendation; very low-quality evidence).[104,105] However, Thombs and colleagues noted that screening is effective if it successfully identifies depressed patients who are not already identified and treated and if the number of people incorrectly labelled as possibly depressed is minimized.[106] In studies in which the screening process was linked to an integrated system of treatment and follow-up, patient outcomes improved. More extensive patient education about depression, alertness and response to symptoms of depression, and targeting of specific at-risk groups, including older adults[107,108] and those individuals in the perinatal period (pregnancy up to one year postpartum)[109] is recommended.

In a cross-sectional study of Canadian women, Lanes, Kuk, and Tamim found that the national prevalence of minor/major and major postpartum depression symptomatology (PPDS) to be 8.46% and 8.69%, respectively.[110] A mother's stress level during pregnancy, the availability of support after pregnancy, and a prior diagnosis of depression were the characteristics that had the strongest significant association with the development of PPDS. Perinatal depression has broad-reaching consequences on the mother, baby, and family. Early detection and treatment can help eliminate or reduce the effects of perinatal depression, particularly for immigrant and adolescent moms found to be a most risk.[110]

Controversial evidence exists regarding the merits of universal screening for perinatal depression. The Canadian Task Force on Preventive Health Care recommended screening for perinatal depression only when symptoms are apparent; admittedly, this was not a strong recommendation because it was based on weak evidence available in the studies that met the review criteria.[105] However, although there is conflict about the value of universal screening, there is consensus about the importance of health care providers being aware of, and alert to, clinical clues and regularly inquiring about depressive symptoms.[109] The 10-item self-report Edinburgh Postnatal Depression Scale (EPDS)[111] is a depression screening tool commonly used worldwide for the perinatal period. It has been specifically validated in perinatal populations, and several studies have demonstrated its acceptability to women. Further assessment by a trained health care provider is required. Notably, a positive screen on the EPDS is not the same as a diagnosis of depression. The gold standard for diagnosis is a diagnostic assessment interview and confirmation of the suspected diagnosis with the DSM-5 criteria. Assessing the risk for suicide and potential risk to the baby are important components of the diagnostic assessment interview.[109]

A number of screening tools for depression are available; however, Dowrick cautioned that the use of screening instruments may encourage practitioners to take a reductionist, biomedical approach, which would divert attention from a broader biopsychosocial–spiritual approach to identifying depression. Instead, a thorough assessment is recommended.[112]

MENTAL HEALTH ASSESSMENT: ADULTS

Patients can perceive the mental health assessment as threatening, even though their cooperation is necessary for its success. Although many nurses find it desirable to establish some degree of rapport first and thereby place the patient at ease, some nurses assess mental health before working with the patient so that the findings can serve as a template against which to measure the accuracy of the rest of the health history; this is not a recommended practice. The successful clinician must develop a style in which much of the mental health assessment is performed through relatively unstructured observations made during history taking and physical examination. The way in which patients relate the history of the current situation and interact in the clinical setting reveals much about their mental health.

Identification/Biographical Information

Note the primary language spoken by the patient, the name the patient prefers to be called, legal name, address, telephone numbers, birthdate and birthplace, gender (remember gender identities include woman, man, trans, genderqueer, nonbinary, femme of centre, and two-spirit—see Chapter 3, Box 3.5), relationship status, ethnocultural background, education, and employment. Usually questions about this information are nonthreatening and thus a safe way to begin.

Reason for Seeking Care

Record the patient's explanation verbatim to describe the reason for the visit. Be knowledgeable of the psychiatric diagnoses (DSM-5) provided by the attending physician/

psychiatrist. Ask what the patient understands about the need to visit your agency.

Past Health

Past Illness, Injury, Hospitalization

Note childhood diseases, surgeries, and trauma (especially if any resulted in concussion or loss of consciousness). Ask about parental use of alcohol and drugs, birth trauma, any pattern of injury suggestive of childhood abuse or neglect, and any obstetrical history. Ask specifically, "Have you ever experienced or witnessed anything that threatened your life or safety or the life and safety of a loved one?" If the answer is "yes," ask for details, keeping in mind that psychological trauma is associated with many mental disorders (e.g., anxiety and depression).

Chronic Illnesses

The stress of chronic illnesses, even when well managed, may affect mental health.

Family Health History

Ask the age and current health of close relatives (e.g., partner, children, parents, siblings, grandparents, aunts, and uncles). If the patient reports a family member's death, ask for the date, the cause, and the effect on the patient. Ask about any illnesses that "run in the family" because many mental disorders are genetically linked and family health history provides information about the patient's risk factors. Ask about any history of postpartum depression because this can induce maternal physical, marital, social, and vocational difficulties; impair maternal–infant interactions; and affect an infant's cognitive and emotional development.[113] Assessing family health identifies sources of social support, family stress, coping ability, and resources.

Current Health

Using a systematic approach to ensure comprehensiveness, sort and cluster information about conditions that affect patient mental health, overall functioning, and quality of life. In addition to asking the patient to describe the critical characteristics of specific concerns outlined in Chapter 5, note the following:

1. Known allergies, type of reaction, and usual treatment and relief measures.
2. Status of immunizations, human immunodeficiency virus (HIV), infection, and hepatitis infection. Persons experiencing mental illness may often dwell in poverty, lack knowledge and supports for health promotion, and have lifestyles that put them at risk for communicable diseases.
3. Current medications. Specify the name of the medication, purpose, usual dose, frequency, effectiveness, adverse effects, name of prescriber, duration of taking the medication, and any over-the-counter and herbal preparations. This information helps identify health maintenance behaviours, medication interactions, and potential knowledge deficits.

DETAILED MENTAL STATUS EXAMINATION

The mental status examination, an integral subset of the comprehensive mental health nursing assessment, involves a sequence of steps that form a *hierarchy* in which the most basic functions (consciousness, language) are assessed first. Accurate assessment of the first steps ensures validity for the steps that follow; that is, if consciousness is clouded, then the patient cannot be expected to have full attention and cooperate with new learning. If language is impaired, subsequent assessment of new learning or abstract reasoning (which requires language functioning) can yield erroneous conclusions. Strive to ask questions that can be corroborated, to enhance reliability.

PREPARATION

Record the exact time and date of the mental status examination because the mental status can change quickly, as in delirium.

EQUIPMENT NEEDED

Pencil, paper, reading material (occasionally)

Normal Range of Findings	Abnormal Findings
Appearance	
Posture. Posture is erect, and position is relaxed.	Sitting on edge of chair or curled in bed, tense muscles, frowning, darting eyes, and restless pacing may occur with anxiety and/or hyperthyroidism. Sitting slumped in chair, walking slowly, and dragging feet may occur with depression and some organic brain diseases.
Body Movements. Body movements are voluntary, deliberate, coordinated, smooth, and even.	Restless, fidgety movements may occur with anxiety. Apathy and psychomotor slowing may occur with depression and organic brain disease. Abnormal posturing and bizarre gestures may occur with schizophrenia. Facial grimaces may be associated with conditions such as cerebral palsy, chorea, hypocalcemia, tetanus, pain, tardive dyskinesia, tic disorder, and Tourette's syndrome.
Dress. Dress is appropriate for setting, season, age, gender, and social group. Clothing fits and is put on appropriately.	Dress can be inappropriate with organic brain syndrome. Eccentric dress combination and bizarre makeup may occur with schizophrenia or manic syndrome.
Grooming and Hygiene. The patient is clean and well-groomed; hair is neat and clean; women have moderate or no makeup; men are shaved, or beard or moustache is well-groomed. Nails are clean (though some jobs leave nails chronically dirty). Use care in interpreting clothing that is dishevelled, bizarre, or in poor repair; piercings; and tattoos, because these sometimes reflect the person's economic status or a deliberate fashion trend (especially among adolescents).	Unilateral neglect (total inattention to one side of body) may occur after stroke. Inappropriate dress, poor hygiene, and lack of concern with appearance occur with depression and severe Alzheimer's disease. Meticulously dressed and groomed appearance and fastidious manner may occur with obsessive–compulsive disorder (OCD). *Note:* A dishevelled appearance in a previously well-groomed patient is significant.
Behaviour	
Level of Consciousness. The patient is awake, alert, and aware of stimuli from the environment and within the self and responds appropriately to stimuli.	Altered levels of consciousness may include coma (unresponsiveness); stupor (responsiveness to pain), and lethargy (drowsiness; see Table 6.2).

Normal Range of Findings	Abnormal Findings

Facial Expression. The expression is appropriate to the situation and changes appropriately with the topic. There is comfortable eye contact unless precluded by cultural norm (e.g., for members of some Indigenous cultures).

Speech. Judge the quality of speech by noting that the patient makes laryngeal sounds effortlessly and makes conversation appropriately. Note whether the voice is raised or muffled, whether the replies to questions are one-word or elaborative, and how fast or slow the patient speaks.

Normally, the pace of the conversation is moderate, and stream of talking is fluent.

Articulation (ability to form words) is clear and understandable.

Word choice is effortless and appropriate to educational level. The patient completes sentences, occasionally pausing to think.

Mood and Affect. Judge this by body language and facial expression and by the answer to the direct question "How do you feel today?" or "How do you feel most days?" Ask about the length of a particular mood, whether the mood has been reactive or not, and whether the mood has been stable or unstable. The affect (expression) should be appropriate to the mood and change appropriately with topics.

Cognitive Functions

Orientation. You can discern orientation through the course of the interview, or you may ask for it directly but tactfully: "Some people have trouble keeping up with the dates while in the hospital. Do you know today's date?" Assess the patient's orientation:

Time: day of week, date, year, season
Place: where person lives, present location, type of building, names of city and province
Person: who examiner is, type of worker
Self: person's own name, age

Many hospitalized patients normally have trouble with the exact date but are fully oriented on the remaining items.

Attention Span. Check ability to concentrate by noting whether the patient completes a thought without wandering. Note any distractibility or difficulty attending to you. An alternative approach is to give a series of directions to follow in a correct sequence of behaviours, such as "Please put this label on your keys, place the keys into the brown envelope, and give the envelope to the clerk for safe keeping during your admission."

Abnormal Findings

Expression may be flat and masklike with parkinsonism and depression.

Dysphonia is abnormal volume and pitch. Patient may monopolize the interview or may remain silent, secretive, or uncommunicative.

Speech may be slow and monotonous with parkinsonism and depression. Speech may be rapid-fire, pressured, and loud with manic syndrome.

Dysarthria is distorted speech. Misuse of words; omitting letters, syllables, or words; and transposing words occur with aphasia.

Unduly long word-finding or failure in word search occurs with aphasia.

Table 6.3 lists mood and affect abnormalities. Wide mood swings occur with manic syndrome. Altered mood states are apparent in schizophrenia. Heightened emotional activity and severely limited emotional or elicited responses (e.g., "OK," "Rough," and "Don't know") necessitate further questioning for clarification of mood.

Disorientation occurs with organic brain disorders, such as delirium and dementia. Orientation is usually lost in this order: first to time, then to place, and rarely to person and self. Disorientation to personal identity is associated with postepileptic seizure states, other dissociative disorders, and agnosia (loss of the ability to recognize sensory inputs).

Attention span is commonly impaired in persons who experience anxiety, fatigue, medication intoxication, or attention-deficit/hyperactivity disorder (ADHD). Impairment is conveyed as confusion, negativism, digression from initial thought, irrelevant replies to questions, or being "stimulus bound" (i.e., any new stimulus quickly draws attention).

Normal Range of Findings	Abnormal Findings

Normal Range of Findings

Immediate Memory. Immediate memory enables making sense of what is going on. For example, it is used during reading to recall what happens sentence by sentence. Assess by asking the patient to recall a statement you just made.

Recent Memory. Assess recent memory in the context of the interview by the 24-hour diet recall or by asking what time the patient arrived at the agency. Ask verifiable questions to screen for the occasional person who confabulates (makes up) answers to fill in the gaps of memory loss.

Remote Memory. In the context of the interview, ask the patient about verifiable past events; for example, ask to describe historical events that are relevant for the patient.

New Learning: The Four Unrelated Words Test. This tests the patient's ability to acquire new memories. It is a highly sensitive and valid memory test that avoids the danger of unverifiable material.

Say to the patient, "I am going to say four words. I want you to remember them. In a few minutes I will ask you to recall them." To be sure that the patient has understood, repeat the words. Pick four words with semantic and phonetic diversity:

1. brown	1. fun
2. honesty	2. carrot
3. tulip	3. ankle
4. eyedropper	4. loyalty

After 5 minutes, ask the patient to recall the four words. To test the duration of memory, ask for a recall at 10 minutes and at 30 minutes. The normal response for persons younger than 60 years of age is an accurate three- or four-word recall after a 5-, 10-, and 30-minute delay.[114]

Additional Testing for Patients With Aphasia

Word Comprehension. Point to articles in the room, and ask the patient to name them.

Reading. An awareness of a patient's reading and writing impairment is important in planning health teaching and rehabilitation. To assess reading, ask the patient to read available print, being careful not to test just literacy.

Writing. Ask the patient to compose and write a sentence. Note coherence, spelling, and parts of speech (the sentence should have a subject and verb).

Abnormal Findings

Head injury, fatigue, anxiety, and strong emotions can affect immediate memory.

The individual affected may demonstrate repetition (e.g., asking the same question) and difficulty finding words during conversation, which may lead to frustration.

Recent memory deficit occurs with organic disorders, such as delirium, dementia, amnesia, or, in chronic alcoholism, Korsakoff's syndrome.

Remote memory is lost when the cortical storage area for that memory is damaged, as in Alzheimer's dementia or any disease that damages the cerebral cortex.

People with Alzheimer's dementia score a zero- or one-word recall. Ability for new learning is also impaired with anxiety (because of inattention and distractibility) and depression (because of a lack of interest or motivation).

Aphasia is the loss of ability to speak or to understand speech, as a result of a stroke.

Speech and language dyslexia, a neurological disorder or learning disability, may create difficulty understanding what other people say (developmental receptive language disorder) or difficulty using spoken language to communicate (developmental expressive language disorder).

Aphasia may limit ability to understand written words. Speech and language dyslexia may create difficulty producing speech sounds (developmental articulation disorder). The individual might mispronounce certain letters or letter combinations. With academic learning dyslexia, the individual cannot identify different word sounds.

Aphasia may limit ability to write coherently. Dyslexia may affect writing abilities, and performance in written language examinations will be very poor. With developmental writing disorder, or dysgraphia, the individual has problems with handwriting or with creating sentences that make sense to others.

| **Normal Range of Findings** | **Abnormal Findings** |

Higher Intellectual Function

Tests of higher intellectual functioning measure problem-solving and reasoning abilities. Results correspond closely to the patient's general intelligence and must be assessed in view of educational and cultural backgrounds. These tests have been widely used to distinguish between organic brain disease and psychiatric disorders; however, there is little evidence that most of these tests validly detect organic dysfunction or have relevance for daily clinical care. Thus, many time-honoured, standard tests of higher intellectual function (such as proverb interpretation) are not discussed here.

Many mental illnesses are associated with varying levels of insight. For example, people with OCD often have relatively good insight that they have a problem and that their thoughts and actions are unreasonable, but they are nonetheless compelled to carry out the thoughts and actions.[115]

Insight and Judgement

Insight is the ability to recognize one's own illness, need for treatment, and consequences of one's behaviour as stemming from an illness.

Patients exercise judgement when they compare and evaluate the alternatives in a situation and reach an appropriate course of action. To assess judgement in the context of the interview, note what the patient says about job plans and social or family obligations; plans for the future; and capacity for violent or suicidal behaviour. Job and future plans should be realistic, in view of the patient's health situation. To assess insight into illness, ask whether patients believe they need help or whether they believe their feelings or conditions are normal.

Further assess insight by asking patients to describe their rationale for personal health care and how they decided about whether to comply with prescribed health regimens. The patient's actions and decisions should be realistic.

Persons with Alzheimer's disease, schizophrenia, or various psychotic conditions tend to have poor awareness that anything is wrong with them.[116] Judgement is impaired (unrealistic or impulsive decisions) with intellectual disability, emotional dysfunction, schizophrenia, and organic brain disease.

Thought Processes, Thought Content, and Perceptions

Thought Processes. Ask yourself, "Does this person make sense? Can I follow what the person is saying?" Note whether the patient responds directly to the questions or deviates from the subject at hand and has to be guided back to the topic more than once.

The *way* a patient thinks should be logical, goal directed, coherent, and relevant. The patient should complete a thought.

Table 6.4 lists examples of abnormal thought processes.

Normal Range of Findings

Thought Content. *What* the patient says should be consistent and logical. To identify any obsessions or compulsions, ask questions such as these:

"How often do you wash your hands or count things over and over?"
"Do you perform specific actions to reduce certain thoughts?"

Explore ritualistic behaviours further to determine the severity of the obsession or compulsion.

To identify any fears that cause the patient to avoid certain situations, ask if he or she has any fears, such as fear of animals, needles, heights, snakes, public speaking, or crowds.

To determine whether a person is having delusions, ask, "Do you have any thoughts that other people think are strange?" or "Do you have any special powers or abilities?"

Perceptions. The patient should be consistently aware of reality, and his or her perceptions should be congruent with yours. Ask the following:

"How do people treat you?"
"Do you feel as if you are being watched, followed, or controlled?"
"Is your imagination very active?"
"Have you heard your name when you're alone?"

If the responses to these questions suggest that a person is experiencing hallucinations, ask some of the following questions: "Do you ever hear voices when no one else is around?" "Can you sometimes see things that no one else can see?" "Do you have other unexplained sensations such as smells, sounds, or feelings?"

If command-type hallucinations are experienced, always ask what the person will do in response. For example, "When the voices tell you to do something, do you obey their instructions or ignore them?"

Abnormal Findings

Persons with OCD often demonstrate both obsessions (obsessive thoughts, ideas, or fears) and compulsions (repetitive rituals to reduce anxiety and stress in response to obsessions). Obsessions are annoying, fearful, at times harmful, and driven by different motives (e.g., fear of being hurt or hurting others, fear of infections or contamination, and need to make everything clean and orderly). Obsessions may have a religious, medical, sexual, or sadistic underpinning. Compulsions bring temporary relief but do not eliminate the obsessions. For example, if a person is afraid of germs and washes hands again and again, every washing does not make the person believe that hands are already clean enough and that there is no danger of receiving germs anymore; thus repeated washing continues. Table 6.5 lists examples of disordered thought content.

Delusions are false beliefs that occur when abnormal significance is attached to a genuine perception without rational or emotional justification. Types of delusions include grandiose (delusions of grandeur, entitlement), religious (belief that one *is* a [or the] deity), persecution (belief that someone wants to cause the patient harm), erotomanic (belief that someone famous is in love with the patient), jealousy (belief that everyone wants what the patient has), thought insertion (belief that someone is putting ideas into the patient's mind), and ideas of reference (belief that everything refers to the patient).

Illusions (misinterpretation of a true optical, auditory, tactile, or olfactory sensation). For example, a brown sock on the floor appears to be a mouse.

Hallucinations (perceptions occurring while the patient is awake and conscious and in the absence of external stimuli): Auditory and visual hallucinations occur with psychiatric and organic brain disease and with ingestion of psychedelic drugs. Tactile hallucinations occur with alcohol withdrawal.

SUPPLEMENTAL MENTAL STATUS EXAMINATION

The Mini-Cog test and the Addenbrooke's Cognitive Examination-Revised (ACE-R) are the best alternative screening tests for dementia, and the MoCA tool is the best alternative screening test for MCI.[117] The Mini-Cog test is brief and takes 3 minutes to administer; it can increase detection of cognitive impairment in older adults. It is useful in detecting Alzheimer's and related dementia. It can be used effectively after brief training in both health care and community settings. It consists of two components: (a) a three-item recall test for memory and (b) a simply scored clock-drawing test. As a screening test, however, it is not a substitute for a complete diagnostic workup.[117]

The Rowland Universal Dementia Assessment Scale (RUDAS), a multicultural cognitive assessment scale, is a short cognitive screening instrument designed to minimize the effects of cultural learning and language diversity on the assessment of baseline cognitive performance. When administering the RUDAS, it is recommended that patients communicate in the language they are most competent and comfortable in. Before administering the RUDAS, health care providers should read the test instructions carefully.[118]

FUNCTIONAL ASSESSMENT (INCLUDING ACTIVITIES OF DAILY LIVING)

Record the dates of the most recent medical examination, eye examination, and dental examination. Ask the patient to describe a typical day and what the patient does on a daily, weekly, and annual basis to promote and maintain health. Assess self-care abilities, including activities of daily living (ADLs) such as bathing, hygiene, dressing, toileting, eating, walking, housekeeping, shopping, cooking, communicating with others, social relationships, finances, and coping. In particular, note the following:

Nutritional patterns. Record the dietary intake recalled by the patient over the past 24 hours (Chapter 12). Ask whether any recent dietary changes have occurred. Note any dissatisfaction with body size, weight, or shape, as well as practices directed at weight loss, particularly if the patient is female, an elite athlete, or engaged in an occupation that emphasizes physical appearance, inasmuch as these factors contribute to eating disorders.

Sleep/rest changes. Ask about sleep onset (how much time it takes to fall asleep), sleep maintenance (frequency of wakening and returning to sleep), early awakening (before the patient needs to be awake), sleep hygiene (measures to promote sleep, such as avoiding caffeine at bedtime), and sleep satisfaction (feeling rested and refreshed). Alterations in sleep are common in many mental disorders (e.g., mania, depression, schizophrenia).

Activity/mobility. Withdrawal from usual activities may signal illness. Avolition (lack of motivational drive and energy) is a symptom of depression, schizophrenia, and chronic marijuana use. Excessive pursuit of physical activity may be associated with mania and eating disorders.

Elimination. Psychotropic medications may lead to constipation and urinary retention. People may misuse laxatives and diuretics in an attempt to lose weight.

Interpersonal relationships and resources. Assess the patient's role in family and social networks to identify sources of stress, support and connectedness. Any withdrawal from usual relationships could indicate declining mental health.

Self-esteem/self-concept. Ask the patient to rate self on a scale from 0 to 10, on which 10 represents the best possible way to feel about self. Ask about values, beliefs, practices, and accomplishments that are most important to the patient.

Spirituality. Ask questions to understand the meaning of faith, spirituality, and religion. For example:

> *"What is it that gives your life meaning? What gives you joy?"*
> *"What, if any, religious activities do you participate in?"*
> *"Do you feel connected with the world?"*
> *"Do you believe in God, the Creator, or a higher power?"*

Coping and stress management. Ask about major stressors to understand and evaluate current coping behaviours. For example:

> *"What stressors would you say are most evident in your life at this time?"*
> *"What are those activities you engage with to alleviate stress?"*
> *"What helps you most to alleviate stress?"*

Smoking, substance use, and problem gambling. Inquire about usual patterns of alcohol use, drug use, and gambling and about any recent changes to those patterns. Ask whether persons close to the patient would believe that alcohol, drug use, or gambling is a problem in the patient's life.

Home and environmental hazards. Ask about safety issues associated with meal preparation, bathing, walking in the home and community, lighting, home heating, transportation to health care clinics, social and commercial services, and social events.

RISK ASSESSMENT

Screen for Suicidal Thoughts

It is difficult to question patients about possible suicidal wishes, especially for novice examiners who may fear invading privacy and may have their own normal discomfort with death and suicide. However, the risk is far greater if you skip these questions; you may be the only health care provider to detect clues of suicide risk.

When the patient expresses sadness, hopelessness, despair, or grief, assess any possible risk that the patient will cause physical self-harm. Begin with more general questions; if you hear affirmative answers, continue with more specific questions. For example:

"Have you ever felt so blue you thought of hurting yourself?"
"Do you feel like hurting yourself now?"
"Do you have a plan to hurt yourself?"
"What would happen if you were dead?"
"How would other people react if you were dead?"

Inquire directly about specific plans, suicide notes, family history (anniversary reaction), and impulse control. Use a matter-of-fact tone of voice and open posture, and attend with interest (e.g., lean toward the person). If you are unsure whether the patient is at high risk for suicide, get help from an experienced health care team leader.

Important clues and warning signs of suicide are as follows:

- A precise suicide plan to take place in the next 24 to 48 hours with the use of a lethal method (constitutes high risk)
- Prior suicide attempts
- Depression, hopelessness
- Social withdrawal, running away
- Self-mutilation
- Hypersomnia or insomnia
- Slowed psychomotor activity
- Anorexia
- Verbal suicide messages (defeat, failure, worthlessness, loss, giving up, desire to kill self)
- Death themes in art, jokes, writing, behaviours
- Saying goodbye (giving away prized possessions)

You are responsible for encouraging the patient to talk about suicidal thoughts and for obtaining immediate help. Determine whether the patient will agree to make a commitment to treatment and living and to contract for safety by agreeing to implement a plan such as calling a crisis hotline or going to the emergency department.

Although you cannot always prevent a suicide, you can often buy time so that the patient can be helped to find an alternative solution to problems. As soon as possible, share with the health care team any concerns you have about a person's suicide ideation.

Screen for Assaultive or Homicidal Ideation

In addition to assessing suicide threat, inquire about past acts of self-harm or violence:

"Do you have any thoughts of wanting to hurt anyone?"
"Do you have any feelings or thoughts that you wish someone were dead?"

If the reply to either question is positive, ask about any specific plans to injure someone and how the patient plans to control these feelings if they occur again.

Screen for Elopement Risk

Elopement from psychiatric facilities increases the risk for injury for patients and others in the community and increases the potential for litigation against the facility.[119] To reduce risk, check the following:

- Are the doors locked? Are they unlocked manually (not electronically) so that the patient does not slip out with visitors?
- Is the patient restricted to the unit, or does the patient have off-unit privileges?
- Does the patient have an adequate understanding of the need for hospitalization?
- Does the family have adequate knowledge of the risk for elopement?
- Should the patient be placed in hospital clothing, with street clothing and shoes removed, to discourage elopement?
- Has the patient been placed on increased observation status?

GLOBAL ASSESSMENT OF FUNCTIONING

The Global Assessment of Functioning is performed by the psychiatrist or qualified clinician. It is used to estimate overall psychological, social, and occupational functioning within any limitations imposed by patient physical and environmental factors. The findings are scored from low functioning (0 to 10) to high functioning (91 to 100); the scores change over time, and scoring is calculated at the start of treatment, during treatment, at discharge, and at any time after (Table 6.6).

Additional content on mental disorders is listed in Tables 6.7 (delirium and dementia), 6.8 (schizophrenia), 6.9 (mood disorders), and 6.10 (anxiety disorders).

ASSESSING PATIENT ATTITUDE TOWARD THE EXAMINER/ASSESSMENT

Record whether the patient appears hostile, defensive, guarded, or uncomfortable. Often, the patient is willing to cooperate and appears interested, friendly, relaxed, or perhaps bored with the interview process. Of note, hostility could be associated with previous negative experiences and even trauma associated with previous health care or other experiences (e.g., stigma and discrimination).

DEVELOPMENTAL CONSIDERATIONS

Normal Range of Findings	Abnormal Findings

Children and Adolescents

Essentially, you will follow the same guidelines (assessing appearance, behaviour, cognition, and thought processes) as for adults, with an emphasis on developmental milestones. Thorough knowledge of developmental milestones, as presented in the online Evolve resources accompanying this book, is critical. Although not exclusive to mental health assessment, the Nipissing District Developmental Screen (NDDS; see Chapter 2) is a screening tool designed to help parents and caregivers monitor children's development from birth to 6 years of age. Areas assessed include vision, hearing, communication, gross motor, fine motor, cognitive, social–emotional, and self-help skills.

Other reliable screening instruments (e.g., the Pediatric Symptom Checklist-17) can be given to the parent to assess emotional and behavioural wellness of children aged 4 to 18 years.[120] It is important to remember anxiety in children often is misdiagnosed as attention-deficit/hyperactivity disorder (ADHD), learning disabilities, or other disorders. For adolescents, continue to follow the same guidelines as described for adults. In consideration of adolescent development patterns, specifically evaluate weight in the appearance assessment; regulation (e.g., self-soothing capacity and anger management skills) in the behaviour assessment; and sleep patterns, eating patterns, interpersonal behaviours (with parents, teachers, and examiner), risk (to self and others), high-risk behaviours (e.g., bullying/fire setting/running away/high-risk sexual activity/cruelty/breaking curfew/lying/stealing/truancy), academic performance (grade, least and most favourite subjects), and substance use with the cognition and thought processes assessments.[5]

Abnormalities are often problems of *omission*; the child does not achieve an expected milestone.

Trust is a particular challenge in working with adolescents. Responses to questions in areas of behaviour risk and personal safety are apt to be guarded unless the examiner has developed rapport with the adolescent. When possible, it is preferred that you interview the adolescent first, before meeting with parents/guardians.

Adults and Older Adults

Always conduct even a brief examination of all older adults. Check sensory status before assessing their mental health. It is recommended that you take time, reduce distractions, and minimize sensory impairments to help older adults maintain their dignity and perform at their actual level of ability.

Age is the greatest risk factor for Alzheimer's disease: 10% of people older than 65 and almost 50% of those older than 85 receive a diagnosis of Alzheimer's disease.[121] By 2021, 17.8% of the total Canadian population will be over 65—that is nearly 7 million people. Canada now has more people aged 65 and older (16.1%) than people younger than 15 (16%).[122]

Follow the guidelines as described for adults with the *additional* considerations listed in the Older Adult Mental Health Assessment (see next description).

More than 33% of older adults admitted to acute care medical and surgical services show varying degrees of confusion.

OLDER ADULT MENTAL HEALTH ASSESSMENT

Normal Range of Findings	Abnormal Findings

Behaviour

Level of Consciousness. Scales such as the Glasgow Coma Scale (see Chapter 25) that give a numerical value to the person's response avoid ambiguity when numerous examiners care for the same person.

Patients with altered levels of consciousness were found to present with stroke or transient ischemic attack (TIA), diabetes, alcohol use, substance use, and seizures.[123]

Normal Range of Findings	Abnormal Findings

Cognitive Functions

Orientation. Older adults may not provide the precise date or complete name of the clinic or setting. You may consider older adults oriented to time if the year and month are correctly stated. Orientation to place is considered acceptable if the patient correctly identifies the type of setting (e.g., the hospital) and the name of the town.

New Learning. In people of normal cognitive function, an age-related decline occurs in performance in the Four Unrelated Words Test described on p. 91. Persons in the eighth decade average two of four words recalled over 5 minutes. Their performance improves at 10 and 30 minutes after being reminded by verbal cues (e.g., "one word was a colour; a common flower in Holland is _____").

Confusion or inability to correctly identify season, name of hometown, name of family members.

In people with Alzheimer's dementia, performance does not improve on subsequent trials.

Supplemental Mental Status Examination

Set Test. The set test was developed specifically for use with older adults. In the original study,[124] people 65 to 85 years of age were tested. It is a quantifiable test, designed to screen for dementia. The test is easy to administer and takes less than 5 minutes. Ask the patient to name 10 items in each of four categories or sets: fruits, animals, colours, and towns (FACT). Do not coach, prompt, or hurry the person. Each correct answer is scored one point. The maximum total score is 40. No one with a score over 25 has been found to have dementia. (Note: Because this is a verbal test, do not use it with persons with hearing impairments or aphasia.)

The set test assesses mental function as a whole instead of examining individual parts of cognitive function. By asking the person to categorize, name, remember, and count the items in the test, you are really assessing this person's alertness, motivation, concentration, short-term memory, and problem-solving ability.

Clock Test. The patient is asked to draw a clock face to depict a specific time, which requires a variety of cognitive functions, including long-term memory, auditory processing, visual–spatial acuity, concentration, numerical knowledge, and abstract thinking. The advantages to this type of screening tool are the short time it takes to administer (approximately 2 minutes), its ability to be used by individuals with little or no experience in cognitive assessment and minimal training in test administration, and its excellent interrater reliability and sensitivity for differentiating patients with mild Alzheimer's disease from patients without Alzheimer's disease when scored by clinicians with expertise in dementia.[125] Clock-drawing tests are not recommended for use as the sole screening tools for dementia because the results are influenced by the severity of the cognitive impairment, limited education, and advanced age.[126]

Set Test scores lower than 15 indicate dementia. Scores between 15 and 24 show less association with dementia and should be evaluated carefully.

Someone with a delirium might exhibit disorganized thinking, poor planning and reasoning ability; poor visuospatial ability; and distractibility while attempting to focus on the task.

DOCUMENTATION AND CRITICAL THINKING

Sample Charting

Appearance: Posture is erect, with no involuntary body movements. Dress and grooming are appropriate for season and setting.

Behaviour: Alert, with appropriate facial expression and fluent, understandable speech. Affect and verbal responses are appropriate.

Cognitive functions: Oriented to time, place, person, and self. Able to attend cooperatively with examiner. Recent and remote memory intact. Can recall four unrelated words at 5-, 10-, and 30-minute intervals. Future plans include returning to home and to local university once individual therapy is established and medication is adjusted.

Thought processes: Perceptions and thought processes are logical and coherent. No suicide ideation.

Focused Assessment: Clinical Case Study

SUBJECTIVE

Mr. Ernie Acte (E.A.) is an 84-year-old First Nations Elder, recently hospitalized for evaluation of increasing memory loss, confusion, and socially unusual behaviour (e.g., wandering into his neighbour's home). His wife Eleanor died 5 years ago and his oldest son died quite suddenly of heart failure 2 years ago. His two other sons, daughter, and one of his granddaughters visit daily, and they concur that E.A.'s hygiene and grooming have decreased (he used to be impeccably dressed); E.A. eats very little, has lost weight, does not sleep through the night, displays angry emotional outbursts that are unlike his former demeanour, and does not recognize the greatgrandchildren with whom he has had very close relationships. According to his children and granddaughter, E.A. has drifted away from the stove while cooking, allowing food to burn on the stovetop. One of his sons who has moved into his house with him (specialization: has found him wandering through the house in the middle of the night, unsure of where he is. He used to go for walks to visit his family (most of whom live close by). However, more recently he has become quite isolated in his home, except on the occasions where he has been found wandering. His son has been wanting him to move in with him. E.A. has been resistant to this idea.*

*Case scenario created in collaboration with Ms. Sukhi Brar, RN, BScN, MScN, Clinical Nurse (Specialization: Geriatric Mental Health), Western University.

OBJECTIVE

During this hospitalization, E.A. underwent a series of medical tests, including related blood work and urinalysis to rule out delirium (e.g., complete blood count [CBC], electrolytes, liver function test [LFT]), a lumbar puncture, electroencephalography, and computed tomography of the head, all of which yielded normal findings. His physician suggests a diagnosis of Alzheimer's type dementia.

Appearance: E.A. is sitting quietly, somewhat slumped, picking at loose threads on his large bulky sweater, which he is wearing over a checkered flannel shirt. His thick grey hair is tucked under his cap.

Behaviour: E.A. is awake and gazing out the window. His son and daughter are in the room with him. However, he is uncommunicative. His expression is flat and vacant. He makes eye contact when called by name, although his gaze quickly shifts back to the window. His speech is a bit slow but articulate; he has some trouble with word finding. No overt signs of agitation are noted.

Cognitive functions: E.A. is oriented to person and place. He can state the season but not the day of the week or the year. He is not able to repeat the correct sequence of complex directions involving lifting and shifting a glass of water to the other hand. He scores a one-word recall on the Four Unrelated Words Test. He cannot tell the examiner how he would plan a grocery-shopping trip, an activity he has been engaged with since his wife died 5 years ago. The RUDAS (as noted on p. 94) should be considered for use with E.A. to assess baseline cognitive performance.

Thought processes: E.A. experiences blocking in train of thought. His thought content is logical. He acts cranky and suspicious with family members. He reports no suicide ideation. His MoCA score is 16.[†74,127]

[†]Scores on the MoCA range from 0 to 30, with a score of 26 and higher generally considered normal. Normal controls in the original study of the MoCA had an average score of 27.4, compared with 22.1 in people with mild cognitive impairment (MCI) and 16.2 in people with Alzheimer's disease.

ASSESSMENT

Examples of Nursing Assessment Statements That May Be Relevant to E.A.

Impaired verbal communication: Cerebral impairment, as demonstrated by altered memory and judgement.

Shifts in abilities related to ADLs: Inattention to hygiene, nutrition, and sleep needs.

Altered nutrition: Reduced intake and weight loss.

Impaired social interaction: Cognitive impairment and withdrawal from others.

Risk for injury: Cognitive impairment, as demonstrated by leaving stove cooking unattended, confusion, and wandering behaviour.

Risk of harm: Related to angry outbursts.

Overall Goals

Help E.A. achieve his highest level of safety and independence in areas such as nutrition, ADLs, grooming, and social interaction by promoting his strengths and remaining capabilities. Family could be an excellent source of collateral information regarding E.A.

Sample Interventions

Ensure that any aids for vision and hearing are positioned correctly and in good working order. Each time you begin a conversation with E.A., make eye contact, identify yourself, and call him by name. Communicate slowly and clearly through short conversations, single-step instructions, and repetition; reduce background distractions such as television. Allow E.A. enough time to process questions and formulate responses. Observe his verbal and nonverbal communications, and show interest in what he is communicating. It would be important to know if E.A. speaks his Indigenous language; use key words from the patient's language of choice. Do not interrupt when E.A. is trying to communicate an idea because this may distract him and cause him to lose his train of thought. Unless you are conducting a supplemental mental status assessment, it may be helpful to supply a word that he is struggling to find. Speak in a low-pitched voice while maintaining an open, calm, and friendly communication manner. Provide cues and gentle reminders. Include family as much as possible if this comforts E.A.

It is important to remember to break down tasks into very basic steps (e.g., [1] Pick up hairbrush, [2] brush front of hair, [3] brush back of hair, [4] put hair brush down).

Assess capabilities regularly; you want to refrain from assuming that current capabilities are based on current status. Also, remember that every behaviour has meaning. It may be E.A.'s way of showing he is in distress or wants something. For example, he may be looking for someone if he is found wandering. It is important to address the underlying reason for the observed behaviours.

Evaluation and Reassessment

Evaluate mental health at least partially during every shift and reassess in full when a change in status is observed.

ABNORMAL FINDINGS

TABLE 6.2   Levels of Consciousness

The terms below are commonly used in clinical practice. To increase clarity when using these terms, also record the following:

1. The level of stimulus used (ranging progressively from the following):
   - Name called in normal tone of voice
   - Name called in loud voice
   - Light touch on person's arm
   - Vigorous shake of shoulder
   - Pain applied
2. The patient's response:
   - Amount and quality of movement
   - Presence and coherence of speech
   - Opening of eyes and making eye contact
3. What the patient does on cessation of your stimulus

Continued

TABLE 6.2	Levels of Consciousness—cont'd

Alert

Awake or readily aroused, oriented, fully aware of external and internal stimuli and responds appropriately, conducts meaningful interpersonal interactions

Lethargic (or Somnolent)

Not fully alert, drifts off to sleep when not stimulated, can be aroused to name when called in normal voice but looks drowsy, responds appropriately to questions or commands but thinking seems slow and fuzzy, inattentive, loses train of thought, spontaneous movements are decreased

Obtunded

(Transitional state between lethargy and stupor)

Sleeps most of time, difficult to arouse: needs loud shout or vigorous shake, acts confused when is aroused, converses in monosyllables, speech may be mumbled and incoherent, requires constant stimulation for even marginal cooperation

Stupor or Semicoma

Spontaneously unconscious, responds only to persistent and vigorous shake or pain; has appropriate motor response (i.e., withdraws hand to avoid pain); otherwise can only groan, mumble, or move restlessly; reflex activity persists

Coma

Completely unconscious, no response to pain or to any external or internal stimuli (e.g., when suctioned, does not try to push the catheter away); in light coma, has some reflex activity but no purposeful movement; in deep coma, has no motor response

Acute Confusional State (Delirium)

Clouding of consciousness (dulled cognition, impaired alertness); inattentive; incoherent conversation; impaired recent memory and confabulatory for recent events; often agitated and having visual hallucinations; disoriented, with confusion worse at night when environmental stimuli are decreased

Adapted from Porth, C. (2007). *Essentials of pathophysiology: Concepts of altered health states.* Hagerstown, MD: Lippincott Williams & Wilkins (p. 835).

TABLE 6.3	Abnormalities of Mood and Affect

Type of Mood or Affect	Definition	Clinical Example
Flat affect (blunted affect)	Lack of emotional response; no expression of feelings; voice monotonous and face immobile	Topic varies, expression does not
Depression	Sad, gloomy, dejected; symptoms may occur with rainy weather, after a holiday, or with an illness; if the situation is temporary, symptoms fade quickly	The patient says, "I've got the blues."
Depersonalization (lack of ego boundaries)	Loss of identity, feeling estranged, perplexed about own identity and meaning of existence	The patient says, "I don't feel real" or "I feel as if I'm not really here."
Elation	Joy and optimism, overconfidence, increased motor activity, not necessarily pathological	The patient says, "I'm feeling very happy."
Euphoria	Excessive well-being, unusually cheerful or elated state that is inappropriate considering physical and mental condition; implies a pathological mood	The patient says, "I am high," "I feel like I'm flying," or "I feel on top of the world."
Anxiety	Worried, uneasy, apprehensive from the anticipation of a danger whose source is unknown	The patient says, "I feel nervous and high strung," "I worry all the time," or "I can't seem to make up my mind."
Fear	Worried, uneasy, apprehensive; external danger is known and identified	Fear of flying in airplanes
Irritability	Annoyed, easily provoked, impatient	Internalizing a feeling of tension, so that a seemingly mild stimulus "sets off" the patient

TABLE 6.3	Abnormalities of Mood and Affect—cont'd	
Type of Mood or Affect	Definition	Clinical Example
Rage	Furious, loss of control	Expressing violent behaviour toward self or others
Ambivalence	The existence of opposing emotions toward an idea, object, person	Feeling love and hate toward another person at the same time
Lability	Rapid shift of emotions	Expressing euphoric, tearful, angry feelings in rapid succession
Inappropriate affect	Affect that is clearly discordant with the content of the person's speech	Laughing while discussing admission for liver biopsy

SPECIAL CONSIDERATIONS FOR ADVANCED PRACTICE

TABLE 6.4	Examples of Abnormalities of Thought Process	
Type of Process	Definition	Clinical Example
Blocking	Sudden interruption in train of thought, seems related to strong emotion	Unable to complete sentence, the patient says, "I forgot what I was going to say."
Confabulation	Fabricating events to fill in memory gaps	The patent gives a detailed description of a long walk around the hospital, although the patient is known to have remained in the patient care room all afternoon.
Neologism	Coining a new word; invented word has no real meaning except for the patient; several words may be condensed	The patient says, "I'll have to turn on my thinkilator."
Circumlocution	Roundabout expression, substituting a phrase when patient cannot think of name of object	The patient says, "the thing you open the door with" instead of "key."
Circumstantiality	Talking with excessive and unnecessary detail, delay in reaching point; sentences have a meaningful connection but are irrelevant (this occurs normally in some people)	The patient says, "When was my surgery? Well I was 28, I was living with my aunt, she's the one with psoriasis, she had it bad that year because of the heat, the heat was worse then than it was the summer of '92 …"
Loosening associations	Shifting from one topic to an unrelated topic; the patient seems unaware that topics are unconnected	The patient says, "My boss is angry with me and it wasn't even my fault. [pause] I saw that movie, too, *Lassie*. I felt really bad about it. But she kept trying to land the airplane and she never knew what was going on."
Flight of ideas	Abrupt change, rapid skipping from topic to topic, practically continuous flow of accelerated speech; topics usually have recognizable associations or are plays on words	The patient says, "Take this pill? The pill is blue. I feel blue. [sings] She wore blue velvet."
Word salad	Incoherent mixture of words, phrases, and sentences; illogical, disconnected, includes neologisms	The patient says, "Beauty, red based five, pigeon, the street corner, sort of."
Perseveration	Persistent repeating of verbal or motor response, even with varied stimuli	The patient says, "I'm going to lock the door, lock the door. I walk every day and I lock the door. I usually take the dog and I lock the door."
Echolalia	Imitation, repeats others' words or phrases, often with a mumbling, mocking, or mechanical tone	[In response to the nurse's request to take a pill] The patient says, mockingly, "Take your pill. Take your pill."
Clanging	Word choice based on sound, not meaning; includes nonsense rhymes and puns	The patient says, "My feet are cold. Cold, bold, told. The bell tolled for me."

TABLE 6.5	Abnormalities of Thought Content	
Type of Content	Definition	Clinical Example
Phobia	Strong, persistent, irrational fear of an object or situation; feeling driven to avoid it	Cats, dogs, heights, enclosed spaces
Hypochondriasis	Morbid worrying about own health; feeling sick with no actual basis for that assumption	Preoccupation with the possibility of having cancer; belief that any symptom or physical sign means cancer
Obsession	Unwanted, persistent thoughts or impulses experienced as intrusive and senseless; logic does not purge them from consciousness	Violence (parent having repeated impulse to kill a loved child); contamination (becoming infected by shaking hands)
Compulsion	Unwanted repetitive act thought to neutralize or prevent discomfort or some dreaded event	Handwashing, counting, checking and rechecking, touching
Delusions	Fixed, false beliefs; irrational beliefs; clinging to delusion despite objective evidence to contrary	Grandiose delusion: belief that one is God, a famous person, a historical figure, a sports figure, or another well-known person Persecution: the patient says, "They are out to get me."

TABLE 6.6	Global Assessment of Functioning Scale

Consider psychological, social, and occupational functioning on a hypothetical continuum of mental health illness. Do not include impairment in functioning caused by physical (or environmental) limitations.

Scoring Range	Description of Level of Functioning
100–91	Superior functioning in a wide range of activities; life's problems never seem to get out of hand; person is sought out by others because of his or her many positive qualities. No symptoms.
90–81	Absent or minimal symptoms (e.g., mild anxiety before an examination); good functioning in all areas; interested and involved in a wide range of activities; socially effective; generally satisfied with life; no more than everyday problems or concerns (e.g., an occasional argument with family members).
80–71	If symptoms are present, they are transient and expectable reactions to psychosocial stressors (e.g., difficulty concentrating after family argument); no more than slight impairment in social, occupational, or school functioning (e.g., temporarily falling behind in school work).
70–61	Some mild symptoms (e.g., depressed mood and mild insomnia) *or* some difficulty in social, occupational, or school functioning (e.g., occasional truancy, or theft within the household), but generally functioning pretty well, has some meaningful interpersonal relationships.
60–51	Moderate symptoms (e.g., flat and circumstantial speech, occasional panic attacks) *or* moderate difficulty in social, occupational, or social functioning (e.g., few friends, conflicts with co-workers).
50–41	Serious symptoms (e.g., suicidal ideation, severe obsessional rituals, frequent shoplifting) *or* any serious impairment in social, occupational, or school functioning (e.g., no friends, unable to keep a job).
40–31	Some impairment in reality testing or communication (e.g., speech is at times illogical, obscure, or irrelevant) *or* major impairment in several areas, such as work or school, family relations, judgement, thinking, or mood (e.g., depressed man avoids friends, neglects family, and is unable to work; child frequently beats up younger children, is defiant at home, and is failing at school).
30–21	Behaviour is considerably influenced by delusions or hallucinations *or* serious impairment in communication or judgement (e.g., sometimes incoherent, acts grossly inappropriately, suicidal preoccupation) *or* inability to function in almost all areas (e.g., stays in bed all day; has no job, home, or friends).
20–11	Some danger of hurting self or others (e.g., suicide attempts without clear expectation of death; frequently violent; manic excitement) *or* occasionally fails to maintain minimal personal hygiene (e.g., smears feces) *or* gross impairment in communication (e.g., largely incoherent or mute).
10–1	Persistent danger of severely hurting self or others (e.g., recurrent violence) *or* persistent inability to maintain minimal personal hygiene *or* serious suicidal act with clear expectation of death.
0	Inadequate information.

From Access Behavioral Health. (n.d.). *Global assessment of functioning.* Retrieved from https://apps.omh.ny.gov/omhweb/childservice/mrt/global_assessment_functioning.pdf.

TABLE 6.7	Comparison of Characteristics of Delirium and Dementia

Delirium is a condition (mild to severe and temporary) in which there is a disturbance in attention and awareness which tends to fluctuate in severity during the course of the day and a disturbance in cognition (e.g., memory deficit, disorientation, visiospatial ability, language or perception). It cannot be explained by a pre-existing or developing neurocognitive disorder. There must be evidence of *direct* physiological consequence of another medical condition, substance intoxication or withdrawal (i.e., due to a drug use or to a medication), or exposure to a toxin, or is due to multiple etiologies.[a]

Dementia (newly named *mild or major neurocognitive disorder* in DSM-5) is a progressive degenerative disease caused by damage to the brain cells. Symptoms include memory loss and a deterioration of cognitive performance and function, physical capacity, and personality features.[b]

Characteristic	Delirium	Dementia
Onset	Sudden; hours to days	Progressive; months to years
Course	Acute; temporary; considered reversible	Chronic, with deterioration over time
Prevalence	Present in 10–30% of hospitalized older adults	Estimated to affect >30% of people older than 85
Distinguishing feature	Presence of an underlying medical disorder (e.g., urinary tract infection, hypoxia)	Age-associated illness with decline in multiple areas of cognitive function, eventually leading to a significant inability to maintain occupational and social performance
Self-awareness	May be aware of changes in cognition; fluctuates	Likely to hide or be unaware of cognitive deficits
Activities of daily living	May be intact or impaired	May be intact early, impaired as disease progresses
Consequences	Contributes to outcomes of longer hospitalization, higher rates of nursing home placement, and possibly higher mortality rate	Major cause of disability, self-neglect, nutrition problems, incontinence, falls, communication difficulties, financial stress from job loss, and caregiver burden and depression[c]

Note: The reader is encouraged to consult the DSM-5 for further details on delirium and dementia.
DSM-5, Diagnostic and Statistical Manual of Mental Disorders (5th ed.).
[a]American Psychiatric Association. (2013). *Desk reference to the diagnostic criteria from DSM-5.* Arlington, VA: Author (p. 292).
[b]American Psychiatric Association. (2013). *Desk reference to the diagnostic criteria from DSM-5.* Arlington, VA: Author (pp. 302–304).
[c]Data from Gagliardi, G. P. (2008). Differentiating among depression, delirium, and dementia in elderly patients. *American Medical Association Journal of Ethics Virtual Mentor, 10*(6), 383–388; and Mental health: Dementia. (n.d.). *Clinical Knowledge Summaries, NHS Evidence.* Retrieved from https://cks.nice.org.uk/.

TABLE 6.8	Diagnostic Criteria for Schizophrenia

Schizophrenia affects a person's cognition (thinking), perception, and affect; the schizophrenic disorders are characterized in general by fundamental and characteristic distortions of thinking and perception, and affects that are inappropriate or blunted. Clear consciousness and intellectual capacity are usually maintained although certain cognitive deficits may evolve in the course of time.

DSM-5	ICD-10 (World Health Organization)
## At Least Two of the Following: • Delusions • Hallucinations • Disorganized speech • Disorganized or catatonic symptoms or negative symptoms (e.g., apathy; reduction in speech; absent, blunted or incongruous emotional responses; social withdrawal; impaired attention; inability to experience pleasure [anhedonia]; sexual problems; lethargy) *And* ## At Least One of the Following: • Delusions • Hallucinations • Disorganized speech	• Thought echo, thought insertion/withdrawal/broadcasting • Delusional perception and delusions control • Influence or passivity • Third-person auditory hallucination with running commentary • Thought disorders and negative symptoms

Continued

TABLE 6.8 **Diagnostic Criteria for Schizophrenia—cont'd**

Duration

Symptoms must persist for at least 6 months, including at least 1 month of active symptoms (or less if successfully treated), with social or occupational deterioration problems occurring over a significant period of time. These problems cannot be attributable to another condition.

The course of schizophrenic disorders can be either continuous or episodic, with progressive or stable deficit, or there can be one or more episodes with complete or incomplete remission.

Note: The reader is encouraged to consult the DSM-5 for further details on schizophrenia. The ICD-11 is the revision of ICD-10 and was released in 2018.
DSM-5, Diagnostic and Statistical Manual of Mental Disorders (5th ed.); *ICD-10,* International Statistical Classification of Diseases and Related Health Problems (10th rev.); *ICD-11,* International Statistical Classification of Diseases and Related Health Problems (11th rev.).
Modified from American Psychiatric Association. (2013). *Desk reference to the diagnostic criteria from DSM-5.* Arlington, VA: Author (pp. 50–52); American Psychiatric Association. (2013). *Diagnostic and statistical manual of mental disorders* (5th ed.). Washington, DC: Author; and World Health Organization. (2016). *International statistical classification of diseases and related health problems* (10th rev.). Geneva, Switzerland: Author.

TABLE 6.9 **Mood Disorders**

Major depressive disorder: According to the DSM-5, major depressive disorder is characterized by one or more depressive episodes lasting at least 2 weeks and accompanied by at least four additional symptoms of depression (e.g., fatigue or loss of energy, insomnia or oversleeping, feelings of worthlessness, significant weight fluctuations—gain or loss).[a]
Bipolar disorders: Bipolar disorder is described in the DSM-5 as Bipolar I or Bipolar II disorders. Bipolar I disorder involves both episodes of mania (e.g., extreme irritability and increased goal-directed activity or energy [accompanied by three or more of the following symptoms: inflated self-esteem or grandiosity, decreased need for sleep, more talkative than usual, flight of ideas, distractibility, increased goal-directed activity or psychomotor agitation, excessive involvement in activities that may or may not be dangerous]) and sometimes hypomania (e.g., irritability and increased energy). Bipolar I also includes depressed mood. Bipolar II disorder involves evidence of episodes of hypomania and depressed mood; there are no episodes of mania.[b]

Note: The reader is encouraged to consult the DSM-5 or a psychiatry textbook for further details on and categories of mood disorders.
DSM-5, Diagnostic and Statistical Manual of Mental Disorders (5th ed.)
[a]American Psychiatric Association. (2013). *Desk reference to the diagnostic criteria from DSM-5.* Arlington, VA: Author (pp. 67–68).
[b]American Psychiatric Association. (2013). *Desk reference to the diagnostic criteria from DSM-5.* Arlington, VA: Author (pp. 65–67).

TABLE 6.10 **Anxiety Disorders**

Anxiety disorders[a] encompass a multitude of disorders whose primary feature is persistent abnormal or inappropriate anxiety. Patients with anxiety experience an increased heart rate, tensed muscles, and other "fight or flight" processes; these symptoms become a problem when they occur without any recognizable stimulus or when the stimulus does not warrant the reaction. There are many types of anxiety disorders (e.g., separation anxiety disorder, selective mutism, specific phobia, social anxiety disorder [social phobia], panic disorder, agoraphobia, and generalized anxiety disorder).[b]

Note: The reader is encouraged to consult the DSM-5 or a psychiatry textbook for further details on and categories of anxiety disorders.
[a]See Heffner, C. L. (n.d.). *Index of psychiatric disorders.* Retrieved from http://allpsych.com/disorders/disorders_alpha.html.
[b]American Psychiatric Association. (2013). *Desk reference to the diagnostic criteria from DSM-5.* Arlington, VA: Author (pp. 115–128).

Summary Checklist: Mental Health Assessment

1. **Health history:**
   Source of information
   Identification/biographic information
   Reason for seeking care (patient's verbatim reason; psychiatric diagnoses [DSM-5])
   Past health (past illness, injury, hospitalization; chronic illnesses)
   Family health history
   Developmental considerations
   Present health (allergies, immunization/HIV/hepatitis status; current medications, including the use of alternative medicines, remedies etc.)

2. **Mental status examination:**
   Appearance
   Behaviour (mood and affect, speech)

Cognitive function (level of consciousness; orientation to time, place, person, self; memory; attention and concentration; comprehension and abstract reasoning)

Thought (perception, content, process, judgement, and insight)

3. **Supplemental mental status examination (if warranted):** Montreal Cognitive Assessment or the Mini-Cog assessment

4. **Functional assessment of ADLs:**
Nutrition patterns
Sleep/rest changes
Activity/mobility
Elimination
Interpersonal relationships and resources
Self-esteem/self-concept
Ethnicity/culture
Spirituality
Coping and stress management

Smoking, alcohol and drug use, problem gambling
Home environmental hazards

5. **Screen for suicidal thoughts, assaultive or homicidal ideation, and elopement risk (when indicated)**

6. **Treatment plan (Global Assessment of Functioning)**

7. **Teaching and health promotion**

ADDITIONAL RESOURCES

Aboriginal Healing Foundation. http://www.ahf.ca

Alzheimer Society Canada. http://www.alzheimer.ca

Canadian Alliance on Mental Illness and Mental Health. http://camimh.ca

Canadian Coalition for Seniors' Mental Health. http://www.ccsmh.ca

Canadian Institute for Health Information. http://www.cihi.ca

Canadian Mental Health Association. http://www.cmha.ca

Centre for Addiction and Mental Health. http://www.camh.ca

Kastner, J. (2013). *Out of sight, out of mind* [Motion picture]. Available from https://www.nfb.ca/film/out_of_mind_out_of_sight/trailer/out_of_mind_out_of_sight_trailer/.

Mental Health Commission of Canada. http://www.mentalhealthcommission.ca

Mood Disorders Society of Canada. http://mdsc.ca

National Eating Disorder Information Centre. http://www.nedic.ca

Partners in Recovery/Uncovering Potential. http://www.psrrpscanada.ca

The Royal's Institute of Mental Health Research—Glossary. http://www.theroyal.ca/research/about-imhr/glossary/

Schizophrenia Society of Canada. http://www.schizophrenia.ca

REFERENCES

1. World Health Organization. (2017). *Mental health: Strengthening our response—Fact sheet.* Retrieved from http://www.who.int/mediacentre/factsheets/fs220/en/.

2. World Health Organization. (2017). *Depression: Fact sheet.* Retrieved from: http://www.who.int/mediacentre/factsheets/fs369/en/.

3. World Health Organization. (2013). *Investing in mental health: Evidence for action.* Geneva, Switzerland (p. 7). Retrieved from http://apps.who.int/iris/bitstream/10665/87232/1/9789241564618_eng.pdf?ua=1.

4. Smetanin, P., et al. (2011). *The life and economic impact of major mental illnesses in Canada: 2011–2041.* Toronto: RiskAnalytica, on behalf of the Mental Health Commission of Canada.

5. Public Health Agency of Canada. (2011). *The mental health status & prevalence of MH problems in Canadian children & adolescents.* Retrieved from http://www.canadianschoolhealth.ca/page/The+Mental+Healt+Status+%26+Prevalence+of+MH+Problems+in+Canadian+Children+%26+Adolescents.

6. Johansen, H., & Finès, P. (2012). *Acute care hospital days and mental diagnosis.* Ottawa: Ministry of Industry, Statistics Canada.

7. Kirmayer, L., Bass, G., Holton, T., et al. (2007). *Suicide among Aboriginal people in Canada.* Ottawa: Aboriginal Healing Foundation.

8. Public Health Agency of Canada. (2006). *The human face of mental health and mental illness in Canada.* Ottawa: Minister of Public Works and Government Services Canada.

9. Public Health Agency of Canada. (2016). *Mental health and wellness.* Retrieved from http://cbpp-pcpe.phac-aspc.gc.ca/public-health-topics/mental-health-and-wellness/.

10. Canadian Mental Health Association. (2008). *Your mental health.* Retrieved from http://www.cmha.ca/bins/content_page.asp?cid=2-267-1319&lang=1.

11. Mind, Mental Health Foundation. (2013). Building resilient communities: Making every contact count for public mental health (p. 3). Retrieved from http://www.thehealthwell.info/node/553608.

12. Rogers, C. R. (1961). *On Becoming a person: A psychotherapists view of psychotherapy.* Boston: Houghton Mifflin.

13. McLeod, S. A. (2014). *Carl Rogers.* Retrieved from http://www.simplypsychology.org/carl-rogers.html.

14. Maslow, A. H. (1943). Hierarchy of needs: A theory of human motivation. *Psychology Review, 50*(4), 370.

15. Chandler, M. J., & Lalonde, C. E. (2008). Cultural continuity as a protective factor against suicide in First Nations youth. *Horizons, 10*(1), 68–72.

16. Chandler, M. J., & Lalonde, C. E. (2009). Cultural continuity as a moderator of suicide risk among Canada's First Nations. In L. J. Kirmayer & G. Valaskakis (Eds.), *Healing traditions: The mental health of First Nations peoples in Canada* (pp. 221–248). Vancouver: UBC Press (p. 238).

17. Auger, M. D. (2016). Cultural continuity as a determinant of Indigenous peoples' health. *The International Indigenous Policy Journal, 7*(4).

18. Greenwood, M. L., & de Leeuw, S. N. (2012). Social determinants of health and the future well-being of Aboriginal children in Canada. *Paediatric & Child Health, 17*(7), 381–384.

19. Loppie Reading, C., & Wien, F. (2009). *Health inequalities and social determinants of Aboriginal peoples' health.* Prince

George, BC: National Collaborating Centre for Aboriginal Health.

20. Richmond, C. A. M., & Ross, N. A. (2009). The determinants of First Nation and Inuit health: A critical population health approach. *Health and Place, 15,* 403–411.

21. Goldner, E. M., Jenkins, E., Palma, J., et al. (2014). *A concise introduction to mental health in Canada* (p. 4). Toronto: Canadian Scholars' Press.

22. Greenwood, M., de Leeuw, S., Lindsay, N. M., et al. (Eds.), (2015). *Determinants of Indigenous peoples' health in Canada: Beyond the social.* Toronto: Canadian Scholars.

23. Bhaloo, S. (2005). *Refugee Women from Sudan and their mental health: Project report.* Hamilton: Funded by the Community Care Research Center and the Arts Research Board at McMaster University.

24. Baya, K., Simich, L., & Bukhari, S. (2008). Women at the centre of changing families: A study of Sudanese women's resettlement experiences. In S. Guruge & E. Collins (Eds.), *Working with immigrant women* (pp. 157–176). Toronto: Centre for Addiction and Mental Health.

25. Health Canada. (2015). *First Nations mental wellness continuum framework* (pp. 1–4). Ottawa: Author. Retrieved from http://nnapf.com/wp-content/uploads/2015/01/24-1 4-1273-FN-Mental-Wellness-Framework-EN05_low.pdf.

26. American Psychiatric Association. (2013). *Diagnostic and statistical manual of mental disorders* (5th ed.). Washington, DC: Author.

27. Perring, C. (2010). Mental illness. E. N. Zalta (Ed.), *The Stanford encyclopedia of philosophy* (Spring 2010 ed.). Retrieved from http://plato.stanford.edu/archives/spr2010/entries/mental-illness/.

28. Huang, K.-L., Su, T.-P., Tzeng-Ji, C., et al. (2009). Comorbidity of cardiovascular diseases with mood and anxiety disorder: A population based four-year study. *Psychiatry and Clinical Neurosciences, 63,* 401–409.

29. Oakley Browne, M. A., Wells, J. E., Scott, K. M. (Eds.), (2006). Te Rau Hinengaro—The New Zealand Mental Health Survey: Summary. Wellington: Ministry of Health, New Zealand.

30. Rodriguez, C., & Thankam, S. (2007). The interplay of comorbidity among patients with medical illness and mental illness: A sociological perspective. *Proceedings of the Annual Meeting of the American Sociological Association.* New York, NY.

31. Statistics Canada. (2011). *Mental comorbidity and its contribution to increased use of acute care hospital services* (Catalogue No. 82-622-X) (p. 20). Ottawa: Author. Retrieved from http://www.statcan.gc.ca/pub/82-622-x/82-622-x2011006-eng.pdf.

32. Kiraly, B., Gunning, K., & Leiser, J. (2008). Primary care issues in patients with mental illness. *American Family Physician, 78*(3), 355–362.

33. Canadian Centre on Substance Abuse. (2010). *Substance abuse in Canada: Concurrent disorders highlights.* Ottawa: Author. Retrieved from http://www.ccsa.ca/Resource%20 Library/ccsa-011813-2010.pdf.

34. Rush, B. (2011). *An update on evidence-informed practices for services and systems for people with concurrent substance use and other mental disorders.* Unpublished report for the Working Group on Concurrent Disorders for the Province of Newfoundland and Labrador.

35. Statistics Canada. (2002). *Canadian community health survey: Mental health and well-being.* Ottawa: Author.

36. Rush, B., Urbanoski, K., Bassani, D., et al. (2008). Prevalence of co-occurring substance use and other mental disorders in the Canadian population. *Canadian Journal of Psychiatry, 53*(12), 800–809.

37. Rush, B. (2015). *Concurrent disorders guidelines: A supplement to the provincial addictions treatment standards.* Unpublished report for the Working Group on Concurrent Disorders for the Province of Newfoundland and Labrador (p. 9). Retrieved from http://www.health.gov.nl.ca/health/mentalhealth/pdf/Concurrent_Disorders.pdf.

38. Canadian Institute for Health Information. (2013). *Hospital mental health services for concurrent mental illness and substance use disorders in Canada: Analysis in brief.* Ottawa: Author.

39. Urbanoski, K. A., Cairney, J., Bassani, D. G., et al. (2008). Perceived unmet need for mental health care for Canadians with co-occurring mental and substance use disorders. *Psychiatric Services, 59*(3), 283–289.

40. Adair, C. (2009). *Concurrent substance use and mental disorders in adolescents: A review of the literature on current science and practice.* Calgary: Alberta Centre for Child, Family, & Community Research.

41. Mental Health Commission of Canada. (2015). *Guidelines for recovery-oriented practice: Hope. Dignity. Inclusion.* Ottawa: Author. Retrieved from https://www.mentalhealthcommission.ca/sites/default/files/2016-07/MHCC_Recovery_Guidelines_2016_ENG.PDF.

42. Goffman, E. (1963). *Stigma: Notes on the management of spoiled identity* (p. 12). Englewood Cliffs, NJ: Prentice-Hall.

43. Link, B. G., & Phelan, J. C. (2001). Conceptualizing stigma. *Annual Review of Sociology, 27,* 363–385.

44. Link, B. G., & Phelan, J. C. (2006). Stigma and its public health implications. *Lancet, 367,* 528–529.

45. Smye, V., Browne, A. J., Varcoe, C., et al. (2011). Harm reduction and methadone maintenance treatment: Intersections of gender, class, race and ability. *Harm Reduction Journal, 8*(17).

46. Canadian Mental Health Association. (2011). *Violence and mental health: Unpacking a complex issue.* Toronto: Author. Retrieved from http://ontario.cmha.ca/wp-content/uploads/2011/09/cmha_on_violence_and_mh_discussion_paper_201109.pdf.

47. Canadian Alliance on Mental Illness and Mental Health. (2007). *Mental health literacy in Canada: Phase one draft report.* Retrieved from http://camimh.ca/wp-content/uploads/2012/04/Mental-Health-Literacy_-_Full-Final-Report_EN.pdf.

48. Canadian Medical Association. (2008). *8th Annual national report on health care.* Retrieved from http://www.bc-psychologist.com/downloads/other/National_Report_Card_EN.pdf.

49. Corrigan, P. W., & Watson, A. C. (2002). Understanding the impact of stigma on people with mental illness. *World Psychiatry, 1*(1), 16–20.

50. Stuart, H. (2006). Mental illness and employment discrimination. *Current Opinion in Psychiatry, 19*(5), 522–526.

51. Stuart, H., Chen, S., Christie, R., et al. (2014). Opening minds in Canada: Targeting change. *Canadian Journal of Psychiatry, 59*(10, Suppl. 1), S13–S18.

52. Knaak, S., Szeto, A., Kassam, A., et al. (2017). Understanding stigma: A pooled analysis of a national program aimed at

health care providers to reduce stigma towards patients with a mental illness. *Journal of Mental Health and Addiction Nursing, 1*(1), e19–e29. Retrieved from http://www.jmhan.org/index.php/JMHAN/article/view/19/27.

53. Ross, C., & Goldner, E. (2009). Stigma, negative attitudes and discrimination towards mental illness within the nursing profession: A review of the literature. *Journal of Psychiatric and Mental Health Nursing, 16*, 558–567.

54. Knaak, S., Mantler, E., & Seto, A. (2017). Mental illness-related stigma in healthcare: Barriers to access and care and evidence-based solutions. *Healthcare Management Forum, 30*(2), 111–116. Retrieved from https://www.mentalhealthcommission.ca/sites/default/files/2017-03/MI%20stigma%20in%20healthcare_barriers%20to%20access%20and%20evidence%20based%20solutions.pdf.

55. Corrigan, P. W., Druss, B., & Perlick, D. (2014). The impact of mental illness stigma on seeking and participating in mental health care. *Psychological Science in the Public Interest, 15*(2), 37–70.

56. Caldwell, T. M., & Jorm, A. F. (2001). Mental health nurses' beliefs about likely outcomes for people with schizophrenia or depression: A comparison with the public and other healthcare professionals. *International Journal of Mental Health Nursing, 10*(1), 42–54.

57. Knaak, S., & Patten, S. (2014). *Building and delivering successful anti-stigma programs for healthcare providers* (p. 13). Ottawa: Mental Health Commission of Canada.

58. Schulze, B. (2007). Stigma and mental health professionals: A review of the evidence on an intricate relationship. *International Review of Psychiatry, 19*(2), 137–155.

59. Stuart, H. (2005). Fighting stigma and discrimination is fighting for mental health. *Canadian Public Policy, 31*(S1), 21–28.

60. Mental Health Commission of Canada. (2012). *Changing directions, changing lives: The mental health strategy for Canada.* Calgary: Author. Retrieved from http://strategy.mentalhealthcommission.ca/pdf/strategy-images-en.pdf.

61. Munn-Rivard, L. (2014). *Current issues in mental health in Canada: Homelessness and access to housing. Legal and Social Affairs Division Parliamentary Information and Research Service: In brief.* Ottawa: Library of Parliament of Canada. Retrieved from http://www.lop.parl.gc.ca/Content/LOP/ResearchPublications/2014-11-e.pdf.

62. Canadian Institute for Health Information. (2007). *Improving the health of Canadians: Mental health and homelessness* (p. 13). Ottawa: Author.

63. Centre for Addiction and Mental Health. (2012). *Road to recovery: Client experiences in supportive housing.* Retrieved from https://www.camh.ca/en/hospital/about_camh/influencing_public_policy/Documents/Road to_Recovery-Client_Experiences_in_Supportive_Housing.pdf.

64. Crowe, C. (2007). *Dying for a home: Homeless activists speak out.* Toronto: Between the Lines.

65. Hartrick Doane, G., & Varcoe, C. (2013). *How to nurse: Relational inquiry with individuals and families in shifting contexts.* Toronto: : Wolters Kluwer.

66. Canadian Nurses Association. (2012). *Professional practice: Canadian Registered Nurse Examination competencies, June 2010–May 2015.* Retrieved from http://www.cna-aiic.ca/CNA/nursing/rnexam/competencies/default_e.aspx.

67. Hamilton, B., Manias, E., Maude, P., et al. (2004). Perspectives of a nurse, a social worker and a psychiatrist regarding patient assessment in acute inpatient psychiatry settings: A case study approach. *Journal of Psychiatric and Mental Health Nursing, 11*, 683–689.

68. O'Brien, A. J. (1999). Negotiating the relationship: Mental health nurses' perceptions of their practice. *Australian and New Zealand Journal of Mental Health Nursing, 8*, 153–161.

69. Registered Nurses' Association of Ontario. (2002). *Establishing therapeutic relationships.* Toronto: Author.

70. Canadian Women's Health Network. (2012). *Health professional guide to memory loss: Mini-Mental State Examination (MMSE).* Retrieved from http://www.cwhn.ca/en/HPmemoryMMSE.

71. Canadian Women's Health Network. (2012). *Health professional guide to memory loss: MoCA, Clock Drawing Test, and other tests.* Retrieved from http://www.cwhn.ca/en/HPmemoryTest.

72. *Instructions for Administering the Mini-Mental State Examination.* (2017). Retrieved from http://gem.rgp.toronto.on.ca/files/MMSE_Test%20(4).pdf.

73. Julayanont, P., Phillips, N., Chertkow, H., et al. (2012). The Montreal Cognitive Assessment (MoCA): Concept and clinical review. In A. J. Larner (Ed.), *Cognitive screening instruments: A practical approach* (pp. 111–152). London: Springer-Verlag. Retrieved from http://www.pphp.concordia.ca/fac/phillips/files/Julayanontetal2013MoCAreview.pdf.

74. Nasreddine, Z. S., Phillips, N. A., Bédirian, V., et al. (2005). The Montreal Cognitive Assessment, MoCA: A brief screening tool for mild cognitive impairment. *Journal of the American Geriatric Society, 53*, 695–699.

75. Nasreddine, Z. S., Phillips, N. A., & Chertkow, H. (2011). *Montreal Cognitive Assessment (MoCA), version 3: Administration and scoring instructions.* Retrieved from http://thehub.utoronto.ca/family/wp-content/uploads/2016/12/MoCA-Instructions-English.pdf.

76. Kidder, K., & Rogers, D. (2004). *Why Canada needs a national youth policy agenda.* Washington, DC: National Children's Alliance. Retrieved from http://www.nationalchildrensalliance.com/nca/pubs/2004/youthpolicypaper.htm.

77. World Health Organization. (2007). *Mental health: Strengthening mental health promotion.* Geneva, Switzerland: Author.

78. Felliti, V. J., Anda, R. F., Nordenberg, D., et al. (1998). Relationship of childhood abuse and household dysfunction to many of the leading causes of death in adults: The Adverse Childhood Experiences (ACE) Study. *American Journal of Preventative Medicine, 14*(4), 245–250.

79. Menzies, P. (2010). Intergenerational trauma from a mental health perspective. *Native Social Work Journal, 7*, 63–85.

80. Knopf, D., Park, M. J., & Mulye, T. P. (2008). *The mental health of adolescents: A national profile.* San Francisco: San Francisco: National Adolescent Health Information Center, University of California.

81. Public Health Agency of Canada. (2008). *Healthy settings for young people in Canada.* Retrieved from http://www.phac-aspc.gc.ca/hp-ps/dca-dea/publications/yjc/index-eng.php.

82. Statistics Canada. (2010). *Table 5.7: Leading causes of death of children and youth, by age group, 2003 to 2005.* Ottawa: Author. Retrieved from http://www.statcan.gc.ca/pub/11-402-x/2010000/chap/c-e/tbl/tbl07-eng.htm.

83. Birkett, M., Espelage, D. L., & Koenig, B. (2009). LGB and questioning students in schools: The moderating effects of homophobic bullying and school climate on negative outcomes. *Journal of Youth and Adolescence, 38*(7), 989–1000.

84. Evenson, J., & Barr, C. (2009). *Youth homelessness in Canada: The road to solutions.* Toronto: Raise the Roof Foundation. Retrieved from http://www.raisingtheroof.org/wp-content/uploads/2015/10/road2sols-FINAL.pdf.

85. Statistics Canada. (2009). *Canadian Community Health Survey, Annual* [Microdata file]. Ottawa: Author.

86. Taylor, C., Peter, T., Schachter, K., et al. (2008). *Youth speak up about homophobia and transphobia: The first national climate survey on homophobia in Canadian schools: Phase one report.* Toronto: Eagle Canada Human Rights Trust.

87. Pearson, C., Janz, T., & Ali, J. (2013). *Health at a glance: Mental and substance use disorders in Canada* (Catalogue no. 82-624-X). Retrieved from http://www.statcan.gc.ca/pub/82-624-x/2013001/article/11855-eng.htm.

88. Boak, A., Jamilton, H. A., Adlaf, E. M., et al. (2016). *The mental health and well-being of Ontario students 1991–2015: Detailed OSDUHS findings* (CAMG Research Document Series No. 43). Toronto: Centre for Addiction and Mental Health.

89. Ontario Human Rights Commission. (2017). *With learning in mind: Inquiry report on systemic barriers to academic accommodation for post-secondary students with mental health disabilities.* Toronto: Author.

90. ACHA-NCHA. (2013). *American College Health Association National College Health Assessment II.* Hanover, MD: Author.

91. ACHA-NCHA. (2016). *American College Health Association National College Health Assessment II.* Hanover, MD: Author.

92. Kwan, M. Y., Arbour-Nicitopoulos, K. P., Duku, E., et al. (2016). Patterns of multiple health risk-behaviours in university students and their association with mental health: Application of latent class analysis. *Health Promotion and Chronic Disease Prevention in Canada: Research, Policy and Practice, 36*(8), 163–170.

93. Berger, J. (2009). Student debt in Canada. In J. Berger, A. Motte, & A. Parkin (Eds.), *The price of knowledge: Access and student finance in Canada* (4th ed., pp. 181–206). Montreal: Millennium Scholarship Foundation.

94. Canadian Council on Learning. (2010). *Tallying the costs of post-secondary education: The challenge of managing student debt and loan repayment in Canada* (Monograph 3). Ottawa: Author. Retrieved from https://files.eric.ed.gov/fulltext/ED525094.pdf.

95. Statistics Canada. (2013). *What has changed for young people in Canada.* Ottawa: Author. Retrieved from http://www.statcan.gc.ca/pub/75-006-x/2013001/article/11847-eng.htm.

96. Oleson, S. C., Butterworth, P., Leach, L. S., et al. (2013). Mental health affects future employment as job loss affects mental health: Findings from a longitudinal population study. *BMC Psychiatry, 13.* Retrieved from https://link.springer.com/article/10.1186/1471-244X-13-144.

97. Schaie, K. W., & Willis, S. L. (2011). *Handbook of the psychology of aging* (7th ed.). Burlingham, MA: Elsevier.

98. Rosenthal, C. J., Matthews, A. M., & Matthews, S. H. (1996). *Caught in the middle? Occupancy in multiple roles and help to parents in a national probability sample of Canadian adults. IESOP Research Paper No. 4.* Retrieved from http://socserv.mcmaster.ca/iesop/papers/iesop_04.pdf.

99. Clark, C. M. (2005). *Relations between social support and physical health.* Retrieved from http://www.personalityresearch.org/papers/clark.html.

100. Neupert, S. D., Almeida, D. M., & Charles, S. T. (2007). Age differences in reactivity to daily stressors: The role of personal control. *Journal of Gerontology. Series B, Psychological Sciences and Social Sciences, 62B*(4), 216–225.

101. Lachman, M. E. (2004). Development in midlife. *Annual Review of Psychology, 55,* 305–331.

102. Birren, J. E., & Schaie, K. W. (Eds.), (2005). *Handbook of the psychology of aging* (6th ed.). San Diego: Academic Press.

103. Tuokko, H., Morris, C., & Ebert, P. (2005). Mild cognitive impairment and everyday functioning in older adults. *Neurocase: The Neural Basis of Cognition, 11*(1), 40–47.

104. Canadian Task Force on Preventive Health Care. (2013). *Depression.* Retrieved from http://canadiantaskforce.ca/portfolios/depression/.

105. Canadian Task Force on Preventive Health Care, Joffries, M., Jaramillo, A., et al. (2013). Recommendations on screening for depression in adults. *Canadian Medical Association Journal, 185*(9), 775–782.

106. Thombs, B. D., Coyne, J. C., Cuijpers, P., et al. (2012). Rethinking recommendations for screening for depression in primary care. *Canadian Medical Association Journal, 184*(4), 413–418.

107. National Collaborating Centre for Mental Health. (2010). *Depression in adults: Recognition and management* (Clinical guideline CG90). Retrieved from https://www.nice.org.uk/guidance/CG90.

108. O'Connor, E. A., Whitlock, E. P., Gaynes, B., et al. (2009). *Screening for depression in adults and older adults in primary care: An updated systematic review* (Report No. 10-05143-EF-1). Rockville, MD: Agency for Healthcare Research and Quality.

109. British Columbia Reproductive Mental Health Program. (2014). *Best practice guidelines for mental health disorders in the perinatal period.* Vancouver: Author. Retrieved from http://www.perinatalservicesbc.ca/Documents/Guidelines-Standards/Maternal/MentalHealthDisordersGuideline.pdf.

110. Lanes, A., Kuk, J. L., & Tamim, H. (2011). Prevalence and characteristics of postpartum depression symptomatology among Canadian women: A cross-sectional study. *BMC Public Health, 11,* 302.

111. Provincial Health Services Authority. (2017). *Edinburgh Postnatal Depression Scale (EPDS).* Retrieved from http://www.perinatalservicesbc.ca/health-professionals/professional-resources/health-promo/edinburgh-postnatal-depression-scale-(epds).

112. Dowrick, C. (2004). *Beyond depression: A new approach to understanding and management.* Oxford, UK: Oxford University Press.

113. Poobalan, A. S., Aucott, L. S., Ross, L., et al. (2007). Effects of treating postnatal depression on mother-infant interaction and child development: Systematic review. *British Journal of Psychiatry, 191,* 378–386.

114. Osaka, N., & Logie, R. H. (2007). *The cognitive neuroscience of working memory.* Oxford, UK: Oxford University Press.

115. Marková, I. S., Jaafari, N., & Berrios, G. E. (2009). Insight and obsessive-compulsive disorder: A conceptual analysis. *Psychopathology, 42*, 277–282.

116. Marková, I. S., Berrios, G. E., & Hodges, J. H. (2004). Insight into memory function. *Neurology, Psychiatry & Brain Research, 11*, 115–126.

117. Tsoi, K. K., Chan, J. Y., Hirai, H. W., et al. (2015). Cognitive test to detect dementia: A systematic review and meta-analysis. *JAMA Internal Medicine, 175*(9), 1450–1458.

118. Storey, J., Rowland, J., Basic, C., et al. (2004). The Rowland Universal Dementia Assessment Scale (RUDAS): A multicultural cognitive assessment scale. *International Psychogeriatrics, 16*(1), 13–31. Retrieved from https://www.fightdementia.org.au/sites/default/files/20110311_2011RUDASAdminScoringGuide.pdf.

119. Jayaram, G. (2009). Elopement: A primer on safety and prevention. In G. Jayaram & A. Herzog (Eds.), *SAFE MD: Practical applications and approaches to safe psychiatric practice* (pp. 16–18). Retrieved from http://suicidepreventioncommunity.files.wordpress.com/2009/01/apa-patientsafety-suicideexcerpt.pdf.

120. Gardner, W., Lucas, A., Kolko, D. J., et al. (2007). Comparison of the PSC-17 and alternative mental health screens in an at-risk primary care sample. *Journal of the American Academy of Child and Adolescent Psychiatry, 46*(5), 611–618.

121. Alzheimer's Association. (2011). *Alzheimer's disease: Facts and figures.* Retrieved from http://www.alz.org/downloads/facts_figures_2011.pdf.

122. Statistics Canada. (2015). *Annual demographic estimates: Canada, provinces and territories* (Catalogue no. 91-215-X). Ottawa: Author. Retrieved from http://www.statcan.gc.ca/pub/91-215-x/91-215-x2015000-eng.pdf.

123. Durant, E., & Sporer, K. A. (2011). Characteristics of patients with an abnormal Glasgow Coma Scale score in the prehospital setting. *Western Journal of Emergency Medicine, 12*(1), 30–36.

124. Isaacs, B., & Kennie, A. (1973). The set test as an aid to the detection of dementia in old people. *British Journal of Psychiatry, 123*, 467–470.

125. Nair, A. K., Gavett, B. E., Damman, M., et al. (2010). Clock drawing test ratings by dementia specialists: Interrater reliability and diagnostic accuracy. *Journal of Neuropsychiatry and Clinical Neurosciences, 22*, 85–92.

126. Lorentz, W., Scanlan, J. M., & Borson, S. (2002). Brief screening tests for dementia. *Canadian Journal of Psychiatry, 47*, 723–733.

127. Rosenzweig, A. (2017). *Montreal Cognitive Assessment (MoCA) test scoring and accuracy.* Retrieved from https://www.verywell.com/alzheimers-and-montreal-cognitive-assessment-moca-98617.

Substance Use and Health Assessment

Written by Colleen Varcoe, PhD, RN, Annette J. Browne, PhD, RN, and Laraine Michalson, MSN, RN

ℯ http://evolve.elsevier.com/Canada/Jarvis/examination/

In a recent study of a health promotion program for Indigenous women who had experienced violence, the majority of the women indicated that they had a **substance use** problem.[1,2] The program did not focus on substance use. Instead, it focused on supporting women with their self-identified health priorities and consisted of nurses working with the women individually and in a group context that included Indigenous Elders who provided cultural and traditional teachings. Throughout the program, the women, nurses, and Elders worked to include women who used substances (ranging from having never used, to years of abstinence, to occasional use, to active and daily use), which meant taking into account how some women's active use negatively affected other women who were trying not to use and disrupted group processes, as well as how some women judged others with detrimental effects. At the end of the program, the women had less depression, less post-traumatic stress disorder (PTSD), and a better quality of life. Although it was not a goal of the program, the women also markedly reduced their substance use, attributing doing so to the nonjudgemental, unconditional positive regard and support offered by the nurses and Elders, and the support of the other women.

The purpose of this chapter is to provide nurse clinicians with knowledge regarding substance use that can be integrated into health assessment across a range of practice contexts with patients of all ages. To help prevent and minimize the harmful effects of substance use, and to develop health-promoting nursing practices that account for a range of substance use practices, nurses must understand the dynamics of substance use, the social and health effects of substance use, the root causes of substance use, harm-reduction principles, and their implications for practice. This is relevant to assessment of *every* patient, regardless of whether substance use issues are immediately apparent. Substance use problems can affect all people, not only people who are disadvantaged. The risks of disclosure of **harmful substance use**, such as job loss, removal of children by protective agencies, and relationship damage, are significant, regardless of social location. This knowledge is necessary for conducting thorough, respectful, and useful health assessments.

SHIFTING SUBSTANCE USE LANGUAGE

Substance use is widespread in Canada; levels of use and acceptability vary according to the type of substance and the community. Our language reflects these shifting levels of acceptability. The lexicon of "misuse," "abuse," or "problematic use" vary by substance, social context, and values. The terms *substance use*, *substance abuse*, *addiction*, and *dependence* are sometimes used interchangeably, which is erroneous. Some of these terms are more pejorative than others; the term *addiction* carries the greatest stigma and is perhaps the most overused. **Addiction** generally refers to compulsion and dependence, and there is considerable disagreement regarding the meaning and usefulness of the term "addiction." As a result, the American Psychiatric Association has replaced the categories of "substance abuse" and "substance dependence" with the category of "**substance use disorder**" in the most recent *Diagnostic and Statistical Manual of Mental Disorders* (DSM-5).[3] In the DSM-5, people with substance use issues receive a diagnosis of mild, moderate, or severe substance use disorder.

This shift in language is intended to reduce the labelling of patients with normal tolerance and withdrawal as "addicts," and, more importantly, to improve the clinical assessment, management, and treatment of pain. The treatment of pain is always relevant to assessment related to substance use because, as is further explored in this chapter, traumatic experiences, pain, and substance use are often interrelated. "Many clinicians believe they lack the knowledge and the necessary communication skills to address the needs of patients with addiction. For this reason, they tend to undertreat pain… owing to misconceptions, biases, morals, and various education system gaps."[4]

It is essential to be clear about the definition of *dependence*. Dependence as a label for compulsive, out-of-control substance use has been problematic, confusing to clinicians, and (as noted earlier) has resulted in patients with normal tolerance and withdrawal being labelled as "addicts." Accordingly, the term **dependence** is limited to physiological dependence, which is a normal response to repeated doses of many medications including beta-blockers, antidepressants, opioids, antianxiety agents, and other drugs. Dependence is characterized by tolerance (needing more amounts of the medication or substance to produce the desired effect) and withdrawal (physiological symptoms that occur when the medication or drug is withdrawn).

Throughout this chapter, the term **substance use** is used in recognition of the controversial, variable, and socially constructed nature of more pejorative terms, including *addiction*, *dependence*, and *misuse*. The term *harmful* is used rather than *problematic* or *misuse* in recognition of the fact that it is generally accepted that substance use becomes a problem when it interferes with a person's relationships or employment, or causes interactions with the legal system. Clinicians are urged to use the term *substance use* and specify the physiological and social effects of such use as they are experienced by individuals.

THE CANADIAN CONTEXT OF SUBSTANCE USE

Like most societies, Canadian society has its particular set of values, beliefs, laws, policies, and practices related to substance use, many of which are contradictory to one another. Awareness of these values, laws, and policies provides clinicians with a "bigger picture" perspective on substance use. In Canada, certain substances, such as alcohol and tobacco, are legal and are the source of government tax revenue, and their use is socially acceptable in many communities. Other substances, such as crack and heroin, are illegal, are the sources of illegal profit-making, and are considered in popular thinking to be extremely dangerous. Moreover, their use is generally deemed socially reprehensible. Still others, such as marijuana, have only recently been made legal for medical usage. Some substances, such as marijuana and Ecstasy, are more socially tolerated and are extremely financially lucrative for those producing and selling them. For example, marijuana will be legal for recreational use in Canada in 2018, which will change the economics of marijuana in Canada.[5]

Finally, some substances, such as solvents and prescription drugs, have legal purposes but are used in ways other than formally intended. The use of substances has intertwined social and health effects that arise not only from the physiological effects of the substance (e.g., reduced or increased anxiety) but also from the social acceptability (e.g., inclusion) and legal consequences of using the substance (e.g., incarceration, impoverishment).

The social, economic, legal, and policy context of substance use in Canada is continually in flux, with shifts in the emphasis on abstinence or harm reduction (Box 7.1). *Abstinence*, which means completely no use of a given substance, is sometimes seen as dichotomous with harm reduction. However, abstinence may be seen as an approach that can work in concert with harm reduction. Abstinence aims to reduce the use of substances entirely, whereas harm reduction aims to reduce the *harms* of substance use, but not to reduce use per se. Programs and individuals may hold the goal of abstinence and, at the same time, seek to reduce

---

BOX 7.1   Harm Reduction and Abstinence

The primary focus of harm reduction is the reduction of the *harms* of substance use, but not the reduction of use. Harm reduction is often contrasted with abstinence, which focuses on the reduction of use toward absolutely no use. It is likely more useful to view harm reduction as being on a continuum with abstinence. For example, on the "harm reduction" end, a managed alcohol program would focus on safe consumption of alcohol, regardless of level of consumption; on the "abstinence" end, an organization such as Alcoholics Anonymous would work toward complete cessation of drinking; and in-between, a program would focus on reducing harms and having fewer drinks or more alcohol-free days.

In Canada, the following three harm-reduction paradigms are in operation:*

1. *Conservative paradigm*, in which harm-reduction measures (e.g., needle exchanges) are seen as temporary, with an ultimate goal of abstinence;
2. *Liberal paradigm*, in which informed choice is supported and a safety net provided; and
3. *Structural paradigm*, in which empowerment, advocacy, and emancipation of people using substances are embraced. The structural paradigm underpins this chapter.

*Cavalieri, W. (2017). *Harm reduction in practice.* Retrieved from http://www.canadianharmreduction.com/node/171.

---

harm. Abstinence underpins many popular approaches such as Alcoholics Anonymous or Narcotics Anonymous, which may be effective for some people.[6]

Until 2015, Canadian policy at the federal level followed that of the United States, moving to an American "War on Drugs" criminalization approach over time. In 1987, the federal government launched Canada's National Drug Strategy, which became "Canada's Drug Strategy" in 1992, when Cabinet regrouped the National Strategy to Reduce Impaired Driving and the National Drug Strategy under one initiative.[7] Funding was significantly cut through the 1990s, but the cornerstone of policy remained the long-term goal of reducing the harms associated with the use of alcohol, tobacco, and other substances to individuals, families, and communities. However, with the modifications to the National Drug Strategy in 2002, and the formation of the 2007 National Anti-Drug Strategy, harm reduction was increasingly washed out of federal policy, with resources funnelled more to enforcement and less to prevention and treatment. Indeed, the National Anti-Drug Strategy included three action plans—preventing illicit drug use; treating patients with dependencies on illicit drugs; and combating the production and distribution of illicit drugs—with no mention of harm reduction.

Researchers, advocates, and people who use substances have worked tirelessly to promote harm reduction. Harm reduction related to substance use includes "downstream" strategies, such as providing access to safe substances (e.g., providing heroin that is not cut with more harmful substances such as fentanyl), safe supplies (such as clean needles or crack pipes that will not cut people's lips), safe places to use substances (such as safe injection sites) and overdose care, such as the public distribution of naloxone (Narcan) kits. Importantly, harm reduction also includes more "upstream" approaches, such as safe housing, income supports, and pain-management services.

Abstinence and harm-reduction approaches have often been seen as being in opposition to one another. For example, North America's first and only legal supervised injection site (Insite) was opened in 2003 as part of a continuum of services aligned with the harm-reduction framework of health service delivery. Under intense scrutiny, and repeated attempts from the Conservative government (2006 to 2015) to shut it down, Insite continues to operate under an exemption to the *Controlled Drugs and Substances Act*. In September 2011, the Supreme Court of Canada declared that Insite saved lives and was effectively improving the health of people who used its services.[8]

With the election of a Liberal federal government in 2015 and in the face of what has been termed "the opioid crisis," harm reduction has been reintroduced as a cornerstone of health care. The opioid crisis in which hundreds of people have died accidentally[9] was sparked by pharmaceutical companies introducing lucrative, powerful drugs such as oxycontin and fentanyl.[10]

Social attitudes toward substance use in general and toward specific substances have shifted along with legal, economic, and policy changes. For example, attitudes toward tobacco use have grown increasingly less tolerant. In contrast, in most communities in Canada, alcohol use has become increasingly acceptable over recent decades,[11,12] with evidence that perception of norms influences use in some populations.[13]

Having an understanding of broad population trends is important so that programs can be developed to target services appropriately. However, at the level of individuals, it is important to remember that *any* person may be experiencing the harms of substance use. Health care providers need to operate with an awareness of population trends without assuming those trends apply to any given person. Indeed, health care providers should anticipate which individuals might expect to be judged incorrectly as using substances at harmful levels, and which individuals might be overlooked as using substances at harmful levels. For example, knowing that alcohol use is trending upward among youth should not lead to assumptions about any specific young person. Guarding against letting untested assumptions influence your practice will help you conduct assessments in ways that are respectful, encourage (rather than inhibit) discussions related to the health effects of substance use, and encourage health care access rather than alienation through shame and stigma.

SUBSTANCE USE IN CANADA

The Canadian Tobacco, Alcohol and Drugs Survey (CTADS) was completed in 2015 and provides the most recent and comprehensive national view of substance use in Canada.[14] According to the CTADS, most Canadians are moderate drinkers. In 2015, 77% reported alcohol beverage consumption in the past year; there was a higher prevalence of alcohol use among males (81%) than females (73%); and the rate of alcohol use was higher in young adults aged 20 to 24 (83%) than youth aged 15 to 19 (59%) and adults 25 years and older (78%). These patterns hold for low- and high-risk alcohol use. In 2015, current cigarette smoking decreased to 13%, which represents the lowest national average ever recorded (it was 25% in 1999, 17% in 2010, and 15% in 2013). According to the 2015 CTADS, cannabis was the most commonly used illicit substance. The prevalence of cannabis use increased from previous surveys, especially for women (from 7% in 2013 to 10% in 2015). In Canada, general population trends show an increase in harmful substance use, especially for Ecstasy and hallucinogens.

Recently, Canada has been facing an unrelenting overdose crisis. Data from 2016 indicate that Western Canada (in particular, Yukon, Northwest Territories, British Columbia, and Alberta) have experienced the worst crises.[15] For example, the rate of illicit drug overdose deaths in British Columbia increased 52% to 31.3 deaths per 100 000 individuals from the 2015 rate of 20.6 deaths per 100 000 individuals.[9] However, rates are increasing in all provinces and territories across Canada.[16] For example, there has been a steady increase in opioid-related harms in Ontario for more than a decade.[17] From 2003 to 2016, the number of opioid-related deaths in Ontario increased by 136%. In 2016, more than 850 Ontarians died from opioid-related causes.[17]

To address this crisis, in December 2016, the federal, provincial, and territorial governments formed a Special Advisory Committee (SAC) on the Epidemic of Opioid Overdoses to focus on urgent issues related to overdoses and deaths linked to the use of opioids, including those laced with fentanyl and carfentanil.[18] The SAC meets monthly to advance discussions on the opioid crisis in three key areas: (a) supporting harm reduction, (b) improving data/surveillance, and (c) addressing prevention and treatment options.

FACTORS INFLUENCING SUBSTANCE USE

Health care providers should know that substance use varies based on social, historical, and economic contexts. Which drugs are used, how much they are used, and how harmful such use is depends on geography (including the local history, what substances are available, and local norms) and income (what is affordable and what is profitable). Clinicians should learn about the particular context in which they are providing care, including cultural and personal histories of trauma and violence, as well as socioeconomic conditions. Understanding how inequities influence substance use can also help health care providers identify potentially successful approaches to addressing substance use.[19] For example, Indigenous people in Canada have gained considerable political power and economic control over their circumstances, which has had a positive effect on their health; in British Columbia, since 2001, they have been consuming less alcohol per capita than the general population.[20]

Four interrelated areas of influence shape substance use. First, social practices and acceptability are the most influential determinants of substance use patterns. In much of Canada, for example, alcohol use is legal, and certain levels of use are socially accepted; for example, daily consumption of wine with meals is acceptable in many communities. However, in other communities, such as certain Christian and Muslim communities, any consumption of alcohol is considered unacceptable. Thus, what is considered "problematic" varies.

Second, affordability is an important determinant of both levels of substance use and types of substances consumed. The importance of affordability has led to the use of pricing as a major policy tool in trying to curb levels of substance use. For example, the opioid crisis has been exacerbated by the relative affordability of certain drugs.[21]

Third, however, regardless of how problematic substance use is defined, substance use with profoundly negative effects on people's health and social well-being has been repeatedly linked to the intertwined issues of trauma, violence, and chronic pain.[22-24] Experiences of trauma (including child maltreatment), sexual assault, and other forms of interpersonal violence have physiological effects that are subsequently associated with substance use.

Finally, mental health and substance use are consistently linked;[25,26] therefore, substance use, violence, and mental health cannot be considered separately. As discussed in Chapters 6 and 8, nurses must understand that histories of trauma are common among people who have problems with substance use and among people with mental health problems such as PTSD and depression.

VIOLENCE, TRAUMA, MENTAL HEALTH, AND SUBSTANCE USE

All forms of interpersonal violence—including intimate partner violence (IPV), child abuse, and sexual assault—consistently have been shown to be related to substance use problems and mental health problems.[27] In a systematic review, Lagdon, Armour, and Stringer reported that robust correlations exist between IPV and depression, PTSD, and anxiety; as well, they noted the frequent co-occurrence of IPV and illicit substance use, which is usually used as a means of self-medication and coping.[28]

The health effects of violence, such as substance use, must be understood in the context of cumulative lifetime abuse rather than as a consequence of one type of violence.[29] For example, in a sample of 4451 Australian women, lifetime prevalence for a substance use disorder was 18.3%; for those who had experienced at least one form of gender-based violence (inclusive of IPV, sexual assault, and stalking), lifetime prevalence for a substance use disorder was 23%, and 57.3% for any mental disorder. For women who had experienced

three or more forms of gender-based violence, the lifetime prevalence for a substance use disorder was 47.1% and the lifetime prevalence for a mental health disorder was 89.4%.[30] These findings, and those of research that suggests violence during childhood or adolescence has more profound effects than violence at later stages of life,[31,32] emphasize the importance of considering experiences of multiple forms and patterns of lifetime violence in relation to substance use. Clinicians must consider substance use within a broader patient history and ensure that their approach to health assessment is "trauma- and violence-informed," wherein practice is based on understanding the relationships among violence, mental health, and substance use.[33] Understanding the relationships among trauma, violence, and substance use helps health care providers understand why certain populations are more likely to experience higher levels of and more harmful substance use. Those who are exposed to higher levels of trauma and violence are more likely to experience harms related to substance use, and those levels are related to social inequities. Trauma- and violence-informed care is discussed further in Chapter 8.

SUBSTANCE USE AND SOCIAL INEQUITIES

Substance use and the impacts of substance use are shaped by social inequities based on gender, age, and income. For example, tobacco use is declining dramatically in Canada, except among low-income populations, where rates are increasing.[14] The increase in low-income populations reflects the stress of living in poverty, limited options for dealing with stress, limited access to tobacco-reduction supports, and health education strategies related to tobacco cessation that are not appropriate or relevant to this population. Social inequities intersect with racism and other forms of discrimination to influence rates of substance use and related problems, including the quality of care received. For example, Indigenous people face greater economic inequity and significantly higher levels of violence of all forms than the rest of the population, and racial stereotypes about Indigenous people are known to influence clinical practice. Moreover, negative health care experiences result in avoidance or delay of care.[34,35] Therefore, in the stereotype-laden field of substance use, it is paramount for clinicians to understand how historical legacies of racism, violence, and dehumanization have led to health inequities for Indigenous people, and how those dynamics are related to substance use and its effects. Similarly, gender nonconforming people face high levels of violence. In a study of lesbian, gay, and bisexual people who use substances, Chow and colleagues demonstrated that sexual minorities are also at greater risk for illicit substance use and related harms than heterosexual populations.[36] Specifically, sexual identity predicted higher usage of Ecstasy, ketamine, and alcohol (but not alcohol-related problems). Significantly, Chow and colleagues found that inadequate housing increased the likelihood of crack cocaine use, highlighting the critical intersections of heterosexism, class, and other social structures in the lived realities of substance use.[36]

THE EFFECTS OF SUBSTANCE USE VARY BY GENDER, CLASS, AGE, AND SEXUALITY

Numerous negative individual, family, and societal outcomes result from high levels of substance use. Harm arises not only from the individual actions but also from the legal and social ramifications of substance use, such as illegal activities, incarceration, child apprehension by the state, and varying levels of stigma that people face, depending on their social position. For example, women with high levels of substance use are at increased risk for incarceration, economic deprivation, human immunodeficiency virus (HIV) infection, acquired immune deficiency syndrome (AIDS), dual diagnoses, depression, PTSD, loss of child custody, and subsequent risk for victimization (including IPV).[37,38] In a study of opioid dependence, Bawor and colleagues found that women experienced a greater burden of disease than men, with respect to medical problems, health outcomes, and social impairment.[39] This finding and the fact that women tend to be introduced to opioids by a physician's prescription point to the need for integrated models of care. Such models of care must consider alternatives to opioid analgesics alongside core social services such as vocational counselling, child care and parenting assistance, medical assistance, relationship or IPV counselling, and smoking-cessation programs. For example, prescribing narcotics to Indigenous people, often in the absence of any alternative pain-management approaches, has become a common and widespread practice by physicians.[40] In our research, a 29-year-old Indigenous woman with a history of violent victimization had suffered persistent abdominal pain since the age of 12, for which she had been prescribed acetaminophen (Tylenol) with codeine.[19] Her pain issues were not actually investigated, however, until she was 28 years old, and no alternatives to opioids were offered in the intervening time. Like many other Indigenous patients in the study, she described how difficult it was for her to not use substances.

The effects of substance use vary with intersecting aspects of social position, such as gender, income, age, sexuality, and ethnicity. Economic and social influences mean that the substance use practices of certain populations are more visible and open to scrutiny. For example, consider two people who use alcohol to the point of being visibly impaired. If one person lives on the street, is homeless, and is unemployed and the other person owns a home and has steady employment, the visibility of their alcohol use will be different and will have different consequences.[41]

Substance use is often viewed as a recreational, indulgent activity in which the participants seek a "high" to enjoy themselves. This limited interpretation can hinder the nurse's understanding of other reasons why people use substances. Many people use substances to feel numb; to stop pain (physical or emotional); or to control anxiety, nightmares, or sadness associated with past, current, and ongoing trauma. Sometimes people use substances to "feel normal" when prescribed therapies have failed. For example, most people using substances on the streets of the Downtown Eastside of Vancouver do not see themselves as "having fun" or enjoying being "high."

Understanding the relationship between patterns of violence across the lifespan, social inequities, and substance use helps health care providers understand substance use as a consequence of multiple influences. Understanding these patterns for both men and women, including different levels of scrutiny and judgement, is critical for improving health care, health policies, ways of approaching health assessment, and, ultimately, patients' health.

As demonstrated by the statistics on substance use in Canada, there is considerable variability with age in relation to the use of particular substances. Furthermore, although substance use occurs throughout the lifespan, some issues are particularly salient for different age groups. For example, for children, the prescription of medications such as methylphenidate (Ritalin) for behaviour problems has become a widespread concern, with controversy regarding the medical diagnoses leading to such prescription.[42] For young people, drinking (and sometimes binge drinking) has increasingly become a rite of passage to adulthood. When pregnant, women who consume substances are more intensely scrutinized. Many older adults take multiple medications and are overmedicated with prescription medications. Health care providers need to have an awareness of the most common problems facing each age group, without making assumptions about particular individuals, to tailor their health assessments most effectively.

UNDERSTANDING SUBSTANCE USE IN THE CONTEXT OF HEALTH CARE

Health care is supposed to be aimed at the promotion of health. However, in relation to substance use, health promotion objectives are often at odds with policies that focus on criminalizing substance use and targeting substance use–related behaviours rather than addressing the causes and factors influencing such use. Health care objectives may be subverted within health care settings by objectives of criminal justice, child welfare, or other organizations. For example, health care providers may participate in the surveillance and monitoring of people's drug use through observed urine tests; such practices may make it difficult to develop the trust needed for an effective health care provider–patient relationship. It is critical that nurses remain focused on health promotion, not law enforcement.

Understanding the links between violence, trauma, pain, mental health, and substance use, and understanding the influence of broader social and policy influences, health care providers can approach health assessments and practice from a comprehensive base. Health care providers must avoid viewing substance use as a primary problem to be targeted; rather, substance use is a symptom of other pre-existing problems and circumstances. Viewing substance use not solely or narrowly as a criminal or health problem but rather as a consequence of other social problems means that nurses should assess substance use in the context of a comprehensive health history, including violence, trauma, and mental health histories, and in the contexts of income, housing, employment, food security, and access to services such as counselling. This broader assessment provides the basis for meaningful interventions to support people in successfully addressing their substance use issues.

INCORPORATING KNOWLEDGE OF SUBSTANCE USE IN HEALTH ASSESSMENT

The understanding of substance use just described suggests that health assessment be based on the following principles:

- *It should be health promoting.* Assessments that involve negative judgements, are intrusive, or are punitive will deter patients from accessing care and, through shame, will increase secrecy and failure to access care, thereby increasing harm to health.
- *It should take the patient's and population's context into account.* Understanding the history, economics, and social conditions (e.g., those of a group of refugees from a war-torn country) will lead practitioners to convey understanding and to focus on salient issues during health assessment.
- *It should be trauma- and violence-informed.* Trauma-informed care is care that takes into account how histories of various forms of abuse shape experiences of substance use.[43] Violence-informed care further accounts for the dynamics of ongoing violence and structural forms of violence, such as policy-structured poverty and racism, and must be integrated with the concept of cultural safety (as discussed in Chapter 3).[34,44,45] Patients' substance use patterns are shaped by their histories of abuse and the patterns are difficult to change when those histories are not addressed and when the patients are facing ongoing violence.
- *It should minimize harm.* Harm reduction in relation to substance use often focuses narrowly on reducing the harms of drug use, such as by reducing overdoses or infections for people who are injecting drugs. A broader understanding of harm reduction recognizes that harms arise from the social, economic, political, and legal context of substance use. Harm reduction also aims to address these contexts by attempting to minimize homelessness, violence, and poverty,[46,47] and aligns with the understanding of harm reduction endorsed by many Canadian nursing organizations such as the Canadian Association of Nurses in HIV/AIDS Care (Box 7.2).

To develop the skills to put these principles into action, we suggest a process of five elements (Box 7.3). We have also developed an online learning module and a harm-reduction tool, which are available at https://equiphealthcare.ca/toolkit/.

Providing evidence-informed care requires that you develop a wide knowledge base. Accurate, current, evidence-informed knowledge about the pharmacological

---

BOX 7.2 Nurses and Harm Reduction

Registered nurses use harm-reduction approaches when they do the following:
- Participate in immunization and health promotion programs
- Provide counselling on safer sex
- Advocate for access to affordable and safe housing
- Develop and implement policies to minimize the risks of surgery
- Provide counselling on smoking cessation
- Administer methadone maintenance treatment
- Share information on the risks associated with alcohol and drug consumption
- Support patients with their daily medications and dietary restrictions
- Reduce the risks of falls in the hospital environment
- Intervene to reduce the adverse consequences of chronic illnesses
- Distribute bleach kits, clean syringes, and condoms
- Develop education material and interventions to reduce the risk for overdose
- Train peers to administer naloxone (Narcan™) for opioid overdose
- Provide preventive and primary care in supervised injection sites

From Canadian Association of Nurses in HIV/AIDS Care. (2015). *Bill C-2: Legislation to amend the Controlled Drugs and Substances Act to allow exemptions for supervised injection sites (and services). Brief for the Standing Senate Committee on Legal and Constitutional Affairs.* Ottawa, Canada (p. 2). Retrieved from http://canac.org/wp-content/uploads/2015/04/BILL-C-2_Brief_CANAC_SENATE.pdf.

BOX 7.3 Five "As" for Integrating Knowledge of Substance Use in Health Assessment

1. **A**cquire knowledge; replace erroneous assumptions. *Know* yourself: your assumptions, attitudes, values, and beliefs.
   Do assume that the majority of your patients use substances and that most feel embarrassed and stigmatized if their use is harmful.
   Do not assume that substance use is a simple choice.
   Do assume that many people who experience harmful substance use also have significant histories of trauma.
2. **A**nticipate harm that may be caused by your practices, reactions, and judgements (e.g., deterring patients from accessing the health care system); harm that may be linked to substance use, such as the social, legal, and economic contexts of use; and harm that may be caused by the substances used.
3. **A**nalyze the impact of policies at the level of organizations (e.g., clinical assessment tools) and society (e.g., what will be the impact of changing legislation related to marijuana be?; how do static social assistance rates in the face of rising costs of living affect substance use?).
4. **A**void social judgement about substance use, such as seeing a person as "bad," deviant, or morally weak.
5. **A**pproach *all* patients respectfully.

actions and physiological effects of different substances is required. Table 7.1 provides a list of possible signs and symptoms of use and withdrawal associated with common substances. However, it is important to bear in mind that over-reliance on such a list can lead to inaccurate assessment and false assumptions and diagnoses for many interrelated reasons. First, there is considerable variation in patient presentation. Second, many street drugs are tainted with unknown substances. People often use multiple substance at once (including prescription medications), so they would not have clearly defined symptoms as listed in the table. Other physical/medical conditions can look like use, intoxication, or withdrawal. For example, the third author of this chapter recently cared for the mother of a young baby. The woman was utterly exhausted from lack of sleep and was slurring her speech, nodding off, and unable to respond quickly during conversation. Because the woman had a history of use, her social worker assumed that she was using drugs. However, other staff were able to provide evidence to the contrary, as well as a urine drug screen test, which exonerated the woman.

Knowledge about promoting safe use is critical for any nurse, because assessment may be accompanied by an opportunity to provide advice. For example, knowing Canada's low-risk alcohol drinking guidelines (Box 7.4) allows you to provide guidance about alcohol use. As with any guidelines, nurses must read and apply them with a critical lens, and adapt them to the patient's or family's specific context. In relation to the use of other substances, learn about where to obtain safe supplies, what new risks are arising (e.g., the current dangers posed by the lacing of various drugs with fentanyl), and how to use safely.

In the process of conducting health assessments, you must be aware of prevalent stereotypes and assumptions related to substance use. To approach assessments related to substance use in a nonjudgemental way, critical self-reflection is crucial (Box 7.5). People who experience persistent, negative social and health effects of substance use are highly sensitive to the attitudes of clinicians. For these reasons and as discussed in Chapter 3, you must be aware of how your attitudes are conveyed through tone of voice, types of questions, and nonverbal behaviours such as facial expressions.

Challenging the Idea of "Choice"

One key assumption that must be challenged is that substance use is simply a matter of individual "choice." Canada has increasingly imported ideas of individualism (that each person is autonomous, making decisions independent of their circumstances), military language (such as "the war on drugs"), and criminalizing approaches to dealing with substance use. These ideas have resulted in pervasive and popularized assumptions that harmful substance use primarily reflects individual choice, which shifts use away from an illness model to an individual choice model.[48] Lewis argued that we should move away from the "choice" model and the "disease" model and, instead, view substance use according to a "developmental" model; in the developmental model, substance use is considered something that is learned and

---

BOX 7.4 Canada's Low-Risk Alcohol Drinking Guidelines

Your Limits

- Reduce your long-term health risks by drinking no more than: 10 drinks* a week for women, with no more than 2 drinks a day most days
- Drink no more than 15 drinks a week for men, with no more than 3 drinks a day most days
- Plan non-drinking days every week to avoid developing a habit.

Special Occasions

- Reduce your risk of injury and harm by drinking no more than 3 drinks (for women) or 4 drinks (for men) on any single occasion. Plan to drink in a safe environment. Stay within the weekly limits outlined above.

When Zero's the Limit

- Do not drink when you are driving a vehicle or using machinery and tools; taking medicine or other drugs that interact with alcohol; doing any kind of dangerous physical activity; living with mental or physical health problems; living with alcohol dependence; pregnant or planning to be pregnant; responsible for the safety of others; making important decisions.

Pregnant? Zero Is Safest

- If you are pregnant or planning to become pregnant, or about to breastfeed, the safest choice is to drink no alcohol at all.

Delay Your Drinking

- Alcohol can harm the way the body and brain develop. Teens should speak with their parents about drinking. If they choose to drink, they should do so under parental guidance; never more than 1–2 drinks at a time, and never more than 1–2 times per week. They should plan ahead, follow local alcohol laws, and consider the "Safer Drinking Tips" listed below.
- Youth in their late teens to age 24 years should never exceed the daily and weekly limits outlined in "Your Limits" above.

Safer Drinking Tips

Set limits for yourself and stick to them; drink slowly; have no more than 2 drinks in any 3 hours. For every drink of alcohol, have one nonalcoholic drink; eat before and while you are drinking; always consider your age, body weight, and health problems that might suggest lower limits. While drinking may provide health benefits for certain groups of people, do not start to drink or increase your drinking for health benefits.

*In these guidelines, a "drink" means: beer (341 mL or 12 oz, 5% alcohol content); cider/cooler (341 mL or 12 oz, 5% alcohol); wine (142 mL or 5 oz, 12% alcohol); distilled alcohol (rye, gin, rum, etc.; 43 mL or 1.5 oz, 40% alcohol).

Modified from Canadian Centre on Substance Abuse and Addiction. (2017). *Canada's low-risk alcohol drinking guidelines.* Retrieved from http://www.ccsa.ca/Eng/topics/alcohol/drinking-guidelines/Pages/default.aspx.

TABLE 7.1 Signs and Symptoms of Use and Withdrawal[a] With Selected Substances

SUBSTANCE	SIGNS AND SYMPTOMS OF USE	WITHDRAWAL
Alcohol	*Appearance:* unsteady gait, incoordination, nystagmus, flushed face *Behaviour:* sedation, relief of anxiety, dulled concentration, impaired judgement, expansive and uninhibited behaviour, talkativeness, slurred speech, impaired memory, irritability, depression, emotional lability	Cessation or reduction in alcohol use, especially after a period of heavy and prolonged drinking, results in **alcohol withdrawal**.[b] The symptoms of alcohol withdrawal syndrome develop within several hours to a few days after an individual stops drinking. Medical attention should be sought immediately. Signs and symptoms of withdrawal can include insomnia; autonomic symptoms such as sweating or racing heart; increased hand tremors (known as "the shakes"); nausea and/or vomiting; psychomotor agitation (feeling physically restless, inability to stop moving); anxiety; seizures; rarely, hallucinations, or perceptual disturbances of the auditory, tactile, or visual type.[b]
Sedatives, hypnotics	Similar to alcohol *Appearance:* unsteady gait, incoordination *Behaviour:* talkativeness, slurred speech, inattention, impaired memory, irritability, emotional lability, sexual aggressiveness, impaired judgement, impaired social or occupational functioning	Anxiety or irritability; nausea or vomiting; malaise; autonomic hyperactivity (tachycardia, sweating); orthostatic hypotension; coarse tremor of hands, tongue, and eyelids; marked insomnia; tonic–clonic seizures
Nicotine	*Appearance:* highly alert, increased systolic blood pressure, increased heart rate, vasoconstriction *Behaviour:* nausea, vomiting, indigestion (first use); loss of appetite, head rush, dizziness, jittery feeling, mild stimulation	Vasodilation, headaches; anger, irritability, frustration, anxiety, nervousness, awakening at night, difficulty concentrating, depression, hunger, impatience or restlessness[c]
Cannabis (marijuana)	*Appearance:* injected (reddened) conjunctivae, tachycardia, dry mouth, increased appetite, especially for "junk" food *Behaviour:* euphoria, anxiety, perception of slowed time, increased sense of perception, impaired judgement, social withdrawal, suspiciousness or paranoid ideation	Cannabis withdrawal syndrome is now officially recognized with defined criteria in the DSM-5. Symptoms include irritability; nervousness; sleep difficulty; decreased appetite; restlessness; depressed mood; physical symptoms and discomfort.[d]
Cocaine	*Appearance:* pupillary dilation, tachycardia or bradycardia, elevated or lowered blood pressure, sweating, chills, nausea, vomiting, weight loss *Behaviour:* euphoria, talkativeness, hypervigilance, pacing, psychomotor agitation, impaired social or occupational functioning, fighting, grandiosity, visual or tactile hallucinations	Dysphoric mood (anxiety, depression, irritability); fatigue, insomnia, or hypersomnia; psychomotor agitation
Amphetamines	Similar to cocaine *Appearance:* pupillary dilation, tachycardia or bradycardia, elevated or lowered blood pressure, sweating or chills, nausea and vomiting, weight loss *Behaviour:* elation, talkativeness, hypervigilance, psychomotor agitation, fighting, grandiosity, impaired judgement, impaired social and occupational functioning	Dysphoric mood (anxiety, depression, irritability); fatigue, insomnia, or hypersomnia; psychomotor agitation
Opiates (morphine, heroin, meperidine)	*Appearance:* pinpoint pupils; decreased blood pressure, pulse, respirations, and temperature *Behaviour:* lethargy; somnolence; slurred speech; initial euphoria followed by apathy, dysphoria, and psychomotor retardation; inattention; impaired memory; impaired judgement; impaired social or occupational functioning	Dysphoric mood; nausea or vomiting; muscle aches; lacrimation or rhinorrhea; pupillary dilation, piloerection, or sweating; diarrhea; yawning; fever; insomnia[e]

DSM-5, *Diagnostic and Statistical Manual of Mental Disorders* (5th ed.).

[a]*Symptoms of use* refer to behavioural and physiological changes resulting from the effects of substances on the central nervous system. *Withdrawal* refers to the physiological symptoms that are produced when use of the substance is discontinued.

[b]Medina, J. (2017). *DSM-5 alcohol withdrawal symptoms.* Retrieved from https://psychcentral.com/disorders/alcohol-withdrawal/.

[c]Baker, T. B., Breslau, N., Covey, L., et al. (2012). DSM criteria for tobacco use disorder and tobacco withdrawal: A critique and proposed revisions for DSM-5. *Addiction, 107*(2), 263–275. doi:10.1111/j.1360-0443.2011.03657.x

[d]Hesse, M., & Thylstrup, B. (2013). Time-course of the DSM-5 cannabis withdrawal symptoms in poly-substance abusers. *BMC Psychiatry, 13*(258). doi: https://doi.org/10.1186/1471-244X-13-258

[e]American Psychiatric Association. (2013). *Diagnostic and statistical manual of mental disorders* (5th ed.). Washington, DC: Author.

TABLE 7.2   Sample Screening Tool

The TWEAK questions[a] help identify at-risk drinking in women, especially pregnant women. Each question is scored on a 7-point scale. A woman who has a total score of 2 or more points is likely to be an at-risk for health related harms.[b]

- **T**olerance: How many drinks does it take to make you feel the first effect?
- **W**orry: Have close friends or relatives worried or complained about your drinking in the past year?
- **E**ye-opener: Do you sometimes take a drink in the morning when you first get up?
- **A**mnesia: Has a friend or family member ever told you about things you said or did that you could not remember?
- K(**C**)ut down: Do you sometimes feel the need to cut down on your drinking?

Scoring

Taking ≥3 drinks to feel high = tolerance.
Score 2 points each for tolerance and worry.
Score 1 point each for the rest.
A low-risk response is ≤1 point.
≥2 points = a likely drinking problem.

[a]Russell, M., Materier, S. S., & Sokol, R. J. (1994). Screening for pregnancy risk drinking. *Alcoholism: Clinical and Experimental Research, 18*(5), 1156–1161.
[b]Carson, G., Cox, L., Crane, J., et al. (2010). Alcohol use and pregnancy consensus clinical guidelines. *Journal of Obstetrics and Gynaecology Canada, 32*(8, Suppl. 3), S1–S31 (p. S16). Retrieved from http://www.sogc.org/guidelines/documents/gui245CPG1008E.pdf.

can be unlearned.[49] Understanding drug use as "choice" draws attention away from the underlying causes and factors influencing substance use and increases the likelihood of blaming and stigmatizing people who use substances beyond dominant social norms. Health care providers can (often unwittingly) communicate blame and shame if they consciously or unconsciously hold assumptions that people "ought to know better," should "pull up their socks and just say no," or are morally weak because they rely on alcohol or drugs. Furthermore, commonly held assumptions that people in specific ethnocultural or social groups use alcohol or drugs more than do people in other groups—despite the evidence to the contrary—can, unless challenged, lead to damaging health care encounters. As discussed in Chapter 3, this in turn can lead to errors in clinical judgement with serious consequences.

Putting Harm-Reduction Principles Into Action

What does it mean to be respectful? How can you gather the information you need in the least invasive, least harmful way?

1. *Learn about the context and population you serve.* What are the most common substance use issues? What are the common histories? What substances are being used? What are the differential effects on particular populations within the communities served? What resources are available? Health care providers who work specifically with people who use substances usually wish to help clinicians who work in more generalist areas acquire new knowledge and skill related to substance use.

2. *Be clear about why you are gathering information,* and convey your reasons to patients you are assessing. For example, if an alcohol screening tool is used in your institution (e.g., the TWEAK screening tool shown in Table 7.2, or the CAGE screening tool described in the footnote on p. 122), you might introduce it by saying, "We know that many people use alcohol, but we ask everyone about their alcohol use so that we can provide better pain management and anticipate reactions to medications and other problems."

3. *Do not gather information that is not needed or will not be used.* When people understand the rationale for being asked about substance use and trust that the information will be used for health reasons, they are more likely to disclose accurate information.

4. *Assess individuals in context.* If you have begun to learn about the context of people's lives in the populations you are serving, you will be better able to listen for and understand individuals' histories. Although you should anticipate that most people use substances of some sort, you should be especially alert when people present with a history of violent victimization, perpetration, or mental health problems.

5. *Start history-taking with the least intrusive questions.* Because alcohol is legal and its use is generally more acceptable than the use of other substances, a person may be more amenable to disclosing information about alcohol use than about other substances. Once you have established a relationship of trust and openness, this may be a good entry point to discussing illicit substance use or prescription medication use. Because many people use multiple substances, this is a logical progression. For example, you may say, "Many people who use alcohol also use cocaine/speed/marijuana and so on to counteract the effects or to enhance the effects. Is that something you have tried?" Ask progressively more detailed questions in the assessment:

- Substances used?
- Amount of substances used? If you do not understand the terms patients use (e.g., "points of heroin"), ask the patient for clarification ("Can you help me understand…?")
- How often?
- By what route ("How do you take that particular drug")?
- For how long have you used these substances?
- When was the last time you used?

This information will guide you in knowing what other tests or assessments are indicated.

Regardless of whether you are using a particular assessment tool, avoid conveying assumptions, and make your questions specific. For example, with regard to alcohol, first ask "Do you drink alcohol?" (people who are targets of racist stereotypes may assume that you are being racist if you simply ask "How much do you drink?"); then ask, "How much do you drink each week [or each day]?" rather than "How much do you drink?" (which is too general). Pose your questions in a way that conveys your knowledge about a given drug. For example, with regard to drugs such as crack, cocaine, or speed, ask "How do you use the drug? Do you smoke it? Inject with needles? Snort?"

If using a standardized assessment tool, you may have to "translate" the wording. For example, for the question "Do you ever have an eye-opener?" a patient might answer, "No" without understanding the meaning of the question. A clearer question, such as "Do you ever have a drink when you wake up, to get you going?" will elicit a more useful answer.

Although it is important to obtain a complete history of substance use, many patients do not trust the clinician adequately to disclose fully, and people who are experiencing the harms of substance use may not want to admit their level of use even to themselves. Consider a lack of disclosure a protective mechanism, and assume that developing trust is your responsibility. If the setting allows, obtain as much information as the patient is willing to share, and then complete the assessment at a later time when you have had time to develop a more trusting relationship.

6. *Use assessment as an opportunity to promote health and offer suggestions for harm reduction.* Discussing the patient's substance use will provide insight into whether the patient views it as harmful. Performing an assessment is also an opportunity to provide brief factual information. Again, start with the least invasive topic; for example, "Cigarette smokers who also use marijuana can decrease the harmful effects of tobacco by not smoking a cigarette while still under the effects of marijuana; the marijuana dilates the lung bed and opens it up more to the toxins from the cigarettes."

Linking your assessment to the person's health emphasizes why you are asking the questions and provides ongoing opportunities to remain focused on promoting health. Explain to the patient that the questions you are asking are important so that appropriate and specific care and testing can be provided: for example, liver function tests for people who use alcohol, skin care/wound care for people who use needles, and testing for infections and respiratory assessment for people who inhale substances. Examples of such explanations are as follows:

> *"People who smoke or snort drugs sometimes have wheezing, or productive coughs, or ulcerations in the nose. Has this been a problem for you?"*
>
> *"If you have ever used needles, then I can offer you blood testing for some infections such as hepatitis C, hepatitis B, and HIV."*

In our practice, we have found that people often are relieved to be offered testing.

7. *Throughout the assessment, avoid making assumptions and being influenced by popularized stereotypes* about people who use drugs or alcohol. This is also crucial during the physical examination. For example, if during a physical examination you notice that there are needle marks on a person's arms, do not assume that the marks are signs of injecting drugs! Many people, including illicit substance users, undergo blood tests for medical reasons. Instead, you might frame your observation neutrally: "I see you've had a needle." If the patient is using needles to inject substances, teaching about hygienic and safer injection techniques, as well as about never injecting when alone, can reduce harm. At the same time, this is an opportunity to ask, "how are you feeling about your use?", and what supports the person might need.

Helping all patients feel accepted and worthy of care, even if they are using illicit substances, is key to building trust. Remember that if people are not able to tell you about their substance use, it is a reflection on your skill at building trust and conveying a nonjudgemental attitude. When a nurse thinks that a patient "lied" about something such as drug use, medications, or diet, the nurse ought to ask, "What did I do to make the patient fear a punitive response for telling the truth?"

The following case example is illustrative:

> I was doing research in an emergency unit, following nurses as they did assessments. One nurse I was following was assigned to a man with chest pain. He was in "bed 1," the first monitor unit nearest the nursing desk reserved for possible myocardial infarction. She took his history: when his symptoms had begun, the nature of the pain, and how had it changed. In the process, she asked him the questions on the CAGE questionnaire.*[50]

---

*The **CAGE questionnaire** (*c*utdown, *a*nnoyed, *g*uilty, *e*ye-opener) takes less than 1 minute to complete and has four straightforward "yes"/"no" questions. The CAGE tests for lifetime alcohol use and dependence, but it does not distinguish past problem drinking from active present drinking.

The man looked distraught but almost relieved as she asked the questions. Yes, he felt he should cut down. Yes, his wife was constantly worrying. Yes, he felt terrible about his drinking. He was up to drinking "a 26er" a day. He wanted to quit.

The nurse ticked the boxes but then hurriedly left the stretcher to get an electrocardiogram on another patient, as the emergency unit filled past capacity. She was darting between about six different stretchers, another patient was vomiting, and I was caught up helping. Twenty minutes later, I noticed bed 1 was empty and asked what happened. "Oh," she replied, "it was just muscle strain, no cardiac problems." "What about the alcohol?" I asked. "We just ask about that in case they are admitted, in case of DTs [delirium tremens]," she said.

Screening tools (such as the TWEAK or CAGE described on pp. 121 and 122, respectively) may be required by your clinical setting and may provide useful ways to initiate a conversation about substance use. However, how such tools are implemented may be harmful (consider the case example just mentioned). Ask yourself:

- What are the practice conditions that might influence how effectively such tools may be used?
- What is required to use such tools in a way that promotes health?
- What is the most important goal of such tools?

Similarly, when biochemical assays such as urine samples are used as part of the physical assessment to screen for particular drugs, collection should be performed in ways that optimize trust, harm reduction, and health promotion. For example, a urine screen to detect the use of specific substances such as cocaine is often required as part of "conditions" for care contracts or child custody and visitation. The principles discussed previously apply directly to the collection of biochemical assays. Treating patients respectfully while they are subject to such surveillance is challenging but can build trust toward a more effective health care provider–patient relationship.

8. *Know and draw on resources.* Learn about your in-house and community resources. Any assessment that suggests harms should lead to action on your part. Depending on where you live, resources may be scarce or plentiful. Learn whether a given resource is more abstinence-based or harm-reduction based, and learn the reputation of a given resource from patients who have accessed the resource.
9. *Advocate for adequate resources for yourself and your patients.* We believe that the conditions of practice should allow nurses to use tools in a health-promoting way. Some of these conditions include taking time to pay attention to patients' answers, acknowledging discomfort (yours and theirs), listening respectfully, following up appropriately, and having resources to offer patients (educational, clinical, and community resources). Nurses can also participate in advocating for and supporting effective resources in their organizations and communities.

Assessing for Withdrawal

Often when patients are admitted to the hospital, their usual patterns of substance use are interrupted. If documentation of the history includes substance use, your health assessment increases the likelihood that you will be alert to the need to assess for and manage withdrawal. Alcohol withdrawal is most likely to be encountered, and all care providers should have a basic knowledge of the signs and symptoms of withdrawal. According to Mirijello and colleagues,[51] withdrawal signs and symptoms may appear within 6 to 12 hours of the abrupt cessation or decrease in alcohol intake. Those signs and symptoms manifest in the following four stages:

- *Stage I, minor withdrawal symptoms (6 to 12 hours):* tremors, diaphoresis, nausea/vomiting, hypertension, tachycardia, hyperthermia, tachypnea
- *Stage II, alcoholic hallucinosis (12 to 24 hours):* dysperceptions—visual (zooscopies), auditory (voices), and tactile (paresthesia)
- *Stage III, alcohol withdrawal seizures (24 to 48 hours):* generalized tonic–clonic seizures (with short or no postictal period)
- *Stage IV, delirium tremens (48 to 72 hours):* delirium, psychosis, hallucinations, hyperthermia, malignant hypertension, seizures, and coma[51]

Clinicians should anticipate such signs and symptoms for people with a history of heavy alcohol use, observe for signs and symptoms, and ensure that treatment is initiated as early as possible. Treatment typically includes various medications, including benzodiazepines. A promising practice being used in community contexts is managed alcohol programs, where the harms of alcohol use are reduced without requiring withdrawal and abstinence.[52,53] Beyond alcohol, clinicians should learn the signs and symptoms of the substances commonly used among the populations they serve, and similarly be alert for those. Again, Table 7.1 lists some possible signs and symptoms of use and withdrawal associated with common substances, but it should only be used as a beginning guide.

SPECIAL CASE: SUBSTANCE USE ASSESSMENT IN PREGNANCY

During pregnancy, women face intense scrutiny related to substance use, including smoking, alcohol use, and use of illegal substances. Societal attitudes can create significant barriers that prevent women from receiving adequate prenatal care. Some women may hide the fact that they are drinking an occasional glass of wine, for example, whereas others may avoid health care altogether, fearing judgement, punitive treatment, or the threat of having their babies removed from their care at birth. Nurses must understand that the fear of punishment is a major concern for many women. In many jurisdictions, because of the belief that use of illicit substances means that a woman is not a fit mother, a positive result of a drug test (in the mother or her newborn) can lead to an apprehension of the child because of "neglect" or "abuse."[54]

A woman who fears that her child may be removed from her care may not seek or may avoid prenatal or other medical or social care. Paradoxically, policies intended to promote healthy pregnancies, births, and children may do the opposite. For example, inadequate nutrition and stress (from poverty, violence, homelessness, and so on) may contribute more to poor obstetrical outcomes than does substance use in pregnancy.[55] Furthermore, good nutrition in pregnancy helps mitigate some of the harmful effects of substance use. However, women avoiding care may miss out on support for nutrition and housing.

Although all health care providers have a duty to report suspected child abuse (as discussed in Chapter 8), in Canada, a fetus is not legally considered a child, and therefore this duty does not apply, despite attempts by lobby groups to define substance use by pregnant women as child abuse. Involvement of child protection services when women are using substances during pregnancy is not appropriate. If a patient discloses substance use and has children in her care, the children are not necessarily at risk for harm. It is appropriate to ask about the safety plan for the children when the patient is using substances. Substance use can be compatible with safe parenting.

Sometimes, with full agreement of the pregnant patient, an early referral to child protection services can be beneficial if supportive services are available to assist the pregnant woman in preparing for birth. When the woman has a history with child protection services (e.g., a child removed from her care in the past), it may be beneficial for her to meet with a child protection worker to demonstrate how well she is doing, what positive changes she has made, and what her plans are for providing a safe environment. This might prevent a removal of the newborn from the mother's care at birth, in contrast to when decisions are based solely on the woman's history. Some jurisdictions are not adequately staffed to carry out investigations before the birth or to provide prenatal support.

Health care providers must have up-to-date and factual information regarding specific substances and their effects on the fetus. Alcohol and tobacco, both legal substances, are known to put the health of the fetus at risk. However, it is important to reassure women that moderate social drinking before confirmation of pregnancy has not been shown to cause birth defects.

Life circumstances that accompany illicit drug use are as detrimental to health as the substances: stigma, poverty, poor nutrition, needle use or sharing, smoking, lung irritants, survival sex work and the illegal activities necessary to obtain enough money to buy drugs, and associated exposure to sexually transmitted infections and violence.

You must recognize the stigma faced by women who use substances while pregnant, and you should provide nonjudgemental, supportive care. Stigma, judgement, and punitive treatment cause harm to the patient. To engage with patients successfully, nurses must actively work to counter such stigma and assure women of confidentiality.[56] Nurses can work to eliminate barriers to care by welcoming the patient and reassuring her that her well-being is the primary goal. By caring for the mother, you are caring for the fetus and infant. For example, some infants prenatally exposed to substances such as opiates, antidepressants, and certain prescription medications may exhibit symptoms of withdrawal in the first hours to days of life; however, when carefully monitored and managed with rooming-in with the mother, skin-to-skin contact, and breastfeeding, most infants do not require medical treatment for withdrawal.[57] There is increasing evidence that people who use illicit drugs can be adequate parents.[58] Most women share concern for the safety of the fetus, and so discussing this with the woman in a nonthreatening way can provide you with the opportunity to offer information about supports in the community (such as prenatal nutrition programs, housing advocates, and food banks).

DOCUMENTATION

Charting about substance use, like all other aspects of care, should be aimed at promoting the health of the patient. Charting should be factual and nonjudgemental, and nonstigmatizing phrasing should be used. Document as accurately as possible the type of drugs used, the amount, the route, and the results of your history and physical assessment.

Nurses and other clinical staff may wonder whether illegal drug use discussed during the process of assessment should be reported to "authorities" (e.g., to police, security officers, supervisors); however, there is no legal requirement to report, and doing so would be a breach of confidentiality if it is done for nonmedical reasons.

Often, efforts must be made to avoid using stigmatizing language and phrasing. For example, avoid labels such as "drug user," which tends to focus on a narrow aspect of a patient's life. Of importance is that the term "addict" not be used, unless to record a patient's statement that they think or have been told that they have "an addiction." Furthermore, people who use alcohol or drugs frequently resume and discontinue substance use as their life circumstances change. An example of less deterministic phrasing is "Uses heroin 2 to 4 times per week for the past year via injection into arm veins. For past year, has been using sterile needles obtained through the local needle-exchange unit."

In some cases, documentation of substance use by women who are pregnant and under surveillance by child welfare authorities can increase the risk that their newborns will be removed from their care or the risk that children who are currently in their custody will be removed from their care. As with the overall approaches to documentation, it is essential to chart only aspects of the history and physical examination that are directly relevant to assessment of the woman's health status. Pay extra attention to avoiding judgemental phrasing when you chart, in view of the extent to which pregnant women who use alcohol or substances are stigmatized in society.

ADDITIONAL RESOURCES

Alcohol and Drug Abuse Institute (University of Washington): http://adai.washington.edu

Canadian Alcohol and Drug Use Monitoring Survey (CADUMS): https://www.canada.ca/en/health-canada/services/health-concerns/drug-prevention-treatment/drug-alcohol-use-statistics.html

Canadian Centre on Substance Use and Addiction: http://www.ccdus.ca

Canadian Harm Reduction Network: http://www.canadianharmreduction.com

Canadian Institute for Substance Use Research (University of Victoria): https://www.uvic.ca/research/centres/cisur/

Coalescing on Women and Substance Use: http://www.coalescing-vc.org

Substance Abuse and Mental Health Services Administration (SAMHSA): http://www.samhsa.gov

Wild, N. (Director). (2007). Bevel up: Drugs'. users and outreach nursing [Video]. Available from https://www.nfb.ca/film/bevel_up_drugs_users_and_outreach_nursing/

REFERENCES

1. Varcoe, C., Browne, A. J., Ford-Gilboe, M., et al. (2017). Reclaiming our spirits: Development and pilot testing of a health promotion intervention for Indigenous women who have experienced intimate partner violence. *Research In Nursing & Health, 40*(3), 237–254.

2. Varcoe, C., Ford-Gilboe, M., Browne, A. J., et al. (in review). The efficacy of a health promotion intervention for Indigenous women: Reclaiming our spirits. *Journal of Interpersonal Violence.*

3. American Psychiatric Association (2013). *Diagnostic and statistical manual of mental disorders* (5th ed.). Washington, DC: Author.

4. O'Brien, C. P. (2014). Managing patients with a history of substance abuse. *Canadian Family Physician, 60*(3), 248–250. (p. 248).

5. Government of Canada. (2017). *Task Force on cannabis legalization and regulation.* Retrieved from http://healthycanadians.gc.ca/task-force-marijuana-groupe-etude/index-eng.php.

6. Kaskutas, L. A. (2009). Alcoholics Anonymous effectiveness: Faith meets science. *Journal of Addictive Diseases, 28*(2), 145–157.

7. Collin, C. (2006). *Substance use issues and public policy in Canada: II Parliamentary action (1987–2005).* Ottawa: Political and Social Affairs Division, Library of Parliament, Canada.

8. Canadian Nurses Association. (2015). *Bill C2: An act to amend the Controlled Drugs and Substances Act (Respect for Communities Act).* Brief for the Standing Senate Committee on Legal and Constitutional Affairs. Ottawa, Canada.

9. British Columbia Coroner's Office. (2017). *Illicit drug overdose deaths in BC: January 1, 2007–October 31, 2017.* Retrieved from http://www2.gov.bc.ca/assets/gov/public-safety-and-emergency-services/death-investigation/statistical/illicit-drug.pdf.

10. Alam, A., & Juurlink, D. N. (2016). The prescription opioid epidemic: An overview for anesthesiologists. *Canadian Journal of Anaesthesia, 63*, 61.

11. Giesbrecht, N. (2008). Recent developments in overall alcohol consumption and high risk drinking: A case for effective population level interventions in Canada. *Adicciones, 20*(3), 207–219.

12. Giesbrecht, N., Ialomiteanu, A., Anglin, L., et al. (2007). Alcohol marketing and retailing: Public opinion and recent policy developments in Canada. *Journal of Substance Use, 12*(6), 389–404.

13. Gilligan, C., Thompson, K., Bourke, J., et al. (2014). "Everybody else is doing it"—Norm perceptions among parents of adolescents. *Journal of Studies on Alcohol & Drugs, 75*(6), 908–918.

14. Government of Canada. (2017). *Canadian Tobacco, Alcohol and Drugs Survey (CTADS): 2015 summary.* Retrieved from https://www.canada.ca/en/health-canada/services/canadian-tobacco-alcohol-drugs-survey.html.

15. Government of Canada. (2018). *National report: Apparent opioid-related deaths in Canada (January 2016 to March 2017).* Retrieved from https://www.canada.ca/en/public-health/services/publications/healthy-living/apparent-opioid-related-deaths-report-2016.html?wbdisable=true#tab1.

16. Public Health Agency of Canada. (2016). *National report: Apparent opioid-related deaths (2016).* Retrieved from https://www.canada.ca/en/health-canada/services/substance-abuse/prescription-drug-abuse/opioids/national-report-apparent-opioid-related-deaths.html#def.

17. Public Health Ontario. (2017). *Opioid-related morbidity and mortality in Ontario.* Retrieved from https://www.publichealthontario.ca/en/dataandanalytics/pages/opioid.aspx.

18. Pan-Canadian Public Health Network. (2017). *Special Advisory Committee on the Epidemic of Opioid Overdoses.* Retrieved from http://www.phn-rsp.ca/sac-opioid-gcs-opioides/index-eng.php.

19. Browne, A., Varcoe, C., & Fridkin, A. (2011). Addressing trauma, violence and pain: Research on health services for women at the intersections of history and economics. In O. Hankivsky (Ed.), *Health inequities in Canada: Intersectional frameworks and practices* (pp. 295–311). Vancouver: UBC Press.

20. British Columbia Provincial Health Officer. (2002). *Report on the health of British Columbians: Provincial health officer's annual report 2001: The health and well-being of Aboriginal people in British Columbia.* Victoria: Ministry of Health Planning.

21. Dasgupta, N., Freifeld, C., Brownstein, J. S., et al. (2013). Crowdsourcing black market prices for prescription opioids. *Journal of Medical Internet Research, 15*(8), e178. doi: http://doi.org/10.2196/jmir.2810.

22. Haskell, L., & Randall, M. (2009). Disrupted attachments: A social context complex trauma framework and the lives of Aboriginal peoples in Canada. *Journal of Aboriginal Health, 5*(3), 48–99.

23. Hwang, S. W., Wilkins, E., Chambers, C., et al. (2011). Chronic pain among homeless persons: Characteristics, treatment, and barriers to management. *BMC Family Practice, 12*, 73.

24. Maxwell, K. (2014). Historicizing historical trauma theory: Troubling the trans-generational transmission paradigm. *Transcultural Psychiatry, 51*(3), 407–435.

25. Catchpole, R. E. H., & Brownlie, E. B. (2016). Characteristics of youth presenting to a Canadian youth concurrent disorders program: Clinical complexity, trauma, adaptive functioning and treatment priorities. *Journal of the Canadian Academy of Child and Adolescent Psychiatry, 25*(2), 106–115.

26. Wu, L.-T., & Blazer, D. G. (2014). Substance use disorders and psychiatric comorbidity in mid and later life: A review.

International Journal of Epidemiology, 43(2), 304–317. doi: http://doi.org/10.1093/ije/dyt173.

27. Mason, R., Wolf, M., O'Rinn, S., et al. (2017). Making connections across silos: Intimate partner violence, mental health, and substance use. *BMC Women's Health, 17,* 29. Retrieved from http://doi.org/10.1186/s12905-017-0372-4.

28. Lagdon, S., Armour, C., & Stringer, M. (2014). Adult experience of mental health outcomes as a result of intimate partner violence victimisation: A systematic review. *European Journal of Psychotraumatology, 5*(1). doi: http://doi.org/10.3402/ejpt.v5.24794.

29. Scott-Storey, K. (2011). Cumulative abuse: Do things add up? An evaluation of the conceptualization, operationalization, and methodological approaches in the study of the phenomenon of cumulative abuse. *Trauma, Violence and Abuse, 12*(3), 135–150.

30. Rees, S., Silove, D., Chey, T., et al. (2011). Lifetime prevalence of gender-based violence in women and the relationship with mental disorders and psychosocial function. *JAMA: The Journal of the American Medical Association, 306*(5), 513–521.

31. McLaughlin, K. A., Green, J. G., Gruber, M. J., et al. (2010). Childhood adversities and adult psychiatric disorders in the National Comorbidity Survey Replication II: Associations with persistence of *DSM-IV* disorders. *Archives of General Psychiatry, 67*(2), 124–132.

32. Smith, C. A., Elwyn, L. J., Ireland, T. O., et al. (2010). Impact of adolescent exposure to intimate partner violence on substance use in early adulthood. *Journal of Studies on Alcohol & Drugs, 71,* 219–230.

33. Ponic, P., Varcoe, C., & Smutylo, T. (2016). Trauma- (and violence-) informed approaches to supporting victims of violence: Policy and practice considerations. *Victims of Crime Research Digest, 9.* Retrieved from http://www.justice.gc.ca/eng/rp-pr/cj-jp/victim/rd9-rr9/p2.html.

34. Goodman, A., Fleming, K., Markwick, N., et al. (2017). "They treated me like crap and I know it was because I was Native": The healthcare experiences of Aboriginal peoples living in Vancouver's inner city. *Social Science & Medicine, 178,* 87–94.

35. Shahram, S. (2016). The social determinants of substance use for Aboriginal women: A systematic review. *Women and Health, 56*(2), 157–176.

36. Chow, C., Vallance, K., Stockwell, T., et al. (2013). Sexual identity and drug use harm among high-risk, active substance users. *Culture, Health & Sexuality, 15*(3), 311–326.

37. Golinelli, D., Longshore, D., & Wenzel, S. L. (2009). Substance use and intimate partner violence: Clarifying the relevance of women's use and partners' use. *Journal of Behavioral Health Services & Research, 36,* 199–211.

38. Schneider, R., Burnette, M. L., Ilgen, M. A., et al. (2009). Prevalence and correlates of intimate partner violence victimization among men and women entering substance use disorder treatment. *Violence and Victims, 24*(6), 744–756.

39. Bawor, M., Dennis, B. B., Varenbut, M., et al. (2015). Sex differences in substance use, health, and social functioning among opioid users receiving methadone treatment: A multicenter cohort study. *Biology of Sex Differences, 6,* 21.

40. Webster, P. C. (2013). Indigenous Canadians confront prescription opioid misuse. *Lancet, 381*(9876), 1447–1448.

41. Robertson, L. A., & Culhane, D. (2005). *In plain sight: Reflections on life in Downtown Eastside Vancouver.* Vancouver: Talonbooks.

42. Visser, J., & Jehan, Z. (2009). ADHD: A scientific fact or a factual opinion? A critique of the veracity of attention deficit hyperactivity disorder. *Emotional & Behavioural Difficulties, 14*(2), 127–140.

43. Covington, S. S. (2008). Women and addiction: A trauma-informed approach. *Journal of Psychoactive Drugs,* (Suppl. 5), 377–385.

44. Pauly, B. B., McCall, J., Browne, A. J., et al. (2015). Toward cultural safety: Nurse and patient perceptions of illicit substance use in a hospitalized setting. *Advances In Nursing Science, 38*(2), 121–135.

45. Varcoe, C., Wathen, C. N., Ford-Gilboe, M., et al. (2016). *VEGA briefing note on trauma- and violence-informed care.* Retrieved from http://projectvega.ca/wp-content/uploads/2016/10/VEGA-TVIC-Briefing-Note-2016.pdf.

46. Pauly, B. (2008). Harm reduction through a social justice lens. *International Journal of Drug Policy, 19*(1), 4–10.

47. Pauly, B. B., Reist, D., Belle-Isle, L., et al. (2013). Housing and harm reduction: What is the role of harm reduction in addressing homelessness?. *International Journal on Drug Policy, 24*(4), 284–290.

48. Cortina, S. C. (2013). Stigmatizing harm reduction through language: A case study into the use of "addict" and opposition to supervised injection sites in Canada. *Journal of Addictions Nursing, 24*(2), 102–107.

49. Lewis, M. (2017). Addiction and the brain: Development, not disease. *Neuroethics, 10*(1), 7–18.

50. Seo, Y. R., Kim, J. S., Kim, S. S., et al. (2016). Development of a simple tool for identifying alcohol use disorder in female Korean drinkers from previous questionnaires. *Korean Journal of Family Medicine, 37*(1), 18–24. Retrieved from http://nationalpaincentre.mcmaster.ca/documents/cage_questionnaire.pdf.

51. Mirijello, A., D'Angelo, C., Ferrulli, A., et al. (2015). Identification and management of alcohol withdrawal syndrome. *Drugs, 75*(4), 353–365.

52. Pauly, B., Gray, E., Perkin, K., et al. (2016). Finding safety: A pilot study of managed alcohol program participants' perceptions of housing and quality of life. *Harm Reduction Journal, 13,* 1–11.

53. Vallance, K., Stockwell, T., Pauly, B., et al. (2016). Do managed alcohol programs change patterns of alcohol consumption and reduce related harm? A pilot study. *Harm Reduction Journal, 13,* 1–11.

54. Niccols, A., Dell, C. A., & Clarke, S. (2010). Treatment issues for Aboriginal mothers with substance use problems and their children. *International Journal of Mental Health and Addiction, 8*(2), 320–335.

55. Boyd, S. C. (2004). *From witches to crack moms: Women, drug law and policy.* Durham, NC: Carolina Academic Press.

56. Radcliffe, P. (2011). Substance-misusing women: Stigma in the maternity setting. *British Journal of Midwifery, 19*(8), 497–506.

57. Abrahams, R. R., MacKay-Dunn, M. H., Nevmerjitskaia, V., et al. (2010). An evaluation of rooming-in among substance-exposed newborns in British Columbia. *Journal of Obstetrics and Gynaecology Canada, 32*(9), 866–871.

58. Shahram, S. Z., Bottorff, J. L., Kurtz, D. L. M., et al. (2017). Understanding the life histories of pregnant-involved young Aboriginal women with substance use experiences in three Canadian cities. *Qualitative Health Research, 27*(2), 249–259.

Interpersonal Violence Assessment

Written by Colleen Varcoe, PhD, RN

http://evolve.elsevier.com/Canada/Jarvis/examination/

Because you are a health care provider (HCP), an acquaintance (Monica) asks you for advice. She has a friend (Evelyn) whose partner is very disrespectful of Evelyn in public. At a recent event associated with their faith community, Monica saw the partner grab Evelyn's 5-year-old son (the partner's stepson) by the back of the neck and throw him on the ground. Monica tried to talk about the incident with Evelyn, but Evelyn said that her partner does not want her talking to Monica any longer. What assumptions do you notice you are making as you read this scenario? What should you advise Monica to do? What should you do? What risks of further violence can you identify?

Interpersonal violence—including intimate partner violence (IPV), sexual assault, child maltreatment, and elder abuse—is a serious problem that HCPs must recognize, assess, and address. In Canada, all provinces have mandatory requirements for reporting child maltreatment, and some provinces have general mandatory reporting requirements within adult legislation that apply to some forms of elder abuse or abuse of people with developmental disabilities. Beyond these legal requirements, all forms of interpersonal violence have significant, long-lasting health consequences and require a meaningful response by HCPs. Importantly, interpersonal violence is continuous with structural forms of violence. **Structural violence** refers to the harmful ways in which society is organized so that people are put at risk, such as through systemic discrimination, poverty sustained by economic arrangements and policies, or other policies that create vulnerabilities for some people. For example, minimum wage legislation and social assistance rates that are insufficient for sustenance create significant risks for health, and expose people to risk—such as through risky transportation options, unsafe housing, or needing to engage in risky work or transactional sex.

A SOCIAL DETERMINANTS OF HEALTH PERSPECTIVE

Violence is a widespread sociocultural problem, but in Western societies, there is a tendency to treat interpersonal violence as a problem of individuals. Rather than social

prevention and intervention, systemic efforts by governments, systems such as justice and health care systems, and organizations that deal with violence are targeted at individuals rather than the social context, often leaving victims responsible for dealing with violence. Furthermore, despite the fact that violence is well-known to occur across all societies and cultural groups, there is a tendency to associate violence with particular groups. To effectively deal with violence, HCPs must take three steps:

1. As argued in earlier chapters, HCPs must evaluate how dominant cultural values and beliefs, including the dominant values operating in health care, affect the care they provide. For example, what is the "common sense" solution to IPV? What common social messages do you encounter about what leads to sexual assault? How well-resourced are health care settings to provide support to people experiencing violence?

2. HCPs must practise based on knowledge and evidence about IPV, sexual assault, child maltreatment,* and elder abuse rather than operate on stereotypes and assumptions. This means understanding all forms of violence as abuses of power and developing knowledge about how the position of children, women, sexual minorities, older adults, people with disabilities, and others in society create vulnerability to violence.

3. HCPs need to consider how ideas about certain groups of people support discrimination in the provision of health care and deter people from seeking health care. For example, what "faith group" came to your mind when you read the opening scenario, and what does that tell you? What groups of people might anticipate being assumed to be abusive toward partners or children? One of the most egregious examples of these dynamics is the situation of Indigenous people. Generations of Indigenous children have been taken from their parents by the state, interfering with their parenting and creating stereotypes about Indigenous parents.[1] These stereotypes play a

---

Child abuse and *child maltreatment* are used interchangeably throughout the literature. In this chapter, unless citing other sources, the term *maltreatment* is used to emphasize the diverse forms, including the most common form, neglect.

role in continued apprehension of children by the state, and deter people from seeking health care.[2]

Rather than assess how experiences of violence are shaped by culture—narrowly defined as ethnicity—it is important to assess how they are shaped by culture in the broader sense. For example, rather than focusing on particular ethnocultural groups, it is more useful to consider how racialization, gender and other forms of discrimination, experiences of immigration, language barriers, and inequitable access to employment and resources shape experiences of violence and access to social support in response to violence.[3]

INTIMATE PARTNER VIOLENCE DEFINED

Intimate partner violence (IPV) encompasses spousal violence and violence committed by current or former dating partners.[4] **Spousal abuse** is physical or sexual violence, psychological violence, or financial abuse within current or former marital or common-law relationships, including spousal relationships between people regardless of sex or gender identity. Johnson has identified three types of IPV.[5] "Intimate partner terrorism" is characterized by coercive control in which one partner tries to control the other; it results in the most severe health consequences[6] and is most commonly perpetrated by men.[5] The second type is called "resistant violence" in which a person who is a victim of intimate terrorism responds with violence. Finally "situational couple violence" is

> *when couple conflicts become arguments that turn to aggression that becomes violent. It is by far the most common form of intimate partner violence, and also the most variable. Somewhere around 40% of the cases identified in general surveys involve only one relatively minor incident, but many cases do involve chronic and/ or serious, even life-threatening, violence. In contrast to intimate terrorism, situational couple violence does not involve an attempt on the part of one partner to gain general control over the other, and unlike intimate terrorism and violent resistance it is roughly gender-symmetric in terms of perpetration.[7]*

Gender is a key risk factor for the types and severity of IPV experienced: "Men's and boys' experiences of violence are different than women's and girls' in important ways. While men are more likely to be injured by strangers in a public or social venue, women are in greater danger of experiencing violence from intimate partners in their own homes. Women are also at greater risk of sexual violence."[4] For example, in 2015, four out of five victims (79%) of police-reported IPV were women. Women were also five times more likely than men to be killed by an intimate partner.[4] Gendered experiences of violence intersect with and are shaped by other forms of marginalization, including racism,[8] ableism,[9] and ageism (Fig. 8.1).[10] Most significantly in Canada, Indigenous women's higher risks of violence are a direct consequence of historical and ongoing colonization.[11,12]

8.1 Women who experience violence are from all backgrounds.

SEXUAL ASSAULT DEFINED

Sexual assault is defined by the Canadian *Criminal Code* as sexual activity in the absence of voluntary agreement, including when consent has not been given, when the person is not capable of giving consent, or when a person initially consented and then withdrew consent.[13] Sexual assault usually occurs either within the context of a partner relationship or by a known assailant, but it may be perpetrated by a stranger. The *Criminal Code* identifies both sexual assault and sexual touching as crimes. There are four levels of **sexual assault**: (a) sexual assault that is forced sexual activity without physical injury; (b) sexual assault with a weapon or verbal threats to a third party; (c) sexual assault causing bodily harm; and (d) aggravated sexual assault, which is forced sexual activity where the attacker seriously injures, wounds, maims, disfigures, or endangers life.

CHILD MALTREATMENT DEFINED

In Canada, child maltreatment and exploitation are prohibited by the *Criminal Code*.[13] Most provinces and territories have child welfare laws that require the public, including HCPs, to report suspected child maltreatment. The Department of Justice Canada defines **child abuse** as follows:

> *the violence, mistreatment or neglect that a child or adolescent may experience while in the care of someone they either trust or depend on, such as a parent, sibling, other relative, caregiver or guardian. Abuse may take place anywhere and most commonly occurs within the child's home and by someone known to the child.*
>
> *There are many different forms of maltreatment, and a child may be subjected to more than one form.[14]*

The 2014 Canadian General Social Survey (GSS) on Victimization reported that 33% of Canadians aged 15 and older experienced some form of maltreatment during childhood.[15] Moreover, child maltreatment and children's exposure to IPV against women often overlap.[16] Box 8.1 lists the Department of Justice Canada's definitions of types of child abuse

BOX 8.1 Types of Child Abuse

Physical Abuse

Physical abuse is the intentional use of force against a child. It can cause physical pain, injury, or injury that may last a lifetime. This type of abuse includes the following:
- Pushing or shoving
- Hitting, slapping, or kicking
- Strangling or choking
- Pinching or punching
- Stabbing or cutting
- Shooting
- Throwing objects at someone
- Holding someone down for someone else to assault
- Locking someone in a room or tying them down
- Killing someone

All of these acts are crimes in Canada.

Sexual Abuse

Child sexual abuse happens when a person takes advantage of a child for sexual purposes. It does not always involve physical contact with a child. For example, it could happen when an adult does the following:
- Makes sexual comments to a child, or
- Watches or films a child for sexual purposes.

Sexual abuse of a child includes the following:
- Any sexual contact between an adult and a child under the age of 16
- Any sexual contact with a child between the ages of 16 and 18 without consent, or
- Any sexual contact that exploits a child under the age of 18.

Any sexual contact between an adult and a child under the age of 16 is a crime. In Canada, the age of consent for sexual activity is 16, but there are some exceptions if the other person is close in age to the child. Child-specific sexual offences are handled differently under provincial and territorial child protection laws. For more information on the age of consent and teenage relationships, visit the Department of Justice link "Age of Consent to Sexual Activity" at http://www.justice.gc.ca/eng/rp-pr/other-autre/clp/faq.html.

In addition, children under the age of 18 cannot legally give their consent to sexual activity that exploits them. Sexual activities that exploit a child include prostitution and pornography. They also include situations where someone in a position of authority or trust, or someone the child depends on, has any kind of sexual activity with the child. A person of authority or trust could be a step-parent, a babysitter, or a coach.

Neglect

Neglect happens when a parent or guardian fails to meet a child's basic needs. Sometimes parents neglect their children on purpose. Sometimes parents do not mean to neglect their children, but they have so many problems themselves that they cannot look after their children properly. Neglect can include the following:
- Not giving a child proper food or warm clothing
- Not providing a child with a safe and warm place to live
- Not making sure a child washes regularly
- Not providing a child with enough health care or medicine
- Not paying any attention to a child's emotional needs
- Not preventing physical harm to a child
- Not making sure a child is supervised properly

Sometimes, neglect can hurt just as much as physical abuse.

Some forms of neglect are crimes in Canada. For example, failing to provide the necessities of life and child abandonment are crimes. The provinces and territories also have laws to protect children from neglect. These laws protect children even if the type of abuse is not a crime.

Emotional Abuse

Emotional abuse happens when a person uses words or actions to control, frighten, isolate, or take away a child's self-respect and sense of worth. Emotional abuse is sometimes called *psychological abuse*. It can include the following:
- Putting a child down or humiliating a child
- Constantly criticizing a child
- Constantly yelling at a child
- Threatening to harm a child or others
- Keeping a child from seeing their family or friends without good reason
- Threatening to move a child out of the home

Based on Department of Justice Canada. (2017). *About family violence.* Retrieved from http://www.justice.gc.ca/eng/cj-jp/fv-vf/about-apropos.html.

(they are consistent with those used in most provincial and territorial laws).

Abuse is a misuse of power and a violation of trust. Child maltreatment arises in relation to the positioning of children as relatively less powerful to adults in society, similar to the abuse of women that arises in relation to their gendered positioning. Thus, it is not surprising that children who are maltreated are usually in a position of dependence on the person who is abusing them. An abuser may use various tactics to exert power and control over the child, and prevent the child from telling anyone about the abuse or seeking support. The abuse may happen once or in a repeated and escalating pattern over months or years, and it may change form over time.

ELDER ABUSE DEFINED

Elder abuse includes interpersonal violence that continues into older adulthood and that arises as persons become more vulnerable with age. IPV may continue as people age, or may begin later in life, or new forms of abuse may arise with increasing vulnerability. The Department of Justice Canada identifies many forms of elder abuse, including psychological, financial, physical, sexual, and spiritual abuses, as well as neglect.[17]

Employment and Social Development Canada notes that elder abuse is perpetrated by people in a wide range of roles: "Elder abuse can be caused by a family member, a friend, someone who provides assistance with basic needs or services, or health care providers in institutional settings. In many situations of elder abuse, the abuser is dependent on the older adult for money, food or shelter."[18] Elder abuse includes violence and/or neglect in the home, in institutions, and self-neglect. McDonald and colleagues noted that research has tended to focus on violence in the home and overlooks institutional abuse, a problem that urgently needs attention given Canada's aging population and increasing institutionalization of older adults.[19] Such abuse may include rough or violent handling during personal care, force feeding or withholding food, and neglect.

The Public Health Agency of Canada estimates that 4% to 10% of older adults experience abuse, and yet only 20% of these report it.[20] Data from the 2015 Uniform Crime Reporting Survey and the 2015 Homicide Survey showed that *police-reported* family violence against older adults is most often perpetrated by an extended family member, grown child, or spouse.[21] Physical assault was the most common form of assault (70%). Of family-related homicides, nearly half of older adult victims were killed by a grown child (47%) and one-third by a spouse (34%). Violence is also related to locale: the highest rates of family-related violence against older adults were in the territories and prairie provinces; for example, Nunavut's rate is 30 times the national rate.

As with any form of interpersonal violence, gender is a risk factor in older adults: that is, older women are at a higher risk than are older men. For example, 6 in 10 of all victimizations of family members were against older women, a rate 26% higher than that against older men.[21] Although age and gender can increase vulnerability, it is important to note that other factors, such as economic dependence, disabilities (e.g., intellectual and physical disabilities), and rural isolation also increase vulnerability to violence as people age. Older adults who become frail and require medical or other health-related services may experience abuse in the form of failure to facilitate their access to medical or health services, failure to provide medical attention, or the conducting of a procedure or treatment without the informed consent of the patient or patient's recognized substitute decision maker.

THE PREVALENCE OF INTERPERSONAL VIOLENCE

IPV, sexual assault, child maltreatment, and elder abuse are significant problems globally and in Canada, although all estimates are widely acknowledged to be underestimates. For example, as of 2018, there has not been a population study specific to violence in Canada since the 1993 Violence Against Women Survey (VAWS). Population estimates have been based on the violence module within the GSS, which does not distinguish situational couple violence from intimate terrorism, and therefore does not take the gendered nature of violence into account.[6] According to the most recent estimates from the 2014 GSS, 4% of women and 4% of men in current or previous spousal relationships reported experiencing some form of spousal violence during the previous 5 years, a decline from the 2004 GSS.[22] However,

violence against women tended to be much more severe; women were twice as likely to have been sexually assaulted, beaten, choked, or threatened with a gun or knife, reflecting the fact that the GSS conflates intimate terrorism with situational couple violence.[23]

Population estimates in Canada do not account well for gender differences, with IPV being grossly under-reported. According to the 2014 GSS, only one in five victims of spousal violence (19%) contact the police to report victimization.[23] However, the gendered nature of spousal violence can be seen in homicide statistics. In 2014, the rate of intimate partner homicide against women was four times higher than that for men, with females 25 to 29 years old being at highest risk (8.2 per 1 million population).[24] In the case of Indigenous women, both in 2014 and 2015, the rate of homicide consistently remained six times that of non-Indigenous women.[25]

Lifetime rates of physical assault by a heterosexual partner have been estimated at 22.4% to 33.6% in English-speaking, middle- to high-income countries.[26] Physical assault is often accompanied by sexual violence or emotional abuse, and many women experience IPV in more than one relationship over their lifetimes.

As reported in the 2014 GSS, victimization rates for all crimes showed a decline over the past decade, with the exception of sexual assault that, at 22 incidents per 1000 people, remained stable for more than a decade, and has remained stable since 1999.[27] In 2015, 21 500 sexual assaults were reported to police in Canada, with the majority of victims being women; this number is estimated to be extremely conservative because close to 95% of sexual assaults are not brought to the attention of the police.[27,28]

The incidence of child maltreatment is also difficult to estimate and often based on *reported* cases. Using data from child welfare authorities, the Canadian Incidence Study of Reported Child Abuse and Neglect—2008 (CIS-2008) estimated a rate of 39.16 investigations of child abuse per 1000 children, a significant jump from 21.47 per 1000 children in 1998, but a slight increase from the 2003 rate of 38.33 per 1000 children.[29] The highest proportion of reported and substantiated child abuse cases involved two primary categories of maltreatment: (a) **exposure to IPV** (34%) and (b) **neglect** (34%), followed by physical abuse (20%), emotional maltreatment (9%), and sexual abuse (3%).[30] Analyses of this report underscore the importance of focusing on understudied categories of maltreatment such as neglect, exposure to IPV, and emotional maltreatment, which researchers have begun to examine.[31] Until recently, emphasis has been on risk assessment and urgent intervention for physical and sexual child abuse but not on the more frequent cases of child neglect. Parenting effectiveness is undermined by socioeconomic status,[32] suggesting that the attention to neglect is important and that HCPs should assess for longer term and broader social support. More research is needed to determine whether providing particular resources such as financial counselling, and adequate and stable housing for lone-parent families and those with child maltreatment histories, could help reduce child neglect and improve functional outcomes for children.[33]

The extent of elder abuse is also difficult to determine. Canadian prevalence data on elder abuse (>65 years) are consistent with international rates: an estimated 4% to 10% of older adults experience some form of abuse, although only 20% of incidents are reported to someone who can help.[21] In 2015, police-reported family violence data indicated that more than 9 900 older adults were victims of violent crime (an increase from 2013). Of these older adults, 33% were victimized by a family member. Moreover, 60% of these older adults were female, and, of these female victims, 33% were victimized by a spouse.[21] Common assault was the most frequently reported form of family violence experienced by older adults (55%), followed by threats (19%), major assaults (15%), and criminal harassment (4%).[21] Older adults experienced a wide range of forms of abuse, with financial and emotional abuse being most prevalent but under-reported. Furthermore, statistics likely under-represent those most vulnerable and marginalized groups of older adults, such as immigrants; refugees; lesbian, gay, bisexual, transgender, queer/questioning, or two-spirited (LGBTQ2) communities; and Indigenous people, who experience both common forms of abuse (physical, sexual, emotional, and financial) as well as other less obvious forms, including disrespect and systemic abuse.[34]

HEALTH EFFECTS OF VIOLENCE

All forms of violence have significant effects on health, and because individuals may experience multiple forms of violence and multiple incidents of violence, the health effects are likely to be cumulative.[35,36] Research, largely focused on women, has established that violent experiences have significant effects on health.[35,37-39]

Health Effects of Intimate Partner Violence

The health consequences of IPV arise from mental and emotional abuse as well as the more obvious consequences of physical and sexual assault, and include the following:

- **Direct effects of physical injuries**, such as bruises and fractures.[38,40] In 2014, one out of three Canadians who had experienced spousal violence reported physical injuries including bruises, cuts, or broken bones.[38] The forced sex that is often part of IPV contributes to gynecological health problems, including chronic pelvic pain, unintended pregnancy, sexually transmitted infections (STIs) (including human immunodeficiency virus [HIV] infection), and urinary tract infections (UTIs).
- **Chronic health problems**, such as chronic pain and arthritis; frequent headaches and migraines; visual problems; unexplained dizziness and fainting; STIs; unwanted pregnancies; gynecological symptoms; hypertension; viral infections such as colds and flus; peptic ulcers; and functional or irritable bowel disease.[37,38]
- **Mental health problems**, including clinical depression; acute and chronic symptoms of anxiety; serious sleep

disturbances; symptoms consistent with post-traumatic stress disorder (PTSD); substance use and dependence; and thoughts of suicide, which are significantly more prevalent among women who have been abused than among women who have not been abused.[41-44]

The most obvious health care problem for women experiencing IPV is injury. IPV injuries have recognizable patterns: head and neck injuries and musculo-skeletal injuries such as sprains and fractures are common. Chronic health problems are less obviously linked to IPV but are significant clinically. In many controlled investigations of women in various health care settings, abused women have been found to have significantly more chronic health problems, including neurological, gastro-intestinal, and gynecological symptoms, as well as chronic pain.[37] Similarly, mental health problems, including depression, suicidal thoughts and attempts, symptoms of PTSD, and substance use are common for women who experience IPV; however, HCPs often do not recognize the underlying causes. Abuse during pregnancy is also a significant health issue, with serious consequences for both the pregnant woman (e.g., antepartum hemorrhage, death, depression, substance use) and the infant (low birth weight, increased risk for child abuse).[45,46] Women who experience IPV visit HCPs more often than women who do not experience IPV, incurring higher health care costs and long-term costs for themselves, their children, and their employers.[47-49] For children, being exposed to abuse (e.g., hearing abuse, directly witnessing abuse), seeing the impact of abuse on their mothers, and living under conditions of chronic stress can lead them to experience a wide range of problems (e.g., physical, behavioural, emotional, and social problems).[16]

While violence against women is a well-known and documented phenomenon, IPV against men has received much less attention. Although the rate of police-reported family violence in Canada for men is half that for women,[50] research evidence shows that male IPV victimization is a significant risk to men's health,[51] with men's experiences, including willingness to report, varying depending on the sex of the perpetrator.[52,53] Among a range of health problems, PTSD, depression, cardiovascular problems, suicide ideation, asthma, and STIs are particular health risks for male victims of IPV and for which they seek help.[51,54]

Health Effects of Elder Abuse

The health effects of elder abuse are not nearly as well studied, but the consequences of IPV can be presumed to be similar for older adults. Like other forms of interpersonal violence, elder abuse is more often financial or emotional than physical, and it can have profound effects on mental and emotional health.[55-57]

The impact of violence on older adults can be compounded by age-related vulnerabilities.[58-60] Complications from intentional injury can range from minor pain and discomfort to life-threatening injuries. Bleeding from intentional trauma can cause significant changes in circulatory homeostasis, leading to marked fluctuations in blood pressure and pulse, shock, and ultimately death. Localized infections can progress to generalized sepsis, even death, in older patients who are immunocompromised. The actual assault or the stress leading up to or after an assault can contribute to cardiac complications. All of the STIs and related complications that are sequelae of abuse in younger women are also present in older women who have been sexually assaulted. In addition, postmenopausal women have more friable vaginal mucosal tissue as a result of estrogen loss, which increases their risk for STIs and vaginal trauma.

Neglect of older adults is common, often co-occurring with other forms of maltreatment, and can be intentional or unintentional.[55] Some family members or caregivers working with older persons consciously and with malice withhold food, water, medication, and appropriate necessities, often concurrently stealing the financial assets of the older, dependent person. This type of neglect is often, by definition, criminal in nature. In other situations, family members or caregivers working with an older adult struggle with their own physical and cognitive health challenges and, perhaps despite good intentions, may profoundly neglect the older person. While unintentional neglect is usually not viewed as a crime, it must be addressed. All caregivers should be assessed for caregiver burden. Finally, self-neglect raises often unanswerable questions about one's right to live autonomously versus society's obligation to care for people who are not able to care for themselves.

Health Effects of Child Maltreatment

Child maltreatment has many possible long-term physical and psychological effects.[32] The immediate consequences of physical abuse can include a spectrum of physical injuries such as bruises, fractures, burns, and lacerations and can involve more severe injury such as head trauma.[29] More severe forms of maltreatment can lead to death or long-term problems such as intellectual disability, blindness, and physical disability. Physical harm has direct effects and often co-occurs with other forms of maltreatment, which also have long-term adverse effects.

Ongoing child maltreatment can lead to changes in brain structure and chemistry, which may lead to long-term physical, psychological, emotional, social, and cognitive dysfunctions in adulthood.[61] All forms of child maltreatment can have effects on a child's development by disrupting the bond between child and caregiver.[62] Research shows that child maltreatment puts children at risk for experiencing depression and PTSD, participating in harmful activities, having difficulties in relationships, and having negative beliefs and attitudes toward others.[63] These effects are often interrelated and increase the likelihood of health problems in adulthood, including substance use, eating disorders, suicide, high-risk sexual behaviours, and sleep disorders,[29,64,65] as well as reduced health-related quality of life, pain, and increased emergency department visits.[65] Child maltreatment may also increase a person's vulnerability to homelessness and victimization through IPV in adulthood, both of which are associated with additional health effects.[66]

RESPONDING TO INTERPERSONAL VIOLENCE: BEGIN WITH TRAUMA- AND VIOLENCE-INFORMED CARE

Given the prevalence of all forms of interpersonal violence, HCPs need to provide an environment that is trauma- and violence-informed; that is, an environment that is safe for people who have previously and are currently experiencing violence.[67,68] Trauma- and violence-informed care (TVIC) builds on the idea of trauma-informed practice by taking into account *ongoing* as well as *historical* violence, and how structural violence (e.g., systemic racism, poverty, discriminatory policies) is related to interpersonal violence. TVIC focuses on creating a safe environment, not on getting a "disclosure"; however, safety (including cultural safety) often leads to disclosure. All care, including assessment, should be informed by knowledge about the dynamics of violence and the effects of violence.[69,70] HCPs can take the following steps:

- Assume that a majority of patients will have a history of abuse of some form.
- Assume that any patient may be currently experiencing abuse.
- Understand that all forms of interpersonal violence are abuses of power; people are primarily abused by those closest to them, including people who may accompany them for health care.
- Provide care that is appropriate for people who have histories of, or are experiencing, abuse, *regardless* of whether abuse has been disclosed. This means anticipating what might be traumatizing—such as touching without permission—and practising as though each person might be an abused person.
- Routinely inquire about how patients' home and work lives are affecting their health.

On the basis of awareness that abuse may be part of any patient's history, and with the use of a relational approach as described in earlier chapters, assessment should routinely include the following:

- *Listening* in a nonjudgemental and accepting manner[71]
- Being alert for "red flags" specific to the age of the person, from children to older adults, and *inquiring directly* about abuse when people present with direct injuries consistent with abuse, chronic health problems associated with abuse (e.g., chronic pain), mental health problems consistent with abuse, or factors known to increase vulnerability (e.g., disabilities, economic dependence, isolation)[72,73]
- Assessing and intervening collaboratively

Responding Safely to Intimate Partner Violence

Despite the wide-ranging and severe health problems associated with IPV and the fact that women who are experiencing IPV access health care more than women who are not abused, primary care providers continue to miss opportunities for offering support.[74] Furthermore, while research shows the prevalence and interconnections between various health problems and IPV, victims of violence often must prioritize presenting one health issue to HCPs and face service delivery silos and institutionalized barriers.[43] Some challenges to providing safe, effective responses to IPV include:

- People who are experiencing violence may not identify their experiences as abuse.
- People who are experiencing violence may be ashamed or anticipate judgement by HCPs.
- Privacy for disclosure may not be available in health care settings.
- People may fear responses from HCPs, including acts that will increase their risks, such as those that increase danger for themselves or family members or increase the risk that their children will be apprehended.
- HCPs inquire more often about IPV with people who are racialized or living in poverty, further perpetuating stereotypes of abuse and underinvestigating the abusive experiences of middle-class and Euro-Canadian people.

To date, the health care response to IPV has been inadequate at best. Over the past several decades, the main recommendation for HCPs was to routinely screen for violence. However, studies repeatedly show that while screening may help identify people experiencing IPV, it does not necessarily benefit abuse victims on a long-term basis by improving their health or reducing violence in their lives.[75–78] In Canada, researchers have found insufficient evidence to justify the implementation of IPV screening programs.[79] However, a TVIC approach and a case-finding approach to all patients are recommended.[77]

Even when abuse is recognized, women's experiences with HCPs tend to be negative.[80,81] Research has shown that women often find health care service responses to abuse unsympathetic, disempowering, coercive, victim-blaming, and focused on physical consequences of violence rather than on the wider effects and the context of women's lives.[82,83] HCPs often lack knowledge about IPV, have attitudes and values that inhibit an effective response, and think they do not have time to respond. HCPs often provide inappropriate or even harmful treatment. A Canadian study of emergency department responses to violence against women showed that nurses' responses were shaped by stereotypical thinking about violence as a problem primarily of poor and racialized people, by judgements of the extent to which women "deserved" help, and by the patterns of practice that required nurses to process cases as quickly as possible.[84]

Assessing for Intimate Partner Violence

Practising in a TVIC manner will foster trust and safe conditions for disclosure.[77,78,85] Women will disclose IPV to HCPs when they feel confident and safe enough to do so.[86] Less is known about what men would find helpful when they experience abuse. However, it is known that seeking help for injuries and health issues arising out of violence (direct or indirect) is not easy for men. Research documents that men face many barriers in the help-seeking process, both internal (such as shame, fear of not being believed or made fun of, internalized gender stereotypes) and external (primarily, lack of supportive and unbiased IPV services for men).[51,87] Thus, a TVIC approach is needed for people of all gender identities, including those who identify as transgender or two-spirit. In line with the 2014 World Health Organization (WHO) guidelines, HCPs should respond to disclosure and assess using the WHO LIVES approach: Listen, Inquire, Validate, Enhance safety, and Support.[77,78,85] This approach can support assessment with or without the patient disclosing a history of IPV.

Listen

Listen without judgement. Because women report that they feel judged and disbelieved by HCPs, it is vital to begin by examining your *own* knowledge and beliefs about IPV. If an HCP thinks that women should "just leave" their partners or that they are responsible for the abuse they experience, or that men cannot be victims, these ideas will be conveyed nonverbally to patients and discourage them from disclosure or seeking further help.

Listening nonjudgementally requires HCPs to evaluate social judgements that are commonly made about people experiencing violence and to acquire sufficient knowledge to counter those negative judgements. Ask yourself the following questions:

- What do I know about IPV? Whom do I hold responsible for IPV? What do I think are the causes of IPV?
- What are my own personal experiences of violence, and how do they shape my understanding?
- What groups do I view as most vulnerable to IPV?
- How might my beliefs about IPV be conveyed to patients in ways that are judgemental or affirming?

Your practice environment also shapes your ability to listen effectively to and assess your patients. Hollingsworth and Ford-Gilboe studied emergency nurses in Ontario and found that those who believed it was futile to assess and respond to women who have experienced abuse were less likely to engage in appropriate clinical practices; those with more positive beliefs about the benefits of assessing and responding to abuse were more likely to engage in appropriate clinical practices.[88] In contrast to literature portraying health providers as unsympathetic and uninterested in providing care to women who have experienced abuse, Hollingsworth and Ford-Gilboe found that the nurses had relatively high levels of positive expectations regarding outcomes. Because *any* of your patients may have a history of abuse, it is critical to listen to *all* patients with that in mind and be confident that you can make a positive difference in their lives. This means routinely using professional interpreters with all patients who speak a different language from you. Questions to ask yourself about your work environment include:

- How is "listening" to patients valued (by colleagues, managers, work expectations)? How much time is available for listening?
- How much privacy is afforded when patients are assessed?
- What is the workplace cultural norm about patients in general (whether you are encouraged to view yourself as the expert), toward women, and toward people who experience violence?

- How do these factors shape your practice? How might you optimize the environment?

Being listened to in a nonjudgemental manner can be reassuring for someone who previously encountered disbelief, blame, or judgement from friends or HCPs[89] and will contribute to building trust so that the person may feel confident enough to disclose abuse.

Expressing interest in the conditions of people's lives beyond the immediate presenting health problem can be a way of conveying openness. For example, with any patient, simple questions such as "How are your work and your home life affecting your health?" can convey interest and acceptance. Inquiring about a person's relationships and their effect on health should be included in the assessment of any person (e.g., "How do the people in your life affect your health?"); the answers provide important information beyond what might be classified as violence or abuse.

Listening (and Observing) for "Red Flags." Listening (and observing) for indicators of violence requires assuming that anyone might be experiencing violence and knowing who might be most vulnerable. It also requires an understanding of the health issues, signs, and symptoms associated with violence. Up to half of your female patients will have experienced at least one incident of physical or sexual assault in their lifetime.[90] However, some patients are more vulnerable to abuse: those who are isolated, economically dependent on others (e.g., immigrants sponsored as spouses, children, and adolescents), or dependent on others for care (e.g., people with disabilities). Actively consider IPV when a person is vulnerable in other ways.

HCPs need to be alert for conditions associated specifically with IPV. Thinking about IPV as a possible contributing factor is important in relation to diverse health issues ranging from substance use to abdominal pain to migraines. In view of the high association of chronic pain with histories of abuse,[35,37] you should have a high index of suspicion for abuse with any person experiencing chronic pain or substance use.[73] For women, especially consider IPV as a possible issue if the person has mental health problems such as depression, symptoms of PTSD (especially problems sleeping and "panic" attacks or problems with "nerves"), substance use, chronic pain (including back pain), or gynecological problems (especially STIs, pelvic pain, or sexual dysfunction). As noted, IPV is often associated with specific injuries (such as fractures, bruises, and sprains), chronic health challenges, and mental health issues. You should identify the factors related to abuse that are most relevant in your specific clinical area.

Inquire

Inquire with a TVIC approach. Research repeatedly shows that women feel disempowered by HCPs, which echoes their experiences of abuse. Thus, it is crucial to foster women's sense of control in decision making, including helping them identify the risks and benefits of seeking help.[91] For people of other genders, including men, it is likely that a similar approach will be effective. To engage men who are

IPV victims and to create a safe environment for disclosure, studies encourage HCPs to use broad questioning techniques (such as asking questions about their children or how things are at home) rather than direct questions about IPV.[92] When beginning most assessments, you do not know patients' abuse histories. Using the relational approach[93] discussed in Chapters 1 and 3, assessment involves several elements:

- *Follow the lead of the patient:* convey trustworthiness and a willingness to listen, allow the patient to take the lead in disclosing (or not), and draw on the patient's knowledge to assess the levels of danger and options.
- *Listen for cues that might suggest abuse.*
- *Self-observe:* pay attention to how your assumptions and biases shape your interactions and how you are reacting.
- *Recognize patterns:* attend to patterns of physical symptoms (e.g., injuries, chronic pain) and health problems (e.g., substance use, sleep problems).
- *Develop knowledge collaboratively:* for example, help individuals recognize connections between health problems and abuse, and help them evaluate levels of danger.
- *Name and support capacity:* focus on strengths and capacities; for example, you might say, "It sounds as though you have been through a lot—you are doing a great job of …"

When you identify social vulnerabilities, health issues commonly associated with abuse, or signs of possible abuse, a thorough assessment of interpersonal violence is needed. Inquire in safe and appropriate ways about patients' needs and concerns followed by appropriate and timely referral.[77,94] Depending on the presentation, use questions that are direct and tailored to the person and situation (e.g., "Often depression is related to violence in a partner relationship—is this the case for you?"). If you are less sure, indirect queries can be used (e.g., "I am concerned about how you are managing your diabetes. Is there any chance that stress at home is contributing to the problem?"). Assessment for abuse is much broader than screening, but questions designed for screening purposes can be used in your assessments; you may suggest that the person's intimate relationships may be negatively affecting health, or you may ask about health problems or circumstances that warrant a high index of suspicion for abuse. For example, an 80-year-old woman, presenting with tachycardia, replied to the nurse's observation that her relationship did not seem to be helping her health with the disclosure that "this [tachycardia] happens every time he gets like that." The nurse was able to clarify the woman's meaning: that the woman's husband battered her frequently.

Even when individuals disclose abuse, they may downplay it, saying "it's only emotional," "it's not that bad," or "we just fight a lot." More abuse may be revealed as you listen. The downplaying is not "denial," but rather the normal minimization that often accompanies trauma from violence. It is important to reinforce that emotional abuse is of concern: for example, you can say, "The stress associated with being treated that way can be just as bad for your physical and mental health as if someone were hitting you."

Validate

The most important response to disclosure is validation of the person's worth. Both women who have experienced abuse and HCPs with experience responding to abuse assert that validation of the woman's worth as a human being and the affirmation that abuse is never deserved are the most important aspects of an effective response and the foundation for a trusting relationship.[71,82,86] Furthermore, if a person "hints" at or discloses abuse, conveying belief in the person's narrative by continuing to be nonjudgemental can be empowering. Sometimes people who are experiencing IPV offer explanations for illnesses or injuries that downplay, overlook, or deny abuse—perhaps because of shame, fear of judgement, or fear of the consequences of disclosure, or because the person has not connected the health problems to abuse. Openly indicating a possible connection to abuse—if done in a nonjudgemental, validating manner—can invite a direct conversation about IPV.

It is appropriate to show that you are concerned and even distressed about the violence. During the assessment, convey the message that the abuse is not the patient's fault. Convey that you are concerned and that help is available: "I am really concerned about your health and the danger you are in, and I would like to help you make a plan for you to be as safe as possible." Still another is that several health problems can occur because of violence: "I am really worried about the amount of pain you are having and the stress you are under. This is very damaging to your health … [add specifics particular to the patient]." In fact, 59% of 265 abused women who accepted a referral to a social worker said they did so because the medical provider expressed concern that their presenting health problem was related to IPV.[95]

Specific clinical contexts have assessment approaches that integrate attention to violence. For example, in the perinatal context, in contrast to the usual assumption that pregnancy is a positive event, it is important to be open to the fact that a pregnant women may be in an abusive relationship.

Assessment related to sexual assault should be based on the same principles as assessment for IPV. The emotional, cultural, and physical safety of the patient should come first, and a validating, nonjudgemental response is essential. The patient should remain in control of care as much as possible, including decisions about calling the police or having forensic evidence collected. Sexual assault victims may be of any gender, and assault may occur within the context of an intimate relationship (e.g., a spousal or dating relationship) or a nonintimate relationship (with a client of a sex worker, or with others such as co-workers, employers, and HCPs). Assault by unknown assailants is much less common.

Survivors may seek treatment immediately, within days, or weeks after the assault. Delaying help-seeking is common. Many survivors are embarrassed and fear being dismissed as undeserving of care, especially those who are victims of date rape, use alcohol or drugs, or for whom the assault is associated with sex work. If the assailant is known, the survivor may fear repercussions for seeking treatment.

Enhance Safety

Any HCP should help a person who has disclosed violence make a safety plan. A safety plan needs to be based on the person's level of danger and specific threats to safety. In the United States, Sharps and colleagues found that 42% of the women killed by their partners had been seen by someone in the health care system (the emergency department in the majority of cases, but also in primary care, prenatal care, and other settings) for some health issue in the year before their murder.[96] These encounters represent missed opportunities for HCPs to identify IPV and intervene to decrease the danger.

Assessing for Danger. Most of what is known about danger assessment is based on research with women.[97,98] This research shows that women do not overestimate but may underestimate their danger. Globally, women are at much greater risk of being killed by an intimate partner than men, and when women kill their partners, they often act in self-defence following ongoing violence and intimidation.[98]

The Danger Assessment (DA) is a tool that helps determine a person's level of danger based on research of predictors of risk for women murdered by their intimate partners.[99] This tool is used extensively by nurses and advocates in various settings. Over the past two decades, it has been refined, translated into several languages, and adapted to various populations and clinical settings, including a shorter version for use in emergency settings.[97,100] The DA is an excellent tool for assessing the frequency and severity of violence. Although the DA does not use cut-off scores, the more the person answers "yes," the more dangerous the person's situation. See the Additional Resources at the end of this chapter for the DA website.

The safety plan should be tailored to the individual's circumstances. There are many comprehensive safety planning tools available to guide you (see the Additional Resources at the end of this chapter). Choose a tool that is closest to the person's needs (where do they live? What is the gender of the partner? Are there children involved?). Typically, safety plans begin with emergency plans, tailored to whether the person is living with the abusive partner or not. Follow the lead of the person, but support a realistic evaluation of danger.

Support

The level of ongoing support you can provide will vary according to your role and practice setting. If you are a nurse practitioner with an ongoing relationship with the person, you can provide consistent support over time. If your relationship is a one-time encounter, such as in an emergency setting, you will need to refer the person to another HCP or social service provider, depending on the resources available. Importantly, referral must be done with the person's full knowledge and consent.

RESPONDING TO ELDER AND VULNERABLE PERSON ABUSE

Older adults face specific barriers to getting help. They may be more vulnerable because of economic dependence, physical and cognitive health challenges, cultural barriers, isolation, and other barriers specific to women.[101,102] Services for IPV rarely are tailored to older adults and thus may not be appropriate for their needs. For women with partners, leaving may not be possible, and services and social expectations are not oriented to the fact that leaving is especially challenging for older women.[103] Thus, assessment must include a broad understanding of the person's life circumstances. Assessing for possible elder abuse can be more complicated than for other forms of IPV if an older adult presents for health care with multiple health, physical, and cognitive challenges. Although some older women have been in abusive relationships for decades, others are experiencing physical and sexual violence for the first time, from previously nonabusive partners who themselves may be afflicted with behaviour-altering neurological illnesses (Alzheimer's disease, organic brain syndromes). An older woman in a long-term abusive relationship may be trying to outlive the abuser, whereas the newly abused older woman may be reluctant to disclose abuse because of embarrassment, shame, and fears that her partner will be institutionalized. Older men and women may be more vulnerable financially, dependent on other people for care, and fearful of retribution. Physical findings inconsistent with the history provided by the patient, family member, or caregiver are significant clues to possible abuse. Again, there are numerous tools to support practice. For example, the National Initiative for the Care of the Elderly offers a brief abuse screen to help identify elder abuse. Elder Abuse Ontario provides many policy and practice supports and tools. See the Additional Resources at the end of this chapter.

Mandatory Reporting of Abuse of Older Adults or Vulnerable Persons

In some provinces, such as Nova Scotia and Newfoundland and Labrador, adult protection legislation includes general mandatory reporting requirements that cover different forms of abuse.[104] The effectiveness of such laws is controversial. The Canadian Network for the Prevention of Elder Abuse has a good summary of the arguments for and against mandatory reporting (see the Additional Resources at the end of this chapter). You should be familiar with your legal obligations. The Canadian Centre for Elder Law's guide to elder abuse and neglect law includes a summary of the laws in each province and territory (see the Additional Resources at the end of this chapter). As with other obligations, however, legal obligations are the minimum standard. HCPs have an ethical obligation to provide a meaningful, health-promoting response whenever abuse is suspected.

RESPONDING TO CHILD MALTREATMENT

In Canada, screening for child maltreatment is not recommended. Because of the high rate of false-positive results of screening tests and the potential for incorrectly labelling individuals as child abusers, the possible harm associated with screening outweighs the benefits.[105] However, reporting suspected child maltreatment is mandatory in most provinces and territories, which means that the identification of child maltreatment relies on careful assessment by HCPs.

It is important that approaches to child maltreatment be similar to those recommended for IPV but modified to (a) take into account that children are highly vulnerable to family members and (b) accommodate the developmental stage of each child. Keep the following in mind:

- "Race" and class stereotypes are widely perpetuated and must be actively countered so that they do not inappropriately influence your assessment. *Any* child may be at risk for some form of abuse, regardless of the ethnicity or income of the family; conversely, no ethnic group is at "greater risk" of perpetrating child maltreatment.
- "Race" and class stereotypes may contribute to the fact that Indigenous families are more often investigated for neglect.[106] According to the CIS-2008, the rate of substantiated child maltreatment investigations is four times higher among Indigenous children compared with non-Indigenous children (49.69 per 1000 Indigenous children versus 11.89 per 1000 non-Indigenous children).[29] Furthermore, research shows that in addition to higher Indigenous caseloads, the out-of-home placements in child maltreatment investigations are also higher, and particularly so when the child welfare agencies are provided by provincial government.[106,107] In Canadian investigations of child maltreatment, at every decision point, Indigenous children are over-represented: investigations are more likely to be substantiated, cases are more likely to be kept open for ongoing services, and children are more likely to be placed in out-of-home care. These dynamics are part of the ongoing overinvolvement with Indigenous parenting by the state as a tool of colonial control.[108]
- Neglect is one of the most common forms of child maltreatment; if you rely only on obvious indicators of physical abuse or look only for cues of sexual abuse, you may overlook abuse and significant harm.
- Parents are not the only possible perpetrators of child maltreatment.
- Many allegations of suspected child maltreatment are unsubstantiated.
- Although some situations warrant removal of children from their parents, this step is stressful for children, and in most cases the children remain in contact with their parents for life.
- The idea that people who are abused as children are more likely to abuse their children is popular, but evidence of this is inconclusive and points to complexities of the situation where simple causal links are hard to draw.[109,110]

- Assessments for child maltreatment are evaluations of parenting and often focus uncritically on evaluating mothers against culturally specific dominant stereotypes of mothering, even when the mother is not the perpetrator.[111,112]
- Ethically, as an HCP, you are obligated to provide "good" care to all, including possible perpetrators of maltreatment.
- Although you must intervene and report suspected child maltreatment, your role as an HCP is not to "rescue" the child at the expense of your relationship with the parents or of the relationship between the child and the parents.

As with any form of abuse, your assumptions and beliefs will be conveyed to children and parents. It is crucial to reflect on your own ideas and experiences and work toward the short- and long-term well-being of all parties. Assessment and intervention for suspected child maltreatment without alienating the parents is possible, regardless of whether the parents are suspected of perpetrating the abuse.

Assessing for Child Maltreatment

Assessing for child maltreatment means integrating awareness of the possibility of child maltreatment into every assessment. Horwath and Morrison have studied the use of a framework for the assessment of children in need and their families in cases of child neglect; this framework can help HCPs focus on broader issues, including the impact of social determinants of health, rather than on dramatic situations of severe physical abuse.[113] The framework focuses on the child's developmental needs, the parent's capacities, and family and environmental factors. The framework attends to the complexity of responding to child neglect, but tensions among these domains must be taken into account to avoid losing focus on the child in question. According to Milot, St-Laurent, and Éthier, a trauma-informed approach to neglect includes the following:

- Taking a detailed assessment of the child's trauma history and characteristics
- Providing a safe environment for the child
- Helping the child build feelings of emotional security
- Offering emotional therapeutic support to the parent[114]

Although physical abuse is less common, it is important to be alert for signs of physical abuse and intentional injury. Carefully evaluate any physical injury within the context of a child's age and developmental stage. Is the injury that is being reported in line with the child's developmental level? For example, the explanation that a 3-week-old child was injured rolling off a bed is not developmentally plausible. Because you may not be able to directly observe the child's motor and cognitive milestones while documenting the history, ask caregivers directly whether the child is crawling, pulling up to stand, or walking, and about other current issues (e.g., tantrums, toilet training).

Responses to known child maltreatment are much more comprehensive than the well-publicized interventions of placing children in out-of-home care. There has been some evidence of the successful support of parents. For example, randomized controlled trials have shown a reduction in the incidence of child maltreatment and outcomes related to physical abuse and neglect among first-time disadvantaged mothers and their infants who received a program of home visitation by nurses from the perinatal period through the children's infancy.[61]

Mandatory Reporting of Child Maltreatment

In Canada, provincial and territorial jurisdictions have the legislative responsibility for child and family services (child welfare). One exception is the federal responsibility for First Nations peoples with status under the *Indian Act*. Each province and territory has specific legislation providing protection for neglected and abused children. Although there is no evidence regarding the effectiveness of mandatory reporting,[115] most provinces and territories have legislation that makes it mandatory for the public, including HCPs, to report child maltreatment. If you are working with children, you should review the specific requirements for the jurisdiction in which you are working. The Canadian Child Welfare Research Portal provides a comprehensive description of policies across Canada, research reports, and contact information for each province and territory (see the Additional Resources at the end of this chapter). If you think a child is being maltreated, you should involve other members of the health care team. Many health care settings have access to social workers who are specifically trained in dealing with child maltreatment. They are often the first point of contact for reporting suspected abuse. It is important to know that you can consult confidentially with child protection social workers before deciding whether the situation warrants a formal report.

Using a respectful, nonjudgemental, and collaborative approach that takes contextual factors into account (such as high levels of stress in the child's family or economic distress), HCPs can make the process of mandatory reporting constructive.[116] Be as transparent as possible with both children and their caregivers regarding what actions you intend to take, as well as your reasons for them.

DOCUMENTING A HISTORY OF INTERPERSONAL VIOLENCE

Depending on your role and the context of practice, an individual's history of abuse may be important to your history taking. If you are providing an immunization and are unlikely to see the person again, you will not need a detailed violence history. If you are providing ongoing care for chronic health problems, it may be useful to learn more about the person's history, given that cumulative abuse has been shown to be associated with more severe mental and physical health problems.[35,37] Balance your "need to know" against the potential traumatic and stigmatizing effects of recounting a violence history. In some cases, a history of traumatic injuries may have an effect on the current health condition. For instance, a woman may have experienced prior episodes of head trauma and strangulation, both of which may be related to chronic but subtle neurological symptoms and problems. Pay particular attention to the most frequent mental health problems associated with violence: depression, suicidal thoughts and attempts, PTSD, substance use, and anxiety. Chapter 6 (mental health assessment) and Chapter 7 (understanding substance use) give direction for conducting this part of the history.

If child maltreatment is suspected and the child is verbal, a history should be obtained from the child separately from the caregivers through open-ended questions or spontaneous statements. It is important to remember that children may have suffered significant trauma but may respond only minimally to open-ended questions.[117] Keeping the questions short and using age-appropriate language and familiar words can help enrich the documentation of the history. Children older than 11 years of age can generally be expected to provide a history at the level of most adults.[117]

The medical history is also an important part of your evaluation. Has the child had previous hospitalizations or injuries, or do they suffer from any chronic medical conditions? Does the child take any medication that may cause easy bruising? Does the child have a history of repeated visits to the hospital? Was there a delay in seeking care for anything other than a minor injury?

PHYSICAL EXAMINATION

Important components of the physical examination of a patient known to have experienced IPV, child maltreatment, or elder abuse include a complete head-to-toe visual examination, especially if the patient is receiving health care services secondary to reported abuse. When the examination reveals physical findings, accurate use of medical terminology to describe injuries is essential.[72] In Canada, it is controversial whether forensic evidence is supportive of women who experience IPV; for example, a study in British Columbia revealed that health records were inaccurate reflections of the woman's experience and were most often used to undermine the woman and her legal claims.[118] However, there is some evidence that forensic examinations do lead to a higher probability of charges and conviction rates in sexual assault cases.[119]

Physical assessment after sexual assault can include the collection of forensic evidence: that is, evidence that can be admitted in court. Such collection usually requires the expert skills of a nurse examiner or physician specially trained in evaluating sexual assault. The details of such evidence collection are beyond the scope of this chapter, but you should be familiar with the protocols and resources available in your area.

Assessment of bruising is often recommended in relation to all forms of abuse. There is no scientific evidence of the accuracy of dating injuries on the basis of the colour of contusions,[120] and children can heal from bruising very quickly. However, a new bruise is usually red and often turns purple or purple-blue 12 to 36 hours after blunt-force trauma. The colour of bruises (and ecchymoses) generally progresses from purple-blue to bluish green to greenish brown to brownish yellow before the bruise fades away.

Bruising is an important sign of elder abuse.[121] Multiple factors can contribute to bruising more readily or more severely in older adults than in younger people. Medications, abnormal blood values related to medications' adverse effects, and underlying hematological disorders can affect ease of bruising or the formation of ecchymosis. Common medications that increase the risk of bruising or bleeding complications include, but are not limited to, Aspirin, ibuprofen (Advil), any nonsteroidal anti-inflammatory medication, warfarin (Coumadin), heparin, and prednisone (Deltasone). Mosqueda, Burnight, and Liao studied older adults who had accidental bruises and found that nearly 90% of their bruises were on their extremities, and no accidental bruises were found on the neck, ears, genitalia, buttocks, or soles of the feet; hence, injuries in the latter areas are suspect for abuse.[122]

Physical Examination of Children

Guidelines for assessing children who have been abused are under development.[123,124] A visual inspection from head to toe is important in any physical examination of a child, particularly when physical abuse is suspected. Significant injuries can be hidden under clothing, diapers, socks, and long hair. Accidental bruising in healthy, active children is common, but the presence of bruises in babies may have significance in evaluating for abuse. Children who are walking with support but not independently "cruising" typically should not have bruises. Bruising in infants who are not yet cruising, usually younger than 9 months of age, should alert you to possible abuse or an underlying medical illness. It is important to know that although some forms of bruising in children may have significance, such as perineal bruising,[125] there is considerable controversy regarding interpretation.[126]

DOCUMENTATION

Documentation of IPV and elder abuse must include objective progress notes, written in unbiased language. Injury maps and photographic documentation may be useful. Histories of IPV and elder abuse need to be recorded directly from the patients within reason. It is clinically unrealistic to document verbatim every statement made by a patient. However, it is critical to document exceptionally poignant statements made by the victim that identify the reported perpetrator and threats of harm made by the reported perpetrator. Other aspects of the abuse history, including reports of past abusive incidents, can be paraphrased with the use of partial direct quotations.

When quoting or paraphrasing the history, you should not sanitize words reportedly heard by the victim. Verbatim documentation of the reported perpetrator's threats interlaced with curses and expletives may be useful in future court proceedings. Also, be careful to use the exact terms an abused patient may use to describe sexual organs or sexually assaultive behaviours.

Photographic documentation in the medical record may be useful. Prior written consent to take photographs should be obtained from all cognitively intact, competent adults. Most health care facilities have standardized consent-to-photograph forms. If a patient is unconscious or cognitively impaired, taking photographs without consent is generally viewed as ethically sound, inasmuch as it is a noninvasive, painless intervention that may help a suspected abuse victim.

When documenting the history and physical findings of child maltreatment and neglect, use the words of the child to describe how any injuries occurred. Remember the possibility that the abuser may be accompanying the child. If the child is nonverbal, use statements from caregivers. It is important to know your employer's or institution's protocol for obtaining history in cases of suspected child maltreatment. Some protocols may delay a full interview until it can be conducted by a forensically trained interviewer.

ADDITIONAL RESOURCES

Canadian Centre for Elder Law. (2011). A practical guide to elder abuse and neglect law in Canada. Vancouver: Author. Retrieved from https://www.bcli.org/sites/default/files/Practical_Guide_English_Rev_JULY_2011.pdf

Canadian Child Welfare Research Portal: http://cwrp.ca

Canadian Network for the Prevention of Elder Abuse: https://cnpea.ca/en/

Danger Assessment: http://www.dangerassessment.org

Department of Justice Canada—Get Help With Family Violence: http://www.justice.gc.ca/eng/cj-jp/fv-vf/help-aide.html

Elder Abuse Ontario: http://www.elderabuseontario.com

Ending Violence Association of BC—Safety Planning: http://endingviolence.org/need-help/safety-planning/

National Initiative for the Care of the Elderly—BASE: Brief Abuse Screen for the Elderly: http://www.nicenet.ca/tools-base-brief-abuse-screen-for-the-elderly

Victim Services of Bruce Grey & Owen Sound. (2013). Safety plan for victims of domestic violence. Owen Sound, ON: Author. Retrieved from http://www.thewomenscentre.org/docs/SafetyPlanVictimsDomesticViolence.pdf

REFERENCES

1. Holmes, C., & Hunt, S. (2017). *Indigenous communities and family violence: Changing the conversation.* Prince George, BC: National Collaborating Center for Aboriginal Health.

2. Denison, J., Varcoe, C., & Browne, A. J. (2014). Aboriginal women's experiences of accessing health care when state apprehension of children is being threatened. *Journal of Advanced Nursing, 70*(5), 1105–1116. doi:10.1111/jan.12271.

3. Stockman, J. K., Hayashi, H., & Campbell, J. C. (2015). Intimate partner violence and its health impact on disproportionately affected populations, including minorities and impoverished groups. *Journal of Women's Health* (15409996), *24*(1), 62–79. doi:10.1089/jwh.2014.4879.

4. Burczycka, M. (2017). Section 3: Police-reported intimate partner violence. *Juristat, 37*(1). Retrieved from https://www.statcan.gc.ca/pub/85-002-x/2017001/article/14698/03-eng.htm.

5. Johnson, M. (2011). Gender and types of intimate partner violence: A response to an anti-feminist literature review. *Aggression and Violent Behaviour, 16*(4), 289–296.

6. Johnson, H. (2015). Degendering violence. *Social Politics, 22*(3), 390–410.

7. Johnson, M. (2011). Gender and types of intimate partner violence: A response to an anti-feminist literature review. *Aggression and Violent Behaviour, 16*(4), 289–296. (p. 290).

8. O'Neal, E. N., & Beckman, L. O. (2017). Intersections of race, ethnicity, and gender. *Violence Against Women, 23*(5), 643–665. doi:10.1177/1077801216646223.

9. Platt, L., Powers, L., Leotti, S., et al. (2017). The role of gender in violence experienced by adults with developmental disabilities. *Journal of Interpersonal Violence, 32*(1), 101–129. doi:10.1177/0886260515585534.

10. Crockett, C., Brandl, B., & Dabby, F. C. (2015). Survivors in the margins: The invisibility of violence against older women. *Journal of Elder Abuse & Neglect, 27*(4/5), 291–302. doi: 10.1080/08946566.2015.1090361.

11. Daoud, N., Smylie, J., Urquia, M., et al. (2013). The contribution of socio-economic position to the excesses of violence and intimate partner violence among Aboriginal versus non-Aboriginal women in Canada. *Canadian Journal of Public Health, 104*(4), e278–e283.

12. Pedersen, J. S., Malcoe, L. H., & Pulkingham, J. (2013). Explaining Aboriginal/non-Aboriginal inequalities in postseparation violence against Canadian women: Application of a structural violence approach. *Violence Against Women, 19*(8), 1034–1058. doi:10.1177/1077801213499245.

13. Department of Justice Canada. (1985). Criminal Code, R.S.C. 1985, c. C-46 (Canada), s. 150.1.

14. Department of Justice Canada. (2007). *Child abuse: A fact sheet from the Department of Justice Canada* (p. 1). Retrieved from http://publications.gc.ca/collections/Collection/J2-295-2002E.pdf.

15. Canadian Centre for Justice Statistics. (2017). *Family violence in Canada.* Retrieved from http://www.statcan.gc.ca/daily-quotidien/170216/dq170216b-eng.htm.

16. MacGregor, J. C. D., Wathen, C. N., & MacMillan, H. L. (2016). *Research brief: Identifying and responding to children's exposure to intimate partner violence.* London, ON: Preventing Violence Across the Lifespan Research Network. Retrieved from http://projectvega.ca/documents/2016/11/prevail-ce-ipv-brief-fall-2016.pdf.

17. Department of Justice Canada. (2012). *Child abuse is wrong: What can I do?* Retrieved from http://www.justice.gc.ca/eng/rp-pr/cj-jp/fv-vf/caw-mei/index.html.

18. Employment and Social Development Canada. (2016). *Elder abuse: It's time to face reality.* Retrieved from https://www.canada.ca/en/employment-social-development/campaigns/elder-abuse/reality.html#d.

19. McDonald, L., Beaulieu, M., Harbison, J., et al. (2012). Institutional abuse of older adults: What we know, what we need to know. *Journal of Elder Abuse & Neglect, 24*(2), 138–160. doi:10.1080/08946566.2011.646512.

20. Public Health Agency of Canada. (2012). *Elder abuse.* Retrieved from http://www.phac-aspc.gc.ca/seniors-aines/ea-mta-eng.php.

21. Conroy, S. (2017). Section 5: Police-reported family violence against seniors. Violence. *Juristat, 37*(1). Retrieved from http://www.statcan.gc.ca/pub/85-002-x/2017001/article/14698/05-eng.htm#r4.

22. Canadian Centre for Justice Statistics. (2016). Family violence in Canada: A statistical profile, 2014. *Juristat, 36*(1). Retrieved from http://www.statcan.gc.ca/pub/85-002-x/2016001/article/14303-eng.pdf.

23. Burczycka, M. (2016). Section 1: Trends in self-reported spousal violence in Canada, 2014. *Juristat, 36*(1). Retrieved from http://www.statcan.gc.ca/pub/85-002-x/2016001/article/14303/01-eng.htm.

24. Ibrahim, D. (2016). Section 3: Police reported intimate partner violence. *Juristat, 36*(1). Retrieved from http://www.statcan.gc.ca/pub/85-002-x/2016001/article/14303/03-eng.htm.

25. Mulligan, L., Axford, M., & Solecki, A. (2016). Homicide in Canada, 2015. *Juristat, 36*(1). Retrieved from http://www.statcan.gc.ca/pub/85-002-x/2016001/article/14668-eng.htm.

26. Desmarais, S. L., Reeves, K. A., Nicholls, T. A., et al. (2012). Prevalence of physical violence in intimate relationships. Part 1: Rates of male and female victimization. *Partner Abuse, 1*(2), 140–169.

27. Perreault, S. (2015). Criminal victimization in Canada, 2014 (Catalogue no. 85-002-X). *Juristat, 35*(1). Retrieved from http://www.statcan.gc.ca/pub/85-002-x/2015001/article/14241-eng.pdf.

28. Allen, M. (2016). *Police-reported crime statistics in Canada, 2015*. Retrieved from http://www.statcan.gc.ca/pub/85-002-x/2016001/article/14642-eng.htm.

29. Public Health Agency of Canada. (2010). *Canadian Incidence Study of Reported Child Abuse and Neglect—2008: Major findings*. Retrieved from http://www.phac-aspc.gc.ca/cm-vee/public-eng.php.

30. Sinha, M. (2012). *Family violence in Canada: A statistical profile, 2010*. Ottawa: Minister of Industry. Retrieved from http://www.statcan.gc.ca/pub/85-002-x/2012001/article/11643-eng.pdf.

31. Potter, D., Nasserie, T., & Tonmyr, L. (2015). A review of recent analyses of the Canadian Incidence Study of Reported Child Abuse and Neglect (CIS). *Chronic Diseases and Injuries in Canada, 35*(8/9).

32. Blumenthal, A. (2015). *Child neglect 1: Scope, consequences, and risk and protective factors*. Retrieved from http://cwrp.ca/sites/default/files/publications/en/141E.pdf.

33. Afifi, T. O., Taillieu, T., Cheung, K., et al. (2015). Substantiated reports of child maltreatment from the Canadian Incidence Study of Reported Child Abuse and Neglect 2008: Examining child and household characteristics and child functional impairment. *Canadian Journal of Psychiatry, 60*(7), 315–323.

34. Ploeg, J., Lohfeld, L., & Walsh, C. A. (2013). What is "elder abuse"? Voices from the margin: The views of underrepresented Canadian older adults. *Journal of Elder Abuse & Neglect, 25*(5), 396–424.

35. Davies, L., Ford-Gilboe, M., Willson, A., et al. (2015). Patterns of cumulative abuse among female survivors of intimate partner violence: Links to women's health and socioeconomic status. *Violence Against Women, 21*(1), 30–48.

36. Scott-Storey, K. (2011). Cumulative abuse: Do things add up? An evaluation of the conceptualization, operationalization, and methodological approaches in the study of the phenomenon of cumulative abuse. *Trauma, Violence and Abuse, 12*(3), 135–150. doi:10.1177/1524838011404253.

37. Dillon, G., Hussain, R., Loxton, D., et al. (2013). Mental and physical health and intimate partner violence against women: A review of the literature. *International Journal of Family Medicine*. doi: http://dx.doi.org/10.1155/2013/313909.

38. Public Health Agency of Canada. (2016). *The Chief Public Health Officer's report on the state of public health in Canada 2016—A focus on family violence in Canada*. Retrieved from https://www.canada.ca/en/public-health/services/publications/chief-public-health-officer-reports-state-public-health-canada/2016-focus-family-violence-canada.html.

39. World Health Organization. (2013). *Global and regional estimates of violence against women: Prevalence and health effects of intimate partner violence and non-partner sexual violence*. Geneva, Switzerland: WHO Press.

40. Anderson, J. C., Stockman, J. K., Sabri, B., et al. (2015). Injury outcomes in African American and African Caribbean women: The role of intimate partner violence. *Journal of Emergency Nursing, 41*(1), 36–42. doi: http://doi.org/10.1016/j.jen.2014.01.015.

41. Lagdon, S., Armour, C., & Stringer, M. (2014). Adult experience of mental health outcomes as a result of intimate partner violence victimisation: A systematic review. *European Journal of Psychotraumatology, 5*(1), doi:10.3402/ejpt.v5.24794.

42. Mason, R., & Du Mont, J. (2015). Advancing our knowledge of the complexity and management of intimate partner violence and co-occurring mental health and substance abuse problems in women. *F1000prime Reports, 7*, 65. doi:10.12703/P7-65.

43. Mason, R., Wolf, M., O'Rinn, S., et al. (2017). Making connections across silos: Intimate partner violence, mental health, and substance use. *BMC Women's Health, 17*(1), 29.

44. Salom, C., Williams, G., Najman, J., et al. (2015). Substance use and mental health disorders are linked to different forms of intimate partner violence victimisation. *Drug Alcohol Dependence, 151*, 121–127.

45. Velonis, A. J., O'Campo, P., Kaufman-Shriqui, V., et al. (2017). The impact of prenatal and postpartum partner violence on maternal mental health: Results from the Community Child Health Network Multisite Study. *Journal of Women's Health, 26*(10).

46. Taillieu, T. L., Brownridge, D. A., Tyler, K. A., et al. (2016). Pregnancy and intimate partner violence in Canada: A comparison of victims who were and were not abused during pregnancy. *Journal of Family Violence, 31*(5), 567–579.

47. Rivara, F. P., Anderson, M. L., Fishman, P., et al. (2007). Healthcare utilization and costs for women with a history of intimate partner violence. *American Journal of Preventive Medicine, 32*(2), 89–96.

48. Rivara, F. P., Anderson, M. L., Fishman, P., et al. (2007). Intimate partner violence and health care costs and utilization for children living in the home. *Pediatrics, 120*, 1270–1277.

49. Varcoe, C., Hankivsky, O., Ford Gilboe, M., et al. (2011). Attributing selected costs to intimate partner violence in a sample of women who have left abusive partners: A social determinants of health approach. *Canadian Public Policy, 37*(3), 359–380.

50. Burczycka, M., & Conroy, S. (2017). *Family violence in Canada: A statistical profile, 2015*. Ottawa: Minister of Industry.

51. Machado, A., Santos, A., Graham-Kevan, N., et al. (2017). Exploring help seeking experiences of male victims of

female perpetrators of IPV. *Journal of Family Violence, 32*(5), 513–523.

52. Nowinski, S., & Bowen, E. (2012). Partner violence against heterosexual and gay men: prevalence and correlates. *Aggression and Violent Behavior, 17*(1), 36–52.

53. Nybergh, L., Enander, V., & Krantz, G. (2016). Theoretical considerations on men's experiences of intimate partner violence: An interview-based study. *Journal of Family Violence, 31*(2), 191–202.

54. Hines, D. A., & Douglas, E. M. (2015). Health problems of partner violence victims: Comparing help-seeking men to a population-based sample. *American Journal of Preventive Medicine, 48*(2), 136–144.

55. McDonald, L., Beaulieu, M., Goergen, T., et al. (2016). *Into the light: National survey on the mistreatment of older Canadians 2015.* Toronto: National Initiative for the Care of the Elderly.

56. Sooryanarayana, R., Choo, W., & Hairi, N. (2013). A review on the prevalence and measurement of elder abuse in the community. *Trauma, Violence and Abuse, 14*(4), 316–325. doi:10.1177/1524838013495963.

57. Wong, J. S., & Waite, L. J. (2017). Elder mistreatment predicts later physical and psychological health: Results from a national longitudinal study. *Journal of Elder Abuse & Neglect, 29*(1), 15–42. doi:10.1080/08946566.2016.1235521.

58. Du Mont, J., Kosa, D., Macdonald, S., et al. (2015). Determining possible professionals and respective roles and responsibilities for a model comprehensive elder abuse intervention: A delphi consensus survey. *PLoS ONE, 10*(12), e0140760. doi:10.1371/journal.pone.0140760.

59. Murphy, K., Waa, S., Jaffer, H., et al. (2013). A literature review of findings in physical elder abuse. *Canadian Association of Radiologists Journal, 64*(1), 10–14.

60. Pillemer, K., Burnes, D., Riffin, C., et al. (2016). Elder abuse: Global situation, risk factors, and prevention strategies. *Gerontologist, 56*(Suppl. 2), S194–S205.

61. MacMillan, H., & Wathen, C. (2014). *Research brief: Interventions to prevent child maltreatment.* London, ON: Preventing Violence Across the Lifespan Research Network.

62. Al Odhayani, A., Watson, W. J., & Watson, L. (2013). Behavioural consequences of child abuse. *Canadian Family Physician, 59*(8), 831–836.

63. Afifi, T. O., MacMillan, H. L., Boyle, M., et al. (2016). Child abuse and physical health in adulthood. *Health Reports, 27*(3), 10.

64. Afifi, T. O., MacMillan, H. L., Boyle, M., et al. (2014). Child abuse and mental disorders in Canada. *Canadian Medical Association Journal, 186*(9), E324–E332.

65. Herrenkohl, T. I., Hong, S., Klika, J. B., et al. (2013). Developmental impacts of child abuse and neglect related to adult mental health, substance use, and physical health. *Journal of Family Violence, 28*(2), doi:10.1007/s10896–012–9474–9.

66. Brownridge, D. A., Taillieu, T., Afifi, T., et al. (2016). Child maltreatment and intimate partner violence among Indigenous and non-Indigenous Canadians. *Journal of Family Violence, 32*(6), 1–13.

67. Ponic, P., Varcoe, C., & Smutylo, T. (2016). *Trauma- (and violence-) informed approaches to supporting victims of violence: Policy and practice considerations.* Retrieved from http://www.justice.gc.ca/eng/rp-pr/cj-jp/victim/rd9-rr9/p2.html.

68. Varcoe, C., Wathen, C. N., Ford-Gilboe, M., et al. (2016). *VEGA briefing note on trauma- and violence-informed care.* Retrieved from http://projectvega.ca/wp-content/uploads/2016/10/VEGA-TVIC-Briefing-Note-2016.pdf.

69. Warshaw, C. (2014). Thinking about trauma in the context of domestic violence: An integrated framework. *Synergy, A Newsletter of the Resource Center on Domestic Violence Child Protection and Custody, 1*(2–8).

70. Wilson, J. M., Fauci, J. E., & Goodman, L. A. (2015). Bringing trauma-Informed practice to domestic violence programs: A qualitative analysis of current approaches. *American Journal of Orthopsychiatry, 85*(6), 586–599.

71. García-Moreno, C., Hegarty, K., d'Oliveira, A. F. L., et al. (2014). The health-systems response to violence against women. *Lancet, 385*(9977), 1567–1579.

72. Etheridge, A., Gill, L., & McDonald, J. (2014). *Domestic violence toolkit for health care providers in BC.* Retrieved from https://www.kpu.ca/sites/default/files/NEVR/DV%20Toolkit%20%20PDF%20August%2024.pdf.

73. Giesbrecht, C. (2012). *Working with women who have experienced violence: A handbook for healthcare professionals in Saskatchewan.* Regina: Provincial association of Transition Houses and Services of Saskatchewan. Retrieved from http://pathssk.org/wp-content/uploads/2011/04/PATHS-Handbook-for-Healthcare-Professionals-Revised-Feb.-20126.pdf.

74. Alvarez, C., Fedock, G., Grace, K. T., et al. (2016). Provider screening and counseling for intimate partner violence a systematic review of practices and influencing factors. *Trauma, Violence and Abuse,* 1–17. doi:10.1177/1524838016637080.

75. Klevens, J., Kee, R., Trick, W., et al. (2012). Effect of screening for partner violence on women's quality of life. *JAMA: The Journal of the American Medical Association, 308*(7), 681–689.

76. O'Doherty, L., Taft, A., Hegarty, K., et al. (2013). Screening women for intimate partner violence in healthcare settings. *Cochrane Database of Systematic Reviews,* (4), Art. No. CD007007, doi:10.1002/14651858.CD007007.pub2.

77. Wathen, C. N., MacGregor, J. C. D., & MacMillan, H. L. (2016). *Research brief: Identifying and responding to intimate partner violence against women.* London, ON: PreVAiL Research Network. Retrieved from http://projectvega.ca/documents/2016/11/prevail-ipv-brief-fall-2016.pdf.

78. PreVAiL. (2017). *Responding safely to intimate partner violence (IPV): We must do better than screening. PreVAiL: Preventing violence across the lifespan research network.* London, ON: Author. Retrieved from http://projectvega.ca/documents/2017/01/ipv-screening-brief.pdf.

79. MacMillan, H. L., Wathen, C., Jamieson, E., et al. (2009). Screening for intimate partner violence in health care settings: A randomized trial. *Journal of the American Medical Association, 302*(5), 493–501.

80. Morse, D. S., Lafleur, R., Fogarty, C. T., et al. (2012). "They told me to leave": How health care providers address intimate partner violence. *Journal of the American Board of Family Medicine, 25*(3), 333–342.

81. Pratt-Eriksson, D., Bergbom, I., & Lyckhage, E. D. (2014). Don't ask don't tell: Battered women living in Sweden encounter with healthcare personnel and their experience of the care given. *International Journal of Qualitative Studies On Health And Well-Being, 9*(1), 23166. doi:10.3402/qhw.v9.23166.

82. Pajak, C., Ahmad, F., Jenney, A., et al. (2014). Survivor's costs of saying no: Exploring the experience of accessing services for intimate partner violence. *Journal of Interpersonal Violence, 29*(14), 2571–2591.

83. Tower, M., Rowe, J., & Wallis, M. (2012). Reconceptualising health and health care for women affected by domestic violence. *Contemporary Nurse: A Journal for the Australian Nursing Profession, 42*(2), 216–225. doi:10.5172/conu.2012.42.2.216.

84. Varcoe, C. (2001). Abuse obscured: An ethnographic account of emergency nursing in relation to violence against women. *Canadian Journal of Nursing Research, 32*(4), 95–115.

85. World Health Organization. (2014). *Health care for women subjected to intimate partner violence or sexual violence: A clinical handbook.* Retrieved from http://apps.who.int/iris/bitstream/10665/136101/1/WHO_RHR_14.26_eng.pdf?ua=1.

86. Bacchus, L., Bullock, L., Sharps, P., et al. (2016). "Opening the door": A qualitative interpretive study of women's experiences of being asked about intimate partner violence and receiving an intervention during perinatal home visits in rural and urban settings in the USA. *Journal of Research in Nursing, 21*(5–6), 345–364.

87. Douglas, E., Hines, D., & McCarthy, S. (2012). Men who sustain female-to-male partner violence: Factors associated with where they seek help and how they rate those resources. *Violence and Victims, 27*(6), 871–894.

88. Hollingsworth, E., & Ford-Gilboe, M. (2006). Registered nurses' self-efficacy for assessing and responding to woman abuse in emergency department settings. *Canadian Journal of Nursing Research, 38*(4), 54–77.

89. Tower, M. (2007). Intimate partner violence and the health care response: A postmodern critique. *Health Care for Women International, 28*, 438–452.

90. Canadian Women's Foundation. (2014). *Moving women out of violence: Fact sheet.* Retrieved from http://www.canadianwomen.org/facts-about-violence.

91. Ford-Gilboe, M., Merritt-Gray, M., Varcoe, C., et al. (2011). A theory-based primary health care intervention for women who have left abusive partners. *Advances in Nursing Science, 34*(3), 198–214.

92. Corbally, M. (2015). Accounting for intimate partner violence: A biographical analysis of narrative strategies used by men experiencing IPV from their female partners. *Journal of Interpersonal Violence, 30*(17), 3112–3132.

93. Doane, G., & Varcoe, C. (2015). *How to nurse: Relational inquiry with individuals and families in changing health and health care contexts.* Philadelphia: Lippincott Williams & Wilkins.

94. World Health Organization. (2013). *Responding to intimate partner violence and sexual violence against women: WHO clinical and policy guidelines.* Geneva, Switzerland: WHO Press.

95. McCaw, B., Berman, W. H., Syme, S. L., et al. (2002). Women referred for on-site domestic violence services in a managed care organization. *Women and Health, 35*(2/3), 23–40.

96. Sharps, P., Koziol-McLain, J., McFarlane, J., et al. (2001). Opportunities for prevention of femicide by health care providers. *Preventive Medicine, 33*, 373–380.

97. Campbell, J. C., Webster, D. W., & Glass, N. (2009). The danger assessment validation of a lethality risk assessment instrument for intimate partner femicide. *Journal of Interpersonal Violence, 24*(4), 653–674.

98. García-Moreno, C., Guedes, A., & Knerr, W. (2012). *Understanding and addressing violence against women: Femicide.* Retrieved from http://apps.who.int/iris/bitstream/10665/77421/1/WHO_RHR_12.38_eng.pdf.

99. Danger Assessment. (2018). Retrieved from https://www.dangerassessment.org.

100. Snider, C., Webster, D., O'Sullivan, C. S., et al. (2009). Intimate partner violence: Development of a brief risk assessment for the emergency department. *Academic Emergency Medicine, 16*(11), 1208–1216. doi:10.1111/j.1553-2712.2009.00457.x.

101. Edwards, P. (2012). *Elder abuse in Canada—A gender-based analysis.* Retrieved from http://www.phac-aspc.gc.ca/seniors-aines/publications/pro/abuse-abus/gba-acs/index-eng.php.

102. Lai, D., Daoust, G., & Li, L. (2014). Understanding elder abuse and neglect in aging Chinese immigrants in Canada. *Journal of Adult Protection, 16*(5), 322–334.

103. Beaulaurier, R., Seff, L., Newman, F., et al. (2007). External barriers to help seeking for older women who experience intimate partner violence. *Journal of Family Violence, 22*, 747–755.

104. Canadian Centre for Elder Law. (2011). *A practical guide to elder abuse and neglect law in Canada.* Retrieved from http://www.bcli.org/project/practical-guide-elder-abuse-and-neglect-law-canada.

105. Gilbert, R., Kemp, A., Thoburn, J., et al. (2009). Recognising and responding to child maltreatment. *Lancet, 373*(9658), 167–180. doi:10.1016/s0140-6736(08)61707-9.

106. Fallon, B., Chabot, M., Fluke, J., et al. (2015). Exploring alternate specifications to explain agency-level effects in placement decisions regarding Aboriginal children: Further analysis of the Canadian Incidence Study of Reported Child Abuse and Neglect Part C. *Child Abuse & Neglect, 49*, 97–106.

107. Fallon, B., Chabot, M., Fluke, J., et al. (2013). Placement decisions and disparities among Aboriginal children: Further analysis of the Canadian incidence study of reported child abuse and neglect part A: Comparisons of the 1998 and 2003 surveys. *Child Abuse & Neglect, 37*(1), 47–60. doi:10.1016/j.chiabu.2012.10.001.

108. McKenzie, H., Varcoe, C., Browne, A., & Day, L. (2016). Disrupting the continuities among residential schools, the Sixties Scoop, and child welfare: An analysis of colonial and neocolonial discourses. *International Indigenous Policy Journal, 7*(2). Retrieved from https://ir.lib.uwo.ca/iipj/vol7/iss2/.

109. Bartlett, J. D., Kotake, C., Fauth, R., et al. (2017). Intergenerational transmission of child abuse and neglect: do maltreatment type, perpetrator, and substantiation status matter? *Child Abuse & Neglect, 63*, 84–94.

110. Widom, C. S., Czaja, S. J., & DuMont, K. A. (2015). Intergenerational transmission of child abuse and neglect: Real or detection bias? *Science, 347*(6229), 1480–1485.

111. Einboden, R., Rudge, T., & Varcoe, C. (2011). Battling the passions: The birth of a conceptual understanding of suspicion for child abuse and neglect. *Aporia—La revue infirmiére/The Nursing Journal, 3*(2), 5–14.

112. Tanner, K., & Turney, D. (2000). The role of observation in the assessment of child neglect. *Child Abuse Review, 9*, 337–348.

113. Horwath, J., & Morrison, T. (2011). Effective inter-agency collaboration to safeguard children: Rising to the challenge

through collective development. *Children & Youth Services Review, 33*(2), 368–375. doi:10.1016/j.childyouth.2010.10.002.

114. Milot, T., St-Laurent, D., & Éthier, L. S. (2016). Intervening with severely and chronically neglected children and their families: The contribution of trauma-informed approaches. *Child Abuse Review, 25*(2), 89–101. doi:10.1002/car.2376.

115. McTavish, J. R., MacMillan, H. L., & Wathen, C. N. (2016). *Briefing note: Mandatory reporting of child maltreatment (VEGA Project and PreVAiL Research Network).* Retrieved from http://projectvega.ca/documents/2016/11/vega-mandatory-reporting-briefing-note-2016.pdf.

116. Pietrantonio, A. M., Wright, E., Gibson, K. N., et al. (2013). Mandatory reporting of child abuse and neglect: Crafting a positive process for health professionals and caregivers. *Child Abuse & Neglect, 37*(2), 102–109.

117. Myers, J. E., Berliner, L., Briere, J., et al. (2002). *The APSAC handbook on child maltreatment.* Thousand Oaks, CA: Sage.

118. Cory, J., Ruebsaat, G., & Hankivsky, O. (2003). *Reasonable doubt: The use of health records in criminal and civil cases of violence against women in relationships.* Retrieved from http://www.bccewh.bc.ca/publications-resources/documents/reasonabledoubt.pdf.

119. Du Mont, J., & White, D. (2013). Barriers to the effective use of medico-legal findings in sexual assault cases worldwide. *Qualitative Health Research, 23*(9), 1228–1239. doi:10.1177/1049732313502396.

120. Langlois, N. E. I., & Greshman, G. A. (2001). The aging of bruises: A review and study of the colour changes with time. *Forensic Science International, 50*, 227–238.

121. Beach, S., Carpenter, C., Rosen, T., et al. (2016). Screening and detection of elder abuse: Research opportunities and lessons learned from emergency geriatric care, intimate partner violence, and child abuse. *Journal of Elder Abuse & Neglect, 28*(4–5), 185–216.

122. Mosqueda, L., Burnight, K., & Liao, S. (2005). The life cycle of bruises in older adults. *Journal of the American Geriatrics Society, 53*, 1339–1343.

123. Campbell, K. A., Olson, L. M., & Keenan, H. I. (2015). Critical elements in the medical evaluation of suspected child physical abuse. *Pediatrics, 136*(1), 35–43. doi:10.1542/peds.2014-4192.

124. Escobar, M. A., Jr., Pflugeisen, B. M., Duralde, Y., et al. (2016). Development of a systematic protocol to identify victims of non-accidental trauma. *Pediatric Surgery International, 32*(4), 377–386. doi:10.1007/s00383-016-3863-8.

125. Pierce, M. C., Kaczor, K., Acker, D., et al. (2017). History, injury, and psychosocial risk factor commonalities among cases of fatal and near-fatal physical child abuse. *Child Abuse & Neglect, 69*, 263–277. doi:10.1016/j.chiabu.2017.04.033.

126. Jackson, J., Miller, M., Moffatt, M., et al. (2015). Bruising in children: Practice patterns of pediatric hematologists and child abuse pediatricians. *Clinical Pediatrics, 54*(6), 563–569. doi:10.1177/0009922814558249.

Assessment Techniques and the Clinical Setting

Written by Carolyn Jarvis, PhD, APN, CNP
Adapted by June MacDonald-Jenkins, RN, BScN, MSc

ⓔ http://evolve.elsevier.com/Canada/Jarvis/examination/

CULTIVATING YOUR SENSES

The health history described in the preceding chapters provides **subjective data** for health assessment: the individual's *own* perception of the health state. **Objective data** are gathered through the use of technical measurements and observations by the health care practitioner.

You will use your senses—sight, smell, touch, and hearing—to gather data during the physical examination. You have always perceived the world through your senses, but now they are focused in a new way. The skills required for the physical examination are inspection, palpation, percussion, and auscultation. They are performed one at a time and in this order.

Inspection

Inspection is concentrated watching. It is close, careful scrutiny, first of the individual patient as a whole and then of each body system. Inspection begins the moment you first meet the patient and develop a "general survey." (Specific data to consider for the general survey are described in Chapter 10.) As you proceed through the examination, start the assessment of each body system with inspection.

Inspection is always performed first. Initially you may feel embarrassed "staring" at the patient without also "doing something." However, do not be too eager to touch the patient. A focused inspection takes time and yields a surprising amount of data. Learn to use each patient as his, her, or their own control by comparing the right and left sides of the body. The two sides are nearly symmetrical. Inspection requires good lighting, adequate exposure, and occasional use of certain instruments (otoscope, ophthalmoscope, penlight, nasal and vaginal specula) to enlarge your view.

Palpation

Palpation follows and often confirms points you noted during inspection. In palpation, you apply your sense of touch to assess texture, temperature, moisture, and organ location and size, as well as any swelling, vibration or pulsation, rigidity or spasticity, crepitation, presence of lumps or masses, and presence of tenderness or pain. Different parts of your hands are best suited for assessing different factors:

- Fingertips: best for fine tactile discrimination such as skin texture, swelling, pulsation, and determining presence of lumps
- A grasping action between the fingers and thumb: best for detecting the position, shape, and consistency of an organ or mass
- The dorsa (backs) of hands and fingers: best for determining temperature because the skin is thinner on the dorsa than on the palms
- Base of fingers (metacarpophalangeal joints) or ulnar surface of the hand: best for vibration

Your palpation technique should be slow and systematic. A patient stiffens when touched suddenly, which makes it difficult for you to feel very much. Use a calm, gentle approach. Warm your hands by kneading them together or holding them under warm water. Identify any tender areas, and palpate them last.

Start with light palpation, using the pads of your fingertips to detect surface characteristics and accustom the patient to being touched. Then perform deeper palpation, perhaps by helping the patient use relaxation techniques such as imagery or deep breathing. Your sense of touch becomes blunted with heavy or continuous pressure. When deep palpation is needed (as for abdominal contents), intermittent pressure is better than one long, continuous palpation. Avoid deep palpation in situations in which it could cause internal injury or pain. Also avoid "digging in" with the ends of your fingers; it will cause pain or discomfort to your patient and may result in increased guarding, by the patient, of the affected areas.

Bimanual palpation requires the use of both of your hands to envelop or detect certain body parts or organs—such as the kidneys, uterus, or adnexa—for more precise delimitation (see Chapters 22 and 27).

Percussion

Percussion is tapping the person's skin with short, sharp strokes to assess underlying structures. The strokes yield a palpable vibration and a characteristic sound that depicts the location, size, and density of the underlying organ. Why learn percussion when an X-ray study is so much more accurate? Because your percussing hands are always available, are

9.1

9.2

easily portable, and give instant feedback. Percussion has the following uses:

- Mapping out the *location* and *size* of an organ by exploring where the percussion note changes between the borders of an organ and its neighbours
- Signalling the *density* (air, fluid, or solid) of a structure by a characteristic note
- Detecting an abnormal mass if it is fairly superficial; the percussion vibrations penetrate about 5 cm deep, and so a deeper mass would yield no change in percussion
- Eliciting pain if the underlying structure is inflamed, as with sinus areas or over the kidneys
- Eliciting a deep tendon reflex with the percussion hammer

Two methods of percussion can be used: (a) *direct* (sometimes called *immediate*) and (b) *indirect* (or *mediate*). In direct percussion, the striking hand contacts the body wall directly. This produces a sound and is used in percussing an infant's thorax or an adult's sinus areas. *Indirect* percussion is used more often and involves both hands. The striking hand contacts the stationary hand, which is fixed on the person's skin. This yields a sound and a subtle vibration. The procedure is as follows:

- *The stationary hand:* Hyperextend the middle finger (the *pleximeter*) of your nondominant hand and place its distal joint firmly against the patient's skin. Avoid the patient's ribs and scapulae; percussing over a bone yields no data because it always sounds "dull." Lift the rest of the stationary hand off the person's skin (Fig. 9.1); otherwise, the stationary hand will dampen the produced vibrations, just as a drummer uses a hand to halt a drum roll.
- *The striking hand:* Use the middle finger of your dominant hand as the *striking finger* (the *plexor*; Fig. 9.2). Hold your forearm close to the patient's skin surface, with your upper arm and shoulder steady. Scan your muscles to make sure they are steady but not rigid. The action is all in the wrist, and it must be relaxed. Spread your fingers,

flick your wrist, and bounce your middle finger off the stationary finger. Aim for just behind the nail bed or at the distal interphalangeal joint; the goal is to hit the portion of the finger that is pushing the hardest into the patient's skin surface. Flex the striking finger so that its tip, not the finger pad, makes contact. It hits directly at right angles to the stationary finger.

Percuss two times in this location, using even, staccato blows. Lift the striking finger off quickly; a resting finger dampens vibrations. Then move to a new body location and repeat, keeping your technique even. The force of the blow determines the loudness of the note. You do not need a very loud sound; use just enough force to achieve a clear note. The thickness of the patient's body wall affects the clarity of the sound. You need a stronger percussion strike for patients who are obese and for those with very muscular body walls.

Percussion can be an awkward technique for beginning examiners. It is often useful to practise on a wall at home and percuss for the placement of the studs along the width of the wall. The changes are distinct and easy to discriminate, enabling you to "establish an ear" for subtle changes in sound, and then transferring that knowledge when examining a patient's body.

Production of Sound

All sound results from vibration of some structure (Fig. 9.3). Percussing over a body structure causes vibrations that produce characteristic waves and are heard as "notes" (Table 9.1). Each of the five percussion notes is differentiated by the following components: (a) **amplitude** (or intensity), loudness or softness of a sound; (b) **pitch** (or frequency), the number of vibrations per second; (c) **quality** (timbre), a subjective difference in a sound's distinctive overtones; and (d) **duration**, the length of time the note lingers.

A basic principle to apply to these components is that a structure with more air (the lungs) produces louder, deeper,

TABLE 9.1	**Characteristics of Percussion Notes**				
CHARACTERISTIC	AMPLITUDE	PITCH	QUALITY	DURATION	SAMPLE LOCATION
Resonant	Medium-loud	Low	Clear, hollow	Moderate	Over normal lung tissue
Hyper-resonant	Louder	Lower	Booming	Longer	Normal finding over a child's lung Abnormal finding in an adult over lungs with increased amount of air, as in emphysema
Tympany	Loud	High	Musical and drumlike (like the kettle drum)	Sustained longest	Over air-filled viscus, such as the stomach or the intestine
Dull	Soft	High	Muffled thud	Short	Relatively dense organ, such as liver or spleen
Flat	Very soft	High	An instant stop of sound, absolute dullness	Very short	When no air is present, over thigh muscles, bone, or tumour

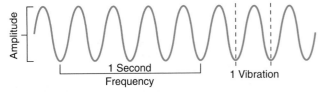

9.3   Sound wave.

and longer sound because it vibrates freely; whereas a denser structure (bone or organs) gives a softer, higher, and shorter sound as it vibrates less easily.

Although Table 9.1 describes five "normal" percussion notes, variations occur in clinical practice. The "note" you hear depends on the nature of the underlying structure, as well as the thickness of the body wall and your technique. The easiest way to learn these differences in sound is to practise with a willing partner.

Auscultation

Auscultation is listening to sounds produced by parts of the body, such as the heart and blood vessels, the lungs, and the abdomen. You have probably already heard certain body sounds with your ear alone: for example, the harsh gurgling of very congested breathing. However, most body sounds are very soft and must be channelled through a **stethoscope** for you to evaluate them. The stethoscope does not magnify sound but does block out extraneous room sounds. Of all the equipment you use, the stethoscope quickly becomes a very personal instrument. Take time to learn its features and to fit one individually to yourself.

The fit and quality of the stethoscope are important. You cannot assess what you cannot hear through a poor-quality instrument. The slope of the earpiece should point forward toward your nose. This matches the natural slope of the normal ear canal and efficiently blocks out environmental sound. If necessary, twist the earpieces to parallel the slope of your ear canals. The earpieces should fit snugly, but if they hurt, they are inserted too far. Adjust the tension, and

experiment with different rubber or plastic earplugs to achieve the most comfort. The tubing should be of thick material, with an internal diameter of 4 mm; standard tubing length is 56 to 69 cm. Be mindful that longer tubing distorts the clarity of low-frequency sounds, such as when auscultating the lungs and diastolic blood pressure, so ensure your stethoscope suits your height and practice preferences.

Choose a stethoscope with two endpieces: a diaphragm and a bell (Fig. 9.4). You use the **diaphragm** most often because its flat edge is best for hearing high-pitched sounds: breath, bowel, and normal heart sounds. Hold the diaphragm against the patient's skin firmly enough to leave a slight ring afterward. The **bell** endpiece has a deep, hollow, cuplike shape. It is best for soft, low-pitched sounds such as extra heart sounds or murmurs. Hold it lightly against the patient's skin, just enough that it forms a perfect seal. Pressing any harder causes the patient's skin to act as a diaphragm, obliterating the low-pitched sounds.

Some newer stethoscopes have one endpiece with a "tunable diaphragm." This enables you to listen to both low- and high-frequency sounds without rotation of the endpiece. To hear low-frequency sounds (traditional bell mode), hold the endpiece very lightly on the patient's skin; to hear high-frequency sounds (traditional diaphragm mode), press the endpiece firmly on the skin.

Before you can evaluate body sounds, it is essential that you eliminate any confusing artifacts:

- Any extra room noise can produce a "roaring" in your stethoscope, and so the examination room must be *quiet*.
- Keep the examination room *warm*. If the patient starts shivering, the involuntary muscle contractions could drown out other sounds.
- *Clean* the stethoscope endpiece with an alcohol wipe, and then warm it by rubbing it against the palm of your hand. Clean the earpieces of your stethoscope as well, especially if it is used by multiple care providers.
- The friction on the endpiece caused by chest hair (on men) causes a crackling sound that mimics an abnormal

9.4 Stethoscope. The endpieces are the diaphragm (on the left) and the bell (on the right).

breath sound called *crackles*. To minimize this problem, wet the hair before auscultating the area.

- *Never listen through a gown.* Reach under a gown to listen, but take care that no clothing rubs on the stethoscope (Fig. 9.5) Prevent your own "artifact," such as breathing on the tubing or the thump from bumping the tubing together.

Auscultation is a skill that beginning examiners are eager to learn, but it is difficult to master. First you must learn the wide range of normal sounds. Once you can recognize normal sounds, you can distinguish the abnormal sounds and extra sounds. Be aware that in some body locations, you may hear more than one sound; this can be confusing. You will need to listen selectively to only one thing at a time. As you listen, ask yourself, "What am I *actually hearing?* What *should* I be hearing at this spot?"

SETTING: CONTEXT OF CARE

The examination environment should be warm and comfortable, quiet, private, and well-lit. An acute care setting is the first environment that many novice practitioners encounter. The majority of nurses and health practitioners never examine a patient in a clinic setting; many practise in the community in patients' homes and in acute and long-term care facilities. Keep in mind that the suggestions for examination are universal, regardless of the setting you are in.

Prior to starting any assessment, it is imperative to ensure the environment is safe. An **environmental scan** of the area you are about to enter is the first step toward patient and practitioner safety. As you enter the patient's room or the practice environment, look at the wider view. What do you see? What devices are attached to the patient? Are there any

9.5

obvious risks when entering the room (e.g., environmental hazards [liquid on floor], biomedical hazards, or patient safety concerns [side rails up])? Do you see and or have the equipment you will need to complete an assessment of the patient (oxygen, suction, vital signs monitor)? Once safety has been established, prepare the setting for the best possible assessment results. Stop or minimize distracting noises—such as humming machinery, radio or television, or people talking—that could make it difficult to hear body sounds. Your time with the individual should be secure from interruptions by other health care personnel. Lighting with natural daylight is best, although it is often not available; artificial light from two sources suffices and prevents shadows. A wall-mounted or gooseneck stand lamp is needed for high-intensity lighting. This provides *tangential* lighting (directed at an angle), which highlights pulsations and body contour better than perpendicular lighting.

Position the patient so that both sides of the body are easily accessible (Fig. 9.6). The examination or bedside table should be at a height at which you can stand without stooping and should be equipped to raise the person's head up to 45 degrees. A roll-up stool is used for the sections of the examination for which you must be sitting. A bedside stand, table, or flat surface is needed to lay out all your equipment.

EQUIPMENT

During the examination, you should not need to search for equipment or leave the room to find an item. Have all your equipment at easy reach and laid out in an organized manner (Fig. 9.7). The following items are usually needed for a screening physical examination:

- Platform scale with height attachment
- Sphygmomanometer (blood pressure monitor)
- Stethoscope with bell and diaphragm endpieces
- Thermometer
- Data collection device (pen and paper, computer)
- Pulse oximeter (in hospital or clinic setting)
- Flashlight or penlight
- Otoscope/ophthalmoscope

9.6

9.7

- Nasal speculum (if a short, broad speculum is not included with the otoscope)
- Tuning fork
- Tongue depressor
- Pocket vision screener
- Skin-marking pen
- Flexible tape measure and ruler marked in centimetres
- Reflex hammer
- Sharp object (split tongue blade)
- Cotton balls
- Clean gloves
- Hand sanitizer or access to a sink
- Lubricant
- Watch or timing device

Those in advanced nursing practice roles may require addition equipment such as vaginal specula, cytology kits, and fecal occult blood-testing materials.

Most of the equipment is described as it comes into use throughout the text. However, the otoscope and ophthalmoscope warrant some greater description as they have uses beyond a simple light source. The **otoscope** funnels light into the ear canal and onto the tympanic membrane. The base serves both as the handle and the battery power source. To attach the head, press it down onto the adaptor end of the base and turn clockwise until you feel it stop. To turn the light on, press the red button rheostat down and clockwise. (Always turn it off after use to increase the life of the bulb and battery.) Five specula, each a different size, are available to attach to the head (Fig. 9.8). (The short, broad speculum is for viewing the nares.) Choose the largest one that will fit comfortably into the patient's ear canal. See Chapter 16 for technique on use of the otoscope.

The **ophthalmoscope** illuminates the internal eye structures. Its system of lenses and mirrors enables you to look through the pupil at the fundus (background) of the eye, much like looking through a keyhole at a room beyond. The ophthalmoscope head attaches to the base adaptor just as the otoscope head does (Fig. 9.9). The head has five different parts:

1. Viewing aperture, with five different aperture sizes
2. Aperture selector dial on the front
3. Mirror window on the front
4. Lens selector dial
5. Lens indicator

Select the aperture to be used (Fig. 9.10).

Rotating the lens selector dial brings the object into focus. The lens indicator shows a number, or *dioptre*, that indicates the value of the lens in position. The black numbers indicate a positive lens, from 0 to +40. The red numbers indicate a negative lens, from 0 to −20. The ophthalmoscope can compensate for myopia (nearsightedness) or hyperopia

9.8   Otoscope

9.9   Ophthalmoscopes.

○   Large (full spot) for dilated pupils

○   Small for undilated pupils

●   Red-free filter — a green beam, used to examine the optic disc for hemorrhage (which looks black) and melanin deposits (which look grey)

⊕   Grid — to determine fixation pattern and to assess size and location of lesions on the fundus

▯   Slit — to examine the anterior portion of the eye and to assess elevation or depression of lesions on the fundus

9.10   Ophthalmoscope apertures.

(farsightedness) in the examiner but does not correct for astigmatism. See Chapter 15 for details on how to hold the instrument and what to inspect.

These are excellent tools that are used regularly by health care providers in advanced practice roles. They are occasionally used during basic assessment, along with some other tools that are specific to the patients' needs, such as the goniometer to measure joint range of motion, the Doppler sonometer to augment pulse or blood pressure measurement, the fetoscope for auscultating fetal heart tones, and the pelvimeter to measure pelvic width. For a child, you also need appropriate pediatric-sized endpieces for the stethoscope and otoscope speculae, materials for developmental assessment, age-appropriate toys, or an infant's soother, if available.

A Clean Field

Do not let your stethoscope become a *"Staph*-oscope"! Stethoscopes and other equipment that are frequently used on many patients can become a common vehicle for transmission of infection. Cleaning instruments with an alcohol swab before use in different patients is an effective control of infection.

Designate "clean" and "used" areas for handling of your equipment. In a hospital setting, you may use the overbed table for your clean surface and the bedside stand for the used equipment surface. In a clinic setting, use two separate areas of the pull-up table. Distinguish the clean area by one or two disposable paper towels. On the towels, place all the new, newly cleaned, or newly alcohol-swabbed equipment that you will use on the current patient. (e.g., your stethoscope endpieces, the reflex hammer, the ruler). As you proceed through the examination, pick up each piece of equipment from the clean area and, after use on the patient, place it in the used area, or (as in the case of tongue blades and gloves) throw it directly in the garbage.

A SAFER ENVIRONMENT

In addition to monitoring the cleanliness of your equipment, take all steps to avoid any possible transmission of infection between patients or between patient and examiner. A **health care–associated infection** (an infection acquired during hospitalization) is a hazard because hospitals have sites that are possible reservoirs for virulent microorganisms. Some microorganisms have become resistant to antibiotics; these include methicillin-resistant *Staphylococcus aureus* (MRSA), vancomycin-resistant *Enterococcus* (VRE), or multidrug-resistant tuberculosis. Other microorganisms include those for which there is currently no known cure, such as the human immunodeficiency virus (HIV).

The single most important step to decrease risk for microorganism transmission is to first establish, through a point-of-care risk assessment (PCRA), what the likelihood of exposure is and then to determine the appropriate actions. The most effective primary intervention continues to be to wash your hands promptly and thoroughly (a) *before* initial patient or patient environment contact; (b) *before* aseptic procedures; (c) *after* contact with blood, body fluids, secretions, and excretions; (4) *after* contact with any equipment contaminated with body fluids; and (5) *after* removing gloves.[1] Using alcohol-based hand rubs takes less time than soap-and-water handwashing; it also kills more organisms more quickly and is less damaging to the skin because of emollients added to the product. Alcohol is highly effective against both Gram-positive and Gram-negative bacteria, *Mycobacterium tuberculosis*, and most viruses, including hepatitis B and C viruses, HIV, and enteroviruses. Use the mechanical action of soap-and-water handwashing when hands are visibly soiled and when patients are infected with spore-forming organisms (e.g., *Clostridium difficile* and noroviruses).

Wear gloves when the potential exists for contact with any body fluids (e.g., blood, mucous membranes, body fluids, drainage, open skin lesions). However, wearing gloves is *not* a protective substitute for washing hands because gloves may have undetectable holes or become torn during use, or hands

---

BOX 9.1   Routine Practices for Use With All Patients

1. *Use point-of-care risk assessment (PCRA)* for each and every patient in the care of your environment. Evaluate the likelihood of exposure, and then choose the appropriate action and personal protective equipment.
2. *Perform hand hygiene* (a) *before* initial patient or patient care environment contact; (b) *before* aseptic procedures; (c) *after* contact with blood, body fluids, secretions, and excretions; (d) after contact with any equipment contaminated with body fluids; and (e) after removing gloves. Alcohol-based hand rub (ABHR) is the preferred method of hand hygiene in all health care settings.
3. *Use personal protective equipment as required.* Perform hand hygiene prior to donning clean gloves when touching blood, body fluids, secretions, excretions, or items contaminated with these materials; mucous membranes; and nonintact skin. Remove gloves promptly after use, before touching noncontaminated items, and before examining another patient, and wash hands immediately.
   a. *Use facial protection.* Wear a mask, face shield, or mask with visor attachment that ensures your eyes, nose, mouth, and chin are covered during procedures and during patient care activities that are likely to generate splashes of blood, body fluids, secretions, and excretions, or that are within 2 m of a coughing patient.
   b. *Wear a gown* (clean, nonsterile, appropriate for activity) to protect uncovered skin and clothing during procedures and during patient care activities that are likely to generate splashes of blood, body fluids, secretions, or excretions. Cuffs of gowns should be covered by gloves.
4. *Apply source control measures* that identify and contain the source of the pathogen. Triage, respiratory hygiene, patient placement and accommodation, patient flow, handling of deceased bodies, and visitor management all fall under source control.
   a. *Place in a private room* any patient who contaminates the environment or who does not or cannot assist in appropriate hygiene or environmental control. Some transmission-based precautions call for providing single accommodations or other negative-pressure–enhanced environments for certain contact and airborne-transmitted pathogens.
   b. *Be especially careful with used patient care equipment* if it is soiled with blood, body fluids, secretions, and excretions; handle it in a manner that prevents skin and mucous membrane exposure, contamination of clothing, and transfer of microorganisms to other patients and environments. Do not use the reusable equipment on another patient until it has been cleaned and reprocessed appropriately. Discard single-use items appropriately.
   c. *Prevent injuries by bloodborne pathogens* when you use or handle needles, scalpels, and other sharp instruments. Never recap used needles, manipulate them with both hands, or direct the point of a needle toward any part of your body; use safety-engineered needles at all times when possible as outlined in the *Safer Needles in Healthcare Workplaces Act* of 2006. Do not remove used needles from disposable syringes by hand, and do not otherwise bend, break, or manipulate used needles by hand. Place used disposable syringes, needles, scalpel blades, and other sharp items in appropriate puncture-resistant containers. Use mouthpieces, resuscitation bags, or other ventilation devices instead of mouth-to-mouth resuscitation methods in areas where the need for resuscitation is predictable.
5. *Follow environmental control policies* for the routine care, cleaning, and disinfection of environmental surfaces, beds, bed rails, bedside equipment, and other frequently touched surfaces. Take care with used linen soiled with blood, body fluids, secretions, and excretions; handle, transport, and process this linen in a manner that prevents skin and mucous membrane exposure.

Adapted from Public Health Agency of Canada. (2013). *Routine practices and additional precautions for preventing the transmission of infection in healthcare settings*. Ottawa: Her Majesty the Queen in Right of Canada. Retrieved from http://publications.gc.ca/collections// collection_2013/aspc-phac/HP40-83-2013-eng.pdf.

---

may become contaminated as gloves are removed. Wear a gown, mask, and protective eyewear when the potential exists for any blood or body fluid spattering (e.g., suctioning, arterial puncture).

The Public Health Agency of Canada's *Routine Practices and Additional Precautions for Preventing the Transmission of Infection in Healthcare Settings* guidelines include the most recent epidemiological information on decreasing infection transmission.[1] The guidelines include two tiers of precautions. **Routine practices** (Box 9.1) are intended for use with *all* patients at *all* times, regardless of their risk for infection or presumed infection status. Routine practices are designed to reduce the risk for transmission of microorganisms from both recognized and unrecognized sources, and they apply to (a) blood; (b) all body fluids, secretions, and excretions except sweat, regardless of whether they contain visible blood; (c) nonintact skin; and (d) mucous membranes.

The second tier is **additional precautions**, which are intended for use when routine practices cannot fully manage the transmissions of the organisms in the health care setting. Routes of transmission have been classified as contact (direct, indirect, and droplet), airborne, common vehicle (single contaminated source, such as food), and vectorborne. The two tiers of precautions may be combined for diseases that have multiple routes of transmission, such as varicella (chicken pox). Vectorborne transmission by insects of a pathogen such as West Nile virus from mosquitoes and Lyme disease from infected ticks have been reported in Canada.

THE CLINICAL SETTING

General Approach

Consider your emotional state and that of the patient being examined. The patient is usually anxious because of the anticipation of being examined by a stranger and the unknown outcome of the examination. If anxiety can be reduced, the patient will feel more comfortable and the data gathered will more accurately reflect the patient's natural state. Anxiety can be reduced by an examiner who is confident and self-assured, as well as considerate and unhurried.

Most beginning examiners feel anything *but* self-assured! Most worry about their technical skill, about missing a significant finding, or about forgetting a step. Many are embarrassed about encountering a partially dressed individual. All of these fears are natural and common. The best way to minimize them is with a lot of practice on a healthy, willing subject, usually a fellow student. You have to feel comfortable with your motor skills before you can absorb what you are actually seeing or hearing in a real patient. This comfort develops with practice under the guidance of an experienced peer or mentor, in an atmosphere in which it is acceptable to make mistakes and to ask questions. Your subject should "act like a patient" so that you can deal with a "real" situation while still in a safe setting. After you feel comfortable in the laboratory setting, join your preceptor or co-assigned nurse during the examination of an actual patient so that you can observe an experienced examiner in the practice setting.

Hands On

With this preparation, it is possible to interact with your own patient in a confident manner. Begin by measuring the patient's height, weight, blood pressure, temperature, pulse, and respiration (see Chapter 10). If necessary, measure visual acuity at this time, using the Snellen eye chart. All of these are familiar, relatively nonthreatening actions; they gradually accustom the patient to the examination. Then ask the patient to change into an examination gown or other clothing that gives you access, leaving underpants on. The patient will feel more comfortable with underpants, and the underpants can easily be removed just before the genital examination. Unless your assistance is needed, leave the room as the patient undresses. Keep in mind that some patients may not wish to disrobe fully or at all, depending on ethnocultural considerations. As you re-enter the room, wash your hands in the patient's presence. Not only is this an infection control measure but also it demonstrates a readiness to provide safe care. Explain each step in the examination and how the patient can cooperate. Encourage the patient to ask questions. Keep your own movements slow, methodical, and deliberate.

Begin by touching the patient's hands, checking skin colour, nail beds, and metacarpophalangeal joints (Fig. 9.11). Again, this is a less threatening way to ease a patient into being touched. Most people are used to having relative strangers touch their hands.

As you proceed through the examination, avoid distractions and concentrate on one step at a time. The sequence of the steps may differ, depending on the age of the patient and your own preference. However, you should establish a system that works for you; stick to it to avoid omissions. Organize the steps so that the patient does not change positions too often. Although proper exposure is necessary, use additional drapes to maintain the patient's privacy and to prevent chilling. Consider possible ethnocultural considerations in regard to touch. As you proceed through the examination,

9.11

ensure that the patient is comfortable with the progression of the assessment.

Do not hesitate to write out the examination sequence and refer to it as you proceed. The patient will accept this as quite natural if you explain you are making brief notations to ensure accuracy. Many agencies use a printed form. You will find that you glance at the form less and less as you obtain experience. Even with a form, you sometimes may forget a step in the examination. When you realize that you have forgotten a step, perform the manoeuvre in the next logical point in the sequence. (See Chapter 28 for the sequence of steps in the complete physical examination.)

As you proceed through the examination, occasionally offer some brief teaching about the patient's body. For example, you might say, "This tapping on your back (percussion) is a little like playing different drums. The different notes I hear tell me where each organ starts and stops. You probably can hear the difference yourself from within your body." Or you might say, "Everyone has two sounds for each heartbeat, something like this: lub-dup. Your own beats sound normal." Do not do this with every single step, or you will be hard pressed to make a comment when you do come across an abnormality. Some sharing of information, however, builds rapport and increases the patient's confidence in you as an examiner. It also gives the patient a little more control in a situation in which it is easy to feel completely helpless.

At some point, you may want to linger in one anatomical location to concentrate on some complicated findings. To avoid causing anxiety, tell the person, "I always listen to heart sounds on a number of places on the chest. Just because I am listening a long time does not necessarily mean anything is wrong." Sometimes, of course, you *will* discover a possible abnormality, and you want another examiner to double-check. You need to give the patient some information, but you should not alarm the person unnecessarily. Say something like, "I do not have a complete assessment of your heart sounds. I want Ms. Wright to listen to you, too."

At the end of the examination, summarize your findings and share the necessary information with the patient. Thank the patient for the time spent. In a hospital setting, apprise the patient of what is scheduled next. Before you leave a hospitalized patient, lower the bed; make the patient comfortable and safe; and return the bedside table, television, or any equipment to the way it was originally. In a clinic or home care setting, your assessment data provide the basis of information needed to develop a collaborative plan of care with your patient.

 ## DEVELOPMENTAL CONSIDERATIONS

Children are different from adults in many ways. Their difference in size is obvious. Their bodies grow in a predictable pattern that is assessed during the physical examination. However, their behaviour is also different. Behaviour develops and changes through predictable stages, just as the body does. Each examiner needs to know the expected emotional and cognitive features of these stages and to perform the physical examination on the basis of developmental principles.[2,3]

With all children, the goal is to increase their comfort in the setting. This approach reveals their natural state as much as possible and will give them a more positive memory of health care providers. Remember that a "routine" examination is anything but routine to children. You can increase their comfort by attending to the developmental principles and approaches discussed in the following sections. The *order* of the developmental stages is more meaningful than the exact chronological age. Each child is an individual, and no child's development fits exactly into one category. For example, if your efforts to "play games" with a preschool-age child are rebuffed, modify your approach to the security measures used with a toddler.

Infants

Erik Erikson defined the major task of infancy as establishing trust. An infant is completely dependent on the parent for basic needs. If these needs are met promptly and consistently, the infant feels secure and learns to trust others.

Position

- A parent always should be present to understand normal growth and development and for the child's feeling of security.
- Place the neonate or young infant supine on a padded examination table (Fig. 9.12). The infant also may be held against the parent's chest for some steps.
- Once the baby can sit without support (at approximately 6 months of age), as much of the examination as possible should be performed while the baby is in the parent's lap.

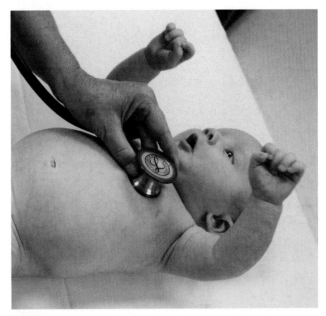

9.12

- By ages 9 to 12 months, the baby is acutely aware of the surroundings. Anything outside the infant's range of vision is "lost," and so the parent must be in full view.

Preparation

- Perform the examination 1 to 2 hours after the baby is fed, when the baby is not too drowsy or too hungry.
- Maintain a warm environment. A neonate may require an overhead radiant heater.
- Infants do not object to being nude. Have the parent remove outer clothing, but leave a diaper on a boy.
- Infants do not mind being touched, but make sure your hands and stethoscope endpieces are warm.
- Use a soft, crooning voice during the examination; babies respond more to the feeling in the tone of the voice than to what is actually said.
- Most infants like eye contact; lock your eyes with the baby's from time to time.
- Smile; a baby prefers a smiling face to a frowning one. (Often beginning examiners are so absorbed in their technique that they look serious or stern.) Take time to play.
- Keep movements smooth and deliberate, not jerky.
- Offer the baby a pacifier for crying or during invasive steps.
- Offer brightly coloured toys for a distraction when an infant is fussy.
- Let an older baby touch the stethoscope or tongue blade.

Sequence

- Seize the opportunity with a sleeping baby to listen to heart, lung, and abdominal sounds first.
- Perform the least distressing steps first. (See the sequence in Chapter 28.) Save the invasive steps of examination of the eye, ear, nose, and throat until last.
- Elicit the Moro, or "startle," reflex at the end of the examination because it may cause the baby to cry.

9.13

Toddlers

Toddlers are at Erikson's stage of developing autonomy. However, the need to explore the world and be independent is in conflict with the basic dependency on the parent. This often results in frustration and negativism. Toddlers may be difficult to examine; do not take this personally. Because they are acutely aware of being in a new environment, toddlers may be frightened and cling to the parents. Also, toddlers fear invasive procedures and dislike being restrained (Fig. 9.13).

Position

- A toddler should be sitting up on the parent's lap for all of the examination. When the toddler must be supine (as in the abdominal examination), move chairs to sit knee-to-knee with the parent. Have the toddler lie in the parent's lap with the toddler's legs in your lap.
- Enlist the aid of a cooperative parent to help position the toddler during invasive procedures. The child's legs can be captured between the parent's legs. The parent can encircle the child's head with one arm, holding it against the chest, and hold the child's arms with the other arm. (See Fig. 17.22.)

Preparation

- Children 1 or 2 years of age can understand symbols, and so a security object, such as a special blanket or teddy bear, is helpful.
- Begin by greeting the child and the accompanying parent by name, but with a child 1 to 6 years old, focus more on the parent. By essentially "ignoring" the child at first, you allow the child to adjust gradually and to size you up from a safe distance. Then turn your attention gradually to the child, at first to a toy or object the child is holding, or perhaps to compliment the child's clothes or hair. If the child is ready, you will note these signals: eye contact with you, smiling, talking with you, or accepting a toy or a piece of equipment.

- A 2-year-old child does not like to be without clothes; have the parent undress the child one part at a time.
- Children 1 or 2 years of age like to say, "No." Do not offer a choice when there really is none. Avoid saying, "May I listen to your heart now?" When the 1- or 2-year-old child says "No," and you go ahead and do it anyway, you lose trust. Instead, use clear firm instructions, in a tone that expects cooperation: "Now it is time for you to lie down so I can check your tummy."
- Also, 1- or 2-year-old children like to make choices. When possible, enhance autonomy by offering a *limited option*: "Shall I listen to your heart next, or your tummy?"
- Demonstrate the procedures on the parent or a plush toy (see Fig. 16.11).
- Praise the child when the child is cooperative.

Sequence

- Collect some objective data while you document the history, which is a less stressful time. While you are focusing on the parent, note the child's gross motor and fine motor skills and gait.
- Begin with "games," such as cranial nerve testing.
- Start with nonthreatening areas. Save distressing procedures—such as examination of the head, ear, nose, or throat—for last.

Preschool-Age Children

Preschool-age children display developing initiative. The preschooler takes on tasks independently, plans the tasks, and follows them through. A child of this age is often cooperative, helpful, and easy to involve. However, children of this age have fantasies and may see illness as punishment for being "bad." The concept of body image is limited. The child fears any body injury or mutilation, and so the child will recoil from invasive procedures (e.g., tongue blade, rectal temperature, injection, and venipuncture).

Position

- With a 3-year-old child, the parent should be present, and the child may be held on the parent's lap during examination (Fig. 9.14).
- A 4- or 5-year-old child usually feels comfortable on the "Big Girl" or "Big Boy" (examining) table, with the parent present.

Preparation

- A preschooler can talk. Verbal communication becomes helpful now, but remember that the child's understanding is still limited. Use short, simple explanations.
- The preschooler is usually willing to undress. Leave underpants on until the genital examination.
- Talk to the child and explain the steps in the examination exactly.
- Do not allow a choice when there is none.
- As with toddlers, enhance the autonomy of preschoolers by offering choice when possible.
- Allow the child to play with equipment to reduce fears.

9.14

9.15

- Preschoolers like to help; have the child hold the stethoscope for you.
- Use games. Have the child "blow out" the light on the penlight as you listen to the breath sounds or pretend to listen to the heart sounds of the child's teddy bear first. One technique that is absorbing to preschoolers is to trace their shape on the examining table paper. You can comment on how big the child is, then fill in the outline with a heart or stomach and listen to the paper doll first. After the examination, the child can take the paper doll home as a souvenir.
- Use a slow, patient, deliberate approach. Do not rush.
- During the examination, give the preschooler needed feedback and reassurance: "Your tummy feels just fine."
- Compliment the child on being cooperative.

Sequence

- Examine the thorax, abdomen, extremities, and genitalia first. Preschoolers are usually cooperative; nevertheless, assess head, eye, ear, nose, and throat last.

School-Age Children

During the school-age period, the major task of children is developing industry. School-age children are developing basic competency in school and in social networks, and they desire the approval of parents and teachers. When successful, children have a feeling of accomplishment. During the examination, school-age children are cooperative and are interested in learning about the body. Language is more sophisticated now, but do not overestimate and treat the school-age child as a small adult. The child's level of understanding may not match that of the child's speech.

Position

- School-age children should be sitting on the examination table.

- Five-year-old children have a sense of modesty. If appropriate in the examination, let an older child (aged 11 or 12 years) decide whether parents or siblings should be present.

Preparation

- Break the ice with small talk about family, school, friends, music, or sports.
- Children should undress on their own, leave underpants on, don a gown, and use a drape.
- Demonstrate equipment; school-age children are curious about how equipment works.
- Comment on the body and how it works (Fig. 9.15). An 8- or 9-year-old child has some understanding of the body and is interested to learn more. It is rewarding to see the child's eyes light up when the child hears the heart sounds.

Sequence

- As with adults, progress from head to toes.

Adolescents

The major task in adolescence is developing a self-identity. This takes shape from various sets of values and different social roles (son or daughter, sibling, and student). In the end, people need to feel satisfied and comfortable with who they are. In the process, adolescents are increasingly self-conscious and introspective. Peer group values and peer acceptance are important.

Position

- An adolescent should be sitting on the examination table.
- Examine the adolescent alone, without a parent or sibling present.

Preparation

- The adolescent's body is changing rapidly. During the examination, the adolescent needs feedback that his, her, or their own body is healthy and developing normally.
- Adolescents have a keen awareness of body image, often comparing themselves with peers. Apprise the adolescent of the wide variation among teenagers on the rate of growth and development (see sexual maturity ratings, Chapters 18, 26, and 27).
- Communicate with some care. Do not treat the teenager like a child, but do not overestimate and treat the teenager like an adult, either.
- Because most adolescents are idealistic, they are amenable to health teaching. Positive attitudes developed now may last throughout adult life. Focus your teaching on ways in which adolescents can achieve their own wellness.

Sequence

- As with the adult, a head-to-toe approach is appropriate. Examine genitalia last, and do so quickly.

Older Adults

During later years, the tasks are developing the meaning of life and one's own existence and adjusting to changes in physical strength and health (Fig. 9.16).

Position

- An older adult should be sitting on the examination table; a frail older adult may need to be supine.
- Arrange the sequence to allow as few position changes as possible.
- Allow rest periods when needed.

Preparation

- For older adults, the pace of the examination may need to be slowed. The slower pace may dictate the ability to implement some techniques. It is better to break the complete examination into a few visits than to rush through the examination and alienate or frighten the patient.
- Use physical touch (unless there is a cultural contraindication). This is especially important with older adults because other senses, such as vision and hearing, may be diminished.
- Do not mistake diminished vision or hearing for confusion. Confusion of sudden onset may signify a disease state. It is manifested by short-term memory loss, diminished thought process, diminished attention span, and labile emotions (see Chapter 6).
- Be aware that the later years contain more of life's stress. Loss is inevitable, including changes in physical appearance of the face and body, declining energy level, loss of job through retirement, loss of financial security, loss of long-time home, and deaths of friends or spouse. How the patient adapts to these losses significantly affects health assessment.

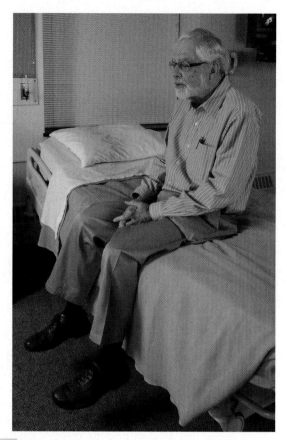

9.16

Sequence

- Use the head-to-toe approach as in younger adults.

Individuals With Acute Health Challenges

For patients in some distress, alter their position during the examination. For example, a patient with shortness of breath or ear pain may want to sit up, whereas a person with faintness or overwhelming fatigue may want to be supine. Initially, it may be necessary just to examine the body areas appropriate to the problem, collecting a **mini-database**. You may resume a complete assessment after the initial distress is alleviated.

REFERENCES

1. Public Health Agency of Canada (2013). *Routine practices and additional precautions for preventing the transmission of infection in healthcare settings.* Ottawa: Her Majesty the Queen in Right of Canada. Retrieved from http://publications.gc.ca/collections//collection_2013/aspc-phac/HP40-83-2013-eng.pdf.
2. Berk, L. E. (2007). *Development through the lifespan* (4th ed.). Boston: Allyn & Bacon.
3. Perry, S., Hockenberry, M., Lowdermilk, D., et al. (2010). *Maternal child nursing care* (4th ed.). St. Louis: Elsevier.

CHAPTER 10

General Survey, Measurement, and Vital Signs

Written by Carolyn Jarvis, PhD, APN, CNP
Adapted by June MacDonald-Jenkins, RN, BScN, MSc

ⓔ http://evolve.elsevier.com/Canada/Jarvis/examination/

OBJECTIVE DATA

The general survey is a study of the whole person, covering the general health state and any obvious physical characteristics. It is an introduction for the physical examination that will follow; it should give an overall impression, a "gestalt," of the patient (see Sample Charting on p. 178). Objective parameters are used to form the general survey, but these apply to the whole person, not just to one body system.

Begin the general survey at the moment you first encounter the patient. What leaves an immediate impression? Does the patient stand promptly as his, her, or their name is called and walk easily to meet you? Or does the patient look ill, rising slowly or with effort, with shoulders slumped and eyes without lustre or downcast? Is the hospitalized patient conversing with visitors, involved in reading or television, or lying still? Even as you introduce yourself and shake hands, you collect data (Fig. 10.1). Does the patient fully extend the arm, shake your hand firmly, make eye contact, or smile? Are the palms dry, or are they damp and clammy? As you proceed through the health history, the measurements, and the vital signs, note the following points that will add up to the general survey. Consider these four areas: (a) **physical appearance**, (b) **body structure**, (c) **mobility**, and (d) **behaviour**.

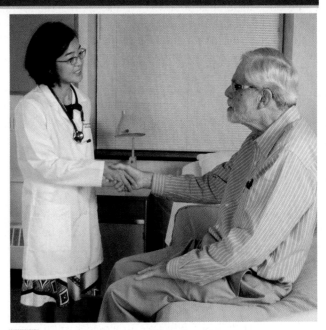

10.1

Normal Range of Findings	Abnormal Findings

The General Survey

Physical Appearance

Age. Appears to be the stated age.

Sex. Sexual development appropriate for gender and age.
Level of Consciousness. Alert and oriented, attending to your questions, and responding appropriately.
Skin Colour. Even colour tone, pigmentation varying with genetic background, and intact skin with no obvious lesions.
Facial Features. Symmetrical with movement.

Appears older than the stated age, as in chronic illness or chronic alcoholism.
Delayed or precocious puberty.
Confused, drowsy, or lethargic (see Table 6.1, p. 84).
Pallor, cyanosis, jaundice, erythema, or any lesions (see Chapter 13).
Immobile, masklike, asymmetrical, or drooping (see Table 14.4, p. 297).

Normal Range of Findings	Abnormal Findings
No signs of acute distress.	Respiratory signs: shortness of breath, wheezing. Pain, indicated by facial grimace and holding the affected body part.

Body Structure

Stature. Height within normal range for age and genetic heritage (see Measurement, p. 155).

Nutrition. Weight within normal range for height and body build; even distribution of body fat.

Symmetry. Body parts equal bilaterally and in relative proportion to each other.

Posture. Standing comfortably erect as appropriate for age; normal "plumb line" through anterior ear, shoulder, hip, patella, and ankle (exceptions: standing toddlers, who have a normally protuberant abdomen ["toddler lordosis"] and older adults, who may be stooped with kyphosis).

Position. Sitting comfortably in a chair, on the bed, or on the examination table; arms relaxed at sides, head turned to examiner.

Body Build, Contour. Normal proportions: (a) arm span (fingertip to fingertip) equals height; (b) body length from crown to pubis approximately equal to length from pubis to sole; obvious physical deformities: note any congenital or acquired defects.

Mobility

Gait. Normally, base width equal to shoulder width; accurate foot placement; smooth, even, and well-balanced walk; and presence of associated movements, such as symmetrical arm swing.

Range of Motion. Full mobility in each joint, and deliberate, accurate, smooth, and coordinated movement (see Chapter 24 for information on more detailed testing of joint range of motion).

Abnormal Findings (right column):

Excessively short or tall (see Table 10.4, p. 179).

Cachectic, emaciated.

Simple obesity, with even fat distribution.

Centripetal (truncal) obesity: fat concentrated in face, neck, trunk, with thin extremities, as in Cushing's syndrome (hyperadrenalism; see Table 10.4, p. 180).

Unilateral atrophy or hypertrophy.

Asymmetrical location of a body part.

Rigid spine and neck; move as one unit (e.g., arthritis).

Patient stiff and tense, ready to spring from chair; fidgety movements.

Slumped shoulders; deflated appearance (e.g., depression).

Tripod: leaning forward with arms braced on chair arms; occurs with chronic pulmonary disease.

Sitting straight up and resisting lying down (e.g., heart failure).

Curled up in fetal position (e.g., acute abdominal pain).

Elongated arm span, arm span greater than height (e.g., Marfan's syndrome, hypogonadism [see Table 10.4, p. 179]).

Missing extremities or digits; webbed digits; shortened limb.

Exceptionally wide base; staggering, stumbling.

Shuffling, dragging, nonfunctional leg.

Limping with injury.

Propulsion: difficulty stopping (see Table 25.5, p. 739).

No observation of involuntary movement.

Limited range of motion in joint.

Paralysis: absence of movement.

Jerky, uncoordinated movement.

Tics, tremors, seizures (see Table 25.4, p. 737).

Normal Range of Findings	Abnormal Findings

Behaviour

Facial Expression. Maintaining eye contact with examiner (unless a cultural consideration exists), expressions appropriate to the situation (e.g., thoughtful, serious, or smiling; note expressions both while the face is at rest and while the patient is talking).

Mood and Affect. Comfortable and cooperative with the examiner and interacting pleasantly.

Speech. Clear and understandable articulation (the ability to form words), as well as the following:

- Fluent stream of talking, with an even pace
- Conveying ideas clearly
- Word choice appropriate to culture and education
- Communicating in native language easily or with an interpreter

Dress. Clothing appropriate for the climate, looks clean and fits the body, and is appropriate for the patient's culture and age group; for example, women of the Hutterite faith may wear nineteenth century–style clothing, and women of Indian descent may wear saris (culturally determined dress should not be labelled as bizarre by Western standards or by adult expectations).

Personal Hygiene. Appearance: clean and groomed appropriately for patient's age, occupation, and socioeconomic group (a wide variation of dress and hygiene is "normal"). Hair: groomed, brushed. Makeup is appropriate for age and culture.

Measurement

Weight

Use a standardized *balance* or electronic standing scale (Fig. 10.2) Instruct the patient to remove shoes and heavy outer clothing before standing on the scale. When a sequence of repeated weights is necessary, aim for approximately the same time of day and the same type of clothing worn each time. Record the weight in kilograms and in pounds.

Show the patient how his, her, or their own weight compares with the recommended range for height. Compare the patient's current weight with that from the previous health visit. A recent weight loss may be explained by successful dieting. A weight gain usually reflects overabundant caloric intake, unhealthy eating habits, sedentary lifestyle, or fluid accumulation.

Abnormal Findings

Flat, depressed, angry, sad, anxious (however, anxiety is common in ill people, and some people smile when they are anxious).

Hostile, distrustful, suspicious, crying.

Dysarthria and dysphonia; speech defect, monotone, garbled speech.

Extremes: few words or constant talking.

Clothing too large and held up by belt: suggestive of weight loss, as does the addition of new holes in belt; belt moved to a looser fit: may indicate weight gain, obesity, or ascites.

Consistent wear of certain clothing may provide clues: long sleeves may conceal needle marks of drug use; broad-brimmed hats may reveal sun intolerance; Velcro fasteners instead of buttons may indicate chronic motor dysfunction.

Body odour, scent of alcohol. Unkempt appearance in an individual who previously was well groomed may indicate depression, illness, or malaise.

An unexplained weight loss may be a sign of a short-term illness (e.g., fever, infection, disease of the mouth or throat) or a chronic illness (endocrine disease, malignancy, or mental health illness).

Unexplained weight gain may indicate fluid retention (e.g., heart failure).[1]

Objective Data

Normal Range of Findings	Abnormal Findings

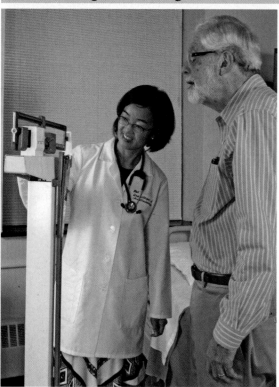

10.2

Height

Use a wall-mounted device or the measuring pole on the balance scale. Align the extended headpiece with the top of the head. The patient should be shoeless, standing straight with gentle traction under the jaw, and looking straight ahead. Feet, shoulders, and buttocks should be in contact with the hard surface.

Body Mass Index

Body mass index (BMI) is a practical marker of optimal weight for height and an indicator of obesity or protein-calorie malnutrition. Evidence supports using BMI in obesity risk assessment because it provides a more accurate measure of total body fat, in comparison with the measure of body weight alone (Fig. 10.3). BMI is calculated as follows:

$$\text{BMI} = \frac{\text{Weight (in kilograms)}}{\text{Height (in metres)}^2} \ Or$$

$$\frac{\text{Weight (in pounds)}}{\text{Height (in inches)}^2} \times 703$$

For a quick determination of BMI, use a straight edge to help locate the point on the chart where height (centimetres or inches) and weight (kilograms or pounds) intersect (see Fig. 10.3). Read the number on the dashed line closest to this point. For example, an individual who weighs 69 kg and is 173 cm tall has a BMI of approximately 23. Many BMI calculators are available online.

BMI interpretation for adults:[2]
<18.5: Underweight
18.5–24.9 Normal weight
25.0–29.9: Overweight
30.0–34.9: Obesity (Class 1)
35–39.9: Obesity (Class 2)
≥40: Extreme obesity (Class 3)

BMI interpretation for children aged 2 to 19 years: 97–99th percentile or beyond = further assessment and intervention is required.[3]

In 2014, 6.2% of Canadians aged 12–17 reported height and weight that classified them as obese.[4]

Normal Range of Findings	Abnormal Findings

10.3 Body mass index (BMI) nomogram.

Waist-to-Hip Ratio

The waist-to-hip ratio reflects body fat distribution as an indicator of health risk. Patients with obesity who have a greater proportion of fat in the upper body, especially in the abdomen, have android obesity; obese patients with most of their fat in the hips and thighs have gynoid obesity. The equation is as follows:

$$\text{Waist-to-hip ratio} = \frac{\text{Waist circumference}}{\text{Hip circumference}}$$

where waist circumference is measured at the smallest circumference below the rib cage and above the iliac crest, and hip circumference is measured at the largest circumference of the buttocks. In addition, **waist circumference** alone can be used to predict greater health risk. Measure at the end of gentle expiration.

In Health Canada's guidelines for body weight classification in adults,[5] BMI and waist circumference serve as indicators of health risk. Use of these measurements is in keeping with internationally adopted recommendations from the World Health Organization (WHO),[6] which are derived from population data. It is important to recognize that weight classification is only a component of a comprehensive health assessment. This classification system is not intended for use with patients younger than 18 years or with pregnant or lactating women.

A waist circumference higher than 88 cm (35 in) in women and higher than 102 cm (40 in) in men places them at risk for type 2 diabetes, coronary heart disease, and hypertension.[5]

Objective Data

Normal Range of Findings	Abnormal Findings

Vital Signs

Temperature

Cellular metabolism requires a mean stable core ("deep body") temperature of 37.2°C (99°F). The body maintains a steady temperature through a thermostat, or feedback mechanism, regulated in the hypothalamus. The thermostat balances heat production (from metabolism, exercise, food digestion, external factors) with heat loss (through radiation, evaporation of sweat, convection, conduction).

The various routes of temperature measurement reflect the body's core temperature. The normal oral temperature in a resting patient ranges from 35.8 to 37.3°C (96.4 to 99.1°F) (mean, 37°C [98.6°F]). The rectal temperature measures 0.4°C to 0.5°C (0.7° to 1°F) higher.

The normal temperature is influenced by the following:

- A diurnal cycle of 1° to 1.5°C, with the trough occurring in the early morning hours, and the peak occurs in late afternoon to early evening.
- The menstruation cycle in women: Progesterone secretion, occurring with ovulation at midcycle, causes a 0.5°C to 1.0°C rise in temperature that continues until menses.
- Exercise: Moderate to strenuous exercise increases body temperature.
- Age: Wider normal variations occur in infants and young children as a result of less effective heat control mechanisms. In older adults, temperature is usually lower than in other age groups, with a mean of 36.2°C (97.2°F).

The **oral temperature** is accurate and convenient. The oral sublingual site has a rich blood supply (from the carotid arteries) that quickly responds to changes in inner core temperature.

The Procedure: Oral Temperature

Shake a mercury-free glass thermometer down to a reading of around 35.5°C (96°F), and place the thermometer at the base of the tongue in either of the posterior sublingual pockets, *not* in front of the tongue. Instruct the patient to keep the lips closed. Leave the thermometer in place 3 to 4 minutes if the patient is afebrile and up to 8 minutes if the patient is febrile. (Measure other vital signs during this time.) Wait 20 minutes before taking the temperature if the patient has just taken hot or iced liquids, and 2 minutes if the patient has just smoked.

The **electronic thermometer** has the advantages of swift and accurate measurement (usually in 20 to 30 seconds) as well as safe, unbreakable, disposable probe covers. The instrument must be fully charged and correctly calibrated. Most children enjoy watching their temperature numbers advance on the box.

The Procedure: Axillary Temperature

The **axillary temperature** is safe and accurate for infants and young children when the environment can be controlled. It is not the method of choice in adults, as it is highly insensitive (see Developmental Considerations, p. 174)

Abnormal Findings

The thermostatic function of the hypothalamus may become disturbed during illness or central nervous system disorders.

Hyperthermia, or fever, is caused by pyrogens secreted by toxic bacteria during infections or as a result of tissue breakdown such as that after myocardial infarction, trauma, surgery, or malignancy. Neurological disorders (e.g., a cerebral vascular accident, cerebral edema, brain trauma, tumour, or surgery) also can reset the thermostat at a higher level, resulting in heat production and conservation.

Hypothermia is usually caused by accidental, prolonged exposure to cold. It also may be purposefully induced to lower the body's oxygen requirements during heart or peripheral vascular surgery, neurosurgery, amputation, or gastro-intestinal hemorrhage.

Normal Range of Findings	Abnormal Findings

The Procedure: Rectal Temperature

Measure the **rectal temperature** only when the other routes are not practical—for example, in comatose or confused patients, those in shock, or those who cannot close the mouth because of breathing or oxygen tubes, wired mandible, or other facial dysfunction—or if no tympanic membrane thermometer equipment is available. Wear gloves, insert a lubricated rectal probe cover on an electronic thermometer, and insert the thermometer only 2 to 3 cm (1 in) into the adult rectum, directed toward the umbilicus. (For a glass thermometer, leave in place for 2.5 minutes.) Disadvantages to the rectal route are patient discomfort and the time-consuming and disruptive nature of the activity.

The Procedure: Tympanic Membrane Temperature

The **tympanic membrane thermometer (TMT)** senses infrared emissions of the tympanic membrane (eardrum). The tympanic membrane shares the same vascular supply that perfuses the hypothalamus (the internal carotid artery), thus making it an accurate measurement of core temperature.

The TMT is a noninvasive, nontraumatic device that is extremely quick and efficient. The probe tip has the shape of an otoscope, the instrument used to inspect the ear. Cover the probe tip with a tip cover, and gently place the probe tip into the patient's ear canal (see Fig. 10.18 on p. 172). Do not force it in, and do not occlude the canal. Activate the device, and you can read the temperature in 2 to 3 seconds.

There is minimal chance of cross-contamination with the tympanic thermometer because the ear canal is lined with skin and not mucous membrane and the tip covers are disposable, one-time use devices.

Conflicting evidence has led to a move away from the use of tympanic thermometry in critical patients and has fallen out of favour in many acute hospital environments.[7]

The Procedure: Temporal Artery Temperature

The newest noninvasive temperature measurement method uses infrared emissions from the temporal artery. The **temporal artery thermometer (TAT)** is used by sliding the probe across the forehead and behind the ear. The thermometer works by taking multiple readings and providing an average. The reading takes approximately 6 seconds. This approach is well tolerated and is more accurate than TMTs; however, there are conflicting reports about its accuracy.[8]

Pulse

With every beat, the heart pumps an amount of blood—the **stroke volume**—into the aorta. This is about 70 mL in adults. The force causes the arterial walls to widen and generates a pressure wave, which is felt in the periphery as the **pulse**. By palpating the peripheral pulse, you can measure the rate and rhythm of the heartbeat, as well as obtain local data on the condition of the artery.

Using the pads of your first three fingers, palpate the radial pulse at the flexor aspect of the wrist laterally along the radius bone (Fig. 10.4). Press until you feel the strongest pulsation. If the rhythm is regular, count the number of beats in 30 seconds and multiply by 2. Although counting in 15 seconds is frequently practised, any one-beat error in counting results in a recorded error of four beats per minute. The 30-second interval is the most accurate and efficient when heart rates are normal or rapid and when rhythms are regular. However, if the rhythm is irregular, as in atrial fibrillation, always count for a full minute (60 seconds). It is more important to establish the rhythm so that you can accurately determine rate. Assess the pulse, including (a) rate, (b) rhythm, (c) force, and (d) equality (when comparing pulses bilaterally). All symmetrical pulses should be assessed simultaneously except for the carotid pulse.

Objective Data

Normal Range of Findings	Abnormal Findings

10.4

Rate

In the adult at physical and mental rest, recent clinical evidence shows the normal resting heart range of 95% of healthy persons at 50 to 95 beats/min. Traditional resting heart rate limits established in the 1950s are 60 to 100 beats/min. This range is still used; however, no research evidence supports it. The rate also varies with gender; after puberty, girls have a slightly faster rate.

In the adult a resting heart rate less than 50 beats/min is **bradycardia**. Heart rates in the 50s/min occur normally in the well-trained athlete whose heart muscle develops along with the skeletal muscles. The stronger, more efficient heart muscle pushes out a larger stroke volume with each beat, thus requiring fewer beats per minute to maintain a stable cardiac output. (Review the equation $CO = SV \times R$, or Cardiac output = Stroke volume × Rate, in Chapter 20.) A more rapid heart rate, variably defined as over 95 beats/min or over 100 beats/min, is **tachycardia**. Rapid rates occur normally with anxiety or with increased exercise to match the body's demand for increased metabolism.[1]

For descriptions of abnormal rates and rhythms, see Table 21.1, p. 559.

Tachycardia occurs with fever, with sepsis, and after myocardial infarction.

Rhythm

The rhythm of the pulse normally has an even tempo. However, one irregularity that is common in children and young adults is **sinus arrhythmia**, in which the heart rate varies with the respiratory cycle, speeding up at the peak of inspiration and slowing to normal with expiration. Inspiration momentarily causes a decreased stroke volume from the left side of the heart; to compensate, the heart rate increases. (See Chapter 20 for a full discussion on sinus arrhythmia.) If any other irregularities are detected, auscultate heart sounds for a more complete assessment (see Chapter 20, p. 519).

Force

The force of the pulse shows the strength of the heart's stroke volume. A "weak, thready" pulse reflects decreased stroke volume (e.g., as occurs with hemorrhagic shock). A "full, bounding" pulse denotes increased stroke volume, as occurs with anxiety, exercise, and some abnormal conditions. The pulse force is recorded on a three-point scale:

3+: Full, bounding
2+: Normal
1+: Weak, thready
0: Absent

Some agencies use a four-point scale; make sure your system is consistent with that used by the rest of your staff. Either scale is somewhat subjective. Experience will improve your clinical judgement. Most healthy adults have a force of 2+.

Objective Data

Normal Range of Findings	Abnormal Findings

Respirations

Normally, a patient's breathing is relaxed, regular, automatic, and silent. Because most people are unaware of their breathing, do not mention that you will be counting the respirations; the patient's awareness that you are doing so may alter the normal pattern. Instead, maintain your position of counting the radial pulse, and unobtrusively count the respirations. Count for 30 seconds or for a full minute if you suspect an abnormality. Avoid the 15-second interval. The result can vary by a factor of ±4, which is significant with such a small number.

When you are documenting respiratory rate, ensure that you count one full cycle (inspiration and expiration) as one respiration. The first rise and fall of the chest is counted as one breath. Note that the respiratory rates presented in Table 10.1 normally are more rapid in infants and children. Also, the ratio of pulse rate to respiratory rate is fairly constant, at approximately 4:1. Normally, both pulse and respiratory rates rise as a response to exercise or anxiety. Respiratory status is described in more detail in Chapter 19.

TABLE 10.1 Normal Respiratory Rates	
AGE	**BREATHS PER MINUTE**
Neonate	30–40
1 year	20–40
2 years	25–32
4 years	23–30
8–10 years	20–26
12–14 years	18–22
16 years	12–20
Adult	10–20

Blood Pressure

Blood pressure (BP) is the force of the blood pushing against the side of the vessel wall. The strength of the push changes with the event in the cardiac cycle. The **systolic pressure** is the maximum pressure felt on the artery during left ventricular contraction, or systole. The **diastolic pressure** is the elastic recoil, or resting, pressure that the blood exerts constantly between each contraction. The **pulse pressure** is the difference between the systolic and diastolic pressures and reflects the stroke volume (Fig. 10.5). The **mean arterial pressure (MAP)** is the pressure forcing blood into the tissues, averaged over the cardiac cycle. This is not an arithmetic average of systolic and diastolic pressures because diastole lasts longer. Rather, it is a value closer to diastolic pressure plus one-third of the pulse pressure.

Objective Data

Normal Range of Findings	**Abnormal Findings**

10.5   A graph of blood pressure from systole through diastole.

The average BP in the young adult is influenced by a variety of factors:
- **Age**: Normally, BP rises gradually through childhood and into the adult years.
- **Sex**: Before puberty, no difference in BP exists between boys and girls. After puberty, girls usually have a lower BP than do male counterparts. After menopause, BP is higher in women than in male counterparts.
- **Ethnocultural considerations**: In Canada, adults of African descent usually have a higher BP than do those of European descent of the same age. The incidence of hypertension is twice as high among those of African descent; reasons for the difference are not fully understood, but it appears to be a result of genetic and environmental factors.
- **Diurnal rhythm**: A daily cycle of a peak and a trough occurs: The BP is highest in late afternoon or early evening and then declines to an early morning low.
- **Weight**: BP is higher in obese patients than in patients of normal weight of the same age (including adolescents).
- **Exercise**: Increasing activity yields a proportionate increase in BP. Within 5 minutes of terminating the exercise, the BP normally returns to baseline.
- **Emotions**: The BP momentarily rises with fear, anger, and pain as a result of stimulation of the sympathetic nervous system.
- **Stress**: The BP is elevated in patients feeling continual tension because of lifestyle, occupational stress, or life problems.

The level of BP is determined by five factors:
1. **Cardiac output.** If the heart pumps more blood into the blood vessels, the pressure on the vessel walls increases (Fig. 10.6).
2. **Peripheral vascular resistance.** Peripheral vascular resistance is the opposition to blood flow through the arteries. When the blood vessels become smaller (i.e., when constricted), greater pressure is needed to push the blood through.
3. **Volume of circulating blood.** The term *volume of circulating blood* refers to how tightly the blood is packed into the arteries. Increasing the volume of blood in the arteries increases the pressure.
4. **Viscosity.** The "thickness" of blood is determined by its formed elements, the blood cells. When the blood is thicker, the pressure increases.
5. **Elasticity of vessel walls.** When the vessel walls are stiff and rigid, more pressure is needed to push the blood through.

Normal Range of Findings	Abnormal Findings

FACTORS CONTROLLING BLOOD PRESSURE

FACTOR	CONDITION		RESULT
Cardiac output	↑ with heavy exercise to meet body demand for increased metabolism		↑BP
	↓ with pump failure (weak pumping action after myocardial infarction, or in shock)		↓BP
Vascular resistance	↑ resistance (vasoconstriction)		↑BP
	↓ resistance (vasodilation)		↓BP
Volume	↓ volume (hemorrhage)		↓BP
	↑ volume (increased sodium and water retention, intravenous fluid overload)		↑BP
Viscosity	↑ viscosity (increased hematocrit in polycythemia)		↑BP
Elasticity of arterial walls	↑ rigidity, hardening as in arteriosclerosis (heart pumping against greater resistance)		↑BP

10.6   (Illustration copyright Pat Thomas, © 2006.)

BP is measured with a stethoscope and an aneroid *sphygmomanometer*. The aneroid gauge is subject to drift; it must be recalibrated at least once each year, and it must rest at zero.

The cuff consists of an inflatable rubber bladder inside a cloth cover. The width of the rubber bladder should equal 40% of the circumference of the patient's arm. The length of the bladder should equal 80% of this circumference. When you use an automated device, ensure that you select the cuff size recommended by the manufacturer.

Cuffs are available in six sizes, ranging from one that fits newborns to one that fits an extra-large adult, as well as tapered cuffs for the cone-shaped obese arm and thigh cuffs. Match the appropriate size cuff to the patient's arm size and shape and not to the patient's age (Fig. 10.7).

The cuff size is important; using a cuff that is too narrow yields a falsely high BP because it takes extra pressure to compress the artery.

Thigh cuff or large arm cuff

Standard adult arm cuff

10.7

Objective Data

Normal Range of Findings	Abnormal Findings

The Procedure: Arm Pressure

A comfortable, relaxed patient yields a valid BP. Many patients are anxious at the beginning of an examination; allow at least a 5-minute rest before measuring the BP. Take three BP measurements separated by 2 minutes; discard the first reading; and average the other two. This procedure is the new recommended Canadian standard.[9]

For each patient, verify BP in both arms once, either on admission or for the first complete physical examination. It is not necessary to continue to check both arms for screening or monitoring. On occasion, a 5- to 10-mm Hg difference may occur in BP in the two arms (if values are different, record the higher value).

> A difference in the two arms of more than 10 to 15 mm Hg may indicate arterial obstruction on the side with the lower reading.

The patient may be sitting or lying, with the bare arm supported at heart level. (If a mercury manometer is used, place it so that it is vertical and at your eye level.) When the patient is sitting, the feet should be flat on the floor because the BP measurement is falsely high when legs are crossed.[9]

Palpate the brachial artery, which is located just above the antecubital fossa, medial to the biceps tendon. Centre the deflated cuff about 2.5 cm (1 in) above the brachial artery, and wrap it evenly around the arm.

Now palpate the brachial or the radial artery (Fig. 10.8). Inflate the cuff until the artery pulsation is obliterated and then 20 to 30 mm Hg beyond. This will prevent missing an **auscultatory gap**, which is a period when Korotkoff's sounds disappear during auscultation (Table 10.2).

> An auscultatory gap occurs in about 5% of people, most often in those with hypertension caused by a noncompliant arterial system.

Deflate the cuff quickly and completely; then wait 15 to 30 seconds before reinflating so the blood trapped in the veins can dissipate. Place the bell of the stethoscope over the site of the brachial artery, making a light but airtight seal (Fig. 10.9). The diaphragm endpiece is usually adequate, but the bell is designed to pick up low-pitched sounds such as the sounds of a BP reading.

Which stethoscope end chosen does not influence measurement error, but for the novice practitioner, using the bell can make the difference between hearing an accurate BP or not hearing it. Thus it is good practice to use the bell while you are acquiring skill for hearing the discrete sounds.

10.8

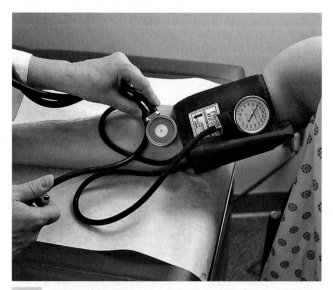

10.9

Normal Range of Findings	Abnormal Findings

TABLE 10.2   Korotkoff's Sounds

PHASE	QUALITY	DESCRIPTION	RATIONALE
Cuff correctly inflated	No sound	—	Cuff inflation compresses brachial artery. Cuff pressure exceeds heart's systolic pressure, occluding brachial artery blood flow.
I	Tapping	Soft, clear tapping, increasing in intensity	The systolic pressure: As the cuff pressure lowers to reach intraluminal systolic pressure, the artery opens, and blood first spurts into the brachial artery. Blood is at very high velocity because of small opening of artery and large pressure difference across opening. This creates turbulent flow, which is audible.
Auscultatory gap	No sound	Silence for 30–40 mm Hg during deflation: an abnormal finding	Sounds temporarily disappear during end of phase I, then reappear in phase II. This is common with hypertension. If it is undetected, systolic reading is falsely low or diastolic reading is falsely high.
II	Swooshing	Softer murmur that follows tapping	Turbulent blood flow through still partially occluded artery.
III	Knocking	Crisp, high-pitched sounds	Duration of blood flow through artery is longer. Artery closes just briefly during late diastole.
IV	Abrupt muffling	Muting of sound to a low-pitched, cushioned murmur; blowing	Artery no longer closes in any part of cardiac cycle. Change is in quality, not intensity.
V	Silence	—	Velocity of blood flow decreases. Streamlined blood flow is silent. The last audible sound (marking the disappearance of sounds) is diastolic pressure. The fifth Korotkoff sound is now used to define diastolic pressure in all age groups.[a]

Brachial artery occluded by cuff, no blood flow

Artery intermittently compressed, blood spurts into artery

Cuff deflated, artery flows free

Auscultatory sound — Silence — I — Clear tapping — IV — Abrupt muffling — V — Silence

[a]Chobanian, A. V., Bakris, G. L., Black, H. R., et al. (2003). The seventh report of the Joint National Committee on Prevention, Detection, Evaluation and Treatment of High Blood Pressure: The JNC 7 report. *Journal of the American Medical Association, 289*, 2560–2572.

Rapidly inflate the cuff to the maximal inflation level that you determined. Then deflate the cuff slowly and evenly, about 2 mm Hg per heartbeat. Note the points at which you hear the first appearance of sound, the muffling of sound, and the final disappearance of sound. These are phases I, IV, and V of **Korotkoff's sounds**, which are the components of a BP reading first described by a Russian surgeon in 1905 (see Table 10.2).

Normal Range of Findings

For all age groups, the fifth Korotkoff phase is now used to define diastolic pressure. However, when the variance is greater than 10 to 12 mm Hg between phases IV and V, record *both* phases along with the systolic reading (e.g., 142/98/80). Seated BPs are used to determine and monitor treatment decisions. Standing BPs are used to diagnose postural hypotension. The Canadian Hypertension Education Program (CHEP) recommends that, on initial assessment of BP, the pressure in both arms is measured.[9] If a significant variance exists (>20 mm Hg), then measurement of bilateral pressures should be continued. Table 10.3 is a list of common errors in BP measurement.

Abnormal Findings

Hypotension is abnormally low BP; **hypertension** is abnormally high BP (see parameters in Table 10.5, p. 181).

TABLE 10.3 Common Errors in Blood Pressure Measurement

COMMON ERROR	RESULT	RATIONALE
Taking blood pressure reading when patient is anxious or angry or has just been active	Falsely high	Sympathetic nervous system stimulation
Faulty arm position		
Above level of heart	Falsely low	Eliminates effect of hydrostatic pressure
Below level of heart	Falsely high	Additional force of gravity added to brachial artery pressure
Patient supports own arm	Falsely high diastolic	Sustained isometric muscular contraction
Faulty leg position (e.g., patient's legs are crossed)	Falsely high systolic and diastolic	Translocation of blood volume from dependent legs to thoracic area
Examiner's eyes are not level with meniscus of mercury column		
Looking up at meniscus	Falsely high	Parallax
Looking down on meniscus	Falsely low	
Inaccurate cuff size (the most common error)		
Cuff too narrow for extremity	Falsely high	Excessive pressure needed to occlude brachial artery
Cuff wrap is too loose or uneven, or bladder balloons out of wrap	Falsely low	Excessive pressure needed to occlude brachial artery
Failure to palpate radial artery while cuff is inflated	Falsely low systolic	Missing initial systolic tapping or tuning in during *auscultatory gap* (tapping sounds disappear for 10–40 mm Hg and then return; common with hypertension)
Poor inflation of the cuff		
Overinflation of the cuff	Pain	
Pushing stethoscope too hard on brachial artery	Falsely low diastolic	Distortion of artery by excessive pressure so that the sounds continue
Deflating cuff		
Too quickly	Falsely low systolic or falsely high diastolic	Insufficient time to hear tapping
Too slowly	Falsely high diastolic	Venous congestion in forearm makes sounds less audible
Halting during descent and reinflating cuff to recheck systolic	Falsely high diastolic	Venous congestion in forearm
Failure to wait 1–2 min before repeating entire reading	Falsely high diastolic	Venous congestion in forearm
Any observer error		
Examiner's haste	Any error	
Faulty technique		
Examiner's digit preference: "hears" more results that end in zero than would occur by chance alone (e.g., 130/80)		
Diminished hearing acuity		
Defective or inaccurately calibrated equipment		

Normal Range of Findings	Abnormal Findings

Normal Range of Findings

Orthostatic (or Postural) Vital Signs

Take serial measurements of pulse and BP when you suspect volume depletion; when the patient is known to have hypertension or is taking antihypertensive medications; or when the patient reports fainting or syncope. Have the patient rest supine for 2 or 3 minutes, take baseline readings of pulse and BP, and then repeat the measurements with the patient sitting and then standing. For a patient who is too weak or dizzy to stand, assess when the patient is first supine and then sitting with legs dangling. When the position is changed from supine to standing, a slight decrease (less than 10 mm Hg) in systolic pressure is normal.

Record the BP by using even numbers. Also record the patient's position, the arm used, and the cuff size, if different from the standard adult cuff. Record the pulse rate and rhythm, noting whether the pulse is regular.

Measurement of Oxygen Saturation

The **pulse oximeter** is a noninvasive method to assess arterial oxygen saturation (SpO_2). A sensor attached to the patient's finger or earlobe has a diode that emits light and a detector that measures the relative amount of light absorbed by oxyhemoglobin and unoxygenated (reduced) hemoglobin. The pulse oximeter compares the ratio of light emitted to light absorbed and converts this ratio into the percentage of SpO_2. Because it measures only light absorption of pulsatile flow, the reading represents arterial SpO_2. A healthy patient with no lung disease and no anemia normally has an SpO_2 of 97 to 99%, but a value of >95% is acceptable in an individual with a normal hemoglobin.[10] Select the appropriate pulse oximeter probe. The finger probe is spring-loaded and feels like a clothespin attached to the finger but does not hurt (Fig. 10.10). An infant has a probe taped to the large toe. If you are using a finger, make sure the hand is warm. At lower oxygen saturation, the earlobe probe is more accurate.[11]

10.10

Electronic Vital Signs Monitor

An automated vital signs monitor is in frequent use in hospital or clinic settings, especially when frequent monitoring is required (Fig. 10.11). The artery pulsations create vibrations that are detected by the electronic sensors. The BP mode is noninvasive and fast and has automatic measurement intervals and a bright numerical display. As with manual BP machines, accuracy depends on cuff selection and placement and on calibration of the equipment.

The electronic BP monitor cannot sense vibrations of low BP or rapidly irregular pulses, as in atrial fibrillation. Do not use it if the patient's systolic BP is less than 90 mm Hg or if the patient has conditions such as shivering, tremors, or seizures. If the numerical display does not correspond to the clinical presentation of the patient, always validate your findings with a manual sphygmomanometer and your stethoscope. Electronic BP measurement is considered the practice device of choice when available, as multiple measures can be taken over a short period of time with greater accuracy.[9] Many of these devices also have probes to measure temperature and heart rate.

Abnormal Findings

Orthostatic hypotension—a drop in systolic pressure of more than 20 mm Hg, or an orthostatic pulse increase of 20 beats per minute (bpm) or more—occurs with a quick change to a standing position. These changes result from abrupt peripheral vasodilatation without a compensatory increase in cardiac output. Orthostatic changes also occur with prolonged bed rest, older age, hypovolemia, and ingestion of some medications.

Objective Data

Normal Range of Findings	Abnormal Findings

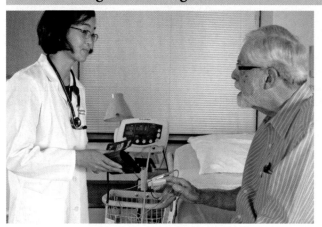

10.11

❖ DEVELOPMENTAL CONSIDERATIONS

Infants and Children

General Survey

Physical Appearance, Body Structure, Mobility. Note the same basic elements as with the adult, with consideration for age and development.

Behaviour. Note the response to stimuli and level of alertness appropriate for age.

Parental Bonding. Note the child's interactions with parents and whether parent and child show a mutual response and are warm and affectionate, appropriate to the child's condition. The parent provides appropriate physical care of child and promotes new learning (see the Promoting Health: Lifestyle Behaviours box, p. 177).

Some signs of child abuse: the child avoids eye contact; the child exhibits no separation anxiety when you would expect it for age; the parent is disgusted by child's odour, sounds, drooling, or stools.

Deprivation of physical or emotional care (see Chapter 8).

Measurement

Weight. Weigh an infant on a platform-type balance scale (Fig. 10.12). To check calibration, set the weight at zero and observe the beam balance. Guard the baby so that the baby does not fall. Weigh to the nearest 10 g (½ oz) for infants and 100 g (¼ lb) for toddlers.

10.12

Objective Data

Normal Range of Findings	Abnormal Findings

By age 2 or 3 years, use the upright scale. Leave underpants on the child. Some young children are fearful of the rickety standing platform and may prefer sitting on the infant scale. Use the upright scale with preschool- and school-age children, maintaining modesty with light clothing (Fig. 10.13).

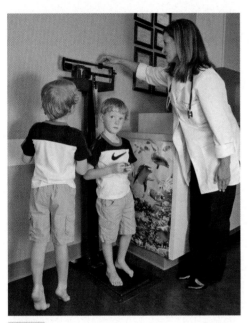

10.13

Length. For a child younger than 2 years, measure the body length when the child is supine by using a horizontal measuring board (Fig. 10.14). Hold the head in the midline. Because infants normally flex their legs, extend the legs momentarily by holding the knees together and pushing them down until the legs are flat on the table. Avoid using a tape measure along the infant's length because this method yields inaccurate results. It is important to measure an infant to the nearest centimetre.

10.14

Objective Data

Normal Range of Findings

By age 2 or 3 years, measure the height by standing the child against the pole on the platform scale or back against a flat ruler taped to the wall (Fig. 10.15). (Sometimes a child will stand more erect against the solid wall than against the narrow measuring pole on the scale.) Encourage the child to stand straight and tall and to look straight ahead without tilting the head. The shoulders, buttocks, and heels should touch the wall. Hold a book or flat board on the child's head at a right angle to the wall. Mark just under the book, noting the measure to the nearest 1 mm (⅛ in).

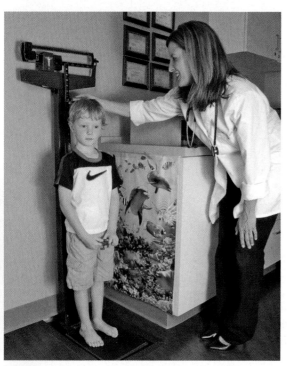

10.15

Physical growth is usually the best index of a child's general health. The child's height and weight are recorded at every health care visit to determine normal growth patterns. The results are plotted on growth charts based on data from the National Center for Health Statistics (NCHS). Normal limits range from the fifth to the ninety-fifth percentile on standardized charts. In 2011, the WHO released a revised set of child growth standards that better reflect the diversity of the global population. These assessment tools—which are based on height, weight, and BMI—minimize variations noted with the NCHS tools, which are based on norms established for American children of European descent. The WHO standards are being accepted globally as a more accurate measure of growth and development.

Healthy childhood growth is continuous but uneven, with rapid growth spurts occurring during infancy and adolescence. Results are more reliable when numerous growth measurements over a long time are compared. These charts are also used to compare an individual child's measurements against those of the general population.

Use your judgement and consider the genetic background of the child who is small for age. Explore the growth patterns of the parents and siblings. Studies have indicated that in Canada, Cree women have a higher prevalence of macrosomia (birth weight >90th percentile) than non-Indigenous women (33% versus 11%). Even after researchers controlled for gestational diabetes, which is known to contribute to higher birth weights, the rates remained significantly higher, indicating potential genetic differences in fetal growth.[12]

Abnormal Findings

Using NCHS Charts

Further explore any growth measurement that

- Falls below the fifth or above the ninety-fifth percentile with no genetic explanation
- Shows a wide percentile difference between height and weight; for example, a tenth-percentile height with a ninety-fifth percentile weight
- Shows that growth has suddenly stopped when it had been steady
- Fails to show normal growth spurts during infancy and adolescence

Using WHO Charts

- A child's score that is far from the median of 0, such as −3 or 3, indicates growth challenges.
- Z-score lines indicate distance from the growth average.

Normal Range of Findings	Abnormal Findings

Head Circumference. Measure the infant's head circumference at birth and at each well-child visit up to age 2 years and then yearly up to 6 years (Fig. 10.16). Circle the tape around the head at the prominent frontal and occipital bones; the widest span is correct. Plot the measurement on standardized growth charts. Compare the infant's head size with that expected for age. A series of measurements is more valuable than a single figure to show the *rate* of head growth.

10.16

The newborn's head measures about 32 to 38 cm (averaging around 34 cm) and is about 2 cm larger than the chest circumference. The chest grows at a faster rate than does the cranium; at some time between 6 months and 2 years, both measurements are about the same, and after 2 years, the chest circumference is greater than the head circumference.

Measurement of the chest circumference is valuable in a comparison with the head circumference, but not necessarily by itself. Encircle the tape around the chest at the nipple line. It should be snug, but not so tight that it leaves a mark (Fig. 10.17).

Head circumference is enlarged with increased intracranial pressure (see Chapter 14).

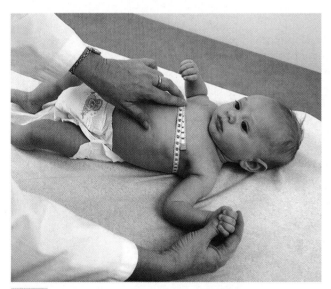

10.17

Objective Data

Normal Range of Findings	Abnormal Findings

Vital Signs

Measure vital signs with the same purpose and frequency as you would in an adult. With an *infant*, reverse the order of vital sign measurement to respiration first and then pulse and temperature. Taking temperature rectally may cause the infant to cry, which will increase the respiratory and pulse rate, thus masking the normal resting values. A *preschooler's* normal fear of body mutilation is increased with any invasive procedure. If recommended, avoid the rectal route and take temperature tympanically. When this is not feasible, use the reverse order and measure the rectal temperature last. Your approach to measuring vital signs with the *adolescent* is much the same as with the adult.

Temperature

Tympanic. TMT and TAT are useful with toddlers who squirm at the restraint needed for the rectal route, and it is useful with preschoolers who are not yet able to cooperate for an oral temperature measurement but fear the disrobing and invasion involved with rectal measurement. These measurement are so rapid that it is usually over before the child realizes it (Fig. 10.18).

10.18

Axillary. The axillary route is safer and more accessible than the rectal route; however, its accuracy and reliability have been questioned. When cold receptors are stimulated, brown fat tissue in the area releases heat through chemical energy, which artificially raises skin temperature. When the axillary route is used, place the tip well into the axilla, and hold the child's arm close to the body.

Oral. Use the oral route when the child is old enough to keep the mouth closed. This is usually at age 5 or 6 years, although some 4-year-old children can cooperate. Use an electronic thermometer when one is available because it is unbreakable and it registers quickly.

Rectal. The Canadian Paediatric Society's 2017 position statement on temperature measurement in the pediatric population is as follows:[14]

Age	Recommended Technique
Birth to 2 years	1. Rectal (definitive)
	2. Axillary (screening low risk children)
From 2 to 5 years	1. Rectal (definitive)
	2. Axillary, tympanic (or temporal artery if in hospital) (screening)
Older than 5 years	1. Oral (definitive)
	2. Axillary, tympanic (or temporal artery if in hospital) (screening)

Febrile seizures usually occur between 3 months and 5 years of age in 2–5% of all children and are associated with fever commonly precipitated by viral infections. They are precipitated by the rate of rise and the rate of decent of the temperature itself.[13]

Normal Range of Findings	Abnormal Findings

The Procedure. An infant may be supine or side-lying, with the examiner's hand flexing the infant's knees up onto the abdomen. (When a baby boy is supine, cover the boy's penis with a diaper.) An infant also may lie prone across the adult's lap. Separate the buttocks with one hand, and insert the lubricated electronic rectal probe no farther than 2.5 cm (1 in). Insertion any deeper increases the risk for rectal perforation because the colon curves posteriorly at 3 cm (1¼ in). (In a glass thermometer, temperature registers by 3 minutes.)

Normally, rectal temperatures measure higher in infants and young children than in adults, with an average of 37.8°C (100°F) at age 18 months. Also, the temperature normally may be elevated in the late afternoon, after vigorous playing, or after eating.

Up to ages 6 to 8 years, children have higher fevers with illness than adults do. Even with minor infections, temperatures may elevate to 40.5°C (105°F).

Pulse. Palpate or auscultate an apical rate with infants and toddlers. (See Chapter 20 for location of apex and technique.) In children older than 2 years, use the radial site. Count the pulse for a full minute to take into account normal irregularities, such as sinus arrhythmia. The heart rate normally fluctuates more in infants and children than in adults in response to exercise, emotion, and illness.

Respirations. Watch the infant's abdomen for movement because the infant's respirations are normally more diaphragmatic than thoracic (Fig. 10.19). Count a full minute because the pattern varies significantly from rapid breaths to short periods of apnea. Note the normal rate in Table 10.1 on page 161.

Tachypnea, or rapid respiratory rate, is >60/min for newborns to 2 months, and >50/min for 2 to 12 months. This occurs with fever and may indicate infection. Tachypnea and laboured respirations may indicate pneumonia.

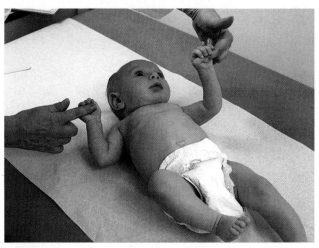

10.19

Blood Pressure. In children aged 3 years and older and in younger children at risk, take a routine BP measurement at least annually. For accurate measurement in children, make some adjustment in the choice of equipment and technique. The most common error is use of the incorrect size cuff. The cuff width must cover two-thirds of the upper arm, and the cuff bladder must encircle it completely.

Objective Data

Normal Range of Findings

Use a pediatric-sized endpiece on the stethoscope to locate the sounds. If possible, allow a crying infant to become quiet for 5 to 10 minutes before measuring the BP; crying may elevate the systolic pressure by 30 to 50 mm Hg. Use the disappearance of sound (phase V Korotkoff's sound) for the diastolic reading in children, as well as in adults.

Note the new guidelines for normal BP values by age groups that are *based on the child's height, age, and sex*. In children, height is more strongly correlated with BP than is age. Children younger than 3 years of age have such small arm vessels that it is difficult to hear Korotkoff's sounds with a stethoscope. Instead, use an electronic BP device that entails *oscillometry* (such as Dinamap) and gives a digital readout for systolic, diastolic, MAP, and pulse. Or, use a *Doppler* ultrasound device to amplify the sounds. This instrument is easy to use and can be used by one examiner. (Note the technique for using the Doppler device in Fig. 10.20 on p. 176.)

Older Adults

General Survey

Physical Appearance. By the eighth and ninth decades, body contour is sharper, with more angular facial features, and body proportions are redistributed.

Posture. A general flexion occurs by the eighth or ninth decade.

Gait. Older adults often use a wider base to compensate for diminished balance; arms may be held out to help balance, and steps may be shorter or uneven.

Measurement

Weight. Older adults appear sharper in contour with more prominent bony landmarks than are found in younger adults. Body weight decreases during the 80s and 90s. This factor is more evident in men, perhaps because of greater muscle shrinkage. The distribution of fat also changes during the 80s and 90s. Even with good nutrition, subcutaneous fat is lost from the face and periphery (especially the forearms), whereas additional fat is deposited on the abdomen and hips.

Height. By the 80s and 90s, many people are shorter than they were in their 70s. This results from shortening in the spinal column, which is caused by thinning of the vertebral discs and shortening of the individual vertebrae, as well as slight flexion in the knees and hips and the postural changes of kyphosis. Because long bones do not shorten with age, the overall body proportion looks different: a shorter trunk with relatively long extremities.

Vital Signs

Temperature. Changes in the body's temperature regulatory mechanism leave older adults less likely to have fever but at greater risk for hypothermia. Thus the temperature is a less reliable index of the older patient's true health state. Sweat gland activity is also diminished.

Pulse. The normal range of heart rate is 60 to 100 bpm, but the rhythm may be slightly irregular. The radial artery may feel stiff, rigid, and tortuous in an older patient, although this condition does not necessarily imply vascular disease in the heart or brain. The increasingly rigid arterial wall needs a faster upstroke of blood, and so the pulse is actually easier to palpate.

Respirations. Aging causes a decrease in vital capacity and a decrease in inspiratory reserve volume. You may note a shallower inspiratory phase and an increased respiratory rate.

Abnormal Findings

Further explore any BP reading that is greater than the ninety-fifth percentile and refer for diagnostic evaluation. For the child whose BP falls between the ninetieth and ninety-fifth percentiles and whose high BP cannot be explained by height or weight, monitor the BP every 6 months. Similar to adults, hypertension in children and adolescents is associated with obesity, dyslipidemia, and diabetes.

Normal Range of Findings	Abnormal Findings

Blood Pressure. The aorta and major arteries tend to harden with age. As the heart pumps against a stiffer aorta, the systolic pressure increases, causing pulse pressure to increase. With many older adults, both the systolic and diastolic pressures increase, which makes it difficult to distinguish normal aging values from abnormal hypertension.

SPECIAL CONSIDERATIONS FOR ADVANCED PRACTICE

Normal Range of Findings	Abnormal Findings

Carotid Compression

Compression of both carotid arteries at the same time results in compromise of blood flow to the brain and is ***never done*** by any nonauthorized practitioner. It can also stimulate the cranial nerve X (vagus nerve), which causes the patient's heart rate to drop rapidly and the eventual loss of consciousness. The "carotid rub or massage" is a manoeuvre executed by cardiologists and clinicians with expertise in the area. In this manoeuvre, the practitioner rubs *only one* carotid artery at a time to slow down rapid irregular heart rates in patients with these identified cardiac considerations. Please keep in mind that this manoeuvre is *not* in the scope of practice of nurses without advanced practice credentials.

The Doppler Technique

In many situations, pulse and BP measurement are enhanced by use of an electronic device, the *Doppler ultrasonic flowmeter.* The Doppler technique works by a principle discovered in the nineteenth century by an Austrian physicist, Johannes Doppler. Sound varies in pitch in relation to the distance between the sound source and the listener; the pitch is higher when the distance is short, and the pitch lowers as the distance increases. Think of a railroad train speeding toward you: the pitch of its train whistle sounds higher the closer it gets, and the pitch of the whistle lowers as the train moves away.

In this case, the sound source is the blood pumping through the artery in a rhythmic manner. A handheld transducer picks up changes in sound frequency and amplifies them as the blood flows and ebbs. The listener hears a whooshing pulsatile beat.

The Doppler technique is used to locate the peripheral pulse sites (see Chapter 21 for further discussion of this technique). For BP measurement, the Doppler technique augments Korotkoff's sounds (Fig. 10.20). Through this technique, you can evaluate sounds that are hard to hear with a stethoscope, such as those in critically ill individuals with a low BP, in infants with small arms, and in obese patients in whom the sounds are muffled by layers of fat. Also, proper cuff placement is difficult on an obese patient's cone-shaped upper arm. In this situation, you can place the cuff on the more even forearm and hold the Doppler probe over the radial artery. For either location, use the following procedure:

- Apply coupling gel to the transducer probe.
- Turn the Doppler flowmeter on.
- Touch the probe to the skin, holding the probe perpendicular to the artery.
- A pulsatile whooshing sound indicates location of the artery. You may need to rotate the probe, but maintain contact with the skin. Do not push the probe too hard or you will obliterate the pulse.

Special Considerations for Advanced Practice

Normal Range of Findings	Abnormal Findings

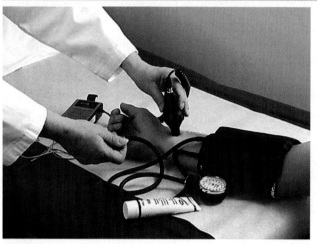

10.20

- Inflate the cuff until the sounds disappear; then inflate by another 20 to 30 mm Hg beyond that point.
- Slowly deflate the cuff, noting the point at which the first whooshing sounds appear. This is the systolic pressure.
- It is difficult to hear the muffling of sounds or a reliable disappearance of sounds that indicates the diastolic pressure (phases IV and V of Korotkoff's sounds). However, the systolic pressure alone is valuable data about the level of tissue perfusion and about blood flow through patent vessels.

Thigh Pressure

When BP measured at the arm is excessively high, particularly in adolescents and young adults, compare it with the thigh pressure to check for **coarctation** of the aorta (a congenital form of narrowing). Normally, the *thigh pressure is higher* than the pressure in the arm. If possible, turn the patient onto the prone position (on the abdomen). (If the patient must remain in the supine position, bend the knee slightly.) Wrap a large cuff, 18 to 20 cm, around the lower third of the thigh, centred over the popliteal artery on the back of the knee. Auscultate the popliteal artery for the reading (Fig. 10.21). Normally, the systolic value is 10 to 40 mm Hg higher in the thigh than in the arm, and the diastolic pressures are the same.

With **coarctation of the aorta**, arm pressures are high. Thigh pressure is *lower* because the blood supply to the thigh is below the constriction.

10.21

PROMOTING HEALTH: LIFESTYLE BEHAVIOURS

Health and Self-Care

As you measure height and weight and record vital signs, it is a good time to begin a teaching plan to help the patient keep these physical signs within normal limits. The Canadian Hypertension Education Program (CHEP) considers the following **health behaviours** to be the foundation of hypertension control. Even if your patient is normotensive and the body weight is within normal limits, the following recommendations help keep blood pressure (BP) under control:

- Engage in physical exercise—walking, jogging, cycling, or swimming 4–7 days per week in addition to the routine activities of daily living (ADLs).
- Maintain a healthy body weight—use height, weight, and waist circumference to determine requirements and lose weight as recommended.
- Limit alcohol intake to no more than two drinks per day: a regular-sized bottle or can of beer, 45 mL (1.5 oz) of hard liquor, or 300 mL (10.5 oz) of wine.
- Cut sodium intake from the average 3 100 mg/day to less than 1 500 mg/day. The recommended adequate intake for sodium is 1 200 to 1 500 mg per day for healthy adults and decreases with age.
- Maintain adequate intake of dietary potassium (approximately 90 mmol/L/day).
- Manage stress—incorporate a healthy balance between work and play.

- Consume a diet that emphasizes fruits, vegetables, low-fat dairy products, dietary and soluble fibre, whole grains, and meat choices low in cholesterol.

One in five Canadians visits a health care provider to manage and/or diagnose hypertension. CHEP recommends that the diagnosis of hypertension be expedited to ensure early intervention. See Fig. 10.22 for Hypertension Canada's hypertension diagnostic algorithm.

Hypertension is diagnosed within one to five visits. The practice of accepting self-administered/home BP measurements has sped up the process of diagnosis significantly. Ambulatory blood pressure measurement (ABPM) is useful for determining readings outside the office setting for patients with suspected office-induced hypertension.

References

Canadian Hypertension Education Program. (2016). Guidelines for blood pressure measurement, diagnosis, assessment of risk, prevention, and treatment of hypertension. *Canadian Journal of Cardiology, 32*(5), 569–588.

Leung, A. A., Daskalopoulou, S. S., Dasgupta, K., et al. (2017). Hypertension Canada's 2017 guidelines for diagnosis, risk assessment, prevention, and treatment of hypertension in adults. *Canadian Journal of Cardiology, 33*(5), 557–576.

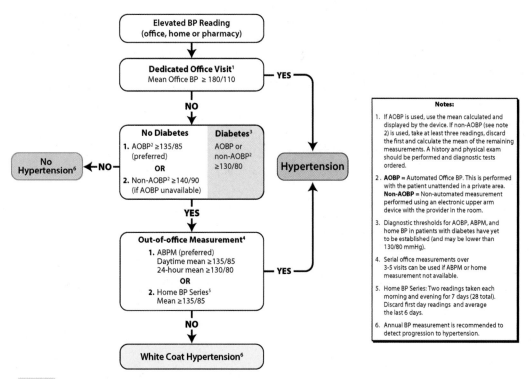

10.22 Hypertension diagnostic algorithm. *ABPM,* Ambulatory blood pressure measurement; *AOBP,* automated office blood pressure; *BP,* blood pressure.

Special Considerations for Advanced Practice

DOCUMENTATION AND CRITICAL THINKING

Sample Charting

Claire Jones is a 47-year-old female of African descent who is a high school principal; well nourished and well developed; appears stated age. Alert, oriented, and cooperative, with no signs of acute distress. Ht, 163 cm (5 ft 4 in); Wt, 57 kg (126 lb); temp, 37°C (98.6°F); pulse, 76 bpm; resp, 14/min; BP, 146/84 mm Hg, right arm, sitting.

Focused Assessment: Clinical Case Study

Rina Grace is a 76-year-old female retired secretary, in previous good health, who is brought to the emergency department by her 83-year-old husband. Both have been ill during the night with nausea, vomiting, abdominal pain, and diarrhea, which they attribute to eating "bad food" at a buffet-style restaurant the night before. Mrs. Grace's husband reports that his condition has improved, but Mrs. Grace's is worse, with severe vomiting, diarrhea, weakness, dizziness, and abdominal pain.

SUBJECTIVE

Mrs. Grace reports extreme fatigue. Weakness and dizziness occur when patient tries to sit or stand up: "Feels like I'm going to black out." Severe nausea and vomiting, thirsty but cannot keep anything down; even sips of water result in "dry heaves." Abdominal pain is moderate aching, intermittent. Diarrhea is watery brown stool, profuse during the night, somewhat diminished now.

OBJECTIVE

Helped to be seated, leg-dangling position; vital signs: BP, 74/52 mm Hg; pulse, 138 bpm, regular rhythm; respirations, 20/min. Skin pale and moist (diaphoretic).

Reports being lightheaded and dizzy in seated position. Returned to supine.

Vital signs: Temp, 37.2°C (99°F); BP (supine), 102/64 mm Hg; pulse (supine), 70 bpm, regular rhythm; resp, 18/min.

Respiratory: Breath sounds clear in all fields; no adventitious sounds.

Cardiovascular: Regular rate (70 bpm) and rhythm when supine, S_1 and S_2 are not accentuated or diminished, no extra sounds. All pulses present, 2+ and equal bilaterally. Carotid pulses 2+ with no carotid bruit.

Abdominal: Bowel sounds hyperactive, skin pale and moist, abdomen soft and mildly tender to palpation. No enlargement of liver or spleen.

Neurological: Level of consciousness: alert and oriented; pupils equal, round, reactive to light and accommodation. Sensory status normal. Mild weakness in arms and legs. Gait and standing leg strength not tested due to inability to stand. Deep tendon reflexes 2+ and equal bilaterally. Babinski reflex → toes curl inward.

ASSESSMENT

Orthostatic hypotension, orthostatic pulse increase, and syncopal symptoms, R/T [related to] hypovolemia
Diarrhea, possibly R/T ingestion of contaminated food
Risk for hyperthermia, R/T dehydration and aging
Deficient fluid volume

Documentation
and Critical Thinking

ABNORMAL FINDINGS

Tables 10.4 and 10.5 list abnormalities in physique and in BP, respectively.

TABLE 10.4	**Abnormalities in Body Height and Proportion**

◀ Hypopituitary Dwarfism

Deficiency in growth hormone in childhood results in developmental delay of growth below the third percentile, delayed puberty, hypothyroidism, and adrenal insufficiency. The 9-year-old girl at left appears much younger than her chronological age, with infantile facial features and chubbiness. The age-matched girl at right shows increased height, more mature facies, and loss of infantile fat.

Acromegaly (Hyperpituitarism)

Excessive secretion of growth hormone in adulthood, after normal completion of body growth, causes overgrowth of bone in the face, head, hands, and feet but no change in height. Internal organs also enlarge, which may result in cardiomegaly or hepatomegaly.

Gigantism

Excessive secretion of growth hormone by the anterior pituitary results in overgrowth of entire body. When this occurs during childhood before closure of bone epiphyses in puberty, it causes increased height (here 2.09 m, or 6 ft 9 in) and in weight and delay in sexual development.

Continued

TABLE 10.4 **Abnormalities in Body Height and Proportion—cont'd**

Achondroplastic Dwarfism

Congenital skeletal malformation caused by a genetic
disorder in converting cartilage to bone. Characterized
by relatively large head with frontal bossing and
midplace hypoplasia, short stature, and short limbs,
and often thoracic kyphosis, prominent lumbar
lordosis, and abdominal protrusion. The mean adult
height is approximately 131.5 cm (51.8 in) in men and
approximately 125 cm (49.2 in) in women.

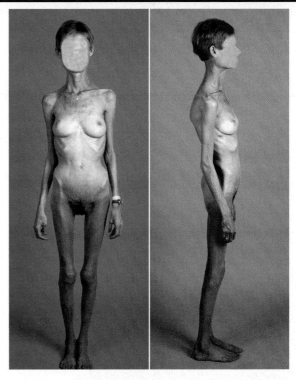

Anorexia Nervosa

A serious psychological disorder characterized by severe
and life-threatening weight loss and amenorrhea in an
otherwise healthy adolescent or young adult. Behaviour
is characterized by fanatic concern about weight, aversion
to food, distorted body image (perceives self as fat despite
skeletal appearance), starvation diets, frenetic exercise
patterns, and striving for perfection.

◄ **Endogenous Obesity: Cushing's Syndrome**

Excessive amounts of adrenocorticotropic hormone
(ACTH)—either administered or produced by the
pituitary gland—stimulates the adrenal cortex to
secrete excess cortisol. This causes Cushing's syndrome,
characterized by weight gain and edema with central
trunk and cervical obesity ("buffalo hump") and round
plethoric face ("moon facies"). Excessive catabolism causes
muscle wasting; weakness; thinness of arms and legs;
reduced height; and thinning and fragility of skin with
purple abdominal striae, bruising, and acne. The obesity
in this condition is markedly different from exogenous
obesity caused by excessive caloric intake, in which body
fat is evenly distributed and muscle strength is intact.

See Illustration Credits for source information.

TABLE 10.5   Abnormalities in Blood Pressure

Hypotension

In normotensive adults: <95/60
In hypertensive adults: < the patient's average reading, but >95/60
In children: < expected value for age

Occurs With	Reason
Acute myocardial infarction	Decreased cardiac output
Shock	Decreased cardiac output
Hemorrhage	Decrease in total blood volume
Vasodilation	Decrease in peripheral vascular resistance
Addison's disease (hypofunction of adrenal glands)	Decrease in aldosterone production

Associated Symptoms and Signs
In conditions of decreased cardiac output, low blood pressure is accompanied by faster pulse, dizziness, diaphoresis, confusion, and blurred vision. The skin feels cool and clammy because the superficial blood vessels constrict to shunt blood to the vital organs. An individual having an acute myocardial infarction may also complain of crushing substernal chest pain, high epigastric pain, and shoulder or jaw pain.

Hypertension

Essential or Primary Hypertension
This has no known cause but is responsible for about 95% of cases of hypertension in adults.
Cardiovascular Risk Stratification in Patients With Hypertension

Major Risk Factors	Target Organ Damage/Clinical Cardiovascular Disease
Smoking	Heart diseases
Dyslipidemia	Left ventricular atrophy
Diabetes mellitus	Angina or prior myocardial infarction
Age >60 years	Prior coronary revascularization
Gender (men and postmenopausal women)	Heart failure
Family history of cardiovascular disease: women aged <65 years	Stroke or transient ischemic attack
or men aged <55 years	Nephropathy
	Peripheral arterial disease
	Retinopathy

REFERENCES

1. McGee, S. (2018). *Evidence-informed physical diagnosis* (4th ed.). Philadelphia: Saunders.
2. World Health Organization. (2017). *BMI classification.* Retrieved from http://www.who.int/bmi/index.jsp?introPage=intro_3.html.
3. Canadian Paediatric Society. (2014). *Promoting optimal monitoring of child growth in Canada: Using the new who growth charts.* Retrieved from http://www.cps.ca/uploads/tools/growth-charts-statement-FULL.pdf.
4. Statistics Canada. (2015). *Overweight and obese youth (self-reported) 2014.* Retrieved from https://www.statcan.gc.ca/pub/82-625-x/2015001/article/14186-eng.htm.
5. Health Canada. (2016). *Canadian guidelines for body weight classifications in adults—quick reference tools for professionals.* Retrieved from http://www.hc-sc.gc.ca/fn-an/nutrition/weights-poids/guide-ld-adult/cg_quick_ref-ldc_rapide_ref-eng.php.
6. World Health Organization. (2000). *Obesity: Preventing and managing the global epidemic: Report of a WHO consultation on obesity.* Geneva, Switzerland: Author.
7. Fountain, C., Goins, L., Hartman, M., et al. (2008). Evaluating the accuracy of four temperature instruments on an adult inpatient oncology unit. *Clinical Journal of Oncology Nursing, 12*(6), 983–987.
8. Holzhauer, J. K., Reith, V., Sawin, K. J., et al. (2009). Evaluation of temporal artery thermometry in children 3–36 months old. *Journal for Specialists in Pediatric Nursing, 14*(4), 239–244.
9. Canadian Hypertension Education Program. (2016). Guidelines for blood pressure measurement, diagnosis, assessment of risk, prevention, and treatment of hypertension. *Canadian Journal of Cardiology, 32*(5), 569–588.
10. American Association of Critical Care Nurses. (2016). *AACN procedure manual for high acuity, progressive and critical care* (7th ed.). St. Louis: Saunders.
11. Grap, M. J. (2002). Pulse oximetry. *Critical Care Nurse, 22*(3), 69.
12. Rodrigues, S., Robinson, E. J., Kramer, M. S., et al. (2000). High rates of infant macrosomia: A comparison of a Canadian native and nonnative population. *Journal of Nutrition, 130,* 806–812.
13. Francis, J., Richmond, P., Lindsay, K., et al. (2016). An observational study of febrile seizures: The importance of viral infection and immunization. *BMC Pediatrics, 16,* 202. doi:10.1186/s12887-016-0740-5.
14. Canadian Paediatric Society. (2017). *CPS position statement: Temperature measurement in pediatrics.* Retrieved from http://www.cps.ca/documents/position/temperature-measurement.

Pain Assessment

Written by Carolyn Jarvis, PhD, APN, CNP
Adapted by Lynn Haslam, RN(EC), MN, NP-Adult

STRUCTURE AND FUNCTION

NEUROANATOMICAL PATHWAY

Pain is a highly complex and subjective experience that originates from the central nervous system (CNS), the peripheral nervous system, or both. Specialized nerve endings called **nociceptors** detect painful sensations from the periphery and transmit them to the CNS. Nociceptors are located within the skin; connective tissue; muscle; and thoracic, abdominal, and pelvic viscera. These nociceptors can be stimulated directly by trauma or injury or secondarily by chemical mediators that are released from the site of tissue damage.

Nociceptors carry the pain signal to the CNS by two primary sensory (or afferent) fibres: **Aδ fibres** and **C fibres** (Fig. 11.1). Aδ fibres are myelinated and larger in diameter, and they transmit the pain signal rapidly to the CNS. Very localized, short-term, and sharp sensations result from Aδ fibre stimulation. In contrast, C fibres are unmyelinated and smaller, and they transmit the signal more slowly, which results in a diffuse and aching sensation.

Peripheral sensory Aδ and C fibres enter the spinal cord by posterior nerve roots within the dorsal horn by the tract of Lissauer. The fibres synapse with **interneurons** located within a specified area of the cord called the **substantia gelatinosa**. A cross-section shows that the grey matter of the spinal cord is divided into a series of consecutively numbered laminae (layers of nerve cells; see Fig. 11.1). The substantia gelatinosa is lamina II, which receives sensory input from various areas of the body. The pain signals then cross over to the other side of the spinal cord and ascend to the brain by the **anterolateral spinothalamic tract**.

NOCICEPTION

Nociception is the term used to describe how noxious stimuli are typically perceived as pain. Nociception can be divided into four phases: (a) transduction, (b) transmission, (c) perception of pain, and (d) modulation (Fig. 11.2).

The first phase, **transduction**, occurs when a noxious stimulus in the form of traumatic or chemical injury, burn, incision, or tumour growth occurs in the periphery. These injured tissues then release a variety of chemicals (neurotransmitters), including substance P, histamine, prostaglandins, serotonin, and bradykinin. The neurotransmitters propagate a pain message, or action potential, along sensory afferent nerve fibres to the spinal cord. These nerve fibres terminate in the dorsal horn of the spinal cord. Because the initial afferent fibres stop in the dorsal horn, a second set of neurotransmitters carries the pain impulse across the synaptic cleft to the dorsal horn neurons. These neurotransmitters include substance P, glutamate, and adenosine triphosphate.

In the second phase, **transmission**, the pain impulse moves from the level of the spinal cord to the brain. Within the spinal cord, at the site of the synaptic cleft, are opioid receptors that can block this pain signalling with endogenous or exogenous opioids. However, if left uninterrupted, the pain impulse moves to the brain via various ascending fibres within the spinothalamic tract that terminate in the brain stem and thalamus. Once the pain impulse moves through the thalamus, the message is dispersed to higher cortical areas via mechanisms that are currently not clearly understood.

The third phase, **perception**, is the conscious awareness of a painful sensation. Cortical structures such as the limbic system account for the emotional response to pain, and somatosensory areas can characterize the sensation. Only when the noxious stimuli are interpreted in these higher cortical structures can this sensation be identified as pain.

Lastly, the pain message is inhibited through the phase of **modulation**. Descending pathways from the brain stem to the spinal cord produce a third set of neurotransmitters that slow down or impede the pain impulse, producing an analgesic effect. These neurotransmitters include serotonin; norepinephrine; neurotensin; γ-aminobutyric acid (GABA); and our own endogenous opioids, β-endorphins, enkephalins, and dynorphins.

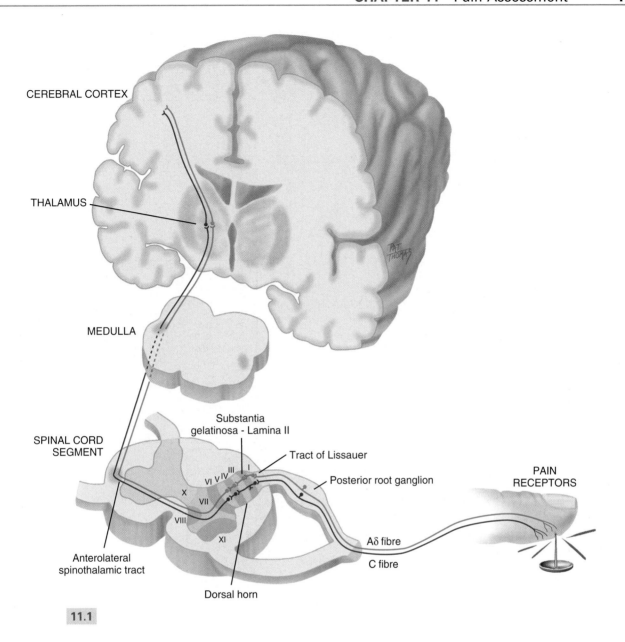

CEREBRAL CORTEX

THALAMUS

MEDULLA

SPINAL CORD SEGMENT

Substantia gelatinosa - Lamina II

Tract of Lissauer

Posterior root ganglion

PAIN RECEPTORS

Aδ fibre

C fibre

Anterolateral spinothalamic tract

Dorsal horn

11.1

SOURCES OF PAIN

Pain is based on its origin, and is classified as nociceptive, neuropathic, or both. **Nociceptive pain** is caused by tissue injury. It is well-localized and often described as aching or throbbing. Nociceptive pain can be further classified as somatic or visceral. **Somatic pain** can be superficial (superficial somatic or cutaneous pain), derived from skin surface and subcutaneous tissues, or deep (deep somatic pain), derived from joints, tendons, muscles, or bone. **Visceral pain** originates from the larger interior organs (e.g., kidney, intestine, gallbladder, and pancreas). The pain can stem from direct injury to the organ or from stretching of the organ as a result of tumour, ischemia, distension, or severe contraction. Visceral pain can be constant or intermittent, and it may be poorly localized or referred to another area of the body. Examples of conditions that cause visceral pain include ureteral colic, acute appendicitis, and pancreatitis.

Neuropathic pain is caused directly by a lesion or a disease affecting the somatosensory nervous system.[1] Neuropathic pain can result from damage to the nerve pathway at any point along the nerve, from the terminals of the peripheral nociceptors to the cortical neurons in the brain. Examples of neuropathic pain may include pain caused by direct nerve trauma (spinal cord injury), infectious diseases (herpes zoster, human immunodeficiency virus [HIV] infection), or metabolic problems (diabetes), or it may be medication-induced (chemotherapy, antiretroviral therapy).[2] Neuropathic pain can be described as burning, shooting, or lancinating, often intensifying at night. Although affected patients may have an identical underlying cause, neuropathic pain manifestations vary between patients.

Referred pain originates in one location but is felt at another site. Both sites are innervated by the same spinal nerve, and it is difficult for the brain to differentiate the point of origin. For example, when the appendix (in the

Structure and Function

11.2

right lower quadrant of the abdomen) is inflamed, pain may be felt in the periumbilical area. It is useful to have knowledge of areas of commonly referred pain (see Table 22.2, p. 599).

TYPES OF PAIN (BY DURATION)

Acute pain is short term and self-limiting, follows a predictable trajectory, and dissipates after an injury heals. Examples of acute pain include that caused by surgery, trauma, and kidney stones. Acute pain serves a self-protective purpose: It warns of actual or potential tissue damage.

In contrast, **persistent pain** (or **chronic pain**) is defined as pain that has been present for 6 months or longer than the time of expected tissue healing.[3] Persistent pain can be categorized as malignant (cancer-related pain) or nonmalignant.

Malignant pain often parallels the pathological process created by the tumour cells. The pain is induced by tissue necrosis or stretching of an organ by the growing tumour. The severity of the pain fluctuates within the course of the disease.

Chronic nonmalignant pain is often associated with musculo-skeletal conditions, such as arthritis, low back pain, and fibromyalgia. Research findings have demonstrated that unrelieved acute pain can lead to chronic pain through two processes: peripheral and central sensitization. Peripheral sensitization is the reduction of the pain threshold and an increased response of the peripheral end of the nociceptors. Central sensitization is an increase in excitability of neurons within the CNS.[3]

DEVELOPMENTAL CONSIDERATIONS

Infants and Young Children

Infants have the same capacity for pain as do adults. By 20 weeks' gestation, ascending fibres, neurotransmitters, and the cerebral cortex are developed and functioning to the extent that the fetus is capable of feeling pain.[4] Inhibitory neurotransmitters are in insufficient supply until birth at full term, which renders preterm infants more sensitive to painful stimuli.

The persistent belief that preverbal infants do not remember pain places them at higher risk for undertreatment of pain. Research indicates that repetitive and poorly controlled pain (e.g., daily heel sticks, venipunctures) can result in life-long adverse consequences, such as neurodevelopmental problems, poor weight gain, learning disabilities, psychiatric disorders, and alcoholism.[4] Toddlers and children older than 2 years of age can report pain and point to its location but are unable to rate pain intensity. It is helpful to ask the parent or caregiver what words their child uses to report pain (e.g., "boo-boo," "owie"). Be aware that some children will try to act "grown up and brave" and often deny having pain in the presence of a stranger, or if they are fearful of receiving a "shot."

Older Adults

No evidence exists to suggest that older adults perceive pain to a lesser degree or that sensitivity is diminished with age. Although pain is a common experience among older adults, it is *not* a normal process of aging. Pain indicates disease or injury. Older adults may express fears about becoming dependent or perceive that they are taking an excessive number of medications. Active listening is the route to understanding the underlying fears that an older patient may have. You should consider the fact that older adults may need more time to respond to an assessment question. The incidence of chronic pain conditions is higher in the older adult population; such conditions include diseases such as arthritis, osteoarthritis, osteoporosis, peripheral vascular disease, peripheral neuropathies, and angina.

Gender Differences

There are gender differences in prevalence rates across painful conditions. Women are more likely to experience migraines with aura, fibromyalgia, irritable bowel syndrome, and rheumatoid arthritis. Men are more likely to experience cluster headaches, gout, coronary artery disease, and duodenal ulcers.[5] According to findings from the Human Genome Project, genetic differences between the sexes may account for the differences in pain perception.[6] The pharmacological treatments for pain, and the related adverse effects, may not be the same for both genders.

⊕ SOCIAL DETERMINANTS OF HEALTH CONSIDERATIONS

Ethnocultural variations are described in Chapter 3. To enhance ethnocultural sensitivity, health care providers need to work with patients and their families so that mutual goals are identified and the patients' understanding and beliefs about pain are taken into account (Box 11.1 discusses pain in relation to Indigenous children and youth). The following

---

BOX 11.1 Truth and Reconciliation: Indigenous Youth and the Expression of Pain

Pain cannot always be objectively assessed. Consider the case of Indigenous children and youth. According to John Sylliboy, community research coordinator with the Aboriginal Children's Hurt and Healing Initiative (ACHH), Indigenous children and youth feel and experience pain just like anyone else, but many tend not to express it outwardly through words, facial expressions, or crying. They just manage it silently and suffer. This response to pain is thought to be a result of cultural traditions and the effects of the residential school system.

At the same time, Indigenous children have higher rates of dental pain, ear infections, and juvenile rheumatoid arthritis. One initiative by the ACHH encouraged young people to share their pain though art. The result was an expression of physical and emotional pain depicted through a mix of dark and hopeful images. Understanding that this population is at a higher risk for pain and is also more likely to be stoic about pain expression should encourage health care providers to have open discussions with Indigenous patients about experiences that may cause them pain—both bodily and spiritually.

Based on Roussy, K. (2016, November 23). Indigenous children, stoic about their pain, are drawn out with art. *CBC News*. Retrieved from http://www.cbc.ca/news/health/aboriginal-youth-art-pain-hurt-healing-1.3852646.

---

are questions you can ask to assess an individual's beliefs about pain:[7]

- Do you have any fears about your pain or pain management options? If so, what do you fear most?
- What traditional remedies have you tried to help you with your pain?
- How do you usually behave when you are in pain? How would other people know you are in pain?
- How do you usually describe your pain?
- What does this pain mean to you? Why do you think you are having pain?
- Who, if anyone, in your family do you talk to about your pain? What is their understanding of your pain? What do you want them to know?
- Do you have family and friends who help you because of your pain? If so, who helps you?

TIMING OF THE PAIN ASSESSMENT

Nurses play a pivotal role in pain management by using current knowledge about pain assessment and relief measures. The ability to measure pain is an important component of a comprehensive or focused assessment. The assessment of pain must be timely, and you must identify variables that are creating or augmenting the pain experience. Rather than signifying a single event, pain screening/recognition and assessment is an ongoing process. Pain is regarded as "the fifth vital sign"; thus a pain assessment should be incorporated when other vital signs are assessed. Similarly, pain should be reassessed at suitable intervals after each pharmacological or nonpharmacological intervention (e.g., 15 to 30 minutes after parenteral administration of medication therapy and 1 hour after oral administration). The acuity of the patient's condition dictates what type of pain assessment you will conduct. For example, if you are in a health promotion type of role, or when you assess chronic pain, a comprehensive pain assessment—for example, the Brief Pain Inventory—is appropriate. In an acutely ill hospitalized patient, an "OPQRSTUV" style of comprehensive assessment can be performed on a daily basis, together with a more frequent unidimensional assessment of the severity of pain (e.g., through the Numerical Rating Scale or the Visual Analogue Scale). See the section Initial Pain Assessment (OPQRSTUV) and the box Critical Findings.

CRITICAL FINDINGS

A comprehensive assessment should also be completed when the patient's pain changes notably from previous findings; sudden changes in pain may signify an underlying pathological process. Nurses at the advanced practice level (e.g., Acute Pain Service nurses) often conduct comprehensive pain assessments on acutely ill patients, to help determine the effectiveness of the interventions.

SUBJECTIVE DATA

"Pain is whatever the experiencing person says it is, existing whenever he says it does."[8] Since pain is a subjective experience, the self-report of pain is the most reliable indicator that an individual is experiencing pain. Complex physiological, genetic, and psychosocial factors contribute to the conversion of neurochemical activity to the pain experience, the individual's reaction to the painful sensation, and any related changes to an individual's mood and behaviour.[3] Optimal use of assessment tools involves engaging both the patient and the health care provider. See the box Promoting Health: Interventions for Pain.

PROMOTING HEALTH: INTERVENTIONS FOR PAIN
Keeping the "Who" in Mind

Understanding the Pain Ladder
Nurses play a key role not only in pain assessment but also in devising front-line intervention plans for optimal pain management. You must understand key elements about treating pain. On the basis of the patient's report, efforts should be directed at reducing or eliminating the pain with appropriate pharmacological and nonpharmacological interventions.

Pharmacological Interventions
Nonopioid analgesics are medications such as acetaminophen (Tylenol) and anti-inflammatory medications.

Acetaminophen has an effect on the central nervous system (CNS), but the mechanism of action is not well understood. Acetaminophen is often an unrecognized player in the pain management plan. Many medications are combined with acetaminophen to achieve a synergistic effect (Percocet, which is acetaminophen and oxycodone; Tylenol 1, 2, and 3, which is acetaminophen with varying amounts of codeine; and Tramacet, which is paracetamol and tramadol). Acetaminophen is well tolerated; however, the maximum daily dosage in a healthy patient should not exceed 4 g per day from all sources combined. The maximum daily dosage is best decreased for older patients and for those with impaired liver function.

A large portion of the anti-inflammatory effect is within the peripheral receptors (site of injury). Anti-inflammatory agents (ibuprofen [Advil], naproxen [Apo-Naproxren]), which are readily available over the counter without a prescription, are generally used for muscular aches, headaches, and menstrual cramp pain. In the acute setting, they are often used to help manage postoperative pain. However, this class of medication is not free of adverse effects, and these medications must be administered with caution to patients with a history of renal insufficiency, gastro-intestinal bleeding, or cardiac disease and in patients about to undergo surgery because they affect clotting ability.

Opioids relieve pain primarily by action in the CNS, binding to opioid receptor sites. There is no "ceiling" dose for opioids; therapy starts at a low dose, which is titrated to effect. All opioids work similarly, but the strength may differ (e.g., hydromorphone [Dilaudid] is five times stronger than morphine; therefore, the hydromorphone dose would be much lower). This concept is referred to as **equianalgesia** (a dose of one opioid whose pain-relieving effects are equivalent to a dose of another opioid). No opioids are safer than others; all opioids have similar adverse effects. Patients taking opioids should be assessed for respiratory quality (rate and depth), level of sedation, and level of consciousness. Opioids should not be mixed with other CNS depressant medications (e.g., benzodiazepines, alcohol), and increased vigilance is required for those patients with underlying respiratory disease, such as obstructive sleep apnea.

Local anaesthetics (peripheral nerve blocks, epidural blocks) can help block the transmission of pain to the periphery, causing "numbness."

The World Health Organization (WHO) developed a pain management ladder for patients experiencing cancer pain; this

PROMOTING HEALTH: INTERVENTIONS FOR PAIN—cont'd

Keeping the Who in Mind

model has also been adopted for *chronic pain*. When patients present with pain, management starts at the bottom of the ladder, with nonopioid analgesics (such as acetaminophen), anti-inflammatory medications, or both. As pain progresses, so too should the treatment therapy. Those on the second step should also receive adjunctive therapy with acetaminophen or anti-inflammatory medications, or both. This method of pain management is often referred to as **multi-modal analgesia**. Before initiating opioid therapy, clinicians need to consider the evidence related to effectiveness of an opioid in those patients with chronic noncancer pain.*

Patients with chronic pain may also be taking many other adjunctive therapy medications, including, but not limited to, gabapentinoids (gabapentin [Apo-Gabapentin], pregabalin [Lyrica]), tricyclic antidepressants (amitriptyline [Elavil], nortriptyline [Apo-Nortriptyline]), and other opioids such as cannabinoid, buprenorphine [Bu-Trans Patch], or methadone.

Nonpharmacological Interventions

Nurses also have a key role to play in advocating for nonpharmacological interventions in the management of pain.

Heat/Ice

The application of ice or heat to relieve pain is a simple but effective tool. Heat can help relax muscles, decrease spasm, and decrease muscle tightness.

Transcutaneous Electric Nerve Stimulation

Transcutaneous electric nerve stimulation (TENS) has been shown to be effective in some acute pain episodes (labour and delivery, postsurgical pain). TENS has also been found to be effective in many conditions involving chronic pain, such as neuropathic pain, rheumatoid arthritis, and osteoarthritis.

Massage Therapy

Massage can be an important component in the management of chronic pain. Results of some studies have suggested that massage in the acute phase can help to decrease pain intensity and pain unpleasantness and to decrease anxiety.[†] Massage therapy can help relieve muscle and soft tissue pain.

Physiotherapy

Many chronic pain syndromes in neurological disorders (e.g., stroke, multiple sclerosis, Parkinson's disease) may be alleviated by implementation of physiotherapy such as hydrotherapy, repositioning, active stretching, and raising limbs, as well as passive range-of-motion exercises.[‡]

Pediatric Strategies

Pediatric nursing often involves potentially painful procedures. Nurses and parents can work together to optimize pain management. In addition to appropriate pharmacological interventions, physical interventions may also include the application of heat or ice, deep breathing, and distraction with activities such as bubble blowing or magic wands, musical toys, books, and video games. Ideally, the techniques should be taught and practised before the procedure, to allow the child to focus on the activity.

There are many other complementary therapies that patients with chronic pain may use. A part of the nursing assessment is to inquire about other therapies that patients may find of benefit and, when possible, to advocate for implementation of these therapies into the pain management plan.

References

*Canadian Guideline for Safe and Effective Use of Opioids for Chronic Non-Cancer Pain. (2017). *2017 Canadian guideline for opioid therapy and chronic non-cancer pain*. Retrieved from http://nationalpaincentre.mcmaster.ca/guidelines.html.

[†]Mitchinson, A., Kim, H., Rosenberg, J., et al. (2007). Acute postoperative pain management using massage as an adjuvant therapy: A randomized trial. *Archives of Surgery*, 142(12), 1158–1167.

[‡]World Health Organization (2006). Neurological disorders: Public health challenges. In *Pain associated with neurological disorders* (Ch. 37). Geneva, Switzerland: Author.

Additional Resources

Adams, M., Holland, L., Bostwick, P., et al. (2010). *Pharmacology for nurses: A pathophysiological approach* (Cdn ed.). Toronto: Pearson Education Canada.

Hattan, J., King, L., & Griffiths, P. (2002). The impact of foot massage and guided relaxation following cardiac surgery. *Journal of Advanced Nursing*, 37(2), 199–207.

Registered Nurses Association of Ontario (2007). *Best practice guideline: Assessment and management of pain*. Toronto: Author.

Rudkin, G. E., & Rudkin, A. K. (2005). Ambulatory surgery acute pain management: A review of the evidence. *Acute Pain*, 7, 41–49.

Subjective Data

Examiner Asks	Rationale

Initial Pain Assessment (OPQRSTUV)

1. O: onset
- When did the pain start?

To identify onset of pain (when active, or resting) or whether pain is acute/chronic.

2. P: provocative/palliative
- Does your pain increase with movement or activity?
- Are the symptoms relieved with rest?
- Were any previous treatments effective?

To identify quality of pain and differentiate between nociceptive and neuropathic pain mechanisms.

To identify alleviating and aggravating factors.

To evaluate effectiveness of current treatment.

3. Q: quality of the pain
- What does your pain feel like?
- What words describe your pain?

To identify mechanism of pain (terms such as "throbbing," "aching," "shooting," and "dull" may provide clues).

4. R: region of the body/radiation
- Where is your pain?
- Does the pain radiate, or move to other areas?

To identify one or more areas of the body that are affected by pain, inasmuch as there may be several.

5. S: severity of pain
- How would you rate your pain on an intensity scale?

To identify intensity (refer to various intensity scales).

To identify degree of impairment and effect on quality of life or ability to perform activities of daily living (ADLs).

6. T: treatment/timing
- What treatments have worked for you in the past?
- Is it a constant, dull, or intermittent pain?

To identify treatments which have been successful in the past.

To identify the timing of the pain so that treatment can be focused on spikes in pain.

7. U: Understanding of pain
- What do you believe is causing the pain?

To understand patient history of pain.

To be able to set achievable pain and function goals when reviewing the plan of care.

8. V: values
- What is your acceptable level for this pain?
- Is there anything else that you would like to say about your pain?
- Are there any other symptoms related to the pain?

To understand and discuss other stressors, spiritual pain.

PAIN ASSESSMENT TOOLS

Pain is multidimensional in scope, encompassing physical, affective, and functional domains. Various tools have been developed to capture unidimensional aspects (e.g., intensity) or multidimensional components (e.g., effect on ADLs and quality of life). Selection of the pain assessment tool is based on its purpose, time involved in administration, and the patient's ability to comprehend and complete the tool. Specialized assessment tools should be used with very young patients, very old patients, patients with cognitive dysfunction, and patients who are unable to self-report.

Educate the patient about the pain assessment tool; this education should include instructions on how to use it, the rationale for the tool when required (e.g., to help identify the effect of pain on daily activities and quality of life), and information about when the tool is likely to be administered again.

In the **Initial Pain Assessment**,[9] the patient answers eight questions concerning location, duration, quality, and intensity of pain; aggravating/relieving factors; and effects of pain on quality of life.

On the **Brief Pain Inventory**,[10] the patient rates the pain within the previous 24 hours, using graduated scales (0 to 10); indicates how much relief the patient has had; and

Brief Pain Inventory

Date:___/___/_____   Time: _____
Name:_____
      Last   First   Middle initial

1. Throughout our lives, most of us have had pain from time to time (such as minor headaches, sprains, and tooth-aches). Have you had pain other than these everyday kinds of pain today?
   1. Yes   2. No

2. On the diagram, shade in the areas where you feel pain. Put an X on the area that hurts the most.

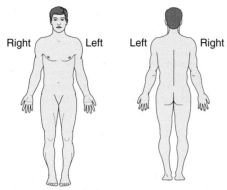

  Right   Left   Left   Right

3. Please rate your pain by circling the one number that best describes your pain at its **worst** in the past 24 hours.

   0 1 2 3 4 5 6 7 8 9 10
   No   Pain as bad as
   pain   you can imagine

4. Please rate your pain by circling the one number that best describes your pain at its **least** in the past 24 hours.

   0 1 2 3 4 5 6 7 8 9 10
   No   Pain as bad as
   pain   you can imagine

5. Please rate your pain by circling the one number that best describes your pain on the **average**.

   0 1 2 3 4 5 6 7 8 9 10
   No   Pain as bad as
   pain   you can imagine

6. Please rate your pain by circling the one number that tells how much pain you have **right now**.

   0 1 2 3 4 5 6 7 8 9 10
   No   Pain as bad as
   pain   you can imagine

7. What treatments or medications are you receiving for your pain?
   _____
   _____

8. In the past 24 hours, how much **relief** have pain treatments or medications provided? Please circle the one percentage that most shows how much relief you have received.

   0% 10 20 30 40 50 60 70 80 90 100%
   No   Complete
   relief   relief

9. Circle the one number that describes how, during the past 24 hours, pain has **interfered** with your:
   A: General activity

   0 1 2 3 4 5 6 7 8 9 10
   Does not   Completely
   interfere   interferes

   B: Mood

   0 1 2 3 4 5 6 7 8 9 10
   Does not   Completely
   interfere   interferes

   C: Walking ability

   0 1 2 3 4 5 6 7 8 9 10
   Does not   Completely
   interfere   interferes

   D: Normal work (includes both work outside the home and housework)

   0 1 2 3 4 5 6 7 8 9 10
   Does not   Completely
   interfere   interferes

   E: Relations with other people

   0 1 2 3 4 5 6 7 8 9 10
   Does not   Completely
   interfere   interferes

   F: Sleep

   0 1 2 3 4 5 6 7 8 9 10
   Does not   Completely
   interfere   interferes

   G: Enjoyment of life

   0 1 2 3 4 5 6 7 8 9 10
   Does not   Completely
   interfere   interferes

Subjective Data

11.3 Brief Pain Inventory.

No pain   Moderate pain   Worst pain

0   1   2   3   4   5   6   7   8   9   10

11.4

Faces Pain Scale — Revised (FPS-R)

In the following instructions, say "hurt" or "pain," whichever seems right for a particular child.

"These faces show how much something can hurt. This face [point to left-most face] **shows no pain. The faces show more and more pain** [point to each from left to right] **up to this one** [point to right-most face] **— it shows very much pain. Point to the face that shows how much you hurt** [right now]**."**

Score the chosen face 0, 2, 4, 6, 8, or 10, counting left to right, so '0' = 'no pain' and '10' = 'very much pain.' Do not use words like 'happy' and 'sad'. This scale is intended to measure how children feel inside, not how their face looks.

Permission for use. Copyright in the FPS-R is held by the International Association for the Study of Pain (IASP) © 2001. This material may be photocopied for non-commercial clinical and research use. To request permission from IASP to reproduce the FPS-R in a publication, or for any commercial use, please e-mail **iaspdesk@iasp-pain.org**. For all other information regarding the FPS-R contact **Tiina.Jaaniste@sesiahs.health.nsw.gov.au** (Pain Medicine Unit, Sydney Children's Hospital, Randwick, NSW 2031, Austrailia).

11.5   Faces Pain Scale—Revised.

describes how the pain interferes with areas such as general activities, mood, walking ability, work, and sleep (Fig. 11.3). In the **Short-Form McGill Pain Questionnaire,**[11] the patient ranks a list of descriptors in terms of their intensity and rates the overall intensity of the pain.

Pain rating scales can be used to ascertain baseline intensity, track changes, and give some degree of evaluation to a treatment modality. The use of unidimensional pain rating scales, such as the **Visual Analogue Scale** or the **Numeric Rating Scale** (from 0 to 10) (Fig. 11.4), is common in clinical practice. On the Numeric Rating Scale, the patient chooses a number to rate the level of pain, wherein 0 represents no pain and 10 indicates the worst possible pain. It can be administered verbally or visually along a vertical or horizontal line.

Pain rating scales can be administered to patients aged 4 or 5 years. The Faces Pain Scale—Revised (FPS-R) tool has six drawings of faces that show pain intensity, from "no pain" on the left (score of 0) to "very much pain" on the right (score of 10) (Fig. 11.5). The child is asked to select the face that best represents his, her, or their pain intensity. Numbers are not shown to children, but the number scoring makes this tool compatible with the widely used 0-to-10 metric for numeric pain scales. This revised drawing has more realistic facial expressions with a furrowed brow and horizontal mouth stretch to rate pain. It avoids smiles or tears, so that children will not confuse pain intensity with happiness or sadness.

Older adults may find the numerical scale too abstract and may respond to scales in which words are used. Such an alternative scale is the simple **Descriptor Scale**, which lists words that describe different levels of pain intensity, such as *no pain*, *mild pain*, *moderate pain*, and *severe pain*.

OBJECTIVE DATA

PREPARATION

The physical examination process can help you understand the nature of the pain. Consider whether this is an acute or chronic condition.

Pain should not be discounted when objective physical evidence of it is not found. According to the American Pain Society:

"In cases in which the cause of acute pain is uncertain, establishing a diagnosis is a priority, but symptomatic treatment of pain should be given while the investigation is proceeding. With occasional exceptions (e.g., the *initial* examination of the patient with an acute condition of the abdomen), it is rarely justified to defer analgesia until a diagnosis is made. In fact, a comfortable patient is better able to cooperate with diagnostic procedures."[12]

EQUIPMENT NEEDED

An assessment tool that is appropriate for the patient; for example, for initial or comprehensive pain assessment, use the Brief Pain Inventory; for acute/in-hospital settings, use the Numeric Rating Scale (0–10) or (for children) the Faces Pain Scale—Revised (FPS-R).

Normal Range of Findings	**Abnormal Findings**

Acute Pain

In the acute phase, patients should report their pain well controlled, with a Numeric Rating Scale intensity of 4 or higher or as "mild to moderate" in severity.

Patients should be able to identify how much pain they can tolerate before it interferes with functioning or rehabilitation exercises; thus, pain management goals for treatment can be set before rehabilitation interventions.

Adverse effects such as nausea, vomiting, or pruritus should also be assessed at time of pain assessment and with pharmacological interventions.

Consider pre-emptive analgesia for procedural pain because patients who are subjected to repetitive painful procedures (e.g., dressing changes, suctioning) may become fearful.

Increased heart rate or blood pressure may indicate pain.

Pain may be a precursor to hypoventilation and hypoxia, inasmuch as patients may not be able to cough effectively.

Joint stiffness may result from limitation secondary to severe pain.

Nausea and vomiting may be present with severe acute pain.

Neuropathic Pain

People with neuropathic pain may have decreased or increased sensation or numbness over the affected area (e.g., as in postherpetic neuralgia).
Inspect the skin and tissues for colour, swelling, and any masses or deformity (e.g., bottoms of feet for diabetic neuropathy).

Changes in sensation may be present; patients may report an increased or decreased sensation of pinprick or cold or loss of sensation of vibration.
Neuropathic pain may increase in severity at night or at times of decreased stimulation.

Lesions, open wounds, tissue damage, change in hair distribution.

Absence of pain sensation (analgesia); increased pain sensation (hyperalgesia); or evoking of a severe pain sensation with a stimulus that does not normally induce pain (allodynia).

Chronic Pain

Pain may be present for an extended period of time after the acute phase. Chronic pain should be manageable through timing of activities (e.g., spacing of tasks) and pain management interventions.

Physical activities should be a regular part of daily activities.

Social support systems should be in place to assist in day-to-day activities.
Financial support and psychosocial support should be in place.

Fear, anxiety, depression, isolation.
Limited mobility and function.
Family distress.
Diminished quality of life.
Possibly decreased ability to complete day-to-day activities; increasing levels of fatigue.

Objective Data

NONVERBAL/BEHAVIOURAL PAIN ASSESSMENT

When a patient cannot verbally communicate pain, you can learn to recognize and assess pain by using a behavioural pain assessment tool. Behavioural pain assessment tools can help you determine the presence of pain, but they cannot help you determine the severity.

Acute Pain Behaviours

Patients may be unable to verbalize the presence of pain for a variety of reasons. However, those who are unable to report their pain are at high risk for the undertreatment of pain. Individuals who are nonverbal but are cognitively intact (e.g., intubated but alert and awake) may be able to indicate the intensity of their pain by using the Numeric Rating Scale, by writing down a description of the quality of their pain, or by pointing to the location of their pain.

Persistent (Chronic) Pain Behaviours

Persons with persistent pain often live with the experience for months and years. A person cannot function physiologically and go on with life in a repetitive state of grimacing, diaphoresis, guarding, and so on. The person adapts over time, and clinicians must not anticipate the same behaviours as in acute pain. Patients with chronic pain may give little indication that they are in pain and therefore are at higher risk for underdetection of pain. Whenever possible, it is best to ask patients how they behave when in pain.

The Unconscious Individual

Individuals who are unconscious for physiological reasons or because they have been given sedative medications also experience pain. Assessment of pain in these individuals may be a challenge, but tools have been created to standardize key areas for assessment. Unconscious individuals experiencing

TABLE 11.1	The Critical-Care Pain Observation Tool		
INDICATOR	**DESCRIPTION**	**SCORE**	
Facial expression	No muscular tension observed	Relaxed, neutral	0
	Presence of frowning, brow lowering, orbit tightening, and levator contraction	Tense	1
	All of the above facial movements plus eyelid tightly closed	Grimacing	2
Body movements	Does not move at all (does not necessarily mean absence of pain)	Absence of movements	0
	Slow, cautious movements, touching or rubbing the pain site, seeking attention through movements	Protection	1
	Pulling tube, attempting to sit up, moving limbs/thrashing, not following commands, striking at staff, trying to climb out of bed	Restlessness	2
Muscle tension			
Evaluation by passive flexion and extension of upper extremities	No resistance to passive movements	Relaxed	0
	Resistance to passive movements	Tense, rigid	1
	Strong resistance to passive movements, inability to complete them	Very tense or rigid	2
and either			
Compliance with the ventilator (intubated patients)	Alarms not activated, easy ventilation	Tolerating ventilator or movement	0
	Alarms stop spontaneously	Coughing but tolerating	1
	Asynchrony: blocking ventilation, alarms frequently activated	Fighting ventilator	2
or			
Vocalization (extubated patients)	Talking in normal tone or no sound	Talking in normal tone or no sound	0
	Sighing, moaning	Sighing, moaning	1
	Crying out, sobbing	Crying out, sobbing	2
Total, range			0–8

From Gélinas, C., Fillion, L., Puntillo, K. A., et al. (2006). Validation of the Critical-Care Pain Observation Tool in adult patients. *American Journal of Critical Care, 15*(4), 420–427. Reprinted with permission.

moderate to intense levels of pain often exhibit grimacing, wincing, moaning, rigidity, arching, restlessness, shaking, or pushing.[13] The Critical-Care Pain Observation Tool[14] was developed to assess pain in patients in the critical care unit. Behaviours assessed include facial expression, body movement, muscle tension, vocalizations, and degree of compliance with ventilation (Table 11.1). The total score ranges between 0 and 8; a higher score is more indicative of pain. Physiological signs (vital signs) should not be used exclusively to rule out or confirm the presence of pain because pulse and blood pressure can also be altered by changes in fluid volume, by medications, and by blood loss.

❖ DEVELOPMENTAL CONSIDERATIONS

Neonates

Because neonates and young infants are preverbal and incapable of self-report, pain assessment is dependent on behavioural and physiological cues. Infants do feel pain; if a procedure or disease process is known to induce pain in adults (e.g., circumcision, surgery, sickle cell disease, cancer), it does induce pain in neonates and infants. Pain measures that include more than one assessment approach within a given instrument are used for measuring pain in neonates and infants. Most measures include both behavioural and physiological indicators, and some also include contextual

factors, such as the gestational age or behavioural sleep/wake state of the infant. Several published measures combine behavioural and physiological indicators for assessing pain in infants with varying degrees of established reliability and validity, such as the Neonatal Pain, Agitation, and Sedation Scale and the Premature Infant Pain Profile.

The Premature Infant Pain Profile is a behavioural measure of pain for premature infants. It was developed at the universities of Toronto and McGill in Canada.[15] Indicators of pain that are assessed include gestational age; behavioural state before painful stimulus; and change in heart rate, change in oxygen saturation, brow bulge, eye squeeze, and nasolabial furrow during painful stimulus.

These measures target acute pain. No biological markers have been identified for long-term chronic pain in infants or children. Therefore, evaluate the whole patient. Look for changes in temperament, expression, and activity.

Intellectual/Cognitive Disability

Although adults may have an intellectual or cognitive disability, their sensory ability to perceive pain is not diminished.[16] Intellectually/cognitively impaired persons may have a limited ability to communicate information about pain, which places them at high risk for undertreatment of pain. Patients who commonly present with a cognitive disability include those with dementia, those with Parkinson's disease, patients after a stroke, and patients with intellectual developmental disabilities. Various pain scales are available for assessment of intellectually/cognitively impaired patients; these include the Pain Assessment in Advanced Dementia (PAINAD) scale[17] and the Abbey scale.[18]

Discussion with the family or other health care team members can help you identify patterns that may indicate that a patient is experiencing pain. A review of medical records can also highlight potential areas for concern (e.g., diabetic neuropathy).

It is important to learn to recognize behavioural cues of pain, by examining facial expressions or changes in appetite, daily activities, involvement in social activities, or sleep/wake cycles. A comprehensive head-to-toe assessment should confirm or rule out any obvious sources of pain, such as skin tears or areas of swelling. Assess any sudden onset of acute confusion or delirium because it may indicate poor control of pain or other competing explanations such as infection or adverse reaction to medications.

DOCUMENTATION AND CRITICAL THINKING

Sample Charting

SUBJECTIVE

Onset within the past 2 weeks; patient states having severe epigastric pain within a half hour of eating greasy fatty foods. Pain is stabbing and squeezing in nature with radiation to right shoulder blade. Patient rates pain as a 10 on a scale of 0 to 10. Nausea accompanies pain. Patient takes antacids, with minimal relief. Pain diminishes after bringing knees to chest and "not moving" for a 1-hour period.

OBJECTIVE

Patient diaphoretic, grimacing, and having difficulty concentrating. Breathless during history. Arms guarding upper abdominal area. Abdomen distended. Severe tenderness noted on light right upper quadrant and epigastric palpation. Bowel sounds hyperactive in all four quadrants.

ASSESSMENT

Acute episodic visceral pain

Focused Assessment: Clinical Case Study 1

Robert Martin (R.M.) is a 20-year-old man with diagnosed sickle cell crisis. Admitted to the emergency department.

SUBJECTIVE

Within the past 48 hours, R.M. reports increasing pain in upper and lower extremity joints and swelling of right knee. States having "stomach flu" 1 week before with periods of vomiting and diarrhea. Pain is aching and constant in nature. Rates pain as 10+ on a scale of 0 to 10. Taking ibuprofen, one to two tablets every 4 hours, and using ice packs, with no relief.

OBJECTIVE

Requires assistance to sit on examination table. Unable to bear weight on right leg. Affect flat, clenches jaw during position changes. Tenderness localized in elbow, wrist, finger, and knee joints. Diminished range of motion in wrists and knees (right knee, 36 cm diameter; left knee, 30 cm). Right knee warm and boggy to touch.

ASSESSMENT

Acute nociceptive pain

Focused Assessment: Clinical Case Study 2

Ann Green (A.G.) is an 85-year-old woman with a 20-year history of osteoarthritis.

Objective Data

Documentation and Critical Thinking

SUBJECTIVE

A.G. reports increased pain and stiffness in her neck, arms, and lower back for the past month. Denies radiation of pain. Denies tingling or numbness in upper or lower extremities.

Having difficulty getting in and out of bathtub and dressing herself. Describes pain as aching, with good and bad days. Becomes frustrated when asked to rate her pain intensity; replies, "I don't know what number to give; it hurts a lot, on and off." Takes acetaminophen extra strength, two tablets, when the pain "really gets the best of me," with some degree of relief. Does not take part in "field trips" offered by assisted living facility because she "hurts too much."

OBJECTIVE

Localized tenderness noted upon palpation to C3 and C4; unable to flex neck to chest. Crepitus noted in both shoulder joints. No swelling noted. Muscle strength 1+ and equal in upper extremities. Lumbar area tender to moderate palpation. Rubs lower back frequently; limited flexion at the waist. Gait slow and unsteady. Facial expression stoic.

ASSESSMENT

Persistent pain

SPECIAL CONSIDERATIONS FOR ADVANCED PRACTICE

SOMATOFORM DISORDERS

Medically unexplained physical symptoms occur in patients with complaints of physical symptoms or signs for which there is inadequate objective pathophysiological evidence to explain the duress.[19]

Acute or persistent pain can be challenging, often necessitating increased pain management (e.g., involvement with Acute Pain Service nurses, as available).

Patients experiencing persistent pain may benefit from referral to chronic pain clinics and from therapies in which pain management involves integration of psychological and pharmacological support.

SICKLE CELL CRISIS

In Canada, it is hard to determine the actual incidence of sickle cell disease because no national hemoglobinopathy program exists, and no "race"-specific health data like that collected in the United States are available. The disease affects not only people of African descent but also people from the Mediterranean, Caribbean, South and Central America, Arabia, and India. It is estimated that approximately 1 per 400 babies of Canadians of African descent are born with sickle cell disease.[20]

Sickle cell disease is characterized by an alteration of hemoglobin and by anemia and tissue injury secondary to vaso-occlusion. Any decrease in oxygenation causes alterations in the shape of the red blood cells, which causes them to stick together and ultimately block small blood vessels. The resulting vaso-occlusion (vaso-occlusive crisis) can cause severe pain, similar to that of a myocardial infarction.

Patients with sickle cell disease can experience any one of a number of pain syndromes:[21]
- Acute regional pain syndrome (chest pain [acute chest syndrome], craniofacial pain, long bone and joint pain, low back pain, muscle pain)
- Persistent pain syndrome (peripheral ulcerations, avascular necrosis, osteomyelitis)
- Other pain syndromes (such as migraines, neuropathic pain, fibromyalgia, and myofascial pain)

Painful sickle cell crises can manifest early in infancy and lead to chronic pain, which can be exacerbated by acute pain in the subsequent vaso-occlusive crises. Vaso-occlusive crises can have psychological causes (e.g., stressful event) or physiological causes (such as infection, dehydration, or overexertion, and sometimes in the postoperative state). Most patients with sickle cell disease experience pain on a daily basis. Management of acute episodic pain begins with a comprehensive pain assessment and documentation of problem areas; you must recognize that many affected patients present to emergency departments with acute pain in addition to their chronic pain. After initial assessment and intervention, these patients require frequent pain reassessments to titrate treatment dosages appropriately, and they would probably benefit from the services of advanced nursing or pain management teams to help control their pain.

Research has shown that many complementary therapies are helpful in limiting the frequency of sickle cell crises, as well as in improving patients' quality of life. Community support is beneficial for patients and their families. Many websites offer a source of online support for patients and health care providers; for example, the Sickle Cell Disease Association of Canada (see the section Additional Resources) offers education and tips for families coping with the disease.

Documentation and Critical Thinking

Special Considerations for Advanced Practice

ADDITIONAL RESOURCES

International Association for the Study of Pain: https://www.iasp-pain.org

Sickle Cell Disease Association of Canada: http://www.sicklecelldisease.ca

The Canadian Pain Society: http://www.canadianpainsociety.ca

REFERENCES

1. Treede, R. D., Jensen, T. S., Campbell, J. N., et al. (2008). Redefinition of neuropathic pain and a grading system for clinical use: Consensus statement on clinical and research diagnostic criteria. *Neurology, 70*, 1630–1635.
2. Gold, M., Chessell, I., Devor, M., et al. (2006). Peripheral nervous system targets: Rapporteur Report. In J. Campbell (Ed.), *Emerging strategies for the treatment of neuropathic pain.* Seattle: IASP Press.
3. Kehlet, H., Jensen, T. S., & Woolf, C. J. (2006). Persistent postsurgical pain: Risk factors and prevention. *Lancet, 367*(9522), 1618–1625.
4. Anand, K. J. S. (2000). Effects of perinatal pain and stress. *Progress in Brain Research, 122*, 117–119.
5. International Association for the Study of Pain. (2007, September). *Differences in pain between women and men.* Retrieved from http://www.iasp-pain.org.
6. Mogil, J. S. (2002). Pain genetics: Pre- and post-genomic findings. *International Association for the Study of Pain Technical Corner Newsletter, 2*, 3–6.
7. Lasch, K. E. (2000). Culture, pain, and culturally sensitive pain care. *Pain Management Nursing, 1*(3, Suppl. 1), 16–22.
8. McCaffery, M. (1968). *Nursing practice theories related to cognition, bodily pain, and man-environment interactions* (p. 95). Los Angeles: University of California, Los Angeles, Students' Store.
9. McCaffery, M., & Pasero, C. (1999). *Pain: Clinical manual* (2nd ed.). St. Louis: Mosby.
10. Daut, R. L., & Cleeland, C. S. (1982). The prevalence and severity of pain in cancer. *Cancer, 50*, 1913–1918.
11. Melzack, R. (1987). The short-form McGill Pain Questionnaire. *Pain, 30*, 191–197.
12. American Pain Society (1992). *Principles of analgesic use in the treatment of acute and cancer pain* (3rd ed., p. 3). Glenview, IL: Author.
13. Puntillo, K. A., Morris, A. B., Thompson, C. L., et al. (2004). Pain behaviors observed during six common procedures: Results from Thunder Project II. *Critical Care Medicine, 32*(2), 421–427.
14. Gélinas, C., Fillion, L., Puntillo, K. A., et al. (2006). Validation of the Critical-Care Observation Tool in adult patients. *American Journal of Critical Care, 15*(4), 420–427.
15. Stevens, B., Johnston, C., Petryshen, P., et al. (1996). Premature Infant Pain Profile: Development and initial validation. *Clinical Journal of Pain, 12*(1), 13–22.
16. Vreeling, F. W., Houx, P. J., Jolles, J., et al. (1995). Primitive reflexes in Alzheimer's disease and vascular dementia. *Journal of Geriatric Psychiatry and Neurology, 8*, 111–117.
17. Warden, V., Hurley, A. C., & Volicer, L. (2003). Development and psychometric evaluation of the Pain Assessment in Advanced Dementia (PAINAD) scale. *Journal of the American Medical Directors Association, 4*, 9–15.
18. Abbey, J., Piller, N., De Bellis, A., et al. (2004). The Abbey pain scale: A 1-minute numerical indicator for people with end stage dementia. *International Journal of Palliative Nursing, 10*(1), 6–13.
19. Neimark, G., Caroff, S., & Stinnett, J. (2005). Medically unexplained physical symptoms. *Psychiatric Annals, 35*(4), 298–306 (p. 296).
20. Health Canada. (2000). *Certain circumstances: Issues in equity and responsiveness in access to health care in Canada.* Retrieved from http://www.hc-sc.gc.ca/hcs-sss/alt_formats/hpb-dgps/pdf/pubs/2001-certain-equit-acces/2001-certain-equit-acces_e.pdf.
21. Tanabe, P., & Todds, K. (2010). Pain in sickle cell disease. In A. Kopf & N. Patel (Eds.), *Guide to pain management in low resource settings.* Seattle: International Association for the Study of Pain.

12 | CHAPTER

Nutritional Assessment and Nursing Practice

Written by Joyce K. Keithley, DNSc, RN, FAAN
Adapted by Ellen Vogel, PhD, RD, FDC;
Andrea Miller, MHSc, RD; and
Christina Vaillancourt, MHSc, RD, CDE

http://evolve.elsevier.com/Canada/Jarvis/examination/

STRUCTURE AND FUNCTION

Healthy eating is a key element of both healthy human development and reducing the risk for many chronic conditions. Nurses, as the first point of contact for patients, collaborate with the multidisciplinary team in the development of the nutritional care plan. Nurses record the patient history, including weight history; assess vital signs; and measure current weight and height. Because nurses frequently initiate patient referrals to dietitians, it is important that they develop knowledge and skills in nutritional screening to ensure that patients' needs are met in an efficient manner. Dietitians and nurses often collaborate to facilitate optimal patient care.

"Registered Dietitian (RD)" (also referred to as *dietitian*) is a protected title across Canada. However, "nutritionist" is a protected title only in some provinces. Dietitians are nutrition experts. Dietitians make it easier for the public to make healthy food choices. The advice and information they provide is tailored to the needs and values of their patients and communities. Dietitians translate complex scientific evidence into practical solutions to promote health and help patients manage special health conditions, including diabetes, heart disease, cancer, food allergies, and obesity. Dietitians work alongside other health care providers, including physicians, nurses, occupational therapists, and pharmacists. Dietitians can be found working in hospitals, health clinics, long-term care facilities, public health agencies, grocery stores, and the food industry; as entrepreneurs; and in education and research.[1]

DEFINING NUTRITIONAL STATUS

Nutritional status is the degree of balance between nutrient intake and nutrient requirements. In addition to genetic predisposition, this balance is affected by income, education, an individual's broad physical and social environments, nutritional literacy, and access to protective foods. For individuals, a lower socio-economic status (education level, income, employment) is often associated with increased obesity among both adults and children. Lower personal income affects affordability of food, which demonstrates the most consistent influence on food consumption. Similarly, individuals living in middle-income to high-income neighbourhoods are more likely to be physically active than their counterparts in lower-income neighbourhoods. Lower-income neighbourhoods are also more likely to contain food vendors that result in a greater access to sources of energy-dense foods (e.g., fast foods) and lower access to supermarkets or other stores stocking healthy foods.[2]

Optimal nutritional status is achieved when nutrients are consumed in amounts that support daily requirements and any increased metabolic demands related to growth, pregnancy, or illness. Individuals who have optimal nutritional status are generally more active, have fewer physical illnesses, and live longer than those who are less well nourished.

Undernutrition occurs when nutritional reserves become depleted or when nutrient intake is inadequate to meet daily requirements or metabolic demands. Certain populations are vulnerable to undernutrition: infants, children, pregnant women, new immigrants, individuals with low incomes, hospitalized people, and older adults. Undernutrition increases the risk for impaired growth and development, lowered resistance to infection and disease, delayed wound healing, longer hospital stays, and higher health-related expenses.

Overnutrition results from the consumption of nutrients—most frequently calories, sodium, and fat—in excess of requirements. Obesity has become one of the world's greatest health concerns and threatens to undo gains made in life expectancy during the twentieth century. An extensive body of research has found associations between excess body weight and numerous chronic conditions, including type 2 diabetes, hypertension, cardiovascular disease, gallbladder disease, and certain types of cancer. Despite cultural norms that stigmatize excess weight, and strong evidence of its adverse health effects, the prevalence of obesity continues to rise.[3]

In its health surveys, Statistics Canada determines obesity using the body mass index (BMI), a relative measure of weight and height. The adjusted prevalence of obesity among Canadians aged 18 years and over was 24.8% in 2011–12. This finding means that one in four adult Canadians, or approximately 6.3 million people, were obese in 2011–12, which is 17.5% more than in 2003. During 2011–12, overall obesity levels were higher for males (26.1%) than for females (23.4%). Males 35 and older had higher levels of obesity than females in that age range. However, among those aged 18 to 34, there were no differences in obesity between the sexes.[3]

Over time, obesity has increased more for men than women. Between 2003 and 2011–12, the prevalence of obesity rose 17.9% among men and 16.8% among women. Age is also related to obesity. Considering both sexes together, those aged 18 to 34 were significantly less likely to be obese than any other age group. Those aged 35 to 64 were most likely to be obese.[3]

Children and youth who are overweight or obese are at an increased risk of remaining obese throughout adulthood. Further, overweight or obese children and youth are at risk for adverse health consequences, including cardiovascular disease, type 2 diabetes, and many cancers (i.e. colorectal, kidney, and oesophageal cancer). Overweight or obese children and youth are also more likely to have a reduced quality of life and are at a greater risk of being teased, bullied, and socially isolated. In 2012–13, 31% of children and youth 5 to 17 years of age were overweight and obese, based on the BMI measured as part of the Canadian Health Measures Survey (CHMS). The prevalence of overweight and obesity differed by age group. Children and youth aged 12 to 17 (37%) were more likely to be overweight or obese than those aged 5 to 11.[4]

The Aboriginal Peoples Survey found that 30% of Inuit aged 18 and over were overweight and 26% were obese, according to their BMI. Among Inuit aged 18 and over living within Inuit Nunangat, 28% of Inuit were overweight and 24% were obese, while outside Inuit Nunangat, 32% were overweight and 31% were obese.[5]

❖ DEVELOPMENTAL CONSIDERATIONS

The nutrients necessary to optimize health over a lifetime are the same for all healthy individuals; however, the amount of each of those nutrients changes based on stages of the life cycle. Nutrition can be viewed as a continuum over the life cycle: a continuum that changes as individuals grow, age, and respond to variations in their environment, physical activity, and health. Optimal nutrition is essential for overall health and well-being and in the prevention of chronic conditions.

Infants and Children

Early nutrition affects later development, and early feedings establish eating habits that influence nutrition throughout life. The time from birth to 4 months of age is the most rapid period of growth in the life cycle. Although infants lose weight during the first few days of life, birth weight is usually regained by the seventh to tenth day after birth. Birth weight doubles by 4 months of age and triples by the age of 1 year. An infant's length changes more slowly, increasing about 25 cm from birth to age 1 year. Growth rate then slows during the second year; an infant typically gains less than 4.5 kg and grows 12.5 cm in the second year. Brain size also increases rapidly during infancy and childhood. By 2 years of age, the brain has reached 50% of its adult size; by age 4, 75%; and by age 8, 100%.

The Canadian Paediatric Society and Health Canada recommend exclusive breastfeeding for full-term infants for the first 6 months of life, for the nutritional, physiological, social, and economic benefits it confers on the infant and mother.[6] Breast milk is ideally formulated to promote normal infant growth and development and natural immunity. With the exception of vitamin D, breast milk provides all the nutrients that a healthy infant needs for the first 6 months of life. It is recommended that all breastfed and partially breastfed, full-term infants in Canada receive a daily vitamin D supplement of 10 mcg (400 IU). After 2 years of age, a vitamin D supplement is no longer recommended.

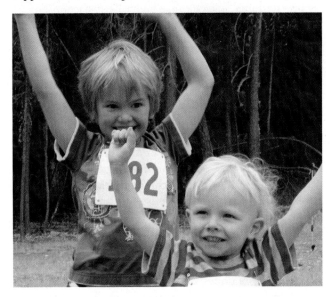

Solid foods can be introduced as the infant becomes physically able to handle them. In healthy full-term infants, the introduction of iron-rich foods, including meat and meat alternatives and iron fortified infant cereals, begins at 6 months of age. Whole cow's milk should *not* be offered until the infant is 9 to 12 months of age, because it is associated with occult blood loss in stool, especially in the first 6 months of life.[6] Lower fat milk (2% or skim) should be avoided until the age of 2 years because it has insufficient fat and calories to support optimal growth and development. It is recommended that children's eating pattern follows *Eating Well With Canada's Food Guide.*[7]

Adolescence

After a period of slower growth in late childhood, adolescence is characterized by rapid physical growth and endocrine and hormonal changes. Energy and protein requirements increase to meet these demands. In addition, because of rapid bone growth and increasing muscle mass (and, in girls, the onset of menarche), calcium and iron requirements increase during adolescence. Careful meal and snack planning is essential to meet the increased nutrient demands of adolescence.

In general, adolescent boys grow taller and accumulate less body fat than do adolescent girls. In girls, body fat increases to about 25% of total body mass; in boys, body fat decreases (replaced by muscle mass) to about 12% of total body mass. In girls, body weight doubles between the ages of 8 and 14 years; in boys, between the ages of 10 and 17 years.

Because of the societal importance placed on physical appearance, many adolescents' can feel pressured to diet to conform to a perceived ideal body image, or they may become dissatisfied with their appearance.[8] Some adolescents have reported pressure to lose weight or have been exposed to body preoccupations and disordered eating at the familial level.[9] Boys increasingly tend to equate their attractiveness with increased muscle definition, mass, and body shape.[9] Research suggests that body dissatisfaction among boys can lead to poor psychological adjustment, disordered eating behaviours (binge eating disorder, bulimia, anorexia, and dysmorphia), steroid use, and exercise dependence.

Pregnancy and Lactation

It is essential that sufficient calories, protein, vitamins, and minerals be consumed to support the synthesis of maternal and fetal tissues during pregnancy. Health Canada has adopted the 2009 U.S. Institute of Medicine's recommendations for gestational weight gain for singleton pregnancies. The Institute of Medicine's recommendations are based on observational data, which consistently show that women who gain within the recommended range experience better pregnancy outcomes.[10]

Recommended weight gain for women whose body weight is *ideal* before pregnancy is 11.5 to 16 kg (25 to 35 lb); for women who are **underweight**, recommended weight gain is 12.5 to 18 kg (28 to 40 lb); for women who begin pregnancy **overweight**, weight gain recommendations are 7 to 11 kg (15 to 24 lb).[10]

Several factors increase nutritional risk for pregnant women. These include age (adolescents are at higher risk for the development of nutrient deficiencies in pregnancy), multiple pregnancies with short (<18-month) intervals between each pregnancy, use of tobacco products, use of alcohol or illicit drugs, twin or triplet (or higher order) pregnancy, restrictive diets (including vegetarianism), and inadequate or excessive weight gain during pregnancy.

In comparison with older mothers, teenage mothers are more likely to experience complications of pregnancy, including anemia, hypertension, pre-eclampsia, renal disease, and depressive disorders. Furthermore, infants born to teenaged mothers may have higher rates of perinatal mortality, higher preterm birth rates, and lower birth weights.[11]

To reduce the risk of neural tube defects in infants, women without personal health risks who are capable of becoming pregnant should take a vitamin supplement containing 400 mcg of folic acid daily. Recommendations include taking folic acid for at least 3 months before pregnancy and continuing throughout pregnancy and the postpartum period (as long as breastfeeding continues).[12,13]

Adulthood

Growth and nutrient requirements stabilize during adulthood. However, lifestyle factors—including use of tobacco products; stress; lack of physical activity; excessive alcohol intake; and diets high in saturated fat, cholesterol, salt, and sugar and low in fibre—contribute to the development of hypertension, obesity, atherosclerosis, some forms of cancer, osteoporosis, and diabetes mellitus. The adult years provide an ideal opportunity for needs-based nutrition education, preserving health and preventing or delaying the onset of chronic disease.

Nutrition counselling is important in the prevention of overweight and obesity. Current recommendations include a diet that is rich in fruits and vegetables, low in total and saturated fat, and high in fibre. Research findings suggest that adults who consume regular meals and snacks manage their weight better than those that have more irregular or erratic eating patterns.[8]

Older Adults

With age, a number of changes take place that make individuals more prone to undernutrition or overnutrition. Poor physical or mental health, social isolation, limited functional ability, poverty, and polypharmacy are risk factors for undernutrition in older adults.[14]

After the age of 50, energy requirements decrease by approximately 5% per decade. Decreasing metabolic rate, combined with an inactive lifestyle, increases the risk for chronic diseases associated with overnutrition, including obesity, type 2 diabetes, hypertension, and cardiovascular disease. Individuals older than 70 years who maintain a BMI between 25 and 32 have been observed to have the lowest mortality risk.

Normal physiological changes of aging directly affecting nutritional status in older adults include poor dentition, decreased visual acuity, decreased saliva production, slowed gastro-intestinal motility, decreased gastro-intestinal absorption, and diminished olfactory and taste sensitivity. Reduced socioeconomic conditions can adversely influence the nutritional status of an older adult. An overall decline in the number of extended families, in addition to the increased mobility of families, reduces available support systems. Access to facilities for meal preparation, availability of a suitable eating environment, access to grocery stores, physical limitations, limited income, and social isolation are all factors that can interfere with the acquisition and preparation of a balanced diet. Medication use must also be considered in older patients. Increasingly, older adults are prescribed multiple medications that may interact with nutrients, vitamin supplements, and other prescription medications.

Finally, with age the synthesis of vitamin D decreases. Health Canada recommended that, in addition to following *Eating Well With Canada's Food Guide*, all individuals older than 50 take a daily vitamin D supplement of 400 IU.[15]

SOCIAL DETERMINANTS OF HEALTH CONSIDERATIONS

At every stage of the life cycle, health is directly or indirectly influenced by key determinants of health such as education and literacy, income and social status, employment and working conditions, and social environments.[16] Increasingly, evidence suggests that "the complex interaction between these determinants can influence health outcomes—both positively and negatively—and, depending on the individual, can result in the individual beginning and progressing through life stages at different times and rates."[16]

Food Security

Food security is described as the condition in which all people, at all times, have access to nutritious, safe, personally acceptable, and culturally appropriate foods, produced in ways that are environmentally sound and socially just.[17] In Canada, income-related *food insecurity* is increasingly acknowledged as a key determinant of nutritional health. Data from Health Canada indicated that in 2007, 961 000 Canadian households (7.7% of the population) were food insecure.[18] The prevalence of household food insecurity was higher in certain groups, including lone-parent families with one or more young children, those receiving social assistance, and Indigenous people living off-reserve. Among off-reserve Indigenous households, approximately one in five (20.9%) households is food insecure, including 8.4% with severe food insecurity. These rates are approximately three times higher than among non-Indigenous households where 7.2% were food insecure, including 2.5% with severe food insecurity.[18]

Individuals and families with lower socioeconomic status are less likely to consume the nutrients needed for proper health and well-being than are those living with higher incomes.[16] Studies have also linked food insecurity to the prevalence of unhealthy weights. Families with lower incomes consume more energy-dense, nutrient-poor diets, whereas families with higher incomes consume more whole grains, lean meats, low-fat dairy products, and fresh vegetables and fruit.

Because foods and eating customs are culturally distinct, each person has a unique cultural heritage that may affect nutritional status. Immigrants commonly maintain traditional eating customs long after the language and manner of dress of an adopted country become routine (especially for holidays and observance of religious customs). Occupation, socioeconomic status, religion, gender, and health awareness also have a great bearing on eating practices.

Dietary Practices and Cultural Diversity

The changing cultural profile in Canada encourages the availability of ethnically diverse foods and cuisines. This aspect of eating in Canada is reflected in updated nutrition education resources, including *Eating Well With Canada's Food Guide*[7] (Fig. 12.1), which has been translated into many different languages (available at the Health Canada website: https://www.canada.ca/en/health-canada).

An example of a new resource designed to complement *Eating Well With Canada's Food Guide* is *Eating Well With Canada's Food Guide—First Nations, Inuit and Métis*, a food guide tailored to reflect the traditions and food choices of those population groups.[7,19] This guide includes both traditional and store-bought foods that are generally available, affordable, and accessible to Indigenous people across Canada.

New immigrants and refugees may be at risk for undernutrition for a variety of reasons. Some individuals come from countries with food supplies that are limited due to poverty, poor sanitation, war, or political strife. General undernutrition, diarrhea, lactose intolerance, osteomalacia (soft bones), scurvy, and dental caries are among the more common nutrition-related problems of new immigrants from developing countries.

Upon arrival in Canada, new immigrants are faced with a new language and a new culture. They may encounter challenges related to new or unfamiliar foods, food storage requirements and facilities, food preparation difficulties, and food-buying habits. Many familiar foods are difficult or impossible to obtain. Limited income may also decrease access to familiar foods. When traditional food habits are disrupted by a new culture, borderline nutrient deficiencies may result. The best way to learn about an individual's eating pattern is to ask about his, her, or their dietary customs. It is important to keep in mind that standard tables of weight for age, height for age, and weight for height may not be appropriate to evaluate growth and development of immigrant children. At present, no reliable standards exist to evaluate every immigrant group. Weight history in these specific population groups may be best assessed through questions related to personal and family weight history.

Lower percentages of immigrant youth and young adults were measured as overweight or obese. For example, 17% of immigrant youth were considered overweight and 5% were obese.[20] Upon arrival in a host country, immigrants often have lower obesity rates than those in the host country, but these rates converge over time. When migrating to countries with high obesity rates, immigrants adopt the host countries' behaviours and ultimately face similar obesity risks.[21]

Important cultural factors to consider in assessing nutritional status include the cultural definition of food; frequency and number of meals eaten away from home; form and content of ceremonial meals; food preparation methods;

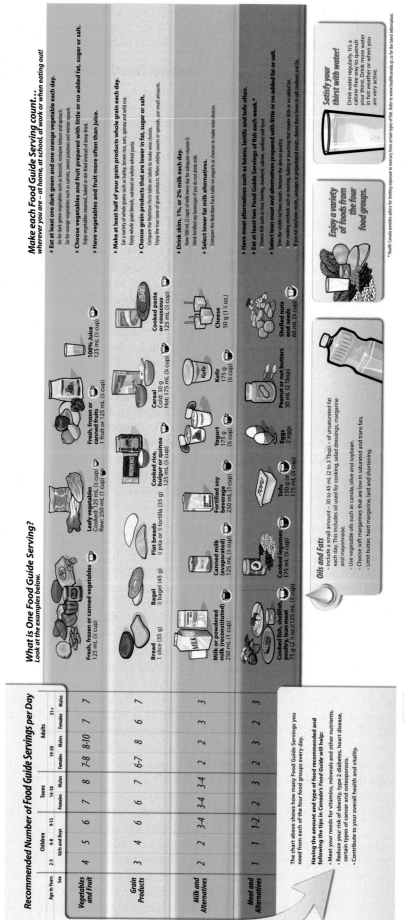

12.1   Extract From *Eating Well With Canada's Food Guide.*

amount and types of foods eaten; and regularity of food consumption. Because of cultural diversity, the 24-hour dietary recall or 3-day food record (traditionally used for nutritional assessment) may be insufficient in assessing nutritional status for people from culturally diverse backgrounds. Traditional nutrition education resources may not provide culture-specific diet information, in as much as nutritional content and exchange tables are generally based on Western diets.

Food itself is only one part of eating. Social interactions during meals are often as meaningful as the food itself. Understanding these social customs is an essential part of completing a nutritional assessment. Questions related to seating and serving styles, eating utensils, and the importance of how much of food served is consumed may facilitate a greater understanding of the cultural diversity of food and eating.

When you work with individuals from other cultures, it is important to avoid **cultural stereotyping**: the tendency to view individuals of common cultural backgrounds similarly and according to a preconceived notion of how they "ought" to behave. Refer to topic-specific nutrition texts for detailed information about culture-specific diets and the nutritional value of ethnic foods.

Cultural food preferences are often interrelated with religious dietary beliefs and practices. Many religious customs involve foods as symbols in celebrations and rituals. Knowing how an individual's religious practices relate to food and eating may enable you to suggest modifications that do not conflict with their customs.

PURPOSES AND COMPONENTS OF NUTRITIONAL ASSESSMENT

Nutrition assessment is a method of collecting and evaluating data to make decisions about a nutrition-related concern or diagnosis. Best practice guidelines suggest that assessment data be compared to evidence-informed standards for evaluation. Nutrition assessment initiates the data-collection process, which provides the framework for nutrition monitoring and evaluation. Nutrition assessment includes subjective data such as medical history; symptoms; dietary intake; psychosocial, behavioural, and functional factors; food and nutrition knowledge; readiness for potential change; and objective data, including anthropometric measurements and biochemical measurements.

Nurses, as part of the multidisciplinary health care team, often initiate the nutrition assessment on admission or with the first clinic visit. The nurse's evaluation and interpretation of the subjective and objective data collected are essential in determining next steps in the nutrition care plan. Individuals identified as being at nutritional risk can be referred to members of the health care team, including the physiotherapist, occupational therapist, speech-language pathologist, and dietitian. Each of these health care providers plays an important role in the comprehensive care of patients.

> ### BOX 12.1 Recommendations for the Best Nutritional Care
>
> 1. Make standardized screening protocols mandatory in hospitals in Canada
> 2. Include an interdisciplinary team in the nutrition care process that starts with nutrition screening, then continues with subjective global assessment and a full nutrition assessment and development of a nutrition care plan by a Registered Dietitian
> 3. Ensure staff (nursing and food/nutrition services) provides patient-focused and protected nutrition through mealtime care that is consistent with the nutrition care plan
> 4. Establish a national standard for menu planning to ensure quality food is provided in hospitals and requires that food services staff provide adequate nutrients to meet the needs of diverse patients, as indicated in their nutrition care plans
> 5. Educate hospital administrators, physicians, nurses, and allied health professionals on the need to integrate nutrition care as part of quality interdisciplinary practice
> 6. Use oral nutrition supplementation, enteral nutrition and parenteral nutrition effectively to prevent and/or treat malnutrition

Based on Canadian Malnutrition Task Force. (2018). *Malnutrition overview.* Retrieved from http://www.nutritioncareincanada.ca/resources/malnutrition-overview.

The purposes of a nutritional assessment are to (a) identify individual nutritional requirements, (b) provide information for designing a nutrition plan of care that will optimize nutrition and meet individual nutrient requirements, and (c) establish baseline data for evaluating the efficacy of nutritional care. Recommendations for the best nutritional care appear in Box 12.1.

Nutrition screening, the first step in assessing nutritional status, can be completed in any setting (e.g., clinic, home, hospital, long-term care facilities). Based on readily obtained data, nutrition screening is an efficient way to identify individuals at nutrition risk, including those who have experienced unintentional weight loss, inadequate food intake, or recent illness. Parameters used for nutrition screening include weight and weight history, diet information, medical history, and routine laboratory data. The Canadian Nutrition Screening Tool (CNST) was rigorously validated and tested for reliability in Canadian hospitals (Fig. 12.2). The tool can be completed at the bedside and does not require any special tools or training.[22]

Assessing Nutritional Intake

Individuals identified as at nutritional risk during screening should be referred, when possible, to a dietitian to undergo a **comprehensive nutritional assessment**, which includes evaluation of dietary history and clinical information, a physical examination, and anthropometric measures.

Various methods for collecting current dietary intake information are available, including the 24-hour recall, the food frequency questionnaire, and the food diary.

Identify patients who are at risk for malnutrition

Ask the patient the following questions*	Date: Admission		Date: Rescreening	
	Yes	No	Yes	No
Have you lost weight in the past 6 months **WITHOUT TRYING** to lose this weight? If the patient reports a weight loss but gained it back, consider it as NO weight loss.				
Have you been eating less than usual **FOR MORE THAN A WEEK**?				
Two "YES" answers indicate nutrition risk†				

* If the patient is unable to answer the questions, a knowledgeable informant can be used to obtain the information. If the patient is uncertain regarding weight loss, ask if clothing is now fitting more loosely.

12.2 Canadian Nutrition Screening Tool (CNST).

Documentation of nutritional intake for hospitalized patients can best be achieved through calorie counts of nutrients consumed or infused.

The 24-Hour Recall

The most common method of obtaining information about dietary intake is the **24-hour recall**. The individual or family member is asked to recall everything eaten within the past 24 hours. It is important to be aware of potential information gaps when this method is used: (a) The individual or family member may not be able to recall type or amount of food eaten; (b) intake within the past 24 hours may be atypical of usual intake; (c) the individual or family member may alter information provided, for a variety of reasons; and (d) snack items and use of condiments may be under-reported.

The Food Frequency Questionnaire

To counter some of the challenges inherent in the 24-hour recall method, a **food frequency questionnaire** may also be completed. The information collected is related to how many times per day, week, or month an individual eats particular foods. The food frequency questionnaire does not quantify amount of food eaten, and, like the 24-hour recall, it relies on the individual's or family member's memory.

The Food Diary

In **food diaries**, the individual or family member records everything consumed for a certain period of time. Three days—two working days and one nonworking day—are often suggested. A food diary is most accurate when the individual records information immediately after eating. Potential challenges with the food diary include (a) nonadherence,

(b) inaccurate recording, (c) atypical intake on the recording days, and (d) conscious alteration of diet during the recording period. Increasingly, mobile devices and applications are being used to assess and monitor intake, including taking photos of meals and tracking weight changes and dietary adherence. Because these technologies are relatively new, their validity is as yet unclear.[23]

Direct Observation

Direct observation of the feeding and eating process can lead to detection of problems not readily identified through standard nutrition interviews. For example, observing the typical feeding techniques used by a parent or caregiver and the interaction between the individual and caregiver can be of value in assessing failure to thrive in children or unintentional weight loss in older adults.

Canada's Food Guide and the Dietary Reference Intakes

Eating Well With Canada's Food Guide[7] and the Dietary Reference Intakes (DRIs) are two tools commonly used to evaluate diet quality. Refer *to Eating Well With Canada's Food Guide* (see Fig. 12.1 or the guide online) for additional information and interactive tools ("My Food Guide") that allow you and your patients to personalize the information found in the guide.

The DRIs include four nutrient-based reference values that are used to assess and plan diets for healthy individuals (Table 12.1). The reference values include (a) the estimated average requirement, (b) the recommended dietary allowance, (c) the adequate intake, and (d) the tolerable upper

TABLE 12.1	Maintaining Healthy Eating Habits

Eating well and being active work together to promote health and well-being and provide benefits such as the following:

- Better overall health
- Lower risk for disease
- A healthy body weight
- Feeling and looking better
- More energy
- Stronger muscles and bones

Steps toward better health and a healthy body weight include the following:

- Eating the recommended amount and types of food each day
- Limiting foods and beverages high in calories, fat, sugar or salt (sodium)
- Being active every day

Following *Eating Well With Canada's Food Guide* will help people do the following:

- Meet their needs for vitamins, minerals, and other nutrients
- Reduce their risk for obesity, type 2 diabetes, heart disease, certain types of cancer, and osteoporosis
- Contribute to their overall health and vitality

Adapted from Health Canada. (2016). *Maintaining healthy habits.* Retrieved from http://www.hc-sc.gc.ca/fn-an/food-guide-aliment/maintain-adopt/index-eng.php; and Health Canada. (2016). *Eating well With Canada's Food Guide.* Retrieved from http://www.hc-sc.gc.ca/fn-an/food-guide-aliment/index-eng.php.

Nutrition Facts
Valeur nutritive

Per 125 mL (87 g) / par 125 mL (87 g)

Amount / Teneur	% Daily Value / % valeur quotidienne
Calories / Calories 80	
Fat / Lipides 0.5 g	1%
Saturated / saturés 0g + Trans / trans 0g	0%
Cholesterol / Cholestérol 0 mg	
Sodium / Sodium 0 mg	0%
Carbohydrate / Glucides 18 g	6%
Fibre / Fibres 2 g	8%
Sugars / Sucres 2 g	
Protein / Protéines 3 g	
Vitamin A / Vitamine A	2%
Vitamin C / Vitamine C	10%
Calcium / Calcium	0%
Iron / Fer	2%

12.3 Nutrition Facts table.

intake level.[24] The DRIs are intended to help individuals optimize their health, prevent disease, and avoid overconsumption of any single nutrient.

The DRIs are designed for health maintenance and disease prevention in healthy individuals. They are not meant for the restoration of health or repletion of nutrients. Under the stress of an acute or chronic condition, an individual may have nutrient needs that are outside of the DRIs. Dietitians can design individualized, therapeutic diets that consider nutrient requirements imposed by acute conditions (burns, surgery) and chronic conditions (diabetes, obesity).

There is considerable scientific and public interest in the use of vitamin supplements for the prevention and management of acute and chronic conditions. Although no nutrient in supplement form can replace a healthy, well-balanced diet, evidence suggests that some supplements are beneficial (e.g., vitamin D). Use caution when you recommend any vitamin or mineral supplement, to ensure that intakes do not exceed tolerable upper intake levels and that there

are no nutrient–medication interactions. Referral to a dietitian may be warranted for patients using multiple nutrient supplements.

Nutrition Labelling in Canada

Nutrition labelling in Canada became mandatory for most prepackaged foods in 2007. Nutrition labelling regulations have been designed to convey information about the nutrient content of food in a standardized format, which allows for comparison among foods. The Nutrition Facts table provides information on energy (calories) and 13 nutrients, based on a stated serving size. The Nutrition Facts table must appear on the label in the prescribed manner. Clear, uniform information can support consumers in making informed food choices to achieve healthy eating goals.[25]

The sample bilingual Nutrition Facts table shown in Fig. 12.3 indicates the core information that must always be included and the order in which it must be presented. Additional nutrition information may also be required in the table or permitted either inside or outside the table, as prescribed.

The percent daily value (%DV) on a nutrition label reflects the needs of a healthy individual who consumes 2 000 to 2 500 calories daily. The %DV is used to express the food's content of nutrients, rather than just serving as a weight measure. The %DV can be used to make comparisons among foods. Refer to UnlockFood.ca (see the section Links to Nutrition Information) for additional information and interactive tools on nutrition labelling.[26]

SUBJECTIVE DATA

When completing a nutrition assessment, the nurse (or other health care provider), must recognize and acknowledge the patient's positive self-management behaviours, such as physical activity, blood glucose monitoring, and nutrition label reading. Rapport and open communication are essential for positive outcomes.

The following list presents potential areas of focus for subjective data collection in a nutrition assessment:

1. Eating patterns
2. Usual weight, recent weight changes
3. Changes in appetite, taste, smell, chewing, swallowing
4. Recent surgery, trauma, burns, infection
5. Chronic conditions

6. Nausea, vomiting, diarrhea, constipation
7. Food allergies or intolerances
8. Medications, nutritional supplements, herbal supplements
9. Self-management behaviours; access to healthy foods
10. Tobacco, alcohol, illegal drug use

11. Exercise and activity patterns
12. Family history
13. Psychological symptoms
14. Physical impairments that limit ability to independently consume foods or liquids

HEALTH HISTORY QUESTIONS

Examiner Asks	Rationale
1. Eating patterns. Number of meals and snacks per day? • Type and amount of food eaten? • Fad, special, or alternative diets? • Where is food eaten? • Food preferences and dislikes? • Religious or cultural considerations? • Usual food preparation methods? • Able to feed self?	Individuals eating fewer than three meals a day may not meet energy or nutrient requirements. Diets that restrict or eliminate entire categories of food are not recommended or supported by data. Ethnicity and religious beliefs, or feeding difficulties, may affect intake of certain foods. Include questions related to food type (e.g., light or low-fat foods); the addition of condiments, salt, or other seasonings; and an estimation of portion sizes and additional servings at meals.
2. Usual weight, recent weight changes. What is your usual weight? • Recent weight change? • How much lost or gained? • Over what time period? • Reason for loss or gain?	Unintentional weight loss and obesity increase nutritional risk. Underweight individuals are vulnerable because their nutrient and energy reserves may be depleted. Obesity increases risk for chronic diseases, including hypertension, type 2 diabetes, and cancer. Protein and calorie needs should not be overlooked in acutely ill, obese individuals. Rapid weight gain over a short period of time may be an indication of a change in fluid status (e.g., edema). It is important to recognize that individuals with obesity can be malnourished and present with unintentional weight loss. Avoid weight bias in nutrition assessment.
3. Changes in appetite, taste, smell, chewing, swallowing. Type of change? • When did change occur? • Any medical conditions and or medications associated with changes?	Poor appetite, alterations in taste and smell, and difficulties in chewing and swallowing can interfere with adequate nutrient intake and increase nutritional risk. Medication adverse effects can lead to changes in taste and appetite. Some medications necessitate alterations in meal timing or the avoidance of specific foods.

Examiner Asks	Rationale
4. Recent surgery, trauma, burns, infection. When did it happen? • Type? • How treated? • Conditions that increase nutrient loss (e.g., draining wounds, effusions, blood loss, dialysis, infection)?	With surgery, trauma, and sepsis, energy and nutrient needs may increase to two or three times greater than normal.
5. Chronic conditions. Type? • When diagnosed? • How managed? • Dietary modifications? • Recent cancer chemotherapy or radiation therapy?	Chronic conditions—including obesity, diabetes, metabolic syndrome, and hypertension—can increase nutrition risk as a result of the combined effects of dietary changes and medication use. Treatment related to cancer (radiation therapy, chemotherapy) can lead to nutrition-related adverse effects, gastro-intestinal (GI) effects, taste changes, loss of appetite, weight loss, etc.
6. Nausea, vomiting, diarrhea, constipation. What was the cause? • How long? • Medication use?	GI symptoms such as nausea, vomiting, diarrhea, and constipation may interfere with nutrient intake or absorption. Many medications interfere with normal GI function. Include a review of prescription and nonprescription medication use. Include a review about any other conditions that lead to GI adverse effects, including recent or chronic antibiotic use.
7. Food allergies or intolerances. Any problematic foods? • Type of reaction? • How long? • How treated/managed? • Related weight changes? • Medication use?	Intolerances related to the inability to digest specific foods, such as lactose in milk products, may result in GI symptoms (i.e., gas, bloating, diarrhea) and lead to nutrient deficiencies. Multiple food allergies or intolerances can lead to the necessary avoidance of many foods. This can result in a nutrient-deficient diet. Referral to a dietitian is warranted in cases of multiple food allergies or intolerances. Not all food intolerances have overt symptoms—a common diagnostic feature of nonceliac gluten sensitivity/celiac disease is iron deficiency. Not all patients present with GI symptoms.
8. Medications, nutritional supplements, herbal supplements. Prescription medications? • Nonprescription medications? • Use over a 24-hour period?	Analgesics, antacids, anticonvulsants, antibiotics, diuretics, laxatives, antineoplastic medications, steroids, and oral contraceptives are among the medications that can interact with nutrients, impairing their digestion, absorption, metabolism, or utilization.

Subjective Data

Examiner Asks	Rationale
• Type of vitamin or mineral supplement? Amount? Frequency and duration of use? • Herbal and botanical products? Probiotic use? Specific type and brand and where obtained? How often used? How does it help you? Any problems? • Recommended by whom, and for what reason?	Vitamin and mineral supplements may be harmful when taken in large amounts. Use of herbal and botanical supplements is commonly under-reported. Discuss use and potential adverse effects, including medication and/or nutrient interactions. Refer to the Natural and Non-prescription Health Products Directorate (NNHPD) website: https://www.canada.ca/en/health-canada/corporate/about-health-canada/branches-agencies/health-products-food-branch/natural-non-prescription-health-products-directorate.html.
9. **Self-management behaviours; access to healthy foods**. Meal preparation facilities? • Transportation for travel to market? • Adequate income for food purchase? • Who prepares meals and does shopping? • Environment during mealtimes? • Current knowledge about healthy eating, label reading?	Socioeconomic factors may interfere with ingestion of adequate amounts of food and nutrients. Food/nutrition literacy (separate from financial status) is an independent risk factor for poor nutrient intake, especially in new immigrants, or those with limited education. Distractions such as television or video games during meals may result in increased energy intake, potentially leading to weight gain.
10. **Tobacco, alcohol, illegal drug use**. When was your last drink of alcohol? • Amount taken that episode? • Amount/type of alcohol each day? Each week? • Duration of use? • Use of other beverages with alcohol (i.e., mixed drinks)? • Use of tobacco products: type, how long, quantity, attempts to quit? (Repeat questions for each substance used.)	These agents are often substituted for nutritious foods and increase requirements for some nutrients. Pregnant women who use tobacco products, drink alcohol, or use illegal drugs give birth to a disproportionate number of infants with low birth weights, failure to thrive, and other serious complications.
11. **Exercise and activity patterns**. Amount? • Type? • Frequency/duration? • Any exercise-related injuries?	Energy and nutrient needs increase with increased physical activity, especially in individuals who participate in competitive sports or perform manual labour. Inactive or sedentary lifestyles increases risk for a number of chronic illnesses.
12. **Family history**. What is your family or personal history of heart disease, osteoporosis, cancer, gout, GI disorders, obesity, or diabetes? • Effect of each on eating patterns? • Effect on activity patterns?	Long-term nutritional deficiencies or excesses may become apparent only when a chronic condition is diagnosed (i.e., calcium and vitamin D deficiency associated with osteoporosis). Early identification of dietary deficits allows for food and activity modifications to be implemented promptly, at a time when the body may recover more fully.

Examiner Asks	Rationale
13. Psychological symptoms. Depression or other mood-altering illness? • Medications that affect mood? • Psychosocial lifestyle factors? • Disordered eating behaviours?	Psychological illness can affect the ability to access and prepare food. Mood can affect food choices and amount of food eaten. Stress, work, and home life issues may also affect eating. Individuals with a history of dieting may be at greater risk for disordered eating behaviours. Distorted body image may increase the risk for eating disorders. Refer individuals with suspected disordered eating to a dietitian.
14. Physical impairments that limit ability to independently consume foods or liquids. Do you have challenges that limit the ability to independently consume foods or liquids? • Chewing or swallowing concerns? • Dentures, dentition, broken or missing teeth?	Conditions that affect coordination (Parkinson's disease) and chewing or swallowing (stroke, dementia) can significantly affect the ability to safely consume a healthy diet. Referral to other members of the health care team—including the speech-language pathologist, occupational therapist, dentist, and dietitian—may be warranted for such patients.

Additional History for Infants and Children

Dietary histories of infants and children are generally obtained from the child's parents or guardian. Asking caregivers to keep a thorough daily food diary and occasionally requesting 24-hour recalls during clinic visits are the most commonly employed techniques for this population group.

Nutrition assessment in infants and children include questions related to feeding (i.e., by whom), use of solid foods, and frequency and type of snacks. Inquire about beverage intake (i.e., milk versus fruit juices) and use of sweetened versus unsweetened foods and beverages. Review food preferences in children, to ensure there is a variety of foods from each food group being consumed on a daily basis.

Regular meal and snack times with few distractions are ideal to promote healthy eating habits and healthy weights in children.

Examiner Asks	Rationale
1. Gestational nutrition. Maternal history of alcohol or illegal medication use? • Maternal weight gain during pregnancy? • Any diet-related complications during gestation (i.e., hyperemesis, food avoidances, etc.)? • Infant's birth weight? • Any evidence of delayed physical or mental growth?	Low birth weight (<2 500 g) is a risk factor in infant morbidity and mortality. Poor gestational nutrition, low maternal weight gain, and maternal alcohol and drug use—all factors in low birth weight—can lead to birth defects and delayed growth and development. Excess weight gain in pregnancy increases risk for a high-birth-weight (<4 500 g) infant, prolonged labour, birth trauma, and Caesarean birth.

Subjective Data

Subjective Data

2. Infant nutrition. Type, frequency, amount, and duration of feeding?
- Any difficulties encountered?
- Timing and method of weaning?

New mothers may experience challenges with breastfeeding or formula feeding or have questions about infant nutrition, the introduction of solid foods, and rate of infant weight gain.

Assess for breast versus formula feeding; assess for alternate milk sources in relation to infant's age. Inquire about Vitamin D supplements in breastfed infants. Assess for introduction of iron-rich foods.

3. Child nutrition. Any special likes or dislikes?
- How much will child eat?
- How do you manage non-nutritious snack foods?
- How do you avoid food aspiration?

Use of small portions, finger foods, simple meals, and nutritious snacks are strategies to improve dietary intake. Avoid foods likely to be aspirated (e.g., hot dogs, nuts, grapes, round candies, popcorn).

Assess for family meals, meal distractions, eating environment (i.e., eating at a table).

Additional History for Adolescents

1. Weight. What would you like to weigh?
- How do you feel about your present weight?
- On any special diet to lose weight?
- Constantly think about "feeling fat"?
- Intentionally vomit or use laxatives or diuretics after eating?

Weight gain, particularly in adolescents, may precipitate dieting and decreased nutrient intake. Because of adolescents' increased body awareness and self-consciousness, they are at increased risk for eating disorders.

Eating disorders are complex psychiatric disorders strongly associated with other mental illness. Referrals to the social worker, psychologist or psychiatrist, and dietitian are warranted in suspected eating disorder cases.

Body weight is not a reliable indicator of the presence or absence of disordered eating. Assess other psychosocial factors.

2. Use of anabolic steroids or other agents to increase muscle size and physical performance. When? Why?
- How much?
- Prescribed by whom?

The use of anabolic steroids and other performance-enhancing agents now extends to junior-high, high-school, and postsecondary males and females. Adverse effects include personality disorders (aggressiveness), and liver and other organ damage.

- Use of caffeinated, energy-boosting drinks? When? Type? Duration?

Energy-boosting drinks contain large amounts of caffeine, other stimulants, or herbal products. Adverse effects include dehydration, dangerously high blood pressure and heart rate, and sleep problems.

3. Overweight and obesity risk factors. What snacks or fast foods do you like to eat?
- When?
- How much?

An accurate dietary history includes between-meal snacks and meals eaten away from home.

Examiner Asks	Rationale
4. Age first started menstruating. What is your menstrual flow like?	Menarche may be delayed in adolescents who are underweight, have very low body fat, or are elite athletes. Scant menstrual flow is associated with nutritional inadequacies.

Additional History for Pregnant Women

1. Number of pregnancies. How many times have you been pregnant?
- When?/Age at first (and subsequent) pregnancies?
- Any problems encountered during previous pregnancies?
- Problems this pregnancy?
- Use of vitamin/mineral/herbal supplements?
- Use of tobacco products?
- Caffeine intake?
- Fish intake?

A multiparous mother with pregnancies occurring less than 1 year apart has an increased risk for depleted nutritional reserves. Note previous complications of pregnancy (excessive vomiting, anemia, or gestational diabetes). Slower GI motility and pressure from the fetus may cause constipation, hemorrhoids, and indigestion. A history of a low-birth-weight infant suggests past nutritional problems. Giving birth to an infant weighing 4500 g (10 lb) or more may signal *latent* diabetes in the mother.

Assess for consumption of fish known to be high in mercury.

2. Food preferences when pregnant. What foods do you avoid?
- Crave any particular foods?

The expectant mother is vulnerable to familial, cultural, and traditional influences for food choices. Cravings for, or aversions to, particular foods are common; evaluate for their potential contribution to, or interference with, dietary intake.

Additional History for Older Adults

1. Diet differences. Has your diet changed in the past year or more?
- How?
- Why?
- What factors affect the way you eat?

Note any physiological, psychological, or socioeconomic changes that may affect nutritional status. Note use of vitamin supplements (specifically, vitamin D).

Subjective Data

Objective Data

OBJECTIVE DATA

PREPARATION

An individual's general appearance—obese, cachectic (fat and muscle wasting), or edematous—can provide clues to overall nutritional status. More specific clinical signs and symptoms suggestive of nutritional deficiencies can be detected through a physical examination and laboratory testing. Laboratory tests for assessment of nutritional status are reviewed later in this chapter.

EQUIPMENT NEEDED

Measurement tape
Pen or pencil
Nutritional assessment data form
Canadian Nutrition Screening Tool (CNST) (see Fig. 12.2)

Normal Range of Findings

Abnormal Findings

Anthropomorphic Measures

Anthropometry is the measurement and evaluation of growth, development, and body composition. The most commonly used anthropometric measures are height, weight, waist–hip ratio, and waist circumference. Measurement of height, weight, and head circumference are described in Chapter 10.

A healthy body weight promotes general health and reduces the risk for some chronic diseases.

Normal Range of Findings	Abnormal Findings

Derived Weight Measures

Two derived weight measures are used to assess changes in body weight. The **percent usual body weight** is calculated as follows:

$$\text{Percent usual body weight} = \frac{\text{Current weight}}{\text{Usual weight}} \times 100$$

Recent weight change is calculated with the following formula:

$$\text{Weight change} = \frac{\text{Usual weight} - \text{Current weight}}{\text{Usual weight}} \times 100$$

A current weight of 85–95% of usual body weight indicates mild malnutrition; 75–84%, moderate malnutrition; and <75%, severe malnutrition.

An unintentional loss of more than 5% of body weight over 1 month, more than 7.5% of body weight over 3 months, or more than 10% of body weight over 6 months is clinically significant.

Body Mass Index

Body mass index (BMI) provides a practical marker of optimal weight for height and an indicator of obesity (see Fig. 10.3, p. 157). It is calculated as follows:

$$\text{BMI} = \frac{\text{Weight (in kilograms)}}{\text{Height (in metres)}^2}$$

$$Or$$

$$\frac{\text{Weight (in pounds)}}{\text{Height (in inches)}^2} \times 703$$

BMI interpretation for adults:[27]

<18.5	Underweight
18.5–24.9	Normal weight
25.0–29.9	Overweight
30.0–39.9	Obesity
≥40	Extreme obesity

BMI interpretation for children aged 2 to 20 years[28] is as follows:

85th to 95th percentiles = risk for overweight

Waist–Hip Ratio

The waist–hip ratio reflects body fat distribution as an indicator of health risk. Obese individuals with a greater proportion of fat in the upper body, especially in the abdomen, have android obesity; obese individuals with most of their fat in the hips and thighs have gynoid obesity. Waist–hip ratio is calculated as follows:

$$\text{Waist} - \text{hip ratio} = \frac{\text{Waist circumference}}{\text{Hip circumferance}}$$

where waist circumference is measured in inches at the smallest circumference below the rib cage and above the umbilicus, and hip circumference is measured in inches at the largest circumference of the buttocks. **Waist circumference** alone can be used to predict increased health risk.

A waist–hip ratio of 1.0 or more in men or 0.8 or more in women is indicative of android (upper body obesity) and increasing risk for obesity-related diseases and early mortality.

A waist circumference exceeding 89 cm (35 in) in women and exceeding 102 cm (40 in) in men increases risk for cardiovascular and metabolic diseases.

❖ DEVELOPMENTAL CONSIDERATIONS

Infants, Children, and Adolescents

Weight. Because longitudinal growth is one of the best indices of nutritional status over time, height and weight should be measured at regular intervals during infancy, childhood, and adolescence. See Chapter 10 for techniques.

Pregnant Women

Weight. Measure weight monthly up to 30 weeks of pregnancy and then every 2 weeks until the last month of pregnancy, at which point weight should be measured weekly.

Consider the expectant mother at nutritional risk if her pre-pregnancy weight was 10% or more below, or 20% or more above, ideal weight.

Normal Range of Findings	Abnormal Findings

Older Adults

Height. Height in men and women declines gradually from the early 30s, which results in an overall loss of height of 2.9 cm in men and 4.9 cm in women.[29,30] Height measures may not be accurate in individuals confined to a bed or wheelchair or in patients with osteoporosis.

Alternative methods for height measurement can be used for patients unable to stand; these methods include knee height, forearm length, and arm span.[31]

Laboratory Studies

Routine laboratory tests can detect preclinical nutritional deficiencies and can be used to confirm or support subjective findings. With older adults, however, use caution in interpreting test results that are outside normal ranges because they may not always indicate a nutritional problem, inasmuch as laboratory standards for older adults have not been firmly established.

Laboratory indicators of nutritional status include hemoglobin, hematocrit, ferritin, cholesterol, triglycerides, total lymphocyte count, and serum albumin measurements. Glucose, low- and high-density lipoproteins, prealbumin, transferrin, and total protein levels also provide meaningful information.

Hemoglobin. Hemoglobin determination is used to detect iron deficiency anemia. Normal values are as follows:

Infants aged 1 to 3 days: 145–225 g/L

Infants aged 2 months: 90–140 g/L

Children aged 6 to 12 years: 115–155 g/L

Male adults: 135–180 g/L

Female adults: 120–160 g/L

Elevated hemoglobin levels suggest hemoconcentration as a result of polycythemia vera or dehydration.

Decreased hemoglobin levels may indicate anemia, recent hemorrhage, or hemodilution caused by fluid retention.

Hematocrit. Hematocrit is a measure of cell volume, as well as an indicator of iron status. Normal values are as follows:

Infants aged 1 to 3 days: 0.44–0.72

Infants aged 2 months: 0.28–0.42

Children aged 6 to 12 years: 0.35–0.45

Male adults: 0.4–0.54

Female adults: 0.38–0.47

Decreased hematocrit indicates insufficient hemoglobin formation. Hematocrit and hemoglobin values should be interpreted together.

Cholesterol. Total cholesterol is measured to evaluate risk for cardiovascular disease. Normal cholesterol concentration is less than 5.2 mmol/L.

Risk for coronary artery disease increases with increasing serum cholesterol level.

Triglycerides. Serum triglycerides are used to screen for dyslipidemia and to determine the risk for coronary artery disease. Normal range is less than 1.7 mmol/L.

Blood Glucose Monitoring. Early identification of prediabetes or diabetes significantly reducing the risk for diabetes-related complications. Screening for type 2 diabetes should be performed every 3 years in individuals older than 40 and more frequently in anyone with one or more risk factor. See https://www.diabetes.ca/about-diabetes/risk-factors/are-you-at-risk for the list of risk factors. Risk can also be assessed by completing the Canadian Diabetes Risk Questionnaire (CANRISK) at http://www.diabetes.ca/take-the-test/.

Glycemic targets to reduce macrovascular complications include a glycated hemoglobin (A_{1C}) value of ≤7.0%.[32]

The Diabetes Canada *Clinical Practice Guidelines* (see the section Links to Nutrition Information at the end of this chapter) contain more detailed information.

Higher serum triglyceride levels are also associated with coronary artery disease.

Diabetes diagnosis criteria are as follows:

FPG ≥7.0 mmol/L (Fasting = no caloric intake for at least 8 hours) or

A_{1C} ≥6.5% (in adults) or

2hPG in a 75 g OGTT ≥11.1 mmol/L or

Random PG ≥11.1 mmol/L (Random = any time of the day, without regard for the interval since the last meal)

All patients with diabetes should be offered timely diabetes education that enhances self-care and behaviours including cognitive-behavioural educational interventions, such as problem solving, goal setting, and self-monitoring of health parameters.[32]

Objective Data

Normal Range of Findings

Total Lymphocyte Count. Tests of immune function include total lymphocyte count (TLC) and skin testing (also called *delayed cutaneous hypersensitivity testing*). TLC is an important indicator of visceral protein status and therefore of cellular immune function. It is an indirect marker of protein-energy malnutrition.

The TLC is derived from the white blood cell (WBC) count and the differential count:

$$\text{TLC} = \text{WBC count} \times \frac{\text{Number of lymphocytes in differential}}{100 \text{ cells}}$$

where TLC is calculated in cells per cubic millimetre.

Normal values for all age categories are between 1 000 and 4 000 cells/mm^3.

Serum Proteins. **Serum albumin** is a measurement of visceral protein status. Because of its relatively long half-life (17 to 20 days) and large body pool (4.0–5.0 g/kg), albumin is not an early indicator of protein malnutrition. Normal serum albumin concentration in infants, in children older than 6 months, and in adults ranges from 35–50 g/L.

Serum transferrin, an iron-transport protein, can be measured directly or by an indirect measurement of total iron-binding capacity. Serum transferrin, which has a half-life of 8 to 10 days, may be a more sensitive indicator of visceral protein status than is albumin.

The normal values for serum transferrin are 1.90–3.35 g/L.

Prealbumin, or thyroxine-binding prealbumin, serves as a transport protein for thyroxine (T_4) and retinol-binding protein. Because its half-life is shorter (48 hours) than that of either albumin or transferrin, prealbumin is sensitive to acute changes in protein status and sudden demands on protein synthesis. Normal prealbumin levels range from 1.5–2.5 g/L.

Nitrogen Balance. Nitrogen balance is also used as an index of protein nutritional status. Nitrogen is released with the catabolism of amino acids and is excreted in the urine as urea. Nitrogen balance therefore indicates whether the person is anabolic (positive nitrogen balance) or catabolic (negative nitrogen balance).

Nitrogen balance is estimated by a formula based on urine urea nitrogen (UUN) excreted during the previous 24 hours:

$$\text{Nitrogen balance} = \text{Nitrogen intake} - \text{Nitrogen excretion}$$
$$= \text{Protein intake}/6.25 - (\text{24-hour UUN} + 4)$$

where nitrogen balance is determined in grams; 24-hour UUN = UUN, measured in grams; and 4 = non-urea nitrogen losses via feces, skin, sweat, and lungs, measured in grams.

❖ DEVELOPMENTAL CONSIDERATIONS

In infancy and childhood, laboratory tests are performed only when undernutrition is suspected or if the child has acute or chronic conditions that affect nutritional status.

Abnormal Findings

Non-nutritional factors that affect TLC include hypoalbuminemia, metabolic stress (e.g., major surgery, trauma, sepsis), infection, cancer, and chronic diseases.

Lymphopenia is a decrease in circulating lymphocytes.

Lymphocytosis is an increase in circulating lymphocytes.

Serum albumin levels are low with protein-calorie malnutrition, altered hydration status, and decreased liver function.

A serum albumin level of 28–35 g/L represents moderate visceral protein depletion, and a level lower than 28 g/L denotes severe depletion.[33]

Levels of 1.5–1.7 g/L suggest mild protein deficiency; 1.0–1.5 g/L, moderate deficiency; and levels less than 1.0 g/L, severe deficiency.[34] Because many clinical conditions can alter serum albumin and transferrin levels, consider the person's history in conjunction with these values for accurate interpretation.

Prealbumin levels are elevated in renal disease and reduced by surgery, trauma, burns, and infection. Prealbumin levels of 1.0–1.5 g/L indicate mild depletion; 0.5–1.0 g/L, moderate depletion; and less than 0.5 g/L, severe depletion.

In response to stress and increased protein demand, the body rapidly mobilizes its protein compartments, which results in increased production of urea and excretion of urea in the urine. With infection, an estimated loss of 9–11 g of UUN per day can be expected. In patients with major burns, 8–12 g of urea nitrogen per day may be expected in the urine.[35]

| **Normal Range of Findings** | **Abnormal Findings** |

During adolescence, unless overt disease is suspected, laboratory evaluation of hemoglobin and hematocrit levels and urinalysis for glucose and protein levels are generally considered adequate for assessment of nutritional status.

During pregnancy, hemoglobin and hematocrit values can be used to detect deficiencies of protein, folacin, vitamin B_{12}, and iron. Urine is frequently tested for glucose and protein (albumin), which can signal diabetes, pre-eclampsia, and renal disease.

In older adulthood, all serum and urine data must be interpreted with an understanding of declining renal efficiency and a tendency for older adults to be overhydrated or underhydrated.

Serial Assessment

Nutritional status in malnourished patients or individuals at risk for malnutrition is monitored through serial measurements of nutritional assessment parameters made at routine intervals. At minimum, weight and dietary intake should be evaluated weekly. Because the other nutritional assessment parameters change more slowly, data on these indicators may be collected biweekly or monthly.

Health Promotion

Essentials of a healthy diet are (a) eating a variety of foods from all food groups to ensure nutrient adequacy; (b) consuming recommended amounts of fruits and vegetables, whole grains, and fat-free or lower-fat dairy products; (c) limiting intake of foods high in saturated fats, trans fats, added sugars, starch, cholesterol, salt, and alcohol; (d) matching calorie intake with calories expended; (e) engaging in 30 to 60 minutes of moderate physical activity most days; and (f) following food safety guidelines for handling, preparing, and storing foods. Canada's physical activity guidelines[36] (https://www.canada.ca/en/public-health/services/health-promotion/healthy-living/physical-activity.html) are designed to help individuals at specific life stages (i.e., children, youth, adults, older adults) make wise choices about physical activity. Research indicates that more than half of Canadian children and youth aged 6 to 19 are not active enough for optimal healthy growth and development.[36] The majority of Canadians are unaware that insufficient physical activity is a serious risk factor for premature death, chronic disease, and disability.[37] According to Health Canada, over 50% of Canadians are inactive.[38]

Approaches to weight loss for people who are overweight or obese must be individualized and reflect cultural sensitivity. They must also account for patients' readiness to lose weight and their health care and self-management behaviours. Weight loss programs involving fewer than 1 000–1 200 calories per day may not provide adequate nutrients. Healthy eating plans that include a balance of foods from all food groups, spread over three meals and two to three snacks, are recommended.

Patients should be discouraged from fad diets, diets that eliminate one or more food groups, and diets promoting weight loss in excess of 0.5–1.0 kg (1–2 lb) per week.

Objective Data

DOCUMENTATION AND CRITICAL THINKING

Sample Charting

SUBJECTIVE: GENERAL ASSESSMENT

No history of diseases or surgery that would alter intake or requirements; no recent weight changes; no appetite changes. Consumes regular meals and snacks, variety of food choices.

Financial resources adequate for healthy eating. No concerns about access to healthy food. Does not use tobacco products; drink alcohol; or use illegal, prescription, or over-the-counter medications. No vitamin/mineral or herbal supplements.

No food allergies or intolerances. Sedentary lifestyle; plays golf once per week.

OBJECTIVE

Dietary intake is adequate to meet protein and energy needs. No clinical signs of nutrient deficiencies (complete physical assessment). Height, weight, BMI, and screening laboratory test results within normal ranges.

Focused Assessment: Clinical Case Study

Namid Gladstone (N.G.) is a 46-year-old female and has type 2 diabetes. She lives at home, on-reserve with her common-law spouse. She has limited income and access to food. She grocery shops once a month; most of her food is package/canned; she has little access to fresh fruit and vegetables.

SUBJECTIVE

N.G. has been unable to access paid employment for over 1 year. Her spouse has recently been laid off from his job. Money is limited. This has led to increased stress, which has made N.G.'s diabetes harder to manage. N.G. has been trying to walk 5 to 7 days a week for 30 minutes to help manage her weight and diabetes.

OBJECTIVE

Inspection: slightly overweight female, looks older than stated age. Current weight: 71.6 kg (158 lb). Height: 162.5 cm (5 ft 4 in). Blood pressure (BP): 137/88 mm Hg. Current medications:

- Metformin (Glucophage): an antidiabetic medication, used to lower blood glucose levels
- Atorvastatin (Lipitor): HMG Co-A reductase inhibitor used to lower cholesterol levels
- Furosemide (Lasix): diuretic used to help lower BP levels
- Venlafaxine (Effexor): antidepressant

Most recent laboratory values:

Test	Result	Reference Range
A_{1C}	0.071	<0.07
FPG [fasting plasma glucose]	10.5 mmol/L	<7.0 mmol/L
LDL [low-density lipoprotein] cholesterol	3.8 mmol/L	<2.0 mmol/L
HDL [high-density lipoprotein] cholesterol	0.89 mmol/L	>1.3 mmol/L
Triglycerides	4.3 mmol/L	<1.7 mmol/L
Total cholesterol	6.6 mmol/L	<4.0 mmol/L

ASSESSMENT

Psychosocial: limited access to food, very limited availability of fresh fruit and vegetables; increased stress resulting from spouse's loss of job, limited income, recent need for social assistance; managing multiple medical concerns. Has started walking to manage weight and diabetes.

Weight: BMI = 27.1: above ideal weight

Laboratory values: elevated FBG, LDL, triglycerides. total cholesterol; low HDL level → increased risk for CVD [cardiovascular disease]

Medication review: appropriate

Diet review: challenges related to decreased income and limited food access, low fruit and vegetable intake, increased intake of processed meats, few whole grains

RECOMMENDATIONS

On this visit, the nurse can discuss a number of potential behaviour changes with N.G. Each of these suggested changes should be negotiated in relation to the planning and implementation of the change. Simply telling patients what they need to do or change has been shown to be ineffective in eliciting positive behaviour change.

Short-term nutritional advice for N.G. may include the following:

- Avoiding simple sugars found in fruit juices, regular soft drinks, and other sweetened beverages. Encouraging water as a primary beverage, in addition to low-fat milk, when available, or using skim milk powder.
- Following guidelines on meal planning and portion control, available from the Diabetes Canada and Health Canada's Aboriginal Diabetes Initiative.[39,40]
- Eating more fruits and vegetables: recommend frozen vegetables and canned (in juice) fruit because they are often more economical and more available.
- Eating lean meats and low-fat dairy products (skim milk, low-fat cheese, and yogourt); using low-fat cooking methods (baking, broiling); and avoiding added salt.
- Continuing positive self-management behaviours (walking).

N.G. should continue to be monitored for BP, blood work, and psychosocial support.

Formal diabetes education is important. However, in remote communities, formal diabetes education may not be readily accessible. Consider initiatives such as Telehealth and video conferencing; investigate local Indigenous diabetes initiatives, such as the Indigenous Diabetes Health Circle (http://soadi.ca).

ABNORMAL FINDINGS

MANAGEMENT OF CHRONIC DISEASE

Obesity

Obesity has been described as a global epidemic. It has been linked to diabetes, hypertension, cardiovascular disease, and some forms of cancer.

Obese individuals more commonly suffer from chronic conditions—including hypertension, diabetes, and heart disease—than do people who are at a healthy weight. Research indicates that more than 70% of obese individuals suffer from at least one other major health problem.

Central Obesity

Even more significant than total body fat is the type and location of fat. Body fat that collects deep within the central abdominal area of the body, called *visceral fat*, is associated with increased risk for diabetes, stroke, hypertension, and cardiovascular disease. The risk for death from all causes may be higher in people with central obesity than in those whose fat accumulates elsewhere in the body. Central obesity can be assessed using the waist–hip ratio and waist circumference (see Chapter 10).

Awareness of the social and economic factors leading to obesity is essential when you complete nutritional screening of patients. Obesity is a complex problem with genetic, environmental, and psychological components. Sensitivity to each of these factors and ensuring that all education is tailored to the individual patient may lead to more positive outcomes.

Diabetes

Diabetes, a chronic condition characterized by elevated blood glucose levels, often leads to other diseases or contributes to their development. The number of people worldwide with diabetes has risen from 108 million in 1980 to 422 million in 2014. The global prevalence of diabetes among adults over 18 years of age has risen from 4.7% in 1980 to 8.5% in 2014.[41] In 2015, diagnosed diabetes affected an estimated 8.9% (3.34 million) of the Canadian population, leading to $3 billion in direct health care costs. In the next 10 years, both prevalence and direct health care costs are projected to grow by over 40%.[42] An aging population, increasing immigration from high-risk populations, and the growth of the Indigenous population will increase the burden of diabetes before 2025. People with diabetes are over 3 times more likely to be hospitalized with cardiovascular disease, 12 times more likely to be hospitalized with end-stage renal disease, and over 20 times more likely to be hospitalized for a nontraumatic lower limb amputation compared with the general population.[42]

Screening for Type 2 Diabetes

It is estimated that 1 in 10 deaths in Canada can be attributed to diabetes.[42] Approximately 1 million Canadians currently have diabetes and have not been diagnosed.[43] Tests for hyperglycemia can identify individuals who may have or be at risk for preventable diabetes complications. Screening for diabetes should be completed every 3 years in individuals that are ≥40 years of age or in individuals at high risk using the Diabetes Canada risk calculator or screening algorithm (http://guidelines.diabetes.ca/screening).[32]

Classification of Diabetes

Type 1 diabetes is the result of pancreatic β cell destruction, of which the cause is unknown. Individuals are at risk for ketoacidosis. Type 1 diabetes is often the result of an autoimmune process for which the β cell destruction is unknown.[44] *Type 2 diabetes* has manifestations ranging from predominant insulin resistance with relative insulin deficiency to a predominant secretory defect with insulin resistance. *Gestational diabetes* is glucose intolerance with onset during pregnancy. The following parameters are diagnostic for diabetes:[44]

- FPG level ≥7.0 mmol/L
- A_{1C} (%) ≥6.5
- Random plasma glucose level ≥11.1 mmol/L plus symptoms of diabetes
- 2-hour plasma glucose level in a 75-g oral glucose tolerance test ≥11.1 mmol/L

Prediabetes places individuals at high risk of developing diabetes and its complications. Not all individuals with prediabetes will necessarily progress to diabetes.[44] Prediabetes: A_{1C} (%) ≥6.0 to 6.4. Optimal glycemic control is fundamental in the management of diabetes. High plasma glucose levels, both fasting and postprandial, increase risk for diabetes-related complications. When you set management goals, it is essential to consider patients' age, prognosis, and presence of complications or comorbid conditions. A_{1C} (previously called *hemoglobin A_{1C}* and *HbA_{1C}*) level reflects glycemia over the 120-day lifespan of erythrocytes (red blood cells). This indicator of treatment effectiveness should be measured approximately every 3 months to ensure that glycemic goals are being met or maintained in individuals with diabetes.

Nutrition counselling with a dietitian is recommended for all individuals with diabetes. Nutrition therapy can reduce A_{1C} by 1.0 to 2.0% and, when used with other components of diabetes management (social work, physiotherapy), can further improve outcomes.[45]

Metabolic Syndrome

Metabolic syndrome is a highly prevalent, multifaceted condition characterized by a distinctive collection of abnormalities, including abdominal obesity, hypertension, dyslipidemia, insulin resistance, and dysglycemia.[44] Individuals with metabolic syndrome are at risk of developing diabetes and cardiovascular disease. Evidence supports an aggressive approach in identifying individuals with metabolic syndrome and managing the associated risk factors.

Consensus regarding operational definitions of metabolic syndrome is lacking. In 1998, the World Health Organization

TABLE 12.2	Clinical Identification of Metabolic Syndrome: ≥3 Measures to Make the Diagnosis
Risk Factor	Defining Level[a]
Elevated FPG	≥ 5.6 mmol/L
Elevated BP	≥ 130/85 mm Hg
Elevated Triglycerides	≥ 1.7 mmol/L
Reduced HDL-C	
Men	< 1.0 mmol/L
Women	< 1.3 mmol/L
Abdominal obesity (waist circumference)	
Men	≥ 102 cm
Women	≥ 88 cm

[a]Metabolic syndrome is diagnosed when three or more of the risk determinants are present.
FPG, Fasting plasma glucose; *BP*, blood pressure; *HDL-C*, high-density lipoprotein cholesterol.
From Canadian Diabetes Association Clinical Practice Guidelines Expert Committee. (2018). Definition, classification and diagnosis of diabetes, prediabetes and metabolic syndrome. *Canadian Journal of Diabetes, 37*, S8–S11. Retrieved from http://guidelines.diabetes.ca/cpg/chapter3. Reprinted with permission.

(WHO) proposed a unifying definition that includes identification of the presence of insulin resistance. More recently, the Diabetes Canada provided an operational definition based on three or more criteria that do not include a measure of insulin resistance (Table 12.2). Results from the 2012–13 CHMS indicate that approximately 21% of adults aged 18 to 79 had metabolic syndrome.[46]

Celiac Disease

Celiac disease is a medical condition in which the absorptive surface of the small intestine is damaged by gluten. This results in an inability of the body to absorb nutrients: protein, fat, carbohydrates, vitamins, and minerals. It is estimated that 1 in 133 persons in Canada are affected by celiac disease. Common symptoms are anemia, chronic diarrhea, weight loss, fatigue, cramps and bloating, and irritability.[47]

Gluten is a protein found in wheat, rye, triticale, and barley. At present there is no cure, but celiac disease is readily treated by following the gluten-free diet.

Until recently, physicians had to rely on clinical signs to suggest the diagnosis and to select which patients should have further investigation to prove the diagnosis. Since these signs may be vague or of varying severity, this may be difficult. Now, blood screening tests are available to help this process.[47] A definitive diagnosis can only be made by a small bowel biopsy. The biopsy is performed by a specialist in the gastro-intestinal field. The biopsy must be done before treatment is started. Celiac disease as yet has no known cure, but can usually be effectively treated and controlled. The treatment of celiac disease is strict adherence to a gluten-free diet, for life. This requires knowledgeable dietetic counselling and frequent "updates" as commercial food contents change.

LINKS TO NUTRITION INFORMATION

Nurses are encouraged to further explore available resources related to nutrition. The Summary Checklist box and the following links include resources and interactive tools for the professional and the consumer. These tools may enhance understandings of the role of nutrition in health and chronic disease prevention and management.

- Diabetes Canada (formally Canadian Diabetes Association): https://www.diabetes.ca
- Dietitians of Canada: http://www.dietitians.ca
- Government of Canada, "Food and Nutrition": https://www.canada.ca/en/services/health/food-nutrition.html
- Public Health Agency of Canada: https://www.canada.ca/en/public-health.html
- UnlockFood.ca (formerly EatRight Ontario): http://www.unlockfood.ca/en/

Summary Checklist: Nutritional Assessment

1. Obtain a **health history** relevant to nutritional status.
2. Elicit **dietary history**, if indicated.
3. **Inspect** skin, hair, eyes, oral cavity, nails, and musculo-skeletal and neurological systems for clinical signs and symptoms suggestive of nutritional deficiencies.
4. **Measure** height, weight, and other anthropometric parameters, as indicated; calculate BMI and waist–hip ratio.
5. Review relevant **laboratory tests**.
6. **Offer health promotion** teaching and referral to a dietitian or other members of the multidisciplinary health care team, as indicated.

REFERENCES

1. Dietitians of Canada. (2016). *Learn about dietitians.* Retrieved from http://www.dietitians.ca/About-Us/About-Dietitians/Learn-about-Dietitians.aspx.
2. Raine, K., Spence, J. C., Church, J., et al. (2008). *State of the evidence review on urban health and healthy weights.* Ottawa: Canadian Institute for Health Information.
3. Navaneelan, T., & Janz, T. (2014). *Adjusting the scales: Obesity in the Canadian population after correcting for respondent bias. Health at a Glance.* Retrieved from http://www.statcan.gc.ca/pub/82-624-x/2014001/article/11922-eng.pdf.
4. Statistics Canada. (2015). *Body mass index of children and youth, 2012 to 2013.* Retrieved from http://www.statcan.gc.ca/pub/82-625-x/2014001/article/14105-eng.htm.
5. Wallace, S. (2015). *Inuit health: Selected findings from the 2012 Aboriginal Peoples Survey.* Retrieved from http://www.statcan.gc.ca/pub/89-653-x/89-653-x2014003-eng.htm.
6. Health Canada. (2015). *Nutrition for healthy term infants: Recommendations from birth to six months.* Retrieved from http://www.hc-sc.gc.ca/fn-an/nutrition/infant-nourisson/recom/index-eng.php.
7. Health Canada. (2016). *Eating well with Canada's food guide.* Retrieved from http://www.hc-sc.gc.ca/fn-an/food-guide-aliment/index-eng.php.
8. Sizer, F. S., Whitney, E., & Piche, L. A. (2014). *Nutrition concepts and controversies* (3rd Cdn ed.). Toronto: Nelson.
9. National Eating Disorder Information Centre. (2014). *Food and weight preoccupation.* Retrieved from http://nedic.ca/know-facts/food-weight-preoccupation.
10. Health Canada. (2010). *Prenatal nutrition guidelines for health professionals; gestational weight gain.* Retrieved from http://www.hc-sc.gc.ca/fn-an/nutrition/prenatal/ewba-mbsa-eng.php.
11. Rao, K., Ramya, K., Batchu, D., et al. (2017). Teenage pregnancy and its obstetric outcome. *Journal of Evidence Based Medicine and Health Care, 4*(15), 901–904.
12. Public Health Agency of Canada. (2012). *Folic acid.* Retrieved from http://www.phac-aspc.gc.ca/hp-gs/guide/02_fa-af-eng.php, http://www.phac-aspc.gc.ca/fa-af/index-eng.php.
13. SickKids Motherisk. (2017). *Taking folic acid before you get pregnant.* Retrieved from http://www.motherisk.org/women/folicAcid.jsp.
14. Favaro-Moreira, N., Krausch-Hofmann, S., Matthys, C., et al. (2016). Risk factors for malnutrition in older adults: A systematic review of the literature based on longitudinal data. *Advances in Nutrition, 7*, 507–522. doi:10.3945/an.115.011254.
15. Health Canada. (2012). *Men and women over the age of 50.* Retrieved from http://www.hc-sc.gc.ca/fn-an/food-guide-aliment/choose-choix/advice-conseil/adult50-eng.php.
16. Public Health Agency of Canada (2011). *The Chief Public Health Officer's report on the state of public health in Canada, 2011: Youth and young adults—Life in transition.* Ottawa: Author. Retrieved from http://www.phac-aspc.gc.ca/cphorsphc-respcacsp/2011/index-eng.php.
17. Fairholm, J. (1999). *Urban agriculture and food security initiatives in Canada: A survey of Canadian non-governmental organizations.* Ottawa: International Development Research Centre.
18. Health Canada. (2012). *Household food insecurity in Canada 2007–2008: Key statistics and graphics.* Retrieved from http://www.hc-sc.gc.ca/fn-an/surveill/nutrition/commun/insecurit/key-stats-cles-2007-2008-eng.php.
19. Health Canada. (2010). *Eating well with Canada's food guide—First Nations, Inuit and Métis.* Retrieved from http://www.hc-sc.gc.ca/fn-an/food-guide-aliment/fnim-pnim/index-eng.php.
20. Statistics Canada. (2007). *Canadian Health Measures Survey, 2007: Cycle 1* [Share Microdata File]. Ottawa, Ontario: Statistics Canada as reported in Public Health Agency of Canada (2011). *The Chief Public Health Officer's report on the state of public health in Canada, 2011: Youth and young*

adults—Life in transition. Ottawa: Public Health Agency of Canada. Retrieved from http://publichealth.gc.ca/CPHOreport.

21. Argys, L. (2015). Consequences of the obesity epidemic for immigrants. *IZA World of Labor, 210,* 1–10. doi:10.15185/izawol.210.

22. Canadian Malnutrition Task Force. (2017). *Tools for your practice.* Retrieved from http://nutritioncareincanada.ca/tools/tools-for-your-practice.

23. Rivera, J., McPherson, A., Hamilton, J., et al. (2016). Mobile apps for weight management: A scoping review. *JMIR mHealth and uHealth, 4*(3), e87. doi: http://doi.org/10.2196/mhealth.5115.

24. Institute of Medicine (2006). *Dietary reference intakes: The essential guide to nutrient requirements.* Washington, DC: National Academies Press.

25. Dietitians of Canada. (2017). *Nutrition labelling.* Retrieved from https://www.dietitians.ca/Dietitians-Views/Food-Regulation-and-Labelling/Nutrition-Labelling.aspx.

26. EatRight Ontario. (2017). *Decoding the nutrition label.* Retrieved from https://www.eatrightontario.ca/en/Articles/Nutrition-Labelling/Decoding-the-Nutrition-Label.aspx.

27. Health Canada. (2012). *Body mass index (BMI) nomogram.* Retrieved from http://www.hc-sc.gc.ca/fn-an/nutrition/weights-poids/guide-ld-adult/bmi_chart_java-graph_imc_java-eng.php.

28. Centers for Disease Control and Prevention. (2015). *Healthy weight; about child and teen BMI.* Retrieved from https://www.cdc.gov/healthyweight/assessing/bmi/childrens_bmi/about_childrens_bmi.html.

29. Gabriella, S. E., & Sinclair, A. J. (1997). Diagnosing undernutrition in elderly people. *Reviews in Clinical Gerontology, 7,* 367–371.

30. Reuben, D. B., Greendale, G. A., & Harrison, G. G. (1995). Nutrition screening in older persons. *Journal of the American Geriatric Society, 43,* 415–425.

31. Froehlich-Grobe, K., Nary, D. E., Van Sciver, A., et al. (2011). Measuring height without a stadiometer: Empirical investigation of four height estimates among wheelchair users. *American Journal of Physical Medicine & Rehabilitation/Association of Academic Physiatrists, 90*(8), 658–666. doi: http://doi.org/10.1097/PHM.0b013e31821f6eb2.

32. Diabetes Canada. (2013). *Screening for type 1 and type 2 diabetes.* Retrieved from http://guidelines.diabetes.ca/executivesummary/ch4.

33. Chernecky, C. C., & Berger, B. J. (2008). *Laboratory tests and diagnostic procedures* (5th ed.). St. Louis: W. B. Saunders.

34. Lee, R. D., & Nieman, D. C. (2003). *Nutritional assessment* (3rd ed.). New York: McGraw-Hill.

35. Blackburn, G. L., Bistrian, B. R., Maini, B. S., et al. (1977). Nutritional and metabolic assessment of the hospitalized patient. *Journal of Parenteral and Enteral Nutrition, 1*(1), 11–22.

36. Government of Canada. (2011). *Physical activity.* Retrieved from https://www.canada.ca/en/public-health/services/health-promotion/healthy-living/physical-activity.html.

37. Statistics Canada. (2015). *Overweight and obese adults, (self-reported) 2014.* Retrieved from http://www.statcan.gc.ca/pub/82-625-x/2015001/article/14185-eng.htm.

38. Statistics Canada. (2015). *Canadian Health Measures Survey: Directly measured physical activity of Canadians, 2012 and 2013.* Retrieved from http://www.statcan.gc.ca/daily-quotidien/150218/dq150218c-eng.htm.

39. Diabetes Canada. (2013). *Just the basics: Aboriginal version.* Retrieved from http://guidelines.diabetes.ca/cdacpg/media/documents/patient-resources/just-the-basics-aboriginal-english.pdf.

40. Health Canada. (2017). *Diabetes: What you eat matters.* http://www.hc-sc.gc.ca/fniah-spnia/alt_formats/pdf/pubs/diseases-maladies/diabete/diabete5-eng.pdf.

41. World Health Organization. (2016). *Diabetes.* Retrieved from http://www.who.int/mediacentre/factsheets/fs312/en/.

42. Diabetes Canada. (2017). *Diabetes statistics in Canada.* Retrieved from http://www.diabetes.ca/how-you-can-help/advocate/why-federal-leadership-is-essential/diabetes-statistics-in-canada.

43. Diabetes Canada. (2011). *Diabetes: Canada at a tipping point. Charting a new path.* Retrieved from http://www.diabetes.ca/CDA/media/documents/publications-and-newsletters/advocacy-reports/canada-at-the-tipping-point-english.pdf.

44. Diabetes Canada. (2013). *Definition, classification and diagnosis of diabetes, prediabetes and metabolic syndrome.* Retrieved from http://guidelines.diabetes.ca/browse/chapter3#sec2.

45. Diabetes Canada. (2013). *Nutrition therapy.* Retrieved from http://guidelines.diabetes.ca/executivesummary/ch11.

46. Statistics Canada. (2015). *Metabolic syndrome in adults 2012 to 2013.* Retrieved from http://www.statcan.gc.ca/pub/82-625-x/2014001/article/14123-eng.htm.

47. Canadian Celiac Association. (2016). *About celiac disease.* Retrieved from http://www.celiac.ca/?page_id=882.

CHAPTER 13

Skin, Hair, and Nails

Written by Carolyn Jarvis, PhD, APN, CNP
Adapted by June MacDonald-Jenkins, RN, BScN, MSc

e http://evolve.elsevier.com/Canada/Jarvis/examination/

STRUCTURE AND FUNCTION

SKIN

Think of the skin as the body's largest organ system. It covers 1.86 square metres of surface area in the average adult. The skin is the sentry that guards the body from environmental stresses (e.g., trauma, pathogens, dirt) and adapts it to other environmental influences (e.g., heat, cold). The skin has two layers: the outer highly differentiated *epidermis* and the inner supportive *dermis* (Fig. 13.1). Beneath these layers is a third layer—the *subcutaneous* layer of adipose tissue.

Epidermis

The *epidermis* is thin but tough. Its cells are bound tightly together into sheets that form a rugged protective barrier. It is stratified into several zones. The inner **basal cell layer** forms new skin cells. Their major ingredient is the tough, fibrous protein *keratin*. The melanocytes interspersed along this layer produce the pigment *melanin*, which gives the skin and hair their brown tones. All people have the same number of melanocytes; however, the amount of melanin they produce varies with genetic, hormonal, and environmental influences.

From the basal layer, the new cells migrate up and flatten into the outer **horny cell layer**. This consists of dead keratinized cells that are interwoven and closely packed. The cells are constantly being shed, or *desquamated*, and are replaced with new cells from below. The epidermis is completely replaced every 4 weeks. On the palms and the soles, skin is thicker because of work and weight bearing. The epidermis is avascular; it is nourished by blood vessels in the dermis below.

Skin colour is derived from three sources: (a) mainly from the brown pigment melanin, (b) from the yellow-orange tones of the pigment carotene, and (c) from the red-purple tones in the underlying vascular bed. All people have skin of varying shades of brown, yellow, and red; the relative proportions of these shades affect the prevailing colour. Skin colour is further modified by the thickness of the skin and by the presence of edema.

Dermis

The *dermis* is the inner supportive layer consisting mostly of connective tissue, or *collagen*. This is the tough, fibrous protein that enables the skin to resist tearing. The dermis also has resilient elastic tissue that allows the skin to stretch with body movements. The nerves, sensory receptors, blood vessels, and lymphatic vessels lie in the dermis. Also, appendages from the epidermis—such as the hair follicles, sebaceous glands, and sweat glands—are embedded in the dermis.

Subcutaneous Layer

The *subcutaneous layer* is adipose tissue, which is made up of lobules of fat cells. The subcutaneous tissue stores fat for energy, provides insulation for temperature control, and aids in protection by its soft, cushioning effect. Also, the loose subcutaneous layer gives skin its increased mobility over structures underneath.

Hair

Hairs are threads of keratin. The hair *shaft* is the visible projecting part, and the *root* is below the surface, embedded in the follicle. At the root, the *bulb matrix* is the expanded area where new cells are produced at a fast rate. Hair growth is cyclical, with active and resting phases. Each follicle functions independently so that while some hairs are resting, others are growing. Around the hair follicle are the muscular *arrector pili*, which contract and elevate the hair so that it resembles "goose bumps" during exposure to cold or in emotional states.

People have two types of hair. Fine, faint **vellus hair** covers most of the body (except the palms and soles, the dorsa of the distal parts of the fingers, the umbilicus, the glans penis, and inside the labia). The other type is **terminal**

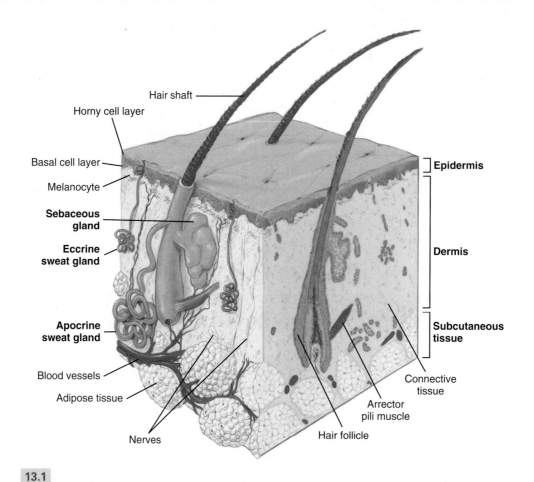

13.1

hair, the darker thicker hair that grows on the scalp and eyebrows and, after puberty, on the axillae, the pubic area, and, in males, the face and chest.

Sebaceous Glands

Sebaceous glands produce a protective lipid substance, *sebum*, which is secreted through the hair follicles. Sebum oils and lubricates the skin and hair and forms an emulsion with water that delays water loss from the skin. (Dryness of skin results from loss of water, not directly from loss of oil.) Sebaceous glands are everywhere except on the palms and soles. They are most abundant in the scalp, forehead, face, and chin.

Sweat Glands

There are two types of sweat glands. The **eccrine** glands are coiled tubules that open directly onto the skin surface and produce a dilute saline solution called *sweat*. The evaporation of sweat reduces body temperature. Eccrine glands are widely distributed through the body and are mature in 2-month-old infants.

The **apocrine** glands produce a thick, milky secretion and open into the hair follicles. They are located mainly in the axillae, anogenital area, nipples, and navel and are vestigial in humans. They become active during puberty, and secretion occurs with emotional and sexual stimulation. Bacterial flora residing on the skin surface react with apocrine sweat to

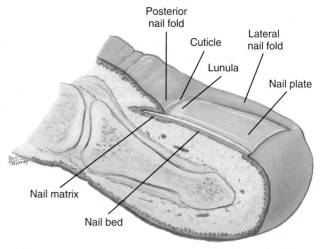

13.2

produce a characteristic musky body odour. The functioning of apocrine glands decreases in older adults.

Nails

The nails are hard plates of keratin on the dorsal edges of the fingers and toes (Fig. 13.2). The nail plate is clear, with fine longitudinal ridges that become prominent in aging. The pink colour of nails is derived from the underlying nail bed of highly vascular epithelial cells. The **lunula** is the white opaque semilunar area at the proximal end of the nail. It lies over the nail matrix, where new keratinized cells are formed. The nail folds overlap the posterior and lateral borders. The cuticle works like a gasket to cover and protect the nail matrix.

FUNCTION OF THE SKIN

The skin is a waterproof, highly resilient covering that has protective and adaptive properties:

- **Protection.** Skin minimizes injury from physical, chemical, thermal, and light wave sources.
- **Prevention of penetration.** Skin is a barrier that stops invasion of micro-organisms and loss of water and electrolytes from within the body.
- **Perception.** Skin is a vast sensory surface holding the sensorineural end organs for touch, pain, temperature, and pressure.
- **Temperature regulation.** Skin allows heat dissipation through sweat glands and heat storage through subcutaneous insulation.
- **Identification.** People identify one another by unique combinations of facial characteristics, hair, skin colour, and even fingerprints. Self-image is often enhanced or deterred by the way each person's perceived characteristics measure up to society's standards of beauty.
- **Communication.** Emotions are expressed in the sign language of the face and in the body posture. Vascular mechanisms such as blushing or blanching also signal emotional states.
- **Wound repair.** Skin allows cell replacement of surface wounds.
- **Absorption and excretion.** Skin allows limited excretion of some metabolic wastes—by-products of cellular decomposition such as minerals, sugars, amino acids, cholesterol, uric acid, and urea.
- **Production of vitamin D.** The skin is the surface on which ultraviolet light converts cholesterol into vitamin D.

 DEVELOPMENTAL CONSIDERATIONS

Infants and Children

The hair follicles develop in the fetus at 3 months' gestation; by midgestation, most of the skin is covered with **lanugo**, the fine downy hair of the newborn infant. In the first few months after birth, this is replaced by fine vellus hair. Terminal hair on the scalp, if present at birth, tends to be soft and to go through a period of a patchy loss, especially at the temples and occiput. Also present at birth is **vernix caseosa**, the thick, cheesy substance made up of sebum and shed epithelial cells.

A newborn's skin is similar in structure to an adult's, but many of its functions are not fully developed. A newborn's skin is thin, smooth, and elastic and is relatively more permeable than that of an adult, and so the infant is at greater risk for fluid loss. Sebum, which holds water in the skin, is present for the first few weeks of life, producing milia (see p. 243) and cradle cap in some babies. Then sebaceous glands decrease in size and production and do not resume functioning until puberty. Temperature regulation is also ineffective. Eccrine sweat glands do not secrete in response to heat until the first few months of life and then only minimally throughout childhood. The skin cannot protect much against cold because it cannot contract and shiver and because the subcutaneous layer is inefficient. In addition, the pigment system is inefficient at birth.

As the child grows, the epidermis thickens, toughens, and darkens, and the skin becomes better lubricated. Hair growth accelerates. At puberty, secretion from apocrine sweat glands increases in response to heat and emotional stimuli, producing body odour. Sebaceous glands become more active; the skin looks oily, and acne develops. Subcutaneous fat deposits increase, especially in females.

Secondary sex characteristics that appear during adolescence are evident in the integument (i.e., skin). In the female the diameter of the areola enlarges and darkens, and breast tissue develops. Coarse pubic hair and then axillary hair develop in boys and girls, and then coarse facial hair develops in males.

Pregnant Women

The change in hormone levels results in increased pigmentation in the areolae and nipples, vulva, and sometimes in the midline of the abdomen (**linea nigra**) or in the face (**chloasma**). Hyperestrogenemia probably also causes the common vascular spiders and palmar erythema. Connective tissue becomes increasingly fragile, which results in **striae gravidarum**, which may develop in the skin of the abdomen, breasts, or thighs. Metabolism is increased in pregnancy; as a way to dissipate heat, the peripheral vasculature dilates, and the sweat and sebaceous glands increase secretion. Fat deposits are laid down, particularly in the buttocks and hips, as maternal reserves for the nursing baby.

Older Adults

The skin is a mirror that reflects aging changes that proceed in *all* organ systems; it just happens to be the one organ that people can view directly. The aging process carries a slow atrophy of skin structures. The aging skin loses its elasticity; it folds and sags. By the 70s to 80s, it looks parchment thin, lax, dry, and wrinkled.

The epidermis's outer layer, the *stratum corneum*, thins and flattens. This allows chemicals easier access into the body. Wrinkling occurs because the underlying dermis also thins and flattens. Elastin, collagen, and subcutaneous fat are lost, as is muscle tone. The loss of collagen increases the risk for shearing and tearing injuries.

Sweat glands and sebaceous glands decrease in number and function, leaving the skin dry. Decreased response of the sweat glands to thermoregulatory demand also puts older adults at greater risk for heat stroke. The vascularity of the skin diminishes while the vascular fragility increases;

a minor trauma may produce dark red discoloured areas, or **senile purpura**.

Sun exposure and cigarette smoking further accentuate aging changes in the skin. Coarse wrinkling, decreased elasticity, atrophy, speckled and uneven colouring, more pigment changes, and a yellowed, leathery texture develop. Chronic sun damage is even more prominent in pale or light-skinned persons.

An accumulation of factors increases older adults' risk for skin disease and breakdown: the thinning of the skin, the decrease in vascularity and nutrients, the loss of protective cushioning of the subcutaneous layer, a lifetime of environmental trauma to skin, the social changes of aging (e.g., less nutrition, limited financial resources), the increasingly sedentary lifestyle, and the chance of immobility. When skin breakdown does occur, subsequent cell replacement is slower, and wound healing is delayed.

In the aging hair matrix, the number of functioning melanocytes decreases, and so the hair turns grey or white and feels thin and fine. A person's genetic script determines the onset of greying and the number of grey hairs. Hair distribution changes. Males may have symmetrical W-shaped balding in the frontal areas. Some testosterone is present in both sexes; as levels decrease with age, the amount of axillary and pubic hair decreases. As the female's estrogen levels also decrease, testosterone is unopposed, and the female may have some bristly facial hairs. Nails grow more slowly. Their surface is lustreless and is characterized by longitudinal ridges that result from local trauma at the nail matrix.

Because the changes of aging in the skin and hair can be viewed directly, their psychological effect is profound. For many people, self-esteem is linked to a youthful appearance. This view is compounded by media advertising in Western society. Although sagging and wrinkling skin and greying and thinning hair are normal processes of aging, they can prompt a loss of self-esteem for many adults.

SOCIAL DETERMINANTS OF HEALTH CONSIDERATIONS

Awareness of normal biocultural differences and the ability to recognize the unique clinical manifestations of disease are especially important for people with dark pigmentation. As described earlier, melanin is responsible for the various colours and tones of skin observed among people from culturally diverse backgrounds. Melanin protects the skin against harmful ultraviolet rays, a genetic advantage that accounts for the lower incidence of skin cancer among individuals of African, Indian, or Indigenous descent with dark skin. The incidence of melanoma is 20 times higher among individuals with lighter skin pigment.

Areas of the skin that are affected by hormones and, in some cases, differ among culturally diverse people, are the sexual skin areas, such as the nipples, areola, scrotum, and labia majora. In general, these areas are darker than other parts of the skin in both adults and children, especially among individuals of African and Asian descent.

The apocrine and eccrine sweat glands are important for fluid balance and for thermoregulation. When apocrine gland secretions are contaminated by normal skin flora, odour results. Inuit people have made an interesting environmental adaptation: In comparison with Canadians of European descent, they sweat less on their trunks and extremities but more on their faces. This adaptation allows for temperature regulation without causing perspiration and dampness of their clothes, which would decrease their ability to self-insulate against severe cold weather and would pose a serious threat to their survival.

Alcohol flush syndrome, mistakenly called "Asian flush" previously, is a condition characterized by a genetic disposition that can cause a range of symptoms such as redness and flushing of the face, heat sensation, splotchy redness of the neck, and accelerated intoxication when alcohol is ingested. It occurs in approximately 90% of individuals of Indigenous and 50% of those of Asian descent. These unpleasant adverse effects sometimes prevent further drinking that could lead to further inebriation, but the symptoms can lead to a misassumption that the people affected are more easily inebriated than others.

SUBJECTIVE DATA

1. Previous history of skin disease (allergies, hives, psoriasis, eczema)
2. Change in pigmentation
3. Change in mole
4. Excessive dryness or moisture
5. Pruritus
6. Excessive bruising
7. Rash or lesion
8. Medications
9. Hair loss
10. Change in nails
11. Environmental or occupational hazards
12. Self-care behaviours

HEALTH HISTORY QUESTIONS

Examiner Asks	Rationale
1. **Previous history of skin disease (allergies, hives, psoriasis, eczema).** Any previous **skin disease** or problem? • How was this treated? • Any family history of allergies or allergic skin problem? • Any known allergies to medications, plants, or animals? • Any birthmarks or tattoos?	Significant familial predisposition: allergies, hay fever, psoriasis, atopic dermatitis (eczema), acne. Identification of offending allergen. Risk for hepatitis C, increased with use of nonsterile equipment to apply tattoos.
2. **Change in pigmentation.** Any **change in skin colour** or **pigmentation**? • Is the colour change generalized (all over), or is it localized?	Hypopigmentation: loss of pigmentation; hyperpigmentation: increase in colour. Generalized change suggestive of systemic illness: pallor, jaundice, cyanosis.
3. **Change in mole.** Any **change in a mole**: colour, size, shape; sudden appearance of tenderness, bleeding, or itching? • Any "sores" that do not heal?	Possible neoplasm in pigmented nevus; person may be unaware of change in nevus on back or buttocks that the person cannot see.
4. **Excessive dryness or moisture.** Any change in the feel of your skin: temperature, **moisture**, or texture? • Any excess **dryness**? Is this seasonal or constant?	Seborrhea: oily. Xerosis: dry.
5. **Pruritus.** Any skin itching? Is this mild (prickling, tingling) or intense (intolerable)? • Does it awaken you from sleep? • Where is the itching? When did it start? • Any other skin pain or soreness? Where?	The most common of skin symptoms; occurs with dry skin, aging, medication reactions, allergy, obstructive jaundice, uremia, lice infestation. Presence or absence of pruritus: possibly significant for diagnosis. Excoriation of primary lesion caused by scratching.
6. **Excessive bruising.** Any excessive **bruising**? Where on the body? • How did this happen? • How long have you had it?	Multiple cuts and bruises, bruises in various stages of healing, bruises above knees and elbows, and illogical explanation: consider the possibility of abuse. Frequent falls: possibly caused by dizziness of neurological or cardiovascular origin. Frequent minor trauma: possibly an adverse effect of alcoholism or other substance use.
7. **Rash or lesion.** Any skin **rash** or **lesion**? • Onset: When did you first notice it? • Location: Where did it start?	Rashes: a common reason for seeking health care. A thorough history is important; it may be an accurate predictor of the type of lesion seen in the examination and its cause. Identification of the primary site; may be clue to cause. Determination of migration pattern, evolution.

Examiner Asks	Rationale
• Extent: Have you noticed it spreading? If so, where?	Spreading pattern: often a clue to the cause of the rash.
• Character or quality: Describe the colour.	
• Texture and odour: Is it raised or flat? Any crust, odour? Does it feel tender, warm?	
• Duration: How long have you had it?	
• Setting: Does anyone at home or work have a similar rash? Have you been camping, acquired a new pet, tried a new food, or taken a new medication? Does the rash seem to come with stress?	Identification of new or relevant exposure, identification of any household or social contacts with similar symptoms.
• Alleviating and aggravating factors: What home care have you tried: bath, lotions, or heat? Do they help, or do they make it worse?	Myriad over-the-counter remedies are available. Many people try them and seek professional help only when they do not see improvement.
• Associated symptoms: Any itching or fever?	
• Significance: What do you think a rash or lesion means?	Assessing person's perception of cause: fear of cancer, illnesses borne by ticks, or sexually transmitted infections.
• Coping strategies: How has the rash or lesion affected your self-care, hygiene, and ability to function at work, at home, and socially?	Assessing effectiveness of coping strategies. Chronic skin diseases may increase risk for loss of self-esteem, social isolation, and anxiety.
• Stress: Any new or increased stress in your life?	Can exacerbate chronic skin illness.
8. Medications. What **medications** do you take?	Medications that may produce allergic skin eruption: Aspirin, antibiotics, barbiturates, some tonics.
• Prescription and over-the-counter?	
• Recent change?	Medications that may increase sunlight sensitivity and produce burn response: sulphonamides, thiazide diuretics, oral hypoglycemic agents, tetracycline.
	Medications that can cause hyperpigmentation: antimalarials, antineoplastic agents, hormones, metals, tetracycline.
• How long have you been taking the medication?	Even after a patient has taken medication for a long time, a sensitivity may develop.
9. Hair loss. Any recent **hair loss**?	**Alopecia** is a significant loss. A full head of hair is equated with vitality in many cultures. If hair loss is treated as a trivial problem, the patient may seek alternative, unproven methods of treatment.
• A gradual or sudden onset? Symmetrical? Associated with fever, illness, increased stress?	
• Any unusual hair growth?	**Hirsutism**: shaggy or excessive hair.
• Any recent change in texture, appearance?	
10. Change in nails. Any **change in nails**: shape, colour, brittleness? Do you tend to bite or chew your nails?	See Table 13.14 (p. 269) for abnormal conditions.
11. Environmental or occupational hazards. Any **environmental** or **occupational** hazards?	Majority of skin neoplasms caused by occupational or environmental agents.
• Any hazard-related problems with your occupation, such as dyes, toxic chemicals, radiation?	People at risk: outdoor sports enthusiasts, farmers, sailors, outdoor workers; or any profession where chemical exposure is possible.
• How about hobbies? Do you perform any household or furniture repair work?	

Examiner Asks	Rationale
• How much sun exposure do you get from outdoor work, leisure activities, sunbathing, or tanning salons? (See the Promoting Health: Tanning/Tanning Beds and Skin Cancer Risk box.)	Unprotected sun exposure, which accelerates aging and produces lesions; at more risk: light-skinned people, and those regularly in sun.
• Have you recently been bitten by an insect: bee, tick, or mosquito? (See the Promoting Health: Lyme Disease Is On the Rise box.) • Any recent exposure to plants or animals in yard work or camping?	Identifying contactants that produce lesions or contact dermatitis. Instruct people with chronic recurrent urticaria (hives) to keep a food diary and environmental exposures list to identify precipitating factors.
12. Self-care behaviours. What do you do to care for your skin, hair, and nails? What cosmetics, soaps, or chemicals do you use? • Do you clip cuticles on nails or use adhesive for false fingernails?	Assessing **self-care** and influence on self-concept: may be important with society's media stress on norms of beauty. Many over-the-counter remedies are costly and exacerbate skin problems.
• If you have allergies, how do you control your environment to minimize exposure? • Do you perform a skin self-examination? • Do you use sunscreen? What number sun protective factor (SPF)?	

Additional History for Infants and Children

1. Birthmarks. Does the child have any birthmarks?	See the discussion on physiological jaundice, p. 243.
2. Change in skin colour. Has there been any change in skin colour as a newborn? • Any jaundice? Which day after birth? • Any cyanosis? What were the circumstances?	
3. Rashes or sores. Have you noted any rash or sores? What seems to bring them on? • Have you introduced a new food or formula? When? Does your child eat chocolate, cow's milk, eggs?	For a generalized rash, consider an allergic reaction to new food. See Table 13.9 (p. 260) for an example of diaper rash. Irritability and general fussiness may indicate the presence of pruritus.
4. Diaper rash. Does the child have any diaper rash? How do you care for this? How do you wash diapers? How often do you change diapers? How do you clean skin?	Occlusive diapers or infrequent changing may cause a rash. Possible allergy to certain detergent or to disposable wipes.
5. Burns or bruises. Does the child have any burns or bruises? • Where? • How did it happen?	A careful history can distinguish expected childhood bumps and bruises from any lesion that may indicate child abuse or neglect: cigarette burns; excessive bruising, especially above knees or elbows; linear whip marks. With abuse, the history often does not coincide with physical appearance and location of lesion.
6. Exposure. Has the child had any exposure to contagious skin conditions (scabies, impetigo, lice), communicable diseases (measles, chicken pox, scarlet fever), or toxic plants (poison ivy)? • Are the child's vaccinations up to date?	

Subjective Data

Examiner Asks	Rationale

7. Self-destructive habits. Does the child have any habits or habitual movements, such as nail-biting, twisting hair, rubbing head on mattress?

8. Sun protection. What steps are taken to protect the child from sun exposure? What about sunscreens and sunblocks? How do you treat a sunburn?

Excessive sun exposure, especially severe or blistering sunburns in childhood, increases risk for melanoma in later life.

Additional History for Adolescents

1. Skin problems. Have you noticed any skin problems such as pimples or blackheads?
- How long have you had them?
- How do you treat this?
- How do you feel about it?

On average, about 85% of the population will have acne by the age of 21.[1] The psychological effects are often more significant than the physical effects; self-treatment is common.

Causes are increased sebum production and epithelial cells that do not desquamate normally.

Additional History for Older Adults

1. Skin changes. What changes have you noticed in your skin in the last few years?

Assessing effect of aging on self-concept; normal aging changes may cause distress.

Many changes attributed to aging result from chronic sun damage.

2. Wound healing. Any delay in wound healing?
- Any skin itching?

Pruritus is common with aging. Consider the adverse effects of medicine or systemic disease (e.g., liver or kidney disease, cancer, lymphoma), but senile pruritus usually results from dry skin (**xerosis**). It is exacerbated by too-frequent bathing or use of soap. Scratching with dirty, jagged fingernails produces excoriations.

3. Skin pain. Any other skin pain?

Some diseases, such as herpes zoster (shingles), produce more intense sensations of pain and itching in older adults. Other diseases (e.g., diabetes) may reduce pain sensation in extremities. Also, some older adults tolerate chronic pain as "part of growing old" and hesitate to "complain."

4. Foot changes. Any change in feet or toenails? Any bunions? Is it possible to wear shoes?

Some older adults cannot reach down to their feet to perform self-care.

5. Falling. Do you experience frequent falls?

Assessing for multiple bruises, trauma from falls.

6. Diabetes and cardiovascular disease. Any history of diabetes, peripheral vascular disease?

Risk for skin lesions in feet or ankles.

Examiner Asks	Rationale
7. Skin care. What do you do to care for your skin?	A bland lotion is important to retain moisture in aging skin. Dermatitis may result from certain cosmetics, creams, ointments, and dyes applied to achieve a youthful appearance. Aging skin has a delayed inflammatory response when exposed to irritants. If the person is not alerted by warning signs (e.g., pruritus, redness), exposure may continue, and dermatitis may ensue.

PROMOTING HEALTH: TANNING/TANNING BEDS AND SKIN CANCER RISK

The Dangers of Tanning Salons and the Sun

People know that prolonged sun exposure can lead to skin cancer, yet why is it that they do not realize the potential dangers of tanning booths? The skin examination is an opportunity for health care providers to educate the public about the dangers of excessive exposure to ultraviolet (UV) rays. As you examine an individual's skin, take the time to ask about the use of tanning salons. Ask about solar exposure and outdoor sun-protective precautions as well.

The popularity of indoor tanning salons appears to be growing, despite public health warnings and increasing evidence of the dangers of artificial UV radiation. The Canadian Cancer Society identified risk factors for the development of skin cancer with prolonged exposure to UV rays.[*] Individuals most at risk are those who have a history of skin cancer, are younger than 18, are fair skinned, have freckles or moles, have a family history of skin cancer, are using medications that increase their sensitivity to UV rays, have a weakened immune system, and have a *CDKN2A* gene mutation.

Many adverse effects of tanning beds have been documented, including acute sunburn, suppression of cutaneous DNA repair and immune functioning, ocular disorders, and increased risk for skin cancer, specifically squamous/basal cell carcinoma and melanoma. The World Health Organization declared tanning beds to be classified as carcinogenic to humans—in the same category as arsenic and asbestos—and declared that, worldwide, no person younger than 18 years old should use a tanning bed.[†‡] Despite these warnings, the tanning industry appears to have convinced the public that indoor tanning is healthy, emphasizing that tanning produces a psychological sense of well-being and can even induce vitamin D production, which is an unproven assumption. Sold as a pre-vacation necessity to assist in the prevention of sunburns, "pretanning" is a particularly dangerous practice because it not only leads to extra UV exposure but also appears to lead to decreased use of subsequent outdoor sun-protective precautions. The Canadian Skin Cancer Foundation recommends the following guidelines for safe exposure once a person heads outside:[§]

- Stay out of the sun between 10 A.M. and 4 P.M. or any time the UV index is 3 or higher.
- Cover arms and legs with loose-fitting, tightly woven, and lightweight clothing.
- Wear a wide-brimmed hat to protect head, face, neck, and ears.
- Stay in the shade: under trees, awnings, or umbrellas.
- Wear sunglasses with UV protection.

Use sunscreen with an SPF of 30 or higher; apply it at least 20 minutes before going into the sun, and reapply every 2 or 3 hours. Although Health Canada regulates manufacturers of indoor tanning equipment and limits the amount of UV radiation that can be emitted, it does not regulate the proportion of UVB radiation emitted. Furthermore, the amount of UVA light received in a tanning salon may be two to three times more than the UVA light received from the sun and is a known risk factor for melanoma. Although one of the sources of vitamin D is exposure to UV light, sources of vitamin D that do not carry an increased risk for skin cancer include vitamin D supplements or food sources supplemented with vitamin D.

Many individuals believe that tanning gives a person a "healthy glow"; on the contrary, the long-term exposure of tanning can lead to something more frightening and deadly.

References

[*] Canadian Cancer Society. (2011). *Indoor tanning—Our position*. Retrieved from http://www.cancer.ca/Canada-wide/Prevention/Sun%20and%20UV/Indoor%20tanning/Indoor%20tanning%20our%20position.aspx?sc_lang=en.

[†] International Agency for Research on Cancer (World Health Organization). (2009, July 29). *Sunbeds and UV radiation* [Press release]. Retrieved from https://www.iarc.fr/en/media-centre/iarcnews/2009/sunbeds_uvradiation.php.

[‡] World Health Organization. (2005, March 17). *The World Health Organization recommends that no person under 18 should use a sunbed* [Press release]. Retrieved from http://www.who.int/mediacentre/news/notes/2005/np07/en/.

[§] Canadian Skin Cancer Foundation. (n.d.). *Skin cancer prevention*. Retrieved from http://www.canadianskincancerfoundation.com/skin-cancer-prevention.html.

Additional Resources

Canadian Cancer Society. (2018). *Be sun safe*. Retrieved from http://www.cancer.ca/en/prevention-and-screening/reduce-cancer-risk/make-healthy-choices/be-sun-safe/?region=on.

Canadian Skin Cancer Foundation. http://canadianskincancerfoundation.com.

World Health Organization. (2003). *Artificial tanning sunbeds: Risks and guidance*. Geneva, Switzerland: Author. Retrieved from http://www.who.int/uv/publications/en/sunbeds.pdf.

SPF, sun protective factor; *UVA,* ultraviolet A; *UVB,* ultraviolet B.

Subjective Data

Objective Data

PROMOTING HEALTH: LYME DISEASE IS ON THE RISE

Protection From Ticks

In 2009, Lyme disease became a nationally reportable disease in Canada. This means that all health care providers should report cases of Lyme disease to the Public Health Agency of Canada through their provincial public health system. From 2009 to 2013, the number of reported cases of Lyme disease has quadrupled across the country, with the greatest increase of cases reported in Nova Scotia and Ontario.*

Borrelia burgdorferi is the bacterium that causes Lyme disease. Small rodents are the most common reservoirs of *B. burgdorferi*, whereas larger animals serve as hosts for ticks. Ticks that transmit Lyme disease thrive in wooded areas and can lurk on the tips of grasses or shrubs, from which they can easily transfer to people or animals as they brush past. In areas where ticks are found, people should know about the risk for Lyme disease and protect themselves.

The risk for exposure to the disease is highest in regions where the ticks that transmit Lyme disease are known to be established. These regions are parts of southern and southeastern Quebec, southern and eastern Ontario, southeastern Manitoba, New Brunswick, Saskatchewan, and Nova Scotia, as well as much of southern British Columbia.

Most cases of human illness with Lyme disease occur in the late spring and summer, when the ticks are most active and human outdoor activity is greatest. The risk for contact with ticks begins in early spring when the weather warms up and lasts until permanent snow cover and subzero temperatures persist. The timing and intensity of these events vary across Canada and thus so does the risk period for exposure to ticks. Ticks may be active in the winter months in provinces with mild seasonal temperatures (4°C and above) and infrequent snow cover.

Personal Precautions to Avoid Infection

- When walking in tick-infested areas, wear long pants, with the legs tucked into boots or socks, and long-sleeved shirts that fit tightly at the wrist to keep ticks from getting to bare skin.
- Wear closed shoes, and avoid sandals.
- Wear light-coloured clothing; ticks will be seen more easily.

- Apply insect repellents containing DEET; they are safe and can effectively repel ticks. Repellents can be applied to clothing, as well as exposed skin, but should not be applied to skin underneath clothing. (*Note:* DEET may damage some materials.)
- Perform a careful self-inspection for attached ticks after being in tick-infested areas. A daily total-body inspection and prompt removal of attached ticks (within 36 hours) can reduce the transmission of *B. burgdorferi* from infected ticks. Black-legged ticks are very small, particularly during the nymph stage, so look carefully. Check children and pets as well.
- Carefully remove attached ticks by using tweezers. Grasp the tick's head and mouth parts as close to the skin as possible and pull slowly until the tick is removed. Do not twist or rotate the tick, and try not to squash or crush the tick during removal.
- After removing ticks, wash the bite site with soap and water, or disinfect it with alcohol or household antiseptic.
- Note the day of the tick bite and try to store the tick in an empty pill vial or double-zippered plastic bag.
- Contact a doctor immediately if you develop symptoms of Lyme disease, especially when you have been in an area where black-legged ticks are found. If you have stored the tick, take it with you to the doctor's office.

The black-legged ticks are primarily found in densely wooded areas and the unmaintained transitional edge habitat between woodlands and open areas. Fewer ticks are found in ornamental vegetation and lawn areas. For recommendations on reducing the risk for ticks inhabiting your surrounding property, see https://www.canada.ca/en/public-health/services/diseases/lyme-disease/prevention-lyme-disease.html#s2.

References

* Public Health Agency of Canada. (2015). *National Lyme disease surveillance in Canada 2013: Web report*. Retrieved from https://www.canada.ca/en/public-health/services/publications/diseases-conditions/national-lyme-disease-surveillance-canada-2013-web-report.html.

DEET, diethyltoluamide.

OBJECTIVE DATA

PREPARATION

Try to control external variables that may influence skin colour and confuse your findings, both in light-skinned and in dark-skinned patients.

Learn to consciously attend to skin characteristics. The danger is one of omission. You grow so accustomed to seeing the skin that you are likely to ignore it as you assess the organ systems underneath. However, the skin demonstrates information about the body's circulation, nutritional status, and signs of systemic diseases, as well as topical data on the integument itself.

Know the patient's normal skin colouring. Baseline knowledge is important for assessing colour or pigment changes. If this is the first time you are examining the patient, ask about the person's usual skin colour and about any self-monitoring practices.

EQUIPMENT NEEDED

Strong direct lighting (natural daylight is ideal for evaluating skin characteristics; halogen light will suffice)
Small centimetre ruler
Penlight
Gloves
Needed for special procedures:
- Wood light (filtered ultraviolet light)
- Magnifying glass, for minute lesions
- Materials for laboratory tests: potassium hydroxide (KOH), glass slide

| Normal Range of Findings | Abnormal Findings |

The Complete Physical Examination. Although it is described alone in this chapter, skin assessment is integrated throughout the complete examination; it is not a separate step. At the beginning of the examination, assessing the patient's hands and fingernails is a nonthreatening way to accustom the patient to your touch. Many people are used to having relative strangers shake their hands or touch their arms. As you proceed through the examination, scrutinize the outer skin surface first before you concentrate on the underlying structures. Separate intertriginous areas (areas with skinfolds)—such as those under large breasts, the obese abdomen, and the groin—and inspect them thoroughly. These areas are dark, warm, and moist and provide the perfect conditions for irritation or infection. Last, always remove the patient's socks and inspect the feet, toenails, and the area between the toes.

In a hospital setting, a more formalized tool may be used to determine factors that may result in putting the patient at risk for skin tears or breakdown. One such scale that is commonly used is the **Braden Scale for Predicting Pressure Sore Risk**. Primarily used in the community and hospital settings, it is an efficient measurement tool for assisting in objective skin risk assessment. Table 13.1 (p. 230) contains the complete scale and interpretation of scores.

The Regional Examination. Ask the patient to remove the clothing to assess the skin and assess the skin as one entity (assist with the removal of the clothing as required). Stand back at first to get an overall impression; this helps reveal distribution patterns. Then inspect lesions carefully. With a skin rash, check all areas of the body because there are some locations that the patient cannot see. Inspect mucous membranes, too, because some disorders produce characteristic lesions here as well.

Inspect and Palpate The Skin

Colour

General Pigmentation. Observe the skin tone. Normally it is consistent with genetic background and varies from pinkish tan to ruddy dark tan or from light to dark brown and may have yellow or olive overtones. Dark-skinned people normally have areas of lighter pigmentation on the palms, nail beds, and lips (Fig. 13.3, *A*).

An acquired condition is **vitiligo**, the complete absence of melanin pigment in patchy areas of white or light skin on the face, neck, hands, feet, and body folds and around orifices (see Fig. 13.3, *B*). Vitiligo occurs in all people, although dark-skinned people are more severely affected and potentially suffer a greater threat to body image.

A

B

13.3

TABLE 13.1 Braden Scale for Predicting Pressure Sore Risk

Patient's Name _____   Evaluator's Name _____

Date of Assessment _____

Indicate Appropriate Numbers Below

SENSORY PERCEPTION	1. COMPLETELY LIMITED	2. VERY LIMITED	3. SLIGHTLY LIMITED	4. NO IMPAIRMENT
Ability to respond meaningfully to pressure-related discomfort	Unresponsive (does not moan, flinch, or grasp) to painful stimuli, due to diminished level of consciousness or sedation. OR Limited ability to feel pain over most of body.	Responds only to painful stimuli. Cannot communicate discomfort except by moaning or restlessness. OR Has a sensory impairment that limits the ability to feel pain or discomfort over $\frac{1}{2}$ of body.	Responds to verbal commands, but cannot always communicate discomfort or the need to be turned. OR Has some sensory impairment which limits ability to feel pain or discomfort in 1 or 2 extremities.	Responds to verbal commands. Has no sensory deficit which would limit ability to feel or voice pain or discomfort.

MOISTURE	1. CONSTANTLY MOIST	2. VERY MOIST	3. OCCASIONALLY MOIST	4. RARELY MOIST
Degree to which skin is exposed to moisture	Skin is kept moist almost constantly by perspiration, urine, etc. Dampness is detected every time patient is moved or turned.	Skin is often, but not always, moist. Linen must be changed at least once a shift.	Skin is occasionally moist, requiring an extra linen change approximately once a day.	Skin is usually dry. Linen only requires changing at routine intervals.

ACTIVITY	1. BEDFAST	2. CHAIRFAST	3. WALKS OCCASIONALLY	4. WALKS FREQUENTLY
Degree of physical activity	Confined to bed.	Ability to walk severely limited or nonexistent. Cannot bear own weight and/or must be assisted into chair or wheelchair.	Walks occasionally during day, but for very short distances with or without assistance. Spends majority of each shift in bed or chair.	Walks outside the room at least twice a day and inside room at least every 2 hours during waking hours.

MOBILITY	1. COMPLETELY IMMOBILE	2. VERY LIMITED	3. SLIGHTLY LIMITED	4. NO LIMITATION
Ability to change and control body position	Does not make even slight changes in body or extremity position without assistance.	Makes occasional slight changes in body or extremity position, but unable to make frequent or significant changes independently.	Makes frequent though slight changes in body or extremity position independently.	Makes major and frequent changes in position without assistance.

TABLE 13.1 Braden Scale for Predicting Pressure Sore Risk—cont'd

NUTRITION	1. VERY POOR	2. PROBABLY INADEQUATE	3. ADEQUATE	4. EXCELLENT
Usual food intake pattern	Never eats a complete meal. Rarely eats more than $\frac{1}{3}$ of any food offered. Eats 2 servings or less of protein (meat or dairy products) per day. Takes fluids poorly. Does not take a liquid dietary supplement. OR Is NPO and/or maintained on clear liquids or IVs for more than 5 days.	Rarely eats a complete meal and generally eats only about $\frac{1}{2}$ of any food offered. Protein intake includes only 3 servings of meat or dairy products per day. Occasionally will take a dietary supplement. OR Receives less than optimum amount of liquid diet or tube feeding.	Eats over half of most meals. Eats a total of 4 servings of protein (meat or dairy products) each day. Occasionally will refuse a meal, but will usually take a supplement if offered. OR Is on tube feedings or TPN regimen, which meets most of nutritional needs.	Eats most of every meal. Never refuses a meal. Usually eats a total of 4 or more servings of meat and dairy products. Occasionally eats between meals. Does not require supplementation.

FRICTION AND SHEAR	1. PROBLEM	2. POTENTIAL PROBLEMS	3. NO APPARENT PROBLEM	
	Requires moderate to maximum assistance in moving. Complete lifting without sliding against sheets is impossible. Frequently slides down in bed or chair, requiring frequent repositioning with maximum assistance. Spasticity, contractures or agitation lead to almost constant friction.	Moves feebly or requires minimum assistance. During a move skin probably slides to some extent against sheets, chair restraints, or other devices. Maintains relatively good position in chair or bed most of the time but occasionally slides down.	Moves in bed and chair independently and has sufficient muscle strength to lift up completely during move. Maintains good position in bed or chair.	

Total Score:

Note:
15 to 18 = At Risk
13 to 14 = Moderate Risk
10 to 12 = High Risk
≤9 = Very High Risk

Assessment Schedule:
Very High to High Risk = minimum monthly
Moderate Risk = q3 months
Low/No Risk = q6 months

Note: Bed and chairbound individuals or those with impaired mobility to reposition should be assessed upon admission for their risk of developing a pressure injury. Patients with established pressure injuries should be reassessed periodically.
IVs, Intravenous feedings; *NPO,* nothing by mouth; *TPN,* total parenteral nutrition.

Normal Range of Findings

General pigmentation is darker in sun-exposed areas. Common (benign) pigmented areas also occur:

- **Freckles** (ephelides): small, flat macules of brown melanin pigment that occur on sun-exposed skin (Fig. 13.4, *A*).
- **Mole** (nevus): a proliferation of melanocytes, tan to brown colour, flat or raised. Acquired nevi are characterized by their symmetry, small size (6 mm or less), smooth borders, and single uniform pigmentation. The **junctional nevus** (see Fig. 13.4, *B*) is macular only and occurs in children and adolescents. In young adults it progresses to the **compound nevi** (see Fig. 13.4, *C*) that are macular and papular. The intradermal nevus (mainly in older age) has nevus cells in only the dermis.
- **Birthmarks**: may be tan to brown in colour.

13.4 **A,** Freckles. **B,** Junctional nevus. **C,** Compound nevus.

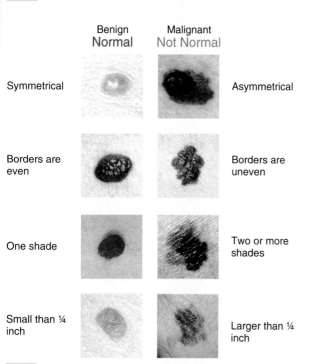

	Benign Normal	Malignant Not Normal	
Symmetrical			Asymmetrical
Borders are even			Borders are uneven
One shade			Two or more shades
Small than ¼ inch			Larger than ¼ inch

13.5 ABCDE mole comparison chart.

Abnormal Findings

Danger signs: abnormal characteristics of pigmented lesions are summarized in the mnemonic **ABCDE:**

Asymmetry (*not* regularly round or oval; two halves of lesion do not look the same)

Border irregularity (notching, scalloping, ragged edges or poorly defined margins)

Colour variation (areas of brown, tan, black, blue, red, white, or combination)

Diameter greater than 6 mm (i.e., the size of a pencil eraser), although early melanomas may be diagnosed at a smaller size

Elevation and **E**volution

Additional symptoms: rapidly changing lesion; a new pigmented lesion; and development of itching, burning, or bleeding in a mole. These signs should raise suspicion of malignant melanoma and warrant referral.

The "ugly duckling" sign is a new technique to help screen for malignant melanoma; the suspicious lesion stands out as looking different compared with neighbouring nevi (see Fig. 13.5).

Objective Data

Normal Range of Findings

Widespread Colour Change. Note any colour change in skin over the entire body, such as pallor (white), erythema (red), cyanosis (blue), and jaundice (yellow). Note whether the colour change is transient and expected or the result of pathology.

Pallor. When the red-pink tones from the oxygenated hemoglobin in the blood are lost, the skin takes on the colour of connective tissue (collagen), which is mostly white. Pallor is common in acute high-stress states, such as anxiety or fear, because of the powerful peripheral vasoconstriction from sympathetic nervous system stimulation. The skin also looks pale with vasoconstriction from exposure to cold and cigarette smoking and in the presence of edema.

Look for pallor in dark-skinned people by the absence of the underlying red tones that normally give brown or black skin its lustre. Generalized pallor can be observed in the mucous membranes, lips, and nail beds. The palpebral conjunctiva and nail beds are preferred sites for assessing the pallor of anemia. When you inspect the conjunctiva, lower the eyelid sufficiently to visualize the conjunctiva near the *outer* canthus as well as the inner canthus. The coloration is often lighter near the inner canthus.

Erythema. Erythema is an intense redness of the skin from excess blood (hyperemia) in the dilated superficial capillaries. This sign is *expected* with fever, local inflammation, or with emotional reactions such as blushing in vascular flush areas (cheeks, neck, and upper chest).

Erythema with fever or localized inflammation is characterized by increased skin temperature from the increased rate of blood flow. Because you cannot see inflammation in dark-skinned persons, it is often necessary to palpate the skin for increased warmth, tautness or tightly pulled surfaces, which may be indicative of edema, and hardening of deep tissues or blood vessels.

Cyanosis. This is a bluish, mottled discoloration that signifies decreased perfusion; the tissues are not adequately perfused with oxygenated blood. Be aware that cyanosis can be a nonspecific sign. A patient who is anemic could have hypoxemia without ever looking blue because not enough hemoglobin is present (either oxygenated or reduced) to colour the skin. In contrast, a patient with polycythemia (an increase in the number of red blood cells) looks ruddy blue at all times and may not necessarily be hypoxemic; this patient is just unable to fully oxygenate the massive numbers of red blood cells. Last, do not confuse cyanosis with the common and normal bluish tone on the lips of dark-skinned persons of Mediterranean origin.

Cyanosis is difficult to observe in a person with dark pigmentation (see Table 13.2, p. 234). Because most conditions that cause cyanosis also cause decreased oxygenation of the brain, other clinical signs—such as changes in level of consciousness and signs of respiratory distress—will be evident.

Jaundice. Jaundice is a yellow discoloration, indicating rising amounts of bilirubin in the blood. Except for physiological jaundice in the newborn (p. 243), jaundice does not occur normally. Jaundice is *first* noted in the junction of the hard and soft palates in the mouth and in the sclera. The scleral yellow of jaundice extends up to the edge of the iris.

Abnormal Findings

In dark-skinned people, the amount of normal pigment may mask colour changes. Lips and nail beds show some colour change, but they vary with the person's skin colour, and the colour change may not always be an accurate sign. The more reliable sites are those with the least pigmentation, such as under the tongue, the buccal mucosa, the palpebral conjunctiva, and the sclera. Table 13.2 (p. 234) lists specific clues to assessment.

Ashen-grey colour in dark skin or marked pallor in light skin occurs with anemia, shock, and arterial insufficiency (see Table 13.2, p. 234).

The pallor of impending shock is accompanied by other subtle manifestations, such as increasing pulse rate, oliguria, apprehension, and restlessness.

Chronic iron-deficiency anemia may present with "spoon" nails, with a concave shape. Fatigue, exertional dyspnea, rapid pulse, dizziness, and impaired mental function accompany most severe anemias.

Erythema occurs with polycythemia, venous stasis, carbon monoxide poisoning, and the extravascular presence of red blood cells (petechiae, ecchymosis, hematoma; see Table 13.2, p. 234, and Table 13.8, p. 260).

Cyanosis indicates hypoxemia and occurs with shock, heart failure, chronic bronchitis, and congenital heart disease.

Jaundice occurs with hepatitis, cirrhosis, sickle cell disease, transfusion reaction, and hemolytic disease of the newborn.

Objective Data

TABLE 13.2   Detecting Colour Changes in Light and Dark Skin

CAUSE	NOTE APPEARANCE	
	LIGHT SKIN	DARK SKIN
Pallor		

Anemia: decreased hematocrit
Shock: decreased perfusion,
  vasoconstriction
	Generalized pallor	Brown skin: appears yellow-brown, dull; black
		  skin: appears ashen grey, dull; skin loses its
		  healthy glow
		Check areas with least pigmentation, such as
		  conjunctivae and mucous membranes

Local arterial insufficiency	Marked localized pallor (e.g., lower
	  extremities, especially when
	  elevated)
		Ashen grey, dull; cool to palpitation

Albinism: total absence of pigment melanin throughout the integument	Whitish pink	Tan, cream, white

Vitiligo: patchy depigmentation from
  destruction of melanocytes
	Patchy milky white spots, often
	  symmetrical bilaterally
		Same as for light skin

Cyanosis		

Increased amount of unoxygenated
  hemoglobin
	Dusky blue	Dark but dull, lifeless; only severe cyanosis is
		  apparent in skin
		Check conjunctivae, oral mucosa, and nail beds

Central: chronic heart and lung disease
  causes arterial desaturation
	Grey coloration	Dark but dull, lifeless; only severe cyanosis is
		  apparent in skin

Peripheral: exposure to cold, anxiety	Nail beds dusky	Hard to detect
Erythema		

Hyperemia: increased blood flow
  through engorged arterioles, such as
  in inflammation, fever, alcohol intake,
  blushing
	Red, bright pink	Purplish tinge, but difficult to see
		Palpate for increased warmth with
		  inflammation, for taut skin, and for hardening
		  of deep tissues

Polycythemia: increased numbers of
  red blood cells, capillary stasis
	Ruddy blue in face, oral mucosa,
	  conjunctiva, hands, and feet
		Well concealed by pigment
		Check for redness in lips

Carbon monoxide poisoning	Bright cherry red in face and upper
	  torso
		Cherry-red colour in nail beds, lips, and oral
		  mucosa

Venous stasis: decreased blood flow
  from area, engorged venules
	Dusky rubor of dependent
	  extremities; a prelude to necrosis
	  with pressure sore
		Easily masked
		Palpate for warmth or edema

Jaundice		

Increased serum bilirubin (>2 to
  3 mg/100 mL) as a result of liver
  inflammation or hemolytic disease,
  such as post–severe burn state and
  some infections
	Yellow in sclera, hard palate, a
	  mucous membranes, then over skin
		Check sclera for yellow near limbus; do not
		  mistake normal yellowish fatty deposits in
		  the periphery under the eyelids for jaundice:
		  jaundice is best noted in junction of hard and
		  soft palate and also palms

Carotenemia: increased serum
  carotene from ingestion of large
  amounts of carotene-rich foods
	Yellow-orange in forehead, palms
	  and soles, and nasolabial folds, but
	  no yellowing in sclera or mucous
	  membranes
		Yellow-orange tinge in palms and soles

Uremia: in renal failure, urochrome
  pigments are retained in the blood
	Orange-green or grey overlying pallor
	  of anemia; ecchymoses and purpura
	  may also be present
		Easily masked
		Rely on laboratory and clinical findings

Brown-Tan		

Addison's disease: increased melanin
  production stimulated by cortisol
  deficiency
	Bronzed appearance, an "eternal
	  tan," most apparent around nipples,
	  perineum, genitalia, and pressure
	  points (inner thighs, buttocks,
	  elbow, axillae)
		Easily masked
		Rely on laboratory and clinical findings

Café au lait spots: caused by increased
  melanin pigment in basal cell layer
	Tan to light brown, irregularly shaped,
	  oval patch with well-defined borders	

Normal Range of Findings	Abnormal Findings

As levels of serum bilirubin rise, jaundice is evident in the skin over the rest of the body. This is best assessed in direct natural daylight. Common calluses on palms and soles often look yellow; do not interpret these as jaundice.

In both light- and dark-skinned people with jaundice, stools are often light or clay-coloured, and urine is often dark golden.

Temperature

Note the temperature of your own hands. Then use the backs (dorsa) of your hands to palpate the person and check bilaterally. The skin should be warm, and the temperature should be equal bilaterally; warmth suggests normal circulatory status. Hands and feet may be slightly cooler in a cool environment.

Hypothermia. Generalized coolness may be induced, such as in hypothermia used for surgery or high fever. Localized coolness is expected with an immobilized extremity, as when a limb is in a cast or with an intravenous infusion.

General hypothermia accompanies central circulatory problem such as shock.

Localized hypothermia occurs in peripheral arterial insufficiency and Raynaud's disease.

Hyperthermia. Generalized hyperthermia occurs with an increase in metabolic rate, as in fever or after heavy exercise. A localized area feels hyperthermic with trauma, infection, or sunburn.

Hyperthyroidism produces an increase in metabolic rate, causing warmth and moistness of skin.

Moisture

Perspiration appears normally on the face, hands, axilla, and skinfolds in response to activity, a warm environment, or anxiety. **Diaphoresis**, or profuse perspiration, accompanies an increase in metabolic rate, as occurs in strenuous activity or fever.

Look for **dehydration** in the oral mucous membranes. Normally there is none, and the mucous membranes look smooth and moist. Be aware that dark skin may normally look dry and flaky, but this does not necessarily indicate systemic dehydration.

Diaphoresis occurs with thyrotoxicosis and with stimulation of the nervous system with anxiety or pain.

With dehydration, mucous membranes look dry and the lips look parched and cracked. With extreme dryness, the skin is fissured, resembling cracks in a dry lake bed.

Texture

Normal skin feels smooth and firm, with an even surface.

Hyperthyroidism: skin feels smoother and softer, like velvet.

Hypothyroidism: skin feels rough, dry, and flaky.

Thickness

The epidermis is uniformly thin over most of the body, although thickened callus areas are normal on palms and soles. A callus is a circumscribed overgrowth of epidermis and is an adaptation to excessive pressure from the friction of work and weight bearing.

Skin is very thin and shiny (atrophic) with arterial insufficiency.

Edema

Edema is fluid that accumulates in the intercellular spaces; it is not present normally. To check for edema, imprint your thumbs firmly against the ankle malleolus or the tibia. Normally, the skin surface resumes its smoothness immediately. If your pressure leaves a dent in the skin, "pitting" edema is present (Fig. 13.6). Its presence is graded on a four-point scale:

1+: Mild pitting, slight indentation, no perceptible swelling of the leg
2+: Moderate pitting, indentation subsides rapidly
3+: Deep pitting, indentation remains for a short time, swelling of leg
4+: Very deep pitting, indentation lasts a long time, gross swelling and distortion of leg

This scale is somewhat subjective; ratings vary among examiners (see further content on this grading scale on p. 552 in Chapter 21).

Edema is most evident in dependent parts of the body (feet, ankles, and sacral areas), where the skin looks puffy and tight. Edema makes the hair follicles more prominent, so you note a pig-skin or orange-peel look (called *peau d'orange*).

Unilateral edema: Consider a local or peripheral cause.

Bilateral edema or edema that is generalized over the whole body *(anasarca)*: Consider a central problem such as heart failure or kidney failure.

Normal Range of Findings	Abnormal Findings

Edema masks normal skin colour and obscures pathological conditions such as jaundice or cyanosis because the fluid lies between the surface and the pigmented and vascular layers. It makes dark skin look lighter.

13.6 Pitting edema.

Mobility and Turgor

Pinch up a large fold of skin on the anterior aspect of the chest under the clavicle. Mobility is the skin's ease of rising, and turgor is its ability to return to place promptly when released. Together, they reflect the elasticity of the skin.

Mobility is decreased when edema is present.

Poor turgor is evident in severe dehydration or extreme weight loss; the pinched skin recedes slowly or "tents" and stands by itself.

Scleroderma, literally "hard skin," is a chronic connective tissue disorder associated with decreased mobility.

Vascularity or Bruising

Cherry (senile) angiomas are small (1–5 mm), smooth, slightly raised bright red dots that commonly appear on the trunk in all adults older than 30 years (Fig. 13.7). They normally increase in size and number with aging and are not significant.

13.7 Cherry angioma.

Normal Range of Findings

Any bruising (ecchymosis) should be consistent with the expected trauma of life. There are normally no venous dilatations or varicosities.

Document the presence of any tattoos (a permanent skin design from indelible pigment) on the person's chart. Advise the person that the use of tattoo needles and tattoo parlour equipment of doubtful sterility increases the risk for hepatitis C.

Lesions

If any lesions are present, note these characteristics:
1. Colour.
2. Elevation: flat, raised, or pedunculated.
3. Pattern or shape: the grouping or distinctness of each lesion; for example, annular, grouped, confluent, or linear. The pattern may be characteristic of a certain disease.
4. Size, in centimetres: Use a ruler to measure. Avoid household descriptions such as "quarter size" or "pea size."
5. Location and distribution on body: Is it generalized or localized to area of a specific irritant; around jewellery, a watchband, eyes?
6. Any exudate: colour and any odour.

Palpate lesions. Wear a glove if you anticipate contact with mucus, blood, any other body fluid, or skin lesion. Roll a nodule between the thumb and index finger to assess depth. Gently scrape a scale to see whether it comes off. Note the nature of its base or whether it bleeds when the scale comes off. Note the surrounding skin temperature. However, the erythema associated with rashes is not always accompanied by noticeable increases in skin temperature.

Does the lesion blanch with pressure or stretch? Stretching the area of skin between your thumb and index finger decreases the normal underlying red tones (blanches), thus providing more contrast and brightening the macules. Red macules from dilated blood vessels do blanch momentarily, whereas those from extravasated blood (petechiae) do not. Blanching also helps you identify a macular rash in dark-skinned patients.

Use a magnifier and light for closer inspection of the lesion (Fig. 13.8). Use a Wood light (i.e., an ultraviolet light filtered through a special glass) to detect fluorescing lesions. With the room darkened, shine the Wood light on the area.

13.8

Abnormal Findings

Multiple bruises at different stages of healing and excessive bruises above knees or elbows should raise concern about physical abuse (see Table 13.7, p. 256).

Needle marks or tracks from intravenous injection of street drugs may be visible on the antecubital fossae, on the forearms, or over any available vein.

Lesions are traumatic or pathological changes in previously normal structures. When a lesion develops on previously unaltered skin, it is **primary**. However, when a lesion changes over time or changes because of a factor such as scratching or infection, it is **secondary**. Table 13.3 (p. 249) lists the shapes and Tables 13.4 (p. 250) and 13.5 (p. 252) list the characteristics of primary and secondary skin lesions. The terms used (e.g., *macule*, *papule*) are helpful for describing any lesion you note.

Note the pattern and characteristics of common skin lesions (see Table 13.10, p. 262) and malignant skin lesions (Table 13.11, p. 265), and lesions associated with acquired immune deficiency syndrome (AIDS; Table 13.12, p. 266).

Lesions with blue-green fluorescence indicate fungal infection, such as tinea capitis (scalp ringworm).

Objective Data

Normal Range of Findings	Abnormal Findings

Inspect and Palpate The Hair

Colour

Hair colour results from melanin production and may vary from pale blond to totally black. Greying normally begins as early as the third decade of life because of reduced melanin production in the follicles. Genetic factors affect the age at onset of greying.

Texture

Scalp hair may be fine or thick and may look straight, curly, or kinky. It should look shiny, although this characteristic may be lost with the use of some beauty products such as dyes, rinses, or perm materials.

Note dull, coarse, or brittle scalp hair.

Grey, scaly, well-defined areas with broken hairs accompany tinea capitis, a ringworm infection found mostly in school-age children (see Table 13.13, p. 266).

Distribution

Fine vellus hair coats the body, whereas coarser terminal hairs grow at the eyebrows, eyelashes, and scalp. During puberty, distribution conforms to normal male and female patterns. At first, coarse curly hairs grow in the pubic area, then in the axillae, and last in the facial area in boys. In the genital area, the female pattern is an inverted triangle; the male pattern is an upright triangle with pubic hair extending up to the umbilicus. In individuals of Asian descent, body hair may be diminished.

Absence or abnormal configuration of genital hair suggests endocrine abnormalities.

Hirsutism: excess body hair. In women, this is characterized by a male pattern of hair distribution on the face and chest and indicates endocrine abnormalities (see Table 13.13, p. 268).

Lesions

Separate the hair into sections and lift it, observing the scalp. When the patient has a history of itching, inspect the hair behind the ears and in the occipital area as well. All areas should be clean and free of any lesions or pest inhabitants. Many people normally have seborrhea (dandruff), which is characterized by loose white flakes.

Head or pubic lice: Distinguish dandruff from nits (eggs) of lice, which are oval, adhere to the hair shaft, and cause intense itching (see Table 13.13, p. 268).

Inspect and Palpate The Nails

Shape and Contour

The nail surface is normally slightly curved or flat, and the posterior and lateral nail folds are smooth and rounded. Nail edges that are smooth, rounded, and clean suggest adequate self-care.

Jagged nails, bitten to the quick, or traumatized nail folds from chronic nervous picking suggest nervous habits.

Chronically dirty nails suggest poor self-care or chronic staining as a result of some occupations.

Clubbing of nails occurs with congenital, chronic, and cyanotic heart disease and with emphysema and chronic bronchitis.

In early clubbing, the angle straightens out to 180 degrees, and the nail base feels spongy on palpation.

The Profile Sign. View the index finger at its profile and note the angle of the nail base; it should be about 160 degrees (Fig. 13.9). The nail base is firm on palpation. Curved nails are a variation of normal with a convex profile. They may look like clubbed nails, but the angle between nail base and nail is normal (i.e., 160 degrees or less).

Objective Data

Normal Range of Findings	**Abnormal Findings**

13.9

Consistency

The surface is smooth and regular, not brittle or splitting.

Nail thickness is uniform.

The nail is firmly adherent to the nail bed, and the nail base is firm on palpation.

Colour

The translucent nail plate is a window to the even, pink nail bed underneath.

Dark-skinned people may have brown-black pigmented areas or linear bands or streaks along the nail edge (Fig. 13.10). All people normally may have white hairline linear markings (leukonychia strata) from trauma or picking at the cuticle (Fig. 13.11). Note any abnormal marking in the nail beds.

13.10 Linear pigmentation.

13.11 Leukonychia striata.

Pits, transverse grooves, or lines may indicate a nutrient deficiency or may accompany acute illness in which nail growth is disturbed (see Table 13.14, p. 269).

With arterial insufficiency, nails are thickened and ridged.

A spongy nail base accompanies clubbing.

Cyanosis or marked pallor.

Brown linear streaks (especially sudden appearance) are abnormal in light-skinned people and may indicate melanoma.

Splinter hemorrhages, transverse ridges, or Beau's lines (see Table 13.14, p. 269).

Objective Data

Objective Data

Normal Range of Findings

Capillary Refill. Depress the nail edge to cause blanching, and then release, noting the return of colour. Normally, colour returns instantly or at least within a few seconds in a cold environment. This indicates the status of the peripheral circulation. A sluggish colour return takes longer than 1 or 2 seconds.
Inspect the toenails. Separate the toes, and note the smoothness of the skin in between.

Promoting Health and Self-Care

Teach Skin Self-Examination

Teach all adults to examine their skin once a month, using the ABCDE rule (see p. 232), to detect warning signals of any suspect lesions: they should use a well-lighted room that has a full-length mirror. It helps to have a small hand-held mirror. They should ask a relative to search skin areas difficult to see (e.g., behind ears, back of neck, back). They should follow the sequence outlined in Fig. 13.12 and report any suspect lesions promptly to the appropriate health care provider.

Abnormal Findings

Cyanotic nail beds or sluggish colour return may be indicative of cardiovascular or respiratory dysfunction.

1. Undress completely. Check forearms, palms, space between fingers. Turn over hands and study the backs.

2. Face mirror; bend arms at elbow. Study arms in mirror.

3. Face mirror and study entire front of body. Start at face, neck, torso, working down to lower legs.

4. Pivot to right side facing mirror. Study sides of upper arms, working down to ankles. Repeat with left side.

5. With back to mirror, study buttocks, thighs, lower legs.

6. Use the handheld mirror to study upper back.

7. Use the handheld mirror to study scalp, lifting the hair. A blow-dryer on a cool setting helps to lift hair.

8. Sit on chair or bed. Study insides of each leg and soles of feet. Use the small mirror to help.

13.12 Skin self-examination.

Normal Range of Findings	Abnormal Findings

 DEVELOPMENTAL CONSIDERATIONS

Infants

Skin Colour: General Pigmentation. Newborns of African descent initially have lighter toned skin than their parents because pigment production is not yet fully functional. Their full melanotic colour is evident in the nail beds and scrotal folds. The **mongolian spot** is a common variation of hyperpigmentation in newborns of Indigenous, African, East Indian, or Hispanic descent (Fig. 13.13). It is a blue-black to purple macular area at the sacrum or buttocks, but sometimes it occurs on the abdomen, thighs, shoulders, or arms. It results from deep dermal melanocytes. It gradually fades during the first year. By adulthood, these spots are lighter but are frequently still visible. Mongolian spots are present in 90% of individuals of African descent and 80% of individuals of Asian or Indigenous descent. If you are unfamiliar with mongolian spots, be careful not to confuse them with bruises. Recognition of this normal variation is particularly important to avoid erroneously identifying children as victims of child abuse.

Bruising is a common soft tissue injury that follows a rapid, traumatic, or breech birth.

Multiple bruises in various stages of healing, or pattern injury, suggest child abuse (see Table 13.7, p. 256).

13.13   Mongolian spot.

The **café au lait spot** is a large round or oval patch of light brown pigmentation (hence, the name, which means "coffee with milk"), which is usually present at birth (Fig. 13.14). Most such patches are normal.

The presence of six or more café au lait macules, each more than 1.5 cm in diameter, is diagnostic of neurofibromatosis, an inherited neurocutaneous disease.

13.14   Café au lait spot.

Normal Range of Findings

Skin Colour Change. Three erythematous states are common variations in the neonate:

1. The newborn's skin has a beefy-red flush for the first 24 hours because of vasomotor instability; then the colour fades to its normal shade.
2. Another finding, the **harlequin colour change**, occurs when the baby is in a side-lying position. The lower half of the body turns red, and the upper half blanches with a distinct demarcation line down the midline. The cause is unknown, and its occurrence is transient.
3. **Erythema toxicum** is a common rash that appears in the first 3 to 4 days of life. Sometimes called the "flea bite" rash or "newborn rash," it consists of tiny, punctate, red macules and papules on the cheeks, trunk, chest, back, and buttocks (Fig. 13.15). The cause is unknown; no treatment is needed.

13.15   Erythema toxicum.

Two temporary cyanotic conditions may occur:

1. **Acrocyanosis** is a bluish colour around the lips, on the hands and fingernails, and on the feet and toenails. This may last for a few hours and disappear with warming.
2. **Cutis marmorata** is a transient mottling in the trunk and extremities in response to cooler room temperatures (Fig. 13.16). It is characterized by a reticulated red or blue pattern over the skin.

13.16   Cutis marmorata.

Abnormal Findings

Persistent generalized cyanosis indicates distress, such as cyanotic congenital heart disease.

Persistent or pronounced cutis marmorata occurs with Down syndrome and prematurity.

Green-brown discoloration of the skin, nails, and umbilical cord occurs with passing of meconium in utero, which produces fetal distress.

Normal Range of Findings

Physiological jaundice is a common variation in about half of all newborns. A yellowing of the skin, sclera, and mucous membranes develops **after the third or fourth day** of life because of the increased numbers of red blood cells that hemolyze after birth. The hemoglobin in the red blood cells is metabolized by the liver and spleen; its pigment is converted into bilirubin.

Carotenemia also produces a yellow-orange colour in light-skinned persons but no yellowing in the sclerae or mucous membranes. It results from ingestion of large amounts of foods containing carotene, a vitamin A precursor. Carotene-rich foods are popular as prepared infant foods, and the absorption of carotene is enhanced by mashing, pureeing, and cooking. The colour is best seen on the palms and soles, the forehead, the tip of the nose and nasolabial folds, and the chin; behind the ears; and over the knuckles. It fades to normal within 2 to 6 weeks after carotene-rich foods are withdrawn from the diet.

Moisture. The vernix caseosa is the moist, white, cream cheese–like substance that covers part of the skin of all newborns. Perspiration is present after 1 month of age.

Texture. A common variation occurring in infants is **milia** (Fig. 13.17). Milia are tiny while papules on the cheeks, forehead, and across the nose and chin caused by sebum that occludes the opening of the follicles. Tell parents not to squeeze the lesions; milia resolve spontaneously within a few weeks.

13.17 Milia.

Thickness. In neonates, the epidermis is normally thin, but you will also note well-defined areas of subcutaneous fat. The baby's skin dimples over joints, but there is no break in the skin. Check for any defect or break in the skin, especially over the length of the spine.

Mobility and Turgor. Test mobility and turgor over the abdomen in an infant.

Vascularity or Bruising. Some vascular markings are common birthmarks in the newborn. A **storkbite** (salmon patch) is a flat, irregularly shaped red or pink patch found on the forehead, eyelid, or upper lip but most commonly at the back of the neck (nuchal area; Fig. 13.18). It is present at birth and usually fades during the first year.

Abnormal Findings

Jaundice on the first day of life may indicate hemolytic disease. Jaundice after 2 weeks of age may indicate biliary tract obstruction.

With meconium staining, vernix is green-tinged.

In children, excessive sweating may accompany hypoglycemia, heart disease, or hyperthyroidism.

Subcutaneous fat may be lacking in premature and malnourished newborns.

A red sacrococcygeal dimple is present with a pilonidal cyst or sinus (see Table 23.2, p. 619).

Poor turgor, or "tenting," indicates dehydration or malnutrition.

More unusual skin marks are port-wine stains, strawberry marks (immature hemangioma), and cavernous hemangiomas (see Table 13.8, p. 257).

Bruising may suggest abuse (see Table 13.7, p. 256).

Objective Data

Normal Range of Findings

Hair. A newborn's skin is covered with fine downy lanugo (Fig. 13.19), especially in a preterm infant. Dark-skinned newborns have more lanugo than do light-skinned newborns. Scalp hair may be lost in the few weeks after birth, especially at the temples and occiput. It grows back slowly.

Nails. A newborn's nail beds may be blue (cyanotic) for the first few hours of life; then they turn pink.

13.18 Storkbite.

Adolescents

The increase in sebaceous gland activity creates increased oiliness and **acne**. Acne is the most common skin problem of adolescence. Almost all teenagers have some acne, even if it is the milder form of open comedones (blackheads; Fig. 13.20, *A*) and closed comedones (whiteheads). Severe acne includes papules, pustules, and nodules (see Fig. 13.20, *B*). Acne lesions usually appear on the face and sometimes on the chest, back, and shoulders. Acne may appear in children as early as 7 to 8 years of age; then the number and severity of the lesions increase, peaking at 14 to 16 years in girls and at 16 to 19 years in boys.

13.19 Lanugo.

Abnormal Findings

The scalp becomes scaly and crusted with seborrheic dermatitis (cradle cap; see Table 13.13, p. 266).

Normal Range of Findings	Abnormal Findings

13.20   **A,** Open comedones. **B,** Severe acne.

Pregnant Women

Striae are jagged linear "stretch marks" coloured silver to pink that appear during the second trimester on the abdomen, breasts, and sometimes thighs. They occur in half of all pregnancies. They fade after delivery but do not disappear. Another skin change on the abdomen is the **linea nigra**, a brownish black line down the midline (see Fig. 30.3, p. 866). **Chloasma** is an irregular brown patch of hyperpigmentation on the face. It may occur with pregnancy or in women taking oral contraceptive pills. Chloasma disappears after delivery or after the woman stops taking the pills. **Vascular spiders** occur in two-thirds of all pregnancies, primarily in Canadians of European descent. These lesions have tiny red centres with radiating branches and occur on the face, neck, upper chest, and arms.

Older Adults

Skin Colour and Pigmentation. **Senile Lentigines.** Called "liver spots," these are small, flat, brown macules that are common variations of hyperpigmentation (Fig. 13.21). These circumscribed areas are clusters of melanocytes that appear after extensive sun exposure. They appear on the forearms and dorsa of the hands. They are not malignant and necessitate no treatment.

13.21   Lentigines.

Keratoses. These lesions are raised, thickened areas of pigmentation that look crusted, scaly, and warty. One type, **seborrheic keratosis**, looks dark, greasy, and "stuck on" (Fig. 13.22). They develop mostly on the trunk but also on the face and hands and on both unexposed and sun-exposed areas. It is uncommon for them to be found as cancerous.

Normal Range of Findings	Abnormal Findings

13.22 Seborrheic keratosis.

Another type, **actinic (senile** or **solar) keratosis,** is less common (Fig. 13.23). These lesions are red-tan scaly plaques that enlarge over the years to become raised and roughened. A silvery white scale may adhere to the plaques. They occur on sun-exposed surfaces and are directly related to sun exposure. They are premalignant and may develop into squamous cell carcinoma.

13.23 Actinic keratosis.

Moisture. Dry skin (xerosis) is common in older adults because of a decline in the size, number, and output of the sweat glands and sebaceous glands. Dry skin itches and looks flaky and loose.

Texture. Variations especially prevalent among older adults are **acrochordons,** or "skin tags," which are overgrowths of normal skin that form a stalk and are polyplike (Fig. 13.24). They occur frequently on eyelids, cheeks, neck, axillae, and trunk.

13.24 Skin tags.

Normal Range of Findings

Abnormal Findings

Sebaceous hyperplasia appears as raised yellow papules with a central depression. They are more common in men, occurring over the forehead, nose, or cheeks. They have a pebbly look (Fig. 13.25).

13.25 Sebaceous hyperplasia.

Thickness. With aging, the skin looks as thin as parchment, and the subcutaneous fat diminishes. Thinner skin is evident over the dorsa of the hands, forearms, lower legs, dorsa of feet, and bony prominences. The skin may feel thicker over the abdomen and chest.

Hair. With aging, the hair growth decreases, and the amount in the axillae and pubic areas decreases. After menopause, women may develop bristly hairs on the chin or upper lip as a result of unopposed androgens. In men, coarse terminal hairs develop in the ears, nose, and eyebrows, although the beard is unchanged. Male-pattern balding, or alopecia, is a genetic trait. It is usually a gradual receding of the anterior hairline in a symmetrical W shape. In men and women, scalp hair gradually turns grey because of the decrease in melanocyte function.

Nails. With aging, the nail growth rate decreases, and local injuries in the nail matrix may produce longitudinal ridges. The surface may be brittle or peeling and sometimes yellowed. Toenails also are thickened and may grow misshapen, almost grotesque. The thickening may be a process of aging, or it may be caused by chronic peripheral vascular disease.

Fungal infections are common in aging, with thickened crumbling toenails and erythematous scaling on contiguous skin surfaces.

Mobility and Turgor. The turgor is decreased (less elasticity), and the skin recedes slowly or "tents" and stands by itself (Fig. 13.26).

13.26

Objective Data

DOCUMENTATION AND CRITICAL THINKING

Sample Charting

SUBJECTIVE

No history of skin disease; no current change in pigmentation or in nevi; no pruritus, bruising, rash, or lesions. Taking no medications. No work-related skin hazards. Uses sunblock cream when outdoors.

OBJECTIVE

Skin: Colour tan-pink, even pigmentation, with no nevi. Warm to touch, dry, smooth, and even. Turgor good, no lesions.
Hair: Even distribution, thick texture, no lesions or pest inhabitants.
Nails: No clubbing or deformities. Nail beds pink with prompt capillary refill.

ASSESSMENT

Warm, dry, intact skin.

Focused Assessment: Clinical Case Study

Ethan Eichel (E.E.) is a 3-year-old boy presenting with his mother, who seeks health care because of Ethan's fever, fatigue, and rash of 3 days' duration.

SUBJECTIVE

2 weeks PTA [prior to arrival]: E.E. was playing with a child in whom chicken pox was subsequently diagnosed.
3 days PTA: Mother reports fever was 37.7°C to 38.3°C (99.9°F to 100.9°F), fatigue, and irritability. That evening noted "tiny blisters" on chest and back.
1 day PTA: Blisters on chest changed to white with scab on top. New eruption of blisters on shoulders, thighs, face. Intense itching and scratching.

OBJECTIVE

Vital signs: Temp, 38.0°C (100.4°F); pulse, 110 bpm; resp, 24/min.
Skin: Generalized vesiculopustular rash covering face, trunk, upper arms, and thighs. Small vesicles on face, pustules and red-honey–coloured crusts on trunk. Otherwise skin is warm and dry, turgor good.
Ears: Tympanic membranes, pearl grey with landmarks intact. No discharge.
Mouth and throat: Mucosa dark pink, no lesions. Tonsils 1+, no exudate. No lymphadenopathy.
Heart: S_1, S_2 normal, not accentuated or diminished, no murmurs or extra sounds.
Lungs: Hyper-resonant to percussion. Breath sounds clear, no adventitious sounds.

ASSESSMENT

Varicella
Impaired skin integrity R/T [related to] infection and scratching

ABNORMAL FINDINGS

TABLE 13.3 Common Shapes and Configurations of Lesions

Annular

Also called *circular*; begins in centre and spreads to
  periphery
Examples: tinea corporis (ringworm), tinea versicolor,
  pityriasis rosea

Confluent

Lesions that merge together
Example: urticaria (hives)

◀ Discrete

Distinct, individual lesions that remain separate
Example: molluscum

Grouped

Clusters of lesions
Example: vesicles of contact dermatitis

Gyrate

Twisted, coiled, spiral, snakelike

Continued

TABLE 13.3 Common Shapes and Configurations of Lesions—cont'd

Target

Also called *iris*; resemble iris of eye, concentric rings of colour in the lesions
Example: erythema multiforme

Linear

A scratch, streak, line, or stripe

Polycyclic

Annular lesions that grow together
Examples: lichen planus, psoriasis

Zosteriform

Linear arrangement along a nerve route
Example: herpes zoster

TABLE 13.4 Primary Skin Lesions[a]

Macule

Patch

Papule

Plaque

Macule

Solely a colour change; flat and circumscribed, <1 cm diameter
Examples: freckles, flat nevi, hypopigmentation, petechiae, measles, scarlet fever

Papule

Palpable: solid, elevated, circumscribed, <1 cm diameter; caused by superficial thickening in the epidermis
Examples: elevated nevus (mole), lichen planus, molluscum, wart (verruca)

TABLE 13.4   Primary Skin Lesions—cont'd

Patch

Macules >1 cm diameter
Examples: mongolian spot, vitiligo, café au lait spot, chloasma, measles rash

Nodule

Tumor

Nodule

Solid, elevated, hard or soft, >1 cm diameter; may extend deeper into dermis than papule
Examples: xanthoma, fibroma, intradermal nevi

Tumour

Larger than a few centimetres in diameter; firm or soft, deeper into dermis; may be benign or malignant, although "tumour" implies "cancer" to most people
Examples: lipoma, hemangioma

Plaque

Papules that coalesce to form surface elevation wider than 1 cm; a plateaulike, disc-shaped lesion
Examples: psoriasis, lichen planus

Wheal

Urticaria

Wheal

Superficial, raised, transient, and erythematous; slightly irregular shape because of edema (fluid held diffusely in the tissues)
Examples: mosquito bite, allergic reaction, dermographism

Urticaria (Hives)

Wheals that coalesce to form extensive reaction; intensely pruritic

Vesicle

Bulla

Vesicle

Bulla

Vesicle

Also called *blister*; elevated cavity containing free fluid, up to 1 cm; clear serum flows if wall is ruptured
Examples: herpes simplex, early varicella (chicken pox), herpes zoster (shingles), contact dermatitis

Cyst

Encapsulated fluid-filled cavity in dermis or subcutaneous layer; tensely elevating skin
Examples: sebaceous cyst, trichilemmal cyst (wen)

Continued

TABLE 13.4   Primary Skin Lesions—cont'd

Bulla

Usually single-chambered (unilocular); superficial in
epidermis; >1 cm diameter; thin-walled, and so it ruptures
easily

Examples: friction blister, pemphigus, burns, contact
dermatitis

Pustule

▶

Cavity filled with turbid fluid (pus); circumscribed and
elevated

Examples: impetigo, acne

ªThe immediate result of a specific causative factor; primary lesions develop on previously unaltered skin.
Line drawings © Pat Thomas, 2010. See Illustration Credits for photo source information.

TABLE 13.5   Secondary Skin Lesionsª

DEBRIS ON SKIN SURFACE

Crust

The thickened, dried-out exudate left when vesicles/pustules
burst or dry up; colour can be red-brown, honeylike,
or yellow, depending on the fluid's ingredients (blood,
serum, pus)

Examples: impetigo (dry, honey-coloured), weeping
eczematous dermatitis, scab after abrasion

Scale

Compact, desiccated flakes of skin, dry or greasy, silvery or
white, from shedding of dead excess keratin cells

Examples: lesions after scarlet fever or medication reaction
(laminated sheets), psoriasis (silver, micalike), seborrheic
dermatitis (yellow, greasy), eczema, ichthyosis (large,
adherent, laminated), dry skin

TABLE 13.5 Secondary Skin Lesions—cont'd

BREAK IN CONTINUITY OF SURFACE

Fissure

Linear crack with abrupt edges, extending into dermis; dry or moist
Examples: cheilosis (at corners of mouth as a result of excess moisture); athlete's foot

Erosion

Scooped-out but shallow depression; superficial; epidermis lost; moist but no bleeding; healing without scar because erosion does not extend into dermis

Ulcer

Deeper depression extending into dermis, irregular shape; may bleed; leaves scar when heals
Examples: stasis ulcer, pressure sore, chancre

Excoriation

Self-inflicted abrasion; superficial; sometimes crusted; scratches from intense itching
Examples: lesions caused by scratching of insect bites, scabies, dermatitis, varicella

Continued

TABLE 13.5   Secondary Skin Lesions—cont'd

Scar

Connective tissue (collagen) that replaces normal tissue
  after a skin lesion is repaired; a permanent fibrotic change
Examples: healed area of surgery or injury, acne

Atrophic Scar

Depression of skin level as a result of loss of tissue; a
  thinning of the epidermis
Example: striae

Lichenification

Thickening of skin with production of tightly packed sets
  of papules, caused by prolonged intense scratching; looks
  like surface of moss (or lichen)

Keloid

A hypertrophic scar; elevation of the resulting skin level
  by excess scar tissue, which is invasive beyond the site of
  original injury; may increase long after healing occurs;
  looks smooth, rubbery, and "clawlike"; has a higher
  incidence among individuals of African descent

Note: Combinations of primary and secondary lesions may coexist in the same person. Such combinations may be termed *papulosquamous*, *maculopapular*, *vesiculopustular*, or *papulovesicular*.
[a]Resulting from a change in a primary lesion from the passage of time; an evolutionary change.
Line drawings © Pat Thomas, 2010. See Illustration Credits for photo source information.

TABLE 13.6   Pressure Injury (Decubitus Ulcer)

In Canada, the prevalence of pressure injury is estimated to be about 4% in an acute care setting compared with 30% in hospital-based, complex-care environments. These estimates are higher than those in most other countries worldwide, perhaps because of issues regarding length of stay in hospital settings and increasing numbers of people with overall level of illness who present in acute and long-term care environments.[2]

Pressure injuries appear on the skin over a bony prominence when circulation is impaired. This occurs when a person is confined to bed or is immobilized. Immobilization impedes delivery of blood, which carries oxygen and nutrients to the skin, and it impedes venous drainage, which carries metabolic wastes away from the skin. These impediments result in ischemia and cell death. Common sites for pressure injury are on the back (heel, ischium, sacrum, elbow, scapula, vertebra) and the side (ankle, knee, hip, rib, shoulder).

Risk factors for pressure injury include impaired mobility, thin fragile skin of aging, decreased sensory perception (which causes inability to perceive pain accompanying prolonged pressure), impaired level of consciousness (which causes inability to respond to pain), moisture from urine or stool incontinence, excessive perspiration or wound drainage, shearing injury (being pulled down or across in bed), poor nutrition, and infection. Learning about risk factors and the prevention of pressure injury is far more easily accomplished than is the treatment of existing wounds. However, once the pressure injury occurs, they are assessed by stage, depending on the pressure ulcer depth:[3]

Stage 1

Intact skin appears red but unbroken. Localized redness in lightly pigmented skin will blanch (turns light with pressure). Affected dark skin appears darker but does not blanch.

Stage 2

Partial-thickness skin erosion causes loss of epidermis or also the dermis. Superficial ulcer looks shallow, like an abrasion or open blister with a red-pink wound bed.

Continued

TABLE 13.6 Pressure Injury (Decubitus Ulcer)—cont'd

Stage 3

Full-thickness pressure injury extends into the subcutaneous tissue and resembles a crater. Subcutaneous fat may be visible, but not muscle, bone, or tendon.

Stage 4

Full-thickness pressure injury involves all skin layers and extends into supporting tissue. Muscle, tendon, and bone may be exposed, and slough (stringy matter attached to wound bed) or eschar (black or brown necrotic tissue).

Unstageable Pressure Injury: Full-thickness skin and tissue loss in which the extent of tissue damage within the injury cannot be confirmed because it is obscured by slough or eschar.

Deep Tissue Pressure Injury: Persistent non-blanchable deep red, maroon or purple discoloration.

These types of injuries required advanced intervention and a wound specialist would most certainly be consulted to intervene with such cases.

See Illustration Credits for source information.

TABLE 13.7 Lesions Caused by Trauma or Abuse

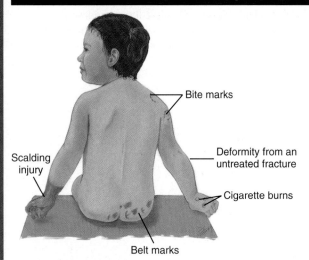

Bite marks

Deformity from an untreated fracture

Scalding injury

Cigarette burns

Belt marks

Scalp petechiae

Hematoma

◀ Pattern Injury

Pattern injury is a bruise or wound whose shape suggests which instrument or weapon caused it (e.g., belt buckle, broomstick, burning cigarette, pinch marks, bite marks, or scalding hot liquid). Inflicted scalding-water immersion burns usually have a clear border, like a glove or sock, indicating that body part was held under water intentionally. Deformity results from an untreated fracture because the bone heals out of alignment.

In a child, these physical signs, together with a history that does not match the severity or type of injury, suggest child abuse and warrant intervention (see Chapter 8).

The Canadian Child Health Welfare Research Portal has a comprehensive description of policies for reporting across Canada. See http://cwrp.ca/child-abuse-neglect.

◀ Hematoma

A hematoma is a bruise that you can palpate. It elevates the skin and is seen as swelling. Multiple petechiae and purpura may occur on the face when prolonged vigorous crying or coughing raises venous pressure.

TABLE 13.7   Lesions Caused by Trauma or Abuse—cont'd

◀ Dog, Cat, and Human Bite Wounds

The dog bite shown here is a crushing injury with puncture wounds and lacerations. Dog bites on adults occur on arms or legs; on children they are more often on the face or scalp. Assess for cosmetic repair and risk for infection. An X-ray image shows bone penetration or tooth fragment left in the wound. Cat bites involve deeply punctured tissue, and over half result in infection. Human bites are even more serious because of abundant micro-organisms in human saliva. All are treated with appropriate antibiotics.[4]

◀ Contusion (Bruise)

A contusion is a large patch of capillary bleeding into tissues. Colour in light-skinned person is usually (1) red-blue or purple immediately after or within 24 hours of trauma, which turns (2) blue to purple and then (3) blue-green, (4) yellow, and (5) brown and then disappears completely. A recent bruise in a dark-skinned person is deep, dark purple. Note that it is *not* possible to date the age of a bruise according to its colour.

Pressure on a bruise does *not* cause it to blanch. Bruises usually occur from trauma, but they are also caused by bleeding disorders and liver dysfunction. Note that a bruise is different from petechiae, ecchymosis, and purpura because these are *not* caused by blunt force trauma.

See Illustration Credits for source information.

TABLE 13.8   Vascular Lesions

Hemangiomas

These are caused by a benign proliferation of blood vessels in the dermis.

◀ Port-Wine Stain (Nevus Flammeus)

This is a large, flat macular patch covering the scalp or face, frequently along the distribution of cranial nerve V. The colour is dark red, bluish, or purplish and intensifies with crying, exertion, or exposure to heat or cold. The marking is formed from mature capillaries. It is present at birth and usually does not fade. The use of yellow-light lasers now makes photoablation of the lesion possible, with minimal adverse effects.

Continued

TABLE 13.8   Vascular Lesions—cont'd

Strawberry Mark (Immature Hemangioma)

This is a raised, bright red area with well-defined borders about 2–3 cm in diameter. It does not blanch with pressure. It is formed from immature capillaries, is present at birth or develops in the first few months, and usually disappears by age 5 to 7 years. It necessitates no treatment, although parental and peer pressure may prompt treatment.

Cavernous Hemangioma (Mature)

This is a reddish blue, irregularly shaped, solid, and spongy mass of blood vessels. It may be present at birth, may enlarge during the first 10 to 15 months, and does not involute spontaneously.

Telangiectases

◀ Telangiectasia

This is the appearance of blood vessels on the skin surface. It is caused by vascular dilatation; the blood vessels are permanently enlarged and dilated.

TABLE 13.8   Vascular Lesions—cont'd

Spider or Star Angioma

This is a fiery red, star-shaped marking with a solid circular centre. Capillary radiations ("legs") extend from the central arterial body. With pressure, note a central pulsating body and blanching of extended "legs." It develops on the face, neck, or chest; may be associated with pregnancy, chronic liver disease, or estrogen therapy; or may be normal.

Venous Lake

This is a blue-purple dilatation of venules and capillaries in a star-shaped, linear, or flaring pattern. Pressure causes them to empty or disappear. They are located on the legs near varicose veins and also on the face, lips, ears, and chest.

Purpuric Lesions

These are caused by blood flowing out of breaks in the vessels. Red blood cells and blood pigments are deposited in the tissues (extravascularly). They are difficult to see in dark-skinned people.

◀ Petechiae

These are tiny punctate hemorrhages, 1–3 mm, round and discrete, and dark red, purple, or brown. They are caused by bleeding from superficial capillaries and do not blanch. They may indicate abnormal clotting factors. In dark-skinned people, petechiae are best visualized in the areas of lighter pigmentation (e.g., the abdomen, buttocks, and volar surface of the forearm). When the skin is black or very dark brown, petechiae cannot be seen in the skin.

Most of the diseases that cause bleeding and microembolism formation—such as thrombocytopenia, subacute bacterial endocarditis, and other septicemias—are characterized by petechiae in the mucous membranes, as well as on the skin. Thus you should inspect for petechiae in the mouth, particularly the buccal mucosa, and in the conjunctivae.

Continued

TABLE 13.8   Vascular Lesions—cont'd

Purpura

This is an extensive patch of confluent petechiae and ecchymoses, >3 mm flat, red to purple, macular hemorrhage. It occurs in generalized disorders such as thrombocytopenia and scurvy. It also occurs in old age as blood leaks from capillaries in response to minor trauma and diffuses through dermis.

Ecchymosis

This is a purplish patch resulting from extravasation of blood into the skin, >3 mm in diameter.

See Illustration Credits for source information.

TABLE 13.9   Common Skin Lesions in Children

Diaper Dermatitis

Red, moist maculopapular patch with poorly defined borders in diaper area, extending along inguinal and gluteal folds. History: infrequent diaper changes or occlusive coverings. Inflammatory disease caused by skin irritation from ammonia, heat, moisture, occlusive diapers.

Intertrigo (Candidiasis)

Scalding red, moist patches with sharply demarcated borders, some loose scales. Usually in genital area, extending along inguinal and gluteal folds. Aggravated by urine, feces, heat, and moisture; *Candida* fungus infects the superficial skin layers.

TABLE 13.9 **Common Skin Lesions in Children—cont'd**

Impetigo

Moist, thin-roofed vesicles with thin, erythematous base. Rupture is followed by formation of thick, honey-coloured crusts. Contagious bacterial infection of skin; most common in infants and children.

Atopic Dermatitis (Eczema)

Erythematous papules and vesicles, with weeping, oozing, and crusting. Lesions usually on scalp, forehead, cheeks, forearms and wrists, elbows, and backs of knees. Paroxysmal and severe pruritus. Family history of allergies.

Measles

Red-purple maculopapular blotchy rash in dark skin (on top) and in light skin (on bottom) appears on third or fourth day of illness. Rash appears first behind ears, spreads over face, and then spreads over neck, trunk, arms, and legs; looks "coppery" and does not blanch. Also characterized by Koplik's spots in mouth: bluish white, red-based elevations of 1–3 mm.

Measles (Rubeola) in Dark Skin

Measles (Rubeola) in Light Skin

Continued

TABLE 13.9   Common Skin Lesions in Children—cont'd

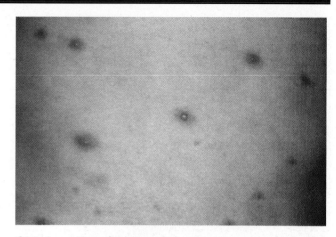

German Measles (Rubella)

Pink papular rash (similar to measles but paler) first appears on face, then spreads. Distinguished from measles by presence of neck lymphadenopathy and absence of Koplik's spots.

Chicken Pox (Varicella)

Small tight vesicles first appear on trunk and then spread to face, arms, and legs (not palms or soles). Shiny vesicles on an erythematous base are commonly described as the "dewdrop on a rose petal." Vesicles erupt in succeeding crops over several days, then become pustules, and then become crusts. Characterized by intense pruritus.

See Illustration Credits for source information.

TABLE 13.10   Common Skin Lesions

Primary Contact Dermatitis

Local inflammatory reaction to an irritant in the environment or an allergy. Characteristic location of lesions often gives clue to diagnosis. Often erythema shows first, followed by swelling, wheals (or urticaria), or maculopapular vesicles, scales. Frequently accompanied by intense pruritus.
Example (in photo): poison ivy

Allergic Medication Reaction

Erythematous and symmetrical rash, usually generalized. Some medications produce urticarial rash or vesicles and bullae. History of medication ingestion.

TABLE 13.10 **Common Skin Lesions—cont'd**

Tinea Corporis (Ringworm of the Body)

Scales are hyperpigmented in white-skinned individuals, depigmented in dark-skinned individuals. On chest, abdomen, and back of arms, forming multiple circular lesions with clear centres.

Tinea Pedis (Ringworm of the Foot)

Also known as "athlete's foot": a fungal infection, first appearing as small vesicles between toes, sides of feet, soles, and then growing scaly and hard. Found in chronically warm, moist feet: children after gymnasium activities, athletes, and older adults who cannot dry their feet well.

Psoriasis

Scaly erythematous patch, with silvery scales on top. Usually on scalp, outside of elbows and knees, low back, and anogenital area.

Tinea Versicolor

Fine, scaling, round patches of pink, tan, or white (hence the name) that do not tan in sunlight; caused by a superficial fungal infection. Usual distribution is on neck, trunk, and upper arms: a short-sleeved turtleneck sweater area. Most common in otherwise healthy young adults. Responds to oral antifungal medication.

Continued

TABLE 13.10   Common Skin Lesions—cont'd

Herpes Simplex (Cold Sores)

Herpes simplex virus infection has a prodrome of skin tingling sensation and sensitivity. Lesion then erupts with tight vesicles, followed by pustules, and then produces acute gingivostomatitis with many shallow, painful ulcers. Common location is upper lip; also in oral mucosa and tongue.

Herpes Zoster (Shingles)

Small grouped vesicles emerge along route of cutaneous sensory nerve, then pustules, then crusts. Caused by the varicella zoster virus, a reactivation of the dormant virus of chicken pox. Acute appearance, almost always unilateral, does not cross midline. Commonly on trunk, but can appear anywhere. If on ophthalmic branch of cranial nerve V, it poses risk to eye. Most common in adults >50 years old. Pain, called *postherpetic neuralgia*, is often severe and long lasting in older adults.

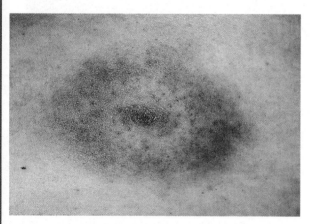

Erythema Migrans of Lyme Disease

The *first* sign of infection is usually a circular rash called *erythema migrans*. This rash occurs in about 70–80% of infected people. It begins at the site of the tick bite after a delay of 3 days to 1 month and can persist for up to 8 weeks. The rash radiates from the site of the tick bite (5 cm or larger), with some central clearing, and is usually located in axilla, midriff, or inguina or behind knee, with regional lymphadenopathy. Rash fades in 4 weeks; untreated individual then may have **disseminated disease** with fatigue, anorexia, fever, chills, and joint or muscle aches. Antibiotic treatment shortens symptoms and decreases risk of progressing to disseminated disease.

Scabies

An intensely pruritic condition caused by the scabies mite. Mites form a linear or curved elevated burrow on the fingers, web spaces of hands, and wrists. Other family members are usually infected. The patient cannot stop scratching.

See Illustration Credits for source information.

TABLE 13.11   Malignant Skin Lesions

Basal Cell Carcinoma

Usually starts as a skin-coloured papule (may be deeply pigmented) with a translucent top and overlying telangiectasia. Then rounded pearly borders develop with central red ulcer, or looks like large open pore with central yellowing. One of the most common forms of skin cancer. It progresses slowly and rarely causes death.

Squamous Cell Carcinoma

Erythematous scaly patch with sharp margins, ≥1 cm. Central ulcer and surrounding erythema develop. Usually on hands or head (areas exposed to solar radiation). As common as basal cell carcinoma in Canada; progresses slowly and is usually removed easily by surgery.

Malignant Melanoma

Half of these lesions arise from pre-existing nevi. Usually brown; can be tan, black, pink-red, purple, or of mixed pigmentation. Often irregular or notched borders. May have scaling, flaking, oozing texture. Common locations are on the trunk and back in men and women, on the legs in women, and on the palms, soles of feet, and the nails in people of African descent. Melanoma represents only 1–2% of all skin cancers but has the highest fatality rate; 20% of all Canadians with diagnosed melanoma die. Occurs earlier in life and progresses rapidly.

Malignant Melanoma

Metastatic Malignant Melanoma

See Illustration Credits for source information.

TABLE 13.12	Skin Lesions Associated With Acquired Immune Deficiency Syndrome

◀ AIDS-Related Kaposi's Sarcoma: Patch Stage

An aggressive form of Kaposi's sarcoma is one of the diseases that characterize AIDS. In the patch stage, multiple early lesions are faint pink on the temple and beard area. They could be mistaken easily for bruises or nevi and be ignored.

AIDS, Acquired immune deficiency syndrome.
See Illustration Credits for source information.

TABLE 13.13	Abnormal Conditions of the Hair

Seborrheic Dermatitis (Cradle Cap)

Thick, yellow to white, greasy, adherent scales with mild erythema on scalp and forehead; very common in early infancy. Resembles eczema lesions except cradle cap is distinguished by absence of pruritus, by "greasy" yellow-pink lesions, and by negative family history of allergy.

Tinea Capitis (Scalp Ringworm)

Rounded patchy hair loss on scalp, leaving broken-off hairs, pustules, and scales on skin. Caused by fungal infection; lesions may fluoresce blue-green under Wood light. Usually seen in children and farmers; highly contagious; routes of transmission include other people, domestic animals, and soil.

TABLE 13.13	Abnormal Conditions of the Hair—cont'd

Toxic Alopecia

Patchy, asymmetrical balding that accompanies severe illness or use of chemotherapy; growing hairs are lost and resting hairs are spared. Regrowth occurs after illness ends or after discontinuation of toxin.

Alopecia Areata

Sudden appearance of a sharply circumscribed, round or oval balding patch, usually with smooth, soft, hairless skin underneath. Unknown cause; when limited to a few patches, person usually has complete regrowth.

Traumatic Alopecia: Traction Alopecia

Linear or oval patch of hair loss along hairline, a part, or with scattered distribution; caused by trauma from hair rollers, tight braiding, tight ponytail, or barrettes.

Trichotillomania

Traumatic self-induced hair loss usually the result of compulsive twisting or plucking. Forms irregularly shaped patch, with broken-off, stublike hairs of varying lengths; does not cause complete baldness. Occurs as child rubs or twists area absently while falling asleep, reading, or watching television. In adults it can be a serious problem and is usually a sign of a personality disorder.

Continued

TABLE 13.13	Abnormal Conditions of the Hair—cont'd

Pediculosis Capitis (Head Lice)

History includes intense itching of the scalp, especially the occiput. The nits (eggs) of lice are easier to see in the occipital area and around the ears, appearing as 2- to 3-mm oval translucent bodies, adherent to the hair shafts. Common among school-age children. Over-the-counter pediculicide shampoos are available; however, nit removal (also called *nit-picking*) by daily combing of wet hair with a fine-tooth metal comb is especially important.

Folliculitis (Razor Bumps)

Superficial infection of hair follicles. Multiple pustules, "whiteheads," with hair visible at centre and erythematous base. Usually on arms, legs, face, and buttocks.

Hirsutism

Excess body hair in women that forms a male sexual pattern (upper lip, face, chest, abdomen, arms, legs); caused by endocrine or metabolic dysfunction; occasionally idiopathic.

Furuncle and Abscess

Red, swollen, hard, tender, pus-filled lesion caused by acute localized bacterial (usually staphylococcal) infection; usually on back of neck or buttocks, occasionally on wrists or ankles. Furuncles result from infection of hair follicles, whereas abscesses result from traumatic introduction of bacteria into the skin. Abscesses are usually larger and deeper than furuncles.

See Illustration Credits for source information.

TABLE 13.14   Abnormal Conditions of the Nails

Paronychia

Red, swollen, tender inflammation of the nail folds. Acute paronychia is usually a bacterial infection; chronic paronychia is most often a fungal infection from a break in the cuticle in those who perform "wet" work.

Beau's Line

Transverse furrow or groove; a depression across the nail that extends down to the nail bed. Occurs with any trauma that temporarily impairs nail formation, such as acute illness, toxic reaction, or local trauma. Dent appears first at the cuticle and moves forward as nail grows.

Splinter Hemorrhages

Red-brown linear streaks, embolic lesions; occur with subacute bacterial endocarditis; also may occur with minor trauma.

Onychomycosis

This is a slow, persistent fungal infection of fingernails and, more often, toenails, common in older adults. Fungus causes change in colour (green where nail plate separates from bed), texture, and thickness, with nail crumbling or breaking and loosening of the nail plate, usually beginning at the distal edge and progressing proximally.

Continued

TABLE 13.14   Abnormal Conditions of the Nails—cont'd

Late Clubbing

Proximal edge of nail elevates; angle >180 degrees. Distal phalanx looks rounder and wider. Occurs with chronic obstructive pulmonary disease and congenital heart disease with cyanosis. Occurs first in thumb and index finger.

Pitting

Sharply defined pitting and crumbling of the nails with distal detachment; often occurs with psoriasis.

Habit-Tic Dystrophy

◄ Depression down middle of nail or multiple horizontal ridges, caused by continuous picking of cuticle by another finger of same hand, which causes injury to nail base and matrix.

See Illustration Credits for source information.

Summary Checklist: Skin, Hair, and Nails Examination

1. **Inspect the skin:**
   Colour
   General pigmentation
   Areas of hypopigmentation or hyperpigmentation
   Abnormal colour changes
2. **Palpate the skin:**
   Temperature
   Moisture
   Texture

   Thickness
   Edema
   Mobility and turgor
   Hygiene
   Vascularity or bruising
3. **Note any lesions:**
   Colour
   Shape and configuration
   Size
   Location and distribution on body

4. **Inspect and palpate the hair:**
   Texture
   Distribution
   Any scalp lesions
5. **Inspect and palpate the nails:**
   Shape and contour
   Consistency
   Colour
6. **Teach skin self-examination and engage in health promotion**

REFERENCES

1. Kundu, R. V., & Patterson, S. (2013). Dermatologic conditions in skin of color: Part I. Special considerations for common skin disorders. *American Family Physician*, 87(12), 850–856. Part II. Disorders occurring predominantly in skin of color. *American Family Physician, 87*(12), 859–865.
2. Denny, K., Lawand, C., & Perry, S. (2014). Compromised wounds in Canada. *Healthcare Quarterly*, 17(1), 7–10. doi:10.12927/hcq.2014.23787.
3. National Pressure Ulcer Advisory Panel. (2016). NPUAP Pressure Injury Stages. http://www.npuap.org/resources/educational-and-clinical-resources/npuap-pressure-injury-stages/.
4. Bower, M. G., 2001). Managing dog, cat, and human bite wounds. *The Nurse Practitioner*, 26(4), 36–47.

CHAPTER 14

Head, Face, and Neck, Including Regional Lymphatic System

Written by Carolyn Jarvis, PhD, APN, CNP
Adapted by June MacDonald-Jenkins, RN, BScN, MSc

 http://evolve.elsevier.com/Canada/Jarvis/examination/

STRUCTURE AND FUNCTION

THE HEAD

The **skull** is a rigid, bony box that protects the brain and special sense organs, and it includes the bones of the cranium and the face (Fig. 14.1). Note the location of these **cranial bones**: frontal, parietal, occipital, and temporal. Use these names to describe any of your findings in the corresponding areas.

The adjacent cranial bones unite at meshed immovable joints called **sutures**. At birth, the bones are not firmly joined, which allows for the mobility and change in shape needed for the birth process. The sutures gradually ossify during early childhood. The **coronal** suture *crowns* the head from ear to ear at the union of the frontal and parietal bones. The **sagittal** suture *separates* the sides of the head lengthwise between the two parietal bones. The **lambdoid** suture separates the parietal bones crosswise from the occipital bone.

The 14 **facial bones** also articulate at sutures (note the nasal bone, zygomatic bone, and maxilla), except for the mandible (the lower jaw). The mandible moves up, down, and sideways from the temporomandibular joints, which are anterior to the ears.

The cranium is supported by the cervical vertebra: C1, the "atlas"; C2, the "axis"; and down to C7. The C7 vertebra has a long spinous process that is palpable when the head is flexed. You can feel this useful landmark, the **vertebra prominens**, on your own neck.

The human **face** has myriad appearances and a large array of facial expressions that reflect mood. The expressions are formed by the facial muscles (Fig. 14.2), which are mediated by cranial nerve VII (the facial nerve). Facial muscle function is symmetrical bilaterally, except for an occasional quirk or wry expression.

Facial structures also are, in general, symmetrical; the eyebrows, eyes, ears, nose, and mouth appear about the same on both sides. The palpebral fissures—the openings between the eyelids—are equal bilaterally. Also, the nasolabial folds—the creases extending from the nose to each corner of the mouth—should be symmetrical. Facial sensations of pain or touch are mediated by the three sensory branches of cranial nerve V (the trigeminal nerve). (Testing for sensory function is described in Chapter 25.)

Two pairs of **salivary glands** are accessible to examination on the face (Fig. 14.3). The **parotid glands** are in the cheeks over the mandible, anterior to and below the ear. They are the largest of the salivary glands but are not normally palpable. The **submandibular glands** are beneath the mandible at the angle of the jaw. A third pair, the **sublingual glands**, lie in the floor of the mouth. (Salivary gland function is described in Chapter 17.) The **temporal artery** lies superior to the temporalis muscle, and its pulsation is palpable anterior to the ear.

THE NECK

The **neck** is delimited above by the base of the skull and inferior border of the mandible and below by the manubrium sterni, the clavicle, the first rib, and the first thoracic vertebra. Think of the neck as a conduit for the passage of many structures, which are lying in close proximity: vessels, muscles, nerves, lymphatic vessels, and viscera of the respiratory and digestive systems. Blood vessels include the common and internal carotid arteries and their associated veins (see Fig. 14.3). The internal carotid artery branches off the common carotid artery and runs inward and upward to supply the brain; the external carotid artery supplies the face, salivary glands, and superficial temporal area. The carotid artery and internal jugular vein lie beneath the sternomastoid muscle. The external jugular vein runs diagonally across the sternomastoid muscle. (Assessment of the neck vessels is discussed in Chapter 20.)

The major **neck muscles** are the **sternomastoid** and the **trapezius** (Fig. 14.4); they are innervated by cranial nerve XI (the spinal accessory nerve). The sternomastoid muscle arises from the sternum and the medial part of the clavicle and extends diagonally across the neck to the mastoid

Structure and Function

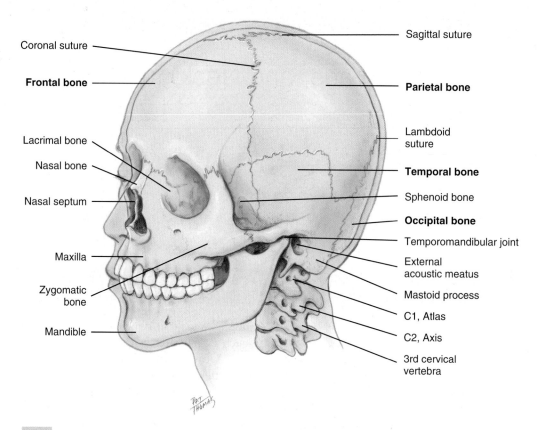

Coronal suture

Sagittal suture

Frontal bone

Parietal bone

Lacrimal bone

Lambdoid suture

Nasal bone

Temporal bone

Nasal septum

Sphenoid bone

Occipital bone

Maxilla

Temporomandibular joint

External acoustic meatus

Zygomatic bone

Mastoid process

C1, Atlas

Mandible

C2, Axis

3rd cervical vertebra

14.1

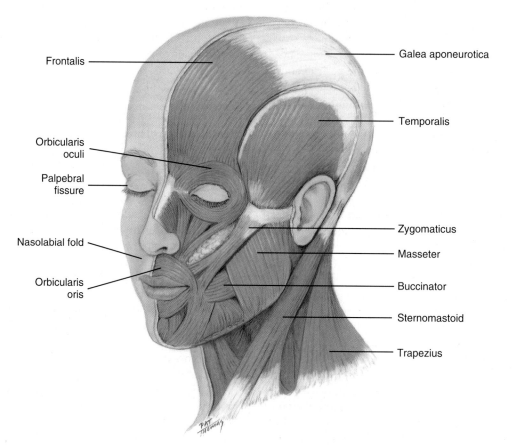

Frontalis

Galea aponeurotica

Temporalis

Orbicularis oculi

Palpebral fissure

Nasolabial fold

Zygomaticus

Orbicularis oris

Masseter

Buccinator

Sternomastoid

Trapezius

14.2 Facial muscles.

Sternomastoid muscle

Internal jugular vein

External jugular vein

Clavicle

Temporal artery

Parotid gland

Submandibular gland

Sublingual gland

External carotid artery

Internal carotid artery

Common carotid artery

14.3

Sternomastoid muscle

Trapezius muscle

Omohyoid muscle

Clavicle

Anterior triangle

Posterior triangle

14.4

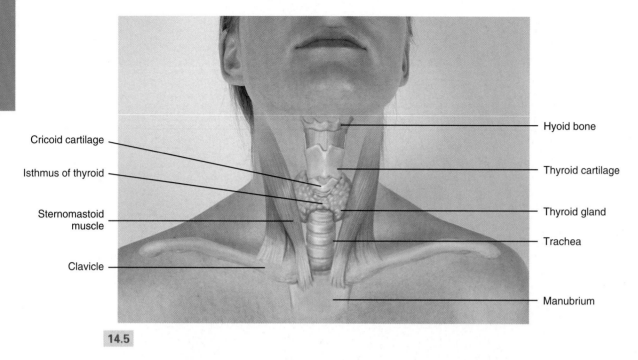

Cricoid cartilage

Isthmus of thyroid

Sternomastoid muscle

Clavicle

Hyoid bone

Thyroid cartilage

Thyroid gland

Trachea

Manubrium

14.5

process behind the ear. It accomplishes head rotation and head flexion. The two trapezius muscles form a trapezoid shape on the upper back. Each arises from the occipital bone and the vertebrae and extends by fanning out to the scapula and clavicle. The trapezius muscles move the shoulders and extend and turn the head.

The sternomastoid muscle divides each side of the neck into two triangles. The **anterior triangle** lies in front, between the sternomastoid and the midline of the body; its base is up along the lower border of the mandible, and its apex is down at the suprasternal notch. The **posterior triangle** is behind the sternomastoid muscle, with the trapezius muscle on the other side; its base is along the clavicle below. It contains the posterior belly of the omohyoid muscle. These triangles are helpful guidelines in describing findings in the neck.

The **thyroid gland** is an important endocrine gland with a rich blood supply. It straddles the trachea in the middle of the neck (Fig. 14.5). This highly vascular endocrine gland synthesizes and secretes thyroxine (T_4) and triiodothyronine (T_3), hormones that stimulate the rate of cellular metabolism. The thyroid has two lobes, both conical in shape, each curving posteriorly between the trachea and the sternomastoid muscle. The lobes are connected in the middle by a thin isthmus lying over the second and third tracheal rings. (Just above the thyroid isthmus, within about 1 cm, is the **cricoid cartilage**, or upper tracheal ring.) The **thyroid cartilage** is above the cricoid cartilage, with a small palpable notch in its upper edge. This notch is the prominent "Adam's apple" in men. The highest structure in the neck is the **hyoid** bone, palpated at the level of the floor of the mouth.

LYMPHATIC SYSTEM

The lymphatic system is discussed more fully in Chapter 21. However, the head and neck have a rich supply of **lymph**

nodes (Fig. 14.6). Note that their labels correspond to adjacent structures:
- *Preauricular:* in front of the ear
- *Posterior auricular* (mastoid): superficial to the mastoid process
- *Occipital:* at the base of the skull
- *Submental:* midline, behind the tip of the mandible
- *Submandibular:* halfway between the angle and the tip of the mandible
- *Tonsillar:* under the angle of the mandible
- *Superficial cervical:* overlying the sternomastoid muscle
- *Deep cervical:* deep under the sternomastoid muscle
- *Posterior cervical:* in the posterior triangle along the edge of the trapezius muscle
- *Supraclavicular:* just above and behind the clavicle, at the sternomastoid muscle

You also should be familiar with the direction of the drainage patterns of the lymph nodes (Fig. 14.7). When nodes are enlarged, check the area in which they drain for the source of the problem. Explore the area proximal (upstream) to the location of the enlarged node. All head and neck structures eventually drain into the cervical chain.

The lymphatic system is a separate vessel system from the cardiovascular system and is a major part of the immune system, whose job is to detect and eliminate foreign substances from the body. The lymphatic vessels gather the clear, watery fluid (lymph) from the tissue spaces into the circulation. Lymph nodes are small, oval clusters of lymphatic tissue that are set at intervals along the lymph vessels, like beads on a string. The nodes slowly filter the lymph and engulf pathogens, preventing harmful substances from entering the circulation. Nodes are located throughout the body but are accessible to examination only in four areas: (a) the head and neck, (b) the arms, (c) the axillae, and (d) the inguinal region. The supply is most extensive in the head and neck.

Posterior auricular

Occipital

Jugulodigastric
(tonsillar)

Superficial cervical

Posterior cervical

Supraclavicular

Preauricular

Submandibular

Submental

Deep cervical chain

14.6

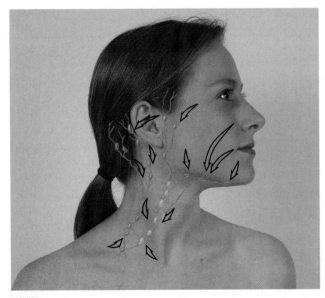

14.7

✣ DEVELOPMENTAL CONSIDERATIONS

Infants and Children

The bones of the neonatal skull are separated by sutures and by **fontanelles**, the spaces where the sutures intersect (Fig. 14.8). These membrane-covered "soft spots" allow for growth of the brain during the first year. They gradually ossify; the triangle-shaped posterior fontanelle is closed by age 1 to 2 months, and the diamond-shaped anterior fontanelle closes between ages 9 months and 2 years.

During the fetal period, head growth predominates. At birth, head size is greater than chest circumference. The head size grows during childhood, reaching 90% of its final size when the child is 6 years old. During infancy, however, trunk growth predominates, so that the proportion of head size to body height changes. Facial bones grow at varying rates, especially nasal and jaw bones. In the toddler, the mandible and maxilla are small and the nasal bridge is low, and so the whole face seems small in comparison with the skull.

Lymphoid tissue is well developed at birth and grows to adult size by the age of 6 years. Lymphatic tissue continues to grow rapidly until age 10 or 11 years, actually exceeding its adult size before puberty. Then the lymphatic tissue slowly atrophies.

In adolescence, facial hair also appears on males first on the upper lip, and last on the chin. The thyroid cartilage enlarges noticeably, and with enlargement, the voice deepens.

Pregnant Women

The thyroid gland enlarges slightly during pregnancy as a result of hyperplasia of the tissue and increased vascularity.

Older Adults

The facial bones and orbits appear more prominent, and the facial skin sags as a result of decreased elasticity, decreased subcutaneous fat, and decreased moisture in the skin. The lower face may look smaller if teeth have been lost.

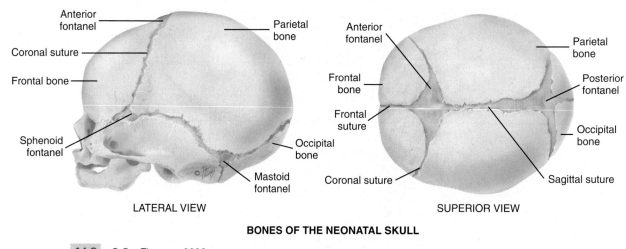

BONES OF THE NEONATAL SKULL

14.8   © Pat Thomas, 2006.

SUBJECTIVE DATA

Record the patient's subjective descriptions of the following abnormalities:

1. Headache
2. Head injury
3. Dizziness
4. Neck pain, limitation of motion
5. Lumps or swelling
6. History of head or neck surgery

HEALTH HISTORY QUESTIONS

Examiner Asks	Rationale

1. Headache. Any unusually frequent or unusually severe **headaches**?
• Onset: When did this *kind* of headache start?
• Gradual, over hours, or a day?
• Or suddenly, over minutes, or less than 1 hour?
 	
• Ever had this *kind* of headache before?
 	
• Location: Where do you feel it: in front, on the sides, behind your eyes, like a band around the head, in the sinus area, or in the occipital area?
 	
• Is pain localized on one side, or is it all over?
 	
• Character: Throbbing (pounding, shooting) or aching (viselike, constant pressure, dull)?
 	
• Is it mild, moderate, or severe?
	This is a more meaningful question than "Do you ever have headaches?" because most people have had at least one headache. Because headache is a symptom in many conditions, a detailed history is important.
	    Of concern is a severe headache in an adult or child who has never had it before.
	    Tension headaches tend to be occipital or frontal, or the sensation is of bandlike tightness; migraines (vascular) tend to be supraorbital, retro-orbital, or frontotemporal; cluster headaches (vascular) produce pain around the eye, temple, forehead, cheek.
	    Unilateral or bilateral pain is a clue to the type of headache (e.g., with cluster headaches, pain is always unilateral and always on the same side of the head).
	    Character is typically viselike with tension headache and throbbing with migraine or temporal arteritis.
	    Pain is often severe with migraine and excruciating with cluster headache.

Examiner Asks	Rationale

- Course and duration: What time of day do the headaches occur: morning, evening? Do they awaken you from sleep?
- How long do they last? Hours, days?
- Have you noted any daily headaches, or several within a time period?

On average, migraines occur at a rate of approximately two per month, each lasting 1 to 3 days; one to two cluster headaches occur per day, each lasting a ½ hour to 2 hours for 1 or 2 months; then complete remission may last for months or years.

- Precipitating factors: What brings it on: activity or exercise, work environment, emotional upset, anxiety, alcohol? (Examiner should also note signs of depression.)

Alcohol ingestion and daytime napping typically precipitate cluster headaches, whereas alcohol, letdown after stress, menstruation, and eating chocolate or cheese precipitate migraines.

- Associated factors: Any relation to other symptoms, such as nausea and vomiting? (Examiner should note which occurred first, headache or nausea.) Any vision changes, pain with bright lights, neck pain or stiffness, fever, weakness, moodiness, stomach problems?

Nausea, vomiting, and visual disturbances are associated with migraines; eye reddening and tearing, eyelid drooping, rhinorrhea, and nasal congestion are associated with cluster headaches; anxiety and stress are associated with tension headaches; nuchal rigidity and fever are associated with meningitis or encephalitis.

- Do you have any other illness?

Hypertension, fever, hypothyroidism, and vasculitis can produce headaches.

- Do you take any medications?

Oral contraceptives, bronchodilators, alcohol, nitrates, and carbon monoxide inhalation can produce headaches.

See Table 14.1, p. 292.

- What makes the pain worse: movement, coughing, straining, exercise?
- Pattern: Any family history of headache?
- What is the frequency of your headaches: once a week? Are your headaches occurring closer together?
- Are they getting worse? Or are they getting better?
- (For women) When do they occur in relation to your menstrual periods?
- Effort to treat: What seems to help: going to sleep, medications, positions, rubbing the area?

Migraines are associated with family history of migraine.

With migraines, people lie down to feel better, whereas with cluster headaches they need to move—even to pace the floor—to feel better.

- Coping strategies: How have these headaches affected your self-care or your ability to function at work, at home, and socially? What do you need to help you to cope?

2. **Head injury.** Any **head injury** or blow to your head?
   - Onset: When? Please describe exactly what happened.
   - Setting: Any hazardous conditions? Were you wearing a helmet or hard hat?
   - How about yourself just before injury: Were you dizzy or lightheaded? Did you have a blackout or a seizure?
   - Did you lose consciousness and then fall? (Note which came first.)
   - Knocked unconscious? Or did you fall and lose consciousness a few minutes later?
   - Any history of illness (e.g., heart trouble, diabetes, epilepsy)?
   - Location: Exactly where did you hit your head?
   - Duration: How long were you unconscious?
   - Any symptoms afterwards: headache, vomiting, projectile vomiting?
   - Any change in level of consciousness (dazed or sleepy) since injury?

Loss of consciousness *before* a fall may have a cardiovascular cause (e.g., heart block).

A change in level of consciousness is of prime importance in the evaluation for a neurological deficit.

Subjective Data

Examiner Asks	Rationale

- Associated symptoms: Any pain in the head or the neck, vision change, or discharge from ear or nose (bloody or watery)? Are you able to move all extremities? Any tremors, staggered walk, numbness, or tingling?
- Pattern: Have symptoms become worse or better, or have they remained unchanged, since injury?
- Effort to treat: Emergency department or hospitalized? Any medications?

3. Dizziness. Experienced any **dizziness**?
- Tell me what you mean by dizziness. Describe it for me (dizziness is a vague term and can be related to many causes). Try not to prompt the person by suggesting descriptors such as spinning, but note their words. "I feel like I am going to faint" suggests presyncope; "I feel like I am spinning" suggests vertigo; "I feel like I am going to fall down" suggests disequilibrium.

Dizziness includes **presyncope**, a light-headed, swimming sensation or a feeling of falling caused by decreased blood flow to the brain or heart irregularity causing decreased cardiac output. **Vertigo** is a sense of true rotational spinning often from a labyrinthine–vestibular disorder in the inner ear. With *objective* vertigo, the person feels like the room is spinning; with *subjective* vertigo, the person feels as if they are spinning. **Disequilibrium** is a shakiness or instability when walking related to musculo-skeletal disorder or multisensory deficits.

- Onset: Abrupt or gradual? After a change in position, such as sudden standing?
- Associated factors: Any nausea and vomiting, pallor, immobility, decreased hearing acuity, or tinnitus along with the dizziness? Any palpitations or shortness of breath?

4. Neck pain, limitation of motion. Any **neck pain**? Limitation of motion?
- Onset: How did the pain start: injury, automobile accident, after lifting, from a fall? Or with fever? Or did it have a gradual onset?
- Location: Does pain radiate? If so, to the shoulders, arms?
- Associated symptoms: Any **limitations to range of motion (ROM)**? Any numbness or tingling in shoulders, arms, or hands?
- Precipitating factors: What movements cause pain? Do you need to lift or bend at work or home?
- Does stress seem to trigger the pain?
- Coping strategies: Are you able to do your work, to sleep?

Acute onset of stiffness with headache and fever occurs with meningeal inflammation.

Pain creates a vicious circle. Tension increases pain and disability, which produces more tension.

5. Lumps or swelling. Any **lumps** or **swelling** in the neck?
- Any recent infection? Any tenderness?
- For a lump that persists, how long have you had it? Has it changed in size?

Tenderness is suggestive of acute infection.

A persistent lump arouses suspicion of malignancy. For patients older than 40 years of age, suspect malignancy until it is proven otherwise.

- Any history of prior irradiation of head, neck, upper chest?

Such irradiation increases risk for salivary and thyroid tumours.

- Any difficulty swallowing?
- Do you smoke? For how long? How many packs a day? Do you chew tobacco?
- When was your last alcoholic drink? How much alcohol do you drink a day?
- Ever had a thyroid problem? Overfunctioning or underfunctioning? How was it treated: surgery, irradiation, any medication?

Dysphagia is the term for this condition. Smoking and chewing tobacco increase the risk for oral and respiratory cancers.
Smoking and large alcohol consumption together increase the risk for cancer.

Examiner Asks	Rationale
6. History of head or neck surgery. Ever had surgery of the head or neck? • For what condition? When did the surgery occur? How do you feel about results?	Surgery for head and neck cancer often is disfiguring and increases the risk for body image disturbance.

Additional History for Infants and Children

1. Prenatal drug exposure. Did the mother use alcohol or street drugs during pregnancy? How often? • How much was used per episode?	Alcohol increases the risk for fetal alcohol spectrum disorder, which is characterized by distinctive facial features (see Table 14.2, p. 294). Cocaine use causes neurological, developmental, and emotional problems.
2. Delivery. Was the **delivery** vaginal or by Caesarean section? Any difficulty? Were forceps used?	Forceps may increase the risk for caput succedaneum, cephalhematoma, and **Bell's palsy**.
3. Growth. What were you told about the **baby's growth**? Was it on schedule? Did the head seem to grow and fontanelles close on schedule? At what age (in months) did the baby achieve head control?	

Additional History for Older Adults

1. Dizziness. If **dizziness** is a problem, how does this affect your daily activities? Are you able to drive safely, manoeuvre about the house safely?	Assess self-care. Assess potential for injury.
2. Pain. If **neck pain** is a problem, how does this affect your daily activities? Are you able to drive, perform at work, do housework, sleep, look down when using stairs?	

Subjective Data

Objective Data

OBJECTIVE DATA

Normal Range of Findings	Abnormal Findings
## The Head ### Inspect and Palpate the Skull **Size and Shape** Note the general size and shape. **Normocephalic** is the term that denotes a round symmetrical skull that is appropriately related to body size. Be aware that "normal" includes a wide range of sizes. To assess shape, place your fingers in the person's hair and palpate the scalp. The skull normally feels symmetrical and smooth. The cranial bones that have normal protrusions are the forehead, the lateral edge of each parietal bone, the occipital bone, and the mastoid process behind each ear. There is no tenderness on palpation.	Deformities: microcephaly (abnormally small head); macrocephaly (abnormally large head), caused by hydrocephaly, or acromegaly (Table 14.4, p. 298). Note lumps, depressions, or abnormal protrusions.
### Temporal Area Palpate the temporal artery above the zygomatic (cheek) bone between the eye and top of the ear. The temporomandibular joint is just below the temporal artery and anterior to the tragus. Palpate the joint as the patient opens the mouth; normal movement is smooth, with no limitation or tenderness.	With **temporal arteritis**, the artery looks more tortuous and feels hardened and tender. Abnormalities include crepitation, limited ROM, and tenderness.

Normal Range of Findings	**Abnormal Findings**

Inspect the Face
Facial Structures

Inspect the face, noting the facial expression and its appropriateness for behaviour or reported mood. Anxiety is common in hospitalized or ill patients.

Although the shape of facial structures may vary somewhat among ethnicities, they should always be symmetrical. Note symmetry of eyebrows, palpebral fissures, nasolabial folds, and sides of the mouth.

Note any abnormal facial structures (coarse facial features, exophthalmos, changes in skin colour or pigmentation) and any abnormal swelling. Also note any involuntary movements (tics) in the facial muscles. Normally, none occur.

Patients may express hostility or aggression.

Tense, rigid muscles may indicate anxiety or pain; a flat affect may indicate depression.

Marked asymmetry may occur with central brain lesion (e.g., cerebrovascular accident) or with peripheral damage to cranial nerve VII (Bell's palsy; see Table 14.4, p. 297).

Edema in the face occurs first around the eyes (periorbital) and the cheeks, where the subcutaneous tissue is relatively loose.

Note grinding of jaws, tics, fasciculations, and excessive blinking.

The Neck

Inspect and Palpate the Neck
Symmetry

Head position is centred in the midline, and the accessory neck muscles should be symmetrical. The head should be held erect and still.

Head tilt occurs with muscle spasm. Rigidity of the head and neck occurs with arthritis.

Range of Motion

Note any limitation of movement during active motion. Ask the patient to touch the chin to the chest, turn the head to the right and left, try to touch each ear to the shoulder (without elevating shoulders), and to extend the neck backward. When the neck is supple, motion is smooth and controlled.

Note pain at any particular movement.

Note ratchety or limited movement from cervical arthritis or inflammation of neck muscles. The arthritic neck is rigid; the affected patient turns at the shoulders rather than at the neck.

Test muscle strength and the status of cranial nerve XI by trying to resist the patient's movements with your hands as the patient shrugs the shoulders and turns the head to each side.

As the patient moves the head, note any enlargement of the salivary glands and lymph glands. Normally, no enlargement is present. Note a swollen parotid gland when the head is extended; look for swelling below the angle of the jaw. Also, note thyroid gland enlargement. Normally, none is present.

Also note any obvious pulsations. The carotid artery runs medial to the sternomastoid muscle, and it has a brisk localized pulsation just below the angle of the jaw. Normally, there are no other pulsations while the patient is in the sitting position (see Chapter 20).

Thyroid enlargement may be a unilateral lump, or it may be diffuse and look like a doughnut lying across the lower neck (Table 14.5, p. 299).

Normal Range of Findings

Lymph Nodes

Using a gentle circular motion of your fingertips, palpate the lymph nodes (Fig. 14.9). (Normally, the salivary glands are not palpable. When symptoms warrant, check for parotid tenderness by palpating in a line from the outer corner of the eye to the lobule of the ear.) Beginning with the preauricular lymph nodes in front of the ear, palpate the 10 groups of lymph nodes in a routine order. Many nodes are closely packed, so you must be systematic and thorough in your examination. Once you establish your sequence, do not vary, or you may miss some small nodes.

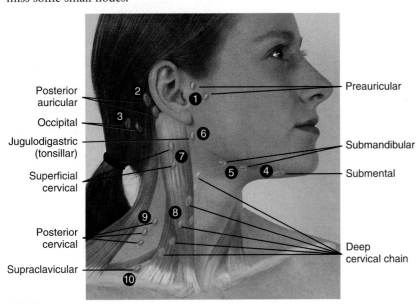

Posterior auricular
Occipital
Jugulodigastric (tonsillar)
Superficial cervical
Posterior cervical
Supraclavicular
Preauricular
Submandibular
Submental
Deep cervical chain

14.9

Palpate gently because strong pressure could push the nodes into the neck muscles. It is usually most efficient to palpate with both hands, so that you can compare the two sides symmetrically. However, the submental gland under the tip of the chin is easier to explore with one hand. When you palpate with one hand, use your other hand to position the person's head. For the deep cervical chain, tip the person's head toward the side being examined to relax the ipsilateral muscle (Fig. 14.10). Then you can press your fingers under the muscle. Search for the supraclavicular node by having the person hunch the shoulders and elbows forward (Fig. 14.11); this relaxes the skin. The inferior belly of the omohyoid muscle crosses the posterior triangle here; do not mistake it for a lymph node.

Abnormal Findings

In mumps, the parotid gland is swollen (see Table 14.3, p. 296).

Parotid enlargement has been found with acquired immune deficiency syndrome (AIDS).

Objective Data

Objective Data

Normal Range of Findings	Abnormal Findings

14.10

14.11

If any nodes are palpable, note their location, size, shape, delimitation (discrete or clumped together), mobility, consistency, and tenderness. Cervical nodes often are palpable in healthy persons, although this palpability decreases with age (Fig. 14.12, *A*). Normal nodes feel movable, discrete, soft, and nontender.

Lymphadenopathy is enlargement of the lymph nodes (>1 cm), caused by infection, allergy, or neoplasm (see Fig. 14.12, *B*, due to mononucleosis).

A

14.12, *A*

B

14.12, *B*

Normal Range of Findings

If nodes are enlarged or tender, check the area they drain for the source of the problem. For example, enlargement or tenderness of those in the upper cervical or submandibular area is often related to inflammation or a neoplasm in the head and neck. Follow up on your findings, or refer the patient to a specialist. An enlarged lymph node, particularly when you cannot find the source of the problem, necessitates prompt attention.

Trachea

Normally, the trachea is midline; palpate for any tracheal shift. Place your index finger on the trachea in the sternal notch, and slip it off to each side (Fig. 14.13). The space should be symmetrical on both sides. Note any deviation from the midline.

14.13

Abnormal Findings

The following criteria are common clues but are not definitive in all circumstances:

- Acute infection: Nodes are bilateral, enlarged, warm, tender, and firm but freely movable.
- Chronic inflammation: Nodes are clumped (e.g., in tuberculosis).
- Cancerous nodes: Nodes are hard, unilateral, nontender, and fixed.
- Human immunodeficiency virus (HIV) infection: Nodes are enlarged, firm, nontender, and mobile. Occipital node enlargement is common with HIV infection.
- Neoplasm in the thorax or abdomen: A single left node may be enlarged, nontender, and hard (Virchow's node).
- Hodgkin's lymphoma: Discrete nodes that are painless and rubbery gradually appear.

Conditions of tracheal shift:

- The trachea is *pushed to the unaffected* (or healthy) side with an aortic aneurysm, a tumour, unilateral thyroid lobe enlargement, and pneumothorax.
- The trachea is *pulled toward the affected* (or diseased) side with large atelectasis, pleural adhesions, or fibrosis.

Tracheal tug is a rhythmic downward pull that is synchronous with systole and that occurs with aortic arch aneurysm. Also noted in pediatric patients in acute respiratory distress.

Normal Range of Findings

Abnormal Findings

Thyroid Gland

The thyroid gland is difficult to palpate; arrange your setting to maximize your likelihood of success. Position a standing lamp to shine tangentially across the neck to highlight any possible swelling. Supply the patient with a glass of water, and first inspect the neck as the patient takes a sip and swallows. Thyroid tissue normally moves up with a swallow.

Auscultate the Thyroid. If the thyroid gland is enlarged, auscultate it for the presence of a **bruit**. This is a soft, pulsatile, whooshing, blowing sound heard best with the bell of the stethoscope. Bruits are not normally present.

Look for diffuse enlargement or a nodular lump.

It is important in a basic assessment to note any visible enlargement of the thyroid. Palpation of the thyroid is considered an advanced practice consideration.

Graves' disease is the most common cause of hyperthyroidism (see Table 14.5, p. 299).

Common signs and symptoms:
- Exophthalmus (bulging eyes)
- Goitre (thickened neck)
- Fatigue, weight loss, and nervousness

Myxedema, also known as hypothyroidism, results from diminished functioning of the thyroid gland (see Table 14.5, p. 299). A bruit occurs with accelerated or turbulent blood flow, which is indicative of hyperplasia of the thyroid (e.g., hyperthyroidism).

SPECIAL CONSIDERATIONS FOR ADVANCED PRACTICE

Normal Range of Findings

Abnormal Findings

Palpation

Posterior Approach to Palpating the Thyroid

To palpate, move behind the person (Fig. 14.14, *A*). Ask the person to sit up very straight and then to bend the head slightly forward and to the right. This will relax the neck muscles. Use the fingers of your left hand to push the trachea slightly to the right.

Curve your right fingers between the trachea and the sternomastoid muscle, retracting it slightly, and ask the patient to take a sip of water. The thyroid moves up under your fingers with the trachea and larynx as the patient swallows. Reverse the procedure for the left side.

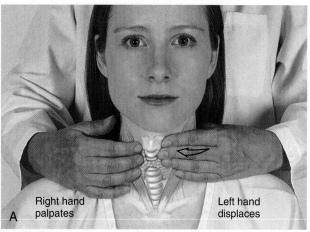

Right hand palpates   Left hand displaces

A

14.14, *A*

Objective Data

Special Considerations for Advanced Practice

Normal Range of Findings

Usually you cannot palpate the normal adult thyroid. In some patients who have a long, thin neck, you can feel the isthmus over the tracheal rings. The lateral lobes are usually not palpable; check them for enlargement, consistency, symmetry, and the presence of nodules.

Anterior Approach to Palpating the Thyroid

This is an alternative method of palpating the thyroid, but it is more awkward to perform, especially for a novice examiner. Stand facing the patient. Ask the patient to tip the head forward and to the right. Use your right thumb to displace the trachea slightly to the patient's right. Hook your left thumb and fingers around the sternomastoid muscle. Feel for lobe enlargement as the patient swallows (Fig. 14.15).

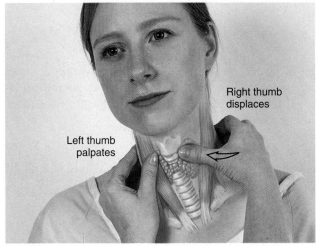

Left thumb palpates

Right thumb displaces

14.15

Abnormal Findings

Abnormalities include enlarged lobes that are easily palpated before swallowing or are tender on palpation (see large goitre in Fig. 14.14, *B*) and the presence of nodules or lumps (see Table 14.3, p. 283).

14.14, *B*

Normal Range of Findings

DEVELOPMENTAL CONSIDERATIONS

Infants and Children
Skull

Measure an infant's **head size** with measuring tape at each visit up to age 2 years, then yearly up to age 6 years. (Measurement of head circumference is described in detail in Chapter 10.)

A newborn's head measures about 32 to 38 cm (average, ≈34 cm) and is 2 cm larger than chest circumference. At age 2 years, both measurements are the same. During childhood, the chest circumference grows to exceed head circumference by 5 to 7 cm.

Abnormal Findings

Note any abnormal increase in head size or failure to grow.

Microcephalic: Head size is below norms for age.
Macrocephalic: Head is large for age or rapidly increasing in size (e.g., as in hydrocephalus [increased cerebrospinal fluid]).

Normal Range of Findings

Observe the infant's head from all angles, not just the front. The contour should be symmetrical. Some racial variation in head shapes is normal; children of Nordic descent tend to have long heads, whereas those of Asian descent have broad heads.

Two common variations in the newborn cause the shape of the skull to look markedly asymmetrical: A **caput succedaneum** is edematous swelling and ecchymosis of the presenting part of the head caused by birth trauma (Fig. 14.16). It feels soft, and it may extend across suture lines. It gradually resolves during the first few days of life, and no treatment is needed.

14.16   Caput succedaneum.

A **cephalhematoma**, a subperiosteal hemorrhage, is also a result of birth trauma (Fig. 14.17, *A* and *B*). It is soft, fluctuant, and well defined over one cranial bone because the periosteum (i.e., the covering over each bone) holds the bleeding in place. It appears several hours after birth and gradually increases in size. No discoloration is present, but it looks bizarre, and so parents need reassurance that the fluid will be reabsorbed during the first few weeks of life without treatment. In rare cases, a large hematoma may persist as long as 3 months.

Abnormal Findings

Frontal bulges, or "bossing," occur with prematurity or rickets.

An infant with cephalhematoma is at greater risk for jaundice as the red blood cells within the hematoma are broken down and reabsorbed.

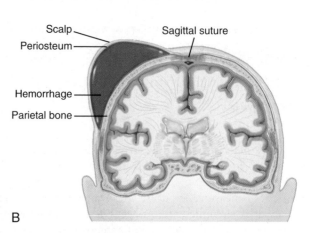

Scalp
Periosteum
Hemorrhage
Parietal bone
Sagittal suture

A   B

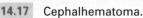

14.17   Cephalhematoma.

Normal Range of Findings

As you palpate the newborn's head, the suture lines feel like ridges. By age 5 to 6 months, they are smooth and not palpable.

A newborn's head may feel asymmetrical and the involved ridges more prominent because of *moulding* of the cranial bones during engagement and passage through the birth canal. Moulding is overriding of the cranial bones; usually, the parietal bone overrides the frontal or occipital bone. Reassure parents that this appearance lasts only a few days or a week. Babies delivered by Caesarean section usually have evenly round heads. Also, *positional moulding* (**positional plagiocephaly**) may occur if the infant continually sleeps on the back which is the recommended position to decrease the incidence of sudden unexpected infant death (SUID). This results in a flattening of the dependent cranial bone, the occiput. Inspection from behind shows a normal-appearing head shape with even horizontally placed ears. Inspection from the top shows a flat side of the occiput with the ear on the side displaced anteriorly, and the ear may fold forward. Head circumference is normal. Teach parents to reposition the baby's head to avoid further deformity.

Gently palpate the skull and **fontanelles** while the infant is calm and some-what in a sitting position (crying, lying down, or vomiting may cause the ante-rior fontanelle to look full and bulging). The skull should feel smooth and fused except at the fontanelles. The fontanelles feel firm, slightly concave, and well defined against the edges of the cranial bones. You may see slight arterial pulsations in the anterior fontanelle.

The posterior fontanelle may not be palpable at birth. If it is, it measures 1 cm and closes by 1 to 2 months. The anterior fontanelle may be small at birth and enlarges to 2.5 cm × 2.5 cm. The diameter is occasionally large (4 to 5 cm) in infants younger than 6 months. A small fontanelle usually is normal. The anterior fontanelle closes between ages 9 months and 2 years. Early closure may be insignificant if head growth proceeds normally.

Note the infant's **head posture** and **head control**. The infant can turn the head side to side by 2 weeks and shows the **tonic neck reflex** when supine and the head is turned to one side (extension of same arm and leg, flexion of opposite arm and leg). The tonic neck reflex disappears between ages 3 and 4 months, and then the head is maintained in the midline. Head control is achieved by age 4 months, when the baby can hold the head erect and steady when pulled to a vertical position. (See Chapters 24 and 25 for further details.)

Face

Check **facial features** for symmetry, appearance, and presence of swelling. Note symmetry of wrinkling when the infant cries or smiles (e.g., both sides of the lips rise and both sides of forehead wrinkle). Children love to comply when you ask them to "make a face." Normally, no swelling is evident. Parotid gland enlargement is most evident when the child sits and looks up at the ceiling; the swelling appears below the angle of the jaw.

Neck

An infant's neck looks short; it lengthens during the first 3 to 4 years. You can see the neck better by supporting the infant's shoulders and tilting the head back a little. This positioning also facilitates palpation of the trachea, which is buried deep in the neck. Feel for the row of cartilaginous rings in the midline or just slightly to the right of the midline.

Abnormal Findings

Sutures palpable when the child is older than 6 months should be investigated.

Marked plagiocephaly (see Table 14.2, p. 295) requires a custom helmet to afford room for brain growth in the flattened area, while moderating growth in the other areas. Used before sutures fuse.

Flattening also occurs in children with rickets.

A fontanelle may be truly tense or bulging with acute increased intracranial pressure.

Fontanelles are depressed and sunken with dehydration or malnutrition.

Pulsations may be markedly noticeable with increased intracranial pressure.

Delayed closure or larger than normal fontanelle size occurs with hydrocepha-lus, Down syndrome, hypothyroidism, and rickets.

A small fontanelle may be a sign of microcephaly, as is early closure.

Persistence of the tonic neck reflex after age 5 months may indicate brain damage.

In children, head tilt occurs with habit spasm, poor vision, and brain tumour.

Head lag after age 4 months may indi-cate intellectual or motor disability.

Unilateral immobility indicates nerve damage (central or peripheral; e.g., note angle of mouth droop on paralyzed side).

Some facies are characteristic of con-genital abnormalities or chronic allergy (see Table 14.2, p. 294).

A short neck or webbing (loose, fanlike folds) may indicate a congenital abnormal-ity (e.g., Down or Turner syndrome), or it may occur alone.

Objective Data

Normal Range of Findings

Assess muscle development with gentle passive ROM. Cradle an infant's head with your hands and turn it side to side, and test forward flexion, extension, and rotation. Note any resistance to movement, especially flexion. Ask an older child to actively move through the ROM, as you would an adult.

During infancy, cervical lymph nodes are normally not palpable. However, an older child's lymph nodes are; they feel more prominent than an adult's until after puberty, when lymphoid tissue begins to atrophy. Palpable nodes smaller than 3 mm are normal. They may be up to 1 cm in size in the cervical and inguinal areas but are discrete, move easily, and are nontender. Children have a higher incidence of infection, and so you should expect a higher incidence of inflammatory adenopathy among children. No other mass should occur in the neck.

The thyroid gland is difficult to palpate in an infant because of the shortness and thickness of the neck. An older child's thyroid may be palpable normally.

Abnormal Findings

Head tilt and limited ROM occur with torticollis (wryneck) or from sternomastoid muscle injury that occurs during birth or as a congenital defect.

Resistance to flexion (nuchal rigidity) and pain on flexion indicate meningeal irritation or meningitis.

Cervical nodes bigger than 1 cm are considered enlarged.

Thyroglossal duct cyst is a cystic lump high up in midline; it is freely movable and rises up during swallowing.

Supraclavicular nodes enlarge with Hodgkin's disease.

SPECIAL CONSIDERATIONS FOR ADVANCED PRACTICE

Normal Range of Findings

Special Considerations for Advanced Practice

Assessment Techniques

These procedures would not be considered part of a basic assessment in an environment in which patients have access to diagnostic testing. In Canada, health care providers may practise in isolated health care environments in which access to computed tomography or magnetic resonance imaging is not readily available. In these environments, the health care practitioner may find the following tests a helpful addition to their toolkit.

Percussion. With an infant, you may directly percuss with your plexor finger against the head surface. This yields a resonant or "cracked pot" sound, which is normal before closure of the fontanelles.

Auscultation. Bruits are common in the skull in children younger than 4 or 5 years or in children with anemia. They are systolic or continuous and are heard over the temporal area.

Pregnant Women

During the second trimester, chloasma may show on the face. This is a blotchy, hyperpigmented area over the cheeks and forehead that fades after delivery. The thyroid gland may be palpable normally during pregnancy.

Abnormal Findings

The sound also occurs with hydrocephalus as a result of separation of cranial sutures (Macewen sign).

After 5 years of age, bruits indicate increased intracranial pressure, aneurysm, or arteriovenous shunt.

Normal Range of Findings	Abnormal Findings

Older Adults

The temporal arteries may look twisted and prominent. In some older adults, a mild rhythmic tremor of the head may be normal. **Senile tremors** are benign and include head nodding (as if saying yes or no) and tongue protrusion. If some teeth have been lost, the lower face looks unusually small, with the mouth sunken in.

The neck may show an increased cervical concave (or inward) curve when the head and jaw are extended forward to compensate for kyphosis of the spine. During the examination, direct the older adult to perform ROM slowly; the older adult may experience dizziness with side movements. An older adult may have prolapse of the submandibular glands, which could be mistaken for a tumour. Drooping submandibular glands feel soft and are present bilaterally.

PROMOTING HEALTH: BRAIN INJURY PREVENTION

Use Your Head: Wear a Helmet

In Canada, helmet use is legislated provincially. Safe Kids Canada joined with Safe Communities Canada, SMARTRISK, and ThinkFirst Canada to create **Parachute**, a national charitable organization dedicated to preventing injury and saving lives. Parachute currently advocates that all provinces adopt the U.S. Consumer Product Safety Commission (CPSP) recommendations in regard to helmet safety standards.

When you buy a helmet in Canada, look for the Canadian Standards Association (CSA), ASTM International, or CPSC standard. The CPSC standard is comparable with the CSA standard. Parachute provides guidelines and information on which helmet to choose for activities to prevent brain and head injury on its website.* Ensure that you are aware of individual provincial helmet legislation, inasmuch as many provinces levy significant fines for nonuse. In the document *Reaching for the Top: A Report by the Advisor on Healthy Children and Youth,* Leitch stated that a pan-Canadian 5-year "National Injury Prevention Strategy" would be implemented.† To date, however, not all provinces in Canada have helmet legislation. Six provinces currently have provincial legislation, but only four of these apply to all ages. In addition, some municipalities have enacted local by-laws requiring cyclists to wear helmets; some of these by-laws cover children only and some cover all ages of cyclists. Municipalities have also introduced all-ages and all-wheel helmet by-laws, which requires mandatory helmet usage for cycling, skateboarding, and in-line skating and nonmotorized scooters. Ensure that you are using the most up-to-date legislated policy to guide your decision making. Visit http://www.parachutecanada.org/downloads/policy/Bike%20Helmet%20Legislation%20Chart-2014.pdf.

In general, all helmets are designed to absorb the impact energy in a collision or fall, protecting the brain from injury and trauma. However, helmets are not created equal. Each type of helmet is specifically designed to protect the head and brain from one or more *specific* types of impact that can take place in the particular sport or activity for which it is intended.

Wearing a properly fitted and safe bicycle helmet can reduce an individual's risk for head injury by 85% and reduce the risk for brain injury by 88%.‡ A helmet needs to be comfortable, snug, and secured. It should not move in any direction when adjusted properly, and the chin strap needs to be securely buckled. A proper fit is as important as wearing the correct helmet. This is particularly important for children. It is important to select a helmet that fits now, not a helmet that a child will grow into.

Children and adults should wear a sport- or activity-specific helmet when participating in the following sports or recreational activities:

- Alpine skiing, snowboarding, and snowmobiling
- ATV riding and go-kart riding
- Baseball and softball
- Bicycling and electronic bicycling (e-biking)
- Football
- Horseback riding
- Ice hockey, rollerskating, and in-line skating
- Lacrosse
- Rock climbing
- Scooter and skateboard riding

Although a helmet has not yet been specifically designed for either ice-skating or sledding, wearing a bicycle, skateboard, or ski helmet may be preferable to wearing no helmet at all. Nova Scotia was the first province in Canada to pass new legislation requiring all skiers (children and adults) to wear CSA-approved helmets on the slopes.

There are also certain activities for which an individual, especially a child, should not wear a helmet: for example, playing on playgrounds or climbing. In these situations, a helmet's chin strap might get caught and pose a risk for strangulation. Furthermore, the helmet itself may also pose an entrapment hazard or risk.

For more information about CPSC standards, visit https://www.cpsc.gov.

References

*Parachute. (2017). *Helmet FAQ.* Retrieved from http://www.parachutecanada.org/injury-topics/topic/C8.

†Leitch, K. (2007). *Reaching for the top: A report by the advisor on healthy children and youth.* Ottawa: Health Canada.

‡Rivara, F. P., Astleuy, S. J., Clarren, S. K., et al. (1999). Fit of bicycle safety helmets and risk of head injuries in children. *Injury Prevention, 5*(3), 194–197.

Special Considerations for Advanced Practice

PROMOTING HEALTH: PLAYING IT SAFE

Use Your Head: Understanding Postconcussion Syndrome

Rowan Stringer was just 17 when she died in 2013, after suffering what proved to be a fatal concussion during a high school rugby game in Ottawa. It was her second concussion within a week. The coroner's inquest that followed cast a harsh light on youth sports organizations, pointing to a lack of protocols that experts say must be addressed to keep our kids safe (Hall, 2017).

On June 7, 2016, Ontario became the first province in Canada to introduce comprehensive legislation called Rowan's Law, aimed at not only preventing and diagnosing head injuries in youth sport, but managing return to play. Several national organizations are lobbying for federal legislation to address this growing concern.

Parachute is a national, charitable organization, formed in July 2012, which united the former organizations of Safe Communities Canada, Safe Kids Canada, SMARTRISK and ThinkFirst Canada into one strong leader in injury prevention. Parachute has responded to this growing concern among amateur and professional athletes with an aggressive awareness program to protect young athletes.

Concussions are brain injuries caused by the impact of the brain with the inside of the skull. The impact causes damage that changes how brain cells function, leading to symptoms that can be physical (headaches, dizziness), cognitive (problems remembering or concentrating), or emotional (feeling depressed). A concussion can result from a blow to the head or body in numerous activities, including sports.

Concussions are common injuries, but because they cannot be detected on radiographs or computed tomographic (CT) scans, they have been difficult to fully investigate and understand. Fortunately, many important advances in knowledge of concussions have been made, including how to identify, manage, and recover from a concussion. Although concussions are often referred to as "mild traumatic head injuries" and often resolve uneventfully, *all* concussions have the potential for serious and long-lasting symptoms, and so each must be treated carefully and in consultation with a health care practitioner. Injuries to the brain are characterized by an altered state of consciousness. The altered state of consciousness is the key finding with any head injury.

Per Parachute Canada (2017), the signs and symptoms of a concussion are as follows:

- Headache
- Dizziness
- Feeling dazed
- Seeing "stars"
- Sensitivity to light
- Ringing in ears
- Tiredness
- Nausea, vomiting
- Irritability
- Confusion, disorientation

Contrary to popular belief, most concussions occur without a loss of consciousness.

It is extremely important to seek medical advice immediately upon receiving a blow to the head or body that results in signs or symptoms of a concussion. Concussions often go untreated, and symptoms may develop days or weeks after the initial injury. Ensure that patients who receive a concussion follow a recommended plan of recovery as outlined by the clinician.

Prevention is always the best approach. Ensure that participants wear a properly fitting CSA-approved helmet that is specific to the sport being played. Advise patients to report any head injuries immediately and to seek medical attention promptly.

Finally, many organizations such as the National Hockey League, local sport organizations, and school athletic programs, are mandating baseline concussion testing on all players to ensure the safety of their participants.

For more information on baseline testing or postconcussion recommendations, visit http://www.parachutecanada.org/injury-topics/item/concussion.

References

Hall, V. (2017). *Rowan's Law*. Retrieved from http://news.nationalpost.com/features/rowans-law.

Parachute Canada. (2017) *Concussion guidelines for physicians*. Retrieved from http://horizon.parachutecanada.org/wp-content/uploads/2014/10/Physicians_Concussion_Guidelines.pdf.

DOCUMENTATION AND CRITICAL THINKING

Sample Charting

SUBJECTIVE

Denies any unusually frequent or severe headache; no history of head injury, dizziness, or syncope; no neck pain, limitation of motion, nodules, or swelling.

OBJECTIVE

Head: Normocephalic, no lumps, no lesions, no tenderness.
Face: Symmetrical, no weakness, or drooping, no involuntary movements.
Neck: Supple with full ROM, no pain. Symmetric, no lymphadenopathy or masses. Trachea midline, thyroid not palpable. No bruits.

ASSESSMENT

Normocephalic symmetrical head and neck

Focused Assessment: Clinical Case Study

Mara is a 19-year-old single female college student with a history of good health and no chronic illnesses; she enters the outpatient clinic today stating, "I think I've had a stroke!"

SUBJECTIVE

1 day PTA [prior to arrival]: First noticed at dinner at college cafeteria when joking with friends, started to stick out tongue and roll tongue and could not do it, right side of tongue was not working. Mara left room to look in mirror and became scared; when smiled, noticed right side was not working. Tried to pucker lips, could not. Could not whistle, could not raise eyebrow: "I looked like a Vulcan." No other movement disorder below neck. Mild pain behind right ear with buzzing in ear. Able to sleep last night, but roommate said Mara's right eyelid did not close completely during sleep.
Today: Still no movement on complete right side of face. Feeling self-conscious in class and during conversations with friends. Now has taste aversion; fluids with high water content taste especially bitter. No hearing loss.

OBJECTIVE

Temp, 37°C (98.6°F); pulse, 64 bpm; resp, 14/min; BP, 108/78 mm Hg.
Forehead appears smooth and immobile on right; patient unable to wrinkle right side. Unable to close right eye; Bell's phenomenon present with attempts to close (right eyeball rolls upward); right palpebral fissure appears wider. No corneal reflex on right. Unable to whistle or puff right cheek. Absent nasolabial fold on right. Mouth droops on right, sags on right when tries to smile. Slight drooling. Left side of face responds appropriately to all these movements. Superficial sensation intact.
Rest of musculo-skeletal system intact: able to hold balance while standing, able to walk, walk heel-to-toe, do knee bend on each knee. Arm strength and ROM intact.

ASSESSMENT

Right-sided facial paralysis, consistent with Bell's palsy
Disturbed body image R/T [related to] effects of loss of facial function
Risk for deficient fluid volume R/T taste aversion and dietary alteration
Risk for sensory deficit, visual impairment, R/T effects of neurological impairment

ABNORMAL FINDINGS

TABLE 14.1	Primary Headaches (Diagnosed by Patient History With No Abnormal Findings in Physical Examination or Laboratory Testing)		
	Tension	**Migraine**	**Cluster**
	Tension	Migraine	Cluster
Definition	Headache (HA) of musculo-skeletal origin; may be a mild-to-moderate, less disabling form of migraine	HA of genetically transmitted vascular origin; headache plus prodrome, aura, other symptoms	HA that is intermittent, excruciating, unilateral, with autonomic signs
Location	Usually both sides, across frontal, temporal, and/or occipital region of head: forehead, sides, and back of head	Commonly one-sided but may occur on both sides Pain is often behind the eyes, the temples, or forehead	Always one-sided Often behind or around the eye, temple, forehead, cheek
Character	Bandlike tightness, viselike Nonthrobbing, nonpulsatile	Throbbing, pulsating	Continuous, burning, piercing, excruciating
Duration	Gradual onset, lasts 30 minutes to days	Rapid onset, peaks 1-2 hr, lasts 4-72 hr, sometimes longer	Abrupt onset, peaks in minutes, lasts 45-90 min
Quantity and severity	Diffuse, dull aching pain Mild-to-moderate pain	Moderate-to-severe pain	Can occur multiple times a day, in "clusters," lasting weeks Severe, stabbing pain
Timing	Situational, in response to overwork, posture	≈2 per month, last 1-3 days ≈1 in 10 patients have weekly headaches	1-2/day, each lasting ½ to 2 hr for 1 to 2 months; then remission for months or years
Aggravating symptoms or triggers	Stress, anxiety, depression, poor posture Not worsened by physical activity	Hormonal fluctuations (premenstrual) Foods (e.g., alcohol, caffeine, MSG, nitrates, chocolate, cheese) Hunger Letdown after stress Sleep deprivation Sensory stimuli (e.g., flashing lights or perfumes) Changes in weather Physical activity	Exacerbated by alcohol, stress, daytime napping, wind or heat exposure

TABLE 14.1	Primary Headaches (Diagnosed by Patient History With No Abnormal Findings in Physical Examination or Laboratory Testing)—cont'd		
Associated symptoms	Fatigue, anxiety, stress Sensation of a band tightening around head, of being gripped like a vice Sometimes photophobia or phonophobia	Aura (visual changes such as blind spots or flashes of light, tingling in an arm or leg, vertigo) Prodrome (change in mood, behaviour, hunger, cravings, yawning) Nausea, vomiting, photophobia, phonophobia, abdominal pain Person looks sick Family history of migraine	Ipsilateral autonomic signs: Nasal congestion or runny nose, watery or reddened eye, eyelid drooping, miosis Feelings of agitation
Relieving factors, efforts to treat	Rest, massage muscles in area, NSAID medication	Lie down, darken room, use eyeshade, sleep, take NSAID early, try to avoid opioid	Need to move, pace floor

Images © Pat Thomas, 2014.
See Illustration Credits for source information.

TABLE 14.2	Pediatric Abnormalities

◀ Hydrocephalus

Obstruction of drainage of cerebrospinal fluid results in excessive accumulation, increasing intracranial pressure, and enlargement of the head. The face looks small in comparison with the enlarged cranium. The increasing pressure also causes dilation of scalp veins, frontal bossing, and downcast or "setting sun" appearance of the eyes (sclera is visible above iris). The cranial bones thin, sutures separate, and percussion yields a "cracked pot" sound (Macewen's sign).

◀ Down Syndrome

Chromosomal aberration (trisomy 21). Head and face characteristics may include up-slanting eyes with inner epicanthal folds, flat nasal bridge, small broad flat nose, protruding thick tongue, ear dysplasia, short broad neck with webbing, and small hands with single palmar crease.

Continued

Abnormal Findings

TABLE 14.2   **Pediatric Abnormalities—cont'd**

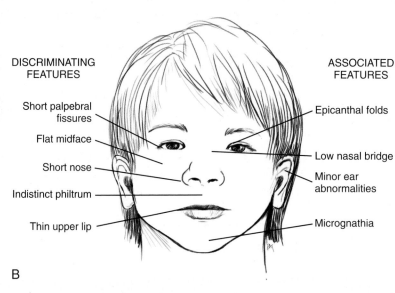

DISCRIMINATING FEATURES

- Short palpebral fissures
- Flat midface
- Short nose
- Indistinct philtrum
- Thin upper lip

ASSOCIATED FEATURES

- Epicanthal folds
- Low nasal bridge
- Minor ear abnormalities
- Micrognathia

A

B

Fetal Alcohol Spectrum Disorder

A pregnant woman who abuses alcohol is at great risk of producing a baby with a wide range of growth and developmental abnormalities. Facial malformations may be recognizable at birth. Characteristic facies include narrow palpebral fissures, epicanthal folds, and midfacial hypoplasia.

Atopic (Allergic) Facies

Children with chronic allergies such as atopic dermatitis often develop characteristic facial features. These include exhausted face, blue shadows below the eyes ("allergic shiners") from sluggish venous return, a double or single crease on the lower eyelids (Morgan's lines), central facial pallor, and open-mouth breathing (allergic gaping). The open-mouth breathing can lead to malocclusion of the teeth and malformed jaw because the child's bones are still forming.

Allergic Salute and Crease

The transverse line on the nose is also a feature of chronic allergies. It is formed when the child chronically uses the hand to push the nose up and back (the "allergic salute") to relieve itching and to free swollen turbinates, which allows air passage.

TABLE 14.2   Pediatric Abnormalities—cont'd

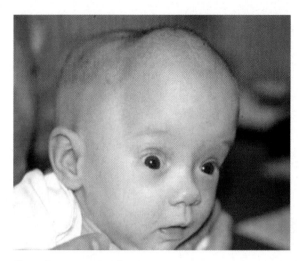

Plagiocephaly

Positional or deformational plagiocephaly has increased dramatically since the "Safe Sleep" campaign started in 1999 to prevent SUID. It is asymmetry of the cranium when seen from the top caused by a positional preference. It is not associated with premature closing of cranial sutures, and growth of the brain proceeds normally. This can be mitigated by "tummy time," when the parent places the infant prone for awake playing. Physical therapy and helmet therapy are further treatments.

Craniosynostosis

Premature closing of one or multiple cranial sutures (shown in the figure) results in a malformed head and a cosmetic deformity. Mechanisms involve genetic mutations coding structural proteins or growth factor receptors. Severe deformities cannot contain the brain, eyes and optic nerves inside the cranial vault, and hypoplasia of the face results, warranting surgery.

SUID, Sudden unexpected infant death.
See Illustration Credits for source information.

TABLE 14.3 Swellings on the Head or Neck

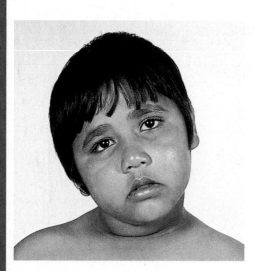

Torticollis (Wryneck)

A shortening or excessive contraction of the sternocleidomastoid muscle in the neck; may be caused by an idiopathic, genetic, or acquired secondary injury that results in a lateral head tilt and chin rotation to the opposite side. Congenital torticollis may be caused by intrauterine malpositioning or by prenatal injury of the muscles or blood supply in the neck. You will feel a firm, discrete, nontender mass in the middle of the muscle on the involved side. This necessitates treatment, or the muscle becomes fibrotic and permanently shortened with permanent limitation of ROM, asymmetry of head and face, and visual problems resulting from the nonhorizontal position of the eyes.

Thyroid: Multiple Nodules

Multiple nodules usually indicate inflammation or a multinodular goitre rather than a neoplasm. However, any rapidly enlarging or firm nodule should be further investigated.

Pilar Cyst (Wen)

Smooth, firm, fluctuant swelling on the scalp. Tense pressure of the contents causes overlying skin to be shiny and taut. It is a benign growth.

Parotid Gland Enlargement

Rapid painful inflammation of the parotid gland occurs with mumps. Parotid swelling also occurs with blockage of a duct, with abscess, and with tumour. Note swelling of anterior to lower ear lobe. Stensen duct obstruction can occur in older adults dehydrated as a result of diuretics or anticholinergics.

ROM, Range of motion.
See Illustration Credits for source information.

TABLE 14.4   Abnormal Facial Appearances With Chronic Illnesses

Parkinson's Syndrome

A deficiency of the neurotransmitter dopamine and degeneration of the basal ganglia in the brain. The immobility of features produces a face that is flat and expressionless, "masklike," with elevated eyebrows, staring gaze, oily skin, and drooling.

Cushing's Syndrome

With excessive secretion of adrenocorticotropic hormone (ACTH) and chronic steroid use, the person develops a plethoric, rounded, moonlike face, prominent jowls, red cheeks, hirsutism on the upper lip, lower cheeks, and chin, and acneiform rash on the chest.

Bell's Palsy (Left Side)

A **lower motor neuron** lesion (**peripheral**), producing cranial nerve VII paralysis, which is almost always unilateral. It has a rapid onset, and the majority of cases are thought to be caused by herpes simplex virus (HSV). Note complete paralysis of one half of the face; person cannot wrinkle forehead, raise eyebrow, close eye, whistle, or show teeth on the right side. Former Canadian Prime Minister Jean Chrétien acquired Bell's palsy in his youth.

Stroke or Cerebrovascular Accident

An **upper motor neuron** lesion (**central**). A "stroke" is an acute neurological deficit caused by an obstruction of a cerebral vessel, as in atherosclerosis, or a rupture in a cerebral vessel. Note paralysis of lower facial muscles, but also note that the upper half of face is not affected because of the intact nerve from the unaffected hemisphere. The person is still able to wrinkle the forehead and close the eyes.

Continued

TABLE 14.4 Abnormal Facial Appearances With Chronic Illnesses—cont'd

Cachectic Appearance

Accompanies chronic wasting diseases such as cancer, dehydration, and starvation. Features include sunken eyes; hollow cheeks; and exhausted, defeated expression.

Acromegaly

Excessive secretion of growth hormone from the pituitary gland after puberty creates an enlarged skull and thickened cranial bones. Note the elongated head, massive face, overgrowth of nose and lower jaw, heavy eyebrow ridge, and coarse facial features.

See Illustration Credits for source information.

TABLE 14.5 Thyroid Hormone Disorders

© Pat Thomas, 2014.

The hypothalamic-pituitary-thyroid axis regulates the production of thyroid hormones by a negative feedback system, much like the thermostat that guides your household furnace. (1) The hypothalamus secretes thyrotropin-releasing hormone (TRH), which (2) acts on the anterior pituitary to secrete thyroid-stimulating hormone (TSH), which (3) directs the thyroid gland to produce T_3 and T_4 hormones. When T_3 and T_4 hormones are high in the bloodstream ("hot" like a furnace), they (4) direct the pituitary and hypothalamus to shut off their signalling hormones. That is the negative feedback. When T_3 and T_4 hormone levels are low (thyroid is like a cold furnace), the pituitary sends out TSH to stimulate new production of T_3 and T_4 hormones. Your body metabolism is most comfortable in a healthy balance of hormone levels.

TABLE 14.5	**Thyroid Hormone Disorders—cont'd**

Hyperthyroidism

Goitre is an increase in the size of the thyroid gland and occurs with hyperthyroidism, Hashimoto's thyroiditis, and hypothyroidism. Graves' disease (shown here) is the most common cause of hyperthyroidism, manifested by goitre and exophthalmos (bulging eyeballs). Symptoms include nervousness, fatigue, weight loss, muscle cramps, and heat intolerance; signs include tachycardia, shortness of breath, excessive sweating, fine muscle tremor, thin silky hair and skin, infrequent blinking, and a staring appearance.

Myxedema (Hypothyroidism)

A deficiency of thyroid hormone, when severe, causes a nonpitting edema or myxedema. Note puffy edematous face, especially around eyes (periorbital edema), coarse facial features, dry skin, and dry coarse hair and eyebrows.

See Illustration Credits for source information.

Summary Checklist: Head, Face, and Neck, Including Examination of Regional Lymphatic System

1. **Inspect and palpate the skull:**
   General size and contour
   Any deformities, lumps, tenderness
   Palpation of temporal artery, temporomandibular joint
2. **Inspect the face:**
   Facial expression
   Symmetry of movement (cranial nerve VII)

Any involuntary movements, edema, lesions
3. **Inspect and palpate the neck:**
   Active ROM
   Enlargement of salivary glands, lymph nodes, thyroid gland
   Position of the trachea

4. **Auscultate the thyroid (if enlarged) for bruit**
5. **Engage in teaching and health promotion**

15 CHAPTER

Eyes

Written by Carolyn Jarvis, PhD, APN, CNP
Adapted by Annette J. Browne, PhD, RN

ⓔ http://evolve.elsevier.com/Canada/Jarvis/examination/

STRUCTURE AND FUNCTION

EXTERNAL ANATOMY

The eye is the sensory organ of vision. Humans are very visually oriented beings. More than half the neocortex is involved with processing visual information.

Because this sense is so important to humans, the eye is well protected by the bony orbital cavity, which is surrounded with a cushion of fat. The **eyelids** are like two movable shades that further protect the eye from injury, strong light, and dust. The upper eyelid is the larger and more mobile one. The eyelashes are short hairs in double or triple rows that curve outward from the eyelid margins, filtering out dust and dirt.

The **palpebral fissure** is the elliptical open space between the eyelids (Fig. 15.1). When the eyes are closed, the eyelid margins approximate completely. When the eyes are open, the upper eyelid covers part of the iris. The lower eyelid margin is just at the **limbus**, the border between the cornea and sclera. The **canthus** is the corner of the eye, the angle where the eyelids meet. At the inner canthus, the **caruncle** is a small fleshy mass containing sebaceous glands.

Within the upper eyelid, **tarsal plates** are strips of connective tissue that give it shape (Fig. 15.2). The tarsal plates contain the **meibomian glands**, modified sebaceous glands that secrete an oily lubricating material onto the eyelids. This stops the tears from overflowing and helps form an airtight seal when the eyelids are closed.

The exposed part of the eye has a transparent protective covering, the **conjunctiva**. The conjunctiva is a thin mucous membrane folded like an envelope between the eyelids and the eyeball. The *palpebral* conjunctiva lines the eyelids and is clear, with many small blood vessels. It forms a deep recess and then folds back over the eye. The *bulbar* conjunctiva overlies the eyeball, with the white sclera showing through. At the limbus, the conjunctiva merges with the cornea. The cornea covers and protects the iris and pupil.

The **lacrimal apparatus** provides constant irrigation to keep the conjunctiva and cornea moist and lubricated (Fig.

15.3). The lacrimal gland, in the upper outer corner over the eye, secretes tears. The tears wash across the eye and are drawn up evenly as the eyelid blinks. The tears drain into the **puncta**, visible on the upper and lower eyelids at the inner canthus. The tears then drain into the nasolacrimal sac, through the centimetre-long nasolacrimal duct, and empty into the inferior meatus inside the nose. A tiny fold of mucous membrane prevents air from being forced up the nasolacrimal duct when the nose is blown.

Extraocular Muscles

Six muscles attach the eyeball to its orbit (Fig. 15.4) and serve to direct the eye to points of the person's interest. These extraocular muscles enable both straight and rotary movements. The four straight, or rectus, muscles are the (a) superior, (b) inferior, (c) lateral, and (d) medial rectus muscles. The two slanting, or oblique, muscles are the (a) superior and (b) inferior oblique muscles.

Each muscle is coordinated, or yoked, with one in the other eye. This ensures that when the two eyes move, their axes always remain parallel (called *conjugate movement*). Parallel axes are important because the human brain can tolerate seeing only one image. Although some animals can perceive two different pictures through each eye, human beings have a binocular, single-image visual system. This occurs because a human's eyes move as a pair. For example, the two yoked muscles that allow looking to the far right are the right lateral rectus and the left medial rectus.

Movement of the **extraocular muscles** (see Fig. 15.4) is stimulated by three **cranial nerves**. Cranial nerve VI, the abducens nerve, *innervates* (carries the nerve impulse that moves a muscle) the lateral rectus muscle (which *abducts* the eye, which means moving it laterally toward the temple); cranial nerve IV, the trochlear nerve, innervates the superior oblique muscle (downward and inward toward the nose); and cranial nerve III, the oculomotor nerve, innervates all the other nerves: the superior, inferior, and medial rectus and the inferior oblique muscles. Note that the superior oblique

Upper eyelid

Palpebral fissure

Lateral canthus

Lower eyelid

Pupil

Iris

Sclera

Medial canthus

Caruncle

Limbus
(border between
cornea and sclera)

15.1   (© Pat Thomas, 2006.)

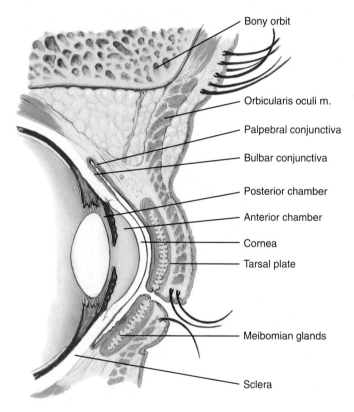

Bony orbit

Orbicularis oculi m.

Palpebral conjunctiva

Bulbar conjunctiva

Posterior chamber

Anterior chamber

Cornea

Tarsal plate

Meibomian glands

Sclera

15.2   (© Pat Thomas, 2006.)

muscle is located on the superior aspect of the eyeball, but when it contracts, it enables the person to look downward and inward.

INTERNAL ANATOMY

The eye is a sphere composed of three concentric coats: (a) the outer fibrous sclera, (b) the middle vascular choroid, and (c) the inner nervous retina (Fig. 15.5). Inside the retina is the transparent vitreous body. The only parts accessible to examination are the sclera anteriorly and the retina through the ophthalmoscope.

The Outer Layer

The **sclera** is a tough, protective, white covering. It is continuous anteriorly with the smooth, transparent cornea, which covers the iris and pupil. The cornea is part of the refracting media of the eye, bending incoming light rays so that they are focused on the retina within.

The **cornea** is very sensitive to touch; contact with a wisp of cotton stimulates a blink in both eyes, called the *corneal reflex*. The trigeminal nerve (cranial nerve V) carries the afferent sensation into the brain, and the facial nerve (cranial nerve VII) carries the efferent message that stimulates the blink.

Structure and Function

The Middle Layer

The **choroid** has dark pigmentation to prevent light from reflecting internally and is heavily vascularized to deliver blood to the retina. Anteriorly, the choroid is continuous with the ciliary body and the iris. The muscles of the ciliary body control the thickness of the lens. The **iris** functions as a diaphragm, varying the opening at its centre, the pupil. This controls the amount of light admitted into the retina. The muscle fibres of the iris contract the pupil in bright light and to accommodate for near vision, and dilate the pupil when the light is dim and for far vision. The colour of the iris varies from person to person, and people with darker irises have darker retinas.

The **pupil** is round and regular. Its size is determined by a balance between the parasympathetic and sympathetic chains of the autonomic nervous system. Stimulation of the parasympathetic branch, through cranial nerve III, causes constriction of the pupil. Stimulation of the sympathetic branch dilates the pupil and elevates the eyelid. As mentioned earlier, the pupil size also reacts to the amount of ambient light and to accommodation (focusing an object on the retina).

The **lens** is a transparent biconvex disc located just behind the pupil. The lens serves as a refracting medium, keeping a viewed object in continual focus on the retina. Its thickness is controlled by the ciliary body; the lens bulges for focusing on near objects and flattens for far objects.

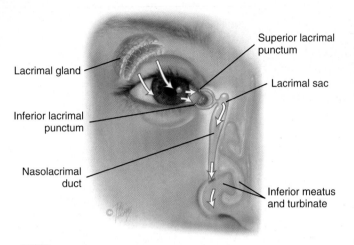

Lacrimal gland

Superior lacrimal punctum

Lacrimal sac

Inferior lacrimal punctum

Nasolacrimal duct

Inferior meatus and turbinate

15.3   (© Pat Thomas, 2006.)

Superior oblique m. (passing through trochlea)

Medial rectus m.

Superior rectus m.

Optic nerve

Lateral rectus m.

Inferior oblique m.

Inferior rectus m.

MUSCLE ATTACHMENTS

A

| Superior rectus m. c.n. III | Inferior oblique m. c.n. III | Inferior oblique m. c.n. III | Superior rectus m. c.n. III |

Lateral rectus m. c.n. VI

Medial rectus m. c.n. III

Lateral rectus m. c.n. VI

| Inferior rectus m. c.n. III | Superior oblique m. c.n. IV | Superior oblique m. c.n. IV | Inferior rectus m. c.n. III |

B   DIRECTION OF MOVEMENT

15.4

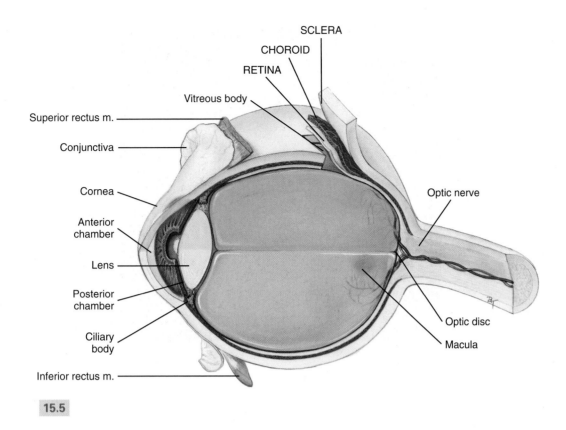

Superior rectus m.
Conjunctiva
Cornea
Anterior chamber
Lens
Posterior chamber
Ciliary body
Inferior rectus m.
Vitreous body
SCLERA
CHOROID
RETINA
Optic nerve
Optic disc
Macula

15.5

The **anterior chamber** is posterior to the cornea and anterior to the iris and lens. The **posterior chamber** lies behind the iris to the sides of the lens. These chambers contain the clear, watery aqueous humor, which is produced continually by the ciliary body. The continuous flow of this fluid serves to deliver nutrients to the surrounding tissues and to drain metabolic wastes. Intraocular pressure is determined by a balance between the amount of aqueous humor produced and resistance to its outflow at the angle of the anterior chamber.

The Inner Layer

The **retina** is the visual receptive layer of the eye in which light waves are changed into nerve impulses. The retina surrounds the soft gelatinous vitreous humor. The retinal structures viewed through the ophthalmoscope are the optic disc, the retinal vessels, the general background, and the macula (Fig. 15.6).

The **optic disc** (or *optic papilla*) is the area in which fibres from the retina converge to form the optic nerve. Located toward the nasal side of the retina, it has these characteristics: a colour that varies from creamy yellow-orange to pink; a round or oval shape; margins that are distinct and sharply demarcated, especially on the temporal side; and a physiological cup, the smaller circular area inside the disc where the blood vessels exit and enter.

The **retinal vessels** normally include a paired artery and vein extending to each quadrant, growing progressively smaller in calibre as they reach the periphery. The arteries appear brighter red and narrower than the veins, and the arteries have a thin sliver of light (the arterial light reflex).

The general background of the fundus varies in colour, depending on the person's skin colour. The **macula** is located on the temporal side of the fundus. It is a slightly darker pigmented region surrounding the **fovea centralis**, the area of sharpest and keenest vision. The macula receives and transduces light from the centre of the visual field (transduction occurs when visual pigments are broken down into neural signals that eventually travel to the visual cortex).

VISUAL PATHWAYS AND VISUAL FIELDS

Objects reflect light. The light rays are refracted through the transparent media (cornea, aqueous humor, lens, and vitreous body) and strike the retina. The retina transforms the light stimulus into nerve impulses that are conducted through the optic nerve and the optic tract to the visual cortex of the occipital lobe.

The image formed on the retina is upside down and reversed from its actual appearance in the outside world (Fig. 15.7); that is, the image of an object in the upper temporal visual field of the right eye is reflected onto the lower nasal area of the retina. All retinal fibres collect to form the optic nerve, but they maintain this same spatial arrangement, with nasal fibres running medially and temporal fibres running laterally.

At the optic chiasm, nasal fibres (from both temporal visual fields) cross over. The left optic tract now has fibres only from the left half of each retina, and the right optic tract contains fibres only from the right half. Thus the right side of the brain looks at the left side of the world.

15.6   The retina.

15.7   Visual pathways (viewed from above).

VISUAL REFLEXES

Pupillary Light Reflex

The **pupillary light reflex** is the normal constriction of the pupils when bright light shines on the retina (Fig. 15.8). It is a subcortical reflex arc (i.e., a person has no conscious control over it); the afferent link is cranial nerve II, the optic nerve, and the efferent path is cranial III, the oculomotor nerve. When one eye is exposed to bright light, a *direct light reflex* occurs (constriction of that pupil), as does a *consensual light reflex* (simultaneous constriction of the other pupil). This happens because the optic nerve carries the sensory afferent message in and then synapses with both sides of the brain. For example, consider the light reflex in a person who is blind in one eye. Stimulation of the normal eye produces both a direct and a consensual light reflex. Stimulation of the blind eye causes no response because the sensory afferent in cranial nerve II is destroyed.

Fixation

This is a reflex direction of the eye toward an object attracting a person's attention. The image is fixed in the centre of the visual field, the fovea centralis. This fixing consists of very rapid ocular movements to put the target back on the fovea, and somewhat slower (smooth pursuit) movements to track the target and keep its image on the fovea. These ocular movements are impaired by medications, alcohol, fatigue, and inattention.

Accommodation

Accommodation is adaptation of the eye for near vision. It is accomplished by increasing the curvature of the lens through movement of the ciliary muscles. Although the lens

CONSENSUAL LIGHT REFLEX
constricts pupil, opposite eye

c.n. III

c.n. II

Afferent nerve

Optic
chiasm

Midbrain

Optic nerve c.n. II

c.n. III

DIRECT LIGHT REFLEX
efferent nerve constricts
pupil, same eye

Key
■ Sensory afferent into brain
■ Motor efferent out to iris

15.8

cannot be observed directly, the components of accommodation that can be observed are convergence (motion toward) of the axes of the eyeballs and pupillary constriction.

 DEVELOPMENTAL CONSIDERATIONS

Infants and Children

At birth, eye function is limited, but it matures fully during the early years. Peripheral vision is intact in the newborn infant. The macula, the area of keenest vision, is absent at birth but is developing by age 4 months and is mature by age 8 months. Eye movements may be poorly coordinated at birth. By 3 to 4 months of age, the infant establishes binocularity and can fixate on a single image with both eyes simultaneously. Most neonates (80%) are born farsighted; this gradually decreases after 7 to 8 years of age.

In structure, the eyeball reaches adult size by 8 years of age. At birth, the iris shows little pigmentation, and the pupils are small. The lens is nearly spherical at birth, becoming flatter throughout life. Its consistency changes from that of soft plastic at birth to that of rigid glass in old age.

Older Adults

Changes in eye structure contribute greatly to the distinct facial changes of older adults. The skin loses its elasticity, causing wrinkling and drooping; fat tissues and muscles atrophy. Lacrimal glands involute, causing decreased tear production and a feeling of dryness and burning.

On the globe itself, the cornea may show an infiltration of degenerative lipid material around the limbus (see discussion of arcus senilis, p. 331). Pupil size decreases. The lens loses elasticity, becoming hard and glasslike, which decreases the lens's ability to change shape to accommodate for near vision; this condition is termed **presbyopia**. The average age at onset of presbyopia is 40 years.[1] By 70 years of age, the normally transparent fibres of the lens begin to thicken and yellow. This is nuclear sclerosis, or the beginning of a "senile cataract."

Inside the globe, debris can accumulate in the vitreous humor (appearing in vision as "floaters") because the vitreous humor is not continuously renewed, as aqueous humor is. Visual acuity may diminish gradually after age 50 years and even more so after age 70 years. Near vision is commonly affected because of the decreased power of accommodation in the lens (presbyopia). As early as the fourth decade, a person may have blurred vision and difficulty reading. Also, older adults need more light to see because of a decreased adaptation to darkness, and this condition may affect the function of night driving.

The prevalence of age-related vision loss is increasing dramatically; there are approximately 1.4 million Canadians living with age-related macular degeneration, and many with significant vision loss.[2] Impaired visual acuity and other problems within the visual system negatively impact functioning and quality of life; in older adults, this has been shown to be associated with decreased participation in social and leisure activities, difficulty in family relationships, depressive symptoms, and injuries from accidents, including falls. They also affect instrumental activities of daily living (IADLs), or ability to work, drive safely, or maintain a driver's licence.[3] When visual acuity declines, it is essential for nurses to assess the increased risk for falls and social isolation, as well as the impact on relationships, and to support individuals and their families or friends.

In the older adult population, the most common causes of decreased visual functioning are as follows:

1. *Macular degeneration*, or the breakdown of cells in the macula of the retina. Loss of central vision, the area of clearest vision, is the most common cause of blindness. **Age-related macular degeneration (AMD)** is the leading cause of blindness in Canada and remains the most common cause of legal blindness in people older than 65.[4] As the population ages, the number of people with AMD is expected to double by 2040. Studies suggest a higher incidence of AMD among women, particularly those with earlier onset of menopause, which suggests that estrogen may play a protective role in minimizing AMD risk.[5,6] The visual symptoms of AMD involve loss of central vision.[7] While peripheral (side) vision is unaffected, with AMD, people lose the sharp, straight-ahead vision necessary for driving, reading, recognizing faces, doing fine manual work such as sewing, and looking at details. Depending on the extent to which the person's activities require close work, loss of central vision may cause great distress.

2. *Cataract formation*, or lens opacity, which results from a clumping of proteins in the lens. Some cataract formation should be expected by 70 years of age. Cataracts represent the second most common cause of correctable visual impairment after the correction of refractive error.[8] Advancing age remains the most common risk factor; progression typically extends over a long time. Other common risk factors include diabetes mellitus, certain medications (steroids), history of ocular trauma, and previous intraocular inflammation or surgery. The prevalence of cataract is more than 50% among people aged 70 to 79 and almost 100% among people older than 90.

3. *Glaucoma,* or increased intraocular pressure. Glaucoma is the second most common cause of vision loss in older adults in Canada.[9] More than 250 000 Canadians have chronic open-angle glaucoma, the most common form of the disease. It involves damage to the optic nerve resulting in a gradual loss of peripheral vision. See the box Promoting Health: Screening for Glaucoma.

4. *Diabetic retinopathy.* This remains the leading cause of visual impairment in people younger than 65.[10] This risk

is highest in diabetic patients with concurrent proteinuria. Patients who are diabetic should be referred regularly for screening by an ophthalmologist for diabetic retinopathy.[11]

To summarize, the number of partially sighted people is rising largely because the proportion of older adults in the population is increasing. The term *partially sighted* refers to vision that is outside normal limits (<20/60) and cannot be improved through medical or surgical means. In Canada, a visual acuity worse than 20/50 disqualifies people from obtaining a driver's licence or restricts their driving to daytime only, as do some visual field deficits.[12] Legal blindness is vision that cannot be corrected to better than 20/200 and peripheral vision that cannot be corrected to better than 20 degrees.

The Canadian Ophthalmological Society's screening recommendations for adults are listed as follows.[13] Screening is done for a variety of purposes: primary screening (e.g., to reduce the occurrence or incidence of disease, to encourage eye protection), secondary prevention (to reduce and control the consequences of existing diseases such as diabetes mellitus, glaucoma, high myopia), and tertiary prevention (e.g., to reduce the harm of a chronic disease, such as reducing intraocular pressure in primary open-angle glaucoma, laser therapy for diabetic retinopathy).[13]

1. Screening intervals in asymptomic low-risk patients:
   - Age 19 to 40 years: at least every 10 years
   - Age 41 to 55 years: at least every 5 years
   - Age 56 to 65 years: at least every 3 years
   - Age older than 65 years: at least every 2 years
2. Screening in symptomatic patients:
   - Any patient noting changes in visual acuity, visual field, colour vision, or physical changes to the eye should be assessed as soon as possible
3. Screening intervals in high-risk patients:
   - Patients at higher risk for visual impairment (e.g., those with diabetes, cataract, macular degeneration, glaucoma [verified or suspected], or a family history of these conditions) should be assessed more frequently and thoroughly
   - Age older than 40 to 50 years: at least every 3 years
   - Age older than 50 to 60 years: at least every 2 years
   - Age older than 60 years: at least annually

PROMOTING HEALTH: SCREENING FOR GLAUCOMA

Preventing Glaucoma

After cataract, glaucoma is the second leading cause of blindness worldwide; it is, however, the number one cause of irreversible vision loss.* Glaucoma is a condition in which the optic nerve is damaged, usually as a result of increasing pressure within the eye. Primary open-angle glaucoma is typically asymptomatic until it is advanced.† People usually do not

report changes until their visual field or acuity is substantially impaired; as a result, glaucoma may be undiagnosed in 50% of patients with the disease. By the time visual symptoms present, irreversible damage to the optic nerve has occurred: once vision has been lost, it cannot be regained. The Canadian Ophthalmological Society recommends glaucoma screening in

PROMOTING HEALTH: SCREENING FOR GLAUCOMA—cont'd

patients at high risk for glaucoma.* Screening for glaucoma is ideal because this condition typically progresses slowly and can be effectively managed.

Health care providers should encourage regular eye examinations, especially for patients with known risk factors. Several risk factors are easily elicited on history-taking.‡ Risk factors for glaucoma include the following:

1. Being older than 60 years: the risk for glaucoma increases with age, but it can occur in anyone in any age group
2. Being of African descent: the prevalence of glaucoma is 4.3 times higher in people of African descent compared with others‡
3. Being a woman: the prevalence of open-angle glaucoma is higher among women than among men†
4. Increased intraocular pressure (IOP) (>21 mm Hg)
5. Family history of glaucoma
6. Steroid use: patients using corticosteroids (topical [ocular], periocular, or systemic) for more than two weeks should have an eye examination to establish a baseline status and undergo regular monitoring to rule out pathological changes (e.g., elevated eye pressure, cataracts)‡
7. Hypertension
8. Eye injury
9. Severe myopia (nearsightedness)
10. Diabetes
11. Use of certain other medications, including antihypertensives, antihistamines, anticholinergics, and antidepressants

There are two main types of glaucoma. To understand the difference, it is helpful to review the basic structure of the eye. The anterior and posterior chambers of the eye are filled with a fluid called *aqueous humor*. This fluid is produced in the posterior chamber and then passes into the anterior chamber through the pupil. The fluid moves out of the eye and into the bloodstream through a drainage area located in front of the iris. This drainage area is located in the angle formed between the iris and the point at which the iris appears to meet the inside of the cornea. If the flow of aqueous humor is blocked, IOP increases. This pressure eventually damages the optic nerve and results in a loss of vision, which is permanent because in the retina, neurons are not regenerated once they are lost.

Open-angle glaucoma is the most common type of glaucoma, accounting for more than 90% of all cases. With open-angle glaucoma, the angle between the iris and the cornea is open, but the fluid is slow to drain, which causes IOP to build. There are virtually no symptoms. Vision loss

begins with the peripheral vision, which often goes unnoticed because affected individuals learn to compensate intuitively by turning their heads. As the condition progresses, the field of peripheral vision decreases until eventually affected patients may not be able to see anything on either side. This condition is referred to as *tunnel vision*.

Closed-angle glaucoma occurs when the space between the cornea and iris is narrower than normal. Anything that causes the pupil to dilate—such as dim light, eye drops, and certain medications—can block the drainage of fluid. Aging and injury also contribute to and can block the drainage of fluid. Closed-angle glaucoma causes sudden increases in IOP that result in blurred vision, sensitivity to light, nausea, and halos around lights. Affected individuals must be treated immediately.

Regular comprehensive eye examinations are extremely important because open-angle glaucoma does not produce symptoms in its early stages. These examinations should include the following:

1. Visual acuity testing
2. Visual field testing
3. Dilated eye examination
4. Tonometry to measure the IOP

Canada has not instituted a population screening program for glaucoma, although it has given serious consideration to doing so in the past.* Screening with simple IOP testing and optic nerve examination tends to yield underestimates of the prevalence of glaucoma. Although visual field testing typically reveals damage, it is usually at a more advanced stage than the very early stage ideal for diagnosis and treatment.

Although individuals who wear glasses appear to have more regular eye examinations, health care providers need to remind all individuals of the risk for glaucoma and the need for regular comprehensive eye examinations.

References

* Canadian Ophthalmological Society Glaucoma Clinical Practice Guideline Expert Committee. (2009). Canadian Ophthalmological Society evidence-based clinical practice guidelines for the management of glaucoma in the adult eye. *Canadian Journal of Ophthalmology*, 44, S7–S93. doi:10.3129/i09.080.
† Vajaranant, T. S., Nayak, S., Wilensky, J. T., et al. (2010). Gender and glaucoma: What we know and what we need to know. *Current Opinion in Ophthalmology*, 21(2), 91–99. doi:10.1097/ICU.0b013e3283360b7e.
‡ Basilious, A., & Buys, Y. M. (2015). A woman with a family history of glaucoma. *Canadian Medical Association Journal*, 187(12), 899. doi:10.1503/cmaj.140685.

 SOCIAL DETERMINANTS OF HEALTH CONSIDERATIONS

Many people in Canada cannot afford vision care costs including vision testing, eye examinations, glasses or contact lenses.[14] A recent Canadian report showed that one-third of paid employees in Ontario do not have employer-provided benefits to offset the costs of vision or dental care.[15] Provincial health care plans typically only provide coverage for eye examinations for children up to age 18 years and adults over age 65 years.[13] None of the Canadian provinces covers the cost of a general/routine eye examination for

individuals between 20 and 64 years old.[16] In four provinces (Saskatchewan, New Brunswick, Newfoundland and Labrador, and Prince Edward Island), people aged 65 years and older are not covered. Eyeglasses are not covered in any of the provinces for any age. In all provinces, to receive low-income vision care assistance, individuals must be in receipt of social assistance. Nurses working in community and acute care need to consider the effect of low income on access to routine eye care and the ability to pay for corrective lenses. People who cannot afford vision testing or corrective lenses must be referred to agencies that can provide those services free of charge or at a reduced cost.

Structure and Function

According to data from large-scale US studies, patients with a predisposition to visual deficits include those who wear glasses or contact lenses, have diabetes, are of African descent, or have a strong family history of glaucoma, AMD, or retinal detachment.[17] For example, research from the United States shows that the rate of primary open-angle glaucoma is three to six times higher among people of African descent than among people of European descent, and the disease is three to six times more likely to cause blindness in people of African descent than in people of European descent.[17] Reasons for these disparities are not known. However, nurses should continue to encourage people to be screened. In Canada, outreach efforts are particularly needed among Indigenous people, in part because the incidence of diabetes can be high in many communities, and also because people may have limited access to facilities offering eye examinations.[18]

Subjective Data

SUBJECTIVE DATA

1. Vision difficulty (decreased acuity, blurring, blind spots)
2. Pain
3. Strabismus, diplopia
4. Redness, swelling
5. Watering, discharge
6. History of ocular problems
7. Glaucoma
8. Use of glasses or contact lenses
9. Self-care behaviours
10. Medications
11. Coping with vision changes or loss

HEALTH HISTORY QUESTIONS

Examiner Asks	Rationale
1. **Vision difficulty (decreased acuity, blurring, blind spots)**. Any **difficulty seeing** or any blurring? Did visual difficulty or change in vision come on suddenly, or develop slowly? In one eye or both? • Is it constant, or does it come and go? • Do objects appear out of focus, or do they look clouded over? Does the problem feel like "greyness" of vision? • Do spots move in front of your eyes? One or many? In one or both eyes?	Any patient who describes a sudden change in vision is experiencing an acute ocular emergency, and should receive immediate ophthalmic evaluation. Floaters are common with myopia or after middle age as a result of condensed vitreous fibres. They are usually not significant, but acute onset of floaters ("shade" or "cobwebs") may occur with retinal detachment.
• Any halos/rainbows around objects? Or rings around lights?	Halos around lights occur with acute narrow-angle glaucoma.
• Any blind spot? Does it move as you shift your gaze? Any loss of peripheral vision?	**Scotoma**, a blind spot in the visual field surrounded by an area of normal or decreased vision, occurs with glaucoma and with disorders of the optic nerve and visual pathway.
• Any night blindness?	Night blindness occurs with optic atrophy, glaucoma, or vitamin A deficiency.
2. **Pain**. Any **eye pain**? Please describe. • Does it come on suddenly?	*Sudden onset* of eye symptoms (pain, floaters, blind spot, loss of peripheral vision) may represent an emergency. Refer the patient immediately to the emergency department or an on-call ophthalmologist. See also the Critical Findings box (p. 332).
• Quality: Is pain burning or itching? • Is it sharp, stabbing pain or pain with bright light? • Is it a foreign body sensation? Or deep aching? Or headache in brow area?	Quality is a valuable diagnostic indicator. **Photophobia** is the inability to tolerate light.

Examiner Asks	Rationale

Note: Some common eye diseases cause no pain (e.g., refractive errors, cataract, glaucoma).

3. **Strabismus, diplopia**. Any history of **crossed eyes**? Now or in the past? Does this occur with eye fatigue?
   - Ever see double? Is this constant, or does it come and go? In one eye or both?

Strabismus is a deviation in the antero-posterior axis of the eye.
Diplopia is the perception of two images of a single object.

4. **Redness, swelling**. Any **redness** or **swelling** in the eyes? In one eye or both? Gradual or sudden onset?
   - Any infections? Now or in the past? When do these symptoms occur? In a particular time of year? Are they seasonal?

5. **Watering, discharge**. Any **watering** or excessive tearing?

   - Any **discharge**? Any matter in the eyes? Is it hard to open your eyes in the morning? What colour is the discharge?
   - How do you remove matter from eyes?

Lacrimation (tearing) and epiphora (excessive tearing) are caused by irritants or obstruction in drainage of tears.
Purulent discharge is thick and yellow. Crusts form at night. Assess the patient's hygiene practices and knowledge of cross-contamination.

6. **History of ocular problems**. Any **history** of injury or surgery to eyes?
   - Any history of allergies?

Allergens (e.g., makeup, contact lens solution) may cause irritation of the conjunctiva or cornea.
Research indicates that the incidence of eye injuries in Canada is extremely high, and they occur at the same rates at home and at work. Encourage the use of eye protection, both at home and at work.[19]

7. **Glaucoma**. Have you ever been tested for **glaucoma**? What were the results?
   - Any family history of glaucoma?

Glaucoma is characterized by increased intraocular pressure.

8. **Use of glasses or contact lenses**. Do you wear **glasses or contact lenses**? How do they work for you?
   - When was your prescription last checked? Was it changed?
   - If you wear contact lenses, are there any problems such as pain, photophobia, watering, or swelling?
   - How do you care for contact lenses? How long do you wear them? How do you clean them? Do you remove them for certain activities?

Assess self-care behaviours for contact lenses.

9. **Self-care behaviours**. When was your **vision last tested**? Who tested it?
   - Has your colour vision ever been tested?
   - Any **environmental conditions** at home or at work that may affect your eyes? For example, flying sparks, metal bits, smoke, dust, chemical fumes? If so, do you wear goggles to protect your eyes?

Assess self-care behaviours for eyes and vision.
Eye disease can be work-related (e.g., by a foreign body from metal working or by radiation damage from welding).

10. **Medications**. What **medications** are you taking? Are they systemic or topical?
    - Do you take any medication specifically for the eyes?

Some medications have ocular adverse effects; for example, prednisone may cause cataracts or increased intraocular pressure.

11. **Coping with vision changes or loss**. If you have experienced a **vision loss**, how do you cope? Do you have books with large print, audiobooks, books printed in Braille?

Examiner Asks	Rationale

- Do you maintain your living environment the same?
- Do you sometimes fear complete loss of vision?

A constant spatial layout eases navigation through the home.

Additional History for Infants and Children

1. Delivery. Any vaginal infections in the mother at time of delivery?

Genital herpes and gonorrheal vaginitis have ocular sequelae for the newborn.

2. Development. Considering the age of the child, which developmental milestones of vision have you (parent) noted?

The parent is most often the one to detect vision problems.

3. Vision testing. Does the child have routine vision testing at school?

4. Safety. Are you (parent) aware of safety measures to protect the child's eyes from trauma? Do you inspect toys?
- Have you taught the child safe care of sharp objects and how to carry and use them?

Additional History for Older Adults

1. Movement. Have you noticed any visual difficulty with climbing stairs or driving? Any problem with night vision?

Assess for any loss of depth perception or central vision.

2. Glaucoma testing. When was the last time you were tested for glaucoma?
- Any aching pain around eyes? Any loss of peripheral vision?
- If you have glaucoma, how do you manage your eyedrops?

Adherence may be a problem if symptoms are absent. Assess the patient's ability to administer eyedrops.

3. Cataracts. Do you have a history of cataracts? Any loss or progressive blurring of vision?

4. Dryness. Do your eyes ever feel dry? Do they burn? What do you do for this?

Tear production may be decreased with aging.

5. Activities. Any decrease in usual activities, such as reading or sewing?

Macular degeneration causes a loss in central vision acuity.

OBJECTIVE DATA

PREPARATION
Position the patient first standing for vision screening and then sitting up with the head at your eye level.

EQUIPMENT NEEDED
Snellen eye chart
Handheld visual screener
Opaque card or occluder
Penlight (some come with a pupil gauge to measure pupil size)
Applicator stick
Ophthalmoscope

Normal Range of Findings	Abnormal Findings

Test Central Visual Acuity

Snellen Eye Chart
The Snellen eye chart is the most commonly used and accurate measure of visual acuity. It has lines of letters arranged in decreasing size.

Normal Range of Findings	Abnormal Findings

Place the Snellen eye chart in a well-lit spot at eye level. Position the patient on a mark exactly 20 ft (6.1 m) from the chart. Hand the patient an opaque card with which to shield one eye at a time during the test; inadvertent peeking may occur if the patient shields the eye with the fingers (Fig. 15.9). If the patient wears glasses or contact lenses, leave them on. Remove only reading glasses because they blur distance vision. Ask the patient to read through the chart to the smallest line of letters possible. Encourage the patient to try the next smallest line in addition. (Note: Use a Snellen picture chart for people who cannot read letters. See pp. 324–325.)

> Note hesitancy, squinting, leaning forward, and misreading letters.

15.9

Record the result by using the numerical fraction at the end of the last line successfully read. Indicate whether the patient missed any letters by noting "minus 1, or minus 2." (Even when patients miss one or two letters on the smallest line they can read, they are still considered to have vision equal to that line.[20]) Also indicate whether corrective lenses were worn: for example, "O.D.* 20/30-1, with glasses."

Normal visual acuity is 20/20. Contrary to some people's impression, the numerical fraction is *not* a percentage of normal vision. Instead, the top number (numerator) indicates the distance the patient is standing from the chart, and the denominator is the distance at which a normal eye could have read that particular line. Thus "20/20" means "You can read at 20 ft [6.1 m] what the normal eye could have read at 20 ft."

If the patient is unable to see even the largest letters, shorten the distance to the chart until the patient can see it, and record that distance (e.g., "10/200"). If visual acuity is even lower, assess whether the patient can count your fingers when they are spread in front of the eyes or distinguish light perception from your penlight.

> The larger the denominator, the poorer the vision. If vision is poorer than 20/30, refer the patient to an ophthalmologist or optometrist. Vision may be impaired as a result of refractive error, opacity in the media (cornea, lens, vitreous), or disorder in the retina or optic pathway.

Near Vision

For patients older than 40 years or for those who report increasing difficulty reading, test near vision with a handheld vision screener with various sizes of print (e.g., a Jaeger card; Fig. 15.10). Instruct the patient to hold the card in good light about 14 in (35 cm) from the eye; at this distance, the print size equals that on the chart used at 20 ft (6.1 m). Test each eye separately, with glasses on. A normal result is "14/14" in each eye, reading without hesitancy and without moving the card closer or farther away. When no vision screening card is available, ask the patient to read from a magazine or newspaper.

> If the patient moves the card farther away, this is a possible sign of presbyopia, the decrease in power of accommodation with aging.

*O.D., *oculus dexter,* or right eye.

Normal Range of Findings	Abnormal Findings

15.10

Test Visual Fields

Confrontation Test

This is a gross measure of peripheral vision. The patient's peripheral vision is compared with your own, if yours is normal. Position yourself at eye level with the patient, about 60 cm away. Direct the patient to cover one eye with an opaque card and to look straight at you with the other eye. Cover your own eye opposite to the patient's covered one (Fig. 15.11, *A*). You are testing the uncovered eye. Hold a pencil or your flicking finger as a target midline between you and the patient, at the periphery of vision, and slowly advance it inward from the periphery in several directions (Fig. 15.11, *B*).

15.11

Normal Range of Findings	Abnormal Findings

Normal Range of Findings

Ask the patient to say "Now" when the patient first sees the target; this location should be the same as when you also see the object. (This works with all but the temporal visual field, with which you would need a 2-m arm to avoid being seen initially! With the temporal direction, start the object somewhat behind the patient.) Estimate the angle between the anteroposterior axis of the eye and the peripheral axis where the object is first seen. Normal results are about 50 degrees upward, 90 degrees temporal, 70 degrees downward, and 60 degrees nasal (Fig. 15.12).

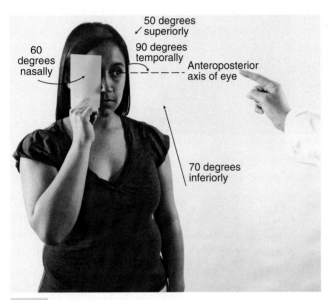

60 degrees nasally

50 degrees superiorly

90 degrees temporally

Anteroposterior axis of eye

70 degrees inferiorly

15.12   Testing range of peripheral vision.

Inspect Extraocular Muscle Function

Corneal Light Reflex (Hirschberg's Test)

Assess the parallel alignment of the eye axes by shining a light toward the patient's eyes. Direct the patient to stare straight ahead as you hold the light about 30 cm away. Note the reflection of the light on the corneas; it should be in exactly the same spot on each eye. See the bright white dots in Fig. 15.30 (p. 329) for symmetry of the corneal light reflex.

Cover-Uncover Test

The **cover-uncover test** detects small degrees of deviated alignment by interrupting the fusion reflex that normally keeps the two eyes parallel. Ask the patient to stare straight ahead at your nose even though the gaze may be interrupted. With an opaque card, cover one eye. As it is covered, note the uncovered eye. A normal response is a steady fixed gaze (Fig. 15.13, *A*).

Meanwhile, the macular image has been suppressed on the covered eye. If muscle weakness exists, the covered eye will drift into a relaxed position.

Now uncover the eye and observe it for movement. It should stare straight ahead (Fig. 15.13, *B*). If it jumps to re-establish fixation, eye muscle weakness exists. Repeat the test by covering the other eye.

Abnormal Findings

If the patient is unable to see the object as you do, the test result suggests peripheral field loss. Refer the patient to an optometrist or ophthalmologist for more precise testing with a tangent screen (see Table 15.5, p. 342).

Asymmetry of the light reflex indicates deviation in alignment as a result of eye muscle weakness or paralysis. If you see this, perform the cover-uncover test.

If the eye jumps to fixate on the designated point, it was out of alignment before.

A **phoria** is a mild weakness noted only when fusion is blocked. **Tropia** is more severe: a constant misalignment of the eyes (see Table 15.1, p. 335).

Normal Range of Findings

Abnormal Findings

 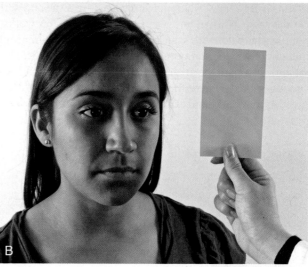

15.13

Diagnostic Positions Test

Leading the eyes through the six cardinal positions of gaze reveals any muscle weakness during movement (Fig. 15.14). Ask the patient to hold the head steady and to follow the movement of your finger, pen, or penlight only with the eyes. Hold the target back about 30 cm so that the patient can focus on it comfortably, and move it to each of the six positions, hold it momentarily, then back to centre. Progress clockwise. A normal response is parallel tracking of the object with both eyes.

Eye movement that is not parallel is abnormal. Failure to follow in a certain direction indicates weakness of an extraocular muscle (EOM) or dysfunction of cranial nerve innervating it.

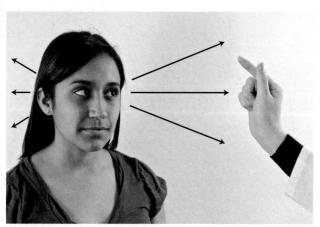

15.14   Diagnostic positions test.

In addition to parallel movement, note any **nystagmus**, a fine oscillating movement best seen around the iris. Mild nystagmus at extreme lateral gaze is normal; nystagmus at any other position is not.

Finally, note that the upper eyelid continues to overlap the superior part of the iris, even during downward movement. You should not see a white rim of sclera between the eyelid and the iris. Such an appearance is termed "*lid lag*."

Nystagmus occurs with disease of the semicircular canals in the ears, a paretic eye muscle, multiple sclerosis, or brain lesions.

Lid lag occurs with hyperthyroidism.

Objective Data

Normal Range of Findings	Abnormal Findings

Inspect External Ocular Structures

Begin with the most external points, and logically work your way inward.

General

Already you will have noted the patient's ability to move around the room, with vision functioning well enough to avoid obstacles and to respond to your directions. Also note the facial expression; a relaxed expression accompanies adequate vision.

Groping with hands.
Squinting or craning forward.

Eyebrows

Normally the eyebrows are present bilaterally, move symmetrically as the facial expression changes, and have no scaling or lesions.

Absence of lateral third of brow occurs with hypothyroidism.
Unequal or absent movement occurs with nerve damage.
Scaling occurs with seborrhea.

Eyelids and Lashes

The upper eyelids normally overlap the superior part of the iris and approximate completely with the lower eyelids when closed. The skin is intact, without redness, swelling, discharge, or lesions.

The palpebral fissures are horizontal or slightly upward in some people of East Asian descent.

Note that the eyelashes are evenly distributed along the eyelid margins and curve outward.

Lid lag occurs with hyperthyroidism.
Incomplete closure creates risk for corneal damage.
Ptosis, drooping of upper eyelid.
Periorbital edema, lesions (see Tables 15.2 and 15.3, pp. 337–338).
Ectropion and entropion (see Table 15.2, p. 338).

Eyeballs

The eyeballs are aligned normally in their sockets with no protrusion or sunken appearance. Some people of African descent normally may have a slight protrusion of the eyeball beyond the supraorbital ridge.

Exophthalmos (protruding eyes) and enophthalmos (sunken eyes) (see Table 15.2, p. 337).

Conjunctiva and Sclera

Ask the patient to look up. Using your thumbs, slide the patient's lower eyelids down along the bony orbital rim. Take care not to push against the eyeball. Inspect the exposed area (Fig. 15.15). The eyeball looks moist and glossy. Numerous small blood vessels normally show through the transparent conjunctiva. Otherwise, the conjunctivae are clear and show the normal colour of the structure below: pink over the lower eyelids and white over the sclera. Note any colour change, swelling, or lesions.

The sclera is china white, although in people with dark skin, it is occasionally grey-blue or "muddy." Also in dark-skinned people, you normally may see small brown macules (like freckles) on the sclera, which should not be confused with foreign bodies or petechiae. Last, some people with dark skin may have yellowish fatty deposits beneath the eyelids away from the cornea. Do not confuse these yellow spots with the overall scleral yellowing that accompanies jaundice.

General reddening (see Table 15.6, p. 343).
Cyanosis of the lower eyelids.
Pallor near the outer canthus of the lower eyelid (may indicate anemia; the inner canthus normally contains less pigmentation).
Scleral icterus (an even yellowing of the sclera extending up to the cornea), indicative of jaundice.
Tenderness, foreign body, discharge, or lesions.

Objective Data

Normal Range of Findings	Abnormal Findings

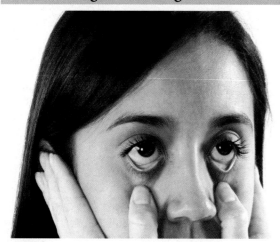

15.15

Eversion of the Upper Eyelid

This manoeuvre is not part of the normal examination, but it is useful when you must inspect the conjunctiva of the upper eyelid, as in cases of eye pain or suspicion of a foreign body. Most patients are apprehensive of any eye manipulation. Enhance their cooperation by using a calm and gentle, yet deliberate, approach.

1. Ask the patient to keep both eyes open and look down. This relaxes the eyelid, whereas closing it would tense the orbicularis muscle.
2. Slide the upper eyelid up along the bony orbit to lift up the eyelashes.
3. Grasp the lashes between your thumb and forefinger and gently pull down and outward.
4. With your other hand, place the tip of an applicator stick on the upper eyelid above the level of the internal tarsal plates (Fig. 15.16, *A*).
5. Gently push down with the stick as you lift the lashes up. This uses the edge of the tarsal plate as a fulcrum and flips the eyelid inside out. Take special care not to push in on the eyeball.
6. Secure the everted position by holding the lashes against the bony orbital rim (see Fig. 15.16, *B*).
7. Inspect for any colour change, swelling, lesion, or foreign body.
8. To return to normal position, gently pull the lashes outward as the patient looks up.

A   B

15.16

Objective Data (side tab)

Normal Range of Findings	**Abnormal Findings**

Lacrimal Apparatus

Ask the patient to look down. With your thumbs, slide the outer part of the upper eyelid up along the bony orbit to expose under the eyelid. Inspect for any redness or swelling.

Normally, the puncta drain the tears into the lacrimal sac. Excessive tearing may indicate blockage of the nasolacrimal duct. Check this by pressing your index finger against the sac, just inside the lower orbital rim, not against the side of the nose (Fig. 15.17). Pressure causes the lower eyelid to evert slightly, but no other response to pressure should occur.

Swelling of the lacrimal gland may manifest as a visible bulge in the outer part of the upper eyelid.

Puncta is red, swollen, and tender to pressure. Watch for any regurgitation of fluid out of the puncta, which confirms duct blockage.

15.17

Inspect Anterior Eyeball Structures

Cornea and Lens

Shine a light from the side across the patient's cornea, and check for smoothness and clarity. This oblique view highlights any abnormal irregularities in the corneal surface. No opacities (cloudiness) should appear in the cornea, the anterior chamber, or the lens behind the pupil. Do not confuse an arcus senilis with an opacity. The arcus senilis is a normal finding in older adults and is illustrated on p. 331.

A corneal abrasion causes irregular ridges in reflected light, producing a shattered appearance with light rays (see Table 15.7, p. 344).

Iris and Pupil

The iris normally appears flat, with a round regular shape and even coloration. Note the size, shape, and equality of the pupils. Normally the pupils appear round, regular, and of equal size in both eyes. In the adult, resting size is from 3 to 5 mm. A small number of people (5%) normally have pupils of two different sizes, which is termed **anisocoria**.

To test the **pupillary light reflex**, darken the room and ask the patient to gaze into the distance. (This dilates the pupils.) Advance a light in from the side* and note the response. Normally you will see (a) constriction of the same-sided pupil (a *direct light reflex*), and (b) simultaneous constriction of the other pupil (a *consensual light reflex*).

Irregular shape.
Although they may be normal, unequal-sized pupils necessitate investigation for central nervous system injury.

Dilated pupils.
Dilated and fixed pupils.
Constricted pupils.
Sluggish pupils.
Unequal or no response to light (see Table 15.4, p. 340).

*Always advance the light in from the *side* to test the light reflex. If you advance from the front, the pupils constrict to accommodate for near vision; thus, you do not know what the pure response to the light would have been.

Normal Range of Findings

In the acute care setting, gauge the pupil size in millimetres, both before and after the light reflex. Recording the pupil size in millimetres is more accurate when many nurses and physicians care for the same patient or when small changes may be significant signs of increasing intracranial pressure. Normally, the resting size is 3, 4, or 5 mm and decreases equally in response to light. An example of a normal response is designated by the following equation:

$$R \frac{3}{1} = \frac{3}{1} L$$

This indicates that both pupils measure 3 mm in the resting state and that both constrict to 1 mm in response to light. A graduated scale printed on a handheld vision screener or taped onto a tongue blade facilitates your measurement (see Fig. 25.59 in Chapter 25).

To test for accommodation, ask the patient to focus on a distant object (Fig. 15.18). This process dilates the pupils. Then have the patient shift the gaze to a near object, such as your finger held about 7 to 8 cm from the nose. A normal response includes (a) pupillary constriction and (b) convergence of the axes of the eyes.

Record the normal response to all these manoeuvres as PERRLA (**p**upils **e**qual, **r**ound, **r**eact to **l**ight, and **a**ccommodation).

Abnormal Findings

Absence of constriction or convergence. Asymmetrical response.

Far vision - pupils dilate

Near vision - pupils constrict

15.18 Testing accommodation. (© Pat Thomas, 2006.)

Inspect the Ocular Fundus

The ophthalmoscope enlarges your view of the eye so that you can inspect the **media** (anterior chamber, lens, vitreous) and the **ocular fundus** (the internal surface of the retina). It accomplishes this by directing a beam of light through the pupil to illuminate the inner structures. Using the ophthalmoscope is thus like peering through a keyhole (the pupil) into an interesting room beyond.

The ophthalmoscope should function as an appendage of your own eye. Using it takes some practice. Practise holding the instrument and focusing at objects around the room before you use it with a real person. Hold the ophthalmoscope right up to your eye, braced firmly against the cheek and brow. Extend your index finger onto the lens selector dial so that you can refocus as necessary during the procedure without taking your head away from the ophthalmoscope to look. Now look about the room, moving your head and the instrument together as one unit. Keep both your eyes open; just view the field through the ophthalmoscope.

Normal Range of Findings

Recall that the ophthalmoscope contains a set of lenses that control the focus (Fig. 15.19). The unit of strength of each lens is the *dioptre*. The black numbers represent positive dioptres; they focus on objects nearer in space to the ophthalmoscope. The red numbers represent negative dioptres and focus on objects farther away.

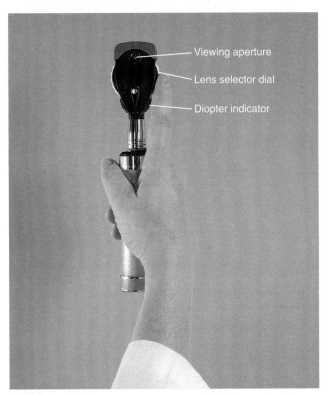

Viewing aperture
Lens selector dial
Diopter indicator

15.19

To examine a patient, darken the room to help dilate the pupils. (Dilating eye drops are not needed during a screening examination. They are used to dilate the pupils for a wider look at the fundus background and macular area. However, eye drops are used only when glaucoma can be completely ruled out because dilating the pupils in the presence of glaucoma can precipitate an acute episode.) Remove your own eyeglasses and the other patient's because they obstruct close movement; you can compensate for their correction by using the dioptre setting. Contact lenses may be left in; they pose no problem as long as they are clean.

Select the large round aperture with the white light for the routine examination. If the pupils are small, use the smaller white light. (Although the instrument has other shape and coloured apertures, as shown in Fig. 15.20, these are rarely used in a screening examination.) The light must have maximum brightness; replace old or dim batteries.

Instruct the patient to keep looking at a light switch (or mark) on the wall across the room, even though your head will get in the way. Staring at a distant fixed object helps dilate the pupils and hold the retinal structures still.

Match sides with the patient; that is, hold the ophthalmoscope in your *right* hand up to your *right* eye to view the patient's *right* eye. You must do this to avoid bumping noses during the procedure. Place your free hand on the patient's shoulder or forehead (Fig. 15.21, *A*). This helps orient you in space, because once you have the ophthalmoscope in position, you have only a very narrow range of vision. Also, your thumb can anchor the patient's upper eyelid and help prevent blinking.

Objective Data

Normal Range of Findings

◯	Large (full spot) for dilated pupils
◯	Small for undilated pupils
◯	Red-free filter — a green beam, used to examine the optic disc for hemorrhage (which looks black) and melanin deposits (which look grey)
⊞	Grid — to determine fixation pattern and to assess size and location of lesions on the fundus
▯	Slit — to examine the anterior portion of the eye and to assess elevation or depression of lesions on the fundus

15.20

15.21

Begin about 25 cm away from the patient at an angle about 15 degrees lateral to the patient's line of vision. Note the red glow filling the patient's pupil. This is the **red reflex**, caused by the reflection of your ophthalmoscope light off the inner retina. Keep sight of the red reflex, and steadily move closer to the eye. If you lose the red reflex, the light has wandered off the pupil and onto the iris or sclera. Adjust your angle to find it again.

Abnormal Findings

Normal Range of Findings

As you advance, adjust the lens to +6 dioptres, and note any opacities in the media. These appear as dark shadows or black dots that interrupt the red reflex. Normally, none are present.

Progress toward the patient until your foreheads almost touch (Fig. 15.21, *B*). Adjust the dioptre setting to bring the ocular fundus into sharp focus. If you and the patient have normal vision, this setting should be at 0. Moving the dioptres compensates for nearsightedness or farsightedness. Use the red lenses for nearsighted eyes and the black for farsighted eyes (Fig. 15.22).

Abnormal Findings

Cataracts appear as opaque black areas against the red reflex (see Table 15.8, p. 345).

NORMAL EYE

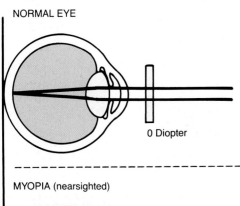

The person's eye and your eye are normal. The 0 diopter (clear glass) will focus sharply on the retina.

0 Diopter

MYOPIA (nearsighted)

In myopia, the globe is longer than normal and light rays focus in *front* of the retina.

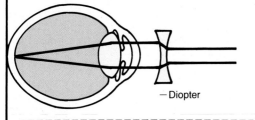

Compensate for myopia in yourself or the other person by using a negative diopter (red number or concave lens). This corrects the focal point onto the retina.

− Diopter

HYPEROPIA (farsighted)

In hyperopia, the globe is shorter than normal. Light rays would focus behind the retina (if they could pass through).

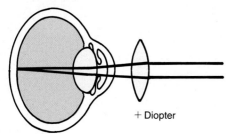

Compensate for hyperopia by using a positive diopter (black number or convex lens). This bends the light rays so the focal point is on the retina.

+ Diopter

15.22

Normal Range of Findings	Abnormal Findings

Normal Range of Findings

By moving in on the 15-degree lateral line, you should bring your view to only the optic disc. If the disc is not in sight, track a blood vessel as it grows larger, and it will lead you to the disc. Systematically inspect the structures in the ocular fundus: (a) optic disc, (b) retinal vessels, (c) general background, and (d) macula. (Fig. 15.23 shows a large area of the fundus. Your actual view through the ophthalmoscope is much smaller: slightly larger than one disc diameter.)

15.23   Normal ocular fundus.

Optic Disc

The most prominent landmark is the optic disc, located on the nasal side of the retina. Explore these characteristics:

1. **Colour**   Creamy yellow-orange to pink
2. **Shape**   Round or oval
3. **Margins**   Distinct and sharply demarcated, although the nasal edge may be slightly fuzzy
4. **Cup–disc ratio** Variable distinctness varies
                       When visible, the physiological cup is a brighter yellow-white than the rest of the disc. Its width is not more than half the disc diameter (Fig. 15.24).

15.24   Normal optic disc.

Abnormal Findings

Pallor, hyperemia.
Irregularity.
Blurred margins.

Cup extending to the disc border (see Table 15.9, p. 346).

Normal Range of Findings

Two normal variations may occur around the disc margins. A **scleral crescent** is a grey-white new moon shape. It is present when pigmentation is absent in the choroid layer, and you can see it by looking directly at the sclera. A **pigment crescent** is black; it is caused by accumulation of pigment in the choroid.

The diameter of the disc (DD) is a standard of measure for other fundus structures (Fig. 15.25). To describe a finding, note its clock-face position, as well as its relationship to the disc in size and distance (e.g., "at 5:00 position, 3 DD from the disc").

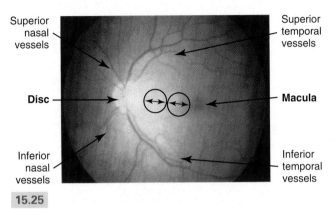

Superior nasal vessels / Superior temporal vessels / Disc / Macula / Inferior nasal vessels / Inferior temporal vessels

15.25

Retinal Vessels

This is the only place in the body where you can view blood vessels directly. Many systemic diseases that affect the vascular system produce signs in the retinal vessels. Follow a paired artery and vein out to the periphery in the four quadrants (see Fig. 15.23), noting these points:

1. **Number** — A paired artery and vein pass through each quadrant. Vessels look straighter at the nasal side.
2. **Colour** — Arteries are brighter red than are veins. Also, they have the arterial light reflex, with a thin stripe of light down the middle.
3. **Artery–vein ratio** — The ratio of the artery width to the vein width is 2:3 or 4:5.
4. **Calibre** — Arteries and veins show a regular decrease in calibre as they extend to periphery.
5. **Arteriovenous crossing** — An artery and vein may cross paths. This is not significant if within 2 DD of disc and if no sign of interruption in blood flow is seen. There should be no indenting or displacing of vessel.
6. **Tortuosity** — Mild vessel twisting when present in both eyes is usually congenital and not significant.
7. **Pulsations** — Pulsations are visible in veins near the disc as their drainage meets the intermittent pressure of arterial systole (often hard to see).

General Background of the Fundus

The colour normally varies from light red to dark brown-red, generally corresponding to the patient's skin colour. Your view of the fundus should be clear; no lesions should obstruct the retinal structures.

Abnormal Findings

Absence of major vessels.

Arteries too constricted.
Veins dilated.
Focal constriction.
Neovascularization.
Crossings more than 2 DD away from disc.
Nicking or pinching of underlying vessel.
Vessel engorged peripheral to crossing (see Table 15.10, p. 347).
Extreme tortuosity or marked asymmetry in two eyes.
Absence of pulsations.

Abnormal lesions: hemorrhages, exudates, microaneurysms.

Normal Range of Findings

Macula

The macula is 1 DD in size and located 2 DD temporal to the disc. Inspect this area last in the funduscopic examination. A bright light on this area of central vision causes some watering and discomfort and pupillary constriction. Note that the normal colour of the area is somewhat darker than the rest of the fundus but is even and homogeneous. Clumping of pigment may occur with aging.

Within the macula, you may note the foveal light reflex. This is a tiny white glistening dot that represents a reflection of your ophthalmoscope's light.

❖ DEVELOPMENTAL CONSIDERATIONS

Infants and Children

The eye examination is often deferred at birth because of transient edema of the eyelids from birth trauma or from the instillation of silver nitrate at birth. The eyes should be examined within a few days and at every well-child visit thereafter.

Visual Acuity

Which screening measures to use depend on the child's age. With a newborn, test visual reflexes and attending behaviours. Test **light perception** by using the blink reflex; the neonate blinks in response to bright light (Fig. 15.26). Also test for the pupillary light reflex, in which the pupils constrict in response to light. These reflexes indicate that the lower portion of the visual apparatus is intact. However, you cannot infer that the infant can *see*; that requires later observation to show that the brain has received images and can interpret them.

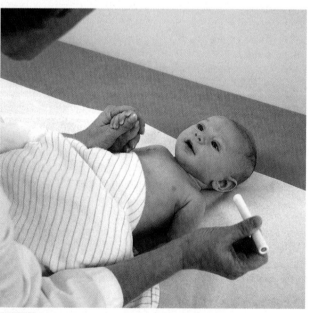

15.26

As you introduce an object to the infant's line of vision, note these normal attending behaviours:

Birth to 2 weeks: Refusal to reopen eyes after exposure to bright light; increasing alertness to object; possible fixation on an object

By 2 to 4 weeks: Fixating on an object

Abnormal Findings

Clumping of pigment occurs with trauma or retinal detachment.

Hemorrhage or exudate in the macula occurs with AMD.

Absence of blinking.

Absence of pupillary light reflex, especially after 3 weeks, which indicates blindness.

Normal Range of Findings

By 1 month: Fixating on and following a light or bright toy
By 3 to 4 months: Fixating on, following, and reaching for the toy
By 6 to 10 months: Fixating and following the toy in all directions

The Canadian Paediatric Society identified the following **clinically useful normal visual development landmarks:**

- Face follow: Birth to 4 weeks of age
- Visual following: Three months of age
- Visual acuity measurable with appropriate chart: 42 months of age[21]

The Allen chart (picture cards) was previously widely used to screen children from 30 to 35 months of age (although it is now thought to be too culturally specific[21]). In some cases, it may be reliable with cooperative toddlers as young as 2 years of age. The test involves seven cards depicting objects that are assumed to be familiar in most (though not all) cases (birthday cake, teddy bear, tree, house, car, telephone, and horse and rider). First, show the pictures up close to the child to make sure that the child can identify them. Then present each picture at a distance of 4.5 m. Results are normal if the child can name three of seven cards within three to five trials.

Use age-appropriate instruments, recognizing that recommendations depend on cognitive ability.[21] The highest level of the chart recognizable by the child should be used. (Many 4-year-olds can recognize Snellen letters and numbers). A Snellen E chart is often used for children between 3 to 6 years. The Snellen E chart shows the capital letter *E* in varying sizes pointing in different directions. The child points the fingers in the direction the "table legs" are pointing. By 6 years of age, when the child is familiar with reading letters, begin to use the standard alphabetical Snellen eye chart. Normally, children achieve 20/20 acuity by 6 to 7 years of age (Fig. 15.27).

The Canadian Paediatric Society recommends periodic screening for infants, children, and youth, outlined as follows:[21]

Newborn to Age 3 Months

- A complete examination of the skin and external eye structures, as well as the conjunctiva, cornea, iris, and pupils, is an integral part of the physical examination of all newborns, infants, and children.
- The **red reflex** should be inspected for lenticular opacities (cataracts) and signs of posterior eye disease (retinoblastoma).
- The red reflex should be equal in brightness and colour, and should fill the pupil completely.
- Corneal light reflex should be tested to detect ocular misalignment.

Ages 6 to 12 Months

- Conduct examination as for newborns.
- Ocular alignment should again be observed to detect strabismus. The corneal light reflex should be central, and the result of the cover-uncover test normal.
- Fixation and following are observed.

Ages 3 to 5 Years

- Conduct examination as for newborns.
- Visual acuity testing with an optotype test (e.g., Snellen E acuity card or Allen chart) should be completed.
- A child with visual acuity of less than 20/30 should be referred to an ophthalmologist.

Ages 6 to 18 Years

- Visual acuity should be assessed every 2 years until age 10 years and then every 3 years thereafter (e.g., with the Snellen eye chart).

Abnormal Findings

Failure of visualization or abnormalities of the red reflex are indications for immediate referral to an ophthalmologist.

The Canadian Paediatric Society recommends:

"School-aged children who pass visual examinations and screenings but have reading difficulties should be referred to a reading specialist educator for further assessment. Any infant or child with abnormalities on examination, or who does not pass visual screening, should be referred for further assessment. Infants and children with risk factors, such as developmental delay, should also be fully examined by a well-trained eye care professional. It is imperative that access to appropriate professional ophthalmological expertise is readily available and provided by the public health care system of Canada."[21]

Objective Data

Normal Range of Findings

Abnormal Findings

15.27

Visual Fields

Assess peripheral vision with the confrontation test in children older than 3 years, when they are able to stay in position. Like adults, children should see the moving target at the same time your normal eyes do. Often a young child forgets to say "now" or "stop" as the moving object is seen. Rather, note the instant the child's eyes deviate or head shifts position to gaze at the moving object. Match this nearly automatic response with your own sighting.

Colour Vision

Colour blindness is an inherited recessive X-linked trait affecting about 8% of male Canadians of European descent. It is less common in male Canadians of African or First Nations descent, and it is rare in female Canadians. "Colour deficient" is a more accurate term because the condition is relative and not disabling. Often, it is just a social inconvenience, although it may affect the patient's ability to discern traffic lights, or it may affect school performance in which colour is a learning tool. Test only boys for colour vision, once between the ages of 4 and 8 years. Use Ishihara's test (a series of polychromatic cards). Each card has a pattern of dots of a specific colour printed against a background of dots of many other colours. Ask the child to identify each pattern. A patient with normal colour vision can see each pattern. A colour blind patient cannot see the letter against the field colour.

Normal Range of Findings	Abnormal Findings

Extraocular Muscle Function

Testing for **strabismus** (squint, crossed eye) is an important screening measure during early childhood. Strabismus causes disconjugate vision because one eye deviates off the fixation point. To avoid diplopia or unclear images, the brain begins to suppress data from the weak eye (a suppression scotoma). Visual acuity in this otherwise normal eye then begins to deteriorate from disuse. Early recognition and treatment are essential for restoring binocular vision. When diagnosed after 6 years of age, strabismus has a poor prognosis. Test misalignment with the corneal light reflex and the cover-uncover test.

Untreated strabismus can lead to permanent visual damage. The resulting loss of vision from disuse is amblyopia ex anopsia.

When performing the cover-uncover test, the uncovered eye should not move. The covered eye should also not reposition when exposed. If any such movement occurs during this test, providing vision is good (fixation is well maintained), the child should be referred immediately for further assessment.[21]

Check the **corneal light reflex** by shining a light toward the child's eyes. The reflection of light should be at exactly the same spot in the two corneas (Fig. 15.28). Some asymmetry (where one light falls off centre) in infants younger than 6 months is normal.

Asymmetry in the corneal light reflex after 6 months of age is abnormal and must be investigated.

15.28

Perform the cover-uncover test on all children as described on p. 313. Some examiners omit the opaque card and place a hand on the child's head. The examiner's thumb extends down and blocks vision over the eye without actually touching the eye. You can use a familiar character puppet to attract the child's attention. The normal results are the same as those listed for adults.

You can assess function of the extraocular muscles during movement in the early weeks of a child's life by watching the child's gaze following a brightly coloured toy as a target. An older infant can sit on the parent's lap as you move the toy in all directions. After the child is 2 years of age, direct the child's gaze through the six cardinal positions of gaze. You may stabilize the child's chin with your hand to prevent the child from moving the entire head.

Normal Range of Findings	Abnormal Findings

External Eye Structures

Inspect the ocular structures as described in the earlier section. A neonate usually holds the eyes tightly shut in response to a bright light. Do not attempt to pry them open; that just increases contraction of the orbicularis oculi muscle. Hold the newborn supine and gently lower the head; the eyes will open. Also, the eyes will open when you hold the infant at arm's length and slowly turn the infant in one direction (Fig. 15.29). In addition to inspecting the ocular structures, this is also a test of the vestibular function reflex: The baby's eyes will look in the direction the body is being turned. When the turning stops, the eyes will shift to the opposite direction after a few quick beats of nystagmus. This reflex, also termed the *doll's-eyes reflex*, disappears by 2 months of age.

15.29

Eyelids and Lashes

Normally the upper eyelids overlie the superior part of the iris. In newborns, the *setting-sun sign* is common. The eyes appear to deviate down, and you see a white rim of sclera over the iris. It may show as you rapidly change the neonate from a sitting to a supine position.

Many infants have an *epicanthal fold,* an excess skinfold extending over the inner corner of the eye, partly or totally overlapping the inner canthus. It is present in many children of East Asian descent and in some children of European descent. In some children, the epicanthal folds disappear as they grow, usually by 10 years of age. While they are present, epicanthal folds give a false appearance of misalignment, termed **pseudostrabismus** (Fig. 15.30). Pseudostrabismus occurs most often when a broad nasal bridge covers the nasal sclera unequally. This can be determined and distinguished from strabismus by the presence of a symmetrical corneal light reflex.[21]

Infants of East Asian descent normally have an upward slant of the palpebral fissures. *Entropion,* a turning inward of the eyelid, is found normally in some children of East Asian descent. If the lashes do not abrade the corneas, it is not significant.

The setting-sun sign also occurs with hydrocephalus as the globes protrude.

Eyes appear blank and sunken with malnutrition, dehydration, and severe illness.

An upward lateral slope, together with epicanthal folds and hypertelorism (abnormally wide spacing between eyes), occurs with Down syndrome.

Normal Range of Findings	Abnormal Findings

15.30   Pseudostrabismus.

Conjunctiva and Sclera

A newborn may have a transient chemical conjunctivitis from the instillation of silver nitrate. This appears within 1 hour and lasts not more than 24 hours after birth. The sclera should be white and clear, although it may have a blue tint as a result of thinness at birth. The lacrimal glands are not functional at birth.

Ophthalmia neonatorum (conjunctivitis of the newborn) is a purulent discharge caused by a chemical irritant or a bacterial or viral agent from the birth canal.

Iris and Pupils

The iris normally is blue or slate grey in light-skinned newborns and brown in dark-skinned newborns. By ages 6 to 9 months, the permanent colour is established. Brushfield's spots, or white specks around the edge of the iris, are occasionally normal.

A searching nystagmus is common just after birth. The pupils are small but constrict to light.

Absence of iris colour occurs with albinism.

Brushfield's spots are usually suggestive of Down syndrome.

Constant nystagmus, prolonged setting-sun sign, marked strabismus, and slow lateral movements are suggestive of vision loss.

The Ocular Fundus

The amount of data gathered during the funduscopic examination depends on the infant's ability to hold the eyes still and on your ability to glean as much data as possible in a brief time.

A complete funduscopic examination is difficult to perform on an infant, but at least check the red reflex when the infant fixates on the bright light for a few seconds. Note any interruption.

Perform a funduscopic examination on an infant between 2 and 6 months of age. Position the infant supine on the table. The fundus appears pale, and the vessels are not fully developed. The foveal light reflection is not present because the macula area is not mature until 1 year of age.

Inspect the fundus of young children and school-age children as described for adults. Allow a child to handle the equipment. Explain why you are darkening the room and that you will leave a small light on. Assure the child that the procedure will not hurt. Direct the young child to look at an appealing picture, or perhaps at a toy or an animal, during the examination.

An interruption in the red reflex indicates an opacity in the cornea or lens. The red reflex is absent in patients with congenital cataracts or retinal disorders.

Papilledema is rare in infants because the fontanelles and open sutures absorb any increased intracranial pressure if it occurs.

Older Adults
Visual Acuity

Perform the same examination as described for adults. Central acuity may be decreased, particularly after 70 years of age. Peripheral vision may be diminished.

Objective Data

Normal Range of Findings

Ocular Structures

The eyebrows may show a loss of the outer one-third to one-half of hair because of a decrease in hair follicles. The remaining brow hair is coarse. As a result of atrophy of elastic tissues, the skin around the eyes may show wrinkles or crow's feet. The upper eyelid may be so elongated as to rest on the lashes, a condition called *pseudoptosis* (Fig. 15.31).

15.31 Pseudoptosis.

The eyes may appear sunken from atrophy of the orbital fat. Also, the orbital fat may herniate, causing bulging at the lower eyelids and inner third of the upper eyelids.

The lacrimal apparatus may decrease tear production, causing the eyes to look dry and lustreless and the patient to feel a burning sensation. **Pingueculae**, which commonly appear on the sclera (Fig. 15.32), are yellowish elevated nodules caused by a thickening of the bulbar conjunctiva as a result of prolonged exposure to sun, wind, and dust. Pingueculae appear at the 3:00 and 9:00 positions: first on the nasal side, then on the temporal side.

15.32 Pinguecula.

Abnormal Findings

Ectropion (lower eyelid dropping away) and entropion (lower eyelid turning in; see Table 15.2, p. 338).

Distinguish pinguecula from the abnormal **pterygium**, which is also an opacity on the bulbar conjunctiva but grows over the cornea (see Table 15.7, p. 344).

Objective Data

Normal Range of Findings	Abnormal Findings

The cornea may look cloudy with age. **Arcus senilis**, commonly seen around the cornea (Fig. 15.33), is a grey-white arc or circle around the limbus; it is caused by deposition of lipid material. As more lipid accumulates, the cornea may look thickened and raised, but the arcus has no effect on vision.

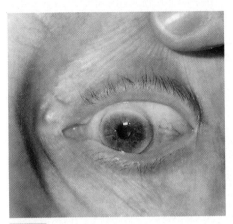

15.33   Arcus senilis.

Xanthelasma are soft, raised yellow plaques on the eyelids at the inner canthus (Fig. 15.34). They commonly occur during the fifth decade of life and more frequently in women. They occur with both high and normal blood levels of cholesterol and have no pathological significance.

15.34   Xanthelasma.

Pupils are small in old age, and the pupillary light reflex may be slowed. The lens loses transparency and looks opaque.

The Ocular Fundus

With age, retinal structures generally have less shine. The blood vessels look paler, narrower, and attenuated. Arterioles appear paler and straighter, with a narrower light reflex. More arteriovenous crossing defects occur.

Normal Range of Findings

A normal development on the retinal surface is **drusen**, or benign degenerative hyaline deposits (Fig. 15.35). They are small, round, yellow dots that are scattered haphazardly on the retina. Although they do not occur in a pattern, they are usually symmetrically placed in the two eyes. They have no effect on vision.

15.35 Drusen.

Abnormal Findings

Drusen are easily confused with *hard exudates*, an abnormal finding that occurs with a more circular or linear pattern (see Table 15.10, p. 348). Also, drusen in the macular area occur with AMD.

SPECIAL CONSIDERATIONS FOR ADVANCED PRACTICE

Assessing for AMD and other common causes of visual impairment in the adult population, including older adults, is an important aspect of advanced practice nursing. Regular examinations are important for determining whether patients may benefit from certain interventions. For example, in relation to AMD, it is recommended that patients older than 55 years with no risk factors receive a comprehensive eye examination every 1 to 2 years.[22] Patients with early-stage disease or a family history of the condition need more frequent follow-up.

Advanced practice nurses frequently encounter patients with a red eye. Most patients with red eye have a benign or self-limited conditions resulting from conjunctivitis (usually viral), blepharitis, small corneal abrasions, dry eye, and subconjunctival hemorrhage.[23] Ominous symptoms or signs that indicate urgent referral to an ophthalmologist are listed in the following Critical Findings box.

CRITICAL FINDINGS

Anyone who reports a sudden change in vision should be referred for urgent, immediate ophthalmic evaluation.[24] Ensure that such a patient is taken to the nearest emergency department; if in hospital, call for an immediate ophthalmology consultation.

For patients with red eye (see examples in Table 15.6, p. 343), immediate, urgent referral to an emergency department or an on-call ophthalmologist is necessary for "a history of severe pain, visual loss, marked pain or decreased vision with the use of contact lenses, trauma, chemical injury and recent eye surgery."[23] On examination, signs necessitating immediate, urgent referral include "decreased visual acuity, pupil irregularity, sluggish pupillary reaction to light, corneal opacification, hyphema … or hypopyon … and elevated intraocular pressure."[23] Patients wearing contact lenses should be told to stop wearing the lenses immediately. Be especially alert when a patient has only one red eye.

DOCUMENTATION AND CRITICAL THINKING

Sample Charting

SUBJECTIVE

Good vision reported with no recent change. No eye pain, no inflammation, no discharge, no lesions. Wears no corrective lenses, vision last tested 1 year PTA [prior to arrival], test result for glaucoma at that time was normal.

OBJECTIVE

Snellen eye chart: O.D. 20/20, O.S. [left eye] 20/20 −1. Fields normal by confrontation. Corneal light reflex symmetrical bilaterally. Diagnostic positions test shows EOMs intact. Brows and lashes present. No ptosis. Conjunctiva clear. Sclera white. No lesions. PERRLA.

Fundi: Red reflex present bilaterally. Discs flat with sharp margins. Vessels present in all quadrants without crossing defects. Retinal background has even colour with no hemorrhages or exudates. Macula has even colour.

ASSESSMENT

Healthy vision function
Healthy eye structures

Focused Assessment: Clinical Case Study 1

Emma Khalin (E.K.) is a 34-year-old woman brought to the emergency department by police after a reported domestic quarrel.

SUBJECTIVE

E.K. states that partner punched her in the face and eyes about 1 hour PTA. "I am having trouble at home. I can't do anything right." Pain in left cheek and both eyes felt immediately and continues. Alarmed at "bright red blood on eyeball." No bleeding from eye area or cheek. Vision intact just after trauma. Now reports difficulty opening eyelids.

OBJECTIVE

Sitting quietly and hunched over, hands over eyes. Voice tired and flat. L [left] cheek swollen and discoloured, no laceration. Lids edematous and discoloured both eyes. No skin laceration. L lid swollen almost shut. L eye—round 1-mm bright red patch over lateral aspect of globe at 3:00 position. No active bleeding out of eye, iris intact, anterior chamber clear. R [right] eye—conjunctiva clear, sclera white, cornea and iris intact, anterior chamber clear. PERRLA. Pupils R 4/1 = 4/1 L. Vision 14/14 both eyes by Jaeger card.

ASSESSMENT

Ecchymoses L cheek and both eyes
Subconjunctival hemorrhage L eye
Pain R/T [related to] inflammation
Chronic low self-esteem R/T effects of domestic violence

Focused Assessment: Clinical Case Study 2

Sam Thibeau (S.T.) is a 63-year-old man admitted to the medical centre for surgery for suspected brain tumour. After postanaesthesia recovery, S.T. is admitted to the neurology critical care unit, awake, lethargic with slowed but correct verbal responses, oriented × 3, moving all four extremities, vital signs stable. Pupils R 4/2 = 4/2 L with sluggish response. Assessments are made q15 min.

Documentation and Critical Thinking

SUBJECTIVE

No response now to verbal stimuli.

OBJECTIVE

Semicomatose: No response to verbal stimuli, does withdraw R arm and leg purposefully to painful stimuli. No movement L arm or leg. Pupils R 5/5 ≠ 4/2 L. Vitals remain stable as noted on graphic sheet.

ASSESSMENT

Unilateral dilated and fixed R pupil
Clouding of consciousness
Focal motor deficit: no movement L side
Ineffective tissue perfusion R/T interruption of cerebral flow

Focused Assessment: Clinical Case Study 3

Trung Quan (T.Q.) is a 4-year-old from Southeast Asia who arrived in Canada 1 month PTA. Lives with parents, two siblings. Speaks only native language; here with mother and uncle, who acts as interpreter.

SUBJECTIVE

Mother seeks care because RN in church sponsoring family noted T.Q. has "crossed eyes." Uncle states vision seemed normal to parents. Plays with toys and manipulates small objects without difficulty. Identifies objects in picture books; does not read.

OBJECTIVE

With uncle interpreting directions for test to T.Q., vision by Snellen E chart: O.D. 20/30, O.S. 20/50 −1. Fields seem intact by confrontation: jerks head to gaze at object entering field.
EOMs: Asymmetrical corneal light reflex with outward deviation L eye. Cover-uncover test: as R eye covered, L eye jerks to fixate, R eye steady when uncovered. As L eye covered, R eye holds steady gaze, L eye jerks to fixate as uncovered. Diagnostic positions: able to gaze in six positions, although L eye obviously misaligned at extreme medial gaze.
Eye structures: Brows and lashes present and normal bilaterally. Upward palpebral slant, epicanthal folds bilaterally: consistent with shape of eyes. Conjunctiva clear, sclera white, iris intact, PERRLA.
Fundi: Discs flat with sharp margins. Observed vessels normal. Unable to see in all four quadrants or to see macular area.

ASSESSMENT

L exotropia
Abnormal vision in L eye
Disturbed visual sensory perception R/T effects of neurological impairment

Focused Assessment: Clinical Case Study 4

Vera Kalu (V.K.) is an 87-year-old woman of African descent who is a widow and homemaker living independently. She is admitted to hospital for observation and adjustment of digitalis medication. Cardiac status has been stable during hospital stay.

SUBJECTIVE

Reports desire to monitor own medication at home but fears problems because of blurred vision. V.K. first noted distant vision blurred 5 years ago but near vision seemed to improve at that time: "I started to read better without my glasses!" Since then, blurring of distant vision has increased, near vision now blurred also.
Able to navigate home environment without difficulty. Fixes simple meals with cold foods. Receives hot meal from Meals On Wheels at lunch. Enjoys TV, although it looks somewhat blurred. Unable to write letters, sew, or read paper, which she regrets.

OBJECTIVE

Vision by Jaeger card: O.D. 20/200, O.S. 20/400 −1, with glasses on. Fields intact by confrontation. EOMs intact. Brow hair: absent lateral third. Upper lids have folds of redundant skin but lids do not droop. Lower lids and lashes intact. Xanthelasma present both inner canthi. Conjunctiva clear, sclera white, iris intact, L pupil looks cloudy, PERRLA, pupils R 3/2 = 3/2 L.

Fundi: Red reflex has central dark spot, both eyes. Discs flat, with sharp margins. Observed vessels normal. Unable to see in all four quadrants or macular area because of small pupils.

ASSESSMENT

Central opacity, both eyes
Central visual acuity deficit, both eyes
Deficient diversional activity R/T poor vision

ABNORMAL FINDINGS

TABLE 15.1	Extraocular Muscle Dysfunction

Symmetrical Corneal Light Reflex

A. *Pseudostrabismus* has the appearance of strabismus because of epicanthic fold but is normal for a young child.

A, Pseudostrabismus.

Asymmetrical Corneal Light Reflex

Strabismus is true disparity of the eye axes. This constant misalignment is also termed *tropia* and is likely to cause amblyopia.
B. Esotropia: inward turn of the eye. C. Exotropia: outward turning of the eyes.

B, Left esotropia.

C, Exotropia.

Continued

TABLE 15.1   Extraocular Muscle Dysfunction—cont'd

Cover-Uncover Test

D. Uncovered eye: If it jumps to fixate on designated point, it was out of alignment before (i.e., when you cover the stronger eye [top], the weaker eye now tries to fixate [bottom]).

Phoria: mild weakness, apparent only with the cover test and less likely to cause amblyopia than a tropia but still possible.

D, Right (uncovered) eye is weaker.

E. Covered eye: If this is the weaker eye, once macular image is suppressed, the eye drifts to relaxed position (top).

As eye is uncovered: If it jumps to re-establish fixation (bottom), weakness exists.

Esophoria: nasal (inward) drift.
Exophoria: temporal (outward) drift.

E, Left (uncovered) eye is weaker.

Diagnostic Positions Test

Paralysis is apparent during movement through six cardinal positions of gaze. This is a test of the ocular muscles: inferior oblique (IO), inferior rectus (IR), lateral rectus (LR), medial rectus (MR), superior oblique (SO), and superior rectus (SR).

Direction That Eye Does Not Turn	Site of Paralysis	Cranial Nerve
Straight nasal	Medial rectus	III
Up and nasal	Inferior oblique	III
Up and temporal	Superior rectus	III
Straight temporal	Lateral rectus	VI
Down and temporal	Inferior rectus	III
Down and nasal	Superior oblique	IV

See Illustration Credits for source information.

TABLE 15.2   Abnormalities in the Eyelids

Periorbital Edema

Eyelids are swollen and puffy. Eyelid tissues are loosely connected, and so excess fluid is easily apparent. This occurs with local infections; with crying; and with systemic conditions such as heart failure, renal failure, allergy, and hypothyroidism (myxedema).

Exophthalmos (Protruding Eyes)

Eyeballs are displaced forward, and palpebral fissures are widened. Note "lid lag"; the upper eyelid rests well above the limbus, and white sclera is visible. Acquired bilateral exophthalmos is associated with thyrotoxicosis.

Enophthalmos (Sunken Eyes; Not Illustrated)

This appearance is of narrowed palpebral fissures, in which the eyeballs are recessed. Bilateral enophthalmos is caused by loss of fat in the orbits and occurs with dehydration and chronic wasting illnesses. For illustration, see Cachectic Appearance in Table 14.4, p. 298.

Ptosis (Drooping Upper Eyelid)

This is a positional defect that gives the patient a sleepy appearance and impairs vision. It is caused by neuromuscular weakness (e.g., myasthenia gravis with bilateral fatigue as the day progresses), oculomotor cranial nerve III damage, or sympathetic nerve damage (e.g., Horner's syndrome).

Upward Palpebral Slant

Although normal in many children, these slants—when combined with epicanthal folds, hypertelorism (wide spacing between the eyes), and Brushfield's spots (light-coloured areas in outer iris)—indicate Down syndrome.

Continued

Abnormal Findings

TABLE 15.2 Abnormalities in the Eyelids—cont'd

Ectropion

The lower eyelid is loose, rolls outward, and does not approximate to eyeball. Puncta cannot siphon tears effectively, and so excess tearing results. The eyes feel dry and itchy because the tears do not drain correctly over the corner and toward the medial canthus. Exposure of palpebral conjunctiva increases risk for inflammation. This occurs with aging as a result of atrophy of elastic and fibrous tissues, but it may result from trauma.

Entropion

The lower eyelid rolls inward because of spasm of eyelids or scar tissue contracting. Constant rubbing of lashes may irritate cornea. The patient feels a "foreign body" sensation.

See Illustration Credits for source information.

TABLE 15.3 Lesions on the Eyelids

Blepharitis (Inflammation of the Eyelids)

Red, scaly, greasy flakes and thickened, crusted eyelid margins occur with staphylococcal infection or seborrheic dermatitis of the eyelid edge. Symptoms include burning sensation, itching, tearing, foreign body sensation, and some pain.

Chalazion

A beady nodule protruding on the eyelid, chalazion is an infection or retention cyst of a meibomian gland. It is a nontender, firm, discrete swelling with freely movable skin overlying the nodule. If it becomes inflamed, it points inside and not on eyelid margin (in contrast to stye).

TABLE 15.3 **Lesions on the Eyelids—cont'd**

Hordeolum (Stye)

Hordeolum is a localized staphylococcal infection of the hair follicles at the eyelid margin. It is painful, red, and swollen: a pustule at the eyelid margin. Rubbing the eyes can cause cross-contamination and development of another stye.

Basal Cell Carcinoma

Carcinoma is rare, but it occurs most often on the lower eyelid and medial canthus. It looks like a papule with an ulcerated centre. Note the rolled-out pearly edges. It should be referred for removal, although metastasis is rare.

Dacryocystitis (Inflammation of the Lacrimal Sac)

Dacryocystitis is infection and blockage of sac and duct. Pain, warmth, redness, and swelling occur below the inner canthus toward the nose. Tearing is present. Pressure on sac yields purulent discharge from puncta.

Dacryoadenitis (Inflammation of the Lacrimal Gland; Not Illustrated)

Dacryoadenitis is an infection of the lacrimal gland. Pain, swelling, and redness occur in the outer third of upper eyelid. It occurs with mumps, measles, and infectious mononucleosis or results from trauma.

See Illustration Credits for source information.

TABLE 15.4 Abnormalities in the Pupil

Location of lesions:

A. Unequal Pupil Size: Anisocoria

Although this exists normally in 5% of the population, consider central nervous system disease.

B. Monocular Blindness

When light is directed to the blind eye (in this illustration, the right eye), no response occurs in either eye. When light is directed to normal (left) eye, both pupils constrict (direct and consensual response to light) as long as the oculomotor nerve is intact.

C. Constricted and Fixed Pupils: Miosis

Miosis occurs with the use of pilocarpine drops for glaucoma treatment, the use of narcotics, with iritis, and with damage of the pons in the brain.

D. Dilated and Fixed Pupils: Mydriasis

Pupils become enlarged with stimulation of the sympathetic nervous system, as a reaction to sympathomimetic medications, with use of dilating drops, and as a result of acute glaucoma and past or recent trauma. Enlarged pupils also herald central nervous system injury, circulatory arrest, or deep anaesthesia.

TABLE 15.4 **Abnormalities in the Pupil—cont'd**

E. Argyll Robertson Pupil

Such pupils have no reaction to light but do constrict with accommodation. They are small and irregular bilaterally. Argyll Robertson pupil occurs with central nervous system syphilis, brain tumour, meningitis, and chronic alcoholism.

F. Tonic Pupil (Adie's Pupil)

This kind of pupil has a sluggish reaction to light and accommodation. It is usually unilateral, a large regular pupil that does react but sluggishly, after a long latent time. It has no pathological significance.

G. Cranial Nerve III Damage

Oculomotor nerve damage causes unilateral pupil dilation with no reaction to light or accommodation. Ptosis may also be present, with eye deviating downward and laterally.

H. Horner's Syndrome

Horner's syndrome, a lesion of the sympathetic nerve, causes unilateral, small, regular pupil that does react to light and accommodation. Ptosis and absence of sweat (anhidrosis) on the same side of the face are also present.

See Illustration Credits for source information.

TABLE 15.5   Visual Field Loss

Location of lesions:

1. Retinal damage
   • Macula: central blind area (e.g., in diabetes)

   • Localized damage: blind spot (scotoma) corresponding to particular area

   • Increasing intraocular pressure: decrease in peripheral vision (e.g., glaucoma); starts with paracentral scotoma

   • Retinal detachment: patient has shadow or diminished vision in one quadrant or one-half of visual field

2. Lesion in globe or optic nerve; injury causes blindness in one eye, or unilateral blindness

3. Lesion at optic chiasm (e.g., pituitary tumour); injury to crossing fibres produces only a loss of nasal part of each retina and a loss of both temporal visual fields; bitemporal (heteronymous) hemianopsia

4. Lesion of outer uncrossed fibres at optic chiasm (e.g., aneurysm of left internal carotid artery exerts pressure on uncrossed fibres); injury produces left nasal hemianopsia

5. Lesion in right optic tract or right optic radiation; visual field loss in right nasal and left temporal fields; loss of same half visual field in both eyes is homonymous hemianopsia

TABLE 15.6 Vascular Disorders of the External Eye

Conjunctivitis

Infection of the conjunctiva ("pink eye") causes vessels at periphery to appear red and beefy, but usually the area around the iris is clearer (although in this illustration it is severe). This is a common symptom of bacterial or viral infection, allergy, or chemical irritation. Purulent discharge accompanies bacterial infection. Preauricular lymph node is often swollen and painful, and patients have a history of upper respiratory infection. Symptoms include itching, burning sensation, foreign body sensation, and eyelids stuck together on awakening.

Subconjunctival Hemorrhage

A red patch on the sclera, subconjunctival hemorrhage looks alarming but is usually not serious. The red patch has clear edges, although in this illustration it is extensive. It is caused by increased intraocular pressure from coughing, sneezing, weight lifting, labour during childbirth, straining at stool, or trauma.

Iritis (Circumcorneal Redness)

Deep, dull red halo around the iris and cornea. Redness is around iris, in contrast to conjunctivitis, in which the redness is more prominent at the periphery. Pupil shape may be irregular from swelling of iris. Patient also has marked photophobia, constricted pupil, blurred vision, and throbbing pain. This condition warrants immediate referral.

Acute Glaucoma

Acute, narrow-angle glaucoma produces a circumcorneal redness around the iris, with dilation of the pupil. Pupil is oval, dilated; cornea looks "steamy"; and anterior chamber is shallow. Acute glaucoma occurs with sudden increase in intraocular pressure caused by blockage of outflow from anterior chamber. The patient experiences a sudden clouding of vision and sudden eye pain and sees halos around lights. This necessitates emergency treatment to prevent permanent vision loss.

TABLE 15.7　Abnormalities on the Cornea and Iris

Pterygium

A triangular opaque wing of bulbar conjunctiva overgrows toward the centre of the cornea. It looks membranous, translucent, and yellow to white; usually invades from nasal side; and may obstruct vision as it covers pupil. It usually results from chronic exposure to hot, dry, sandy climate, which stimulates the growth of a pinguecula (p. 330) and development into a pterygium.

Corneal Abrasion

This is the most common result of a blunt eye injury, but irregular ridges are usually visible only when fluorescein stain reveals yellow-green branching. Top layer of corneal epithelium is removed, from scratches or poorly fitting or overworn contact lenses. Because the area is rich in nerve endings, the patient feels intense pain and a foreign body sensation and exhibits lacrimation, redness, and photophobia.

Normal Anterior Chamber (for Contrast)

A light directed across the eye from the temporal side illuminates the entire iris evenly because the normal iris is flat and creates no shadow.

Shallow Anterior Chamber

The iris is pushed anteriorly because of increased intraocular pressure. Because direct light is received from the temporal side, only the temporal part of iris is illuminated; the nasal side is shadowed (the "shadow sign"). This may be a sign of acute angle-closure glaucoma; the iris looks bulging because aqueous humor cannot circulate.

TABLE 15.7   Abnormalities on the Cornea and Iris—cont'd

Hyphema

Blood in anterior chamber is a serious result of blunt trauma (a fist or a baseball) or spontaneous hemorrhage. Suspect scleral rupture or major intraocular trauma. Note that gravity causes blood to settle.

Hypopyon

Purulent matter in anterior chamber occurs with iritis and with inflammation in the anterior chamber.

See Illustration Credits for source information.

TABLE 15.8   Opacities in the Lens

Senile Cataracts

Central Grey Opacity: Nuclear Cataract

Nuclear cataract shows as an opaque grey surrounded by black background as it forms in the centre of lens nucleus. Through the ophthalmoscope, it looks like a black centre against the red reflex. It begins after age 40 years and develops slowly, gradually obstructing vision.

Star-Shaped Opacity: Cortical Cataract

Cortical cataract appears as asymmetrical, radial, white spokes with black centre. Through ophthalmoscope, black spokes are evident against the red reflex. This forms in outer cortex of lens, progressing faster than nuclear cataract.

See Illustration Credits for source information.

TABLE 15.9 Abnormalities in the Optic Disc

Papilledema   Retinal hemorrhages

Optic Atrophy (Disc Pallor)

Optic atrophy is a white or grey colour of the disc as a
  result of partial or complete death of the optic nerve. This
  results in decreased visual acuity, decreased colour vision,
  and decreased contrast sensitivity.

Papilledema (Choked Disc)

Increased intracranial pressure causes venous stasis in the
  globe, producing redness, congestion, and elevation of
  the disc; blurred margins; hemorrhages; and absence of
  venous pulsations. This is a serious sign of intracranial
  pressure, usually caused by a space-occupying mass (e.g., a
  brain tumour or hematoma). Visual acuity is not affected.

◄ Excessive Cup–Disc Ratio

With primary open-angle glaucoma, the increased intraocular pressure
  decreases blood supply to retinal structures. The physiological cup enlarges
  to more than half of the disc diameter, vessels appear to plunge over edge of
  cup, and the vessels are displaced nasally. This is asymptomatic, although the
  patient may have decreased vision or visual field defects in the late stages of
  glaucoma.

See Illustration Credits for source information.

TABLE 15.10	Abnormalities in Retinal Vessels and Background

Macular star   Retinal folds   Disc edema

Arteriovenous Crossing (Nicking)

Arteriovenous crossing with interruption of blood flow. When vein is occluded, it dilates distal to crossing. The patient whose fundus is pictured here also has disc edema and hard exudates in a macular star pattern that occur with acutely elevated (malignant) hypertension. With hypertension, the arteriole wall thickens and becomes opaque so that no blood is seen inside it (silver wire arteries).

Age: 14 Yrs   Age: 61 Yrs

Narrowed (Attenuated) Arteries

This is a generalized decrease in diameter. The light reflex also narrows. It occurs with severe hypertension (right), with occlusion of the central retinal artery, and with retinitis pigmentosa.

Diabetic Retinopathy

Intraretinal Hemorrhages

Dot-shaped hemorrhages are deep intraretinal hemorrhages that look like splattering on the fundus. They may be distinguished from microaneurysms by the blurred irregular edges. Flame-shaped hemorrhages are superficial retinal hemorrhages that look linear and spindle shaped. They occur with hypertension.

Microaneurysms

Microaneurysms are round, punctate red dots that are localized dilatations of a small vessel. Their edges are smooth and discrete. The vessel itself is too small to view with the ophthalmoscope; only the isolated red dots are seen. This occurs with diabetes.

Continued

TABLE 15.10	Abnormalities in Retinal Vessels and Background—cont'd

◀ **Exudates**

Soft exudates, or cotton wool spots, look like fluffy grey-white cumulus clouds. They are arteriolar microinfarctions that envelop and obscure the vessels. They occur with diabetes, hypertension, subacute bacterial endocarditis, lupus, and papilledema of any cause. Hard exudates are numerous small yellow-white spots that have distinct edges and a smooth, solid-looking surface. They often form a circular pattern, clustered around a venous microinfarction. They also may form a linear or star pattern. (This is in contrast with drusen, which have a scattered haphazard location [see Fig. 15.35, p. 332]).

See Illustration Credits for source information.

Summary Checklist: Eye Examination

1. **Test visual acuity:**
   Snellen eye chart
   Near vision (in patients older than 40 years of age or those having difficulty reading)
2. **Test visual fields: confrontation test**
3. **Inspect extraocular muscle function:**
   Corneal light reflex (Hirschberg's test)
   Cover-uncover test
   Diagnostic positions test

4. **Inspect external eye structures:**
   General
   Eyebrows
   Eyelids and lashes
   Eyeball alignment
   Conjunctiva and sclera
   Lacrimal apparatus
5. **Inspect anterior eyeball structures:**
   Cornea and lens
   Iris and pupil
   Size, shape, and equality
   Pupillary light reflex
   Accommodation

6. **Inspect the ocular fundus:**
   Optic disc (colour, shape, margins, cup–disc ratio)
   Retinal vessels (number, colour, artery–vein ratio, calibre, arteriovenous crossings, tortuosity, pulsations)
   General background (colour, integrity)
   Macula
7. **Engage in teaching and health promotion**

Abnormal Findings

ADDITIONAL RESOURCES

Canadian National Institute for the Blind (CNIB): http://www.cnib.ca

Canadian Ophthalmological Society—Canadian Ophthalmological Society guidelines: http://www.cos-sco.ca/clinical-practice-guidelines/

Canadian Paediatric Society—Vision Screening in Infants, Children and Youth: https://www.cps.ca/en/documents/position/children-vision-screening

REFERENCES

1. Canadian National Institute for the Blind. (2017). *Aging eyes (presbyopia)*. Retrieved from http://www.cnib.ca/en/your-eyes/eye-conditions/aging-eyes/Pages/default.aspx.

2. Canadian National Institute for the Blind. (2017). *Fast facts about vision loss*. Retrieved from http://www.cnib.ca/en/about/media/vision-loss/.

3. Pillay, J., Freeman, E., MacGregor, T., et al. (2016). *Screening for impaired visual acuity and vision-related functional limitations in adults 65 years and older in primary health care: Protocol for evidence review*. Edmonton: Evidence Review Synthesis Centre. Retrieved from http://canadiantaskforce.ca/ctfphcguidelines/overview/.

4. Canadian National Institute for the Blind (2009). *The cost of vision loss in Canada: summary report*. Toronto: Author. Retrieved from http://www.cnib.ca/eng/cnib%20document%20library/research/summaryreport_covl.pdf.

5. Canadian National Institute for the Blind. (2012). *Age-related macular degeneration (AMD)*. Retrieved from http://www.cos-sco.ca/vision-health-information/conditions-disorders-treatments/retinal-diseases/amd/.

6. Rudnicka, A. R., Zakariya, J., Wormald, R., et al. (2011). Age and gender variations in age-related macular degeneration prevalence in populations of European ancestry: A meta-analysis. *Ophthalmology, 119*(3), 571–580. doi:10.1016/j.ophtha.2011.09.027.

7. Canadian Ophthalmological Society. (2017). *Age-related macular degeneration (AMD)*. Retrieved from http://www.cos-sco.ca/vision-health-information/conditions-disorders-treatments/retinal-diseases/amd/.

8. Canadian Ophthalmological Society Clinical Practice Guideline Expert Committee. (2008). Canadian Ophthalmological Society evidence-based clinical practice guidelines for cataract surgery in the adult eye. *Canadian Journal of Ophthalmology, 43*(Suppl. 1), 1–64.

9. Canadian National Institute for the Blind. (2017). *Glaucoma*. Retrieved from http://www.cnib.ca/en/your-eyes/eye-conditions/glaucoma/Pages/default.aspx.

10. Canadian National Institute for the Blind. (2017). *About diabetic retinopathy*. Retrieved from http://www.cnib.ca/en/your-eyes/eye-conditions/eye-connect/DR/About/Pages/default.aspx.

11. Canadian Diabetes Association Clinical Practice Guidelines Expert Committee. (2013). Clinical practice guidelines for the prevention and management of diabetes in Canada: Retinopathy. *Canadian Journal of Diabetes, 37*(Suppl. 1), 137–141. doi:10.1016/j.jcjd.2013.01.038.

12. Canadian National Institute for the Blind. (2015). *How AMD affects vision*. Retrieved from http://www.cnib.ca/en/your-eyes/eye-conditions/amd/risk-factors/.

13. Canadian Ophthalmological Society Clinical Practice Guideline Expert Committee. (2007). Canadian Ophthalmological Society evidence-based clinical practice guidelines for the periodic eye examination in adults in Canada. *Canadian Journal of Ophthalmology, 42*, 39–45, pp. 40, 41, 43.

14. Jin, Y.-P., & Trope, G. E. (2011). Eye care utilization in Canada: Disparity in the publicly funded health care system. *Canadian Journal of Ophthalmology, 46*(2), 133–138. doi:10.3129/i10-120.

15. Barnes, S., Abban, V., & Weiss, A. (2015). *Low wages, no benefits: Expanding access to health benefits for low income Ontarians*. Toronto: Wellesley Institute.

16. Hong, C. J., Trope, G. E., Buys, Y. M., et al. (2014). Does government assistance improve utilization of eye care services by low-income individuals? *Canadian Journal of Ophthalmology, 49*(4), 320–325. doi:10.1016/j.jcjo.2014.03.006.

17. Zhang, X., Cotch, M. F., Ryskulova, A., et al. (2012). Vision health disparities in the United States by race/ethnicity, education, and economic status: Findings from two nationally representative surveys. *American Journal of Ophthalmology, 154*(6), S53–S62, e1. doi:10.1016/j.ajo.2011.08.045.

18. National Collaborating Centre for Aboriginal Health. (2014). *Promoting health vision for children*. Retrieved from http://www.nccah-ccnsa.ca/415/Promoting_Healthy_Vision_for_Children.nccah.

19. Gordon, K. D. (2012). The incidence of eye injuries in Canada. *Canadian Journal of Ophthalmology, 47*(4), 351–353. doi:10.1016/j.jcjo.2012.03.005.

20. U.S. National Library of Medicine. (2012). *Visual acuity test*. Retrieved from http://www.nlm.nih.gov/medlineplus/ency/article/003396.htm.

21. Canadian Paediatric Society. (2016). *Vision screening in infants, children and youth* (Position statement). Retrieved from https://www.cps.ca/en/documents/position/children-vision-screening.

22. Noble, J., & Chaudhary, V. (2010). Age-related macular degeneration. *Canadian Medical Association Journal, 182*(16), 1759. doi:10.1503/cmaj090378.

23. Noble, J., & Lloyd, J. C. (2011). The red eye. *Canadian Medical Association Journal, 183*(1), 81. doi:10.1503/cmaj.090379.

24. Noble, J., & Chaudhary, V. (2010). Age-related macular degeneration. *Canadian Medical Association Journal, 182*(16), 1759. doi:10.1503/cmaj090378.

16 | CHAPTER

Ears

Written by Carolyn Jarvis, PhD, APN, CNP
Adapted by June MacDonald-Jenkins, RN, BScN, MSc

ⓔ http://evolve.elsevier.com/Canada/Jarvis/examination/

STRUCTURE AND FUNCTION

EXTERNAL EAR

The ear is the sensory organ for hearing and maintaining equilibrium. The ear has three parts: the (a) external, (b) middle, and (c) inner ears (Fig. 16.1). The external ear is called the **auricle, or pinna,** and consists of movable cartilage and skin. The external ear has a characteristic shape and serves to funnel sound waves into its opening, the **external auditory canal**. The canal is a cul-de-sac that is 2.5 to 3 cm long in adults and terminates at the **eardrum**, or **tympanic membrane**. The canal is lined with glands that secrete cerumen, a yellow waxy material that lubricates and protects the ear. The wax forms a sticky barrier that helps keep foreign bodies from entering and reaching the sensitive eardrum. Cerumen migrates out to the meatus by the movements of chewing and talking.

The outer third of the canal is cartilage; the inner two-thirds consists of bone covered by thin sensitive skin. The canal has a slight S-shaped curve in the adult. The outer third curves up and toward the back of the head, whereas the inner two-thirds angle down and forward toward the nose.

The tympanic membrane separates the external ear and middle ear and is tilted obliquely to the ear canal, facing downward and somewhat forward. It is a translucent, pearly grey membrane in which a prominent cone of light in the anteroinferior quadrant is the reflection of the otoscope light (Fig. 16.2). The eardrum is oval and slightly concave, pulled in at its centre by one of the middle ear ossicles, the **malleus**. The parts of the malleus show through the translucent eardrum; these are the **umbo**, the **manubrium** (handle), and the **short process**. The small, slack, superior section of the tympanic membrane is called the **pars flaccida**. The remainder of the eardrum, which is thicker and more taut, is the **pars tensa**. The **annulus** is the outer fibrous rim of the drum.

Lymph fluid of the external ear drains into the parotid, mastoid, and superficial cervical nodes.

MIDDLE EAR

The middle ear is a tiny air-filled cavity inside the temporal bone (see Fig. 16.1). It contains tiny ear bones, or auditory ossicles: the **malleus, incus,** and **stapes.** The middle ear has several openings. Its opening to the outer ear is covered by the eardrum. The openings to the inner ear are the oval window at the end of the stapes and the round window. Another opening is the **eustachian tube**, which connects the middle ear with the nasopharynx and allows passage of air. The tube is normally closed, but it opens with swallowing or yawning.

The middle ear has three functions: (a) It conducts sound vibrations from the outer ear to the central hearing apparatus in the inner ear; (b) it protects the inner ear by reducing the amplitude of loud sounds; and (c) its eustachian tube allows equalization of air pressure on each side of the eardrum so that the membrane does not rupture (e.g., during altitude changes in an airplane).

INNER EAR

The inner ear is embedded in bone. It contains the **bony labyrinth**, which holds the sensory organs for equilibrium and hearing. Within the bony labyrinth, the **vestibule** and the **semicircular canals** constitute the vestibular apparatus, and the **cochlea** (Latin for "snail shell") contains the central hearing apparatus. Although the inner ear is not accessible to direct examination, its functions can be assessed.

HEARING

Note the landmarks of the auricle, and use these terms to describe your findings (Fig. 16.3). The mastoid process, the bony prominence behind the lobule, is not part of the ear but is an important landmark.

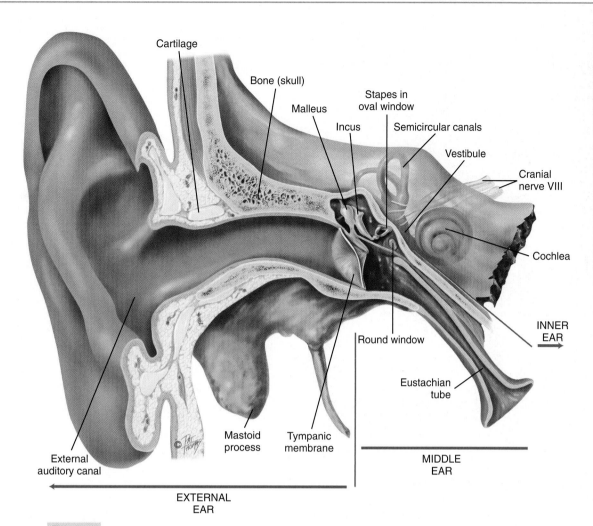

Fig. 16.1 © Pat Thomas, 2010.

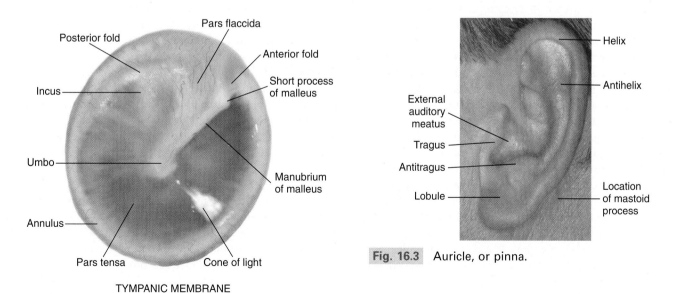

TYMPANIC MEMBRANE

Fig. 16.2 Tympanic membrane (eardrum).

Fig. 16.3 Auricle, or pinna.

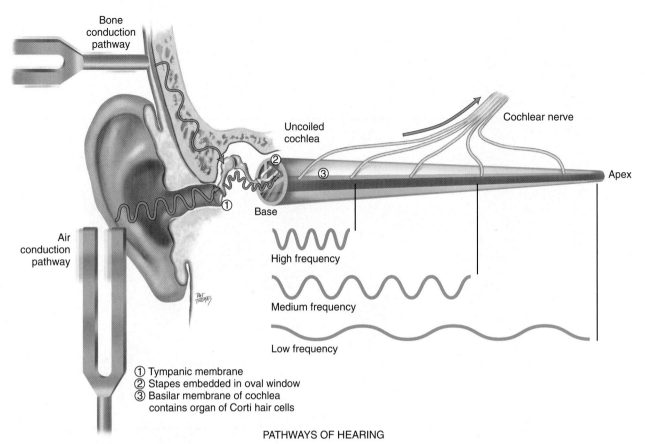

Fig. 16.4 © Pat Thomas, 2006.

The function of hearing involves the auditory system at three levels: (a) peripheral, (b) brain stem, and (c) cerebral cortex. At the peripheral level, the ear transmits sound and converts its vibrations into electrical impulses, which can be analyzed by the brain. For example, suppose you hear an alarm bell ringing. Its sound waves travel instantly to your ears. The *amplitude* is how loud the alarm is; its *frequency* is the pitch (in this case, high), or the number of cycles per second. The sound waves produce vibrations on your eardrum. These vibrations are carried by the middle ear ossicles to the oval window. Then the sound waves travel through the cochlea, which is coiled like a snail's shell, and are dissipated against the round window. Along the way, the **basilar membrane** vibrates at a point specific to the frequency of the sound. In this case, the alarm's high frequency stimulates the basilar membrane at its base near the stapes (Fig. 16.4). The numerous fibres along the basilar membrane are the receptor hair cells of the **organ of Corti**, the sensory organ of hearing. As the hair cells bend, they mediate the vibrations into electric impulses. The electrical impulses are conducted by the auditory portion of cranial nerve VIII to the brain stem.

The function at the brain stem level is *binaural interaction*, which enables a person to locate the direction of a sound in space, as well as identifying the sound. How does this work? Each ear is actually one-half of the total sensory organ. The ears are located on each side of a movable head.

The cranial nerve VIII from each ear sends signals to both sides of the brain stem. Areas in the brain stem are sensitive to differences in intensity and timing of the messages from the two ears, depending on the way the head is turned.

The function of the cortex is to interpret the meaning of the sound and begin the appropriate response. All this happens in the split second it takes you to react to the alarm.

Pathways of Hearing

The normal pathway of hearing is air conduction, described previously; it is the most efficient. An alternative route of hearing is by bone conduction, in which the bones of the skull vibrate. These vibrations are transmitted directly to the inner ear and to cranial nerve VIII.

Hearing Loss

Anything that obstructs the transmission of sound impairs hearing. A **conductive hearing loss** involves a mechanical dysfunction of the external or middle ear. It is a partial loss because the person is able to hear if the sound amplitude is increased enough to reach normal nerve elements in the inner ear. Conductive hearing loss may be caused by impacted cerumen, foreign bodies, a perforated eardrum, pus or serum in the middle ear, or otosclerosis (a decrease in mobility of the ossicles).

Sensorineural hearing loss (or *perceptive loss*) signifies pathology of the inner ear, cranial nerve VIII, or the auditory areas of the cerebral cortex. A simple increase in amplitude may not enable the person to understand words. Sensorineural hearing loss may be caused by *presbycusis*, a gradual nerve degeneration that occurs with aging, and by ototoxic medications, which affect the hair cells in the cochlea. A **mixed loss** is a combination of conductive and sensorineural types in the same ear.

Equilibrium

The three semicircular canals, or labyrinth, in the inner ear constantly feed information to the brain about the body's position in space. They work like plumb lines to determine verticality or depth. The plumb lines of the ear register the angle of your head in relation to gravity. If the labyrinth ever becomes inflamed, it feeds the wrong information to the brain, creating a staggering gait and a strong, spinning, whirling sensation called *vertigo*.

 DEVELOPMENTAL CONSIDERATIONS

Infants and Children

The inner ear starts to develop early in the fifth week of gestation. In early development, the ear is posteriorly rotated and low set; later it ascends to its normal placement around eye level. If maternal rubella infection occurs during the first trimester, it can damage the organ of Corti and impair hearing.

An infant's eustachian tube is relatively shorter and wider and its position is more horizontal than an adult's, and so it is easier for pathogens from the nasopharynx to migrate to the middle ear (Fig. 16.5). The lumen is surrounded by lymphoid tissue, which increases during childhood; thus, the lumen is easily occluded. These factors place infants at greater risk for middle ear infections than adults. The infant's and young child's inner ear canals are shorter and have a slope opposite to that of the adult's.

Adults

Otosclerosis is a common cause of conductive hearing loss in young adults between the ages of 20 and 40 years. It is a gradual hardening that causes the footplate of the stapes to become fixed in the oval window, which impedes the transmission of sound and causes progressive deafness.

Older Adults

In older adults, the cilia lining the ear canal become coarse and stiff. This may cause a decrease in hearing because it impedes sound waves travelling toward the eardrum. It also causes cerumen to accumulate and oxidize, which greatly reduces hearing. The cerumen itself is drier because of atrophy of the apocrine glands. Also, a life history of frequent ear infections may result in scarring on the drum.

Impacted cerumen is common in aging adults (up to 57%) and other at-risk groups (e.g., people with mental disabilities),[1] who may under-report the associated hearing loss. Cerumen impaction also blocks conduction in those wearing hearing aids. Cerumen should be removed when it leads to conductive hearing loss or interferes with full assessment of the ear. Ceruminolytics are wax-softening agents that expedite removal with electric or manual irrigators. After removal, over half of those with impaction passed the whispered voice test.[1] A person living in a noise-polluted area (e.g., near an airport or a busy highway) has a greater risk for hearing loss. However, **presbycusis** is a type of hearing loss that occurs with aging, even in people living in a quiet environment. It is a gradual sensorineural loss caused by nerve degeneration in the inner ear or auditory nerve. More than 50% of all Canadians older than 65 years of age have hearing loss. The person first notices a high-frequency tone loss; it is harder to hear consonants than vowels. Much speech information is lost, and words sound garbled. The ability to localize sound is also impaired. This communication dysfunction is

INFANT
Horizontal eustachian tube

ADULT
Sloped eustachian tube

Fig. 16.5

accentuated when unfavourable background noise is present (e.g., with music, with dishes clattering, or at a large, noisy party).[2]

Speech-Language and Audiology Canada recommends that hearing be tested every 3 years, starting at age 2, or earlier if language skills are not developing.[3] Individuals who listen to very loud music (see the box Promoting Health: Use of Digital Music Players), work with high levels of industrial noise, or are older than 65 years of age should see an audiologist annually. There is significant evidence that neonatal hearing screening should be implemented as routine practice; however, it currently is only in common practice in four provinces in Canada. British Columbia has the most comprehensive infant hearing screening program in the country.[3]

PROMOTING HEALTH: USE OF DIGITAL MUSIC PLAYERS

Earbuds and Hearing Loss

Today, there is growing concern about the potential for hearing loss in young people who use digital music players and earbud headphones. Unlike earphones, which are placed over the ear, earbuds are placed directly in the ear canal, which causes the sound to be placed closer to the eardrum. Furthermore, because the sound is digital, there is virtually no distortion, no matter how loud one turns up the volume. Probably of most significance is that because digital music players can hold thousands of songs and can play for hours without recharging, users tend to listen continuously for hours at a time.

Hearing loss occurs slowly and often goes unnoticed until it is quite extensive; therefore, early prevention is the key. The risk for hearing loss increases as sound is played louder and for longer durations. For this reason, current research proposes the 60–60 rule: that individuals use their digital music players and earbuds for no more than 60 minutes a day at levels below 60% of maximum volume. Many experts are suggesting that digital music players be designed to prevent the playing of music above 90 dB, or about 60% of the maximum volume (≈120 dB) of the typical digital music player today. Simply put, it means dialling down the volume to a "6" or lower and taking a break at least every hour. Other ways to avoid hearing loss include using larger headphones that rest *over* the ear opening and noise-cancelling headphones that eliminate background noise so that listeners do not have to increase the volume as high. It is often difficult to explain this to young people who abound with youthful optimism and tend not to worry about future damage. However, listening with earbuds boosts sound signals by as much as 6 to 9 dB, about the difference between the sound of a vacuum cleaner and a motorcycle.

The decibel scale is logarithmic; for example, 40 dB is 100 times as intense as 20 dB. Normal conversation takes place around 60 dB, whereas a chainsaw typically registers at 100 dB and a rock concert at 120 dB. Government minimum safety standards in Canada dictate that 85 dB for 8 hours daily is the limit for occupational exposure to noise. Adopted by several provinces across the country, these standards exist to protect workers from hearing loss in the workplace. As the decibel level increases, exposure time needs to be cut significantly.

Although people know not to look into the sun because its intense rays damage the eyes, people do not seem to realize that blasting their ears with intense sound is going to do damage, too. There is a certain irony in the appearance of young people donning sunglasses and earbuds.

References
Gilliver, M., Carter, L., Macoun, D., et al. (2012). Music to whose ears? The effect of social norms on young people's risk perceptions of hearing damage resulting from their music listening behavior. *Noise and Health, 14*(57), 47–51. doi:10.4103/1463-1741.95131.
Health Canada. (2017). *Noise induced hearing loss.* Retrieved from http://www.hc-sc.gc.ca/hl-vs/iyh-vsv/environ/hearing_loss-perte_audition-eng.php.

Additional Resources
Selvin, J. (2005, September 22). *Play it loud and you may pay for it. SF Gate.* Retrieved from https://www.sfgate.com/entertainment/article/Play-it-loud-and-you-may-pay-for-it-A-warning-2607307.php.
Statistics Canada. (2015). *Prevalence of hearing loss among Canadians aged 20 to 79: Audiometric results from the 2012/2013 Canadian Health Measures Survey.* Retrieved from http://www.statcan.gc.ca/pub/82-003-x/2015007/article/14206-eng.pdf.

Local audiologists can test hearing and may refer patients to other health care providers on the basis of their findings. Every year in Canada, over 1 000 children are born with permanent hearing loss. There is significant evidence to indicate that children who receive early diagnosis and intervention (screening by 1 month, diagnosis by 3 months and intervention by 6 months of age) have better communication, literacy, and cognitive ability than children with delayed diagnoses.[3]

SOCIAL DETERMINANTS OF HEALTH CONSIDERATIONS

Otitis media (middle ear infection) results from obstruction of the eustachian tube or of passage of nasopharyngeal secretions into the middle ear. Otitis media is one of the most common illnesses in children. Otitis media is so common in childhood that 50% of all children under the age of 2 years will have at least one episode, and 13% will experience multiple episodes.[4] In Canada, for years the incidence and severity of otitis media in Indigenous children was higher than in non-Indigenous children. It was believed that the higher incidence in Indigenous children was primarily associated with shorter and wider eustachian tubes and increased cerumen development. This belief has proven to be unsubstantiated. For example, a 2016 study of ear infections in rural school-aged children in Canada found that non-Indigenous children have a higher incidence of otitis media than their Indigenous counterparts.[5] The study results indicated that the following factors are significant determinants of otitis media: being a young age, having had tonsillitis and asthma, having a respiratory allergy, being first born, and ethnicity (being non-Indigenous or Indigenous).

Besides the anatomy of the infant eustachian tube, the following risk factors predispose children to acute otitis media: absence of breastfeeding in the first 3 months of age, exposure to **second-hand tobacco smoke**, day care attendance, male sex, pacifier use, low birth weight, low socioeconomic status, and formula feeding in the supine position. Instruct parents to not prop the bottle or let the baby take a bottle to bed. Encouraging breastfeeding helps prevent this problem.

In Canada, ambulatory visits for acute otitis media have decreased by 60% over the past 20 years.[4] This decrease is best explained by a concurrent increase in the number of smoke-free households, public awareness of the dangers of second-hand smoke, and provincial legislation banning smoking in vehicles with children.

The most important adverse effect of acute otitis media is the persistence of fluid in the middle ear after treatment. This middle ear effusion can impair hearing, increasing the child's risk for delayed cognitive development.

Cerumen is genetically determined and comes in two major types: (a) dry cerumen, which is grey, flaky, and frequently forms a thin mass in the ear canal, and (b) wet cerumen, which is honey brown to dark brown and moist. Among individuals of Asian or Indigenous descent, the frequency of dry cerumen exceeds 80%, whereas among individuals of African or Euro-Canadian descent, the frequency of wet cerumen exceeds 97%.[5] The presence and composition of cerumen are not related to poor hygiene. Take caution to avoid mistaking the flaky, dry cerumen for eczematous lesions.

Almost one in four of all adult Canadians report some level of hearing loss, although about 10% of those identify themselves as "culturally deaf," "oral deaf," "deafened," or "hard of hearing."[6] Hearing loss is the third most prevalent chronic condition in older adults. The Canadian Hearing Society has produced a series of position statements regarding the social and ethical dilemmas faced by Canadians with hearing loss (see the website for the Canadian Hearing Society in the section Additional Resources at the end of this chapter). *Audism* is a form of discrimination based on a person's ability to hear or behave in the manner of people who hear. This is one of the primary issues faced by people with a hearing impairment.

SUBJECTIVE DATA

1. Earache
2. Infections
3. Discharge
4. Hearing loss
5. Environmental noise
6. Tinnitus
7. Vertigo
8. Self-care behaviours

HEALTH HISTORY QUESTIONS

Examiner Asks	Rationale
1. Earache. Any **earache** or other pain in ears? • Location: Does it feel close to the surface or deep in the head? • Does it hurt when you push on the ear? • Character: Is it dull and aching or sharp and stabbing? Is it constant, or does it come and go? Is it affected by changing position of head? Ever had this kind of pain before? • Any accompanying cold symptoms or sore throat? Any problems with sinuses or teeth? • Ever been hit on the ear or on the side of the head, or had any sport injury? Ever had any ear trauma from a foreign body? • What have you tried to relieve pain?	**Otalgia** (ear pain) may be caused directly by ear disease or may represent referred pain from a problem in the teeth or oropharynx. A virus/bacterium that causes upper respiratory tract infection may migrate up the eustachian tube to involve the middle ear. Trauma may rupture the eardrum. Assess effect of coping strategies.

Examiner Asks	Rationale
2. Infections. Any ear **infections**? In adulthood or in childhood? • How frequent were they? How were they treated? • How effective was treatment?	A history of chronic ear problems suggests possible sequelae. Repeated infections in childhood can result in progressive loss of hearing. The insertion of "tubes" (tympanoplasty) continues to be a procedure that is recommended, despite little evidence to support its benefit over nonsurgical topical/systemic treatment approaches.[7]
3. Discharge. Any **discharge** from your ears? • Does it look like pus, or is it bloody? • Any odour to the discharge? • Any relationship between the discharge and the ear pain?	Otorrhea (discharge) suggests infection of the canal or a perforated eardrum. For example: • *External otitis:* purulent, sanguineous, or watery discharge • *Acute otitis media with perforation:* purulent discharge • *Cholesteatoma:* dirty yellow or grey discharge with foul odour With perforation: ear pain typically occurs first and stops with a popping sensation; then drainage occurs.
4. Hearing loss. Ever had any **trouble hearing**? • Onset: Did the loss come on slowly or all at once? • Do you have a family history of otosclerosis? • Character: Has all your hearing decreased, or just your hearing of certain sounds? • In what situations do you notice the loss: conversations, using the telephone, watching television, at a party? • Do people seem to shout at you? • Do ordinary sounds seem hollow, as if you are hearing in a barrel or under water? • Have you recently travelled by airplane? • Any family history of hearing loss? • Effort to treat: Have you tried any hearing aid or other device? Anything to help hearing? • Coping strategies: How does the loss affect your daily life? Any job problem? Do you feel embarrassed? Frustrated? How do your family and friends react?	The onset of presbycusis is gradual (over years), whereas hearing loss caused by trauma is often sudden. Refer any sudden loss in one or both ears that is *not* associated with upper respiratory tract infection. The onset of otosclerosis is generally during the second and third decades of life and is diagnosed on the basis of symptoms of conductive hearing loss. **Conductive hearing loss** is caused by fixation of the stapes (bone of the inner ear) and is present in approximately 10% of all cases. The amount of hearing loss is related directly to the degree of immobilization of the stapedial footplate (i.e., the more rigid the eardrum, the greater the hearing loss). The hearing loss may not be noticed in the early stages of otosclerosis. Loss is apparent when competition from background noise is present, as at a party. *Recruitment:* a condition in which loss is marked when sound is initially at low intensity but actually becomes painful when repeated loudly. Character of hearing loss is affected when cerumen expands and becomes impacted, as after swimming or showering. Hearing loss can cause social isolation and can lessen pleasure in leisure activities.

Examiner Asks	Rationale

Note to examiner: During history documentation, note these clues from normal conversation with a patient that indicate possible hearing loss:

1. Lip reading or watching your face and lips closely rather than your eyes
2. Frowning or straining forward to hear
3. Posturing of head to catch sounds with better ear
4. Misunderstanding your questions or frequently asking you to repeat what you said
5. Acting irritable or showing startle reflex when you raise your voice (recruitment)
6. Speech sounding garbled; possible distortion of vowel sounds
7. Inappropriately loud voice
8. Flat, monotonous tone of voice

5. Environmental noise. Any **loud noises** at home or on the job? For example, do you live in a noise-polluted area, near an airport, or near a busy traffic area? Now, or in the past?

- Are you near other noises, such as heavy machinery, loud persistent music, gunshots (e.g., while hunting)?
- Coping strategies: Have you taken any steps to protect your ears, such as using headphones or ear plugs?

Old trauma to hearing initially goes unnoticed but results in further decibel loss in later years.

6. Tinnitus. Ever felt **ringing**, crackling, or buzzing in your ears? When did this occur?

- Does it seem louder at night?
- Are you taking any medications?

Tinnitus originates within the person; it accompanies some hearing or ear disorders.

Tinnitus seems louder when there is no competition from environmental noise.

Many medications have ototoxic sequelae: Aspirin, aminoglycosides (streptomycin [Streptomycin SteriMax], gentamicin [Garamycin], neomycin [Neosporin]), ethacrynic acid [Edecrin], furosemide [Lasix], indomethacin [Indocin], naproxen [Apo-Naproxren], quinine [Pro-Quinine], vancomycin [pms-Vancomycin], and local anaesthetic.

7. Vertigo. Ever felt **vertigo**? That is, do you feel the room spinning around or yourself spinning? (Vertigo is a true sensation of twirling.)

A true sensation of rotational spinning occurs with dysfunction of the labyrinth. In **objective vertigo**, people feel as if the room is spinning. In **subjective vertigo**, people feel as if they are spinning.

Distinguish true vertigo from dizziness or lightheadedness.

- Ever felt dizzy, as if you are not quite steady, like falling or losing your balance? Giddy, lightheaded?

8. Self-care behaviours. How do you **clean your ears**?

Assess potential trauma from invasive instruments. Cotton-tipped applicators can cause impaction of cerumen, resulting in hearing loss.

- When was the last time you had your hearing checked?
- If a hearing loss was noted, did you obtain a hearing aid? How long have you had it? Do you wear it? How does it work? Any trouble with upkeep, cleaning, or changing batteries?

Prescribe frequency of hearing assessment according to the patient's age or risk factors.

Examiner Asks	Rationale

Additional History for Infants and Children

1. Ear Infections. At what age was the child's first episode?
- How many ear infections in the last 6 months? How many total? How were these treated? How effective was the treatment?
- Has the child had any surgery, such as insertion of ear tubes or removal of tonsils?
- How effective was the surgical intervention?

- Are the infections increasing in frequency, in severity, or staying the same?
- Does anyone in the home smoke cigarettes?
- Is there a wood-burning stove in your home?
- Is the child breast or formula fed? Does the child use a soother?
- Does your child receive child care outside your home? In a day care centre or someone else's home? How many children in the group?

A first episode that occurs in the first 3 months of life increases the risk for recurrent otitis media. Recurrent otitis media is three episodes in the past 3 months or four within the past year.[8] Children with recurrent otitis media are often prescribed low-dose long-term antibiotics for treatment, or tympanoplasty is indicated.

Removal of environmental factors is very effective in diminishing repeated infection.

The following factors are known to exacerbate infection:
- Soothers
- Formula feeding
- Wood-burning homes
- Second-hand and gestational smoke
- Being in day care
- Exposure to cold (child should wear a hat)

2. Hearing. Does the child seem to be hearing well?
- Have you noticed that the infant startles with loud noise? Did the infant start babbling at approximately 6 months of age? Does the infant talk? At what age did talking start? Was the speech intelligible?
- Ever had the child's hearing tested? If there was a hearing loss, did it follow any diseases in the child or in the mother during pregnancy?

Children at risk for hearing deficit include those exposed to maternal rubella, syphilis, cytomegalovirus, toxoplasmosis, or maternal ototoxic medications in utero; premature infants; infants of low birth weight; infants who suffered trauma or hypoxia at birth; and infants with congenital liver or kidney disease.

In children, an episode of meningitis, measles, mumps, otitis media, and any illness with persistent high fever may increase risk for hearing deficit.

On the basis of the available evidence, the Canadian Paediatric Society recommends hearing screening for all newborns.[9]

3. Injury. Does the child tend to put objects in the ears? Is the older child or adolescent active in contact sports?

These children are at increased risk for trauma.

OBJECTIVE DATA

PREPARATION

An adult should be sitting up straight with the head at your eye level. On occasion, the ear canal is partially filled with cerumen, which obstructs your view of the eardrum. If the membrane is intact and no current infection is present, a preferred method of cleaning the adult canal is to soften the cerumen with a warmed solution of mineral oil and hydrogen peroxide. Then, with a bulb syringe or a low-pulsatile dental irrigator (Waterpik), irrigate the canal with warm water (body temperature). Direct water to the posterior wall. Leave space around the irrigator tip for water to escape. Do not irrigate if the history or the examination findings suggest perforation or infection.

EQUIPMENT NEEDED

Otoscope with bright light (fresh batteries give off white—not yellow—light)

Pneumatic bulb attachment, sometimes used with infants or young children

Normal Range of Findings	Abnormal Findings

Normal Range of Findings

Inspect and Palpate the External Ear

Size and Shape

The ears are of equal size bilaterally with no swelling or thickening. Ears of unusual size and shape may be a normal familial trait with no clinical significance.

Skin Condition

The skin colour is consistent with the patient's facial skin colour. The skin is intact, with no lumps or lesions. On some people you may note **Darwin's tubercle**, a small painless nodule at the helix. This is a congenital variation and is not significant (Fig. 16.6).

— Darwin's tubercle

Fig. 16.6

Tenderness

Move the pinna and push on the tragus. They should feel firm, and movement should produce no pain. Palpating the mastoid process should also produce no pain.

The External Auditory Meatus

Note the size of the opening to direct your choice of speculum for the otoscope. No swelling, redness, or discharge should be present.

Some cerumen is usually present. The colour varies from grey-yellow to light brown and black, and the texture varies from moist and waxy to dry and desiccated. A large amount of cerumen obscures visualization of the canal and eardrum.

Abnormal Findings

Microtia: ears smaller than 4 cm vertically.

Macrotia: ears larger than 10 cm vertically.

Edema.

Reddened, excessively warm skin indicates inflammation (see Table 16.1, p. 369).

Crusts and scaling occur with otitis externa, eczema, contact dermatitis, and seborrhea.

Enlarged, tender lymph nodes in the region indicate inflammation of the pinna or mastoid process.

Red-blue discoloration indicates frostbite.

Sebaceous cyst, tophi, chondrodermatitis, keloid, and carcinoma are discussed in Table 16.2, p. 370.

Pain with movement occurs with otitis externa and furuncle.

Pain at the mastoid process may indicate mastoiditis or lymphadenitis of the posterior auricular node.

Atresia: absence or closure of the ear canal.

Sticky yellow discharge accompanies otitis externa or may indicate otitis media if the eardrum has ruptured.

Impacted cerumen is a common cause of conductive hearing loss. (See Table 16.3, p. 372.)

Objective Data

Normal Range of Findings

Inspect With the Otoscope

As you inspect the external ear, note the size of the auditory meatus. Then choose the largest speculum that will fit comfortably in the ear canal, and attach it to the otoscope. Tilt the patient's head slightly away from you toward the opposite shoulder. This method brings the obliquely sloping eardrum into better view.

Pull the pinna up and back on adults or older children; this helps straighten the S-shaped curve of the canal (Fig. 16.7). (Pull the pinna down on infants and children younger than 3 years of age [see Fig. 16.14, p. 365]). Hold the pinna gently but firmly. Do not release traction on the ear until you have finished the examination and the otoscope is removed.

Fig. 16.7

Hold the otoscope upside down along your fingers, and have the dorsa (back) of that hand along the patient's cheek braced to steady the otoscope (Fig. 16.8). This position may feel awkward to you at first. It soon will feel natural, and you will find it useful in preventing forceful insertion. Also, your stabilizing hand acts as a protecting lever if the patient suddenly moves the head.

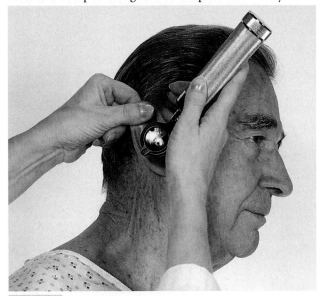

Fig. 16.8

Abnormal Findings

Use caution when introducing the otoscope into an ear. Do not push the otoscope into the canal; this causes extreme pain for the patient and may result in damage to the canal. The otoscope should just "sit" in the canal. For better visualization, adjust the pinna to straighten out the canal.

Normal Range of Findings

Insert the speculum slowly and carefully along the axis of the canal. Watch the insertion; then put your eye up to the otoscope. Avoid touching the inner (bony) section of the canal wall, which is covered by a thin epithelial layer and is sensitive to pain. Sometimes you cannot see anything but canal wall. If that is the case, try to reposition the patient's head, apply more traction on the pinna, and re-angle the otoscope to look forward toward the patient's nose.

Once it is in place, you may need to rotate the otoscope slightly to visualize all of the eardrum; do this gently. Perform the otoscopic examination before you test hearing; when ear canals have impacted cerumen, the hearing test will yield erroneous findings of pathological hearing loss.

The External Canal

Note any redness and swelling, lesions, foreign bodies, or discharge. If any discharge is present, note the colour and odour. (Also, clean any discharge from the speculum before examining the other ear, to avoid contamination with possibly infectious material.) For a patient with a hearing aid, note any irritation on the canal wall from poorly fitting ear moulds.

The Tympanic Membrane
Colour and Characteristics

Systematically explore the eardrum's landmarks (Fig. 16.9). The normal eardrum is shiny and translucent, with pearly grey coloration. The cone-shaped light reflex is prominent in the anteroinferior quadrant (at the 5:00 position in the right eardrum and at the 7:00 position in the left eardrum). This light reflex is the reflection of your otoscope light. Sections of the malleus are visible through the translucent eardrum: the umbo, manubrium, and short process. (Infrequently, you also may see the incus behind the eardrum; it shows as a whitish haze in the upper posterior area.) At the periphery, the annulus looks whiter and denser.

Fig. 16.9 Normal tympanic membrane (right ear).

Abnormal Findings

Redness and swelling occur with otitis externa; the canal may be completely closed by swelling.

Purulent otorrhea suggests otitis externa or otitis media if the eardrum has ruptured.

Frank blood or clear, watery drainage (cerebrospinal fluid) after trauma suggests basal skull fracture and warrants immediate referral. Other abnormalities include foreign body, exostosis, furuncle, and polyp (see Table 16.4, p. 373).

Yellow-amber eardrum discoloration occurs with otitis media with effusion (serous).

Redness occurs with acute otitis media.

Absent or distorted landmarks.

Air/fluid level or air bubbles behind eardrum indicate otitis media with effusion (see Tables 16.5 and 16.6, p. 375).

Normal Range of Findings	Abnormal Findings

Position

The eardrum is flat and slightly pulled in at the centre.

Integrity of Membrane

Inspect the eardrum and the entire circumference of the annulus for perforations. The normal tympanic membrane is intact. Some adults may show scarring, which is a dense white patch on the drum. This is a sequela of repeated ear infections.

Test Hearing Acuity

Your screening for a hearing deficit begins during the history: "Do you have difficulty hearing now?" If the answer is *yes*, perform audiometric testing or refer for audiometric testing. If the answer is *no*, screen using the whispered voice test described next.

A pure tone audiometer gives a precise quantitative measure of hearing by assessing the person's ability to hear sounds of varying frequency. This is a battery-powered, lightweight, handheld instrument that is available in most outpatient settings. With the patient sitting, prop the patient's elbow on the armrest of the chair with the hand making a gentle fist. Tell the patient, "You will hear faint tones of different pitches. Please raise your finger as soon as you hear the tone; then lower your finger as soon as you no longer hear the tone." Choose tones of random loudness in decibels on the audioscope. Each tone is on for 1.5 seconds and off for 1.5 seconds. Test each ear separately and record the results. An audiometer gives a precise quantitative measure of hearing by assessing the person's ability to hear sounds of varying frequency.

Whispered Voice Test

Stand arm's length (half a metre, or 2 feet) behind the person. Test one ear at a time while masking hearing in the other ear to prevent sound transmission around the head. This is done by placing one finger on the tragus and pushing it in and out of the auditory meatus. Move your head to about half a metre (2 feet) from the person's ear. Exhale fully and whisper slowly a set of three random numbers and letters, such as "5, B, 6." Normally the person repeats each number/letter correctly after you say it. If the response is not correct, repeat the whispered test using a different combination of 3 numbers and letters. A passing score is correct repetition of at least three of a possible six numbers/letters.[10] Assess the other ear using yet another set of whispered items, such as "4, K, 2."

Tuning Fork Tests

Tuning fork tests are used to measure hearing by air conduction or by bone conduction, in which the sound vibrates through the cranial bones to the inner ear. The air conduction route through the ear canal and middle ear is usually the more sensitive route. Traditionally, these tests have been taught for physical examination, but evidence shows that both the Weber and the Rinne tuning fork tests do not yield precise or reliable data. Thus, these tests should not be used for general screening.

Abnormal Findings

Retracted eardrum is caused by vacuum in middle ear with obstructed eustachian tube.

Bulging eardrum is caused by increased pressure in otitis media.

Eardrum hypomobility is an early sign of otitis media (see Table 16.6, p. 376).

Perforation shows as a dark oval area or a larger opening on the eardrum (see Table 16.6, p. 376).

This single question in people over 50 years of age has an 83 to 90% agreement with hearing loss documented by audiometric testing.

Inability to hear whispered words (a whisper is a high-frequency sound and is used to detect high-tone loss).

Normal Range of Findings	Abnormal Findings

The Vestibular Apparatus

The **Romberg test** is an assessment of the ability of the vestibular apparatus in the inner ear to help maintain standing balance. Because the Romberg test is also used to assess intactness of the cerebellum and proprioception, it is discussed in Chapter 25 (see Fig. 25.18, p. 706).

 DEVELOPMENTAL CONSIDERATIONS

Infants and Young Children

Examination of the external ear of an infant or a young child is similar to that described for an adult, with the addition of examination of position and alignment on head.

Note the ear position. The top of the pinna should be horizontally aligned with the corner of the eye to the occiput. Also, the ear should be positioned within 10 degrees of vertical (Fig. 16.10).

Low-set ears or deviation in alignment may indicate intellectual disability or a genitourinary malformation.

Normal alignment

Fig. 16.10 © Pat Thomas, 2006.

Low-set ears and deviation in alignment

Otoscopic Examination

In addition to its role in the complete examination, eardrum assessment is mandatory for any infant or child requiring care for illness or fever. For infants and young children, it is best to perform the otoscopic examination toward the end of the complete examination. Many young children protest vigorously during this procedure no matter how well you prepare, and it is difficult to re-establish cooperation afterwards. Save the otoscopic examination until last. Then the parent can hold and comfort the child.

To help prepare the child, let the child hold your funny-looking "flashlight." You may wish to have the child look in the parent's or a plush toy's ear as you hold the otoscope (Fig. 16.11).

Ear pain and ear rubbing are associated with acute otitis media, as are a cloudy, bulging eardrum and a distinctly red eardrum.[11]

Objective Data

Normal Range of Findings	Abnormal Findings

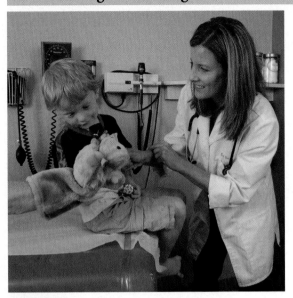

Fig. 16.11

Positioning of a child is important. You need a clear view of the canal. You should avoid harsh restraint, but you must protect the eardrum from injury in case of sudden head movement (Fig. 16.12). Enlist the aid of a cooperative parent. Prop an infant upright against the parent's chest or shoulder, with the parent's arm around the upper part of the head A toddler can be held in the parent's lap or may lie on the examining table with the arms gently secured. As you pull down on the pinna, gently push in on the child's tragus to ease insertion of the speculum tip. This sometimes helps avoid startling the child with a poke of the speculum tip.

Remember to pull the pinna straight down on an infant or a child younger than 3 years of age. This method will help match the slope of the ear canal (Fig. 16.13).

Fig. 16.12

Normal Range of Findings

Abstract

ADULT   YOUNG CHILD

Adult—pull
pinna up and back

Infant/child under 3—pull
pinna straight down

Fig. 16.13

At birth, the patency of the ear canal is determined, but the otoscopic examination is not performed because the canal is filled with amniotic fluid and vernix caseosa. After a few days, the eardrum is examined. During the first few days, the eardrum often looks thickened and opaque. It may look infected and have a mild redness from increased vascularity. The eardrum also looks infected in infants after crying.

The position of the eardrum is more horizontal in the neonate, which makes it more difficult to see completely and harder to differentiate from the canal wall. By 1 month of age, the eardrum is in the oblique (more vertical) position, as in older children, and examination is a bit easier.

When you examine an infant or young child, use a pneumatic bulb attachment on the otoscope to direct a light puff of air toward the eardrum to assess **vibratility** (Fig. 16.14). For a secure seal, choose the largest speculum that will fit in the ear canal without causing pain. A rubber tip on the end of the speculum gives a better seal. Give a small pump to the bulb (positive pressure), then release the bulb (negative pressure). Normally, the eardrum moves inward with a slight puff and outward with a slight release.

Atresia: absence or closure of the ear canal.

Eardrums can turn pink when a child or an infant is crying. Use of the pneumatic bulb is the most reliable way to detect otitis media because with otitis media, there is little to no movement of the eardrum.

An abnormal response is no movement. Eardrum hypomobility indicates effusion or a high vacuum in the middle ear. For the newborn's first 6 weeks, eardrum immobility is the best indicator of middle ear infection.

Fig. 16.14

Objective Data

Normal Range of Findings

Normally the eardrum is intact. In a child being treated for chronic otitis media, you may note the presence of a tympanostomy tube in the central part of the eardrum. This is inserted surgically to equalize pressure and drain secretions. In addition, it is common, although not normal, to note a foreign body in a child's canal, such as a small stone or a bead.

Test Hearing Acuity

Use the developmental milestones mentioned in this section to assess hearing in an infant. Also, attend to the parents' concern over the infant's inability to hear; their assessment is usually well founded. The room should be silent and the baby contented. Make a loud sudden noise (clap hands or squeeze toy) out of the baby's peripheral range of vision of about 30 cm. You may need to repeat a few times, but you should note the following responses:

- Newborn: startle (Moro) reflex, acoustic blink reflex
- Ages 3 to 4 months: acoustic blink reflex; stopping movement and appearing to listen; halting sucking; quieting if crying, crying if quiet
- Ages 6 to 8 months: turning head to localize sound, responding to own name
- Preschool- and school-age children: must be screened with audiometry

Note that a young child may be unaware of a hearing loss because the child does not know what "ought" to be heard. Note these behavioural manifestations of hearing loss:

1. The child is inattentive in casual conversation.
2. The child reacts more to movement and facial expression than to sound.
3. The child's facial expression is strained or puzzled.
4. The child frequently asks to have statements repeated.
5. The child confuses words that sound alike.
6. The child has an accompanying speech problem: Speech is monotonous or garbled; the child mispronounces or omits sounds.
7. The child appears shy and withdrawn and "lives in a world of his or her own."
8. The child frequently complains of earaches.
9. The child hears better at times when the environment is more conducive to hearing.

Older Adults

An older adult may have pendulous earlobes with linear wrinkling because of loss of elasticity of the pinna. Coarse, wiry hairs may be present at the opening of the ear canal. During otoscopy, the eardrum normally may appear whiter, more opaque, and duller than in the younger adult. It also may look thickened. A high-tone frequency loss is apparent for those affected with presbycusis, the hearing loss that occurs with aging. Note any difficulty hearing in the whispered voice test and hearing consonants during conversational speech. Many older adults believe that other people are "mumbling," and they feel isolated in family or friendship groups.

Abnormal Findings

Chronic otitis media relieved by tympanostomy tubes (see Table 16.6, p. 376).

Foreign body (see Table 16.4, p. 373).

Absence of alerting behaviour may indicate congenital deafness.

Failure to localize sound.

No intelligible speech by 2 years of age.

DOCUMENTATION AND CRITICAL THINKING

Sample Charting

SUBJECTIVE

States hearing is good; no earaches, infections, discharge, hearing loss, tinnitus, or vertigo.

OBJECTIVE

Pinna: Skin intact with no masses, lesions, tenderness, or discharge.
Otoscope: External canals are clear with no redness, swelling, lesions, foreign body, or discharge. Both eardrums are pearly grey in colour, with light reflex and landmarks intact, no perforations.
Hearing: Responds appropriately to conversation.

ASSESSMENT

Healthy ear structures
Hearing accurate

Focused Assessment: Clinical Case Study 1

Jamal Kabira is a 9-month-old infant of African descent who was brought to the clinic by his mother because he "feels hot and was up crying all night."

History: Jamal is the third child of Mr. and Mrs. Kabira. Mrs. Kabira received regular prenatal care. Jamal was born at 37 weeks' gestation; labour and delivery were uncomplicated. Jamal weighed 3 200 g at birth, and was discharged 2 days after delivery. Jamal has been fed formula, with solids introduced at 5 months. Well-baby care has been regular; immunizations are up to date. Jamal has had two prior episodes of otitis media, and no other illnesses.

Social History: Jamal lives with his family in a two-bedroom apartment over their grocery store and shares a bedroom with a 4-year-old brother and a 2-year-old brother. Mr. Kabira works full time in their grocery store; Mrs. Kabira provides child care in her home for her children and for her sister's two young children. Both parents smoke cigarettes, one to two packs per day.

SUBJECTIVE

1 day PTA [prior to arrival]: Mrs. Kabira put Jamal down for nap with a bottle of juice, as is usual. Jamal woke up in the middle of the nap crying furiously. Quieted somewhat when held upright but still fussy. Took juice from bottle, refused solid baby food. Temperature 38°C (100.4°F) rectally. Crying and fussy all night. Mrs. Kabira has given no medications to Jamal.

OBJECTIVE

Vital signs: Temp 38.4°C (101.1°F) (tympanic), pulse 152 bpm, resp 36/min, Wt 9.2 kg, Ht 74 cm.
General: Alert, active, crying, and fussy. Developmentally appropriate for age.
Skin: Warm and dry, no rashes or lesions.
Head: Anterior fontanelle flat, 1 × 1.5 cm, posterior fontanelle closed.
Eyes: No exudate, conjunctivae clear, sclerae white, red reflex present bilaterally.
Ears: Both eardrums dull red and bulging, no light reflex, no mobility on pneumatic otoscopy.
Mouth/throat: Oral mucosa pink, no lesions or exudate, tonsils 1+.
Neck: Supple, no lymphadenopathy.
Heart: Regular rate and rhythm, no murmurs.
Lungs: Breath sounds clear and equal bilaterally, unlaboured.
Abdomen: Bowel sounds present, abdomen soft, nontender.

ASSESSMENT

Acute otitis media, both ears
Pain R/T [related to] inflammation in eardrums

Risk for ear infection injury R/T supine formula feeding, group child care, second-hand smoke

Deficient knowledge (parents) R/T lack of exposure to risk factors for otitis media

Focused Assessment: Clinical Case Study 2

Todd Ray is a 15-year-old high school student who comes to the health centre to seek care for "cough off and on all winter and earache since last night."

SUBJECTIVE

Six weeks PTA: Nonproductive cough throughout day, no fever, no nasal congestion, no chest soreness. Todd's father gave him an over-the-counter decongestant, which helped, but cough continued off/on since. Does not smoke.

One day PTA: Intermittent cough continues, nasal congestion and thick white mucus. Also earache R (right) ear, treated self with recommended dose of acetaminophen [Tylenol], pain unrelieved. Pain is moderate, not deep and throbbing. Says R ear feels full, "hollow headed," voices sound muffled and far away, switches telephone to L (left) ear to talk. No sore throat, no fever, no chest congestion or soreness.

OBJECTIVE

Vital signs: Temp 37°C (98.6°F) (oral), pulse 76 bpm, BP 106/72 mm Hg

Ears: L ear, canal, eardrum normal, R ear and canal normal, R eardrum retracted, with multiple air bubbles, eardrum colour is yellow/amber. No sinus tenderness.

Nose: Turbinates bright red and swollen, mucopurulent discharge.

Throat: Not reddened, tonsils 1+.

Neck: One R anterior cervical node enlarged, firm, movable, tender. All others not palpable.

Lungs: Breath sounds clear to auscultation, resonant to percussion throughout.

ASSESSMENT

Serous otitis media, R ear, with mild upper respiratory tract infection

Transient conductive hearing loss

Disturbed sensory perception (auditory) R/T excessive fluid in middle ear

Pain R/T middle ear pressure

Focused Assessment: Clinical Case Study 3

Emma Schmidt, 78 years old, has a medical diagnosis of angina pectoris, which has responded to nitroglycerine prn [as needed] and periods of rest between activity. She has been independent in her own home, is coping well with activity restrictions through help from neighbours and family. Now hospitalized for evaluation of acute chest pain episode; MI [myocardial infarction] has been ruled out, pain diagnosed as angina, to be released to own home with a β-blocking medication and nitroglycerine prn.

Just before this hospitalization, Mrs. Schmidt received a hearing aid after evaluation by an audiologist. Mrs. Schmidt was born in Germany, immigrated to Canada at age 5 years, considers English her primary language.

SUBJECTIVE

Since this hospitalization, feels "irritable and nervous." Relates this to worry about heart and also, "I get so mixed up in here, this room is so strange, and I just can't hear the nurses. They talk like cavemen, 'oo-i-ee-uou.'" Tried using her new hearing aid but no relief. "It just kept screeching in my ear, and it made the monitor beep so loud it drove me crazy." States no tinnitus, no vertigo.

OBJECTIVE

Ears: Pinna with elongated lobes but no tenderness to palpation, no discharge, no masses or lesions. Both canals clear of cerumen. Both eardrums appear grey-white, slightly opaque, and dull, although all landmarks visible. No perforation.

Hearing: Difficulty hearing room conversation. Unable to hear whispered voice bilaterally.

ASSESSMENT

Chest pain/angina pectoris
Deficient knowledge R/T lack of teaching about hearing aid
Disturbed sensory perception (auditory) R/T effects of aging
Anxiety R/T change in cardiovascular health status and inability to communicate effectively

ABNORMAL FINDINGS

TABLE 16.1   Abnormalities of the External Ear

From the Clinical Slide Collection on the Rheumatic Diseases, © 1991, 1995, 1997. Used by permission of the American College of Rheumatology.

Frostbite

Reddish-blue discoloration and swelling of pinna after exposure to extreme cold. Vesicles or bullae may develop, the patient feels pain and tenderness, and ear necrosis may ensue.

Otitis Externa (Swimmer's Ear)

An infection of the outer ear, with severe pain on movement of the pinna and tragus, redness and swelling of pinna and canal, scanty purulent discharge, scaling, itching, fever, and enlarged tender regional lymph nodes. Hearing is normal or slightly diminished. More common in hot, humid weather. Swimming causes canal to become waterlogged and swell; skinfolds are set up for infection. Prevent by using rubbing alcohol or 2% acetic acid eardrops after every swim.

◄ Branchial Remnant and Ear Deformity

A facial remnant or leftover of the embryological branchial arch usually appears as a skin tag; in the infant pictured, it contains cartilage. These tags occur most often in the preauricular area, in front of the tragus. When bilateral, there is increased risk for renal anomalies.

Continued

TABLE 16.1	Abnormalities of the External Ear—cont'd

Cerebrospinal Fluid Otorrhea (Not Illustrated)

Skull fracture of temporal bone causes cerebrospinal fluid to leak from ear canal and pool in concha when the patient is supine. Cerebrospinal fluid feels oily and tests positive for glucose.

Cellulitis

Inflammation of loose, subcutaneous connective tissue. It manifests as thickening and induration of pinna with distorted contours.

See Illustration Credits for source information.

TABLE 16.2	Lumps and Lesions on the External Ear

From the Clinical Slide Collection on the Rheumatic Diseases, © 1991, 1995, 1997. Used by permission of the American College of Rheumatology.

Sebaceous Cyst

Location is commonly behind lobule, in the postauricular fold. A nodule with central black punctum indicates blocked sebaceous gland. It is filled with waxy sebaceous material and is painful if it becomes infected. Often are multiple.

Tophi

Small, whitish-yellow, hard, nontender nodules in or near helix or antihelix; contain greasy, chalky material of uric acid crystals and are a sign of gout.

TABLE 16.2	Lumps and Lesions on the External Ear—cont'd

Chondrodermatitis Nodularis Helicis

Painful nodules that develop on the rim of the helix (which has no cushioning subcutaneous tissue) as a result of repetitive mechanical pressure or environmental trauma (sunlight). Small, indurated, dull red, poorly defined, and very painful.

Keloid

Overgrowth of scar tissue, which invades original site of trauma. It is more common in dark-skinned people, although it also occurs in individuals with light skin. In the ear it is most common at lobule at the site of an ear piercing. Keloid shown here is unusually large.

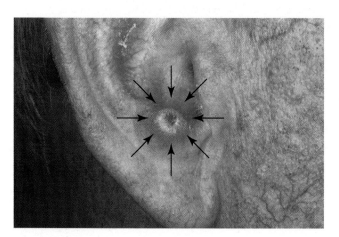

Carcinoma

Ulcerated crusted nodule with indurated base that fails to heal. Bleeds intermittently. Must refer for biopsy. Usually occurs on the superior rim of the pinna, which has the most sun exposure. May occur also in ear canal and exude chronic discharge that is either serosanguineous or bloody.

Battle Sign

Trauma to the side of the head may lead to a basilar skull fracture involving the temporal bone. This shows as ecchymotic discoloration just posterior to the pinna and over the mastoid process. A look inside the ear canal may show hemotympanum as well (see Table 16.6, p. 377).

See Illustration Credits for source information.

TABLE 16.3   Hearing Loss

CONDUCTIVE   SENSORINEURAL

Cholesteatoma

Otosclerosis
Ossification of
stapes

Foreign body

Cerumen

Otitis externa

Exostosis

Perforated tympanic
membrane

Tympanosclerosis

Otitis media with
effusion

Eustachian tube
blockage

Trauma - temporal
bone fracture

Ménière disease

Infection (meningitis,
labyrinthitis)

Tumor (acoustic
neuroma)

Noise
trauma
Medications -
ototoxicity

© Pat Thomas, 2014.

Hearing loss may be sensorineural, conductive, or mixed. Age-related sensorineural loss (presbycusis) affects 63% of those over 70 years of age[a] and 80% of those over 85 years of age[b]; the incidence will increase as current baby boomers age. Despite its prevalence, loss is underscreened and undertreated. This leads to social isolation, diminished quality of life, and even cognitive impairment and depression. Hearing aids can improve this loss. Note other causes of sensorineural loss in the figure. Conductive hearing loss blocks sound transmission somewhere in the external auditory canal, tympanic membrane, or middle ear.

[a]Pacala, J., & Yueh, B. (2012). Hearing deficits in the older patient: "I didn't notice anything." *JAMA: The Journal of the American Medical Association, 307*(11), 1185–1194.
[b]Walling, A., & Dickson, G. (2012). Hearing loss in older adults. *American Family Physician, 85*(12), 1150–1156.

TABLE 16.4 Abnormalities in the Ear Canal

Excessive Cerumen

Excessive cerumen is produced or is impacted because canal is narrow and tortuous or as a result of poor cleaning method. May appear as round ball partially obscuring eardrum or totally occluding canal. Even when canal is 90–95% blocked, hearing stays normal; when last 5–10% is totally occluded (when cerumen expands after swimming or showering), patient has sensation of ear fullness and sudden hearing loss.

Otitis Externa

Severe swelling of canal, inflammation, tenderness. In this illustration, canal lumen is narrowed to one-fourth of normal size. (See complete description in Table 16.1, p. 369.)

Osteoma

Single, stony hard, rounded nodule that obscures the eardrum; nontender; overlying skin appears normal. Attached to inner third (the bony part) of canal. Benign, but should be referred for removal.

Foreign Body

Usually children are the patients who place a foreign body in the ear (here, an obstruction completely occludes the canal), which is later noted on routine examination. Common objects are beans, corn, breakfast cereals, jewellery beads, small stones, and sponge rubber. Cotton is most common in adults and becomes impacted from cotton-tipped applicators. A trapped live insect is uncommon but makes the patient especially frantic.

Continued

TABLE 16.4   Abnormalities in the Ear Canal—cont'd

Exostosis

More common than osteoma. Small, hard, rounded nodules of hypertrophic bone, covered with normal epithelium. They arise near the eardrum but usually do not obstruct the view of the eardrum. They are usually multiple and bilateral. They may occur more frequently in cold-water swimmers. The condition needs no treatment, although it may cause accumulation of cerumen, which blocks the canal.

Furuncle

Exquisitely painful, reddened, infected hair follicle. In this illustration, it is on the tragus, but it also may be on cartilaginous part of ear canal. Regional lymphadenopathy often accompanies a furuncle.

◀ Polyp

Arises in canal from granulomatous or mucosal tissue; redder than surrounding skin and bleeds easily; bathed in foul purulent discharge; indicates chronic ear disease. Benign, but should be referred for excision.

TABLE 16.5	Abnormal Findings Seen on Otoscopy	
Appearance of Eardrum	Indicates	Suggested Condition
Yellow-amber colour	Serum or pus	Serous otitis media or chronic otitis media
Prominent landmarks	Retraction of eardrum	Negative pressure in middle ear from obstruction of eustachian tube
Air/fluid level or air bubbles	Serous fluid	Serous otitis media
Absence or distortion of light reflex	Bulging of eardrum	Acute otitis media
Bright red colour	Infection in middle ear	Acute purulent otitis media
Blue or dark red colour	Blood behind eardrum	Trauma, skull fracture
Dark, oval areas	Perforation	Eardrum rupture
White, dense areas	Scarring	Sequelae of infections
Diminished or absence of landmarks	Thickened eardrum	Chronic otitis media
Black or white dots on eardrum or canal	Colony of growth	Fungal infection

Adapted from Sherman, J. L., & Fields, S. K. (1988). *Guide to patient evaluation* (5th ed.). New York: Medical Examination Publishing. Reprinted by permission of Elsevier, Inc.

TABLE 16.6	Abnormal Tympanic Membranes

Retracted Eardrum

Landmarks look more prominent and well defined. Malleus handle looks shorter and more horizontal than normal. Short process is very prominent. Light reflex is absent or distorted. The eardrum is dull and lustreless and does not move. These signs indicate negative pressure and middle ear vacuum caused by obstruction of eustachian tube and serous otitis media.

Otitis Media With Effusion

An amber-yellow eardrum suggests serum in middle ear that transudates to relieve negative pressure from the blocked eustachian tube. Air/fluid level may be present with fine black dividing line or air bubbles visible behind eardrum. Symptoms are sensation of fullness, transient hearing loss, popping sound with swallowing. Also called *serous otitis media, glue ear.*

Early stage

Later stage

Continued

TABLE 16.6 Abnormal Tympanic Membranes—cont'd

Acute (Purulent) Otitis Media

This results when the middle ear fluid is infected. Absence of light reflex as a result of increasing middle ear pressure is an early sign. Redness and bulging are first noted in superior part of eardrum (pars flaccida; in *A*), along with earache and fever. Then, fiery redness and bulging of entire eardrum (in *B*), deep throbbing pain, fever, and transient hearing loss occur. Pneumatic otoscopy reveals eardrum hypomobility.

◀ Perforation

If the acute otitis media is not treated, the eardrum may rupture as a result of increased pressure. Perforations are also caused by trauma (e.g., a slap on the ear). Usually the perforation appears as a round or oval darkened area on the eardrum, but in this photo, the perforation is very large. *Central* perforations occur in the pars tensa. *Marginal* perforations occur at the annulus. When marginal perforations occur in superior part of the eardrum (the pars flaccida), they are called *attic perforations.*

Insertion of Tympanostomy Tubes

Polyethylene tubes are inserted surgically into the eardrum to relieve middle ear pressure and promote drainage of fluid from chronic or recurrent middle ear infections. Number of acute infections tends to decrease because of improved aeration. Tubes are extruded spontaneously in 12–18 months.

Cholesteatoma

An overgrowth of epidermal tissue in the middle ear or temporal bone may result over the years after a marginal tympanic membrane perforation. It has a pearly white, cheesy appearance. Growth of cholesteatoma can erode bone and produce hearing loss. Early signs include otorrhea, unilateral conductive hearing loss, and tinnitus.

TABLE 16.6 Abnormal Tympanic Membranes—cont'd

Scarred Eardrum

Dense white patches on the eardrum are sequelae of repeated ear infections. They do not necessarily affect hearing.

Blue Eardrum (Hemotympanum)

This indicates the presence of blood in the middle ear, as occurs when trauma results in skull fracture.

Bullous Myringitis

Small vesicles containing blood on the eardrum accompany *Mycoplasma pneumoniae* and virus infections. Affected patients may have blood-tinged discharge and severe otalgia.

Fungal Infection (Otomycosis)

Colony of black or white dots on eardrum or canal wall suggests a yeast or fungal infection.

See Illustration Credits for source information.

Summary Checklist: Ear Examination

1. **Inspect external ear:**
   Size and shape of pinna
   Position and alignment on head
   Skin condition: colour, lumps, lesions
   Movement of pinna and tragus (check for tenderness)
   External auditory meatus: size, swelling, redness, discharge, cerumen, lesions, foreign bodies

2. **Perform otoscopic examination:**
   External canal
   Cerumen, discharge, foreign bodies, lesions
   Redness or swelling of canal wall

3. **Inspect eardrum:**
   Colour and characteristics
   Position (flat, bulging, retracted)
   Integrity of membrane

4. **Test hearing acuity:**
   Behavioural response to conversational speech
   Voice test

5. **Engage in teaching and health promotion**

ADDITIONAL RESOURCES

Canadian Hearing Society: http://www.chs.ca

REFERENCES

1. Weener, D., Zacharek, M., & Malani, P. (2010). Evaluation and management of hearing loss in older adults. *Clinics in Geriatric Medicine, 18*(9), 20–26.

2. Kane, R. L., Ouslander, J. G., & Abrass, I. E. (2013). *Essentials of clinical geriatrics* (7th ed.). New York: McGraw-Hill.

3. Speech-Language and Audiology Canada. (2016). *Position statement on Early Hearing Detection and Intervention (EHDI): Canadian Infant Hearing Task Force.* Retrieved from https://www.sac-oac.ca/sites/default/files/resources/2016_EHDI_CIHTF_Position_Statement.pdf.

4. Le Saux, N., Robinson, J. L., & Canadian Paediatric Society. (2016). Position statement: Management of acute otitis media in children six months of age and older. *Paediatrics & Child Health, 21*(1), 39–44. Retrieved from https://www.cps.ca/en/documents/position/acute-otitis-media.

5. Karunanayake, C., Albritton, W., Rennie, D., et al. (2016). Ear infection and its associated risk factors in First Nations and rural school-aged Canadian children. *International Journal of Pediatrics, 2016*, 1–10. doi:org/10.1155/2016/1523897.

6. Canadian Hearing Society. (2013). *Facts and figures.* Retrieved from http://www.chs.ca/facts-and-figures.

7. Roland, P. S. (2017, March 15). *Chronic suppurative otitis media treatment & management.* Retrieved from https://emedicine.medscape.com/article/859501-treatment.

8. Carlson, L. (2005). Otitis media: New information on an old disease. *The Nurse Practitioner, 30*, 31–43.

9. Patel, H., & Feldman, M. (2011). Universal newborn hearing screening. *Paediatrics & Child Health, 16*(5), 301–305. Retrieved from http://www.cps.ca/english/statements/CP/cp11-02.htm#Recommendations.

10. Walling, A., & Dickson, G. (2012). Hearing loss in older adults. *American Family Physician, 85*(12), 1150–1156.

11. Schilder, A. G., Chonmaitree, T., Cripps, A. W., et al. (2016). Otitis media. *Nature Reviews. Disease Primers, 2*, doi:10.1038/nrdp.2016.63.

CHAPTER 17

Nose, Mouth, and Throat

Written by Carolyn Jarvis, PhD, APN, CNP
Adapted by Barbara Wilson-Keates, PhD, RN

ⓔ http://evolve.elsevier.com/Canada/Jarvis/examination/

STRUCTURE AND FUNCTION

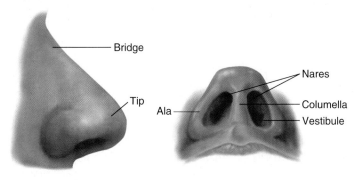

17.1 External nasal structures. (© Pat Thomas, 2006.)

NOSE

The **nose** is the first segment of the respiratory system. It warms, moistens, and filters inhaled air, and is the sensory organ for smell. The external nose is triangular with one side attached to the face (Fig. 17.1). On its leading edge, the superior part is the *bridge*, and the free corner is the *tip*. The oval openings at the base are the *nares*; just inside, each naris widens into the *vestibule*. The *columella* divides the two nares and is continuous inside with the nasal septum. The *ala* is the lateral outside wing of the nose on either side. The upper third of the external nose is made up of bone; the rest is cartilage.

Inside, the **nasal cavity** is much larger than the external size of the nose would indicate (Fig. 17.2). It extends back over the roof of the mouth. The anterior edge is lined with numerous coarse nasal hairs (*vibrissae*). The rest of the cavity is lined with a blanket of ciliated mucous membrane. Nasal hairs filter coarse matter from inhaled air, whereas the mucous blanket filters out dust and bacteria. Nasal mucosa appears redder than oral mucosa because of the rich blood supply present to warm the inhaled air.

The nasal cavity is divided medially by the **septum** into two slitlike passages. The anterior part of the septum holds a rich vascular network, *Kiesselbach's plexus*, the most common site of nosebleeds. In many people, the nasal septum may deviate to one side.

The lateral walls of each nasal cavity contain three parallel bony projections: the (a) superior, (b) middle, and (c) inferior **turbinates**. They increase the surface area so that more blood vessels and mucous membranes are available to warm, humidify, and filter inhaled air. Underlying each turbinate is a cleft, the **meatus**, named for the turbinate above. The sinuses drain into the middle meatus, and tears from the nasolacrimal duct drain into the inferior meatus.

Olfactory receptors (hair cells) lie at the roof of the nasal cavity and the upper one-third of the septum. These smell receptors merge into the olfactory nerve, cranial nerve I, which transmits impulses to the temporal lobe of the brain. Although not necessary for human survival, the sense of smell enhances the pleasure and taste of food.

The **paranasal sinuses** are air-filled pockets within the cranium (Fig. 17.3). They communicate with the nasal cavity and are lined with the same type of ciliated mucous membrane. They lighten the weight of the skull bones, serve as resonators for sound production, and provide mucus, which drains into the nasal cavity. The sinus openings are narrow

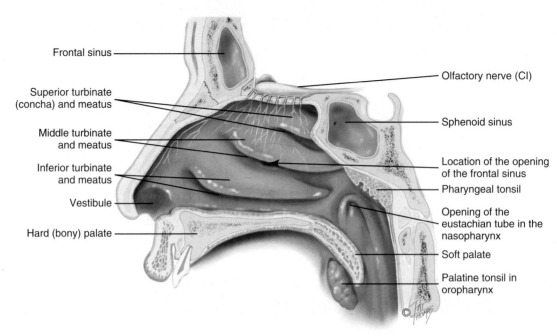

Frontal sinus

Olfactory nerve (CI)

Superior turbinate
(concha) and meatus

Sphenoid sinus

Middle turbinate
and meatus

Location of the opening
of the frontal sinus

Inferior turbinate
and meatus

Pharyngeal tonsil

Vestibule

Opening of the
eustachian tube in the
nasopharynx

Hard (bony) palate

Soft palate

Palatine tonsil in
oropharynx

RIGHT LATERAL WALL - NASAL CAVITY

17.2 © Pat Thomas, 2006.

and easily occluded, which may cause inflammation or sinusitis.

Two **frontal sinuses**, in the frontal bone above and medial to the orbits, and two **maxillary sinuses**, in the maxilla (cheekbone) along the side walls of the nasal cavity, are accessible to examination. The other two sets are smaller and deeper: the **ethmoid sinuses**, between the orbits, and the **sphenoid sinuses**, deep within the skull in the sphenoid bone.

Only the maxillary and ethmoid sinuses are present at birth. The maxillary sinuses reach full size after all permanent teeth have erupted. The ethmoid sinuses grow rapidly between 6 and 8 years of age and after puberty. The frontal sinuses are absent at birth, fairly well developed between 7 and 8 years of age, and reach full size after puberty. The sphenoid sinuses are minute at birth and develop after puberty.

MOUTH

The **mouth** is the first segment of the digestive system and an airway for the respiratory system. The **oral cavity** is a short passage bordered by the lips, palate, cheeks, and tongue. It contains the teeth and gums, tongue, and salivary glands (Fig. 17.4).

The **lips** are the anterior border of the oral cavity: the transition zone from the outer skin to the inner mucous membrane lining the oral cavity. The palate is the arching roof of the mouth and is divided into two parts. The anterior **hard palate** is made up of bone and is a whitish colour. The posterior **soft palate** is a pinker and mobile arch of muscle. The **uvula** is the free projection hanging down from the middle of the soft palate. The **cheeks** are the side walls of the oral cavity.

The floor of the mouth consists of the horseshoe-shaped mandible bone, the tongue, and underlying muscles. The **tongue** is a mass of striated muscle arranged in a crosswise pattern so it can change shape and position. The **papillae** are rough, bumpy elevations on its dorsal surface. Note the larger **vallate papillae** in an inverted V shape across the posterior base of the tongue, and do not confuse them with abnormal growths. Underneath, the ventral surface of the tongue is smooth, shiny and has prominent veins. The **frenulum** is a midline fold of tissue connecting the tongue to the mouth floor.

The tongue's ability to change shape and position enhances its functions in mastication, swallowing, cleansing the teeth, and speech. The tongue also functions in taste sensation. Microscopic taste buds are in the papillae at the back and sides of the tongue and on the soft palate.

The mouth contains three pairs of **salivary glands** (Fig. 17.5). The largest, the **parotid gland**, lies within the cheeks in front of the ear and extend from the zygomatic arch down to the angle of the jaw. Its duct, Stensen's duct, runs forward to open on the buccal mucosa opposite the second molar. The **submandibular gland**, the size of a walnut, lies beneath the mandible at the angle of the jaw. Wharton's duct runs up and forward to the floor of the mouth opening at either side of the frenulum. The smallest salivary gland, the almond-shaped **sublingual gland**, lies within the floor of the mouth. It has many small openings along the sublingual fold under the tongue.

The glands secrete saliva, clear fluid that moistens and lubricates the food bolus, starts digestion, and cleans and protects the mucosa.

Adults have 32 **permanent teeth**, 16 in each arch. Each tooth has three parts: the crown, the neck, and the root. The **gums** (gingivae) collar the teeth. They are thick fibrous

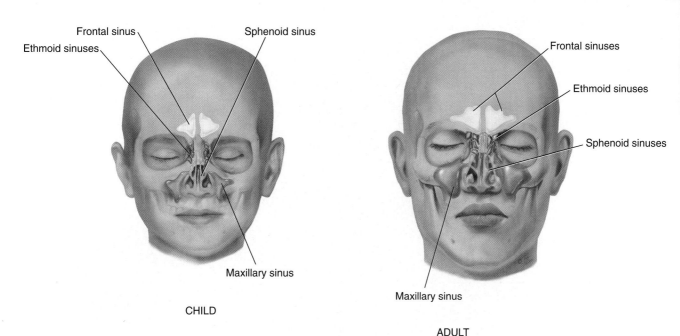

Frontal sinus

Sphenoid sinus

Ethmoid sinuses

Maxillary sinus

CHILD

Frontal sinuses

Ethmoid sinuses

Sphenoid sinuses

Maxillary sinus

ADULT

Ethmoid sinuses

Frontal sinus

Maxillary sinus

Sphenoid sinus

 17.3 Paranasal sinuses. © Pat Thomas, 2006.

tissues covered with mucous membrane. The gums are different from the rest of the oral mucosa because of their pale pink colour and stippled surface.

THROAT

The **throat**, or **pharynx**, is the area behind the mouth and nose. The **oropharynx** is separated from the mouth by the anterior tonsillar pillars—two folds of tissue, one on each side. Behind the folds are the **tonsils**, each a mass of lymphoid tissue the same colour as surrounding mucous membrane, but which look more granular and have deep crypts visible on their surface. Tonsillar tissue enlarges during childhood until puberty, then decreases in size and function. The posterior pharyngeal wall behind these structures may have visible small blood vessels.

The **nasopharynx** is continuous with the oropharynx, above the oropharynx and behind the nasal cavity. The pharyngeal tonsils (adenoids) and eustachian tube openings are located here (see Fig. 17.2).

The oral cavity and throat have a rich lymphatic network (review Chapter 14), which is important to keep in mind when you evaluate the mouth.

❖ DEVELOPMENTAL CONSIDERATIONS

Infants and Children

In infants, salivation starts at 3 months of age. Babies drool periodically for a few months before learning to swallow the saliva. Drooling does not herald the eruption of teeth, as many parents believe.

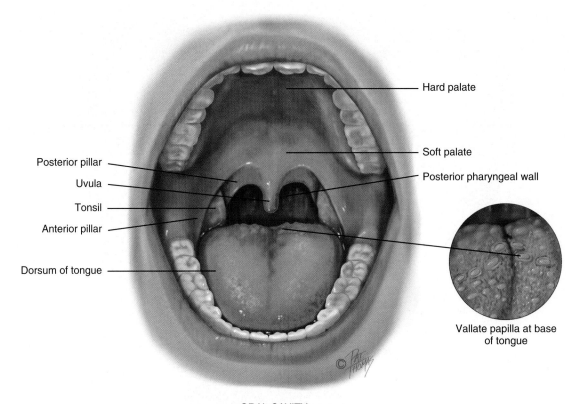

Hard palate

Soft palate

Posterior pharyngeal wall

Posterior pillar

Uvula

Tonsil

Anterior pillar

Dorsum of tongue

Vallate papilla at base
of tongue

ORAL CAVITY

17.4 © Pat Thomas, 2010.

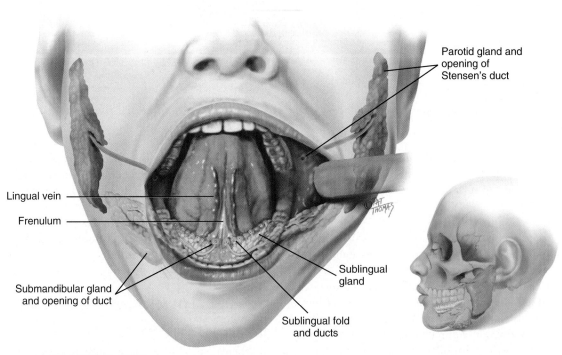

Parotid gland and
opening of
Stensen's duct

Lingual vein

Frenulum

Submandibular gland
and opening of duct

Sublingual
gland

Sublingual fold
and ducts

SALIVARY GLANDS

17.5 © Pat Thomas, 2006.

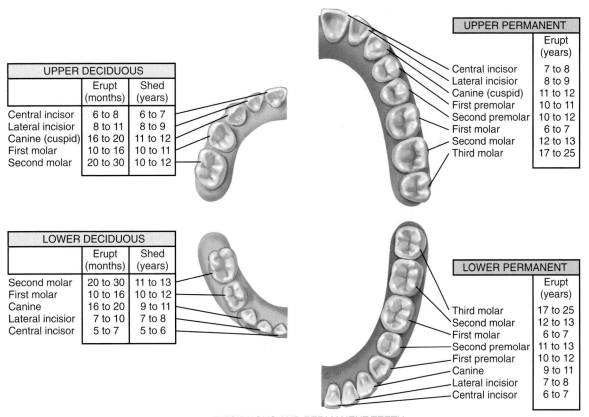

UPPER DECIDUOUS		
	Erupt (months)	Shed (years)
Central incisor	6 to 8	6 to 7
Lateral incisior	8 to 11	8 to 9
Canine (cuspid)	16 to 20	11 to 12
First molar	10 to 16	10 to 11
Second molar	20 to 30	10 to 12

UPPER PERMANENT	
	Erupt (years)
Central incisor	7 to 8
Lateral incisior	8 to 9
Canine (cuspid)	11 to 12
First premolar	10 to 11
Second premolar	10 to 12
First molar	6 to 7
Second molar	12 to 13
Third molar	17 to 25

LOWER DECIDUOUS		
	Erupt (months)	Shed (years)
Second molar	20 to 30	11 to 13
First molar	10 to 16	10 to 12
Canine	16 to 20	9 to 11
Lateral incisior	7 to 10	7 to 8
Central incisor	5 to 7	5 to 6

LOWER PERMANENT	
	Erupt (years)
Third molar	17 to 25
Second molar	12 to 13
First molar	6 to 7
Second premolar	11 to 13
First premolar	10 to 12
Canine	9 to 11
Lateral incisior	7 to 8
Central incisor	6 to 7

DECIDUOUS AND PERMANENT TEETH

17.6   © Pat Thomas, 2006.

Both sets of teeth begin development in utero. Children have 20 temporary **deciduous teeth**. These erupt between 6 and 24 months of age. All 20 teeth should appear by 2½ years of age. The deciduous teeth are lost between ages 6 to 12 years. They are then replaced by permanent teeth, starting with the central incisors (Fig. 17.6), which appear earlier in girls than boys.

The nose develops during adolescence, along with secondary sex characteristics. This growth starts at age 12 or 13 years, reaching full growth at age 16 years in girls and 18 years in boys.

Pregnant Women

Nasal stuffiness and nosebleeds, or *epistaxis*, may occur during pregnancy as a result of increased vascularity in the upper respiratory tract. The gums may be hyperemic and softened and may bleed with normal tooth brushing. Contrary to folklore, no evidence shows that pregnancy causes tooth decay or loss.

Older Adults

Subcutaneous fat is gradually lost during later middle adult years, making the nose appear more prominent in some people. Nasal hairs grow coarser and stiffer and may not filter the air as well. The hairs protrude and may cause itching and sneezing. Many older adults clip these hairs, thinking them unsightly, but this practice may cause infection. The sense of smell may diminish because of a decreased number of olfactory nerve fibres. It decreases progressively after age 60 years.

In the oral cavity, soft tissues atrophy and the epithelium thins, especially in the cheek and tongue, which results in loss of taste buds and about 80% reduction in taste functioning. Further impairments in taste include decreased salivary secretion, which is needed to dissolve flavouring agents, and the presence of upper dentures, which cover secondary taste sites.

Atrophic tissues ulcerate easily, increasing older adults' risk for oral yeast infections, also known as *thrush* or *candidiasis*. The risk for malignant oral lesions is also increased.

With aging, tooth surfaces are abraded, gums begin to recede, and teeth begin to erode at the gum line. A smooth V-shaped cavity forms around the neck of the tooth, exposing the nerve and making the tooth hypersensitive. Some tooth loss may result from bone resorption (osteoporosis), which decreases the inner tooth structure and its outer support. Natural tooth loss is exacerbated by years of inadequate dental care, decay, poor oral hygiene, and tobacco use.

If tooth loss occurs, the remaining teeth drift, causing upper or lower incisors to protrude, known as **malocclusion**. The stress of chewing with misaligned teeth causes further problems: (a) excessive bone resorption, resulting in further tooth loss; (b) muscle imbalance resulting from misalignment of the mandible and maxilla, producing muscle spasms, tenderness of muscles of mastication, and chronic headaches; and (c) increased stress on the temporomandibular joint leading to osteoarthritis, pain, and inability to fully open the mouth.

Diminished senses of taste and smell decrease older adults' appetite and may contribute to malnutrition. Saliva production decreases; saliva helps move food around the mouth. Decreased saliva also reduces the mouth's self-cleaning property. The major cause of decreased saliva flow is not the aging process itself but use of medications that have anticholinergic effects. More than 250 medications have an adverse effect of dry mouth.

Because of the absence of some teeth and trouble with mastication, many older adults eat soft foods (usually high in carbohydrates) and decrease meat and fresh vegetable intake producing a risk for nutritional deficits in protein, vitamins, and minerals.

 ## SOCIAL DETERMINANTS OF HEALTH CONSIDERATIONS

The incidence of **cleft palate** is similar across ethnic groups, but Indigenous people have a higher occurrence of **cleft lip** and combined cleft lip/cleft palate. Torus palatinus, a bony ridge running down the middle of the hard palate, is also more common in Indigenous people and people of Asian descent. **Leukoedema**, a greyish-white benign lesion occurring on the buccal mucosa, may be present in people of African descent. Oral hyperpigmentation, usually absent at birth, increases with age. It is more common among people of African descent and is believed to be caused by a lifetime accumulation of postinflammatory oral changes.

As oral health care is not covered under the Canadian health care system, access to comprehensive dental health care is a major barrier to oral health promotion and maintenance and places vulnerable populations at risk. Coverage by employer-provided or privately-purchased dental insurance plans is directly related to employment status, earnings, and wealth. Thirty-two percent of Canadians lack adequate dental insurance and may not be able to pay oral care expenses.[1]

In Canada, Indigenous people and individuals living in remote communities reported worse oral health status and greater frequency of oral pain as compared with non-Indigenous or people living in urban areas.[2] A lack of access to comprehensive oral health care services is a key factor affecting those living in remote or isolated areas. For Indigenous people, higher rates of dental disease are also the result of a change from a traditional diet to one higher in processed and sugary foods and the lack of access to fluoridated water. Indigenous preschoolers are eight times more likely to undergo general anaesthesia for dental caries compared with non-Indigenous children. Also, 23% of Indigenous children required restorative care for dental caries.[3] More dental disease is treated by extractions and results in a higher rate of being toothless, also known as *edentulism*, among Indigenous people. Given that many northern communities lack a resident oral care practitioner, practitioners from southern Canada fly into the communities on an irregular basis to treat serious cases and dental emergencies. Consequently, restorative dental care, such as fillings and extractions, are more prevalent than oral health promotion and preventive measures.[3]

Recent refugees and immigrants also face obstacles accessing oral health care for many reasons, including limited financial resources, poor language skills, a fear of dentists, history of inadequate care, embarrassment about their oral condition, and differences in cultural approaches and concepts for oral health care prevention and treatment. Individuals from lower income households have a greater prevalence of edentulism, periodontal disease, dental pain, and chewing difficulties. Also, they report poorer oral health-related quality of life than Canadians from higher income groups.[2] In addition, many refugees and immigrants are from Africa and Asia, where the prevalence of dental caries is increasing. Consequently, new Canadians experience inferior oral health when compared with other Canadians.[4]

People with disabilities may experience challenges in maintaining oral health, preventing disease, and accessing oral health care. Barriers include physical and equipment limitations, personal social challenges (fear, anxiety, embarrassment, stigma, or discrimination), and cost.[5]

Body piercing, a type of body modification practised in many cultures, is the establishment of an unnatural tract through tissue held open by artificial means. The nose is the most common site for oral piercing, followed by the mouth, and tongue. Most prevalent among women between 20 and 30 years of age, main motivators for oral piercings are fashion, expression of individuality or personal values, and sexual expression. Infection is the most frequent complication of piercings (which provide a route of entry for micro-organisms), with infection rates ranging from 9% to 35%. Additional complications include abnormal tooth wear, tooth chipping/cracking, tooth loss, and periodontal disease.[6]

SUBJECTIVE DATA

Nose

1. Discharge
2. Frequent colds (upper respiratory infections)
3. Sinus pain
4. Trauma
5. Epistaxis (nosebleeds)
6. Allergies
7. Altered smell

Mouth and Throat

1. Sores or lesions
2. Sore throat
3. Bleeding gums
4. Toothache
5. Sugar consumption

6. Bruxism (teeth grinding)
7. Hoarseness
8. Dysphagia
9. Altered taste
10. Tobacco consumption

11. Alcohol consumption
12. Sleep apnea
13. Self-care behaviours
    Oral care pattern
    Dentures or appliances

HEALTH HISTORY QUESTIONS

Examiner Asks	Rationale

Nose

1. **Discharge.** Any **nasal discharge** or runny nose? Continuously?
   - Is the discharge watery, purulent, mucoid, bloody?

   Rhinorrhea (nasal discharge) occurs with colds, allergies, sinus infection, or trauma.

2. **Frequent colds (upper respiratory infections).** Any unusually frequent or severe colds? How often do these occur?

   Most people have occasional colds; asking this more precise question yields more meaningful data.

3. **Sinus pain.** Any **sinus pain** or sinusitis? How is this treated?
   - How did you respond to treatment?
   - Do you have chronic postnasal drip?

4. **Trauma.** Ever had any **trauma** or a blow to the nose? (See Critical Findings box.)
   - Can you breathe through your nose? Is either side obstructed?

   Trauma and cocaine use may cause a deviated septum, which may cause nares to be obstructed.

CRITICAL FINDINGS

Trauma to teeth, mouth, tongue, nose, and throat necessitate immediate assessment and attention. Prompt care is required for patients with slurred speech, difficulty speaking or swallowing, jaw pain, or swelling in their throats. These findings suggest stroke, cardiac problems, dysphagia, or anaphylaxis. Choanal atresia in both nostrils warrants immediate insertion of an oral airway to ensure a patent airway, given that newborns are obligate nose breathers. Epistaxis lasting longer than 20 minutes necessitates urgent intervention because it may indicate life-threatening hypertension, a bleeding disorder, or a skull fracture from head trauma. Unrelenting tooth pain that accompanies facial or neck swelling, redness, or bleeding necessitates prompt attention. It may suggest a dental abscess with systemic implications if left untreated.

5. **Epistaxis (nosebleeds).** Any **nosebleeds**? How often?
   - How much bleeding—a teaspoonful, or does it pour out?
   - Colour of the blood—red or brown? Clots?
   - From one nostril or both?
   - Aggravated by nose picking or scratching?
   - How do you treat the nosebleeds? Are they difficult to stop?

   Epistaxis occurs with trauma, vigorous nose blowing, foreign body, or cocaine use.

   The patient should sit up with head tilted forward, and pinch the nose between thumb and forefinger for 5 to 15 minutes.

6. **Allergies.** Any **allergies** or hay fever? To what are you allergic (e.g., pollen, dust, pets)?
   - How was this determined?
   - What type of environment makes it worse? Can you avoid exposure?
   - What are your symptoms?

   Allergic rhinitis is "seasonal" if caused by pollen and "perennial" if the allergen is dust.
   Common oral symptoms include sneezing, itchy/runny/blocked nose, and swollen lips and tongue.

Subjective Data

Examiner Asks	Rationale

- Do you use inhalers, nasal spray, nose drops? How often? Which type?
- How long have you used this?

Misuse of over-the-counter nasal medications irritates the mucosa and causes rebound swelling, a common problem.

7. Altered smell. Any change in sense of smell?

Sense of smell diminishes with cigarette smoking, chronic allergies, and aging.

Mouth and Throat

1. **Sores or lesions.** Noticed any **sores** or **lesions** in the mouth or on the tongue or gums?
   - How long have you had it? Ever had this lesion before?
   - Is it single or multiple?
   - Is it associated with stress, season change, food?
   - How have you treated the sore? Applied any local medication?
   - How did you respond to treatment?

The patient's history helps determine whether oral lesions have infectious, traumatic, immunological, or malignant causes.

2. **Sore throat.** How frequently do you get a sore throat? Have a sore throat now? When did it start?
   - Is it associated with cough, fever, fatigue, decreased appetite, headache, postnasal drip, or hoarseness?
   - Is it worse when you arise? What is the humidity level in the room where you sleep? Any dust or smoke inhaled at work?
   - Do you usually get a throat culture for sore throats? Were any documented as "strep throat"? (streptococcal infections)
   - How have you treated this sore throat: medication, gargling? How effective are these? Have your tonsils or adenoids been removed?

Untreated streptococcal infections may lead to complication of rheumatic fever.

3. **Bleeding gums.** Any **bleeding gums**? How long have you had this?

A little bleeding is normal if a patient is just starting to floss. More frequent bleeding from brushing or flossing may indicate periodontal disease or a clotting disorder.

4. **Toothache.** Any **toothache**? Are your teeth sensitive to hot, cold? Have you lost any teeth?

5. **Sugar consumption.** How many **sugar-sweetened soft drinks, juices or sweets** do you drink/eat each day?

Sugar is a main factor in tooth decay and periodontal disease, with the average Canadian consuming 13 tsp of added sugar daily.[7]

6. **Bruxism (teeth grinding).** Has a family member or bed partner informed you that you **grind your teeth** at night? If yes, do you wear a mouthguard when sleeping?
   - Do you have jaw pain or tenderness?

Teeth grinding occurs when upper and lower teeth are clenched together and then forcefully moved in a forward and backward motion. Usually caused by dental problems or stress, it happens more frequently at night during sleep but may also occur during the day. Grinding may result in fractured or flattened teeth, and pain or tenderness in temporomandibular joints (TMJ), face, or ear.

7. **Hoarseness.** Any **hoarseness**, voice change? For how long?
   - Do you feel like you have to clear your throat? Or have a "lump in your throat"?
   - Do you use your voice a lot at work, recreation?
   - Does the hoarseness seem associated with a cold or a sore throat?

Hoarseness of the larynx has many causes: overuse of the voice, upper respiratory infection, chronic inflammation, lesions, or neoplasm.

Examiner Asks	Rationale

8. Dysphagia. Any **difficulty swallowing**? How long have you had it?
- Do you feel as if food gets stopped at a certain point?
- Do you cough while drinking or eating?
- Does your voice sound "wet" or hoarse when you eat or drink?
- Any drooling or leakage of food or liquid while eating?
- Does any food get stuck in your mouth (pocketing) or in your throat?
- What have you done to improve swallowing? How effective was it?
- Any pain with this?

Dysphagia may be oropharyngeal in origin (difficulty in safe transfer of liquid or food bolus from mouth to the esophagus), or esophageal dysphagia (difficulty in passing food down the esophagus to the stomach). At least 30% of individuals with acute stroke have dysphagia.[8] Other causes of dysphagia are head, neck, and esophageal cancers, head trauma, decreased alertness, and progressive neurological diseases.

Untreated dysphagia increases risk for aspiration pneumonia, malnutrition, and dehydration, and may reduce quality of life.

Nursing care includes screening with a reliable and validated tool such as TOR-BSST©, designed specifically for stroke patients (Fig. 17.7). Patients who fail dysphagia screening can be referred for a comprehensive assessment to a speech language pathologist, who may suggest dietary modification, good oral care, and resting at least 30 minutes after meal in an upright position.

Odynophagia (pain upon swallowing), may be burning or sharp, indicating mucosal inflammation, or a cramping, squeezing pain that suggests a muscular cause.

9. Altered taste. Any change in sense of **taste**?

10. Tobacco consumption.

Do you **smoke**? Pipe or cigarettes? How many packs a day? For how many years?
- Do you currently want to quit smoking?
- Have you tried quitting? Were you successful? What helped you quit?
- Do you vape or use e-cigarettes? What substance do you vape? How long have you vaped?
- Do you use smokeless tobacco? (See the box Promoting Health: Oral Health)

Chronic tobacco use can lead to tooth loss, coronal and root caries, periodontal disease, and oral and pharyngeal cancers.

Individual intention to quit is a major factor in successful smoking cessation programs and interventions.

11. Alcohol consumption. When was your last **alcoholic drink**? How much alcohol did you drink that time? How much do you usually drink?

Chronic heavy alcohol consumption increases risk for oral and pharyngeal cancers.

Subjective Data

TOR-BSST©
The Toronto Bedside Swallowing
Screening Test©

(addressograph)

DATE: _____ *(mm/dd/yyyy)*   TIME: _____ *(hh/mm)*

A) Before water intake: (Mark either abnormal or normal for each task.)

	Abnormal	*Normal*
1. Have patient say 'ah' and judge voice quality	☐	☑
2. Ask patient to stick their tongue out and then move it from side to side.	☐	☑

B) Water intake: Have the patient **sit upright** and give water. Ask patient to **say "ah"** after each intake. Mark as abnormal if you note any of the following signs: **coughing, change in voice quality** or **drooling.** If abnormal, stop water intake and advance to 'D'.

1) One Tsp Swallows	**Cough during/after swallow**	**Voice change after swallow**	**Drooling during/after swallow**	**Normal**
Swallow 1	☐	☐	☐	☐
Swallow 2	☐	☐	☐	☐
Swallow 3	☐	☐	☐	☐
Swallow 4	☐	☐	☐	☐
Swallow 5	☐	☐	☐	☐
Swallow 6	☐	☐	☐	☐
Swallow 7	☐	☐	☐	☐
Swallow 8	☐	☐	☐	☐
Swallow 9	☐	☐	☐	☐
Swallow 10	☐	☐	☐	☐
2) Cup drinking	☐	☐	☐	☐

C) After water intake: (Administer at least a minute after you finish Section B.)

	Abnormal	*Normal*
1. Have patient say 'ah' again and judge voice quality.	☐	☐

D) Results: ☐ **Passed**   ☐ **Failed → Initiate referral to SLP**
                    (no abnormal signs)   (1 or more abnormal signs)

TOR-BSST© Screener's Signature: _____

June 2007 version

17.7   Toronto Bedside Swallowing Screening Test (TOR-BSST©). Note: Screeners may be health care providers, such as nurses, who have received proper training using the standardized 4-hour training program. (© 2003. The TOR-BSST© form is copyrighted. It may not be altered, sold, translated, or adapted without the permission of Rosemary Martino, rosemary.martino@utoronto.ca.)

PROMOTING HEALTH: ORAL HEALTH

E-Cigarettes and Smokeless Tobacco

An electronic cigarette (e-cigarette) is a handheld electronic device that creates an aerosol which vapourizes a flavoured nicotine and propylene glycol liquid. As tobacco is absent, the user inhales vapour into the lungs and not smoke. Using e-cigarettes is sometimes called **vaping**. A survey of Canadian youth and young adults reported that 16% of individuals had previously vaped and almost 45% were aware of e-cigarettes. Former and current smokers were more likely to have vaped than nonsmokers.[*]

The long-term health risks of e-cigarettes are uncertain. Although, no serious adverse effects have been reported in trials, less serious adverse effects include throat and mouth irritation, vomiting, nausea, and coughing. As smoke and its carcinogens are not inhaled, users believe e-cigarettes are a safer choice than regular cigarettes. Proponents also feel e-cigarettes can help some smokers quit; however, no research has provided evidence to support these claims. When used by nonsmokers, e-cigarettes have been linked to nicotine addiction and commencement of smoking.[†]

Known as "snuff," or "chew," smokeless tobacco (SLT) carries significant health risks and is not a safe substitute for smoking. Two types of SLT are common in Canada: *chewing tobacco* comes in loose leaves and is chewed, and *snuff* is finely ground tobacco that is placed between the gingival and buccal mucosa. The user sucks on the tobacco and spits out the juices. Many SLT brands are heavily sweetened with sugars and flavouring salts. The sugar is held in the mouth next to the teeth, promoting periodontal disease, tooth decay, and delayed wound healing while flavouring salts contribute to hypertension and kidney disease. Furthermore, the gritty materials scratch soft tissues, allowing nicotine and other chemicals to directly enter the bloodstream.

Over 3 000 chemicals, including nicotine and 28 carcinogens, have been identified in SLT. Holding one pinch of SLT in your mouth for 30 minutes typically delivers as much nicotine as four cigarettes. Nicotine may play a role in disease development, including coronary artery and peripheral vascular diseases, hypertension, peptic ulcer disease, and fetal mortality and morbidity.

Use of any form of tobacco or nicotine increases the risk for oral cancer. Use of SLT is associated with a greater risk for oral cancer than regular cigarettes.[†] As pain is rarely an early symptom of oral cancer, a thorough examination of the mouth is important.

Early signs of oral cancer include:
- An ulcer or sore that does not heal
- White or red patches
- Prolonged sore throat or feeling that something is in the throat
- Difficulty chewing
- Unexplained bleeding
- Numbness or tingling
- Restricted movement of tongue or jaw
- Small lump or thickening in the lip, tongue, floor or roof of mouth, cheeks, gums, tonsil

References

*Czoli, A., Hammond, D., & White, C. (2014). Electronic cigarettes in Canada: Prevalence perceptions of use among youth and young adults. *Canadian Journal of Public Health*, 105(2), e97–e102. Retrieved from http://citeseerx.ist.psu.edu/viewdoc/download?doi=10.1.1.689.5275&rep=rep1&type=pdf.

†Canadian Cancer Society. (2017). *Any tobacco use can hurt your body.* Retrieved from http://www.cancer.ca/en/prevention-and-screening/live-well/smoking-and-tobacco/any-tobacco-use-can-hurt-your-body/?region=ab??2??.

Examiner Asks	Rationale
12. Sleep Apnea. Has your bed partner told you that you **snore loudly**? For example, is it louder than talking? Heard through two closed doors? • Do you **stop breathing** when asleep? • Do you have excessive daytime sleepiness?	Characterized by complete or partial upper airway closure causing periods of not breathing, or *apnea*, during sleep, obstructive sleep apnea (OSA) affects up to 26% of the population. Risk factors include obesity, aging, and chronic use of alcohol and tobacco. Treatment involves weight loss, use of a positive pressure airway machine (e.g., continuous positive airway pressure [CPAP] machine) to help keep airway open, and other breathing devices. Untreated OSA results in increased risks for postoperative complications and cardiovascular events, greater morbidity and mortality rates, and higher chance of work-related or driving accidents. Use of the STOP-Bang Questionnaire, a preoperative bedside screening tool, identifies individuals with undiagnosed OSA.[9]

Examiner Asks	Rationale
13. Self-care behaviours. Tell me about your daily **dental care**. How often do you use a toothbrush and floss? • Do you have oral health care benefits? • When was your last dental examination? Do dental problems affect which foods you eat? • Do you have a dental appliance: braces, bridge, headgear? • Do you wear dentures? All the time? How long have you had this set? How do they fit?	Assess self-care behaviours for oral hygiene. Regular dental screening, usually every 6 months, is necessary for promotion and maintenance of oral health. More frequent checkups may be recommended, depending on oral and overall health; however, dental benefit plans may provide coverage for dental screening and cleaning only every 9 months. One-third of Canadians do not have oral health care coverage, which may adversely affect self-care behaviours.[5]
• Any sores or irritation of palate or gums? • Any problems with talking: Do the dentures whistle or drop? Can you chew all foods with them? How do you clean them?	Lesions may arise from ill-fitting dentures, or the presence of dentures may mask eruption of new lesions.

Additional History for Infants and Children

Examiner Asks	Rationale
1. Mouth disease. Does the child have any mouth infections or sores, such as thrush or chancre sores? How frequently do these occur?	
2. Throat disease. Does the child have frequent sore throat or tonsillitis? How often? How are these treated? • Have they ever been documented as "strep throat" (streptococcal infections)?	
3. Tooth development. Did the child's teeth erupt about on time? Do the teeth seem straight to you? • Is the child using a bottle? How often during the day? Does the child go to sleep with a bottle at night? • Sugar consumption: How many sugar-sweetened soft drinks or juices does your child drink each day? How many sugar-sweetened sweets does your child eat each day? • Have you noticed any thumb-sucking after the child's secondary teeth came in? • Have you noticed the child grinding the teeth? Does this happen at night?	Prolonged bottle use increases the risk for tooth decay and middle ear infections. Sugar is the main factor in tooth decay and periodontal disease in children. Prolonged thumb-sucking (after age 6 to 7 years) may affect occlusion. Bruxism usually occurs in sleep and results from dental problems or stress.
4. Self-care behaviours. How are the child's dental habits? Does the child use a toothbrush regularly? How often does the child see a dentist? • Do you use fluoridated water or a fluoride supplement?	Evaluate child's self-care. When baby teeth have erupted (age 2 to 3 years), begin regular 6-month dental checkups to evaluate self-care and identify potential problems. To prevent fluorosis, adults should brush teeth of children younger than 3 years, using a smear of toothpaste. Children 3 to 6 years of age should brush with a pea-sized portion of toothpaste.
• Does the child wear a mouth protector or mouthguard when participating in sports?	Mouth protectors and mouthguards reduce the risk for damage to teeth, cheeks, lips, and tongue during sports or recreational activities.

Examiner Asks	Rationale
Additional History for Older Adults	
1. Mouth dryness. Any dryness in the mouth? How do you treat the dryness? • Are you taking any medications? What medications are you currently taking? (Note prescribed, herbal, and over-the-counter medications.)	**Xerostomia** (dry mouth) is an adverse effect of many medications: antidepressants, anticholinergics, antispasmodics, antihypertensives, antipsychotics, and bronchodilators.
2. Teeth. Have you lost any teeth? Can you chew all types of food?	Note a decrease in eating meat, fresh vegetables, and tooth-cleansing foods such as apples.
3. Mouth care. Are you able to care for your own teeth or dentures?	Self-care may be decreased by physical disability (arthritis), vision loss, confusion, or depression.
4. Taste and smell. Have you noticed a change in your sense of taste or smell?	Some people add extra salt and sugar to enhance food when taste begins to wane. Diminished smell may decrease ability to detect food spoilage, natural gas leaks, or smoke from a fire.

Subjective Data

OBJECTIVE DATA

PREPARATION
Position the patient sitting up straight with head at your eye level. If the patient wears dentures, offer a paper towel and ask the patient to remove them.

EQUIPMENT NEEDED
Otoscope with short, wide-tipped nasal speculum attachment
Penlight
Two tongue blades
Cotton gauze pad (10 × 10 cm)
Gloves*
Occasionally: long-stem light attachment for otoscope

---

*Always wear gloves to examine mucous membranes, in accordance with routine practices, to prevent spread of communicable diseases.

Objective Data

Normal Range of Findings	Abnormal Findings

Inspect and Palpate the Nose

External Nose

Normally, the nose is midline, symmetrical, and in proportion to other facial features (Fig. 17.8). Inspect for deformity, asymmetry, inflammation, or lesions. If injury reported or suspected, palpate gently for any pain or break in contour.

17.8

Test patency of nostrils by pushing each nasal wing shut with your finger while asking the person to sniff inward through the other naris. This reveals any obstruction, which later is explored using the nasal speculum. Sense of smell, mediated by cranial nerve I, is usually not tested in a routine examination. The procedure for assessing smell is described with cranial nerve testing in Chapter 25.

Absence of sniff indicates obstruction (e.g., common cold, nasal polyps, and rhinitis).

Nasal Cavity

Attach the short wide-tipped speculum to the otoscope head and insert this combined apparatus into the nasal vestibule, avoiding pressure on the nasal septum. Gently lift up the tip of the nose with your finger before inserting.

Normal Range of Findings

View each nasal cavity with the patient's head erect and then tilted back. Inspect the nasal mucosa, noting its normal red colour and smooth moist surface (Fig. 17.9). Note any swelling, discharge, bleeding, or foreign body.

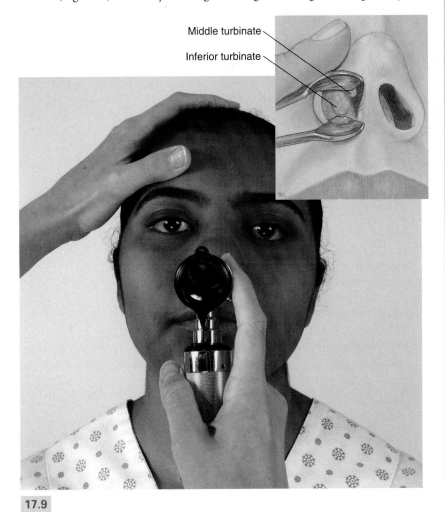

Middle turbinate

Inferior turbinate

17.9

Abnormal Findings

Nasal mucosa is swollen and bright red with rhinitis and upper respiratory infection.

Discharge is common with rhinitis and sinusitis, varying from watery and copious to thick, purulent, and green-yellow.

With chronic allergy, mucosa looks swollen, boggy, pale, and grey.

Objective Data

Normal Range of Findings

Observe the nasal septum for deviation (Fig. 17.10), which is common and only significant if air flow is obstructed. (If present in a hospitalized patient, document the deviated septum in the event the patient needs nasal suctioning or a nasogastric tube.) Also note any perforation or bleeding in the septum.

17.10   Deviated septum.

Inspect the turbinates, the bony ridges curving down from the lateral walls. The superior turbinate is not in view, but the middle and inferior turbinates appear the same light red colour as nasal mucosa. Note any swelling, but do not try to push the speculum past it. Turbinates are quite vascular and tender if touched.

Note any polyps, benign growths that accompany chronic allergy, and distinguish them from normal turbinates.

Palpate the Sinus Areas

Using your thumbs, press over the frontal sinuses below the eyebrows (Fig. 17.11, *A*) and over the maxillary sinuses below the cheekbones (see Fig. 17.11, *B*). Take care not to palpate below the bony orbitals (eye sockets) to avoid pressing the eyeballs. The patient should feel firm pressure but no pain.

A   B

17.11

Abnormal Findings

A deviated septum looks like a hump or shelf in one nasal cavity.

Perforation is visible as a spot of light from the penlight shining in the other naris and occurs with cocaine use.

Epistaxis commonly originates from the anterior septum (see Table 17.1, p. 406).

Polyps are smooth, pale grey, avascular, mobile, and nontender (see Table 17.1, p. 408).

Sinus areas are tender to palpation with chronic allergies and acute infection (sinusitis).

Normal Range of Findings	**Abnormal Findings**

Inspect the Mouth

Begin with anterior structures, and move posteriorly. Use a tongue blade to retract structures and a bright light for optimal visualization.

Lips

Inspect lips for colour, moisture, cracking, and lesions. Retract lips, and note their inner surface (Fig. 17.12). Individuals with darker complexions may normally have bluish lips and a dark line on the gingival margin.

In light-skinned people, whiteness around the lips (circumoral pallor) occurs with shock and anemia; bluish lips (cyanosis) with hypoxemia and chilling; and cherry red lips with carbon monoxide poisoning.

Cheilitis (perlèche): cracking at the corners.

Herpes simplex, other lesions (see Table 17.2, p. 408).

17.12

Teeth and Gums

The condition of the teeth is an index of the patient's general health. Your examination should not replace regular dental examination, but note any diseased, absent, loose, or abnormally positioned teeth. Teeth normally look white, straight, evenly spaced, and clean and free of debris or decay.

Compare the number of teeth with the number expected for the patient's age. Ask the patient to bite as if chewing something, and note alignment of upper and lower jaw. In normal occlusion in the back, the upper teeth rest directly on the lower teeth; in the front, the upper incisors slightly override the lower incisors.

Periodontal disease is linked to cardiovascular disease, diabetes, pulmonary infections, kidney disease, and osteoporosis.

Discoloured teeth appear brown with excessive fluoride use, and yellow with tobacco use.

Grinding down of tooth surface.

Plaque: soft debris.

Caries: decay.

Enamel erosion: eating disorder.

Malocclusion: protrusion of upper or lower incisors (see Table 17.3, p. 410).

Normal Range of Findings

Normally, the gums look pink or coral with a stippled (dotted) surface. Gum margins at the teeth are tight and well defined (Fig. 17.13). Check for swelling, retraction of gingival margins, and spongy, bleeding, or discoloured gums. Darker-skinned patients may normally have a dark melanotic line along the gingival margin.

17.13

Tongue

Check the tongue for colour, surface characteristics, and moisture. The colour is pink and even. The dorsal surface is normally roughened from the papillae. A thin white coating may be present (Fig. 17.14). Ask the patient to touch the tongue to the roof of the mouth. Its ventral surface looks smooth, glistening, and shows veins. Saliva is present.

A   B

17.14

Abnormal Findings

Gingival hyperplasia (see Table 17.3, p. 411), crevices between teeth and gums, pockets of debris.

Bleeding of gums with slight pressure indicate gingivitis.

Dark line on gingival margins occurs with lead and bismuth poisoning.

Tongue appears beefy red and swollen; some areas may be smooth and glossy (see Table 17.5, p. 414).

Enlargement of the tongue (macroglossia) occurs with allergic and anaphylactic reactions, hypothyroidism, and acromegaly. The tongue may be small with malnutrition.

Dry mouth occurs with dehydration, fever; tongue has deep vertical fissures.

Saliva is decreased by anticholinergic and other medications.

Excess saliva and drooling occur with gingivostomatitis and neurological dysfunction.

Normal Range of Findings	**Abnormal Findings**

With a glove and a cotton gauze pad for traction, gently pull out the tongue and move it to each side (Fig. 17.15). Inspect for white patches or lesions: normally, none are present. If any are present, palpate these lesions for firmness, or induration.

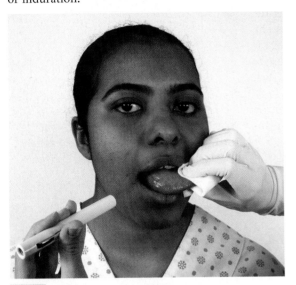

17.15

Inspect carefully the entire U-shaped area under the tongue behind the teeth. Oral malignancies are most likely to develop there. Note any white patches, nodules, or ulcerations. If lesions are present, or in any patient older than 50 years of age or with a positive history of smoking or alcohol use, use your gloved hand to palpate the area. Place your other hand under the jaw to stabilize the tissue and detect any abnormality (Fig. 17.16). Note any firmness or induration.

Any lesion or ulcer persisting for more than 2 weeks must be investigated.

A hardened area may be a mass or lymphadenopathy, and must be investigated.

17.16

Buccal Mucosa

Hold cheek open with a wooden tongue blade, and check buccal mucosa for colour, nodules, and lesions. It normally looks pink, smooth, and moist, although patchy hyperpigmentation is common and normal in dark-skinned people.

Dappled brown patches are present with Addison's disease (chronic adrenal insufficiency).

Normal Range of Findings

An expected finding is **Stensen's duct**, the opening of the parotid salivary gland. It looks like a small dimple opposite the upper second molar. You also may see a raised occlusion line on the buccal mucosa parallel with the level at which the teeth meet, caused by the teeth closing against the cheek.

Leukoedema, a benign greyish opaque area that may be present along the buccal mucosa, is more common in people of African or South Asian descent. When mild, the patch disappears as you stretch the cheeks. The severity of the condition increases with age, looking greyish white and thickened. The cause of the condition is unknown. Do not mistake leukoedema for oral infections such as candidiasis (thrush).

Fordyce's granules are small, isolated white or yellow papules on the mucosa of the cheeks, tongue, and lips (Fig. 17.17). These little sebaceous cysts are painless and not significant.

17.17 Fordyce's granules.

Palate

Shine your light on the roof of the mouth. The more anterior hard palate is white with irregular transverse rugae. The posterior soft palate is pinker, smooth, and upwardly movable. A normal variation is a nodular bony ridge, called a **torus palatinus**, down the middle of the hard palate (Fig. 17.18). This benign growth arises after puberty and is more common in Indigenous people and people of African or Asian descent.

Abnormal Findings

In mumps, the orifice of Stensen's duct becomes red.

Koplik's spots (see Table 17.4, p. 412) are an early prodromal (early warning) sign of measles.

Leukoplakia, a chalky white raised patch, is abnormal (see Table 17.4, p. 412).

Candida infection will usually rub off, leaving a clear or raw denuded surface.

With jaundice, the hard palate appears yellow. In dark-skinned people with jaundice, it may look yellow, muddy yellow, or green-brown.

Oral Kaposi's sarcoma is the most common early lesion in people with acquired immune deficiency syndrome (AIDS; see Table 17.6, p. 416).

Torus in upper hard palate

Upper lip

Mirror

17.18 Torus palatinus (viewed in a mirror).

Normal Range of Findings

Observe the uvula; it normally looks like a fleshy pendant hanging in the midline (Fig. 17.19). Ask the patient to say "ahhh," and note the soft palate and uvula rise in the midline. This is a test of one function of cranial nerve X, the vagus nerve.

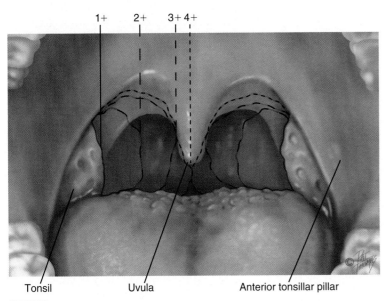

Tonsil   Uvula   Anterior tonsillar pillar

17.19 (© Pat Thomas, 2006.)

Notice any breath odour (halitosis). This is common and usually has a local cause, such as poor oral hygiene, consumption of odoriferous foods, alcohol consumption, heavy smoking, or dental infection. On occasion, it indicates systemic disease.

Inspect the Throat

With your light, observe the oval, rough-surfaced tonsils behind the anterior tonsillar pillar (see Fig. 17.19). Their colour is the same pink as the oral mucosa, and their surface is peppered with indentations, or crypts. In some people the crypts collect small plugs of whitish cellular debris. This does not indicate infection. Tonsils are graded in size as follows:

1+: Visible
2+: Halfway between tonsillar pillars and uvula
3+: Touching the uvula
4+: Touching each other

You may normally see grade 1+ or grade 2+ tonsils in healthy people, especially in children, because lymphoid tissue is proportionately enlarged until puberty.

Abnormal Findings

A **bifid uvula** looks as if it is split in two; it is more common in Indigenous people (see Table 17.6, p. 415).

Any deviation to the side or absence of movement indicates nerve damage, which also occurs with poliomyelitis and diphtheria.

Diabetic ketoacidosis produces a sweet, fruity breath odour; this acetone smell also occurs in children with malnutrition or dehydration. Other breath odours include ammonia, which occurs with uremia; a musty odour, with liver disease; a foul, fetid odour, with dental or respiratory infections; and an alcohol odour, with ingestion of alcohol or chemicals.

With acute infection, tonsils are bright red and swollen and may have exudates or large white spots.

A white membrane covering the tonsils may accompany infectious mononucleosis, leukemia, and diphtheria.

Tonsils are enlarged to 2+, 3+, or 4+ with an acute infection.

Objective Data

Normal Range of Findings

Enlarge your view of the posterior pharyngeal wall by depressing the tongue with a tongue blade (Fig. 17.20). Push down halfway back on the tongue; if you push on its tip, the tongue will hump up in back. Press slightly off-centre to avoid eliciting the gag reflex.

17.20

Scan the posterior wall for colour, exudate, or lesions. When you are finished, discard the tongue blade.

Although eliciting the gag reflex is usually not done in the screening examination, you can do so by touching the posterior wall with the tongue blade. This is a test of cranial nerves IX and X, the glossopharyngeal and vagus nerves.

Test cranial nerve XII, the hypoglossal nerve, by asking the patient to stick out the tongue. It should protrude in the midline. Children enjoy this request. Note any tremor, loss of movement, or deviation to the side.

❖ DEVELOPMENTAL CONSIDERATIONS

Infants and Children

Because the oral examination is intrusive for infants or young children, timing is best toward the end of the complete examination, along with the ear examination. If any crying episodes occur earlier, however, seize the opportunity to examine the open mouth and oropharynx.

As with the ear examination, let the parent help position the child. Place the infant supine on the examining table, with arms restrained (Fig. 17.21).

Older infants and toddlers may sit on the parent's lap, with one of the parent's hands holding the arms down and the other hand securing the child's head against the parent's chest. Although it is not often needed, the parent's leg can be used to reach over and hold the child's legs between the parent's own (Fig. 17.22).

Abnormal Findings

You can help patients with an easily triggered gag reflex by offering to let them depress their tongue with the tongue blade. (Some people can lower their own tongue, so the tongue blade is not needed.) If the tongue blade does not help to visualize the posterior wall, the patient should be asked to say "ahhh" to help.

With cranial nerve XII damage, the tongue deviates *toward* the paralyzed side.

A fine tremor of the tongue occurs with hyperthyroidism; a coarse tremor, with cerebral palsy and alcoholism.

Objective Data

| **Normal Range of Findings** | **Abnormal Findings** |

17.21

17.22

Use a game to help prepare the young child. Encourage preschool-age children to use a tongue blade to look into a puppet's mouth, or place a mirror so they can look into the mouth while you do. School-age children are usually cooperative and love to show off missing or new teeth (Fig. 17.23).

17.23

Be discriminating in your use of the tongue blade. It may be necessary for a full view of oral structures, but it produces a strong gag reflex in infants. You may avoid the tongue blade completely with cooperative preschool-age and school-age children. Try asking a young child to open the mouth "as big as a lion" and to move the tongue in different directions. To enlarge your view of the oropharynx, ask the child to stick out the tongue and "pant like a dog."

With an uncooperative young child who clenches the teeth and refuses to open the mouth, you can slide the tongue blade along the buccal mucosa and turn it between the back teeth. Push down to depress the tongue, stimulating the gag reflex. The child opens the mouth wide for a few seconds, allowing a *brief* look at the throat.

Objective Data

Normal Range of Findings	Abnormal Findings

Nose

The newborn may have milia across the nose. The nasal bridge may be flat in Indigenous children and in children of Asian or African descent. There should be no nasal flaring or narrowing with breathing.

It is essential to determine patency of the nares in the immediate newborn period because most newborns are obligate nose breathers. Nares blocked with amniotic fluid are suctioned gently with a bulb syringe. If obstruction is suspected, a small-lumen (5 to 10 Fr) catheter is passed down each naris to confirm patency.

Avoid using the nasal speculum with infants and young children. Instead, gently push up the tip of the nose with your thumb while using your other hand to shine the light into the naris. With a toddler, be alert for the possibility of a foreign body lodged in the nasal cavity (see Table 17.1, p. 406).
Palpate the sinus areas in children older than 8 years of age. In younger children, sinus areas are too small for palpation.

Mouth and Throat

A normal finding in infants is the **sucking tubercle**, a small pad in the middle of the upper lip from friction of breastfeeding or bottle-feeding. Note the number of teeth and whether this number is appropriate for the child's age. Also note pattern of eruption, position, condition, and hygiene. Use this guide for children younger than age 2 years: the child's age in months minus the number 6 should equal the expected number of deciduous teeth. Normally, all 20 deciduous teeth are in by age 2½ years. Saliva is present at 3 months of age and shows in excess with teething children.

Mobility should allow the tongue to extend at least as far as the alveolar ridge.

Note any bruising or laceration on buccal mucosa or gums of an infant or a young child.
On the palate, **Epstein pearls** are a normal finding in newborns and infants (Fig. 17.24). They are small, whitish, glistening, pearly papules on the hard palate and gums, where they look like teeth. They are small retention cysts and disappear in the first few weeks.
Bednar aphthae are traumatic areas or ulcers on the posterior hard palate on either side of the midline. They result from abrasions during sucking.

17.24   Epstein pearls.

Abnormal Findings

Nasal flaring in the infant indicates respiratory distress.

Many children with a chronic allergy have a transverse ridge across the nose, caused by wiping the nose upward with the palm (see Table 14.2, p. 294). Nasal narrowing on inhalation is seen with chronic nasal obstruction and mouth breathing.

Inability to pass a catheter through the nasal cavity indicates choanal atresia, which necessitates immediate intervention (see Table 17.1, p. 406).

No teeth by age 1 year is abnormal.

Discoloured teeth appear yellow or yellow-brown in infants taking tetracycline or whose mothers took the medication during the last trimester; they appear green or black with excessive iron ingestion, although this reverses when the iron is stopped. White specks may indicate that a child getting too much fluoride (fluorosis). It is a cosmetic condition, not health threatening.

Ankyloglossia, a short lingual frenulum, can limit tongue protrusion and impair speech development (see Table 17.5, p. 413).

Trauma may indicate forced feeding of bottle or spoon, which may be child abuse.

A high-arched palate is usually normal in newborns, but a very narrow or very high arch also occurs with Turner's syndrome, Ehlers-Danlos syndrome, Marfan's syndrome, and Treacher Collins syndrome. It also develops in mouth-breathers with chronic allergies, and from thumb-sucking.

Nursing bottle caries are brown discolorations on upper front teeth (see photo in Table 17.3, p. 410).

Normal Range of Findings	Abnormal Findings

Tonsils are not visible in newborns. They gradually enlarge during childhood, remaining proportionately larger until puberty. Tonsils appear even larger in an infant who is crying or gagging. Normally, newborns can produce a strong, lusty cry.

Insert your gloved finger into the baby's mouth and palpate the hard and soft palates as the baby sucks. The sucking reflex can be elicited in infants up to 12 months of age.

As teeth begin to erupt in the older infant and child, check age at eruption, sequence, and condition. Teeth should emerge straight up or down from the gums, and enamel should be clear white and smooth. Lift the upper lip to check for dental caries (tooth decay); normally there are none.

Pregnant Women

Gum hypertrophy (surface looks smooth and stippling disappears) may occur normally at puberty or during pregnancy (pregnancy gingivitis; Fig. 17.25). Gums may bleed as a result of increased hormone production, which causes increased vascularity and fragility. Proper oral hygiene and healthy food choices help prevent pregnancy gingivitis.

17.25   Early gingivitis.

Older Adults

The nose may appear more prominent on the face from loss of subcutaneous fat. In edentulous patients, the mouth and lips fold in, giving a "purse-string" appearance. Teeth may look slightly yellowed, although the colour is uniform, as dentin becomes visible through worn enamel. The surface of incisors may show vertical cracks from a lifetime of exposure to extreme temperatures. Teeth may look longer as gum margins recede (Fig. 17.26).

Tooth surfaces look worn down or abraded. Old dental work deteriorates, especially at gum margins. Teeth loosen with bone resorption and may move with palpation.

The tongue looks smoother due to papillary atrophy. An older adult's buccal mucosa is thinned and may look shinier, as though it were varnished.

17.26   Receded gums.

Objective Data

DOCUMENTATION AND CRITICAL THINKING

Sample Charting

SUBJECTIVE

Nose: No history of discharge, sinus problems, obstruction, epistaxis, allergy, or altered smell. Colds: one to two per year, mild. Nose fractured during high school sports, treated by MD.

Mouth and throat: No pain, lesions, bleeding gums, toothache, teeth grinding, hoarseness, dysphagia, altered taste, or sleep apnea. Occasional sore throat with colds. Tonsillectomy, age 8. Drinks 1 diet pop daily. Smokes cigarettes 1 PPD × 9 years. Alcohol: one to two drinks socially, about 2×/month. Visits dentist annually, dental hygienist 2×/year, flosses daily. No dental appliance.

OBJECTIVE

Nose: Symmetrical, no deformity or skin lesions. Nares patent. Mucosa pink; no discharge, lesions, or polyps; no septal deviation or perforation. Sinuses: no tenderness to palpation.

Mouth: Can clench teeth. No malocclusion. Lips: pink and moist with no lesions. Mucosa and gingivae pink, no masses or lesions. Teeth are all present, straight, and in good repair. Tongue smooth, pink, no lesions, protrudes in midline, no tremor.

Throat: Mucosa pink, no lesions or exudate. Uvula rises in midline on phonation. Tonsils out. Gag reflex present.

ASSESSMENT

Structures intact and appear healthy

Focused Assessment: Clinical Case Study 1

Brad Mikwabi (B.M.), a 34-year-old First Nations man, seeks care for "sore throat for 2 days."

SUBJECTIVE

2 days PTA [prior to arrival]: B.M. experienced sudden onset of sore throat, swollen glands, fever 38.6°C (101°F), occasional shaking chills, extreme fatigue.

Today: Symptoms remain. Cough productive of yellow sputum. Treated self with Aspirin with minimal relief. Unable to eat past 2 days because "throat on fire." Taking adequate fluids, on bed rest. Not aware of exposure to other sick persons. Does not smoke.

OBJECTIVE

Nose: No discharge. Mucosa pink, no swelling.
Mouth: Mucosa and gingivae pink, no lesions.
Throat: Tonsils 3+. Pharyngeal wall bright red with yellow-white exudate; exudate also on tonsils.
Neck: Enlarged anterior cervical nodes bilaterally, painful to palpation. No other lymphadenopathy.
Chest: Resonant to percussion throughout. Breath sounds clear anterior and posterior. No adventitious sounds.

DIAGNOSTIC TESTS

Throat swab taken for throat culture and sensitivity was positive for group A β-hemolytic *Streptococcus* species.

ASSESSMENT

Bacterial pharyngitis
Pain R/T [related to] inflammation
Imbalanced nutrition: less than body requirements R/T dysphagia

Focused Assessment: Clinical Case Study 2

Yousef Abadi (Y.A.), a 53-year-old recent refugee from Syria, is in hospital awaiting coronary bypass surgery for coronary artery disease. He is allergic to dust and animal hair. He does not smoke or drink alcohol. As part of a preoperative teaching plan for coughing and deep breathing, a respiratory assessment is performed.

SUBJECTIVE

Through a translator, Y.A. states understanding of reason for admission and extent of coronary artery disease. Unaware of details of surgical procedure and postoperative care. Interested: "I do better when I know what I'm dealing with." History of exertional angina after walking one short block or climbing one flight of stairs, treats self with nitroglycerine. Does not smoke. Chronic watery nasal discharge, "comes and goes, but present most of the time." Denies dysphagia, sleep apnea, or bleeding gums.

OBJECTIVE

Nose: Only R [right] naris patent. Mucosa grey and boggy bilaterally. L [left] naris has mobile, grey, nontender mass, obstructing view of turbinates and rest of nasal cavity.
Mouth and throat: Mucosa pink, no lesions. Uvula midline, rises on phonation. Tonsils absent. No lumps or lesions on palpation.
Chest: Thorax symmetrical, AP [anteroposterior] < transverse diameter, resp 18/min, effortless. Resonant to percussion. Breath sounds are clear. No adventitious sounds.

ASSESSMENT

L nasal mass, possibly polyp
Deficient knowledge for surgery and expected postoperative course R/T lack of exposure

Focused Assessment: Clinical Case Study 3

Elaine Valieri (E.V.) is a 61-year-old professor who was admitted to hospital for chemotherapy for carcinoma of the breast. On her fifth day in hospital, an oral assessment is performed and she complains of "soreness and a white coating" in the mouth.

SUBJECTIVE

Felt soreness on tongue and cheeks during night. Now pain persists, and E.V. can see a "white coating" on tongue and cheeks. "I'm really worried. I hope this isn't more cancer."

OBJECTIVE

E.V. appears restless and apprehensive.
Oral mucosa is pink. Large white, cheesy patches covering most of dorsal surface of tongue and buccal mucosa. Scrapes off with tongue blade, revealing red eroded area beneath.
Bleeds with slight contact. Posterior pharyngeal wall pink, no lesions. Patches soft to palpation. No palpable lymph nodes.

ASSESSMENT

Oral lesion, appears as candidiasis
Impaired oral mucous membrane R/T effects of chemotherapy
Pain R/T infectious process
Restlessness R/T threat to health status

Documentation
and Critical Thinking

ABNORMAL FINDINGS

TABLE 17.1 Abnormalities of the Nose

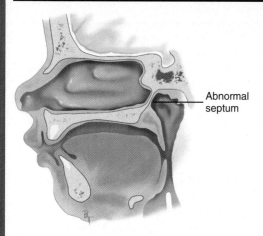

Abnormal septum

Choanal Atresia

A bony or membranous septum between the nasal cavity and pharynx of the newborn. When the condition is bilateral, an oral airway must be established immediately to prevent asphyxia because most newborns are obligate nose breathers. When the condition is unilateral, the infant may have no symptoms until onset of first respiratory infection.

Epistaxis

The most common site of a nosebleed is Kiesselbach's plexus in the anterior septum. It may be spontaneous from a local cause or a sign of underlying illness. Causes include nose picking, forceful coughing or sneezing, fracture, foreign body, rhinitis, heavy exertion, or coagulation disorder. Bleeding from the anterior septum is easily controlled and rarely severe. Posterior hemorrhage is less common (<10% of cases) but more profuse, harder to manage, and more serious.

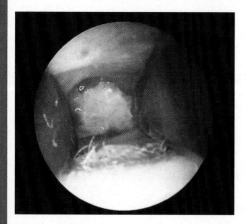

Foreign Body

Children are particularly apt to put an object up the nose (here, yellow plastic foam), which leads to unilateral mucopurulent drainage and foul odour. Because of some risk for aspiration, removal should be prompt.

Perforated Septum

A hole in the septum, usually in the cartilaginous part, may be caused by snorting cocaine, chronic infection, trauma from continual picking of crusts, or nasal surgery. It is seen directly or as a spot of light when a penlight is directed into the other naris.

TABLE 17.1 **Abnormalities of the Nose—cont'd**

(Reprinted from Fireman, P. (1995). *Atlas of allergies* (2nd ed.). St. Louis: Mosby, by permission of the publisher.)

Furuncle

A small boil located in the skin or mucous membrane; appears red and swollen and is quite painful. Avoid any manipulation or trauma that may spread the infection.

Acute Rhinitis

The first sign is a clear, watery discharge—rhinorrhea—which later becomes purulent. This is accompanied by sneezing and swollen mucosa, which causes nasal obstruction. Turbinates are dark red and swollen.

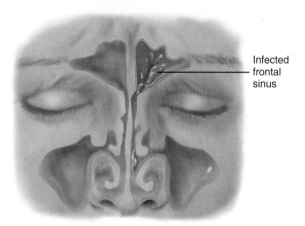

Infected frontal sinus

Allergic Rhinitis

Rhinorrhea, itching of nose and eyes, lacrimation, nasal congestion, and sneezing are present. Note serous edema and swelling of turbinates to fill the air space. Turbinates are usually pale (but may appear violet), and their surface looks smooth and glistening. May be seasonal or perennial, depending on allergen. Affected individual often has strong family history of seasonal allergies.

Sinusitis

Facial pain, after upper respiratory infection; signs include red swollen nasal mucosa, swollen turbinates, and purulent discharge. Patient also has fever, chills, and malaise. With maxillary sinusitis, dull throbbing pain occurs in cheeks and teeth on the same side, and pain with palpation is present. With frontal sinusitis, pain is above the supraorbital ridge.

Continued

TABLE 17.1	Abnormalities of the Nose—cont'd

◀ Nasal Polyps

Smooth, pale grey nodules, which are overgrowths of mucosa, most commonly caused by chronic allergic rhinitis. May be stalked. A common site is protrusion from the middle meatus. Often multiple, they are mobile and nontender in contrast to turbinates. They may obstruct air passageways as they enlarge. Symptoms include absence of a sense of smell and a "valve that moves" in the nose as the patient breathes.

See Illustration Credits for source information.

TABLE 17.2	Abnormalities of the Lips

Cleft Lip

Maxillofacial clefts are the most common congenital deformities of the head and neck. Incidence varies widely among ethnocultural groups, with a higher frequency among Indigenous people than people of European descent.[a] Early treatment preserves functions of speech, language formation, and deglutition (swallowing).

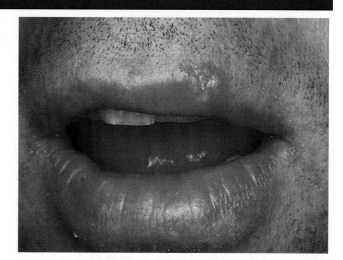

Herpes Simplex 1

"Cold sores" are groups of clear vesicles with a surrounding indurated erythematous base. These evolve into pustules, which rupture, weep, crust, and heal in 4–10 days. The most likely site is the lip–skin junction; infection often recurs in same site. Caused by herpes simplex virus (HSV-1), the lesion is highly contagious and spreads by direct contact. Recurrent herpes infections may be precipitated by sunlight, fever, colds, and allergy. It is very common, affecting 50% of adults.

TABLE 17.2	**Abnormalities of the Lips—cont'd**

Angular Cheilitis (Stomatitis, Perlèche)

Erythema, scaling, and shallow, painful fissures at the corners of the mouth occur with excess salivation and *Candida* infection. Cheilitis is often seen in edentulous patients and those with poorly fitting dentures, causing the corners of the mouth to fold in, creating a warm, moist environment favourable for the growth of yeast.

Carcinoma

The initial lesion is round and indurated, then becomes crusted and ulcerated with an elevated border. The majority occur between the outer and middle thirds of the lip. Any lesion unhealed after 2 weeks should be investigated.

◄ Retention "Cyst" (Mucocele)

A round, well-defined translucent nodule that may be very small or up to 2 cm in diameter. It is a pocket of mucus that forms when a duct of a minor salivary gland ruptures. The benign lesion also may occur on the buccal mucosa, on the floor of the mouth, or under the tip of the tongue.

[a]Bluestone, C. D., Simons, J. P., and Healy, G. B. (2014). *Pediatric otolaryngology* (5th ed.). Shelton, CT: PMPH USA. See Illustration Credits for source information.

TABLE 17.3 Abnormalities of the Teeth and Gums

Baby Bottle Tooth Decay

Destruction of numerous deciduous teeth may occur in older infants and toddlers who take a bottle of milk, juice, or sweetened drink to bed and prolong bottle-feeding past 1 year of age. Liquid pools around the upper front teeth. Mouth bacteria act on carbohydrates in the liquid, especially sucrose, forming metabolic acids. Acids break down tooth enamel and destroy its protein.

Malocclusion

Upper or lower dental arches are not in alignment, and incisors protrude as a result of a developmental problem of the mandible or maxilla or because of incompatibility between jaw size and tooth size. The condition increases risk for facial deformity, negative body image, chewing problems, and speech dysfluency.

Dental Caries

Progressive destruction of tooth. Decay initially looks chalky white. Later, it turns brown or black and forms a cavity. Early decay is apparent only on radiographs. Susceptible sites are tooth surfaces where food debris, bacterial plaque, and saliva collect.

Epulis

A nontender, fibrous nodule of the gum, seen emerging between the teeth (*arrow*); an inflammatory response to injury or hemorrhage.

TABLE 17.3   **Abnormalities of the Teeth and Gums—cont'd**

Gingival Hyperplasia

Painless enlargement of the gums, sometimes overreaching the teeth. It occurs with puberty, pregnancy, leukemia, and long-term therapeutic use of phenytoin (Dilantin).

Gingivitis

Gum margins are red and swollen, and bleed easily. This case is severe; gingival tissue has desquamated, exposing roots of teeth. Inflammation is usually a result of poor dental hygiene or vitamin C deficiency. The condition may occur in pregnancy and puberty because of changing hormonal balance.

◀ Meth Mouth

Illicit methamphetamine abuse ("crystal meth," "meth ice") leads to extensive dental caries, gingivitis, tooth cracking, and tooth loss. Methamphetamine causes vasoconstriction and a decrease in saliva, and it increases the urge to consume sugars and starches and to neglect oral hygiene. Absence of the buffering saliva leads to increased acidity in the mouth, and increased plaque encourages bacterial growth. These conditions and presence of carbohydrates set up an oral environment prone to caries, cracking of enamel, and the damage seen here.

See Illustration Credits for source information.

TABLE 17.4 Abnormalities of the Buccal Mucosa

Aphthous Ulcers

Also called *chancre sore*; they are vesicles at first and then become small, round, "punched-out" ulcers with a white base surrounded by a red halo. They are quite painful and last for 1 to 2 weeks. The cause is unknown, although they are associated with stress, fatigue, and food allergy. They are common, affecting 20–60% of the population.

Koplik's Spots

Small blue-white spots with irregular red halo that are scattered over mucosa opposite the molars. They are an early sign, and pathognomonic, of measles.

Leukoplakia

Chalky white, thick, raised patch with well-defined borders. The lesion is firmly attached and cannot be scraped off. It may occur on the lateral edges of tongue. It is caused by chronic irritation and occurs more frequently with heavy smoking and heavy alcohol use. Lesions are precancerous, and the patient should be referred. Here, the lesion is associated with squamous carcinoma.

Candidiasis or Monilial Infection

A white, cheesy, curdlike patch on the buccal mucosa and tongue. It scrapes off, leaving a raw, red surface that bleeds easily. Termed *thrush* in newborns. It is an opportunistic infection that occurs after the use of antibiotics or corticosteroids and in immunosuppressed patients.

TABLE 17.4   Abnormalities of the Buccal Mucosa—cont'd

◀ **Herpes Simplex 1**

Herpes infection on the hard palate (see discussion in Table 17.2, p. 408).

See Illustration Credits for source information.

TABLE 17.5   Abnormalities of the Tongue

Ankyloglossia

Also known as *tongue-tie.* A short lingual frenulum, here fixing the tongue tip to the floor of the mouth and gums. This limits mobility and will affect speech (pronunciation of *a, d, n*) if the tongue tip cannot be elevated to the alveolar ridge. A congenital defect.

Fissured or Scrotal Tongue

Deep furrows divide the papillae into small irregular rows. The condition occurs in 5% of the general population and in Down syndrome. The incidence increases with age. (Vertical, or longitudinal, fissures also occur with dehydration because of reduced volume of the tongue.)

Continued

TABLE 17.5 **Abnormalities of the Tongue—cont'd**

Geographic Tongue (Migratory Glossitis)

Pattern of normal coating interspersed with bright red, shiny, circular bald areas with raised pearly borders. The pattern resembles a map that changes as lesions heal in one area and migrate to a different area of the tongue. Not significant, and its cause is not known.

Smooth, Glossy Tongue (Atrophic Glossitis)

The surface is slick and shiny; the mucosa thins and looks red as a result of decreased papillae. Accompanied by dryness of tongue and burning sensation. Occurs with vitamin B_{12} deficiency (pernicious anemia), folic acid deficiency, and iron-deficiency anemia. Here, also note angular cheilitis.

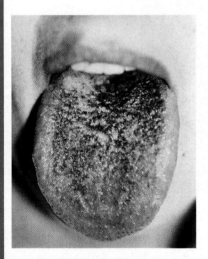

Black Hairy Tongue

The black appearance is not really hair but the elongation of filiform papillae and painless overgrowth of mycelial threads of fungus infection on the tongue. Colour varies from black-brown to yellow. It occurs after use of antibiotics, which inhibit normal bacteria and allow proliferation of fungus.

Enlarged Tongue (Macroglossia)

The tongue is enlarged and may protrude from the mouth. The condition is not painful but may impair speech development. Here, it occurs with Down syndrome; it also occurs with cretinism, myxedema, and acromegaly. Also, a transient swelling can occur with local infections.

TABLE 17.5	Abnormalities of the Tongue—cont'd

◄ Carcinoma

An ulcer with rolled edges; indurated. It occurs particularly at sides, base, and under the tongue. When it is in the floor of the mouth, it may cause tongue movement to be painful or limited. Risk for early metastasis is high because of rich lymphatic drainage. Heavy smoking and heavy alcohol use increase the risk.

See Illustration Credits for source information.

TABLE 17.6	Abnormalities of the Oropharynx

Cleft Palate

A congenital defect involving the failure of fusion of the maxillary processes. Wide variation occurs in the extent of cleft formation: from upper lip only, palate only, or uvula only to clefts of the nostril and the hard and soft palates.

Bifid Uvula

The uvula looks partly severed. May indicate a submucous cleft palate, which feels like a notch at the junction of the hard and soft palates. The submucous cleft palate may affect speech development because it prevents necessary air trapping. The incidence of bifid uvula is higher among Indigenous people.

Continued

Abnormal Findings

TABLE 17.6	Abnormalities of the Oropharynx—cont'd

Oral Kaposi's Sarcoma

Bruiselike, dark red or violet, confluent macule, usually on the hard palate, may be on soft palate or gingival margin. Oral lesions may be the earliest lesions to develop with AIDS.

Acute Tonsillitis and Pharyngitis

Bright red throat; swollen tonsils; white or yellow exudate on tonsils and pharynx; swollen uvula; and enlarged, tender anterior cervical and tonsillar nodes. Accompanied by severe sore throat, painful swallowing, and fever (temperature >38.3°C [101°F]) of sudden onset.

Caution: Bacterial infection cannot be distinguished from viral infection on the basis of clinical data alone; all patients with sore throats need a throat culture. Bacterial pharyngitis caused by group A β-hemolytic *Streptococcus* species, if untreated, may lead to the complication of rheumatic fever. This is a serious, complex illness characterized by fever, malaise, swollen joints, rash, and scarring of heart valves.

AIDS, Acquired immune deficiency syndrome.
See Illustration Credits for source information.

Summary Checklist: Nose, Mouth, and Throat Examination

Nose
1. **Inspect external nose:**
   Symmetry
   Any deformity
   Lesions
2. **Palpate nostrils:**
   Patency of each nostril
3. **Inspect internal nose with nasal speculum:**
   Nasal mucosa: colour, integrity

Septum: any deviation, perforation, bleeding
Turbinates: colour, exudates, swelling, polyps
4. **Palpate sinus areas:**
   Tenderness

Mouth and Throat
1. **Inspect with penlight:**
   Lips, teeth, gums, tongue, buccal mucosa: colour; whether structures are intact; any lesions

Palate and uvula: integrity, mobility as patient phonates
Tonsils: grade tonsils
Pharyngeal wall: colour, exudate, lesions
2. **Palpate the mouth:**
   When indicated in adults, palpate mouth bimanually
   With the neonate, palpate for integrity of palate, and to assess sucking reflex

REFERENCES

1. Duncan, L., & Bonner, A. (2014). Effects of income and dental insurance need for dental care in Canada. *Journal of Canadian Dental Association, 80*, e6. Retrieved from http://www.jcda.ca/article/e6.
2. Canadian Academy of Health Sciences. (2014). *Improving access to oral health care for vulnerable people living in Canada.* Retrieved from http://cahs-acss.ca/wp-content/uploads/2015/07/Access_to_Oral_Care_FINAL_REPORT_EN.pdf.
3. Schroth, R. J., Quinonez, C., Shwart, L., et al. (2016). Treating early childhood caries under general anesthesia: A national review of Canadian data. *Journal of Canadian Dental Association, 82*, g20. Retrieved from http://www.jcda.ca/g20.
4. Reza, M., Amin, M. S., Sgro, A., et al. (2016). Oral health status of immigrant and refugee children in North America: A scoping review. *Journal of Canadian Dental Association, 82*, g3. Retrieved from http://www.jcda.ca/article/g3.
5. Federal, Provincial and Territorial Dental Working Group. (2014). *Reducing dental disease: A Canadian oral health framework 2013–2018.* Retrieved from https://www.caphd.ca/sites/default/files/FrameworkOctober%202014%20-%20FINAL%20English.pdf.
6. Duval Smith, F. (2016). Caring for surgical patients with piercings. *Association of Perioperative Nurses Journal, 103*(6), 584–593. doi:10.1016/j.aorn.2016.04.005.
7. Brisebois, T. D., Marsden, S., Anderson, G. H., et al. (2014). Estimated intakes and sources of total and added sugars in the Canadian diet. *Nutrients, 6*(5), 1899–1912.
8. Flowers, H. L., Silver, F. L., Fang, J., et al. (2013). The incidence, co-occurrence, and predictors of dysphagia, dysarthria, and aphasia after first-ever acute ischemic stroke. *Journal of Communication Disorders, 46*(3), 238–248. doi: https://doi.org/10.1016/j.jcomdis.2013.04.001.
9. Yang, Y., & Chung, F. (2013). A screening tool of obstructive sleep apnea: STOP-Bang questionnaire. *Sleep Medicine Clinics, 8*(1), 65–72. doi:10.1016/j.jsmc.2012.11.004.

18 | CHAPTER

Breasts and Regional Lymphatic System

Written by Carolyn Jarvis, PhD, APN, CNP
Adapted by Erin Wilson, PhD, MSN, NP(F)

ⓔ http://evolve.elsevier.com/Canada/Jarvis/examination/

The assessment of breast health is always performed in the context of health promotion; it offers a prime opportunity for teaching about health promotion and preventive health care practices related to women's health in general, as well as breast health more specifically. Most women and some men are well aware of the prevalence of breast cancer and are motivated to have regular breast examinations and to follow their health practitioner's health promotion and disease prevention recommendations.

STRUCTURE AND FUNCTION

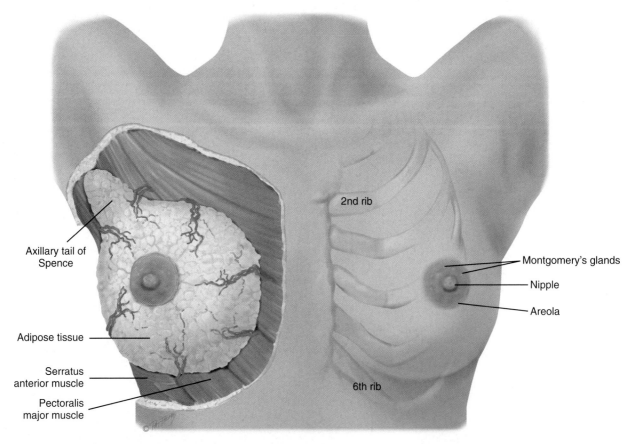

18.1   (© Pat Thomas, 2010.)

18.2

The breasts, or mammary glands, are present in both women and men, although in men they are rudimentary throughout life. The female breasts are accessory reproductive organs with a function of producing milk for nourishing the newborn.

SURFACE ANATOMY

The **breasts** lie anterior to the pectoralis major and serratus anterior muscles (Fig. 18.1). The breasts are located between the second and sixth ribs, extending from the side of the sternum to the midaxillary line. The superior lateral corner of breast tissue, called the axillary **tail of Spence**, projects up and laterally into the axilla.

The **nipple** is just below the centre of the breast. It is rough, round, and usually protuberant; its surface looks wrinkled and is indented with tiny milk duct openings. The **areola** surrounds the nipple for a 1- to 2-cm radius. In the areola are small elevated sebaceous glands, called Montgomery's glands. These glands secrete a protective lipid material during lactation. The areola also has smooth muscle fibres that cause nipple erection when stimulated. Both the nipple and areola are more darkly pigmented than the rest of the breast surface; the colour varies from pink to brown, depending on the person's skin colour and parity.

INTERNAL ANATOMY

The breast is composed of (a) glandular tissue; (b) fibrous tissue, including the suspensory ligaments; and (c) adipose tissue (Fig. 18.2). The **glandular tissue** contains 15 to 20 lobes radiating from the nipple, and these are composed of lobules. Within each lobule are clusters of **alveoli** that produce milk. Each lobe empties into a **lactiferous** duct. The 15 to 20 lactiferous ducts form a collecting duct system that converges at the nipple. There, the ducts form ampullae, or lactiferous sinuses, behind the nipple, which are reservoirs for storing milk.

The suspensory ligaments, or **Cooper's ligaments**, are fibrous bands extending vertically from the surface to attach on chest wall muscles. These support the breast tissue. They become contracted in cancer of the breast, which produces pits or dimples in the overlying skin.

The lobes are embedded in **adipose tissue**. These layers of subcutaneous and retromammary fat actually provide most of the bulk of the breast. The relative proportions of glandular, fibrous, and fatty tissue vary, depending on age, cycle, pregnancy, lactation, and general nutritional state.

The breast may be viewed as four quadrants, with imaginary horizontal and vertical lines intersecting at the nipple (Fig. 18.3). This mapping is convenient for describing clinical findings. The upper outer quadrant includes the axillary tail of Spence, the cone-shaped breast tissue that projects up into the axilla, close to the pectoral group of axillary lymph nodes. The upper outer quadrant is the site of most breast tumours.

LYMPHATIC SYSTEM

The breast has extensive lymphatic drainage. Lymph is a protein rich fluid that passes into the interstitium via oncotic

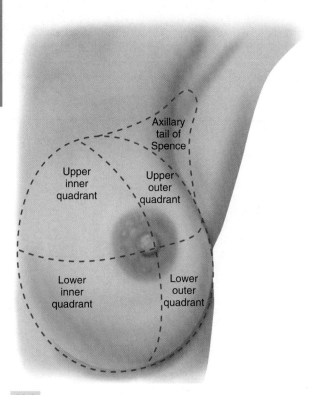

18.3

and hydrostatic pressures, and unidirectional flow of lymph once in the lymphatic system is dependent on valves.[1] Most of the lymph, more than 75%, drains into the ipsilateral (same side) axillary nodes. Four groups of axillary nodes are present (Fig. 18.4):

1. **Central axillary nodes**: high up in the middle of the axilla, over the ribs and serratus anterior muscle. These receive lymph from the other three groups of nodes.
2. **Pectoral** (anterior): along the lateral edge of the pectoralis major muscle, just inside the anterior axillary fold.
3. **Subscapular** (posterior): along the lateral edge of the scapula, deep in the posterior axillary fold.
4. **Lateral**: along the humerus, inside the upper arm.

From the central axillary nodes, lymph flows up to the infraclavicular and supraclavicular nodes.

A smaller amount of lymph does not drain through these channels but flows directly up to the infraclavicular group, deep into the chest, or into the abdomen, or directly across to the opposite breast.

❖ DEVELOPMENTAL CONSIDERATIONS

During embryonic life, ventral epidermal ridges, or "milk lines," are present; these curve down from the axilla to the

18.4

Supernumerary nipple

18.5

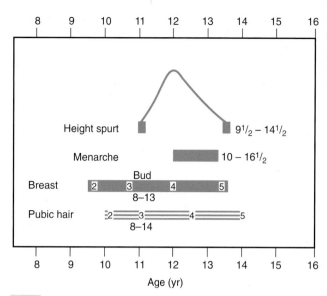

18.6 Relationship of puberty events in girls.

groin bilaterally (Fig. 18.5). The breast develops along the ridge over the thorax, and the rest of the ridge usually atrophies. On occasion, a **supernumerary nipple** (i.e., an extra nipple) persists and is visible somewhere along the track of the mammary ridge (see Fig. 18.8 on p. 431).

At birth, the only breast structures present are the lactiferous ducts within the nipple. No alveoli have developed. Little change occurs until puberty.

Adolescents

At puberty, the estrogen hormones stimulate breast changes. The breasts enlarge, mostly as a result of extensive fat deposition. The duct system also grows and branches, and masses of small, solid cells develop at the duct endings. These are potential alveoli.

On occasion, one breast grows faster than the other, which results in a temporary asymmetry. This may cause some distress; reassurance is necessary that this is a normal finding. Tenderness in the developing breasts is also common. Although the age at onset varies widely, the breasts develop in five stages according to the classic description of sexual maturity rating, or **Tanner staging** (Table 18.1).

Full development from stage 2 to stage 5 takes an average of 3 years, although the range is 1.5 to 6 years. During this time, pubic hair appears, and axillary hair appears 2 years after the appearance of pubic hair. **Thelarche**, the beginning of breast development, precedes **menarche** (beginning of menstruation) by about 2 years. Menarche occurs during breast development stage 3 or 4, usually just after the peak of the adolescent growth spurt, at approximately 12 years of age. Note the relationship of these events (Fig. 18.6). This aids in assessing the development of adolescent girls and increases their knowledge about their own development.

Breasts of nonpregnant women change with the ebb and flow of hormones during the monthly menstrual cycle. Nodularity increases from midcycle up to menstruation. During the 3 to 4 days before menstruation, the breasts feel full, tight, heavy, and occasionally sore. The breast volume is smallest on days 4 to 7 of the menstrual cycle.

Pregnant Women

During pregnancy, breast changes start during the second month and are an early sign of pregnancy for most women. Pregnancy stimulates the expansion of the ductal system and supporting fatty tissue, as well as development of the true secretory alveoli. Thus the breasts enlarge and feel more nodular. The nipples are larger, darker, and more erectile, and the areolae become larger and darken as pregnancy progresses. (The colour fades after lactation, but the areolae never return to the original colour.) The tubercles become more prominent. A venous pattern is prominent over the skin surface (see Fig. 30.4 on p. 867).

After the fourth month, **colostrum** may be expressed. This thick yellow fluid is the precursor of milk, containing the same amount of protein and lactose but practically no fat. The breasts produce colostrum for the first few days after delivery. It is rich with antibodies that protect the newborn against infection, and is one reason that breastfeeding is important. Milk production (lactation) begins 1 to 3 days postpartum. The whitish colour of the milk is caused by the presence of emulsified fat and calcium caseinate.

Older Women

After menopause, ovarian secretion of estrogen and progesterone decreases, which causes the breast glandular tissue to atrophy. This is replaced with fibrous connective tissue. The fat envelope also atrophies, beginning in the middle years and becoming marked in the eighth and ninth decades. These changes decrease breast size and elasticity, so that the breasts may droop or sag. Drooping is accentuated by the kyphosis in some older women.

Structure and Function

TABLE 18.1 Sexual Maturity Rating in Girls		
Stage 1 (preadolescent): Only a small elevated nipple is present.		
Stage 2 (breast bud stage): A small mound of breast and nipple develops; the areola widens.		
Stage 3: The breast and areola enlarge; the nipple is flush with the breast surface.		
Stage 4: The areola and nipple form a secondary mound over the breast.		
Stage 5 (mature breast): Only the nipple protrudes; the areola is flush with the breast contour (the areola may continue as a secondary mound in some normal women).		

See Illustration Credits for source information.

As a result of decreased breast size, the inner structures become more prominent. A breast lump that may have been present for years but not detected becomes palpable. Around the nipple, the lactiferous ducts are more palpable and feel firm and stringy because of fibrosis and calcification. The axillary hair decreases.

THE MALE BREAST

The male breast is a rudimentary structure consisting of a thin disc of undeveloped tissue underlying the nipple. The areola is well developed, although the nipple is relatively very small. During adolescence, it is common for the breast tissue to temporarily enlarge; such enlargement represents **gynecomastia** (see Fig. 18.21 on p. 438). This condition is usually unilateral and temporary. Reassurance is necessary for adolescent boys, to whom body image is extremely important. Gynecomastia may reappear in older men and may be a result of testosterone deficiency.

🌎 SOCIAL DETERMINANTS OF HEALTH CONSIDERATIONS

Few health initiatives across Canada have been taken up by the public in the way that women's breast screening has. Breast cancer is being diagnosed at earlier stages of cancer

TABLE 18.2 Risk Factors for Breast Cancer

UNMODIFIABLE RISK FACTORS	MODIFIABLE RISK FACTORS	POSSIBLE RISK FACTORS[a]
Female sex, age between 50 and 69 years	Nulliparity or first child after age 30 years	Physical inactivity
Personal history of breast cancer	Hormonal contraceptive use	Adult weight gain
Family history of breast cancer	Hormone replacement therapy	Smoking and second-hand smoke exposure
Dense breasts	Alcohol intake of ≥1 drink daily	
BRCA gene mutation	Obesity	High birth weight
Ashkenazi Jewish ancestry	High socioeconomic status	Night shift work
Specific rare genetic conditions		Certain benign breast conditions
Early menarche (before age 11 years) or late menopause (age 55 or older)		
Exposure to ionizing radiation		
Atypical hyperplasia		
Tall adult height		

[a]Although possible risk factors have some association with breast cancer, evidence at the time of publication is insufficient to identify these as known risk factors.

Data adapted from Canadian Cancer Society. (2018). *Risk factors for breast cancer.* Retrieved from http://www.cancer.ca/en/cancer-information/cancer-type/breast/risks/?region=on.

development with more than 80% of female breast cancers diagnosed at either Stage I or II.[2] Combined with increased screening mammography, more effective therapies after breast surgery, and a decline in women using hormone replacement therapy, the incidence of breast cancer has remained relatively stable and mortality has declined.[3] Despite these successes, breast cancer remains the most common cancer in women.[3]

The lifetime risk for breast cancer in Canada is approximately 1 per 8, and 1 per 30 women may be expected to die from breast cancer. The five year survival rate is 87%.[3] Incidence and mortality rates for breast cancer, and related risk factors, are heavily influenced by socioeconomic level, ethnocultural background, rural location, and inequities in access to health services. For example, women of higher socioeconomic status have a slightly increased risk for breast cancer; researchers speculate that this may be related to an average older age at childbearing, having fewer children, or a greater likelihood of receiving postmenopausal hormone replacement therapy.[3] However, researchers and health care providers are focusing increasingly on how social determinants of health, such as low socioeconomic level, education, living in a rural or remote area, and ethnocultural background, along with an identified lack of culturally safe health service options, present barriers to women's access to and use of health care resources.

Globally, cancer mortality among Indigenous peoples is increasing, but these populations, including Indigenous women in Canada, commonly underuse cancer-screening services.[4] Factors that contribute to the underscreening of Indigenous women include difficulty accessing services in rural or remote locations, past negative experiences with the health care system, and a lack of understanding or apprehension about the procedure. Similarly, research shows that many South Asian immigrant women in Canada are underscreened in relation to mammography because of language barriers, lack of transportation options, and lack of familiarity with the procedure.[5,6] Peer leaders and lay health educators can be effective in helping women navigate language barriers and increase women's sense of comfort and ease with mammography services.[6] Providing linguistic support and accompaniment to group screening sessions have been identified as particularly crucial to increase screening rates. These strategies are likely to be applicable to other groups of women who are also underscreened.

The growing obesity "epidemic" in Canada has important implications for breast cancer risk: obesity is an identified risk factor for breast cancer (Table 18.2). Although obesity is an identified breast cancer risk factor, and increased body mass index is associated with poor prognosis for breast cancer,[7] the relationship of breast cancer to dietary fat is not yet clear. It is clear, however, that the relationship between obesity, high-fat diets, and breast cancer has implications for Canadians who consume a "typical" high-fat North American–style diet and, in particular, for those who lack the socioeconomic resources to eat more nutritious foods. For example, Indigenous people living in northern and remote communities may not be able to make more nutritious food choices because of both the high cost and the lack of availability of such foods in their communities.

SUBJECTIVE DATA

Breast

1. Pain	5. Swelling	8. Surgery
2. Lump	6. Trauma	9. Self-care behaviours
3. Discharge	7. History of breast disease, and	Perform breast self-examination
4. Rash	breast cancer risk factors	Last mammogram

Axilla

1. Tenderness, lump, or swelling
2. Rash

In Western culture, the female breasts signify more than their primary purpose of lactation. Women are surrounded by messages that feminine norms of beauty and desirability are enhanced by and dependent on the size of the breasts and their appearance. Women leaders have tried to refocus this attitude, stressing women's self-worth as individual human beings, not as stereotyped sexual objects. The intense cultural emphasis is gradually changing, but the breasts still are crucial to many women's self-concept and their perception of their femininity. Matters pertaining to the breast affect a woman's body image and generate deep emotional responses.

This emotionality may take strong forms that you observe as you discuss the woman's history. One woman may be acutely embarrassed talking about her breasts, as evidenced by lack of eye contact, minimal response, nervous gestures, or inappropriate humour. Another woman may talk wryly and disparagingly about the size or development of her breasts.

A young adolescent is acutely aware of her own development in relation to her peers.

Transgender individuals may also have strong emotions about breast development and appearance. Individuals may bind their breasts or express interest in gender-affirming surgery, whether that is chest surgery (masculinizing surgery) or breast construction (feminizing surgery). Acknowledging a person's preferred name and pronoun is essential in helping to establish a safe environment for transgendered individuals to seek care about their breasts.

A woman who has found a breast lump may exhibit fear, high anxiety, and even panic. Although many breast lumps are benign, women initially assume the worst possible outcome: cancer, disfigurement, and death. While you are collecting the subjective data, be attuned to cues for these behaviours, which necessitate a straightforward and reasoned attitude on your part.

HEALTH HISTORY QUESTIONS

Examiner Asks	Rationale
Breast	
1. Pain. Any **pain** or tenderness in the breasts? When did you first notice it? • Where is the pain? Localized or all over? • Is the painful spot sore to touch? Do you feel a burning or pulling sensation? • Is the pain cyclical? Any relation to your menstrual period? • Is the pain brought on by strenuous activity, especially involving one arm; a change in activity; manipulation during sex; part of an underwire bra; or exercise?	**Mastalgia (breast pain)** occurs with trauma, inflammation, infection, and benign breast disease. Cyclical pain is common with normal breasts, oral contraceptives, and benign breast disease. Determine whether pain is related to specific cause.
2. Lump. Ever noticed a **lump** or **thickening** in the breast? Where? • When did you first notice it? Has it changed at all since then? • Does the lump have any relation to your menstrual period? • Have you noticed any change in the overlying skin: redness, warmth, dimpling, swelling?	Carefully explore the presence of any lump. A lump present for many years and exhibiting no change may not be serious but still should be investigated. Approach any recent change or new lump with suspicion.

Examiner Asks	Rationale

3. Discharge. Any **discharge** from the nipple?
- When did you first notice this?
- What colour is the discharge?
- Consistency: Is it thick or runny?
- Does it have an odour?

Galactorrhea refers to the secretion of milky-white discharge from one or both breasts in a man, or in a woman who is neither pregnant nor breastfeeding.

Note medications that may cause clear nipple discharge: oral contraceptives, phenothiazines, diuretics, digitalis, steroids, methyldopa (Aldomet), calcium channel blockers.

Bloody or blood-tinged discharge should always be investigated. Any discharge with a lump should be investigated.

4. Rash. Any **rash** on the breast?
- When did you first notice this?
- Where did it start? On the nipple, areola, or surrounding skin?

Paget's disease starts with a small crust on the nipple apex and then spreads to the areola (see Table 18.6, p. 444).

Eczema or other dermatitis rarely starts at nipple unless it is caused by breastfeeding. It usually starts on the areola or surrounding skin and then spreads to the nipple.

5. Swelling. Any **swelling** in the breasts? In one spot or all over? Unilateral or bilateral?
- Related to your menstrual period, pregnancy, or breastfeeding?
- Any change in bra size?

6. Trauma. Any **trauma** or injury to the breasts?
- Did it result in any swelling, lump, or break in skin?

A lump from an injury is caused by local hematoma or edema and should resolve shortly. Trauma may also cause a woman to feel the breast and find a lump that really was there before.

7. History of breast disease, and breast cancer risk factors. Do you have any personal **history of breast disease**?
- What type? How was this diagnosed? For example, has a health care provider ever told you that you have "dense" breasts or "atypical hyperplasia" of your breasts?
- When did this occur?
- How is it being treated?
- Any breast cancer in your family? In whom: sister, mother, maternal grandmother, maternal aunts, daughter?
- At what age did this relative have breast cancer?
- At what age did your menses start?
- (If postmenopausal) What was your age at menopause?
- Have you experienced any changes in your weight?
- Have you had any exposure to ionizing radiation (e.g., chest radiographs, computed tomography [CT])? What is your alcohol intake? Do you have Ashkenazi Jewish ancestry or any genetic conditions?
- Reproductive history: How many times have you been pregnant? How old were you when your first child was born? Have you used hormonal contraceptives or (if perimenopausal) hormone replacement therapy?

Past breast cancer increases the risk for recurrent cancer (see Table 18.2, p. 423).

The presence of benign breast disease makes the breasts more difficult to examine; the general lumpiness conceals a new lump.

Women who have a first-degree relative with breast cancer have approximately double the lifetime risk of developing breast cancer.[8] Genetic factors are also implicated as risk factors but to a lesser extent: only 5–10% of cancers are characterized by an identifiable breast cancer gene (*BRCA1* or *BRCA2*; see Table 18.2, p. 423).

Examiner Asks	Rationale
8. Surgery. Have you ever had **surgery** on your breasts? Was this a biopsy? • What were the biopsy results? • Did you undergo mastectomy? Have you undergone mammoplasty (augmentation or reduction)?	
9. Self-care behaviours. Have you ever discussed your breast cancer risk and screening recommendations with a health care provider? • Do you ever examine your own breasts? Have you ever been taught **breast self-examination (BSE)**? • (If yes) I would like you to show me your technique after I complete your examination. • (If no) If you decide you would like to practise BSE after a discussion of the benefits and risks, I will teach you the technique. • Have you ever had **mammography**, a screening X-ray examination of the breasts? (If yes) How often? Have you ever been prescribed hormone therapy? • Do you have your breasts examined by a trained health care provider as part of your routine health checkup?	
Axilla	
1. Tenderness, lump, or swelling. Any **tenderness** or **lump** in the underarm area? • Where? When did you first notice this?	Breast tissue extends up into the axillae. Also, the axillae contain many lymph nodes, where the lymphatics of the breast drain.
2. Rash. Any **axillary rash**? Please describe it. • Does it seem to be a reaction to deodorant?	
Additional History for Preadolescents	
1. Female breast changes. Have you noticed your breasts changing? • How long has this been happening?	Developing breasts are the most obvious sign of puberty and the focus of attention for most girls, especially in comparison with peers. Assess each girl's perception of her own development, and provide teaching and reassurance as indicated.
2. Other pubertal changes. Many girls notice other changes in their bodies, too, that come with growing up. What changes have you noticed? • What do you think about all this?	
Additional History for Pregnant Women	
1. Breast changes. Have you noticed any enlargement or fullness in the breasts? • Is there any tenderness or tingling? • Are your nipples **inverted** or everted?	Breast changes are expected and normal during pregnancy. Assess the woman's understanding, and provide reassurance. **Inverted** nipples (i.e., that are depressed or invaginated) may need special care in preparation for breastfeeding.
2. Breastfeeding. Are you planning to breastfeed your baby?	Breastfeeding provides complete nutrition and antibodies for the baby, decreases the risk for ear infections, promotes bonding, and provides relaxation.
Additional History for Menopausal Women	
1. Breast changes. Have you noticed any change in the breast contour, size, or firmness? (Note: Change may not be as apparent to obese women or to the woman whose earlier pregnancies already have produced breast changes.)	Decreased estrogen level causes decreased firmness. Rapid decrease in estrogen level causes actual shrinkage.

Examiner Asks	Rationale

Special Considerations for Advanced Practice

The breast health history offers an ideal opportunity to provide information about risk assessment and counselling related to hormone therapy in perimenopausal women. Many women are afraid to broach the question of hormone therapy with health practitioners because of concerns about its safety. Reassure women that risk assessment and counselling about using hormone therapy is an individual matter; with adequate risk analysis and by following evidence-informed guidelines, many women may safely use hormone therapy for the relief of uncomfortable perimenopausal symptoms, such as hot flashes.[9] See the box Promoting Health: Breast Cancer.

PROMOTING HEALTH: BREAST CANCER

Best Practices for Breast Cancer Risk Assessment and Screening Recommendations

Breast cancer is the second major cause of death from cancer in women. However, early detection and improved treatment have increased survival rates. The 5-year net survival for breast cancer across Canada is 87%.* The net survival is "survival probability that would be observed in the hypothetical situation where the cancer of interest is the only possible cause of death."*

Health assessment offers an opportunity to review the patient's knowledge about breast cancer risk and screening. It is also an opportunity to assess the patient's breast cancer risk, offer education and counselling about current breast cancer screening recommendations, and, in collaboration with the patient, develop a breast cancer screening plan customized to the patient's level of risk and her individual preferences about screening methods.[†]

The best way to detect a patient's risk for breast cancer is by asking the correct history questions. Table 18.2 (p. 423) highlights risk factors for breast cancer, and from these you can fashion your questions. Be aware that most breast cancers occur in women with no identifiable risk factors, other than gender and age. Just because a woman does not report the cited risk factors does not mean that you or she should fail to consider breast cancer seriously.

According to the recommendations by the Canadian Task Force on Preventive Health Care (CTFPHC), Tonelli, Connor Gorber, and colleagues[‡] for breast cancer screening (see Box 18.1), neither breast self-examination (BSE) nor clinical breast examination (CBE) is now routinely recommended to Canadian women who have an average or low risk for breast cancer. Note that new guidelines are being released from the CTFPHC in 2018. Current evidence suggests that these procedures lack specificity and result in excessive benign or false-positive results of biopsies, lead to overdiagnosis and overtreatment, and create anxiety. In other words, the harms

outweigh the benefits. However, of importance is that these guidelines are directed only to women between the ages of 40 and 74 years and of average risk. *Average risk* is defined by the guideline as having (a) no previous history of breast cancer, (b) no history of breast cancer in a first-degree relative, (c) no known *BRCA/BRCA2* gene mutations, and (d) no previous exposure of the chest wall to radiation. Also of importance is that the recommendations are considered *weak*, being informed by moderate- or low-quality evidence. Thus your assessment of individual risk directs how you implement the guideline in clinical practice with any individual patient.

The value of early detection of breast cancer is clear. Although screening mammography is available for many groups of women in developed countries, BSE is available to virtually all women. BSE is valuable to women who are younger or older than the ages recommended for screening mammography or who have barriers to accessing mammography. BSE has no cost, is noninvasive, can be accomplished without a visit to a health care provider, and enhances self-care action.

The Canadian Cancer Society continues to recommend that it is important for all women to be familiar with their own breasts, regardless of their risk for breast cancer or what screening protocol is followed.[§] The seeming discrepancy between the evidence-informed guideline of the CTFPHC and colleagues[‡] and the Canadian Cancer Society's recommendation[§] underscores what is *most important* about counselling and teaching women about BSE: the decision to do BSE is an *individual* informed decision made by each woman based on her *individual* breast cancer risk assessment, and a comprehensive discussion with her health care provider about the risks and benefits to her as an *individual* of breast cancer screening (both BSE and CBE).

Continued

BSE, Breast self-examination; *CBE*, clinical breast examination.

SPECIAL CONSIDERATIONS FOR ADVANCED PRACTICE

BREAST CANCER SCREENING TOOLS

The use of breast cancer risk assessment tools in the clinical setting (Box 18.1) supports more effective early detection programs for individuals at high risk for breast cancer. The Gail Model, a breast cancer risk assessment tool, is widely used for calculating individual risk estimates for breast cancer. This model takes into account identified risk factors, including current age, age at menarche, age at first live birth, and family history of breast cancer in first-degree relatives. It also calculates 5-year and lifetime cumulative absolute risk estimates for the individual. It is easy to complete, and many computer-based data programs are available to clinicians (e.g., see the Halls MD "Detailed Breast Cancer Risk Calculator" listed in the section Additional Resources at the end of this chapter). The U.S. National Cancer Institute also provides an interactive online tool that is based on the Gail Model to assist health care providers in estimating a woman's risk of developing breast cancer (see the section Additional Resources at the end of this chapter).

However, the Gail Model may underestimate the breast cancer risk in the subgroup of women with family cancer histories suggestive of hereditary breast cancer syndromes, such as those caused by the oncogenes *BRCA1* and *BRCA2*.

The Pedigree Assessment Tool (PAT) was developed to identify this subgroup of women and can be used along with the Gail Model to screen for breast cancer risk. The PAT score is calculated by adding the points assigned to every

---

BOX 18.1 **Summary of Breast Cancer Screening Recommendations for Clinicians and Policymakers**

Recommendations are presented for the use of mammography, magnetic resonance imaging (MRI), breast self-examination, and clinical breast examination to screen for breast cancer. These recommendations apply only to women at average risk for breast cancer aged 40–74 years. They do not apply to women at higher risk because of personal history of breast cancer, history of breast cancer in first-degree relatives, known mutations of the *BRCA1/BRCA2* genes, or previous exposure of the chest wall to radiation. No recommendations are made for women aged 75 years and older, given the lack of data available for this group.

Mammography
* For women aged 40–49 years, we recommend not routinely screening with mammography. (*Weak recommendation; moderate-quality evidence.*)
* For women aged 50–69 years, we recommend routinely screening with mammography every two to three years. (*Weak recommendation; moderate-quality evidence.*)

* For women aged 70–74 years, we recommend routinely screening with mammography every two to three years. (*Weak recommendation; low-quality evidence.*)

Magnetic Resonance Imaging
* We recommend not routinely screening with MRI scans. (*Weak recommendation; no evidence.*)

Clinical Breast Examination
* We recommend not routinely performing clinical breast examinations alone or in conjunction with mammography to screen for breast cancer. (*Weak recommendation; low-quality evidence.*)

Breast Self-Examination
* We recommend not advising women to routinely practise breast self-examination. (*Weak recommendation; moderate-quality evidence.*)

From Canadian Task Force on Preventive Health Care, Tonelli, M., Connor Gorber, S., et al. (2011). Recommendations on screening for breast cancer in average-risk women aged 40–74 years. *Canadian Medical Association Journal, 183*(17), 1991–2001 (p. 1995). doi:10.1503/cmaj.110334 family member, including second- and third-degree relatives, with a breast or ovarian cancer diagnosis. Additional points for each individual are calculated for bilateral disease, the occurrence of both breast and ovarian cancers, and for the age at diagnosis. A separate score is calculated for the individual's maternal and paternal family histories. The higher of the two scores is used. The specific inclusion of both sides of a woman's family is important because many women often disregard or overlook paternal lineage altogether when thinking about or reporting family history of breast cancer. For more information about the Gail Model and PAT risk assessments, as well as instructions on calculating a PAT score, see the section Additional Resources at the end of this chapter.

Although breast cancer screening tools such as the Gail Model and PAT provide useful information to health practitioners, it is important to remember the limitations of each tool. Screening tools provide additional valuable assessment data that must be considered critically and within the context of the whole assessment, to best counsel a woman about her individual breast cancer risk.

OBJECTIVE DATA

PREPARATION

The woman is sitting up and facing the examiner. An alternative draping method is to use a short gown, open at the back, and lift it up to the woman's shoulders during inspection. During palpation, when the woman is supine, cover one breast with the gown while examining the other. Be aware that many women are embarrassed to have their breasts examined; use a sensitive but matter-of-fact approach.

EQUIPMENT NEEDED

Small pillow
Ruler marked in centimetres

Special Considerations for Advanced Practice

Objective Data

Normal Range of Findings

Inspect The Breasts

General Appearance

Note symmetry of size and shape (Fig. 18.7). It is common and normal to have a slight asymmetry in size; often the left breast is slightly larger than the right.

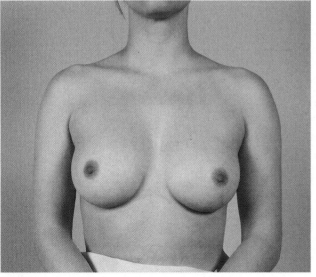

18.7

Abnormal Findings

A sudden increase in the size of one breast signifies inflammation or new growth.

Normal Range of Findings

Abnormal Findings

Skin

The skin is normally smooth and of even colour. Note any localized areas of redness, bulging, or dimpling. Also, note any skin lesions or focal vascular pattern. A fine blue vascular network is normally visible during pregnancy. Pale linear **striae**, or stretch marks, often follow pregnancy or periods of weight gain/loss.

Normally, no edema is present. Edema exaggerates the hair follicles, giving an "orange-peel" look (also called *peau d'orange*).

Lymphatic Drainage Areas

Observe the axillary and supraclavicular regions. Note any bulging, discoloration, or edema.

Nipple

The nipples should be symmetrical, on the same plane on the two breasts. Nipples usually protrude, although some are flat and some are inverted. They tend to stay in their original condition over time. Distinguish a recently retracted nipple from one that has been inverted for many years or since puberty. Normal nipple inversion may be unilateral or bilateral, and usually the nipple can be pulled out (i.e., it is not fixed).

Note any dry scaling, any fissure or ulceration, and bleeding or other discharge.

A supernumerary nipple is a normal and common variation (Fig. 18.8). An extra nipple along the embryonic "milk line" on the thorax or abdomen (see Fig. 18.5 on p. 421) is a congenital occurrence. Usually, it is 5–6 cm below the breast near the midline and has no associated glandular tissue. It looks like a mole, although a close look reveals a tiny nipple and areola. It is not significant; merely distinguish it from a mole.

Hyperpigmentation.
Redness and heat with inflammation.
Unilateral dilated superficial veins in a nonpregnant woman.

Edema (see Table 18.3, p. 441).

Deviation in nipple pointing (see Table 18.3, p. 442).
Recent nipple retraction: signifies acquired disease (see Table 18.3, p. 442).

Explore any discharge, especially in the presence of a breast mass. (See the Critical Findings box.)

CRITICAL FINDINGS

Unexplained discharge or bleeding from nipples, open or ulcerating nontraumatic lesions, or a breast mass in a patient with previously diagnosed cancer indicate further investigation on an urgent basis. Patients with these conditions may require referral to a practitioner who can requisition the appropriate diagnostic tests (such as a nurse practitioner, physician, or surgeon). Tests may include diagnostic mammography, ultrasonography, biopsy, or magnetic resonance imaging (MRI), depending on the specific findings and the patient's history (see Table 18.6, p. 444).

In rare cases, additional glandular tissue, called a *supernumerary breast*, is present.

Normal Range of Findings	Abnormal Findings

18.8 Supernumerary nipple and areolar complex.

Manoeuvres to Screen for Retraction

Direct the woman to change position while you check the breasts for skin retraction signs. First, ask her to lift the arms slowly over the head. Both breasts should move up symmetrically (Fig. 18.9).

18.9 Retraction manoeuvre.

Next, ask her to push her hands onto her hips (Fig. 18.10) and then to push her two palms together (Fig. 18.11). These manoeuvres contract the pectoralis major muscle. Both breasts are lifted slightly.

Retraction signs result from fibrosis in the breast tissue, usually caused by growing neoplasms. The fibrosis shortens with time, causing signs that are in contrast to the normally loose breast tissue.

Note a lag in movement of one breast.

Note a dimpling or a pucker, which indicates skin retraction (see Table 18.3, p. 442).

Objective Data

Normal Range of Findings	Abnormal Findings

18.10

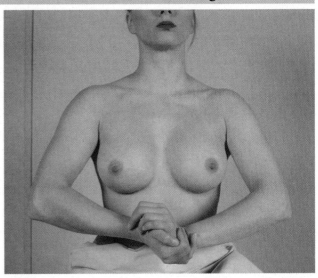

18.11

Ask a woman with large, pendulous breasts to lean forward while you support her forearms. Note the symmetrical free-forward movement of both breasts (Fig. 18.12).

Note fixation to chest wall or skin retraction (see Table 18.3, p. 442).

18.12

| **Normal Range of Findings** | **Abnormal Findings** |

Inspect and Palpate The Axillae

Examine the axillae while the woman is sitting. Inspect the skin, noting any rash or infection. Lift the woman's arm and support it yourself, so that her muscles are loose and relaxed. Use your right hand to palpate the left axilla for tenderness or palpable lymph nodes (Fig. 18.13). Reach your fingers high into the axilla. Move them firmly down in four directions: (a) down the chest wall in a line from the middle of the axilla, (b) along the anterior border of the axilla, (c) along the posterior border, and (d) along the inner aspect of the upper arm. Move the woman's arm through the range of motion to increase the surface area you can reach.

18.13

Usually nodes are not palpable, although you may feel a small, soft, non-tender node in the central group. Expect some tenderness when palpating high in the axilla. Note any enlarged and tender lymph nodes.

Nodes enlarge with any local infection of the breast, arm, or hand, and with breast cancer metastases.

Palpate The Breasts

Help the woman to a supine position. Tuck a small pad under the side to be palpated and raise her arm over her head. These manoeuvres will flatten the breast tissue and displace it medially. Any significant lumps will then feel more distinct (Fig. 18.14).

18.14

Normal Range of Findings

Use the pads of your first three fingers, and make a gentle rotary motion on the breast. Vary your pressure so you are palpating light, medium, and deep tissues in each location. The vertical strip pattern (Fig. 18.15, *A*) currently is recommended as the best to detect a breast mass, but two other patterns are in common use: from the nipple palpating out to the periphery, as if following spokes on a wheel, and in concentric circles out to the periphery (see Fig. 18.15, *B* and *C*).

Abnormal Findings

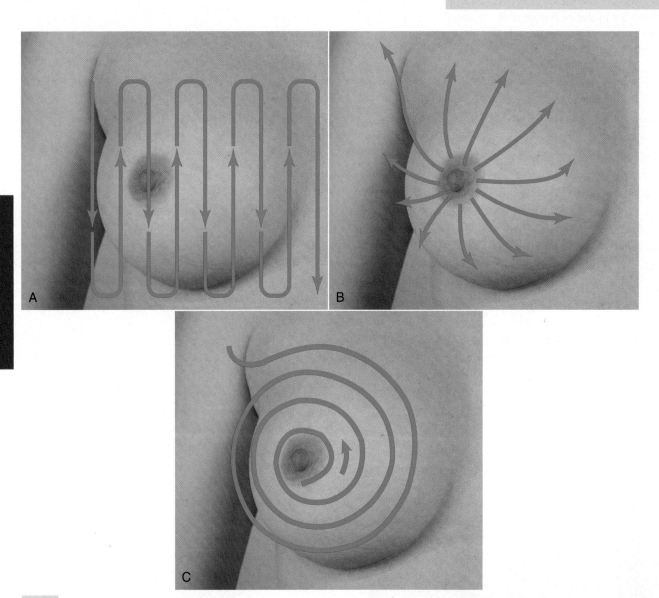

18.15 Patterns of breast palpation. **A,** Vertical strip pattern. **B,** Spokes-on-a-wheel pattern. **C,** Concentric circles pattern.

For the vertical strip pattern, start high in the axilla and palpate down just lateral to the breast. Proceed in overlapping vertical lines, ending at the sternal edge. In every pattern, take care to palpate every square centimetre of the breast and to examine the tail of Spence high into the axilla. Be consistent and thorough in your approach to each woman.

Normal Range of Findings

In nulliparous women, normal breast tissue feels firm, smooth, and elastic. After pregnancy, the tissue feels softer and looser. Premenstrual engorgement from increasing progesterone is normal. This consists of a slight enlargement, tenderness to palpation, and a generalized nodularity; the lobes feel prominent and their margins more distinct.

Also, normally you may feel a firm transverse ridge of compressed tissue in the lower quadrants. This is the **inframammary ridge**, and it is especially noticeable in large breasts. Do not confuse it with an abnormal lump.

After palpating over the four breast quadrants, palpate the nipple (Fig. 18.16). Note any induration or subareolar mass. With your thumb and forefinger, gently depress the nipple tissue into the well behind the areola. The tissue should move inward easily. If the woman reports spontaneous nipple discharge, press the areola inward with your index finger; repeat from a few different directions. If any discharge appears, note its colour and consistency.

18.16

For the woman with large, pendulous breasts, you may palpate by using a bimanual technique (Fig. 18.17). The woman should sit up and lean forward. Support the inferior part of the breast with one hand. Use your other hand to palpate the breast tissue against your supporting hand.

18.17

Abnormal Findings

In women who are not lactating and not postpartum, heat, redness, and swelling in the breasts indicate inflammation.

Except during pregnancy and lactation, discharge is abnormal (see Table 18.6, p. 444). Note the number of discharge droplets and the quadrant or quadrants producing them. Blot the discharge on a white gauze pad to ascertain its colour. Test any abnormal discharge for the presence of blood.

Objective Data

Normal Range of Findings	Abnormal Findings

If the woman mentions a breast lump that she has discovered herself, examine the unaffected breast first to learn a baseline of normal consistency for this woman. If you do feel a lump or mass, note these characteristics (Fig. 18.18):

1. **Location:** Using the breast as a clock face, describe the distance in centimetres from the nipple (e.g., "7:00 position, 2 cm from the nipple"). Or diagram the breast in the woman's record and mark in the location of the lump.
2. **Size:** Judge in centimetres in three dimensions: width × length × thickness.
3. **Shape:** State whether the lump is oval, round, lobulated, or indistinct.
4. **Consistency:** State whether the lump is soft, firm, or hard.
5. **Movable:** Note whether the lump is freely movable or is fixed when you try to slide it over the chest wall.
6. **Distinctness:** Note whether the lump is solitary or multiple.
7. **Nipple:** Determine whether the lump is displaced or retracted.
8. **Note the skin over the lump:** Is it erythematous, dimpled, or retracted?
9. **Tenderness:** Note whether the lump is tender to palpation.
10. **Lymphadenopathy:** Determine whether any regional lymph nodes are palpable.

See Tables 18.4 and 18.5 (pp. 442–443) for descriptions of common breast lumps with these characteristics.

18.18

Teach Breast Self-Examination

According to the Canadian Cancer Society, "There really isn't a right or wrong way for women to examine their breasts. They just need to know the whole area of their breast tissue well enough to notice changes. This includes the entire breast area up to the collarbone and under the armpits, as well as the nipples."[10] Reinforce to patients that self-examination will familiarize them with their own breasts and their normal variation. Emphasize the absence of lumps (not the presence of them). However, do encourage women to report any unusual finding promptly.

While teaching women about the importance of being familiar with their own breasts, focus on the positive aspects of breast self-examination. Avoid citing frightening mortality statistics about breast cancer. This may generate excessive fear and denial that actually obstructs a woman's self-care action. Rather, be selective in your choice of factual material:

- The majority of women never get breast cancer.
- The great majority of breast lumps are benign.
- Early detection of breast cancer is important; if the cancer is not invasive, the survival rate is close to 100%.

Normal Range of Findings	Abnormal Findings

Emphasize self-care through knowledge of risk factors and early referral for any suspect findings.

Keep your teaching simple! The simpler the plan, the more likely the patient is to comply. Suggest that women inspect their breasts in front of a mirror while disrobed to the waist. Encourage women to learn how their breasts feel while in the shower, where soap and water assist palpation, and while lying supine so that breast tissue is flattened. Encourage each woman to palpate her own breasts while you are there to monitor her technique. Many examiners use a breast model (Fig. 18.19), so that the woman can palpate a simulated "lump." Pamphlets are also helpful reinforcers. Use the return demonstration to assess the patient's technique and understanding of the procedure.

18.19

The Breast Examination In Men

Your examination of the male breast can be much more abbreviated, but do not omit it. Combine the breast examination with that of the anterior thorax. Inspect the chest wall, noting the skin surface and any lumps or swelling. Palpate the nipple area for any lump or tissue enlargement (Fig. 18.20). It should feel even, with no nodules. Palpate the axillary lymph nodes.

Of all new cases of cancer in men per year, breast cancer represented 0.2% in 2017.[3]

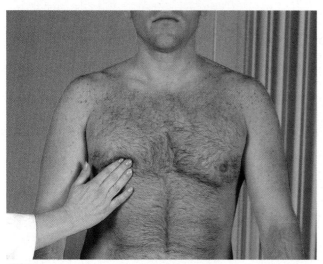

18.20

Normal Range of Findings

The normal male breast has a flat disc of undeveloped breast tissue beneath the nipple. Gynecomastia is an enlargement of this breast tissue, which makes it clinically distinguishable from the other tissues in the chest wall (Fig. 18.21). It feels like a smooth, firm, movable disc. This occurs normally during puberty. It usually affects only one breast and is temporary. Male adolescents are acutely aware of body image. Reassure them that this change is normal, common, and temporary. In contrast, an obese adolescent boy has an increase of fatty, not glandular, tissue.

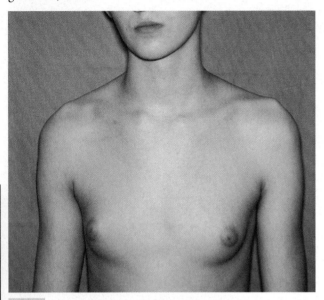

18.21 Adolescent gynecomastia.

❖ DEVELOPMENTAL CONSIDERATIONS

Infants and Children

In neonates, the breasts may be enlarged and visible as a result of maternal estrogen crossing the placenta. They may secrete a clear or white fluid, called "witch's milk." These signs are not significant and are resolved within a few days to a few weeks.

Note the position of the nipples on the prepubertal child. They should be symmetrical, just lateral to the midclavicular line, between the fourth and fifth ribs. The nipple is flat, and the pigmentation of the areola is darker than that of the surrounding skin.

Adolescents

Adolescent breast development begins, on average, between 8 and 10 years of age. Expect some asymmetry during growth as a normal finding. (Distinguish breast development from extra adipose tissue present in obese children.) Record the stage of development by using Tanner staging,[11] described in Table 18.1 on p. 422. Use the chart to teach the adolescent normal developmental stages and to assure her of her own normal progress.

With maturing adolescents, palpate the breasts as you would with the adult. The breasts normally feel firm and uniform. Note any mass.

Abnormal Findings

Gynecomastia also occurs with use of anabolic steroids, some medications, and some disease states (see Table 18.8, p. 446).

Premature thelarche is early breast development with no other hormone dependent signs (pubic hair, menses).

Note precocious development, which occurs before age 8 years. It is usually normal but also occurs with thyroid dysfunction, stilbestrol ingestion, or ovarian or adrenal tumour.

Note delayed development, which occurs with hormonal failure, anorexia nervosa beginning before puberty, or severe malnutrition.

At this age, a mass is almost always a benign **fibroadenoma** or a cyst (see Table 18.4, p. 443).

Objective Data

Normal Range of Findings	**Abnormal Findings**

Pregnant Women

A delicate blue vascular pattern is visible over the breasts. The breasts increase in size, as do the nipples. Jagged linear stretch marks, or striae, may develop if breast size increases significantly. The nipples also become darker and more erectile. The areolae widen; grow darker; and contain the small, scattered, elevated Montgomery's glands. On palpation, the breasts feel more nodular, and thick yellow colostrum can be expressed after the first trimester.

Lactating Women

Colostrum changes to milk production around the third postpartum day. At this time, the breasts may become engorged, appearing enlarged, reddened, and shiny and feeling warm and hard. Frequent nursing helps drain the ducts and sinuses and stimulate milk production. Nipple soreness is normal, occurring after the baby feeds for approximately the first 20 times, lasting 24–48 hours, then disappearing rapidly. The nipples may look red and irritated. They may even crack but will heal rapidly if kept dry and exposed to air. Frequent nursing is also the best treatment for nipple soreness.

> If one section of the breast surface appears red and tender, a duct is plugged (see Table 18.7, p. 445).

Older Women

On inspection, the breasts look pendulous, flattened, and sagging. Nipples may be retracted but can be pulled outward. On palpation, the breasts feel more granular, and the terminal ducts around the nipple feel more prominent and stringy. Thickening of the inframammary ridge at the lower breast is normal, and it feels more prominent with age.

Reinforce the value of routine breast health behaviours. Women older than 50 years have an increased risk for breast cancer. Older women may have problems with arthritis, limited range of motion, or decreased vision that may inhibit self-care. Suggest aids to the self-examination; for example, talcum powder helps fingers glide over skin.

> Because atrophy causes shrinkage of normal glandular tissue, cancer detection is somewhat easier in older women. Any palpable lump that cannot be positively identified as a normal structure should be investigated.

DOCUMENTATION AND CRITICAL THINKING

Sample Charting: Female

SUBJECTIVE

52-year-old woman. States no breast pain, lump, discharge, rash, swelling, or trauma. No history of breast disease herself; mother does have benign breast disease. No history of breast surgery. Never been pregnant. Hormonal contraceptive use aged 20 through 40 years. Perimenopausal but no hormone replacement. Last CBE, 1 year ago. Mammogram q2 years, due next month.

OBJECTIVE

Inspection: Breasts symmetrical. Skin smooth with even colour and no rash or lesions. Arm movement shows no dimpling or retractions. No nipple discharge, no lesions.
Palpation: Breast contour and consistency firm and homogeneous. No masses or tenderness. No lymphadenopathy.

ASSESSMENT

Healthy breast structure
Knowledgeable regarding breast screening recommendations

Sample Charting: Male

SUBJECTIVE

No pain, lump, rash, or swelling.

OBJECTIVE

No masses or tenderness. No lymphadenopathy.

Focused Assessment: Clinical Case Study 1

Jane Giorgio (J.G.) is a 32-year-old female high school teacher, married, with no children. She reports good health until finding "lump in my right breast 2 weeks ago."

SUBJECTIVE

2 weeks PTA [prior to arrival]: J.G. noticed lump in R [right] breast while showering. Lump firm, nonmovable area "the size of a quarter," in upper outer quadrant of breast, tender on touch only. No skin changes, no nipple discharge, on no medications. No history of breast disease in self or family. Gravida 0. No known genetic risk factors. CXR [chest radiograph] age 15 (chest infection). Menarche age 13. Hormonal contraceptive use, ages 21–30 years. Moderate alcohol use, 2 glasses of wine a week.

2 days PTA: J.G. saw MD, who confirmed presence of lump and recommended biopsy as outpatient. Last menstrual period 1/25 (2½ weeks PTA). States that the last 2 days she has been so nervous that she has been unable to sleep well or to concentrate at work: "I just know it's cancer."

OBJECTIVE

Voice trembling and breathless during history. Sitting posture stiff and rigid. BP 148/78 mm Hg. Temp 37°C (98.6°F), pulse 92 bpm, resp 16/min.

Inspection: Breasts symmetrical, nipples everted. No skin lesions, no dimpling, no retraction, no fixation.

Palpation: Left breast firm, no mass, no tenderness, no discharge. Right breast firm, with 2 cm × 2 cm × 1 cm mass at 10:00 position, 5 cm from the nipple. Lump is firm, oval, with smooth discrete borders, nonmovable, tender to palpation. No other mass. No discharge. No lymphadenopathy.

ASSESSMENT

Lump in R breast
Anxiety

Focused Assessment: Clinical Case Study 2

Dana Bachman (D.B.) is a 62-year-old female bank comptroller, married, with no children. History of hypertension, managed by diuretic medication and diet. No other health problems until yearly company physical examination 3 days PTA, when NP [nurse practitioner] "found a lump in my right breast."

SUBJECTIVE

3 days PTA: NP noted lump in R breast during yearly physical examination. NP did not describe lump but told D.B. it was "serious" and needed immediate biopsy. D.B. has not felt it herself. States has noted no skin changes, no nipple discharge. No previous history of breast disease. Mother died aged 54 years of breast cancer; no other relative with breast disease. *BRCA/BRCA2* status unknown. D.B. has had no term pregnancies; two spontaneous abortions, ages 28 and 31 years. Menarche age

11, menopause completed at age 52 years. No hormone replacement. No hormonal contraceptive use. No alcohol use. No history of chest wall irradiation.

Married 43 years. States husband supportive, but "I just can't talk to him about this. I can't even go near him now."

OBJECTIVE

Inspection: Breasts symmetrical when sitting, arms down. Nipples flat. No lesions, no discharge. As lifts arms, left breast elevates, right breast stays fixed. Dimple in right breast, 9:00 position, apparent at rest and with muscle contraction. Leaning forward reveals left breast falls free, right breast flattens.

Palpation: Left breast feels soft and granular throughout, no mass. Right breast soft and granular, with large, stony hard mass in upper outer quadrant. Lump is 5 cm × 4 cm × 2 cm, at 9:00 position, 3 cm from nipple. Borders irregular, mass fixed to tissues, no pain with palpation.

One firm, palpable lymph node in centre of right axilla. No palpable nodes on the left.

ASSESSMENT

Lump in R breast
Situational stress R/T [related to] breast lump

ABNORMAL FINDINGS

TABLE 18.3	Signs of Retraction and Inflammation in the Breast

Dimpling

The shallow dimple (also called a *skin tether*) shown in this photo is a sign of skin retraction. Cancer causes fibrosis, which contracts the suspensory ligaments. The dimple may be apparent at rest, with compression, or with lifting of the arms. Also note the distortion of the areola in this photo as the fibrosis pulls the nipple toward it.

Edema (Peau d'Orange)

Lymphatic obstruction produces edema. This thickens the skin and exaggerates the hair follicles, which produces a pig-skin or orange-peel look. This condition suggests cancer. Edema usually begins in the skin around and beneath the areola, the most dependent area of the breast. Also note nipple infiltration in this photo.

Continued

Documentation
and Critical Thinking

Abnormal Findings

TABLE 18.3	Signs of Retraction and Inflammation in the Breast—cont'd

Nipple Retraction (Not Illustrated)

The retracted nipple looks flatter and broader, like an underlying crater. A recent retraction suggests cancer, which causes fibrosis of the whole duct system and pulls in the nipple. It also may occur with benign lesions such as ectasia of the ducts. Do not confuse retraction with the normal longstanding type of nipple inversion, which has no broadening and is not fixed.

Fixation

Asymmetry, distortion, or decreased mobility with the elevated arm manoeuvre. As cancer becomes invasive, the fibrosis fixes the breast to the underlying pectoral muscles. In this photo, note that the right breast is held against the chest wall.

Deviation in Nipple Pointing

An underlying cancer causes fibrosis in the mammary ducts, which pulls the nipple angle toward it. In this photo, note the swelling behind the right nipple and that the nipple tilts laterally.

See Illustration Credits for source information.

TABLE 18.4	Breast Lump

◄ Benign Breast Disease

Multiple tender masses. Formerly called *fibrocystic breast disease;* this is a meaningless term because it covers too many entities. Actually, six diagnostic categories exist, based on symptoms and physical findings:[12]
- Swelling and tenderness (cyclical discomfort)
- Mastalgia (severe pain, both cyclical and noncyclical)
- Nodularity (significant lumpiness, both cyclical and noncyclical)
- Dominant lumps (including cysts and fibroadenomas)
- Nipple discharge (including intraductal papilloma and duct ectasia)
- Infections and inflammations (including subareolar abscess, lactational mastitis, breast abscess, and Mondor's disease)

About 50% of all women have some form of benign breast disease. Nodularity occurs bilaterally; regular, firm nodules that are mobile, well demarcated, and feel rubbery, like small water balloons. Pain may be dull, heavy, and cyclical or just before menses as nodules enlarge. Some women have nodularity but no pain, and some vice versa. Cysts are discrete, fluid-filled sacs. Dominant lumps and nipple discharge must be investigated carefully, and biopsy may be needed to rule out cancer. Nodularity itself is not premalignant but may cause difficulty in detecting truly cancerous lumps.

TABLE 18.4	**Breast Lump—cont'd**

Cancer

Solitary unilateral nontender mass. Single focus in one area, although it may be interspersed with other nodules. Solid, hard, dense, and fixed to underlying tissues or skin as cancer becomes invasive. Borders are irregular and poorly delineated. Grows constantly. Often painless, but may cause pain. Most common in upper outer quadrant. Usually found in women 30–80 years of age; risk increases at ages 50–69 years. As cancer advances, signs include firm or hard irregular axillary nodes; skin dimpling; and nipple retraction, elevation, and discharge.

Fibroadenoma

Solitary nontender benign mass. Most common between 15 and 30 years of age but can occur up to age 55 years; is most commonly self-detected in late adolescence. Solid, firm, rubbery, and elastic. Round, oval, or lobulated; 1–5 cm. Freely movable, slippery; fingers slide it easily through tissue. Usually no axillary lymphadenopathy. Grows quickly and constantly. Diagnosis is based on history, physical examination, ultrasonography; suspect tumours (i.e., large, rapidly growing, or other suspect findings) may necessitate biopsy, surgical excision, or both.[13]

TABLE 18.5	**Differentiating Breast Lumps**		
Characteristic	Fibroadenoma	Benign Breast Disease	Cancer
Likely age	15–30 years; can occur up to 55 years	30–55 years; conditions tend to decrease after menopause	30–80 years; risk increases after 50 years
Shape	Round, lobular	Round, lobular	Irregular, star-shaped
Consistency	Usually firm, rubbery	Firm to soft, rubbery	Firm to stony hard
Demarcation	Well demarcated, clear margins	Well demarcated	Poorly defined
Number	Usually single	Usually multiple, may be single	Single
Mobility	Very mobile, slippery	Mobile	Fixed
Tenderness	Usually none	Present, usually increases before menses, may be noncyclical	Usually none but may be present
Skin retraction	None	None	Usually
Pattern of growth	Grows quickly and constantly	Size may increase or decrease rapidly	Grows constantly
Risk to health	None; they are benign and must be diagnosed through biopsy	Benign, although general lumpiness may mask other cancerous lump	Serious, necessitates early treatment

TABLE 18.6	Abnormal Nipple Discharge

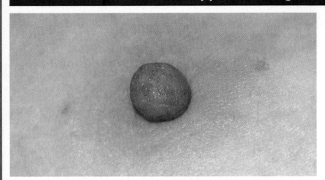

Mammary Duct Ectasia

Pastelike matter in subareolar ducts produces sticky, purulent discharge that may be white, grey, brown, green, or bloody. A light green, single duct discharge is shown in this photo. Caused by stagnation of cellular debris and secretions in the ducts, leading to obstruction, inflammation, and infection. Occurs in women who have lactated; usually occurs in perimenopausal period.

Itching, burning sensation, or pulling pain occurs around nipple. May have subareolar redness and swelling. Ducts are palpable as rubbery, twisted tubules under areola. May have palpable mass, soft or firm, poorly delineated. Not malignant, but biopsy is needed to rule out cancer.

Intraductal Papilloma

Serous or serosanguineous discharge, which is spontaneous, unilateral, or from a single duct. Lesion consists of tiny tumours, 2–3 mm in diameter. Often there is a palpable nodule in the underlying duct (highlighted by black marker in this photo). Papillomas affect women 40–60 years of age; most are benign. Refer any patient with bloody discharge for careful evaluation, including biopsy, to rule out cancer.

Carcinoma

Bloody nipple discharge that is unilateral and from a single duct necessitates further investigation. Although there was no palpable lump associated with the discharge shown in this photo, mammography revealed a 1-cm, centrally located, ill-defined mass.

Paget's Disease (Intraductal Carcinoma)

Early lesion has unilateral, clear, yellow discharge and dry, scaling crusts, friable at nipple apex. Spreads outward to areola with erythematous halo on areola and crusted, eczematous, retracted nipple. In later stages of lesion, nipple is reddened, excoriated, and ulcerated, with bloody discharge when surface is eroded, and an erythematous plaque surrounds the nipple. Symptoms include tingling sensation, burning sensation, itching.

Except for the redness and occasional cracking from initial breastfeeding, any dermatitis of the nipple area must be carefully explored and investigated immediately.

See Illustration Credits for source information.

TABLE 18.7 **Disorders Occurring During Lactation**

Plugged Duct

A fairly common and not serious condition. One milk duct is clogged. One section of the breast is tender and may be reddened. No infection. It is important to keep breast as empty as possible and milk flowing. The woman should nurse frequently, on affected side first to ensure complete emptying, and manually express any remaining milk. A plugged duct usually resolves in less than 1 day.

Mastitis

This is uncommon; an inflammatory mass before abscess formation. Usually occurs in single quadrant. Area is red, swollen, tender, very hot, and hard; in this photo, redness is forming outward from areola upper edge, in right breast. The woman in this photo also has a headache, malaise, fever, chills and sweating, increased pulse, and flulike symptoms. Mastitis may occur during first 4 months of lactation from infection or from stasis from plugged duct. Treat with rest, local heat to area, antibiotics, and frequent nursing to keep breast as empty as possible. Weaning must not be undertaken now, or the breast will become engorged and the pain will increase. Antibiotic administered to mother is not harmful to infant. Condition usually resolves in 2–3 days.

◀ Breast Abscess

A rare complication of generalized infection (e.g., mastitis) if untreated. A pocket of pus accumulates in one local area. This photo shows extensive nipple edema, and abscess is "pointing" at the 3:00 position on the areolar margin. Nursing on affected breast must be discontinued temporarily; manually express milk and discard. Continue to nurse on unaffected side. Treat with antibiotics, and refer patient for surgical incision and drainage.

See Illustration Credits for source information.

TABLE 18.8   Abnormalities in the Male Breast

◀ Gynecomastia

Benign enlargement of male breast that occurs when estrogen concentration exceeds testosterone levels. It is a mobile disc of tissue located centrally under the nipple-areola. At puberty, it is usually mild and transient. In older men, it is bilateral, tender, and firm but not as hard as breast cancer. Gynecomastia occurs with Cushing's syndrome, liver cirrhosis (because estrogens cannot be metabolized), adrenal disease, hyperthyroidism, and numerous substances: alcohol and marijuana; estrogen treatment for prostate cancer; antibiotics (metronidazole [Flagyl], isoniazid [Rifater]); spironolactone [Aldactone], digoxin [Toloxin], angiotensin-converting enzyme (ACE) inhibitors; and psychoactive drugs (diazepam [Apo-Diazepam], tricyclic antidepressants).[14]

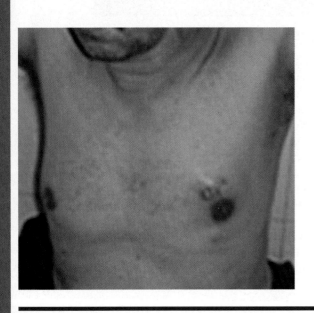

◀ Breast Carcinoma in Men

About 1% of breast cancers occur in men.[15] There is no standard screening mammography; thus it is detected by clinical symptoms. It presents as a painless palpable mass—hard, irregular, nontender, fixed to the area; may have nipple retraction. Nipple discharge, with or without a palpable mass, is a significant warning of early breast cancer.[16] Note retraction and ulceration shown here. Early spread to axillary lymph nodes occurs because of minimal breast tissue. Because of lack of screening and general awareness, men are diagnosed 10 years later than women and at later stages, with the mean age between 60 and 70 years. The stage at diagnosis is the most important indicator for survival.

See Illustration Credits for source information.

Summary Checklist: Breasts and Regional Lymphatic Examination

1. **Inspect breasts** as the woman sits, raises arms overhead, pushes hands on hips, and leans forward
2. **Inspect** the **supraclavicular** and **infraclavicular areas**
3. **Palpate** the **axillae** and **regional lymph nodes**
4. With woman supine, **palpate the breast tissue**, including tail of Spence, the nipples, and areolae
5. **Engage in teaching and health promotion**

ADDITIONAL RESOURCES

Breast Cancer Society of Canada: http://www.bcsc.ca

Canadian Cancer Society—What Is Breast Cancer?: http://www.cancer.ca/en/cancer-information/cancer-type/breast/breast-cancer/?region=on

Canadian Task Force on Preventive Health Care—Breast Cancer: https://canadiantaskforce.ca/guidelines/published-guidelines/breast-cancer/

Halls MD—Detailed Breast Cancer Risk Calculatior—The Gail Model: http://halls.md/breast/risk.htm

Moose & Doc—Breast Cancer: http://breast-cancer.ca/riskytools/

The North American Menopause Society: http://www.menopause.org

U.S. National Institutes of Health, National Cancer Institute—Breast Cancer Risk Assessment Tool: https://www.cancer.gov/bcrisktool/

U.S. Preventive Services Task Force, Final Recommendation Statement: BRCA-Related Cancer—Risk Assessment, Genetic Counseling, and Genetic Testing: https://www.uspreventiveservicestaskforce.org/Page/Document/RecommendationStatementFinal/brca-related-cancer-risk-assessment-genetic-counseling-and-genetic-testing#table-4-pedigree-assessment-tool

REFERENCES

1. Avraham, T., Daluvoy, S. V., Kueberuwa, E., et al. (2010). Anatomical and surgical concepts in lymphatic regeneration. *The Breast Journal*, 16(6), 639–643. doi:10.1111/j.1524-4741.2010.00978.x.

2. Canadian Cancer Statistics Advisory Committee. (2018). *Canadian Cancer Statistics 2018*. Toronto, ON: Canadian Cancer Society. Available at: cancer.ca/Canadian-Cancer-Statistics-2018-EN.

3. Canadian Cancer Statistics Advisory Committee. (2017). *Canadian Cancer Statistics 2017*. Toronto, ON: Canadian Cancer Society. Available at: cancer.ca/Canadian-Cancer-Statistics-2018-EN. (Accessed 7 July 2018).

4. Kolahdooz, F., Jang, S. L., Corriveau, A., et al. (2014). Knowledge, attitudes, and behaviours towards cancer screening in Indigenous populations: A systematic review. *Lancet Oncology*, 15(11), e504–e516. doi:10.1016/S1470-2045(14)70508-X.

5. Ahmad, F., Mahmood, S., Pietkiewicz, I., et al. (2012). Concept mapping with South Asian immigrant women: Barriers to mammography and solutions. *Journal of Immigrant and Minority Health*, 14, 242–250. doi:10.1007/s10903-011-9472-7.

6. Dunn, S. F., Lofters, A. K., Ginsburg, O. M., et al. (2017). Cervical and breast cancer screening after CARES: A community program for immigrant and marginalized women. *American Journal of Preventive Medicine*, 52(5), 589–597. doi:10.1016/j.amepre.2016.11.023.

7. Widschwendter, P., Friedl, T. W. P., Schwentner, L., et al. (2015). The influence of obesity on survival in early, high-risk breast cancer: Results from the randomized SUCCESS A trial. *Breast Cancer Research*, 17, 129. doi:10.1186/s13058-015-0639-3.

8. Canadian Cancer Society. (2018). *Risk factors for breast cancer*. Retrieved from http://www.cancer.ca/en/cancer-information/cancer-type/breast/risks/?region=sk.

9. North American Menopause Society. (2017). *Clinical care recommendations: Estrogen therapy and estrogen-progesterone therapy*. Retrieved from http://www.menopause.org/publications/clinical-care-recommendations/chapter-8-prescription-therapies.

10. Canadian Cancer Society. (2017). *Screening for breast cancer*. Retrieved from http://www.cancer.ca/en/cancer-information/cancertype/breast/screening/?region=bc.

11. Tanner, J. M. (1962). *Growth at adolescence* (2nd ed.). Oxford, UK: Blackwell Scientific.

12. Love, S., & Lindsey, K. (2015). *Dr. Susan Love's breast book* (6th ed.). Cambridge, MA: Da Capo Lifelong Books.

13. Jayasinghe, Y. & Simmons, P. S. (2009). Fibroadenomas in adolescence. *Current Opinion in Obstetrics & Gynecology*, 21(5), 402–406. doi:10.1097/GCO.0b013e32832fa06b.

14. Dickson, G. (2012). Gynecomastia. *American Family Physician*, 85(7), 716–722.

15. Canadian Cancer Society. (2018). *Male breast cancer*. Retrieved from http://www.cbcf.org/central/AboutBreastCancerMain/FactsStats/Pages/Male-Breast-Cancer.aspx.

16. Farooq, A., & Horgan, K. (2011). Male breast cancer presenting as nipple discharge. *Case Reports in Surgery*. doi:10.1155/2011/804843.

Thorax and Lungs

Written by Carolyn Jarvis, PhD, APN, CNP
Adapted by June MacDonald-Jenkins, RN, BScN, MSc

(e) http://evolve.elsevier.com/Canada/Jarvis/examination/

STRUCTURE AND FUNCTION

ANTERIOR THORACIC CAGE

19.1 Anterior thoracic cage. © Pat Thomas, 2010.

POSITION AND SURFACE LANDMARKS

The **thoracic cage** is a bony structure with a conical shape, which is narrower at the top (Fig. 19.1). It is defined by the sternum, 12 pairs of **ribs**, and 12 thoracic **vertebrae**. Its "bottom" is the **diaphragm**, a musculotendinous septum that separates the thoracic cavity from the abdomen. The anterior aspects of the first seven ribs attach directly to the sternum via their costal cartilages; those of ribs 8, 9, and 10 attach to the costal cartilage above; and those of ribs 11 and 12 are "floating," with free palpable tips. The **costochondral junctions** are the points at which the ribs join their cartilages. They are not palpable.

Anterior Thoracic Landmarks

Surface landmarks on the thorax are signposts for underlying respiratory structures. Knowledge of landmarks will help you localize a finding and will facilitate communication of your findings to other professionals.

Suprasternal Notch. Feel this hollow U-shaped depression just above the sternum, in between the clavicles.

Sternum. The **sternum**, or "breastbone," has three parts: (a) the manubrium, (b) the body, and (c) the xiphoid process. Walk your fingers down the manubrium a few centimetres until you feel a distinct bony ridge, the manubriosternal angle.

Sternal Angle. The sternal angle, often called the *angle of Louis*, is the articulation of the manubrium and body of the sternum, and it is continuous with the second rib. The angle of Louis is a useful place to start counting ribs, which helps localize a respiratory finding horizontally. Identify the angle of Louis, palpate lightly to the second rib, and slide down to the second intercostal space. Each intercostal space is numbered by the rib above it. Continue counting down the ribs in the middle of the hemithorax, not close to the sternum, where the costal cartilages lie too close together to count. You can palpate easily down to the tenth rib.

The angle of Louis also marks the site of tracheal bifurcation into the right and left main bronchi; it corresponds with the upper border of the atria of the heart, and it lies above the fourth thoracic vertebra on the back.

Costal Angle. The right and left costal margins form an angle where they meet at the xiphoid process. Usually 90 degrees or less, this angle increases when the rib cage is chronically overinflated, as in emphysema.

Posterior Thoracic Landmarks

Counting ribs and intercostal spaces on the back is a bit harder because of the muscles and soft tissue surrounding the ribs and spinal column (Fig. 19.2).

Vertebra Prominens. Start at the base of your neck. Flex your head and feel for the most prominent bony protrusion there. This is the spinous process of C7. If two bumps seem equally prominent, the upper one is C7 and the lower one is T1.

Spinous Processes. Count down the vertebrae, which stack together to form the spinal column. Note that the spinous processes align with their same-numbered ribs only down to T4. After T4, the spinous processes angle downward from their vertebral bodies, and each overlies the vertebral body and rib below.

Inferior Border of the Scapula. The scapulae are located symmetrically in each hemithorax. The lower tip is usually at the level of the seventh or eighth rib.

Twelfth Rib. Palpate midway between the spine and the patient's side to identify the free tip of the twelfth rib.

Reference Lines

Use the reference lines to pinpoint a finding vertically on the chest. On the chest, note the **midsternal line** and the **midclavicular line**. The midclavicular line bisects the centre of each clavicle at a point halfway between the palpated sternoclavicular and acromioclavicular joints (Fig. 19.3).

The posterior chest wall can be demarcated by the **vertebral line** (or *midspinal line*) and the **scapular line**, which extends through the inferior angle of the scapula when the arms are at the sides of the body (Fig. 19.4).

Lift up one of the patient's arms 90 degrees, and observe the lateral chest. It can be demarcated by three lines: (a) the **anterior axillary line** extends down from the anterior

POSTERIOR THORACIC CAGE

19.2 Posterior thoracic cage. © Pat Thomas, 2010.

19.3

19.5

19.4

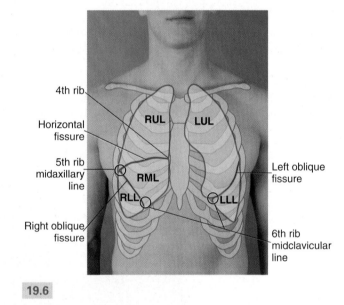

19.6

axillary fold, where the pectoralis major muscle inserts; (b) the **posterior axillary line** continues down from the posterior axillary fold, where the latissimus dorsi muscle inserts; and (c) the **midaxillary line** runs down from the apex of the axilla and lies between and parallel to the other two (Fig. 19.5).

THE THORACIC CAVITY

The **mediastinum** is the middle section of the thoracic cavity, and it contains the esophagus, trachea, heart, and great vessels. The right and left **pleural cavities**, on either side of the mediastinum, contain the lungs.

Lung Borders. In the anterior chest, the **apex**, or highest point, of lung tissue is 3 or 4 cm above the inner third of the clavicles. The **base**, or lower border, rests on the diaphragm

at about the sixth rib in the midclavicular line. Laterally, lung tissue extends from the apex of the axilla down to the seventh or eighth rib. Posteriorly, the location of C7 marks the apex of lung tissue, and T10 usually corresponds to the base. Deep inspiration expands the lungs, and their lower border drops to the level of T12.

Lobes of the Lungs

The lungs are paired but not precisely symmetrical structures (Fig. 19.6). The right lung is shorter than the left lung because of the underlying liver. The left lung is narrower than the right lung because the heart bulges to the left. The right lung has three lobes, and the left lung has two lobes. These lobes are not arranged in horizontal bands like dessert layers in a parfait glass; rather, they stack in diagonal sloping segments and are separated by **fissures** that run obliquely through the chest.

19.7

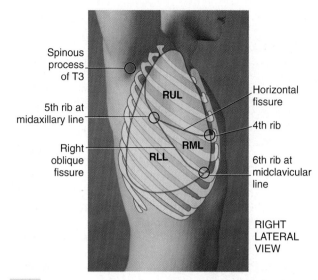

19.8

Anterior. On the anterior chest, the **oblique fissure** (the major or diagonal fissure) crosses the fifth rib in the midaxillary line and terminates at the sixth rib in the midclavicular line. The right lung also contains the **horizontal fissure** (minor fissure), which divides the right upper and middle lobes. This fissure extends from the fifth rib in the right midaxillary line to the third intercostal space or fourth rib at the right sternal border. The anterior chest contains primarily upper and middle lobes.

Posterior. The most remarkable point about the posterior chest is that it is almost all lower lobe (Fig. 19.7). The upper lobes occupy a smaller band of tissue from their apices at T1 down to T3 or T4. At this level, the lower lobes begin, and their inferior border reaches down to the level of T10 on expiration and to T12 on inspiration. Note that the right middle lobe does not project onto the posterior chest at all. If the patient abducts the arms and places the hands on the back of the head, the division between upper and lower lobes corresponds to the medial border of the scapulae.

Lateral. Laterally, lung tissue extends from the apex of the axilla down to the seventh or eighth rib. The right upper lobe extends from the level of the apex of the axilla down to the level of the horizontal fissure at the fifth rib (Fig. 19.8). The right middle lobe extends from the level of the horizontal fissure down and forward to the level of the sixth rib at the midclavicular line. The right lower lobe continues from the level of the fifth rib to that of the eighth rib in the midaxillary line.

The left lung contains only two lobes, upper and lower (Fig. 19.9). These appear laterally as two triangular areas separated by the oblique fissure. The left upper lobe extends from the level of the apex of the axilla down to the level of the fifth rib at the midaxillary line. The left lower lobe continues down to the level of the eighth rib in the midaxillary line.

Using these landmarks, try determining the outline of each lobe on a willing partner. Take special note of the three points that commonly confuse beginning examiners:

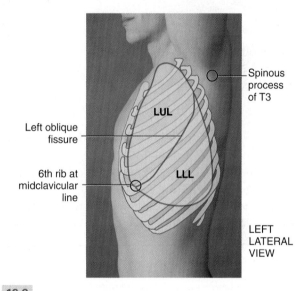

19.9

1. The left lung has no middle lobe.
2. The anterior chest contains mostly upper and middle lobe with very little lower lobe.
3. The posterior chest contains almost all lower lobe.

Pleurae

The thin, slippery **pleurae** form an envelope between the lungs and the chest wall (Fig. 19.10). The **visceral pleura** lines the outside of the lungs, dipping down into the fissures. It is continuous with the **parietal pleura**, which lines the inside of the chest wall and diaphragm.

The inside of the envelope, the pleural cavity, is a potential space filled only with a few millilitres of lubricating fluid. It normally has a vacuum, or negative pressure, which holds the lungs tightly against the chest wall. The lungs slide smoothly and noiselessly up and down during respiration, lubricated by a few millilitres of fluid. Think of this as similar to two glass slides with a drop of water between them; although it

CROSS-SECTION OF THORAX

- Left lung
- Parietal pleura (lines chest cavity)
- Visceral pleura (encloses lung)
- Heart

ACINUS

- Pulmonary artery
- Pulmonary vein
- Bronchiole
- Alveolus
- Interalveolar septum
- Alveolar sac

PLEURAE AND TRACHEOBRONCHIAL TREE

- Thyroid cartilage
- Cricoid cartilage
- Cut edge of parietal pleura
- Right upper lobe
- Right bronchial tree
- Right middle lobe
- Right lower lobe
- Costodiaphragmatic recess
- Diaphragm
- Esophagus
- Trachea
- Left upper lobe
- Tracheal bifurcation
- Left bronchial tree
- Left lower lobe
- Parietal pleura (intact, enclosing lung)

19.10 Pleurae and tracheobronchial tree. (© Pat Thomas, 2006.)

is difficult to separate the slides, they slide smoothly back and forth. The pleurae extend about 3 cm below the level of the lungs, forming the **costodiaphragmatic recess**. This is a potential space; when it abnormally fills with air or fluid, it compromises lung expansion.

Trachea and Bronchial Tree

The **trachea** lies anterior to the esophagus and is 10 to 11 cm long in the adult. It begins at the level of the cricoid cartilage in the neck and bifurcates just below the sternal angle into the right and left main bronchi. Posteriorly, tracheal bifurcation is at the level of T4 or T5. The right main bronchus is shorter, wider, and more vertical than the left main bronchus.

The **trachea** and **bronchi** transport gases between the environment and the lung parenchyma. They constitute the *dead space*, or space that is filled with air but is not available for gaseous exchange. In adults, its capacity is approximately 150 mL. The bronchial tree also protects alveoli from small particulate matter in the inhaled air. The bronchi are lined with goblet cells, which secrete mucus that entraps the particles, and with cilia, which sweep the particles upward where they can be swallowed or expelled.

An **acinus** is a functional respiratory unit that consists of the bronchioles, alveolar ducts, alveolar sacs, and the alveoli. Gaseous exchange occurs across the respiratory membrane in the alveolar duct and in the millions of alveoli. The alveoli are clustered like grapes around each alveolar duct. As a result, there are millions of interalveolar septa (walls) that tremendously increase the working space available for gas exchange. This bunched arrangement creates a surface area for gas exchange that is as large as a tennis court.

MECHANICS OF RESPIRATION

The respiratory system has four major functions: (a) supplying oxygen to the body for energy production, (b) removing carbon dioxide as a waste product of energy reactions, (c) maintaining homeostasis (acid–base balance) of arterial blood, and (d) maintaining heat exchange (less important in humans).

By supplying oxygen to the blood and eliminating excess carbon dioxide, respiration maintains the pH, or the acid–base balance, of the blood. The body tissues are bathed by blood, whose normal acceptable pH has a narrow range. Although a number of compensatory mechanisms regulate the pH, the lungs help maintain the balance by adjusting the level of carbon dioxide through respiration; that is, hypoventilation (slow, shallow breathing) causes carbon dioxide to build up in the blood, and hyperventilation (rapid, deep breathing) causes carbon dioxide to be blown off.

Control of Respirations

Normally, a person's breathing pattern changes, without the person's awareness, in response to cellular demands. This

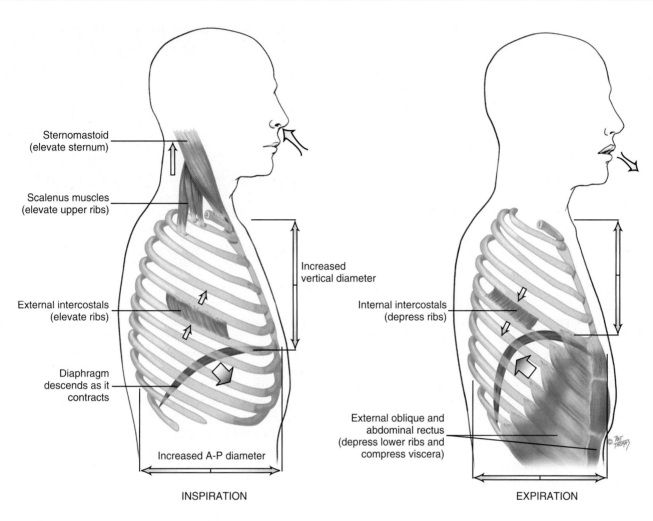

Sternomastoid
(elevate sternum)

Scalenus muscles
(elevate upper ribs)

Increased
vertical diameter

External intercostals
(elevate ribs)

Internal intercostals
(depress ribs)

Diaphragm
descends as it
contracts

External oblique and
abdominal rectus
(depress lower ribs and
compress viscera)

Increased A-P diameter

INSPIRATION

EXPIRATION

19.11   © Pat Thomas, 2010.

involuntary control of respiration is mediated by the respiratory centre in the brain stem (pons and medulla). The major feedback loop is humoral regulation, or the change in carbon dioxide and oxygen levels in the blood and, of less importance, the hydrogen ion level. The *normal stimulus to breathe* for most people is an increase of carbon dioxide in the blood, or **hypercapnia**. A decrease of oxygen in the blood (**hypoxemia**) also increases respirations but is less effective than hypercapnia.

Changing Chest Size

Respiration is the physical act of breathing; air rushes into the lungs as the chest size increases (inspiration) and is expelled from the lungs as the chest recoils (expiration). The mechanical expansion and contraction of the chest cavity alters the size of the thoracic container in two dimensions: (a) the vertical diameter lengthens or shortens, which is accomplished by downward or upward movement of the diaphragm, and (b) the anteroposterior diameter increases or decreases, which is accomplished by elevation or depression of the ribs (Fig. 19.11).

In inspiration, increasing the size of the thoracic container creates a slightly negative pressure in relation to the atmosphere, and so air rushes in to fill the partial vacuum. The major muscle responsible for this increase is the diaphragm. During inspiration, contraction of the bell-shaped diaphragm causes it to descend and flatten. This lengthens the vertical diameter. Intercostal muscles lift the sternum and elevate the ribs, making them more horizontal. This increases the anteroposterior diameter.

Expiration is primarily passive. As the diaphragm relaxes, elastic forces within the lung, thoracic cage, and abdomen cause it to expand upward and form a dome. All this squeezing creates a relatively positive pressure within the alveoli, and the air flows out.

In forced inspiration, such as that after heavy exercise or occurring pathologically with respiratory distress, the accessory neck muscles are used to heave up the sternum and rib cage. These neck muscles are the sternomastoid, scalene, and the trapezius muscles. In forced expiration, the abdominal muscles contract powerfully to push the abdominal viscera forcefully in and up against the diaphragm, causing it to expand upward as a dome and squeeze against the lungs.

❖ DEVELOPMENTAL CONSIDERATIONS

Infants and Children

During the first 5 weeks of fetal life, the primitive lung bud emerges; by 16 weeks, the conducting airways reach the same number as in the adult; at 32 weeks, **surfactant**, the complex lipid substance needed for sustained inflation of the air sacs, is present in adequate amounts; and by birth, the lungs have 70 million primitive alveoli ready to start the job of respiration.

Breath is life. When the newborn inhales the first breath, the lusty cry that follows reassures anxious parents that their baby is all right (Fig. 19.12). The baby's body systems all develop in utero, but the respiratory system alone does not function until birth. Birth necessitates its instant performance.

When the umbilical cord is cut, blood is cut off from the placenta, and it gushes into the pulmonary circulation. Relatively less resistance exists in the pulmonary arteries than in the aorta, and so the foramen ovale in the heart closes just after birth. (See the discussion of fetal circulation in Chapter 20, p. 501.) The ductus arteriosus (linking the pulmonary artery and the aorta) contracts and closes several hours later, and pulmonary and systemic circulation become functional.

Respiratory development continues throughout childhood, with increases in the diameter and length of airways and in the size and number of alveoli, reaching the adult range of 300 million by adolescence.

19.12

The relatively smaller size and immaturity of children's pulmonary systems and the presence of people who smoke result in enormous vulnerability and increased risks to child health. Prenatal exposure results in chronic hypoxia and low birth weight. Also, it sensitizes the fetal brain to nicotine, which increases risk for addiction when the child is exposed to nicotine at a later age.[1] Postnatal exposure to environmental tobacco smoke is linked to increased rates of otitis media, sudden infant death syndrome, lower respiratory tract infections, and childhood asthma.[2] (See the box Promoting Health: Environmental Tobacco Smoke.)

PROMOTING HEALTH: ENVIRONMENTAL TOBACCO SMOKE

Second/Third-Hand Smoke: There Is No Risk-Free Level of Exposure!

Second-hand smoke, also referred to as *environmental tobacco smoke*, is a mixture of *sidestream smoke* (the smoke from the burning end of a cigarette, pipe, or cigar) and *mainstream smoke* (the smoke exhaled from the lungs of the smoker). According to Health Canada, there is *no safe level* of exposure to the carcinogens in cigarette smoke.* Exposure to second-hand smoke, which is primarily involuntary, increases the risk for adverse health effects. Furthermore, exposure to second-hand smoke, for the general public (both smokers and others) is much higher than most people realize.

Because children breathe faster than adults, they are particularly vulnerable to environmental tobacco smoke. Parents who smoke increase the chances that their children will develop asthma by 200% to 400%. Children exposed to second-hand smoke are also more likely to develop ear infections and later become smokers themselves; it can be seen as socially acceptable when parents are role models for this behaviour. In 2016, 16.9% of Canadians aged 12 and older (roughly 5.2 million people) smoked either daily or occasionally. This percentage is a decrease from 2014 (18.1%) and is the lowest smoking rate reported since 2001.† Ontario and British Columbia have the lowest smoking rates in Canada, while the territories and Nunavut have the highest smoking rates. Since 2001, provincial legislation in Canada has been implemented to restrict smoking in the workplace. Not all provinces have enacted 100% smoke-free legislation, but provinces such as Alberta and British Columbia have implemented some of the most aggressive nonsmoking laws in the country.

Second-hand smoke contains hundreds of chemicals known to be toxic or carcinogenic, including formaldehyde, benzene, vinyl chloride, arsenic, and cyanide. Smoke can linger in the air for hours long after the cigarette, cigar, or pipe has been extinguished and is involuntarily inhaled by nonsmokers.‡ **Third-hand smoke** is a new name for an old problem: the toxic chemicals in smoke that linger in the air, even after the smoker has put out the cigarette, cigar, or pipe. Third-hand smoke gets trapped in hair, skin, fabric, carpet, furniture, and toys, and it builds up over time.

Exposure to second-hand smoke places nonsmokers at risk for the same diseases that active smoking does. Nonsmokers exposed to second-hand smoke are 25% more likely to have heart disease and 20% more likely to have lung cancer than are nonsmokers not exposed to smoke. Separating smokers from nonsmokers, cleaning the air indoors, and ventilating buildings do not eliminate the exposure risk to nonsmokers. However, eliminating smoking in indoor spaces does fully protect the nonsmoker.‡

PROMOTING HEALTH: ENVIRONMENTAL TOBACCO SMOKE—cont'd

Second-Hand/Third-Hand Smoke: There Is No Risk-Free Level of Exposure!

In Canada, 20- to 24-year-olds represent the single largest group of smokers in the country. In Ontario, since 2000, Leave the Pack Behind campaigns and programs have applied evidence-informed tobacco-control strategies to support reduced tobacco use among young Canadians. This program has a large presence on university and college campuses as well as centres that support adolescents and young adults.[§]

Other provincial and national prevention programs include a tax increase on tobacco products to make it more difficult to sustain the habit; greater availability of cessation programming; and national tobacco products labelling regulations that require packaging to visually depict the harmful effects of tobacco on humans.

How do you reduce exposure to second-hand/third-hand smoke? First, do not smoke or allow smoking in your home. Tell smokers that you do mind if they smoke indoors, and ask them to go outside while they smoke. It is important to protect children from the harmful effects of tobacco smoke, inasmuch as research has demonstrated that children have an especially high risk for health problems from exposure. Children breathe in more air than do adults in relation to their body weight—which means they absorb more tobacco smoke—and their immune systems are less developed; moreover, they have less power and ability to complain about being around tobacco smoke. The Canadian Lung Association launched a national strategy to ban smoking in vehicles with children. Smoking with anyone younger than 16 present in a vehicle is currently banned in all provinces. Legislation is pending in the territories and Nunavut. In Nova Scotia, smoking is banned in vehicles when persons younger than 19 are present.[¶]

For more information about smoking cessation, visit the Canadian Lung Association website at https://www.lung.ca/lung-health/smoking-and-tobacco.

References

*Health Canada. (2012). *Tobacco products labelling regulations (cigarettes and little cigars)*. Retrieved from http://www.hc-sc.gc.ca/hc-ps/tobac-tabac/legislation/reg/label-etiquette/index-eng.php.

†Statistics Canada. (2017). *Smoking, 2016*. Retrieved from https://www150.statcan.gc.ca/n1/pub/82-625-x/2017001/article/54864-eng.htm.

‡Health Canada. (2016). *Smoke-free public places: You can get there*. Ottawa: Author.

§Leave the Pack Behind. (2017). *About*. Retrieved from https://www.leavethepackbehind.org.

¶Health Canada. (2015). *Dangers of second-hand smoke*. Retrieved from https://www.canada.ca/en/health-canada/services/smoking-tobacco/avoid-second-hand-smoke/second-hand-smoke/dangers-second-hand-smoke.html.

Pregnant Women

The enlarging uterus elevates the diaphragm 4 cm during pregnancy. This decreases the vertical diameter of the thoracic cage, but this decrease is compensated for by an increase in the horizontal diameter. The increase in estrogen level relaxes the thoracic cage ligaments. This allows an increase in the transverse diameter of the thoracic cage by 2 cm, and the costal angle widens. The total circumference of the thoracic cage increases by 6 cm. Although the diaphragm is elevated, it is not fixed. It moves with breathing even more during pregnancy, which results in a 40% increase in tidal volume.[3]

The growing fetus increases the oxygen demand on the mother's body. This demand is met easily by the increasing tidal volume (deeper breathing). Little change occurs in the respiratory rate. An increased awareness of the need to breathe develops, even early in pregnancy. This **physiologic dyspnea** affects close to 75% of women; it does not alter activities of daily living (ADLs) and is not associated with cough, wheezing, or exercise.[4]

Older Adults

In older adults, the costal cartilages become calcified, which reduces the mobility of the thorax. Respiratory muscle strength declines after age 50 years and continues to decrease into the 70s. A more significant change is the decrease in elastic properties within the lungs, which makes them less distensible and lessens their tendency to contract and recoil. In summary, the aging lung is a more rigid structure that is harder to inflate.

These changes result in an increase in small airway closure, and that causes a *decreased vital capacity* (the maximum amount of air that a person can expel from the lungs after first filling the lungs to maximum) and an *increased residual volume* (the amount of air remaining in the lungs even after the most forceful expiration).

With aging, histological changes (i.e., a gradual loss of intra-alveolar septa and a decrease in the number of alveoli) also occur, so that less surface area is available for gas exchange. Also, the lung bases become less ventilated as a result of the closing off of a number of airways. This increases the risk for shortness of breath with exertion beyond an older person's usual workload.

The histological changes also increase older persons' risk for postoperative pulmonary complications. That is, older persons have a greater risk for postoperative atelectasis and infection as a result of a decreased ability to cough, a loss of protective airway reflexes, and increased secretions.

SOCIAL DETERMINANTS OF HEALTH CONSIDERATIONS

Tuberculosis (TB) is a major global health problem. In 2016, an estimated 10.4 million new cases were reported worldwide. A total of 1 639 of these new cases were from Canada, which represented a small increase from the preceding year (1 614). The number of reported cases of active TB disease has remained relatively stable in Canada. The western provinces, the territories, and Nunavut have the highest incidence in the country; foreign-born individuals and Indigenous people are disproportionately represented among reported cases of TB. Pulmonary TB remains the most commonly reported site of disease. Low socioeconomic conditions, the number of household inhabitants, and access to health care resources all impact both the ability to diagnose and the subsequent treatment of the condition. A full 84% of all Canadians diagnosed in 2015 were successfully treated. *Mycobacterium tuberculosis*, which causes this disease, is an airborne pathogen. Therefore, the isolation of infected individuals and early diagnosis are essential for minimizing spread of the disease.[5]

In 2014, 2.4 million people reported that they had been diagnosed with asthma by a health care provider. This rate has remained fairly consistent since 2001. The two most important preventable risk factors for respiratory disease are tobacco smoke (both personal and second-hand) and poor air quality (indoor and outdoor). From 2011 to 2014, asthma was a contributing factor in approximately 10% of the hospital admissions of children younger than age 5 years and in 8% of those aged 5 to 14 years.[6]

Respiratory diseases, including lung cancer, are a major cause of death in Canada. Lung cancer remains the leading cause of cancer death in both men and women. In 2017, the Canadian Cancer Society estimated that 1 in 11 Canadian men would develop lung cancer during his lifetime, and 1 in 14 would die of it. It also estimated that 1 in 14 women would develop lung cancer during her lifetime, and 1 in 17 were expected to die from it.[7] The incidence rate among women, although still elevated, appears to be stabilizing. In men, the incidence has been decreasing.[8]

Women and Chronic Obstructive Pulmonary Disease

With regard to chronic obstructive pulmonary disease (COPD), a national report called for increased awareness, screening, and advocacy.[9] Spirometry in women should be as routine as mammography for breast screening.[10] Women seem to incur greater lung damage from exposure to environmental tobacco smoke than do men. Despite a decrease in COPD nationally, younger women still are the greatest area of increased incidence since 2011. Moreover, the percentage of women who undergo appropriate screening for the disease is unacceptably low.[11]

SUBJECTIVE DATA

1. Cough
2. Shortness of breath
3. Chest pain with breathing
4. History of respiratory infections
5. Smoking history
6. Environmental exposure
7. Self-care behaviours

HEALTH HISTORY QUESTIONS

Examiner Asks	Rationale
1. Cough. Do you have a **cough**? When did it start? Gradual or sudden? • How long have you had it? • How often do you cough? At any special time of day or just on arising? Does the cough wake you up at night?	Acute cough lasts less than 2 or 3 weeks; chronic cough lasts more than 2 months. In some conditions, the timing of a cough is characteristic: • Continuous throughout day: acute illness (e.g., respiratory infection) • Afternoon/evening: may reflect exposure to irritants at work • Night: postnasal drip, sinusitis • Early morning: chronic bronchial inflammation of smokers
• Do you cough up any phlegm or sputum? How much? What colour is it?	Chronic bronchitis is characterized by a history of productive cough for 3 months of the year for 2 years in a row.

Examiner Asks	Rationale
• Cough up any blood (**hemoptysis**)? Does this look like streaks or frank blood? Does the sputum have a foul odour?	In some conditions, sputum production is characteristic: • White or clear mucoid: colds, bronchitis, viral infections • Yellow or green: bacterial infections • Rust coloured: tuberculosis, pneumococcal pneumonia • Pink, frothy: pulmonary edema, some sympathomimetic medications (adverse effect of pink-tinged mucus)
• How would you describe your cough: hacking, dry, barking, hoarse, congested, bubbling?	Some conditions are accompanied by a characteristic cough: • *Mycoplasma* pneumonia: hacking • Early heart failure: dry • Croup: barking • Colds, bronchitis, pneumonia: congested
• Does the cough seem to come with anything: activity, position (lying), fever, congestion, talking, anxiety? • Does activity make it better or worse? • What treatment have you tried: prescription or over-the-counter medications, vaporizer, rest, position change? • Does the cough bring on anything: chest pain, ear pain? Is it tiring? Are you concerned about it?	Assess effectiveness of coping strategies. Note severity.
2. **Shortness of breath**. Ever had any **shortness of breath** or a hard-breathing spell? What brings it on? How severe is it? How long does it last? • Is it affected by position, such as lying down?	Determine how much activity precipitates the shortness of breath; state specific number of blocks walked, number of stairs. **Orthopnea** is difficulty breathing in the supine position. State number of pillows needed to achieve comfort (e.g., "two-pillow orthopnea").
• Does it occur at any specific time of day or night?	**Paroxysmal nocturnal dyspnea** is awakening from sleep with shortness of breath and needing to be upright to achieve comfort. This condition is diaphoresis. The bluish colour is cyanosis.
• Are the episodes associated with night sweats? • Are they associated with cough, chest pain, or bluish colour around lips or nails? Wheezing sound? • Do episodes seem to be related to food, pollen, dust, animals, season, or emotion? • What do you do in a hard-breathing attack: take a special position, or use pursed-lip breathing? Use any oxygen, inhalers, or medications? • How does the shortness of breath affect your work or home activities? Is it getting better or worse, or is it staying about the same?	Asthma attacks may be associated with a specific allergen, extreme cold, or anxiety. Assess effect of coping strategies and the need for more teaching. Assess effect on ADLs.
3. **Chest pain with breathing**. Any **chest pain with breathing**? Please point to the exact location. • When did it start? Is it constant, or does it come and go? • Describe the pain: burning, stabbing? • Is it brought on by respiratory infection, coughing, or trauma? Is it associated with fever, deep breathing, or unequal rising and falling of the chest? • What have you done to treat it? Medication or heat application?	Chest pain of thoracic origin occurs with muscle soreness from coughing or from inflammation of pleura overlying pneumonia. Distinguish this from chest pain of cardiac origin (see Chapter 20) or from heartburn of stomach acid.

Examiner Asks	Rationale
4. History of respiratory infections. Any **past history of breathing trouble or lung diseases** such as bronchitis, emphysema, asthma, pneumonia?	Consider sequelae after these conditions.
• Have you had unusually frequent or unusually severe colds?	Because most people have had some colds, it is more meaningful to ask about excess number or severity.
• Any family history of allergies, tuberculosis, or asthma?	Assess possible risk factors.
5. Smoking history. Do you **smoke** cigarettes or cigars? At what age did you start? How many packs per day do you smoke now? For how long?	State number of packs per day and the number of years smoked.
• Have you ever tried to quit? What helped? Why do you think it did not work? What activities do you associate with smoking?	Most people who smoke already know they should quit smoking. Instead of admonishing, assess smoking behaviour and ways to modify daily smoking activities, identify triggers, and manage withdrawal.
• Do you live with someone who smokes?	
6. Environmental exposure. Are there any **environmental conditions** that may affect your breathing? Where do you work: at a factory, chemical plant, coal mine, farm, outdoors in a heavy traffic area?	Pollution exposure. Farmers may be at risk for grain inhalation and pesticide inhalation. "Farmer's lung" (**extrinsic allergic alveolitis**) occurs in about 2% to 10% of farm workers, depending on the region. The disease is most common in Canada in regions with wet weather at harvest time. Coal miners have a risk for pneumoconiosis. Stone cutters, miners, and potters are at risk for silicosis. Other irritants include asbestos and radon.
• Do you do anything to protect your lungs, such as wear a mask or have the ventilatory system checked at work? Do you do anything to monitor your exposure? Do you have periodic examinations, pulmonary function tests, radiographic examinations?	Assess **self-care** measures.
• Do you require treatment devices to support your breathing? Home oxygen? **Continuous positive airway pressure (CPAP)** machine?	Low dose home oxygen via nasal prongs is noted in some individuals with chronic respiratory conditions such as COPD or pulmonary fibrosis.[12] CPAP is a form of positive airway pressure ventilator that applies mild air pressure on a continuous basis to keep the airways open in individuals who have obstructive sleep apnea.[13]
• Do you know what specific symptoms to note that may signal breathing problems?	General symptoms: cough, shortness of breath. Some gases produce specific symptoms: • Carbon monoxide: dizziness, headache, fatigue • Sulphur dioxide: cough, congestion
7. Self-care behaviours. When was your most recent tuberculosis skin test, chest radiographic study, pneumonia immunization, or influenza immunization?	"Flu" vaccine is modified yearly; it is recommended for adults with chronic medical conditions, for residents of nursing homes, for health care workers, and for people who are immunosuppressed.

Subjective Data

Examiner Asks	Rationale

Additional History for Infants and Children

1. Illness. Has the child had any frequent or very severe colds?

No more than four to six uncomplicated upper respiratory infections per year are expected in early childhood.

2. Allergy. Is there any history of allergy in the family?
- For a child younger than age 2 years: At what age were new foods introduced? Was the child breastfed or formula-fed?

Consider new foods or formula as possible allergens.

3. Chronic respiratory illness. Does the child have a cough? Seem congested? Have noisy breathing or wheezing? (Further questions similar to those listed in the section on adults.)

Document onset, and follow course of childhood chronic respiratory problems: asthma, bronchitis.

4. Safety. What measures have you taken to childproof your home and yard? Is there any risk that the child could inhale or swallow toxic substances?
- Has anyone taught you emergency care measures in case of accidental choking or a hard-breathing spell?

Young children are at risk for accidental aspiration, poisoning, and injury.
Assess knowledge level of parents and caregivers.

5. Environmental tobacco smoke. Any smokers in the home or in the car with the child?

Environmental tobacco smoke increases the risk for acute and chronic ear and respiratory infections in children.[1,2]

Additional History for Older Adults

1. Changes. Have you noticed any shortness of breath or fatigue with your daily activities?

In older adults, the respiratory system is less efficient (decreased vital capacity, less surface area for gas exchange), and so they have less tolerance for activity.

2. Physical activity. Tell me about your usual amount of physical activity.

Older patients may have reduced capacity to perform exercise because of pulmonary function deficits of aging.
Sedentary or bedridden people are at risk for respiratory dysfunction.

3. History of respiratory conditions. For patients with a history of COPD, lung cancer, or tuberculosis: How are you getting along each day? Any weight change in the last 3 months? How much?
- How about energy level? Do you tire more easily? How does your illness affect you at home? At work?

Assess coping strategies.

Activities may decrease because of increasing shortness of breath or pain.

4. Chest pain with breathing. Do you have any chest pain with breathing?

- Any chest pain after a bout of coughing? After a fall?
For people with a frequent productive cough and/or a long smoking history, use the following questionnaire. This is a simple, short tool to identify persons who will need spirometry testing to confirm the diagnosis of COPD.[14]

Some older adults feel pleuritic pain less intensely than do younger adults.
When pain is precisely localized and sharp (patient points to it with one finger), consider fractured rib or muscle injury.

Subjective Data

Examiner Asks	Rationale

Lung Function Questionnaire

Do you suffer from breathing problems and/or frequent cough?

These questions ask about your breathing problems and/or frequent cough. As you answer these questions, think about how you feel physically when you experience these symptoms. For each question, choose the one answer that best describes your symptoms. Share the answers with your healthcare provider.

Step 1: Answer each question and write the score in the box next to it.
Step 2: Add together the scores in each box to get your total score.
Step 3: Take the test to your provider to talk about your score.

1. How often do you cough up mucus?

   Never (5) Rarely (4) Sometimes (3) Often (2) Very often (1)   SCORE ☐

2. How often does your chest sound noisy (wheezy, whistling, rattling) when you breathe?

   Never (5) Rarely (4) Sometimes (3) Often (2) Very often (1)   ☐

3. How often do you experience shortness of breath during physical activity (walking up a flight of stairs or walking up an incline without stopping to rest)?

   Never (5) Rarely (4) Sometimes (3) Often (2) Very often (1)   ☐

4. How many years have you smoked?

   Never smoked (5) 10 years or less (4) 11-20 years (3) 21-30 years (2) More than 30 years (1)   ☐

5. What is your age?

   Less than 40 years (5) 40-49 years (4) 50-59 years (3) 60-69 years (2) 70 years or older (1)   ☐

Step 4: If your score is <u>18 or less</u>, you may be at risk for Chronic Obstructive Pulmonary Disease (COPD). COPD includes chronic bronchitis, emphysema, or both.   TOTAL ☐

OBJECTIVE DATA

PREPARATION

Ask the patient to sit upright and to leave the gown on and open at the back. When you examine the anterior chest, lift up the gown and drape it on the patient's shoulders, rather than removing it completely. This promotes comfort by giving the patient the feeling of being somewhat clothed. To ensure further comfort, use a warm room and a warm diaphragm endpiece, and provide private examination time with no interruptions.

Perform the inspection, palpation, percussion, and auscultation on the posterior and lateral thorax. Then move to face the patient, and repeat these four manoeuvres on the anterior chest. This avoids repetitiously moving front to back around the patient.

Finally, clean your stethoscope endpiece with an alcohol wipe. Because your stethoscope touches many people, it could be a possible vector for both aerobic and anaerobic bacteria. Cleaning with an alcohol wipe is very effective.

EQUIPMENT NEEDED
Stethoscope
Small ruler, marked in centimetres
Marking pen
Alcohol wipe

Normal Range of Findings	Abnormal Findings

Inspect the Posterior Chest

Thoracic Cage

Note the **shape and configuration** of the chest wall. The spinous processes should appear in a straight line. The thorax is symmetrical, in an elliptical shape, with downward sloping ribs, angled at approximately 45 degrees in relation to the spine. The scapulae are symmetrically placed in each hemithorax.

Skeletal deformities may limit thoracic cage excursion: scoliosis, kyphosis (see Table 19.4, p. 480).

Normal Range of Findings

The anteroposterior diameter (AP) should be less than the transverse diameter. The normal ratio of anteroposterior diameter to transverse diameter is approximately 1:2.

The neck muscles and trapezius muscles should have developed normally for age and occupation.

Note the **position** the patient takes to breathe. This includes a relaxed posture and the ability to support one's own weight with arms comfortably at the sides or in the lap.

Assess the **skin colour** and **condition**. Colour should be consistent with the patient's genetic background, with allowance for sun-exposed areas on the chest and the back. No cyanosis or pallor should be present. Note any lesions. Inquire as to any change in a nevus in a place where the patient may have difficulty monitoring, such as on the back (see Chapter 13).

Palpate the Posterior Chest

Symmetrical Expansion

Confirm **symmetrical chest expansion** by placing your warmed hands on the patient's posterolateral chest wall, with your thumbs at the level of T9 or T10. Slide your hands medially to pinch up a small fold of skin between your thumbs (Fig. 19.13).

19.13

Abnormal Findings

AP diameter equals transverse diameter ("barrel chest"). Ribs are horizontal, chest appears as if held in continuous inspiration. This occurs in chronic emphysema as a result of hyperinflation of the lungs (see Table 19.4, p. 479).

Neck muscles are hypertrophied in COPD as a result of aiding in forced respirations.

Patients with COPD often sit in a tripod position, leaning forward with arms braced against their knees, chair, or bed. This gives them leverage so that their rectus abdominis, intercostal, and accessory neck muscles all can aid in expiration.

Cyanosis occurs with tissue hypoxia.

Normal Range of Findings	Abnormal Findings

Ask the patient to take a deep breath. Your hands serve as mechanical amplifiers; as the patient inhales deeply, your thumbs should move apart symmetrically. Note any lag in expansion.

Tactile Fremitus

Assess **tactile** (or **vocal**) **fremitus**. Fremitus is a palpable vibration. Sounds generated from the larynx are transmitted through patent bronchi and through the lung parenchyma to the chest wall, where you feel them as vibrations.

Use either the palmar base (the ball) of the fingers or the ulnar edge of one of your hands, and touch the patient's chest while the patient repeats the words "ninety-nine" or "blue moon." These are resonant phrases that generate strong vibrations. Start over the lung apices, and palpate from one side to another (Fig. 19.14).

19.14

Symmetry is most important; the vibrations should feel the same in the corresponding area on each side. Avoid palpating over the scapulae because bone damps sound transmission.

The following factors affect the normal intensity of tactile fremitus:

- Fremitus is most prominent between the scapulae and around the sternum, sites where the major bronchi are closest to the chest wall. It normally decreases as you progress down because more and more tissue impedes sound transmission.
- Fremitus feels greater over a thin chest wall than over an obese or heavily muscular one, in which thick tissue damps the vibration.
- A loud, low-pitched voice generates more fremitus than does a soft, high-pitched one.

Note any areas of abnormal fremitus. Sound is conducted better through a uniformly dense structure than through a porous one, which changes in shape and solidity (as does the lung tissue during normal respiration). Thus conditions that increase the density of lung tissue make a better conducting medium for sound vibrations and increase tactile fremitus.

Abnormal Findings

Chest expansion is unequal with marked atelectasis or pneumonia; with thoracic trauma such as fractured ribs; and with pneumothorax.

Pain accompanies deep breathing when the pleurae are inflamed.

Decreased fremitus occurs when anything obstructs transmission of vibrations (e.g., obstructed bronchus, pleural effusion or thickening, pneumothorax, or emphysema). Any barrier between the sound and your palpating hand decreases fremitus.

Increased fremitus occurs with compression or consolidation of lung tissue (e.g., lobar pneumonia). This occurs only when the bronchus is patent and when the consolidation extends to the lung surface. Note that only gross changes increase fremitus. Small areas of early pneumonia do not significantly affect it.

Normal Range of Findings

Using the fingers, gently **palpate the entire chest wall**. This enables you to note any areas of tenderness, to note skin temperature and moisture, to detect any superficial lumps or masses, and to explore any skin lesions noted on inspection.

Percuss the Posterior Chest

Lung Fields

Determine the **predominant note over the lung fields**. Start at the apices and percuss the band of normally resonant tissue across the tops of both shoulders (Fig. 19.15). Then, percussing in the interspaces, make a side-to-side comparison all the way down the lung region. Percuss at 5-cm intervals. Avoid the damping effect of the scapulae and ribs.

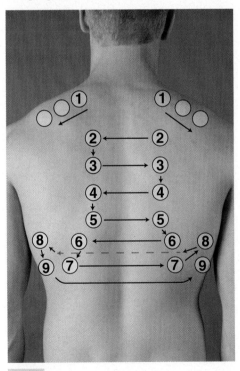

19.15

Resonance is the low-pitched, clear, hollow sound that predominates in healthy lung tissue in adults (Fig. 19.16). However, resonance is a relative term and has no constant standard. The resonant note may be modified somewhat in an athlete with a heavily muscular chest wall and in an obese adult, in whom subcutaneous fat produces scattered dullness.

The depth of penetration of percussion has limits. Percussion sets into motion only the outer 5 to 7 cm of tissue. It does not penetrate to reveal any change in density deeper than that. Also, any abnormal tissue must be 2 to 3 cm wide to yield an abnormal percussion note. Lesions smaller than that are not detectable by percussion.

Abnormal Findings

Rhonchal fremitus is palpable with thick bronchial secretions.

Pleural friction fremitus is palpable with inflammation of the pleura (see Table 19.6, p. 482).

Crepitus is a coarse crackling sensation palpable over the skin surface. It occurs in subcutaneous emphysema when air escapes from the lung and enters the subcutaneous tissue, as after open thoracic injury or surgery.

Hyper-resonance is a lower-pitched, booming sound found when too much air is present, as in emphysema or pneumothorax.

A **dull note** (soft, muffled thud) signals abnormal density in the lungs, as with pneumonia, pleural effusion, atelectasis, or tumour.

Normal Range of Findings

Abnormal Findings

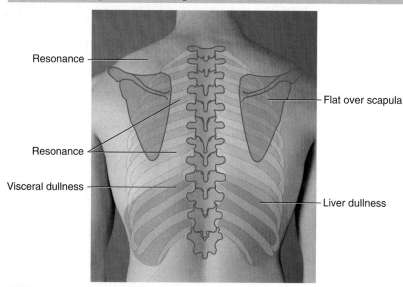

Resonance

Flat over scapula

Resonance

Visceral dullness

Liver dullness

19.16 Expected percussion notes.

Auscultate the Posterior Chest

The passage of air through the tracheobronchial tree creates a characteristic set of noises that are audible through the chest wall.

Breath sounds are changed by obstruction within the respiratory passageways or by changes in the lung parenchyma, the pleura, or the chest wall.

Breath Sounds

Evaluate the presence and quality of **normal breath sounds**. The patient should be sitting, leaning forward slightly, with arms resting comfortably across the lap. Instruct the patient to breathe through the mouth, a little bit deeper than usual, but to stop if the patient begins to feel dizzy. Be careful to monitor the breathing throughout the examination and allow times for the patient to rest and breathe normally. Many patients are willing to comply with your instructions in an effort to please you and to be a "good patient." Watch that the patient does not hyperventilate to the point of fainting.

Clean the flat diaphragm endpiece of the stethoscope and hold it firmly on the patient's chest wall. Listen to at least one full respiration in each location. Side-to-side comparison is most important.

Do not confuse background noise with lung sounds. Become familiar with these extraneous noises that may be confused with lung pathology if not recognized:

1. Examiner's breathing on stethoscope tubing
2. Stethoscope tubing bumping together
3. Patient shivering
4. Patient's hairy chest: Movement of hairs under stethoscope sounds like crackles (rales) (see Table 19.7, p. 483); minimize this movement by pressing harder or by wetting the hair with a damp cloth
5. Rustling of paper gown or paper drapes

Crackles are abnormal lung sounds (see Table 19.7, p. 483).

| **Normal Range of Findings** | **Abnormal Findings** |

While standing behind the patient, listen to the following lung areas: posterior from the apices at C7 to the bases (around T10) and laterally from the axilla down to the seventh or eighth rib. Use the sequence illustrated in Fig. 19.17.

19.17 Sequence for auscultation.

Continue to visualize approximate locations of the lobes of each lung so that you correlate your findings to anatomical areas. As you listen, think about (a) what you are hearing over this spot and (b) what you should expect to be hearing. You should expect to hear three types of normal breath sounds in adults and older children: (a) **bronchial** (sometimes called *tracheal* or *tubular*), (b) **bronchovesicular**, and (c) **vesicular**. Study the characteristics of these normal breath sounds in Table 19.1.

TABLE 19.1 Characteristics of Normal Breath Sounds

TYPE OF BREATH SOUND	PITCH	AMPLITUDE	DURATION	QUALITY	NORMAL LOCATION
BRONCHIAL (TRACHEAL)	High	Loud	Inspiration < expiration	Harsh, hollow, tubular	Trachea and larynx
BRONCHOVESICULAR	Moderate	Moderate	Inspiration = expiration	Mixed	Over major bronchi, where fewer alveoli are located: posterior, between scapulae (especially on right); anterior, around upper sternum in first and second intercostal space
VESICULAR	Low	Soft	Inspiration > expiration	Rustling, like the sound of the wind in the trees	Over peripheral lung fields, where air flows through smaller bronchioles and alveoli

Normal Range of Findings

Note the normal location of the three types of breath sounds on the chest wall of adults and older children (Figs. 19.18 and 19.19).

19.18

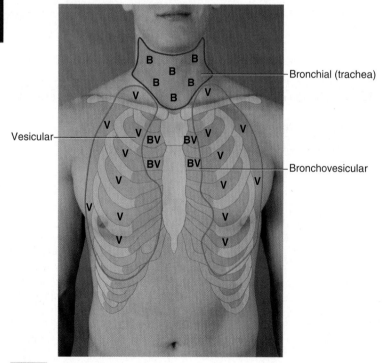

19.19

Abnormal Findings

Decreased or **absent breath sounds** are indications of the following situations:

1. Obstruction of the bronchial tree at some point by secretions, mucus plug, or a foreign body
2. Emphysema, as a result of loss of elasticity in the lung fibres and decreased force of inspired air; also, because the lungs are already hyperinflated, the inhaled air does not make as much noise
3. Obstruction of the transmission of sound between the lung and your stethoscope, as in pleurisy or pleural thickening or by air (pneumothorax) or fluid (pleural effusion) in the pleural space

A silent chest means no air is moving in or out, which is an ominous sign.

Increased breath sounds mean that sounds are louder than they should be (e.g., bronchial sounds heard over an abnormal location, the peripheral lung fields, are abnormal). They have a high-pitched, tubular quality, with a prolonged expiratory phase and a distinct pause between inspiration and expiration. They sound very close to your stethoscope, as if they were right *in* the tubing close to your ear. They occur when consolidation (e.g., pneumonia) or compression (e.g., fluid in the intrapleural space) increases the density in a lung area, which enhances the transmission of sound from the bronchi. When the inspired air reaches the alveoli, it hits solid lung tissue that conducts sound more efficiently to the surface.

Normal Range of Findings	Abnormal Findings

Adventitious Sounds

Note the presence of any **adventitious sounds**. These are additional sounds that are *not* normally heard in the lungs. If present, they are heard as being superimposed on the breath sounds. They are caused by the collision of moving air with secretions in the tracheobronchial passageways or by the popping open of previously deflated airways. Sources differ as to the classification and nomenclature of these sounds, but **crackles** (or rales) and **wheeze** (or rhonchi) are terms commonly used by most examiners. If you hear adventitious sounds, be sure to describe whether they are on inspiration or expiration; loudness; pitch; and location on the chest wall.

Study Table 19.7, p. 483, for a complete description of these abnormal adventitious breath sounds.

One type of adventitious sound, **atelectatic crackles**, is not pathological. These are short, popping, crackling sounds that sound like fine crackles but do not last beyond a few breaths. When sections of alveoli are not fully aerated (as in people who are asleep or in older adults), they deflate slightly and accumulate secretions. Crackles are heard when these sections are expanded by a few deep breaths. Atelectatic crackles are heard only in the periphery, usually in dependent portions of the lungs, and disappear after the first few breaths or after a cough.

During normal tidal flow, high-pitched wheeze occurs with asthma.

Charting of normal breath sound would include notes of both air entry and adventitia. Thus, when breath sounds are normal, your notes will read as follows: "Good bilateral A/E [air entry] with no adventitia noted."

Inspect the Anterior Chest

Note the **shape and configuration** of the chest wall. The ribs are sloping downward with symmetrical interspaces. The costal angle is within 90 degrees. Development of abdominal muscles is as expected for the patient's age, weight, and athletic condition.

Barrel chest is characterized by horizontal ribs and a costal angle exceeding 90 degrees.

Hypertrophy of abdominal muscles occurs in chronic emphysema.

Note the patient's **facial expression**. The facial expression should be relaxed and benign, indicating unconscious effort of breathing.

Facies appear tense, strained, and tired in COPD.

The patient with COPD may purse the lips in a whistling position. By exhaling slowly and against a narrow opening, the pressure in the bronchial tree remains positive, and fewer airways collapse.

Assess the **level of consciousness**. The patient should be alert and cooperative.

Cerebral hypoxia may be manifested by excessive drowsiness or by anxiety, restlessness, and irritability.

Note skin **colour and condition**. The lips and nail beds are free of cyanosis or unusual pallor. The nails are of normal configuration. Explore any skin lesions.

Clubbing of the distal phalanx occurs with chronic respiratory disease.

Cutaneous angiomas (spider nevi) associated with liver disease or portal hypertension may be evident on the chest.

Assess the quality of **respirations**. Normal relaxed breathing is automatic and effortless, regular and even, and produces no noise. The chest expands symmetrically with each inspiration. Note any localized lag on inspiration.

Breathing may be noisy with severe asthma or chronic bronchitis.

Chest expansion is unequal when part of the lung is obstructed or collapsed, as with pneumonia, or in guarding, to avoid postoperative incisional pain or pleurisy pain.

Normal Range of Findings

No retraction or bulging of the interspaces should occur on inspiration.

Normally, accessory muscles are not used to augment respiratory effort. However, with very heavy exercise, the accessory neck muscles (scalene, sternomastoid, trapezius) are used momentarily to enhance inspiration.

The respiratory rate is within normal limits for the patient's age (see Table 10.1, p. 167), and the pattern of breathing is regular. Occasional sighs normally punctuate breathing.

Palpate the Anterior Chest

Palpate for **symmetrical chest expansion**. Place your hands on the anterolateral wall with the thumbs along the costal margins and pointing toward the xiphoid process (Fig. 19.20).

19.20

Ask the patient to take a deep breath. Watch your thumbs move apart symmetrically, and note smooth chest expansion with your fingers. Any limitation in thoracic expansion is easier to detect on the anterior chest because the range of motion is greater with breathing here.

Assess **tactile (vocal) fremitus**. Begin palpating over the lung apices in the supraclavicular areas (Fig. 19.21). Compare vibrations from one side to the other as the patient says, "ninety-nine." Avoid palpating over female breast tissue because breast tissue normally damps sounds.

Abnormal Findings

Retraction suggests obstruction of the respiratory tract or that increased inspiratory effort is needed, as in atelectasis. Bulging indicates trapped air, as in forced expiration associated with emphysema or asthma.

Accessory muscles are used in acute airway obstruction and massive atelectasis.

In COPD, the rectus abdominis and internal intercostal muscles are used to force expiration.

Tachypnea and hyperventilation, bradypnea and hypoventilation, and periodic breathing are abnormal (see Table 19.5, p. 481).

With emphysema, the costal angle is abnormally wide, and little inspiratory variation occurs.

A lag in expansion occurs with atelectasis, pneumonia, and postoperative guarding.

A palpable grating sensation with breathing indicates pleural friction fremitus (see Table 19.6, p. 482).

Objective Data

Normal Range of Findings	Abnormal Findings

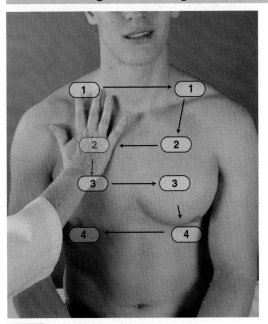

19.21   Assess tactile fremitus.

Palpate the anterior chest wall to note any tenderness (normally none is present) and to detect any superficial lumps or masses (again, normally none is present). Note skin mobility and turgor, and note skin temperature and moisture.

If any lumps are found in male breast tissue, refer the man to a specialist.

Percuss the Anterior Chest

Begin percussing the apices in the supraclavicular areas. Then, percussing the interspaces and comparing one side with the other, move down the anterior chest.

Interspaces are easier to palpate on the anterior chest than on the back. Do not percuss directly over female breast tissue because this would produce a dull note. Shift the breast tissue over slightly with the edge of your stationary hand. In women with large breasts, percussion may yield little useful data. With all people, use the sequence illustrated in Fig. 19.22.

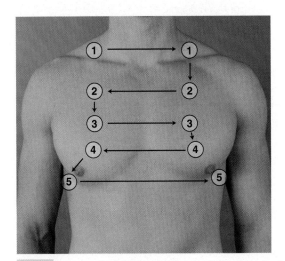

19.22   Sequence for percussion and auscultation.

Objective Data

Normal Range of Findings

Note the borders of cardiac dullness normally found on the anterior chest, and do not confuse these with suspected lung pathology (Fig. 19.23). In the right hemithorax, the upper border of liver dullness is located in the fifth intercostal space in the right midclavicular line. On the left, tympany is evident over the gastric space.

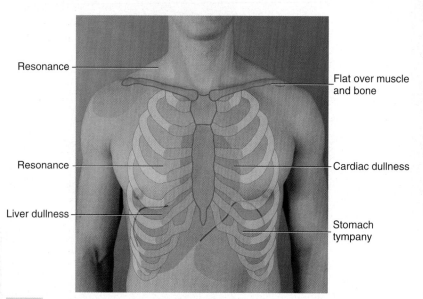

Resonance

Resonance

Liver dullness

Flat over muscle and bone

Cardiac dullness

Stomach tympany

19.23 Expected percussion notes.

Auscultate the Anterior Chest

Breath Sounds

Auscultate the lung fields over the anterior chest from the apices in the supraclavicular areas down to the sixth rib. Progress from side to side as you move downward, and listen to one full respiration in each location. Use the sequence indicated for percussion. Do not place your stethoscope directly over the female breast. Displace the breast and listen directly over the chest wall.

Evaluate normal breath sounds, noting any abnormal breath sounds and any adventitious sounds. If the situation warrants, assess the voice sounds on the anterior chest.

The Lateral Chest

Often forgotten—but equally important in the inspection, palpation, percussion, and auscultation of the thorax—is including the lateral chest wall. It is an extension of the vesicular lung field that wraps around the sides of the patient. The only way to ensure that you are aware what is happening in the right middle lobe is to extend your assessment into the lateral chest area.

Abnormal Findings

Lungs are hyperinflated with chronic emphysema; therefore, you would hear hyper-resonance where you would expect cardiac dullness.

Study Table 19.8, pp. 485–491, for a complete description of abnormal respiratory conditions.

Women, in particular, are prone to accumulating excretions into the right middle lobe secondary to postural drainage and the size of their breast tissue, which can impede movement of the chest wall. It is a common site of pneumonia and often the forgotten lobe, because it is the small third lobe of the right lung.

Normal Range of Findings	Abnormal Findings

Measurement of Pulmonary Function Status

The **pulse oximeter** is a noninvasive method of assessing arterial oxygen saturation (SpO_2) and is described in Chapter 10. A healthy person with no lung disease and no anemia normally has an SpO_2 of 97 to 98%. However, every SpO_2 value must be evaluated in the context of the patient's hemoglobin level, acid–base balance, and ventilatory status.

CRITICAL FINDINGS

- SpO_2 of less than 93% on room air must be attended to immediately. Sit the patient up and have the patient take a few deep breaths to see whether this brings the SpO_2 saturation back to a normal range.
- Apply O_2 as indicated in standing orders or clinician orders for the acute area in which you are working.
- Ensure that your patient is not a CO_2 retainer (such patients may have COPD or other obstructive or restrictive disorder). Normal O_2 levels for such patients range from 88 to 92%, and many are receiving low-flow O_2 (1–2 L/min).
- If you are unsure of how to help your patient with a dropping SpO_2 level, *go and find help* from a health care provider who is capable of determining the best course of action.

The **6-minute walk test (6MWT)** is a safer, simple, inexpensive, clinical measure of functional status in aging adults.[15] The 6MWT is used as an outcome measure for patients in pulmonary rehabilitation because it mirrors conditions that are used in everyday life. Locate a flat-surfaced corridor that has little foot traffic, is wide enough to enable comfortable turns, and has a controlled environment. Ensure that the patient is wearing comfortable shoes. Equip the patient with a pulse oximeter to monitor oxygen saturation. Ask the patient to walk at his, her, or their own pace to cover as much ground as possible in 6 minutes, and assure the patient that it is all right to slow down or to stop to rest at any time. Use a stopwatch to time the walk. A patient who walks more than 300 m in 6 minutes is more likely to engage in ADLs.[16]

Ask the patient to stop the walk if the SpO_2 is below 85 to 88% or if extreme breathlessness occurs.

 ### DEVELOPMENTAL CONSIDERATIONS

Infants and Children

To prepare, let the parent hold an infant supported against the chest or shoulder. Do not let the usual sequence of the physical examination restrain you; seize the opportunity with a sleeping infant to inspect and then to listen to lung sounds. This way you can concentrate on the breath sounds before the baby wakes up and possibly cries. The crying does not have to be a problem for you, however, because it actually enhances palpation of tactile fremitus and auscultation of breath sounds.

A child may sit upright on the parent's lap. Offer the stethoscope and let the child handle it. This reduces any fear of the equipment. Promote the child's participation; school-age children usually are delighted to hear their own breath sounds when you place the stethoscope properly. While you listen to breath sounds, ask the young child to take a deep breath and "blow out" your penlight while you hold the stethoscope with your other hand. Time your letting go of the penlight button so the light goes off after the child blows. Or, ask the child to "pant like a dog" while you auscultate.

Objective Data

Normal Range of Findings

Inspection. In infants, the thorax is rounded, and the anteroposterior-to-transverse ratio is 1 (Fig. 19.24). By age 6 years, the thorax reaches the adult ratio of 1:2. The newborn's chest circumference is 30 to 36 cm and is 2 cm smaller than the head circumference until 2 years of age. The chest wall is thin, with little musculature. The ribs and the xiphoid process are prominent; you can both see and feel the sharp tip of the xiphoid process. The thoracic cage is soft and flexible.

19.24 Round thorax in an infant.

The newborn's first respiratory assessment is part of the **Apgar scoring system** to measure the success of transition to extrauterine life (Table 19.2). The five standard parameters are scored at 1 minute and at 5 minutes after birth. A 1-minute total Apgar score of 7 to 10 indicates that the newborn is in good condition, needing only suctioning of the nose and mouth and otherwise routine care.

Abnormal Findings

A barrel shape that persists after age 6 years may develop with chronic asthma or cystic fibrosis.

In the immediate neonatal period, respirations may be depressed as a result of maternal medications, interruption of the uterine blood supply, or obstruction of the tracheobronchial tree by mucus or fluid.

A 1-minute total Apgar score of 3 to 6 indicates that the newborn's status is moderately depressed and that more resuscitation and subsequent close observation are needed. A score of 0 to 2 indicates severe depression and necessitates full resuscitation, ventilatory assistance, and subsequent critical care.

TABLE 19.2	**Apgar Scoring System**			
CHARACTERISTIC	**2**	**1**	**0**	**SCORE**
Heart rate	Over 100	Slow (below 100)	Absent	_____
Respiratory effort	Good, sustained cry; regular respiration	Slow, irregular, shallow	Absent	_____
Muscle tone	Active motion, spontaneous flexion	Some flexion of extremities; some resistance to extension	Limp, flaccid	_____
Reflex irritability (response to catheter nares)	Sneeze, cough, cry	Grimace, frown	No response	_____
Colour	Completely pink	Body pink, extremities pale	Cyanotic, pale	_____
				Total score _____

Normal Range of Findings

Infants breathe through the nose rather than the mouth and are obligate nose breathers until age 3 months. Slight flaring of the lower costal margins may occur with respirations, but normally no flaring of the nostrils and no sterna retractions or intercostal retractions occur. The **diaphragm** is the newborn's major respiratory muscle. Intercostal muscles are not well developed. Thus you observe the abdomen bulge with each inspiration but see little thoracic expansion.

Count the respiratory rate for 1 full minute. Normal rates for the newborn are 30 to 40 breaths per minute but may spike up to 60 per minute. The respiratory rate is counted most accurately when the infant is asleep; when awake, infants reach rapid rates with very little excitation. The respiratory pattern may be irregular with extremes in room temperature or during feeding or sleeping. Brief periods of apnea lasting less than 10 or 15 seconds are common. This periodic breathing is more common in premature infants.

Palpation. Palpate symmetrical chest expansion by encircling the infant's thorax with both hands. Further palpation should reveal no lumps, masses, or crepitus, although you may feel the costochondral junctions in some normal infants.

Auscultation. Auscultation normally reveals bronchovesicular breath sounds in the peripheral lung fields of infants and young children up to ages 5 to 6 years. Their relatively thin chest walls with underdeveloped musculature do not damp the sound as do the thicker walls of adults; thus breath sounds are louder and harsher.

Fine crackles are the adventitious sounds commonly heard in the immediate neonatal period as a result of the opening of the airways and clearing of fluid. Because the newborn's chest wall is so thin, transmission of sounds is enhanced, and sound is heard easily all over the chest; thus localization of breath sounds is difficult. Even bowel sounds are easily heard in the chest. Try using the smaller pediatric diaphragm endpiece of a stethoscope, or place the bell of the stethoscope over the infant's interspaces and not over the ribs. Use the pediatric diaphragm on an older infant or toddler (Fig. 19.25).

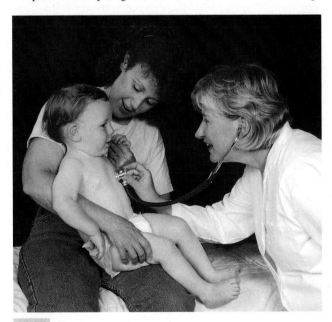

19.25

Abnormal Findings

Marked retractions of sternum and intercostal muscles indicate increased inspiratory effort, as in atelectasis, pneumonia, asthma, and acute airway obstruction.

Respiratory rates are rapid in pneumonia, fever, pain, heart disease, and anemia.

In an infant, tachypnea (rate of 50 to 100 per minute) during sleep may be an early sign of heart failure.

Asymmetrical expansion occurs with diaphragmatic hernia or pneumothorax.

Crepitus is palpable around a fractured clavicle, which may occur with difficult forceps delivery.

Breath sounds are diminished with pneumonia, atelectasis, pleural effusion, and pneumothorax.

Persistent fine crackles that are scattered over the chest occur with pneumonia, bronchiolitis, or atelectasis.

Crackles only in upper lung fields occur with cystic fibrosis; crackles only in lower lung fields occur with heart failure.

Expiratory wheezing occurs with lower airway obstruction (e.g., asthma or bronchiolitis). When unilateral, it may be caused by foreign body aspiration.

Persistent peristaltic sounds with diminished breath sounds on the same side may indicate diaphragmatic hernia.

Stridor is a high-pitched inspiratory crowing sound heard without the stethoscope, occurring with upper airway obstruction (e.g., croup, foreign body aspiration, or acute epiglottitis).

Objective Data

Normal Range of Findings	Abnormal Findings

Pregnant Women

The thoracic cage may appear wider, and the costal angle widens by about 50%. Respirations may be deeper, with a 40% increase in tidal volume.

Older Adults

The thoracic cage commonly has an increased anteroposterior diameter, which produces a round barrel shape, and **kyphosis**, an outward curvature of the thoracic spine (see Table 19.4, p. 480). The patient compensates by holding the head extended and tilted back. You may palpate marked bony prominences because of decreased subcutaneous fat. Chest expansion may be somewhat decreased in an older patient, although it still should be symmetrical. The costal cartilages become calcified with aging, resulting in less mobility of the thorax.

Older patients may fatigue easily, especially during auscultation when deep mouth breathing is required. Take care that such patients do not hyperventilate and become dizzy. Allow brief rest periods or quiet breathing. If a patient does feel faint, instruct the patient to hold the breath for a few seconds; this will restore equilibrium.

Acutely Ill Patients

Ask a second examiner to hold the patient's arms and to support the patient in the upright position. If a second examiner is not available, you need to roll the patient from side to side, examining the uppermost half of the thorax. This obviously prevents you from comparing findings from one side to another. Also, side flexion of the trunk alters percussion findings because the ribs of the upward side may flex closer together.

SPECIAL CONSIDERATIONS FOR ADVANCED PRACTICE

Normal Range of Findings	Abnormal Findings

Voice Sounds

Determine the quality of **voice sounds** or **vocal resonance**. The spoken voice can be auscultated over the chest wall just as it can be felt in tactile fremitus described earlier. Ask the patient to repeat a phrase such as "ninety-nine" while you listen over the chest wall. Normal voice transmission is soft, muffled, and indistinct; you can hear sounds through the stethoscope but cannot distinguish exactly what is being said. Disease that increases lung density enhances transmission of voice sounds.

Voice sounds are usually *not* elicited in routine examination. Rather, this testing consists of supplemental manoeuvres that are performed if you suspect lung disease on the basis of earlier data. When they are performed, you are testing for possible presence of **bronchophony, egophony,** and **whispered pectoriloquy** (see Table 19.3, p. 475).

If Not Now, When?

The voice test is not considered part of a basic health assessment; however, it can be used to further investigate abnormal findings noted in the traditional auscultation, as a method of confirming your findings.

Voice sounds are assessed primarily in advanced practice settings. One caution in using the voice test: if the patient has sustained a facial injury or has a chronic upper respiratory issue with the nasal cavity, all voice sounds coming through the oropharyngeal area are distorted because the test sounds, such as "ninety-nine," are nasally generated.

It may be more beneficial in this case to use egophony or whispered pectoriloquy.

Normal Range of Findings	**Abnormal Findings**
	Consolidation or compression of lung tissue will enhance the voice sounds, making the words more distinct.

TABLE 19.3 Voice Sounds

TECHNIQUE	NORMAL FINDING	ABNORMAL FINDING
Bronchophony Ask the patient to repeat "ninety-nine" while you listen with the stethoscope over the chest wall; listen especially if you suspect disease.	Normal voice transmission is soft, muffled, and indistinct; you can hear sound through the stethoscope but cannot distinguish exactly what is being said.	Disease that increases lung density enhances transmission of voice sounds; when auscultating, you clearly hear the words "ninety-nine." The words are more distinct than normal and sound close to your ear.

Egophony[a] Auscultate the chest while the patient phonates a long "eeeeeeee" sound.	Normally, you should hear "eeeeeeee" through your stethoscope.	Over area of consolidation or compression, the spoken "eeeeeeee" sounds like a bleating, long "aaaaa."
Whispered Pectoriloquy Ask the patient to whisper a phrase such as "one-two-three" as you auscultate.	Normal voice transmission is faint, muffled, and almost inaudible.	With only small amounts of consolidation, the whispered voice is transmitted very clearly and distinctly, although it is still somewhat faint; it sounds as if the patient is whispering, "one-two-three" right into your stethoscope.

[a]From Greek, referring to the voice of a goat.

Special Considerations for Advanced Practice

| **Normal Range of Findings** | **Abnormal Findings** |

Diaphragmatic Excursion

Determine **diaphragmatic excursion**, a measurement of distance between the base of the lungs on inspiration and expiration as the diaphragm recoils. Percuss to map out the lower lung border, both in expiration and in inspiration. First, ask the patient to "exhale and hold it" briefly while you percuss down the scapular line until the sound changes from resonant to dull on each side (Fig. 19.26, *A*). This helps you estimate the level of the diaphragm where the lungs are separated from the abdominal viscera. It may be somewhat higher on the right side (about 1 to 2 cm) because of the presence of the liver. Mark the spot.

19.26

Now ask the person to "take a deep breath and hold it." Continue percussing down from your first mark, and mark the level where the sound changes to dull on this deep inspiration. Measure the difference. This diaphragmatic excursion should be equal bilaterally and measure about 3 to 5 cm in adults, although it may be up to 7 to 8 cm in well-conditioned patients (Fig. 19.26, *B*).

Often beginning examiners become so involved in the subtle differences of percussion notes that they extend the patient's limits of breath-holding. Always hold your own breath when you ask your patient to. When you run out of air, the other person surely has, too, especially if that person has a respiratory problem.

If Not Now, When?

Not traditionally considered part of a basic assessment for beginning practitioners. The procedure is done in advanced practice settings when access to diagnostic imaging tools is not readily available. However, it is an excellent tool when the stethoscope is not an option for the practitioner, such as transporting a patient in a helicopter.

Note any abnormally high level of dullness and absence of diaphragmatic excursion. These characterize pleural effusion (fluid in the space between the visceral and parietal pleura) and atelectasis of the lower lobes.

Normal Range of Findings	Abnormal Findings

Measurement of Pulmonary Function Status

The **forced expiratory time** is the number of seconds it takes for the patient to exhale from total lung capacity to residual volume. It is a screening measure of airflow obstruction. Although the test usually is *not* performed in the respiratory assessment, it is useful when you wish to screen for pulmonary function.

Ask the patient to inhale the deepest breath possible and then to blow it all out hard, as quickly as possible, with the mouth open. Listen with your stethoscope over the sternum. The normal time for full expiration is 4 seconds or less. In the ambulatory care setting, a handheld **spirometer** is used to measure lung health in chronic conditions, such as asthma. Ask the patient to inhale deeply and then exhale into the spirometer as fast as possible, until the most air is exhaled. The **forced vital capacity (FVC)** is the total volume exhaled. The **forced expiratory volume in 1 second (FEV$_1$)** is the volume exhaled in the first measured second. A normal finding is a FEV$_1$/FVC ratio of 75% to 80% or greater, meaning that no significant obstruction of airflow is present.

If Not Now, When?

Measuring forced expiratory time is not a part of the basic assessment for beginning practitioners. However, an understanding of pulmonary function is helpful in certain situations:

- As a means of identifying early pulmonary disease
- As a means of testing FVC before discharge from hospital
- As a means of monitoring ongoing chronic respiratory disease in the community setting

With obstructive lung disease, forced expiration takes 6 seconds or more. In such cases, refer patients for more precise pulmonary function studies.

The ratio of FEV$_1$ to FVC is an indication of the severity of airflow obstruction:

- Mild obstruction of airflow: FEV$_1$/FVC = 60 to 70%
- Moderate obstruction of airflow: FEV$_1$/FVC = 50 to 60%
- Severe obstruction of airflow: FEV$_1$/FVC<50%

Special Considerations for Advanced Practice

DOCUMENTATION AND CRITICAL THINKING

Sample Charting

SUBJECTIVE

No cough, shortness of breath, or chest pain with breathing. No history of respiratory diseases. Has "one or no" colds per year. Has never smoked. Works in well-ventilated office; smoking by co-workers is restricted to lounge. Last TB [tuberculin] skin test: 4 years PTA [prior to arrival], negative. Never had chest radiography.

OBJECTIVE

Inspection: AP [anteroposterior] < transverse diameter. Respirations: 16/min, relaxed and even.
Palpation: Chest expansion: symmetrical. Tactile fremitus: equal bilaterally. No tenderness to palpation. No lumps or lesions.
Percussion: Resonant to percussion over lung fields. Diaphragmatic excursion: 5 cm bilaterally.
Auscultation: Vesicular breath sounds: clear over lung fields. No adventitious sounds.

ASSESSMENT

Intact thoracic structures
Lung sounds clear

Documentation and Critical Thinking

Focused Assessment: Clinical Case Study

Thomas George (T.G.) is a 58-year-old, thin, male traffic patrol officer who appears older than stated age. Face is anxious and tense, although in no acute distress at this time. Seeks care for "increasing shortness of breath and fatigue in last couple months."

SUBJECTIVE

1 year PTA: T.G. noticed more "winded" than usual when walking >3–4 blocks. Early morning cough present daily × 10 years, but now increased sputum production to 2 T per morning, frothy white.

6 months PTA: Had a "cold" with severe harsh coughing, productive of "½ cup" thick white sputum per day. Noted midsternal chest pain (mild) with cough. Lasted 2 weeks. Treated self with humidifier and OTC [over-the-counter] cough syrup—minimal relief.

3 months PTA: Noticed increasing SOB [shortness of breath] with less activity. Fatigue and SOB when working outside during traffic rush hours. Unable to take evening walks (usually 2–3 blocks) because of SOB and fatigue. Has two-pillow orthopnea. Wakes 3–4 times during night.

Now: Feels he is "worse and needs some help." Continues with two-pillow orthopnea. Unable to walk >2 blocks or climb >1 flight stairs without resting. Unable to blow out birthday candles on cake last week. Morning cough productive of "¼ cup" thin white sputum, cough continues sporadically during day.

No chest pain, hemoptysis, night sweats, or paroxysmal nocturnal dyspnea. No history of allergies, hospitalizations, or injuries to chest. No family history of TB [tuberculosis], allergies, asthma, or cancer. Smokes cigarettes 2 packs per day × 30 years. Alcohol: <1 six-pack beer/week, summer months only.

OBJECTIVE

Inspection: Sitting on side of bed with arms propped on bedside table. Resp. resting: 24/min, regular, shallow with prolonged expiration; resp. ambulating: 34/min. Increased use of accessory muscles, AP = transverse diameter (barrel chest) with widening of costal angle, slightly flushed face, tense expression.

Palpation: Minimal but symmetrical chest expansion. Tactile fremitus = bilaterally. No lumps, masses, or tenderness to palpation.

Percussion: Diaphragmatic excursion is 1 cm. Hyper-resonance over lung fields.

Auscultation: Breath sounds diminished. Expiratory wheeze throughout posterior chest, R [right]>L [left]. No crackles.

ASSESSMENT

Chronic and increasing SOB

Ineffective airway clearance R/T [related to] bronchial secretions and obstruction

Activity intolerance R/T imbalance between oxygen supply and demand

Insomnia R/T dyspnea and decreased mobility

Anxiety R/T change in health status

ABNORMAL FINDINGS

TABLE 19.4   Configurations of the Thorax

Normal Adult (for Comparison)

The thorax has an elliptical shape with an anteroposterior-to-transverse ratio of 1:2 to 5:7.

Barrel Chest

Note equal anteroposterior-to-transverse ratio and that ribs are horizontal instead of the normal downward slope. This is associated with normal aging and also with chronic emphysema and asthma as a result of hyperinflation of lungs.

Pectus Excavatum

A markedly sunken sternum and adjacent cartilages (also called *funnel breast*). Depression begins at second intercostal space, becoming depressed most at junction of xiphoid process with body of sternum. More noticeable on inspiration. Congenital, usually not symptomatic. When severe, sternal depression may cause embarrassment and a negative self-concept. Surgery may be indicated.

Pectus Carinatum

A forward protrusion of the sternum, with ribs sloping back at either side, and vertical depressions along costochondral junctions (pigeon breast). Less common than pectus excavatum, this minor deformity necessitates no treatment. If severe, surgery may be indicated.

Continued

Abnormal Findings

TABLE 19.4	Configurations of the Thorax—cont'd

Scoliosis

A lateral S-shaped curvature of the thoracic and lumbar spine, usually with involved vertebrae rotation. Note unequal shoulder and scapular heights, unequal hip levels, and rib interspaces flared on convex side. Onset is more prevalent in adolescent age groups, especially girls. Mild deformities are asymptomatic. If deviation is severe (>45 degrees), scoliosis may reduce lung volume; then the patient is at risk for impaired cardiopulmonary function. Primary impairment is cosmetic deformity, negatively affecting self-image. Refer early for treatment, which is often surgery.

Kyphosis

An exaggerated posterior curvature of the thoracic spine (humpback) that causes significant back pain and limited mobility. Severe deformities impair cardiopulmonary function. If the neck muscles are strong, patient compensates by hyperextension of head to maintain level of vision.

Kyphosis has been associated with aging, especially in cases of "dowager's hump" in postmenopausal women with osteoporosis. However, it is common well before menopause. It is related to physical fitness; women with adequate exercise habits are less likely to have kyphosis.

TABLE 19.5	Respiration Patterns[a]

Inspiration Expiration

Normal Adult (for Comparison)

Rate: 10–20 breaths per minute.
Depth: 500–800 mL.
Pattern: even.
Depth: air moving in and out with each respiration.
The ratio of pulse to respirations is fairly constant, about 4 : 1. Both values increase as a normal response to exercise, fear, or fever.

Sigh

Occasional sighs punctuate the normal breathing pattern and help expand alveoli. Frequent sighs may indicate emotional dysfunction. Frequent sighs also may lead to hyperventilation and dizziness.

TABLE 19.5	Respiration Patterns—cont'd

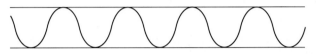

Tachypnea

Rapid, shallow breathing. Increased rate is more than 24 per minute. This is a normal response to fever, fear, or exercise. Rate also increases with respiratory insufficiency, pneumonia, alkalosis, pleurisy, and lesions in the pons.

Hyperventilation

Increase in both rate and depth. Normally occurs with extreme exertion, fear, or anxiety. Also occurs with diabetic ketoacidosis (Kussmaul's respirations), hepatic coma, salicylate overdose (hyperventilation produces a respiratory alkalosis to compensate for the metabolic acidosis), lesions of the midbrain, and alteration in blood gas concentration (either an increase in carbon dioxide or decrease in oxygen). Hyperventilation causes the level of carbon dioxide in the blood to decrease (alkalosis).

Bradypnea

Slow breathing. A decreased but regular rate (<10 per minute), as in drug-induced depression of the respiratory centre in the medulla, increased intracranial pressure, and diabetic coma.

Hypoventilation

An irregular, shallow pattern caused by an overdose of narcotics or anaesthetics. May also occur with prolonged bed rest or conscious splinting of the chest to avoid respiratory pain.

Cheyne-Stokes Respiration

A cycle in which respirations gradually wax and wane in a regular pattern, increasing in rate and depth and then decreasing. The breathing periods last 30 to 45 seconds, with periods of apnea (20 seconds) alternating the cycle. The most common cause is severe heart failure; other causes are renal failure, meningitis, drug overdose, and increased intracranial pressure. Occurs normally in infants and older adults during sleep.

Biot's Respiration

Similar to Cheyne-Stokes respiration, except that the pattern is irregular. A series of normal respirations (three to four) is followed by a period of apnea. The cycle length is variable, lasting anywhere from 10 seconds to 1 minute. Occurs with head trauma, brain abscess, heat stroke, spinal meningitis, and encephalitis.

◀ **Chronic Obstructive Breathing**

Normal inspiration and prolonged expiration to overcome increased airway resistance. In a patient with chronic obstructive lung disease, any situation calling for increased heart rate (exercise) may lead to dyspneic episode (air trapping) because then the patient does not have enough time for full expiration.

Normal inspiration   Prolonged expiration   Air trapping

ᵃAssess (a) rate, (b) depth (tidal volume), and (c) pattern.

TABLE 19.6 Abnormal Tactile Fremitus

Increased Tactile Fremitus

Occurs with conditions that increase the density of lung tissue, thereby making a better conducting medium for vibrations (e.g., compression or consolidation [pneumonia]). For increased fremitus to be apparent, at least one bronchus must be patent, and consolidation must extend to lung surface.

Decreased Tactile Fremitus

Occurs when anything obstructs transmission of vibrations (e.g., an obstruction in bronchus, pleural effusion or thickening, pneumothorax, and emphysema).

Rhonchal Fremitus

Vibration felt when inhaled air passes through thick secretions in the larger bronchi. This may decrease somewhat after coughing.

Pleural Friction Fremitus

Produced when inflammation of the parietal or visceral pleura causes a decrease in the normal lubricating fluid. Then the opposing surfaces make a coarse grating sound when rubbed together during breathing. Although this sound is best detected by auscultation, it may sometimes be palpable and feels like two pieces of leather grating together. It is synchronous with respiratory excursion. Also called a *palpable friction rub*.

TABLE 19.7   Adventitious Lung Sounds

Sound	Description	Mechanism	Clinical Example

Discontinuous Sounds

These are discrete, crackling sounds.

Sound	Description	Mechanism	Clinical Example
Crackles—fine (formerly called *rales*) *Inspiration — Expiration*	Discontinuous, high-pitched, short crackling, popping sounds heard during inspiration that are not cleared by coughing; you can simulate this sound by rolling a strand of hair between your fingers near your ear, or by moistening your thumb and index finger and separating them near your ear.	Inhaled air collides with previously deflated airways; airways suddenly pop open, creating crackling sound as gas pressures between the two compartments equalize.[17]	*Late inspiratory crackles* occur with restrictive disease: pneumonia, heart failure, and interstitial fibrosis. *Early inspiratory crackles* occur with obstructive disease: chronic bronchitis, asthma, and emphysema. *Posturally induced crackles* (PICs) are fine crackles that appear with a change from sitting to the supine position or with a change from supine to supine with legs elevated. PICs that appear after acute myocardial infarction have been associated with increased mortality.[18]
Crackles—coarse (coarse rales)	Loud, low-pitched, bubbling and gurgling sounds that start in early inspiration and may be present in expiration; may decrease somewhat after suctioning or coughing but will reappear shortly; sounds like opening a Velcro fastener.	Inhaled air collides with secretions in the trachea and large bronchi.	Pulmonary edema, pneumonia, pulmonary fibrosis, and a depressed cough reflex in terminally ill patients.
Atelectatic crackles (atelectatic rales)	Sound like fine crackles but do not last and are not indications of disease; disappear after the first few breaths; heard in axillae and bases (usually dependent) of lungs.	When sections of alveoli are not fully aerated, they deflate and accumulate secretions. Crackles are heard when these sections re-expand with a few deep breaths.	Occur in older adults, bedridden patients, and in patients just aroused from sleep.

Continued

TABLE 19.7   Adventitious Lung Sounds—cont'd

Sound	Description	Mechanism	Clinical Example
Pleural friction rub	A very superficial sound that is coarse and low-pitched; it has a grating quality as if two pieces of leather are being rubbed together; sounds just like crackles, but *close* to the ear; sounds louder if you push the stethoscope harder onto the chest wall; sound is inspiratory and expiratory.	Caused when pleurae become inflamed and lose their normal lubricating fluid; their opposing roughened pleural surfaces rub together during respiration; heard best in anterolateral wall, where lung mobility is greatest.	Pleuritis, accompanied by pain with breathing (rub disappears after a few days if pleural fluid accumulates and separates pleurae).

Continuous Sounds

These are connected, musical sounds.

Sound	Description	Mechanism	Clinical Example
Wheeze—high-pitched (sibilant)	High-pitched, musical squeaking sounds that sound polyphonic (multiple notes as in a musical chord); predominate in expiration but may occur in both expiration and inspiration.	Air squeezed or compressed through passageways narrowed almost to closure by collapsing, swelling, secretions, or tumours; the passageway walls oscillate in apposition between the closed and barely open positions; the resulting sound is similar to that from a vibrating reed.[17]	Diffuse airway obstruction from acute asthma or chronic emphysema.
Wheeze—low-pitched (sonorous rhonchi)	Low-pitched; monophonic single note, musical snoring, moaning sounds; they are heard throughout the cycle, although they are more prominent on expiration; may clear somewhat after coughing.	Airflow obstruction as described by the vibrating reed mechanism for high-pitched wheeze; the pitch of the wheeze cannot be correlated with the size of the passageway that generates it.	Bronchitis, single bronchus obstruction from airway tumour.
Stridor	High-pitched, monophonic, inspiratory, crowing sound, louder in neck than over chest wall.	Originating in larynx or trachea; upper airway obstruction from swollen, inflamed tissues or lodged foreign body.	Croup and acute epiglottitis in children, foreign body inhalation, and obstructed airway (all may be life-threatening).

TABLE 19.8	**Assessment of Common Respiratory Conditions**

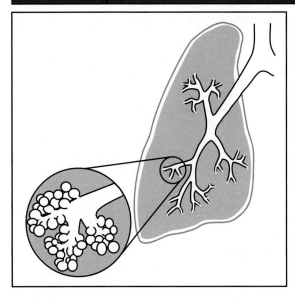

◀ Normal Lung (for Comparison)

Inspection: Anteroposterior < transverse diameter, relaxed posture, normal musculature; rate 10–18 breaths per minute, regular, no cyanosis or pallor.

Palpation: Symmetrical chest expansion. Tactile fremitus present and equal bilaterally, diminishing toward periphery. No lumps, masses, or tenderness.

Percussion: Resonant. Diaphragmatic excursion 3 to 5 cm and equal bilaterally.

Auscultation: Vesicular over peripheral fields. Bronchovesicular parasternally (anterior) and between scapulae (posterior). Infants and young children: bronchovesicular throughout.

Adventitious sounds: None.

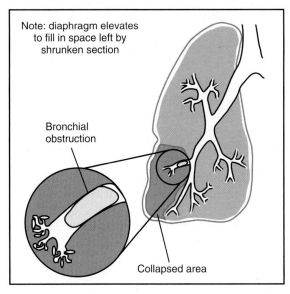

Note: diaphragm elevates to fill in space left by shrunken section

Bronchial obstruction

Collapsed area

◀ Atelectasis (Collapse)

Condition: Collapsed shrunken section of alveoli, or an entire lung, as a result of (a) airway obstruction (e.g., the bronchus is completely blocked by thick exudate, aspirated foreign body, or tumour): the alveolar air beyond it is gradually absorbed by the pulmonary capillaries, and the alveolar walls cave in; (b) compression on the lung; and (c) lack of surfactant (hyaline membrane disease).

Inspection: Cough. Lag on expansion on affected side. Increased respiratory rate and pulse. Possible cyanosis.

Palpation: Chest expansion decreased on affected side. Tactile fremitus decreased or absent over area. With large collapse, tracheal shift toward affected side.

Percussion: Dull over area (remainder of thorax sometimes having hyper-resonant note).

Auscultation: Vesicular decreased or absent over area. Voice sounds variable, usually decreased or absent over affected area.

Adventitious sounds: None if bronchus is obstructed. Occasional fine crackles if bronchus is patent.

Continued

TABLE 19.8 Assessment of Common Respiratory Conditions—cont'd

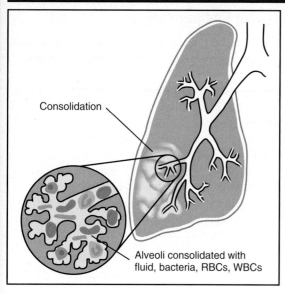

Consolidation

Alveoli consolidated with
fluid, bacteria, RBCs, WBCs

◄ Lobar Pneumonia

Condition: Infection in lung parenchyma leaves alveolar membrane edematous and porous, and so red blood cells (RBCs) and white blood cells (WBCs) pass from blood to alveoli. Alveoli progressively fill up (become consolidated) with bacteria, solid cellular debris, fluid, and blood cells, all of which replace alveolar air. This results in decreased surface area of the respiratory membrane, which causes hypoxemia.

Inspection: Increased respiratory rate. Guarding and lag on expansion on affected side. Children: sternal retraction, nasal flaring.

Palpation: Chest expansion decreased on affected side. Tactile fremitus increased if bronchus patent, decreased if bronchus obstructed.

Percussion: Dull over lobe.

Auscultation: Breath sounds louder with patent bronchus, as if coming directly from larynx. Voice sounds have increased clarity; bronchophony, egophony, whispered pectoriloquy present. Children: diminished breath sounds may occur early in pneumonia.

Adventitious sounds: Crackles, fine to medium.

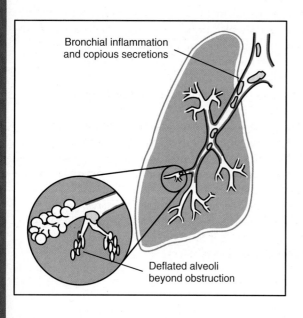

Bronchial inflammation
and copious secretions

Deflated alveoli
beyond obstruction

◄ Bronchitis

Condition: Proliferation of mucous glands in the passageways, resulting in excessive mucus secretion. Inflammation of bronchi with partial obstruction of bronchi by secretions or constrictions. Sections of lung distal to obstruction may be deflated. Bronchitis may be acute or chronic with recurrent productive cough. Chronic bronchitis is usually caused by cigarette smoking.

Inspection: Hacking, rasping cough productive of thick mucoid sputum. Chronic: dyspnea, fatigue, cyanosis, possible clubbing of fingers.

Palpation: Tactile fremitus normal.

Percussion: Resonant.

Auscultation: Normal vesicular. Voice sounds normal. Chronic: prolonged expiration.

Adventitious sounds: Crackles over deflated areas. Wheeze may be present.

TABLE 19.8 **Assessment of Common Respiratory Conditions—cont'd**

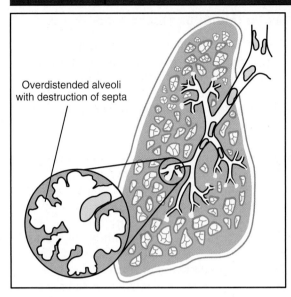

Overdistended alveoli with destruction of septa

◄ Emphysema

Condition: Caused by destruction of pulmonary connective tissue (elastin, collagen); characterized by permanent enlargement of air sacs distal to terminal bronchioles and rupture of interalveolar walls. Airway resistance is increased, especially on expiration, which causes hyperinflation of the lung and an increase in lung volume. Cigarette smoking accounts for 80%–90% of cases of emphysema.

Inspection: Increased anteroposterior diameter. Barrel chest. Use of accessory muscles to aid respiration. Tripod position. Shortness of breath, especially on exertion. Respiratory distress. Tachypnea.

Palpation: Decreased tactile fremitus and chest expansion.

Percussion: Hyper-resonant. Decreased diaphragmatic excursion.

Auscultation: Decreased breath sounds. Expiration may be prolonged. Muffling of heart sounds as a result of overdistension of lungs.

Adventitious sounds: Usually none; occasionally, wheeze.

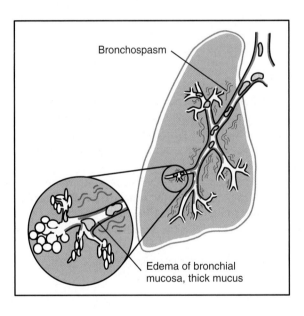

Bronchospasm

Edema of bronchial mucosa, thick mucus

◄ Asthma (Reactive Airway Disease)

Condition: An allergic hypersensitivity to certain inhaled allergens (pollen), irritants (tobacco, ozone), micro-organisms, stress, or exercise that produces a complex response characterized by bronchospasm, inflammation, edema in walls of bronchioles, and secretion of highly viscous mucus into airways. These factors greatly increase airway resistance, especially during expiration, and produce the symptoms of wheezing, dyspnea, and sensation of tightness in the chest.

Inspection: During severe attack: increased respiratory rate, shortness of breath with audible wheeze, use of accessory neck muscles, cyanosis, apprehension, retraction of intercostals spaces. Expiration laboured, prolonged. When asthma is chronic, barrel chest may develop.

Palpation: Tactile fremitus decreased; tachycardia.

Percussion: Resonant. May be hyper-resonant if asthma is chronic.

Auscultation: Diminished air movement. Breath sounds decreased, with prolonged expiration. Voice sounds decreased.

Adventitious sounds: Bilateral wheezing on expiration; sometimes inspiratory and expiratory wheezing.

Continued

TABLE 19.8 Assessment of Common Respiratory Conditions—cont'd

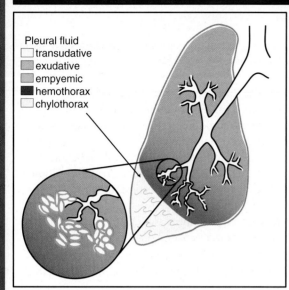

Pleural fluid
☐ transudative
☐ exudative
☐ empyemic
■ hemothorax
☐ chylothorax

◀ **Pleural Effusion (Fluid) or Thickening**

Condition: Collection of excess fluid in the intrapleural space, with compression of overlying lung tissue. Effusion may contain watery capillary fluid (transudative), protein (exudative), purulent matter (empyemic), blood (hemothorax), or milky lymphatic fluid (chylothorax). Gravity settles fluid in dependent areas of thorax. Presence of fluid subdues all lung sounds.

Inspection: Increased respirations, dyspnea; patient may have dry cough, tachycardia, cyanosis, abdominal distension.

Palpation: Tactile fremitus decreased or absent. Tracheal shift away from affected side. Chest expansion decreased on affected side.

Percussion: Dull to flat. No diaphragmatic excursion on affected side.

Auscultation: Breath sounds decreased or absent. Voice sounds decreased or absent. When remainder of lung is compressed near the effusion, bronchial breath sounds may be heard over the compression along with bronchophony, egophony, whispered pectoriloquy.

Adventitious sounds: None.

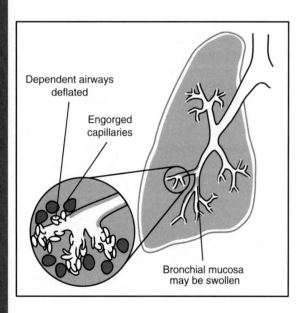

Dependent airways deflated

Engorged capillaries

Bronchial mucosa may be swollen

◀ **Heart Failure**

Condition: Pump failure with increasing pressure of cardiac overload causes pulmonary congestion or an increased amount of blood present in pulmonary capillaries. Dependent air sacs are deflated. Pulmonary capillaries engorged. Bronchial mucosa may be swollen.

Inspection: Increased respiratory rate, shortness of breath on exertion, orthopnea, paroxysmal nocturnal dyspnea, nocturia, ankle edema, pallor in light-skinned people.

Palpation: Skin moist, clammy. Tactile fremitus normal.

Percussion: Resonant.

Auscultation: Normal vesicular. Heart sounds include S_3 gallop.

Adventitious sounds: Crackles at lung bases.

TABLE 19.8 Assessment of Common Respiratory Conditions—cont'd

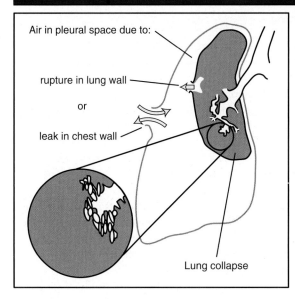

Air in pleural space due to:

rupture in lung wall

or

leak in chest wall

Lung collapse

◀ **Pneumothorax**

Condition: Free air in pleural space causes partial or complete lung collapse. Air in pleural space neutralizes the usual negative pressure present; thus lung collapses. Usually unilateral. Pneumothorax can be (a) *spontaneous* (air enters pleural space through rupture in lung wall), (b) *traumatic* (air enters through opening or injury in chest wall), or (c) *tension* (trapped air in pleural space increases, compressing lung and shifting mediastinum to the unaffected side).

Inspection: Unequal chest expansion. If pneumothorax is large, patient may have tachypnea, cyanosis, apprehension, bulging in interspaces.

Palpation: Tactile fremitus decreased or absent. Tracheal shift to opposite side (unaffected side). Chest expansion decreased on affected side. Tachycardia, decreased blood pressure.

Percussion: Hyper-resonant. Decreased diaphragmatic excursion.

Auscultation: Breath sounds decreased or absent. Voice sounds decreased or absent.

Adventitious sounds: None.

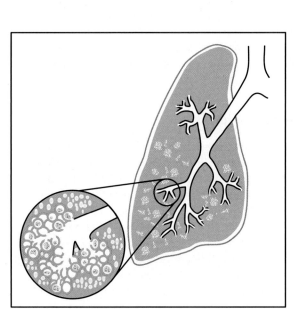

◀ *Pneumocystis jiroveci* **Pneumonia**

Condition: This virulent form of pneumonia is a protozoal infection associated with AIDS. The parasite *P. jiroveci* (formerly known as *Pneumocystis carinii*) is common in Canada and harmless to most people except in immunocompromised patients, in whom a diffuse interstitial pneumonitis ensues. More than 75% of children are seropositive by the age of 4, which suggests a high rate of background exposure to the organism. Cysts containing the organism and macrophages form in alveolar spaces, alveolar walls thicken, and the disease spreads to bilateral interstitial infiltrates of foamy, protein-rich fluid.

Inspection: Anxiety, shortness of breath, dyspnea on exertion, malaise are common; also tachypnea; fever; a dry, nonproductive cough; intercostal retractions in children; cyanosis.

Palpation: Decreased chest expansion.

Percussion: Dull over areas of diffuse infiltrate.

Auscultation: Breath sounds may be diminished.

Adventitious sounds: Crackles may be present but often are absent.

Continued

TABLE 19.8 Assessment of Common Respiratory Conditions—cont'd

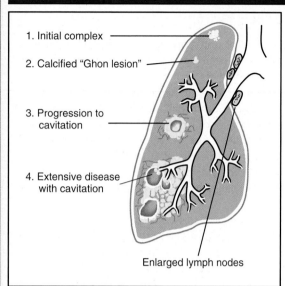

1. Initial complex
2. Calcified "Ghon lesion"
3. Progression to cavitation
4. Extensive disease with cavitation

Enlarged lymph nodes

◄ Tuberculosis

Condition: Inhalation of tubercle bacilli into the alveolar wall starts course of disease: (a) Initial complex is acute inflammatory response; macrophages engulf bacilli but do not kill them. Tubercle forms around bacilli. (b) Scar tissue forms, and lesion calcifies and is visible on radiograph. (c) Previously healed lesion is reactivated. Dormant bacilli now multiply, producing necrosis, cavitation, and caseous lung tissue (cheeselike appearance). (d) Extensive destruction occurs as lesion erodes into bronchus, forming air-filled cavity. Apex usually has the most damage.

Subjective data: Initially no symptoms, manifests as positive result of skin test or on radiograph. Progressive tuberculosis involves weight loss, anorexia, easy fatigability, low-grade afternoon fevers, night sweats. Patient may have pleural effusion, recurrent lower respiratory infections.

Inspection: Cough initially nonproductive, later productive of purulent, yellow-green sputum, may be blood-tinged. Dyspnea, orthopnea, fatigue, weakness.

Palpation: Skin moist at night from night sweats.

Percussion: Resonant initially. Dull over any effusion.

Auscultation: Normal or decreased vesicular breath sounds.

Adventitious sounds: Crackles over upper lobes common, persist after full expiration and cough.

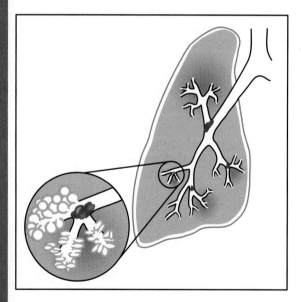

◄ Pulmonary Embolism

Condition: Undissolved materials (e.g., thrombus, air bubbles, fat globules), originating in legs or pelvis, detach and travel through venous system, returning blood to right heart and lodging to occlude pulmonary vessels. More than 95% arise from deep vein thrombi in lower legs as a result of stasis of blood, vessel injury, or hypercoagulability. Pulmonary occlusion results in ischemia of downstream lung tissue, increased pulmonary artery pressure, decreased cardiac output, and hypoxia. In rare cases, a saddle embolus in bifurcation of pulmonary arteries leads to sudden death from hypoxia. More often, small to medium pulmonary branches occlude, leading to dyspnea. These may resolve by fibrolytic activity.

Subjective data: Chest pain, worse on deep inspiration, dyspnea.

Inspection: Apprehensiveness, restlessness, anxiety, mental status changes, cyanosis, tachypnea, cough, hemoptysis, PaO_2<80 on pulse oximetry. Arterial blood gases show respiratory alkalosis.

Palpation: Diaphoresis, hypotension.

Auscultation: Tachycardia, accentuated pulmonic component of S_2 heart sound.

Adventitious sounds: Crackles, wheezes.

TABLE 19.8	Assessment of Common Respiratory Conditions—cont'd

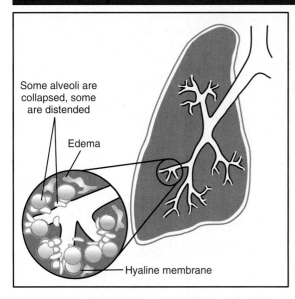

Some alveoli are collapsed, some are distended

Edema

Hyaline membrane

◄ Acute Respiratory Distress Syndrome (ARDS)

Condition: An acute pulmonary insult (trauma, gastric acid aspiration, shock, sepsis) damages alveolar capillary membrane, leading to increased permeability of pulmonary capillaries and alveolar epithelium, and to pulmonary edema. Gross examination (autopsy) would show dark red, firm, airless tissue, with some alveoli collapsed, and hyaline membranes lining the distended alveoli.

Subjective: Acute onset of dyspnea, apprehension.

Inspection: Restlessness; disorientation; rapid, shallow breathing; productive cough; thin, frothy sputum; retractions of intercostal spaces and sternum. Decreased PaO_2; blood gases show respiratory alkalosis; radiographs show diffuse pulmonary infiltrates; a late sign is cyanosis.

Palpation: Hypotension.

Auscultation: Tachycardia.

Adventitious sounds: Crackles, rhonchi.

AIDS, Acquired immune deficiency syndrome; *PaO₂,* arterial partial pressure of oxygen.

Summary Checklist: Thorax and Lung Examination

1. **Inspect:**
   Assess thoracic cage
   Measure respirations
   Assess skin colour and condition
   Evaluate patient's position
   Observe patient's facial expression
   Assess level of consciousness
2. **Palpate:**
   Confirm symmetrical expansion
   Assess tactile fremitus
   Detect any lumps, masses, tenderness
3. **Percuss:**
   Percuss over lung fields
   Estimate diaphragmatic excursion
4. **Auscultate:**
   Assess normal breath sounds
   Note any abnormal breath sounds
   If breath sounds are abnormal, perform bronchophony, whispered pectoriloquy, and egophony
   Note any adventitious sounds
5. **Engage in teaching and health promotion**

Abnormal Findings

REFERENCES

1. Best, D. (2009). Technical report: Secondhand and prenatal tobacco smoke exposure. *Pediatrics, 124*(5), e1017–e1044.
2. Håberg, S. E., Bentdal, Y. E., London, S. J., et al. (2010). Prenatal and postnatal parental smoking and acute otitis media in early childhood. *Acta Paediatrica, 99*(1), 99–105.
3. Cunningham, F. G., Leveno, K., Bloom, S., et al. (2010). *Williams obstetrics* (23rd ed.). New York: McGraw-Hill Professional.
4. Bobrowski, R. A. (2010). Pulmonary physiology in pregnancy. *Clinical Obstetrics and Gynecology, 53*(2), 285.
5. Gallant, V., Duccuri, V., & McGuire, M. (2017). Tuberculosis in Canada—summary 2015. *Canada Communicable Disease Report, 43*(3), 77–82. Retrieved from https://www.canada.ca/content/dam/phac-aspc/migration/phac-aspc/publicat/ccdr-rmtc/17vol43/dr-rm43-3-4/assets/pdf/17vol43_3_4-ar-04-eng.pdf.
6. Tarlo, S. M., & Lemiere, C. (2014). Occupational asthma. *New England Journal of Medicine, 370*(7), 640–649.
7. Canadian Cancer Society. (2017). *Lung cancer statistics.* Retrieved from http://www.cancer.ca/en/cancer-information/cancer-type/lung/statistics/?region=on.
8. Public Health Agency of Canada (2014). *Asthma, by age group and sex.* Ottawa: Minister of Health.
9. Lung Association (2006). *Women & COPD: A national report.* Ottawa: Author. Retrieved from http://www.lung.ca/_resources/Women_COPD_Report_2006.pdf.
10. Doucet, M., Rochette, L., & Hamel, D. (2016). Incidence, prevalence, and mortality trends in chronic obstructive pulmonary disease over 2001 to 2011: A public health point of view of the burden. *Canadian Respiratory Journal, 2016,* 7518287. doi:dx.doi.org/10.1155/2016/7518287.
11. Nantel-Smith, R., Olivenstein, R., Martin, J., et al. (2016). A population based assessment of asthma and the asthma chronic obstructive pulmonary disease overlap syndrome (ACOS): A Canadian perspective. *American Journal of Respiratory and Critical Care Medicine, 193,* A4444.
12. Yusen, R. D., Criner, G. J., Sternberg, A. L., et al. (2018). The long-term oxygen treatment trial for chronic obstructive

pulmonary disease: Rationale, design, and lessons learned. *Annals of the American Thoracic Society, 15*(1), 89–101. doi:doi.org/10.1513/AnnalsATS.201705-374SD.

13. McEvoy, R. D., Antic, N. A., Heeley, E., et al. (2016). CPAP for prevention of cardiovascular events in obstructive sleep apnea. *New England Journal of Medicine, 375*, 919–931.

14. Hanania, N. A., Mannino, D. M., Yawn, B. P., et al. (2010). Predicting risk of airflow obstruction in primary care: Validation of the lung function questionnaire (LFQ). *Respiratory Medicine, 104*(8), 1160–1170.

15. Du, H., Newton, P. J., Salamonson, Y., et al. (2009). A review of the six-minute walk test. *European Journal of Cardiovascular Nursing, 8*(1), 2–8.

16. Prescher, S., Schoebel, C., Koehler, K., et al. (2016). Prognostic value of serial six-minute walk tests using tele-accelerometry in patients with chronic heart failure: A pre-specified sub-study of the TIM-HF-trial. *European Journal of Preventive Cardiology, 23*(2S), 21–26. doi:10.1177/2047487316671438.

17. Forgacs, P. (1978). The functional basis of pulmonary sounds. *Chest, 73*, 399–405.

18. Deguchi, F., Hirakawa, S., Gotoh, K., et al. (1993). Prognostic significance of posturally induced crackles: Long term follow-up of patients after recovery from acute myocardial infarction. *Chest, 103*, 1457–1462.

CHAPTER 20

Heart and Neck Vessels

Written by Carolyn Jarvis, PhD, APN, CNP
Adapted by June MacDonald-Jenkins, RN, BScN, MSc

ⓔ http://evolve.elsevier.com/Canada/Jarvis/examination/

STRUCTURE AND FUNCTION

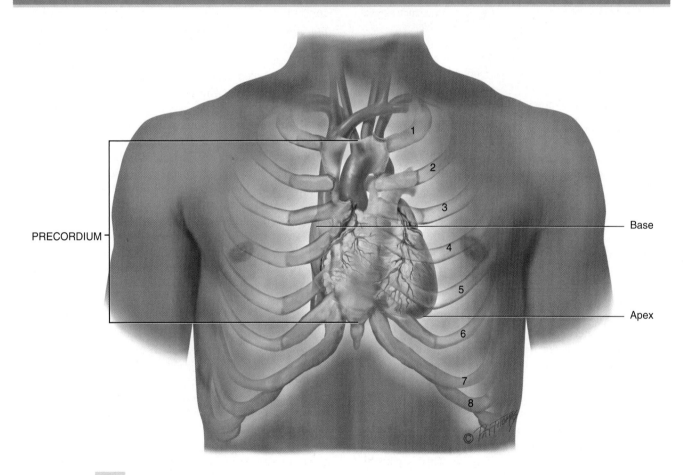

PRECORDIUM

1
2
3
Base
4
5
Apex
6
7
8

20.1 © Pat Thomas, 2006.

POSITION AND SURFACE LANDMARKS

The cardiovascular (CV) system consists of the **heart** (a muscular pump), and the **blood vessels**. The **precordium** is the area on the anterior chest overlying the heart and great vessels (Fig. 20.1). The great vessels are the major arteries and veins connected to the heart. The heart and the great vessels are located between the lungs in the middle third of the thoracic cage (in the area called the **mediastinum**). The heart extends from the levels of the second to the fifth intercostal spaces and from the right border of the sternum to the left midclavicular line.

Inside the body, the heart is positioned so that its right side is anterior and its left side is mostly posterior. Of the heart's four chambers, the right ventricle is immediately behind the sternum and forms the greatest area of anterior

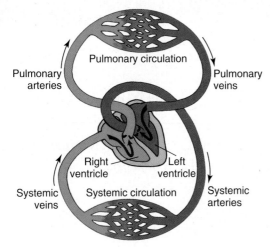

Pulmonary circulation

Pulmonary arteries

Pulmonary veins

Right ventricle

Left ventricle

Systemic veins

Systemic circulation

Systemic arteries

20.2   Two loops—separate but interdependent.

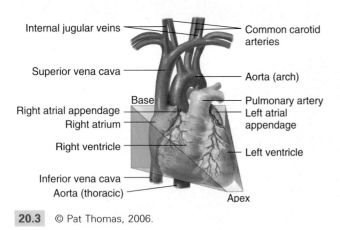

Internal jugular veins

Common carotid arteries

Superior vena cava

Aorta (arch)

Base

Right atrial appendage

Pulmonary artery

Left atrial appendage

Right atrium

Right ventricle

Left ventricle

Inferior vena cava

Aorta (thoracic)

Apex

20.3   © Pat Thomas, 2006.

cardiac surface. The left ventricle lies behind the right ventricle and forms the apex and slender area of the left border. The right atrium lies to the right and above the right ventricle and forms the right border. The left atrium is located posteriorly, with only a small portion, the left atrial appendage, showing anteriorly.

The blood vessels are arranged in two continuous loops: the *pulmonary circulation* and the *systemic circulation* (Fig. 20.2).

Think of the heart as an upside-down triangle in the chest. The "top" of the heart is the broader *base*, and the "bottom" is the *apex*, which points down and to the left (Fig. 20.3). During contraction, the apex beats against the chest wall, producing an apical impulse. This is palpable in most people, normally at the fifth intercostal space, 7 to 9 cm from the midsternal line. The **great vessels** lie bunched above the base of the heart. The **superior** and **inferior venae cavae** return unoxygenated venous blood to the right side of the heart. The **pulmonary artery** leaves the right ventricle, bifurcates, and carries the venous blood to the lungs. The **pulmonary veins** return the freshly oxygenated blood to the left side of the heart, and the **aorta** carries it out to the body. The aorta ascends from the left ventricle, arches back at the level of the sternal angle, and descends behind the heart.

HEART WALL, CHAMBERS, AND VALVES

The **heart wall** has numerous layers. The **pericardium** is a tough, fibrous, double-walled sac that surrounds and protects the heart (Fig. 20.4). It has two layers that contain a few millilitres of serous *pericardial fluid*. This ensures smooth, friction-free movement of the heart muscle. The pericardium is adherent to the great vessels, esophagus, sternum, and pleurae and is anchored to the diaphragm. The **myocardium** is the muscular wall of the heart; it does the pumping. The **endocardium** is the thin layer of endothelial tissue that lines the inner surface of the heart chambers and valves.

The common metaphor is to think of the heart as a pump. However, the heart is actually *two* pumps: the right side of the heart pumps blood into the lungs, and the left side of the heart simultaneously pumps blood into the body. The two pumps are separated by an impermeable wall, the septum. Each side has an atrium and a ventricle. The **atrium** (Latin for "anteroom") is a thin-walled reservoir for holding blood, and the thick-walled **ventricle** is the muscular pumping chamber.

The four **chambers** are separated by swinging-door–like structures, called *valves*, whose main purpose is to prevent backflow of blood. The valves are unidirectional; they can open only one way. The valves open and close *passively* in response to pressure gradients in the moving blood.

There are four **valves** in the heart (see Fig. 20.4). The two **atrioventricular (AV) valves** separate the atria and the ventricles. The right AV valve is the **tricuspid valve**, and the left AV valve is the bicuspid or **mitral valve**. The valves' thin leaflets are anchored by collagenous fibres (**chordae tendineae**) to papillary muscles embedded in the ventricle floor. The AV valves open during the heart's filling phase (diastole) to allow the ventricles to fill with blood. During the pumping phase (systole), the AV valves close to prevent regurgitation of blood back up into the atria. The papillary muscles contract at this time, so that the valve leaflets meet and unite to form a perfect seal without turning themselves inside out.

The **semilunar valves** are located between the ventricles and the pulmonary arteries. Each semilunar valve has three cusps that look like half moons. The semilunar valves are the **pulmonic valve** in the right side of the heart and the **aortic valve** in the left side of the heart. They open during pumping, or systole, to allow blood to be ejected from the heart.

Note that there are no valves between the venae cavae and the right atrium, nor between the pulmonary veins and the left atrium. For this reason, abnormally high pressure in the left side of the heart produces symptoms of pulmonary congestion, or heart failure, and abnormally high pressure in the right side of the heart manifests as distension of neck veins and abdomen.

DIRECTION OF BLOOD FLOW

Think of an unoxygenated red blood cell being drained downstream into the venae cavae. It is swept along with the

Aorta (arch)

Cut edge of pericardium

Pulmonary veins

Left atrium

Aortic valve

Mitral (AV) valve

Chordae tendineae

Left ventricle

Papillary muscle

Endocardium

Myocardium

Superior vena cava

Pulmonary artery

Pulmonary veins

Pulmonic valve

Right atrium

Tricuspid (AV) valve

Inferior vena cava

Right ventricle

20.4   © Pat Thomas, 2006.

flow of venous blood and follows the route illustrated in Fig. 20.5:

1. Blood flows from liver to right atrium through inferior vena cava.

   Superior vena cava drains venous blood from the head and upper extremities.

   From right atrium, venous blood travels through tricuspid valve to right ventricle.

2. From right ventricle, venous blood flows through pulmonic valve to pulmonary artery.

   Pulmonary artery delivers unoxygenated blood to lungs.

3. Lungs oxygenate blood.

   Pulmonary veins return fresh blood to left atrium.

4. From left atrium, arterial blood travels through mitral valve to left ventricle.

   Left ventricle ejects blood through aortic valve into aorta.

5. Aorta delivers oxygenated blood to body.

   Remember that the circulation is a continuous loop. The blood is kept moving along by continually shifting pressure gradients. The blood flows from an area of higher pressure to one of lower pressure.

CARDIAC CYCLE

The rhythmic movement of blood through the heart is the **cardiac cycle**. It has two phases: (a) diastole and (b) systole.

In **diastole**, the ventricles relax and fill with blood. This takes up two-thirds of the cardiac cycle. During **systole**, the heart's contraction, blood is pumped from the ventricles and fills the pulmonary and systemic arteries. This takes up one-third of the cardiac cycle.

Diastole

In diastole, the ventricles are relaxed, and the AV valves (i.e., the tricuspid and mitral valves) are open (Fig. 20.6). (Opening of the normal valve is acoustically silent.) The pressure in the atria is higher than that in the ventricles, and so blood pours rapidly into the ventricles. This first passive filling phase is called **early** or **protodiastolic filling**.

Toward the end of diastole, the atria contract and push the last amount of blood (about 25% of stroke volume) into the ventricles. This active filling phase is called **presystole**, or **atrial systole**, sometimes referred to as the *atrial kick*. It causes a small rise in left ventricular pressure. (Note that atrial systole occurs during ventricular diastole, a confusing but important point.)

Systole

At this point, a large volume of blood has been pumped into the ventricles. This volume raises ventricular pressure so that it is finally higher than that in the atria, and the mitral and tricuspid valves swing shut. The closure of the AV

to head
and neck

to arms

to arms

to abdomen
and lower
extemities

20.5

valves contributes to the first heart sound (S_1) and signals the beginning of systole. The AV valves close to prevent any regurgitation of blood back up into the atria during contraction.

For a very brief time, all four valves are closed. The ventricular walls contract. This contraction against a closed system works to build pressure inside the ventricles to a high level (**isometric contraction**). Consider first the left side of the heart. When the pressure in the ventricle finally exceeds pressure in the aorta, the aortic valve opens and blood is ejected rapidly.

After the ventricle's contents are ejected, its pressure falls. When pressure falls below pressure in the aorta, some blood flows backward toward the ventricle, causing the aortic valve to swing shut. This closure of the semilunar valves causes the second heart sound (S_2) and signals the end of systole.

Diastole Again

At this point in the cardiac cycle, all four valves are closed and the ventricles relax (called **isometric** or **isovolumic relaxation**). Meanwhile, the atria have been filling with blood delivered from the lungs. Atrial pressure is now higher than the relaxed ventricular pressure. The mitral valve drifts open, and diastolic filling begins again.

Events in the Right and Left Chambers

The same events are happening in the right side of the heart, but pressures in the right chambers of the heart are much lower than those of the left chambers because less energy is needed to pump blood to its destination, the pulmonary circulation. Also, events occur just slightly later in the right side of the heart because of the route of myocardial depolarization. As a result, each of the heart sounds has two distinct components, and sometimes you can hear them separately. In S_1, closure of the mitral valve (M_1) can be heard just before tricuspid valve closure (T_1). In S_2, aortic valve closure (A_2) occurs slightly before pulmonic valve closure (P_2).

HEART SOUNDS

Events in the cardiac cycle generate sounds that can be heard through a stethoscope over the chest wall. These include normal heart sounds and, on occasion, extra heart sounds and murmurs (Fig. 20.7).

Normal Heart Sounds

The **first heart sound (S_1)** occurs with closure of the AV valves and thus signals the beginning of systole. The mitral component of the first sound (M_1) slightly precedes the tricuspid component (T_1), but you usually hear these two components fused as one sound. You can hear S_1 over all the precordium, but it is usually loudest at the apex.

The **second heart sound (S_2)** occurs with closure of the semilunar valves and signals the end of systole. The aortic component of the second sound (A_2) slightly precedes the pulmonic component (P_2). Although it is heard over all the precordium, S_2 is loudest at the base.

Effect of Respiration

The volumes of right and left ventricular systole are just about equal, but this balance can be affected by respiration. To learn this, consider the following mnemonic:

Mo**R**e to the **R**ight,

Less to the **L**eft

That means that during inspiration, intrathoracic pressure is decreased. This pushes more blood into the venae cavae, increasing venous return to the right side of the heart, which increases right ventricular stroke volume. The increased volume prolongs right ventricular systole and delays pulmonic valve closure.

Meanwhile on the left side, a greater amount of blood is sequestered in the lungs during inspiration. This momentarily decreases the amount returned to the left side of the heart, decreasing left ventricular stroke volume. The decreased volume shortens left ventricular systole and allows the aortic valve to close a bit earlier. When the aortic valve closes significantly earlier than the pulmonic valve, you can hear the two components separately. This is a *split S_2*.

Pressure Changes in Left Heart

THE CARDIAC CYCLE

20.6

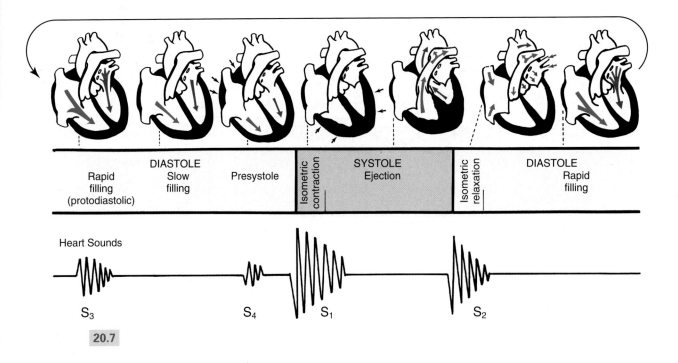

DIASTOLE			Isometric contraction	SYSTOLE	Isometric relaxation	DIASTOLE
Rapid filling (protodiastolic)	Slow filling	Presystole		Ejection		Rapid filling

Heart Sounds

S_3 S_4 S_1 S_2

20.7

Extra Heart Sounds

Third Heart Sound (S_3)

Normally diastole is a silent event. However, in some conditions, ventricular filling creates vibrations that can be heard over the chest. These vibrations constitute the S_3. The S_3 is heard when the ventricles are resistant to filling during the early rapid filling phase (protodiastole). This occurs immediately after S_2, when the AV valves open and atrial blood first pours into the ventricles. (See a complete discussion of S_3 in Table 20.7, p. 530.)

Fourth Heart Sound (S_4)

The S_4 occurs at the end of diastole, at presystole, when the ventricle is resistant to filling. The atria contract and push blood into a noncompliant ventricle. This creates vibrations that are heard as S_4. The S_4 occurs just before S_1.

Murmurs

Blood circulating through normal cardiac chambers and valves usually makes no noise. However, some conditions create turbulence in blood flow and collision currents. These result in a murmur, much like the sound of noisy water flow created by a pile of stones or a sharp turn in a stream. A murmur is a gentle, blowing, swooshing sound that can be heard on the chest wall.

The following conditions result in a murmur:
1. Increases in velocity of blood flow (flow murmur; e.g., in exercise, thyrotoxicosis)
2. Decreases in viscosity of blood (e.g., in anemia)
3. Structural defects in the valves (narrowed valve, incompetent valve) or unusual openings in the chambers (dilated chamber, septal defect)

Characteristics of Sound

All heart sounds are described by four characteristics:
1. Frequency (pitch): heart sounds are described as high pitched or low pitched, although these terms are relative because all are low-frequency sounds, and you need a high-quality stethoscope to hear them
2. Intensity (loudness): loud or soft
3. Duration: very short for heart sounds; silent periods are longer
4. Timing: systole or diastole

CONDUCTION

Of all organs, the heart has a unique ability: automaticity. The heart can contract by itself, independently of any signals or stimulation from the body. The heart contracts in response to an electrical current conveyed by a conduction system (Fig. 20.8). Specialized cells in the sinoatrial node near the superior vena cava initiate an electrical impulse. (Because the sinoatrial node has an intrinsic rhythm, it is the "pacemaker.") The current flows in an orderly sequence, first across the atria to the AV node low in the atrial septum. At the AV node, it is delayed slightly so that the atria have time to contract before the ventricles are stimulated. Then the impulse travels to the bundle of His, a collection of heart muscle cells specialized for electrical conduction. The bundle of His transmits the electrical impulses to the point of the apex of the fascicular branches, called the right and left bundle branches, and then through the ventricles.

The electrical impulse stimulates the heart to do its work, which is to contract. A small amount of electricity spreads to the body surface, where it can be measured and

SA node

Bundle of His

AV node

R

P   **T**

Q

S

CONDUCTION SYSTEM

ELECTROCARDIOGRAPH
(ECG) WAVE

20.8   © Pat Thomas, 2006.

PRELOAD

AFTERLOAD

20.9   © Pat Thomas, 2006.

recorded on the electrocardiogram (ECG). The ECG waves are arbitrarily labelled *PQRST*, which stand for the following elements:

P wave: depolarization of the atria

P–R interval: the interval from the beginning of the P wave to the beginning of the QRS complex (the time necessary for atrial depolarization plus time for the impulse to travel through the AV node to the ventricles)

QRS complex: depolarization of the ventricles

T wave: repolarization of the ventricles

Electrical events slightly *precede* the mechanical events in the heart. The phases of the cardiac cycle are labelled on an illustration of the ECG in Fig. 20.8.

PUMPING ABILITY

In the resting adult, the heart normally pumps between 4 and 6 L of blood per minute throughout the body. This **cardiac output (CO)** equals the volume of blood in each systole (called the *stroke volume* [SV]) times the number of beats per minute (*rate* [R]); that is,

$$CO = SV \times R$$

The heart can alter its cardiac output to adapt to the metabolic needs of the body. Preload and afterload affect the heart's ability to increase cardiac output.

Preload is the venous return that builds during diastole. It is the length to which the ventricular muscle is stretched at the end of diastole just before contraction (Fig. 20.9).

Right external jugular vein

Right common carotid artery

Sternomastoid muscle

Left external jugular vein

Left common carotid artery

Left internal jugular vein

Sternomastoid muscle and clavicle cut

Superior vena cava

Aorta

NECK VESSELS

20.10

When the volume of blood returned to the ventricles is increased (as when exercise stimulates skeletal muscles to contract and force more blood back to the heart), the muscle bundles are stretched beyond their normal resting state to accommodate it. The force of this switch is the preload. According to the Frank–Starling law, the greater the stretch, the stronger is the heart's contraction. This increased contractility results in an increase in the volume of blood ejected (increased stroke volume).

Afterload is the opposing pressure that the ventricle must generate to open the aortic valve against the higher aortic pressure. It is the resistance against which the ventricle must pump its blood. Once the ventricle is filled with blood, the ventricular end-diastolic pressure is 5 to 10 mm Hg, whereas that in the aorta is 70 to 80 mm Hg. To overcome this difference, the ventricular muscle *tenses* (isovolumic contraction). After the aortic valve opens, rapid ejection occurs.

THE NECK VESSELS

CV assessment includes the survey of vascular structures in the neck: the carotid artery and the jugular veins (Fig. 20.10). These vessels reflect the efficiency of cardiac function.

Carotid Artery Pulse

Chapter 10 describes the pulse as a pressure wave generated by each systole as blood is pumped into the aorta. The carotid artery is a central artery; that is, it is close to the heart. The timing of the carotid artery pulse closely coincides with

S_1 S_2 S_1 S_2

Phonocardiogram (apex)

D   D

Carotid artery pulse tracing

QRS   QRS

P   T U   P   T U

ECG

ARTERIAL PULSE

20.11

ventricular systole. (Assessment of the peripheral pulses is described in Chapter 21, and blood pressure assessment is described in Chapter 10.)

The **carotid artery** is located in the groove between the trachea and the sternomastoid muscle, medial to and alongside that muscle. Note the characteristics of its waveform (Fig. 20.11): a smooth rapid upstroke, a summit that is rounded and smooth, and a downstroke that is more gradual

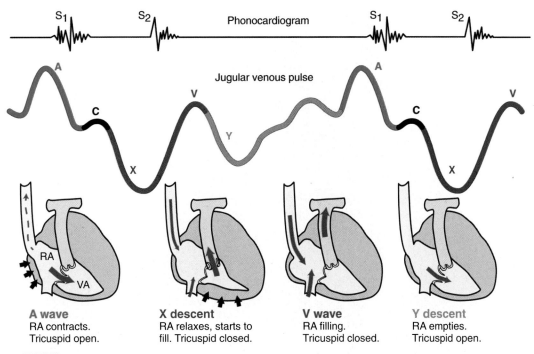

A wave
RA contracts.
Tricuspid open.

X descent
RA relaxes, starts to
fill. Tricuspid closed.

V wave
RA filling.
Tricuspid closed.

Y descent
RA empties.
Tricuspid open.

   Note: Match colour on waveform with its description.

and that has a dicrotic notch caused by closure of the aortic valve (marked *D* in the figure).

Jugular Venous Pulse and Pressure

The **jugular veins** empty unoxygenated blood directly into the superior vena cava. Because no cardiac valve exists to separate the superior vena cava from the right atrium, the jugular veins give information about activity on the right side of the heart. Specifically, they reflect filling pressure and volume changes. When the right side of the heart fails to pump efficiently, the volume and pressure increase, as exposed by the jugular veins.

Two jugular veins are present in each side of the neck (see Fig. 20.10). The larger **internal jugular vein** lies deep and medial to the sternomastoid muscle. It is usually not visible, although its diffuse pulsations may be seen in the sternal notch when the person is supine. The **external jugular vein** is more superficial; it lies lateral to the sternomastoid muscle, above the clavicle.

Although an arterial pulse is caused by a forward propulsion of blood, the jugular vein pulse is different. The jugular vein pulse results from movement of a waveform backward as a result of events upstream. The jugular vein pulse has five components, as shown in Fig. 20.12.

The five components of the jugular vein pulse occur because of events in the right side of the heart. The A wave reflects atrial contraction because some blood flows backward to the vena cava during right atrial contraction. The C wave, or ventricular contraction, is backflow from the bulging upward of the tricuspid valve when it closes at the beginning of ventricular systole (not from the neighbouring carotid artery pulsation). Next, the X descent shows atrial relaxation when the right ventricle contracts during systole

and pulls the bottom of the atria downward. The V wave occurs with passive atrial filling because of the increasing volume in the right atria and increased pressure. The Y descent reflects passive ventricular filling when the tricuspid valve opens and blood flows from the right atrium to the right ventricle.

DEVELOPMENTAL CONSIDERATIONS

Infants and Children

The fetal heart functions early; it begins to beat at the end of 3 weeks' gestation. The lungs are nonfunctional, but the fetal circulation compensates for this (Fig. 20.13). Oxygenation takes place at the placenta, and the arterial blood is returned to the right side of the heart. There is no point in pumping all this freshly oxygenated blood through the lungs; it is therefore rerouted in two ways. First, about two-thirds of it is shunted through an opening in the atrial septum, the **foramen ovale**, into the left side of the heart, where it is pumped out through the aorta. Second, the rest of the oxygenated blood is pumped by the right side of the heart out through the pulmonary artery, but it is detoured through the **ductus arteriosus** to the aorta. Because they are both pumping into the systemic circulation, the right and left ventricles are equal in weight and muscle wall thickness.

Inflation and aeration of the lungs at birth produces circulatory changes. The blood is oxygenated through the lungs rather than through the placenta. The foramen ovale closes within the first hour after birth because of the new pressure in the right side of the heart, which is lower than in the left side. The ductus arteriosus closes later, usually within 10 to 15 hours of birth. The left ventricle has the greater workload

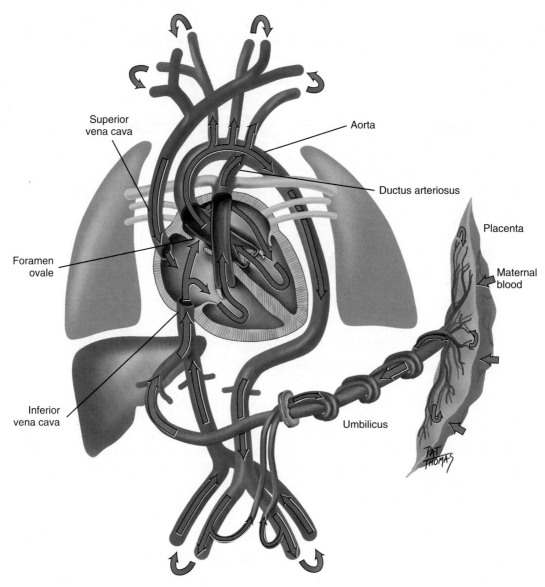

Superior vena cava

Aorta

Ductus arteriosus

Placenta

Maternal blood

Foramen ovale

Inferior vena cava

Umbilicus

PAT THOMAS

FETAL CIRCULATION

20.13

of pumping into the systemic circulation, so that when the baby has reached 1 year of age, the left ventricle's mass increases to reach the adult proportion; the ratio of the left ventricle to right ventricle is 2:1.

The heart's position in the chest is more horizontal in the infant than in the adult; thus the apex is higher, located at the fourth left intercostal space (Fig. 20.14). It reaches the adult position by 7 years of age.

Pregnant Women

Blood volume increases by 30 to 40% during pregnancy; the expansion is most rapid during the second trimester. This expansion causes an increase in stroke volume and cardiac output and an increase in pulse rate by 10 to 15 beats per minute. The pulse rate rises in the first trimester and peaks in the third, and returns to baseline within the first 10 days postpartum. Despite the increase in cardiac output, arterial

blood pressure decreases in pregnancy as a result of peripheral vasodilation. The blood pressure drops to its lowest point during the second trimester and then rises.

Older Adults

It is difficult to isolate the "aging process" of the CV system because it is so closely interrelated with lifestyle, habits, and pathology. We know that lifestyle modifies the development of cardiovascular disease (CVD); smoking, diet, alcohol use, exercise patterns, and stress have an immense influence. Lifestyle also affects the aging process; cardiac changes once thought to be caused by aging result partially from the increasingly sedentary lifestyle accompanying aging.

Hemodynamic Changes With Aging

- With aging systolic blood pressure increases. This is caused by the thickening and stiffening of the large

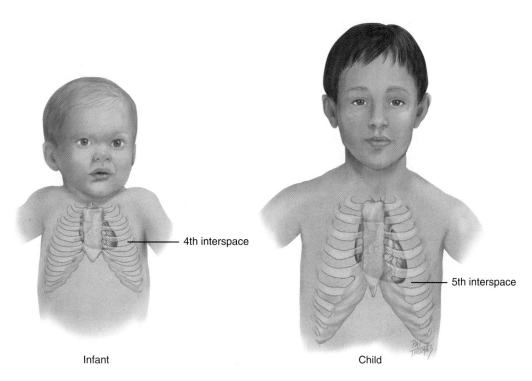

4th interspace

5th interspace

Infant   Child

HEART'S POSITION IN THE CHEST

20.14

arteries, which, in turn, is caused by collagen and calcium deposits in vessel walls and loss of elastic fibres. This stiffening (arteriosclerosis) creates an increase in pulse wave velocity because the less compliant arteries cannot store the volume ejected.

- The overall size of the heart does not increase with age, but left ventricular wall thickness increases. This is an adaptive mechanism to accommodate the vascular stiffening mentioned earlier that creates an increased workload on the heart.
- Diastolic blood pressure may decrease after the sixth decade. Together with a rising systolic pressure, this increases the pulse pressure (the difference between the two).
- No change in resting heart rate occurs with aging.
- Cardiac output at rest is not changed with aging.

There is a decreased ability of the heart to augment cardiac output with exercise. This is shown by a decreased maximum heart rate with exercise and a diminishing of sympathetic response. Noncardiac factors also cause a decrease in maximum work performance with aging: decrease in skeletal muscle performance, increase in muscle fatigue, and increased sense of dyspnea. Persistent exercise conditioning modifies many of the aging changes in CV function.[1]

Dysrhythmias. The presence of supraventricular and ventricular arrhythmias increases with age. Ectopic beats are common in older adults; although these are usually asymptomatic in healthy older adults, they may compromise cardiac output and blood pressure when disease is present.

Tachydysrhythmias may not be tolerated as well by older adults. The myocardium is thicker and less compliant, and

early diastolic filling is impaired at rest. Thus it may not tolerate a tachycardia as well because of shortened diastole. Also, tachydysrhythmias may further compromise a vital organ whose function has already been affected by aging or disease.[2]

Electrocardiograph. Age-related changes in the ECG occur as a result of histological changes in the conduction system. These changes include:

- Prolonged P–R interval (first-degree AV block) and prolonged Q–T interval; the QRS interval is unchanged
- Left axis deviation from mild age-related left ventricle (LV) hypertrophy and fibrosis in the left bundle branch
- Increased incidence of bundle branch block

Although the hemodynamic changes associated with aging alone do not seem severe or portentous, the fact remains that the incidence of CVD increases with age. CVD is the second leading cause of death in Canada for individuals over the age of 65 years. The incidence of hypertension (systolic, >140 mm Hg; diastolic, >90 mm Hg) and heart failure also increases with age. Lifestyle habits (smoking, chronic alcohol use, lack of exercise, poor diet) play a significant role in the acquisition of heart disease. Increasing the physical activity of older adults—even at a moderate level—shows a reduction in the risk for death from CVD and respiratory illnesses. Thus, health teaching is a crucial treatment parameter.[3]

SOCIAL DETERMINANT OF HEALTH CONSIDERATIONS

In 2014, Canadians with the lowest household incomes were more likely than those with the highest household incomes to report living with a CVD.[4] Income, cultural food choices, and employment security are some of the influencing factors that inhibit one's ability to manage CVD. Indigenous people in Canada report higher than normal national averages for the development of CVD over the age of 20 years.[5] Social determinants (versus genetics) are the greatest influencing factor.[6]

The prevalence of death from CVD is sharply decreasing on an annual basis, and yet the incidence of CVD itself continues to increase. Better medications, early intervention, and public health awareness are some of the factors contributing to the reduction in deaths. Men and women in Canada have almost equal rates of death from CVD, a trend noted since 2000.[7] However, men are two times more likely to suffer a heart attack than women.[7] Interestingly, early heart attack signs were missed in 78% of women, resulting in delay in treatment and greater injury to the myocardium associated with initial misdiagnosis.[8] In 2015, heart disease was the second leading cause of death for Canadians, at 20% of all deaths, while cancer remains the leading cause of death, at 29% of all deaths.[9] The prevalence of heart disease and stroke is higher among adults of African descent than in any other ethnic group.[10] The prevalence rates of CVD for Indigenous people and Canadians of African descent show the crucial need to improve early detection, screening, and treatment in these populations.

Socioeconomic factors also influence the incidence of CVD in Canadians. Concerns about food security continue to be in the forefront of arguments for action to diminish heart disease. "*Food security* is described as the condition in which all people, at all times, have access to nutritious, safe, personally acceptable, and culturally appropriate foods, produced in ways that are environmentally sound and socially just" (this was discussed in Chapter 12).[11] A lack of food security as a result of economic or geographical barriers, as in most northern communities, is a significant determinant of health and an important heart health issue for many. Income and employment, access to resources, and extended health care plans also influence the ability to support a heart-healthy lifestyle. The major risk factors for heart disease and stroke are high blood pressure, smoking, high cholesterol levels, obesity, physical inactivity, and diabetes. Additionally, the use of hormone replacement therapy (HRT) increases the risk of heart disease for postmenopausal women.

High blood pressure. In 2014, 5.3 million Canadians (17.7%) aged 12 and older reported being diagnosed with **hypertension**.[3] The incidence rate of high blood pressure has increased year over year since 2001, with no significant differences based on sex. The 2014 rate is lower than the self-reported value reported in the 2010 Canadian Community Health Survey (19.4%).[12] This discrepancy could reflect the number of Canadians self-managing their hypertension without pharmaceutical intervention. The Atlantic provinces continue to have the highest prevalence of hypertension in the nation; the western and the northern provinces (Yukon, British Columbia, and Northwest Territories) have the lowest rates.[13]

Smoking. The Canadian Tobacco Use Monitoring Survey revealed a 9% decline in the overall prevalence of smoking in Canada from 1999 to 2012.[14] In 2016, 16.9% of Canadians aged 12 and older (roughly 5.2 million people) smoked either daily or occasionally.[15] Provincial and national smoking-prevention programs (discussed in Chapter 19) highlight the country's desire to manage this contributing factor. Smoking-cessation programs are available at public health units and on college and university campuses.

Serum cholesterol. During childhood (ages 4 to 19), children and adolescents of African descent have higher levels of total cholesterol, low-density lipoprotein cholesterol (the "bad" cholesterol), and high-density lipoprotein cholesterol (the "good" cholesterol) than do children and adolescents of Euro-Canadian descent. These differences reverse during adulthood, so that individuals of African descent have lower serum cholesterol levels than do those of Euro-Canadian descent.

Obesity. *Overweight* is defined by a body mass index (BMI) of 25 to 29.9 kg/m^2 and *obesity* by a BMI of 30 kg/m^2 or higher. These problems have reached epidemic proportions in Canada. Currently, 59% of adult Canadians are either classified as overweight or obese, with the Atlantic provinces reporting the highest incidence.[16] Overweight and obesity among children are of national concern. Between 1978/79 and 2004, the combined prevalence of overweight and obesity among those aged 2 to 17 years increased from 15 to 26%. Increases were highest among youth, aged 12 to 17 years, with overweight and obesity more than doubling for this age group, from 14 to 29%.[17] There is significant evidence that obesity is at least partly genetic.[16] Certain ethnic groups are more vulnerable to obesity and obesity-related disorders. Genome-wide association studies show that some genes are associated with a higher BMI. However, genes are not the whole story: the significant change in obesity rates since the 1990s is evidence against genetic drift and in favour of strong environmental influences interacting with existing genes.

Children are particularly vulnerable to their environment because they have less ability to shape it. Children's eating habits and physical activity patterns tend to be similar to those of their parents, which is one environmental reason why obesity and obesity-related disorders often run in families. There is growing evidence that the environment in the womb helps to "program" a child's metabolism. Exposure to gestational diabetes or maternal obesity, high birth weight, and intrauterine growth delay with rapid catch-up growth are all associated with obesity later on. In contrast, breastfeeding in infancy may reduce the risk for obesity, as may other health practices, such as getting enough sleep, and eating only in response to appetite cues.

Diabetes. More than 9 million Canadians live with diabetes or are prediabetic. It is estimated that the prevalence will increase significantly by 2025, in part because the population is aging, obesity rates are rising, Canadian lifestyles are increasingly sedentary, and nearly 80% of all new Canadians belong to Hispanic, Asian, South Asian, and African populations, which are at increased risk of developing type 2 diabetes. The personal cost of diabetes may include a reduced quality of life and an increased likelihood of complications, such as heart disease, stroke, kidney disease, blindness, need for amputation, and erectile dysfunction. Medical costs for individuals with diabetes are two to three times higher than those for individuals without the disease. By 2020, it is estimated that diabetes will cost the Canadian health care system $16.9 billion annually.[18]

In Canada, the following federal programs have been instituted to address the growing incidence of diabetes and the socioeconomic factors that influence care provision:

- Canadian Diabetes Strategy (CDS): The strategy focuses on promoting health; preventing chronic disease by reducing risks for Canadians at risk; and supporting early detection and management of chronic diseases.
- Aboriginal Diabetes Initiative (ADI): The ADI focuses on increasing awareness of diabetes among Indigenous populations to reduce the prevalence and incidence of diabetes in these high-risk communities. The ADI supports over 600 programs for Indigenous people living with diabetes in Canada.
- Canadian Chronic Disease Surveillance System (CCDSS): The CCDSS is a collaborative network of provincial and territorial surveillance systems, supported by the Public Health Agency of Canada. Starting with diabetes surveillance, the CCDSS is expanding to include other chronic disease conditions.
- Healthy Weights: In 2010, federal, provincial, and territorial ministers of health endorsed *Curbing Childhood Obesity: A Federal, Provincial, and Territorial Framework for Action to Promote Healthy Weights*. Through the framework, the ministers agreed to make childhood obesity a collective priority.
- In 2011, Canada endorsed a United Nations Declaration on preventing and controlling noncommunicable diseases. The Declaration acknowledges the four main noncommunicable diseases as (a) cancer, (b) diabetes, (c) chronic respiratory diseases, and (d) CVD.[19,20]

SUBJECTIVE DATA

1. Chest pain
2. Dyspnea
3. Orthopnea
4. Cough
5. Fatigue
6. Cyanosis or pallor
7. Edema
8. Nocturia
9. Cardiac history
10. Family cardiac history
11. Personal habits (cardiac risk factors)

HEALTH HISTORY QUESTIONS

Examiner Asks	Rationale
1. Chest pain. Any **chest pain** or tightness? • Onset: When did it start? How long have you had it this time? Have you had this type of pain before? How often? • Location: Where did the pain start? Does the pain radiate to any other spot? • Character: How would you describe it: crushing, stabbing, burning, viselike? (Allow the patient to offer adjectives before you suggest them. Note whether the patient uses a clenched fist to describe pain.) • Is the pain brought on by activity (what type), rest, emotional upset, eating, sexual intercourse, or cold weather? • Do you have any associated symptoms: sweating, ashen grey or pale skin, heart skipping a beat, shortness of breath, nausea or vomiting, heart racing? • Is the pain made worse by moving the arms or neck, by breathing, or by lying flat? • Is the pain relieved by rest or nitroglycerine? How many sprays?	Angina, an important cardiac symptom, occurs when heart's vascular supply cannot keep up with metabolic demand. Chest pain also may be of pulmonary, musculo-skeletal, or gastro-intestinal origin; it is important to differentiate. A squeezing "clenched fist" sign is characteristic of angina, but the symptoms listed below may be anginal equivalents in the absence of chest pain. Diaphoresis, cold sweats, pallor, greyness. Palpitations, dyspnea, nausea, tachycardia, fatigue. Try to differentiate pain of cardiac versus noncardiac origin.

Examiner Asks	Rationale
2. Dyspnea. Any **shortness of breath**? • What type of activity, and how much, brings on shortness of breath? How much activity brought it on 6 months ago? • Onset: Does the shortness of breath come on unexpectedly? • Duration: Constant, or does it come and go? • Seems to be affected by position: lying down? • Awakens you from sleep at night? • Does the shortness of breath interfere with activities of daily living (ADLs)?	**Dyspnea** on exertion (DOE): quantify exactly (e.g., DOE after walking two level blocks). Paroxysmal dyspnea. Constant or intermittent dyspnea. Recumbent dyspnea. Paroxysmal nocturnal dyspnea occurs with heart failure. Lying down increases volume of intrathoracic blood, and the weakened heart cannot accommodate the increased load. Affected patients classically awaken after 2 hours of sleep with the perception of needing fresh air. See Table 20.2, p. 526, for a clinical portrait of heart failure.
3. Orthopnea. How many **pillows do you use** when sleeping or lying down?	*Orthopnea* is the need to assume a more upright position to breathe. Note the exact number of pillows used.
4. Cough. Do you have a **cough**? • Duration: How long have you had it? • Frequency: Is it related to time of day? • Type: Is it dry, hacking, barky, hoarse, or productive? • Do you cough up mucus? What colour is it? Any odour? Blood-tinged (hemoptysis)? • Is the cough associated with activity, position (lying down), anxiety, talking? • Does activity make it better or worse (sit, walk, exercise)? • Is it relieved by rest or medication?	Sputum production, mucoid or purulent. Hemoptysis is often a pulmonary disorder but also occurs with mitral stenosis.
5. Fatigue. Do you seem to **tire easily**? Are you able to keep up with your family and co-workers? • Onset: When did fatigue start? Was it sudden or gradual? Has any *recent* change occurred in energy level? • Is fatigue related to time of day: all day, morning, evening?	Fatigue from decreased cardiac output is worse in the evening, whereas fatigue from anxiety or depression is present all day or is worse in the morning.
6. Cyanosis or pallor. Ever noted your facial skin **turn blue or ashen**?	**Cyanosis** or **pallor** occurs with myocardial infarction or low cardiac output states as a result of decreased tissue perfusion.
7. Edema. Any **swelling of your feet and legs**? • Onset: When did you first notice this? • Any recent change? • What time of day does the swelling occur? Do your shoes feel tight at the end of day? • How much swelling would you say there is? Are both legs equally swollen? • Does the swelling go away with rest, with elevation, or after a night's sleep? • Do you have any associated symptoms, such as shortness of breath? If so, does the shortness of breath occur before leg swelling or after?	**Edema** is dependent when caused by heart failure. Cardiac edema is worse at evening and better in morning after legs are elevated all night. Cardiac edema is bilateral; unilateral swelling has a local vein cause.

Examiner Asks	Rationale
8. **Nocturia.** Do you **awaken at night with an urgent need to urinate**? How long has this been occurring? Any recent change?	Recumbency at night promotes fluid reabsorption and excretion; **nocturia** occurs with heart failure in patients who are ambulatory during the day.
9. **Cardiac history.** Do you have any **history** of hypertension, elevated cholesterol or triglyceride levels, heart murmur, congenital heart disease, rheumatic fever or unexplained joint pains in childhood or youth, recurrent tonsillitis, anemia, or diabetes? • Ever had heart disease? When was this? Was it treated by medication or heart surgery? • Have you ever had a heart attack? If so, when, and what treatment or intervention did you receive? (See the box Promoting Health: Women and Heart Attacks.) • When was your most recent ECG, stress ECG, serum cholesterol measurement, or other heart tests?	

Subjective Data

PROMOTING HEALTH: WOMEN AND HEART ATTACKS

The Heart Truth

When someone complains of chest pain or pain radiating down the left arm, the person almost always thinks "heart attack." After all, these are the typical symptoms, correct? Well, yes and no. In the past it was believed that women experienced different warning signs than men. The Heart and Stroke Foundation noted that this may not actually be the case.* Both women and men may experience typical or atypical symptoms, such as nausea; sweating; pain in the arm, throat, or jaw; or pain that is unusual. However, women may describe their pain differently than men. Nevertheless, the most common symptom in women is still chest pain.

Many of the symptoms that women experience are easily attributable to something else, other than the heart, and are therefore often ignored. According to the Heart and Stroke Foundation of Canada, while both men and women typically experience chest pain as their primary sign, women describe their pain differently, which can impact their diagnosis and treatment.* Women tend to use descriptors such as "pressure" or "tightness," with associated signs and symptoms such as nausea, unusual fatigue, or jaw pain—not always an elephant sitting on their chest or pain radiating down the left arm. The Heart and Stroke Foundation also noted:

Women and their doctors are slow to identify the early signs of an impending heart attack. According to a retrospective study published in Circulation, *early heart attack signs were missed in 78% of women in the study group of women, even though these signs occurred repeatedly over a period of weeks or months. These early signs are subtle— shortness of breath, weakness, fatigue, dizziness—but are strong indicators of an impending heart attack. At the same time, they were often missed (or dismissed) by women themselves or when they sought medical assistance.**

Heart disease is the second most common cause of death in Canadian women. Women tend to be safeguarded from heart disease before menopause because of the protective effect of naturally occurring estrogen.†

Some factors directly influence a woman's risk for cardiovascular disease. During a woman's reproductive life cycle, from approximately ages 12 to 50, the naturally occurring estrogen provides a protective effect on women's cardiovascular health. However, estrogen's protective effect can change, depending on a variety of factors and conditions.

Oral contraceptives are much safer now than the forms used in the past and are not associated with significant risk any longer unless combined with other risk factors, such as smoking.

During the menopausal transition, which occurs around age 51, a woman's risk for heart disease and stroke increases. During this period, the ovaries slowly decrease the production of the hormone estrogen, which will result in an increase in serum cholesterol and a tendency toward developing higher blood pressure. Reduced estrogen levels may also increase body fat above the waist, which has harmful effects on the way blood clots and affects the way the body metabolizes sugar (which can be a precursor to diabetes).

Until the 2000s, it was thought that hormone replacement therapy (HRT) could help reduce the risk for cardiac disease in menopausal women. However, studies have shown that taking certain types of hormones (estrogen with progestin) can actually increase the risk for heart attack, stroke, blood clots, and breast cancer for some women. As a result of these studies, HRT is no longer recommended for the prevention of heart disease, although it may be helpful for some women in treating other symptoms of menopause, such as hot flashes. Women should always consult their physician for recommendations regarding HRT.

Naturally occurring estrogen also helps to keep cholesterol levels in a healthy range. After menopause, as estrogen levels drop, the incidence of high cholesterol increases. A health care provider should be consulted about how often cholesterol levels should be checked.

In Canada, blood cholesterol rises steadily with increasing age. Whereas 23% of 18- to 39-year-olds have elevated blood cholesterol, in the 65-to-74 age group, the prevalence is 65%.‡

Exercise and weight control are paramount for mitigating the risk for heart disease. Inactive women have twice the risk of developing heart disease than do active women. Thirty

Continued

Subjective Data

PROMOTING HEALTH: WOMEN AND HEART ATTACKS—cont'd

The Heart Truth

minutes of physical activity, four to six times a week, helps to keep the heart strong and prevent heart disease. Even losing a small amount of extra weight can also help reduce the risk.

The Heart Truth is a national public health education campaign to raise awareness that heart disease and stroke is a common killer of women in Canada. The Heart and Stroke Foundation of Canada adopted this US-based initiative in 2008 because of its overwhelming success. The Heart Truth campaign introduced the red dress as the national symbol for women and heart disease awareness. Since its introduction, many women have taken ownership of the symbol. Each year, the red dress is featured on runways as top Canadian fashion designers create original red dress creations, modelled by some of Canada's most celebrated women.[§]

For more information on women and heart disease, consult the following websites:

*   Heart and Stroke Foundation of Canada: http://www .heartandstroke.ca
*   Women with Heart Disease: Living a Good Life: https:// www.canada.ca/en/public-health/services/chronic -diseases/cardiovascular-disease/women-heart-disease -living-a-good-life.html

References

*Heart and Stroke Foundation of Canada. (2017). *Ms.Understood: Heart & Stroke 2018 heart report* (p. 6). Retrieved from http://www .heartandstroke.ca/-/media/pdf-files/canada/2018-heart-month/ hs_2018-heart-report_en.ashx?la=en&hash=3BBC7F1DD1DA3 EDC6B2B0E9BB31E855268C051EB.

†Heart and Stroke Foundation of Canada. (2018). *Heart: Women's unique risk factors*. Retrieved from http://www.heartandstroke.ca/ heart/risk-and-prevention/womens-unique-risk-factors.

‡Statistics Canada. (2015). *Cholesterol levels of adults, 2012 to 2013*. Retrieved from http://www.statcan.gc.ca/pub/82-625-x/2014001/ article/14122-eng.htm.

§Clark, M. I., McGannon, K. R., Berry, T. R., et al. (2016). Taking a hard look at the Heart Truth campaign in Canada: A discourse analysis. *Journal of Health Psychology*, doi:10.1177/1359105316669581.

 Women & Heart Disease

Examiner Asks	Rationale

10. Family cardiac history. Any **family history** of hypertension, obesity, diabetes, coronary artery disease (CAD), sudden death at a young age?

11. Personal habits (cardiac risk factors)
*   Nutrition: Please describe your usual daily diet. (Note whether this diet is representative of the basic food groups, and note the amount of calories, cholesterol, and any additives such as salt.) What is your usual weight? Has it changed recently?
*   Smoking: Do you smoke cigarettes or other tobacco? At what age did you start? How many packs per day? For how many years? Have you ever tried to quit? If so, how did this go?
*   Alcohol: How much alcohol do you usually drink each week or each day? When was your most recent drink? What was the number of drinks that episode? Have you ever been told you had a drinking problem?
*   Exercise: What is your usual amount of exercise each day or week? What type of exercise (state type or sport)? If a sport, what is your usual amount (light, moderate, heavy)?
*   Medications: Do you take any antihypertensives, β-blockers, calcium channel blockers, digoxin, diuretics, Aspirin/anticoagulants, over-the-counter medications, or street drugs?
*   Stress: Tell me about stress in your life. What are the main causes? How do you manage it? How does it affect you?

Risk factors for CAD: Collect data regarding elevated cholesterol level, elevated blood pressure, random plasma glucose level value in excess of 11.1 mmol/L or known diabetes mellitus, obesity, cigarette smoking, low activity level, and, for postmenopausal women, length of any hormone replacement therapy for postmenopausal women.

Additional History for Infants

1. Maternal health. How was the mother's health during pregnancy? Any unexplained fever, rubella during first trimester, other infection, hypertension, medications taken?

2. Feeding. Have you noted any cyanosis while the baby is nursing or crying? Is the baby able to eat, nurse, or finish bottle without tiring?

To screen for heart disease in an infant, note fatigue during feeding. Infants with heart failure take fewer ounces each feeding; become dyspneic with sucking; may be diaphoretic and then fall into exhausted sleep; and awaken after a short time hungry again.

Examiner Asks	Rationale

3. Growth. Has the baby grown as expected by growth charts and about the same as siblings or peers?

Poor weight gain.

4. Activity. Were the baby's motor milestones achieved as expected? Is the baby able to play without tiring? How many naps does the baby take each day? How long does a nap last?

Additional History for Children

1. Growth. Has the child grown as expected by growth charts?

Poor weight gain.

2. Activity. Is the child able to keep up with siblings or age mates? Is the child willing or reluctant to go out to play? Is the child able to climb stairs, ride a bike, walk a few blocks? Does the child squat to rest during play or to watch television, or assume a knee-chest position while sleeping? Have you noted "blue spells" during exercise?

Fatigue: Record specific limitations. Cyanosis.

3. Joint pain and fever. Has the child had any unexplained joint pains or unexplained fever?

4. Headache and nosebleed. Does the child have frequent headaches or nosebleeds?

5. Respiratory disease. Does the child have frequent respiratory infections? How many per year? How are they treated? Have any of these proved to be streptococcal infections?

6. Family history. Does the child have a sibling with heart defect? Is anyone in the child's family known to have chromosomal abnormalities, such as Down syndrome?

Additional History for Pregnant Women

1. High blood pressure. Have you had any high blood pressure during this or earlier pregnancies?
  - What was your usual blood pressure level before pregnancy? How has your blood pressure been monitored during the pregnancy?
  - If high, what blood pressure treatment has been started?
  - Any associated symptoms: weight gain; protein in urine; swelling in feet, legs, or face?

2. Faintness or dizziness. Have you had any faintness or dizziness with this pregnancy?

Additional History for Older Adults

1. Disease. Do you have any known heart or lung disease: hypertension, CAD, chronic emphysema, or bronchitis?
  - What efforts to treat this have been started?
  - Have your usual symptoms changed recently? Does your illness interfere with ADLs?

2. Medications. Do you take any medications for your heart, such as water pills, blood pressure pills, or heart pills? Are you aware of adverse effects? Have you recently stopped taking your medication? Why?

Nonadherence to a treatment regimen may be related to adverse effects or lack of finances.

3. Environment. Does your home have any stairs? How often do you need to climb them? Does this have any effect on ADLs?

Subjective Data

OBJECTIVE DATA

PREPARATION

To evaluate the carotid arteries, the patient can be sitting up. To assess the jugular veins and the precordium, the patient should be supine with the head and chest elevated between 30 and 40 degrees.

Stand on the patient's right side; this will facilitate your hand placement and viewing of the neck veins and auscultation of the precordium.

The room must be warm; a chilly room makes the patient uncomfortable, and shivering interferes with heart sounds. Take scrupulous care to ensure *quiet*; heart sounds are very soft, and any ambient room noise masks them.

Ensure privacy by keeping the chest draped. A woman's left breast overrides part of the area you need to examine. Gently displace the breast upward, or ask the woman to hold it out of the way.

Perform a **regional cardiovascular assessment** in this order:
1. Pulse and blood pressure (see Chapter 10)
2. Extremities (see Chapter 21)
3. Neck vessels
4. Precordium

The logic of this order is that you will begin observations peripherally and move in toward the heart. For choreography of these steps in the complete physical examination, see Chapter 28.

EQUIPMENT NEEDED

Marking pen
Small centimetre ruler
Stethoscope with diaphragm and bell
  endpieces
Alcohol wipe (to clean endpiece)

Normal Range of Findings

The Neck Vessels

Auscultate the Carotid Artery

For middle-aged or older patients or patients who show symptoms or signs of CVD, auscultate each carotid artery for the presence of a **bruit** (pronounced *bru'-ee*; Fig. 20.15). This is a blowing, swishing sound indicating blood flow turbulence; normally none is present.

20.15

Abnormal Findings

A bruit indicates turbulence with a local vascular cause, such as atherosclerotic narrowing.

CRITICAL FINDINGS

The importance of auscultating the carotids prior to palpating is to determine the presence of a bruit. Bruits can be indicators of narrowed arteries secondary to atherosclerotic plaque buildup. Palpation may result in the dislodging of the plaque or a sudden drop in blood pressure and heart rate secondary to carotid hypersensitivity or established CVD in the area. If unsure what you are hearing, have it checked by another health care provider.

Normal Range of Findings	Abnormal Findings

Normal Range of Findings

Keep the neck in a neutral position. Lightly apply the bell of the stethoscope over the carotid artery at three levels: (1) the angle of the jaw, (2) the midcervical area, and (3) the base of the neck (see Fig. 20.15). Avoid compressing the artery because this could create an artificial bruit, and it could compromise circulation if the carotid artery is already narrowed by atherosclerosis. Ask the patient to take a breath, exhale, and hold still briefly without breathing while you listen so that tracheal breath sounds do not mask or mimic a carotid artery bruit. (Holding the breath on inhalation will also tense the levator scapulae muscles, which makes it hard to hear the carotid arteries.) Sometimes you can hear normal heart sounds transmitted to the neck; do not confuse these with a bruit.

Palpate the Carotid Artery

Located central to the heart, the carotid artery yields important information about cardiac function.

Palpate each carotid artery medial to the sternomastoid muscle in the neck (Fig. 20.16). Avoid excessive pressure on the carotid sinus area higher in the neck; excessive vagal stimulation here could slow down the heart rate, especially in older adults. Take care to palpate gently. To avoid compromising arterial blood flow to the brain, **palpate only one carotid artery at a time**.

20.16

Feel the contour and amplitude of the pulse. Normally the contour is smooth with a rapid upstroke and slower downstroke, and the normal strength is moderate. The findings should be the same bilaterally.

Inspect the Jugular Venous Pulse

From the jugular veins, you can assess the **central venous pressure (CVP)** and thus judge the heart's efficiency as a pump. Although the external jugular vein is easier to see, the internal (especially the right) jugular vein is attached more directly to the superior vena cava and thus is more reliable for assessment. You cannot see the internal jugular vein itself, but you can see its pulsation.

Position the patient supine at a 30- to a 45-degree angle, wherever you can best see the pulsations. In general, the higher the venous pressure is, the higher the position you need. Remove the pillow to avoid flexing the neck; the head should be in the same plane as the trunk. Turn the patient's head slightly away from the examined side, and direct a strong light tangentially onto the neck to highlight pulsations and shadows.

Abnormal Findings

A carotid bruit is audible when the lumen is half to two-thirds occluded. Bruit loudness increases as the atherosclerosis worsens until the lumen is two-thirds occluded. After that, bruit loudness decreases. When the lumen is completely occluded, the bruit disappears. Thus absence of a bruit does not ensure absence of a carotid lesion.

A murmur sounds much the same but is caused by a cardiac disorder. Some aortic valve murmurs (aortic stenosis) radiate to the neck and must be distinguished from a local bruit.

Carotid sinus hypersensitivity is the condition in which pressure over the carotid sinus leads to a decrease in heart rate, a decrease in blood pressure, and cerebral ischemia with syncope. This may occur in older adults with hypertension or occlusion of the carotid artery.

Diminished pulse feels small and weak (decreased stroke volume).

Increased pulse feels full and strong (hyperkinetic states; see Table 20.3, p. 526).

This inspection is considered by many authorities to be an advanced skill for practitioners in the cardiopulmonary environments in particular. It is not considered part of the basic cardiac assessment when no other abnormal cardiac findings are evident.

Objective Data

Normal Range of Findings

Note the external jugular veins overlying the sternomastoid muscle. In some patients, the veins are not visible at all, whereas in others they are full in the supine position. As the patient is raised to a sitting position, these external jugular veins flatten and disappear, usually at 45 degrees.

Now look for pulsations of the internal jugular veins in the area of the suprasternal notch or around the origin of the sternomastoid muscle around the clavicle. You must be able to distinguish pulsation of the internal jugular vein from that of the carotid artery. It is easy to confuse them because they lie close together. Use the guidelines shown in Table 20.1.

Abnormal Findings

Unilateral distension of external jugular veins has a local cause (kinking or aneurysm).

Full distended external jugular veins above 45 degrees signify increased CVP, as with heart failure.

TABLE 20.1	Characteristics of Jugular Versus Carotid Pulsations	
CHARACTERISTIC	**INTERNAL JUGULAR PULSE**	**CAROTID PULSE**
Location	Lower, more lateral, under or behind the sternomastoid muscle	Higher and medial to this muscle
Quality	Undulant and diffuse; two visible waves per cycle	Brisk and localized; one wave per cycle
Respiration	Varies with respiration; its level descends during inspiration when intrathoracic pressure is decreased	Does not vary
Palpability	None	Yes
Pressure	Light pressure at the base of the neck easily obliterates	No change
Position of patient	Level of pulse drops and disappears as the patient is brought to a sitting position	Unaffected

The Precordium

Inspect the Anterior Chest

Arrange tangential lighting to accentuate any flicker of movement.

Pulsations. You may or may not see the **apical impulse**, the pulsation created as the left ventricle rotates against the chest wall during systole. When visible, it appears at the level of the fourth or fifth intercostal space, at or inside the midclavicular line. It is easier to see in children and in patients with thin chest walls.

A **heave** or **lift** is a sustained forceful thrusting of the ventricle during systole. It occurs with ventricular hypertrophy as a result of increased workload. A right ventricular heave is seen at the sternal border; a left ventricular heave is seen at the apex (see Table 20.8, p. 532).

Palpate the Apical Impulse

Locate the apical impulse precisely by using one finger pad (Fig. 20.17, *A*). Asking the patient to "exhale and then hold it" aids the examiner in locating the pulsation. You may need to roll the patient midway to the left to find it; note that this also displaces the apical impulse farther to the left (see Fig. 20.17, *B*).

20.17 Checking the apical impulse. **A,** With the patient supine. **B,** With the patient rolled laterally.

Normal Range of Findings

Note the following characteristics:

- Location: The apical impulse should occupy only one interspace, the fourth or fifth, and be at or medial to the midclavicular line
- Size: Normally 1 × 2 cm
- Amplitude: Normally a short, gentle tap
- Duration: Short; normally occupies only first half of systole

The apical impulse is palpable in the supine position in 25 to 40% of adults and in the left lateral position in 50 to 73% of adults. It is not palpable in obese patients or in patients with thick chest walls. In states of high cardiac output (anxiety, fever, hyperthyroidism, anemia), the apical impulse increases in amplitude and duration.

Palpate Across the Precordium

Using the palmar aspects of your four fingers, gently palpate over the apex, the left sternal border, and the base, searching for any other pulsations (Fig. 20.18). Normally none are felt. If any are felt, note the timing. Use the carotid artery pulsation as a guide, or auscultate as you palpate.

20.18

Percussion*

*Percussion to outline the cardiac borders has been replaced with chest radiographic image or echocardiogram. Studies show that percussed heart borders are only moderately accurate, and therefore not considered best practice. As well, it has limited usefulness in women, as breast mass interferes with meaningful assessment.

Abnormal Findings

Cardiac enlargement is characterized as follows:

- Left ventricular dilatation (volume overload) displaces impulse down and to left and increases size more than one space.
- Increased force and duration but no change in location occurs with left ventricular hypertrophy and no dilatation (pressure overload; see Table 20.8, p. 532).

Cardiac enlargement: Left ventricular dilation (volume overload) displaces impulse down and to the left and increases size more than one costal vertebral space (from fifth to sixth intercostal space). This occurs with heart failure and cardiomyopathy.

Left ventricular hypertrophy presents with a sustained impulse with increased force and duration, but no change in location (see Table 20.8, p. 532).

A **thrill** is a palpable vibration. It feels like the throat of a purring cat. The thrill signifies turbulent blood flow and accompanies loud murmurs. Absence of a thrill, however, does not necessarily rule out the presence of a murmur.

Accentuated first and second heart sounds and extra heart sounds also may cause abnormal pulsations.

Objective Data

Normal Range of Findings	Abnormal Findings

Auscultation

Identify the auscultatory areas where you will listen. These include the four traditional valve "areas" (Fig. 20.19). The valve areas are not over the actual anatomical locations of the valves but are the sites on the chest wall where sounds produced by the valves are best heard. The sound radiates with the direction of blood flow. The valve areas are as follows:

• Second right interspace: aortic valve area
• Second left interspace: pulmonic valve area
• Fifth intercostal space at left lower sternal border: tricuspid valve area
• Fifth interspace at around left midclavicular line: mitral valve area

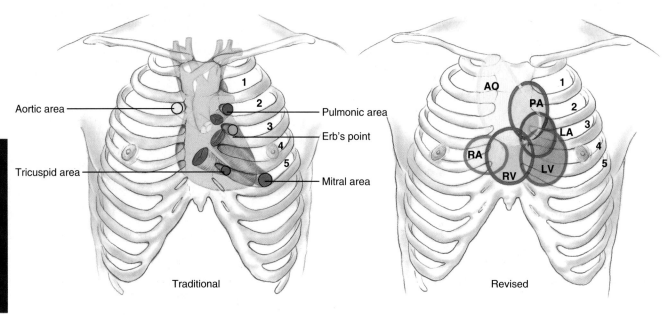

AUSCULTATORY AREAS

20.19 Auscultatory areas.

Do not limit your auscultation to only four locations. Sounds produced by the valves may be heard all over the precordium. (For this reason, many experts even discourage the naming of the valve areas.) Thus learn to inch your stethoscope in a rough Z pattern, from the base of the heart across and down, then over to the apex. Or start at the apex and work your way up. Include the sites shown in Fig. 20.19.

Recall the characteristics of a high-quality stethoscope (see Chapter 9). Clean the earpiece and endpiece with an alcohol wipe; you will use both. Although all heart sounds are low frequency, the diaphragm is for relatively higher pitched sounds, and the bell is for relatively lower pitched ones.

Before you begin, alert the patient: "I always listen to the heart in a number of places on the chest. Just because I am listening a long time, it does not necessarily mean that something is wrong."

After you place the stethoscope, try closing your eyes briefly to tune out any distractions. Concentrate, and listen selectively to *one* sound at a time. Consider that at least two, and perhaps three or four, sounds may be happening in less than 1 second. You cannot process everything at once. Begin with the diaphragm endpiece and use the following routine: (a) Note the rate and rhythm, (b) identify S_1 and S_2, (c) assess S_1 and S_2 separately, (d) listen for extra heart sounds, and (e) listen for murmurs.

Normal Range of Findings

Note the Rate and Rhythm. The rate ranges normally from 60 to 100 beats per minute. (Review the full discussion of the pulse in Chapter 10 and the normal rates across age groups.) The rhythm should be regular, although **sinus arrhythmia** occurs normally in young adults and children. With sinus arrhythmia, the rhythm varies with the patient's breathing, increasing at the peak of inspiration and slowing with expiration. Note any other irregular rhythm. If one occurs, check whether it has any pattern or if it is totally irregular.

When you notice any irregularity, check for a **pulse deficit** by auscultating the apical beat while simultaneously palpating the radial pulse. Count a serial measurement (one after the other) of apical beat and radial pulse. Normally, with every beat you hear at the apex, the pulse should perfuse to the periphery and be palpable. The two counts should be identical. When they are different, subtract the radial rate from the apical rate, and record the remainder as the pulse deficit.

Identify S_1 and S_2. This is important because S_1 is the start of systole and thus serves as the reference point for the timing of all other cardiac sounds. Usually, you can identify S_1 instantly because you hear a pair of sounds close together (lub-dup), and S_1 is the first of the pair. The guideline works except in the cases of the tachydysrhythmias (rates >100 beats/min). Diastolic filling time is shortened, and the beats are too close together to distinguish. Other guidelines to distinguish S_1 from S_2 are as follows:

- S_1 is louder than S_2 at the apex; S_2 is louder than S_1 at the base.
- S_1 coincides with the carotid artery pulse. Feel the carotid pulse gently as you auscultate at the apex; the sound you hear as you feel each pulse is S_1 (Fig. 20.20).
- S_1 coinciding with the R wave (the upstroke of the QRS complex) if the person is on an ECG monitor.

20.20

Listen to S_1 and S_2 Separately. Note whether each heart sound is normal, accentuated, diminished, or split. Inch your diaphragm across the chest as you do this.

Abnormal Findings

Premature beat: An isolated beat is early, or a pattern occurs in which every third or fourth beat sounds early.

Irregularly irregular: Sounds have no pattern; beats come rapidly and at random intervals.

A **pulse deficit** signals a weak contraction of the ventricles; it occurs with atrial fibrillation, premature beats, and heart failure.

Objective Data

Normal Range of Findings

First Heart Sound (S₁). Caused by closure of the AV valves, S_1 signals the beginning of systole. You can hear it over the entire precordium, although it is loudest at the apex (Fig. 20.21). (Sometimes the two sounds are equally loud at the apex because S_1 is lower pitched than S_2.)

S₁   S₂

APEX

LUB — dup

20.21

You can hear S_1 with the diaphragm of the stethoscope when the patient is in any position and equally well during inspiration and expiration. A split S_1 is normal, but it is rare. A split S_1 means you are hearing the mitral and tricuspid components separately. It is audible in the tricuspid valve area (the left lower sternal border). The split is very rapid, with the two components only 0.03 second apart.

Second Heart Sound (S₂). The S_2 is associated with closure of the semilunar valves. You can hear it with the diaphragm over the entire precordium, although S_2 is loudest at the base (Fig. 20.22).

S₁   S₂

BASE

lub — DUP

20.22

Splitting of S₂. A split S_2 is a normal phenomenon that occurs toward the end of inspiration in some people. Recall that closure of the aortic and pulmonic valves is nearly synchronous. Because of the effects of respiration on the heart described earlier, inspiration separates the timing of closure of the two valves, and the aortic valve closes 0.06 seconds before the pulmonic valve. Instead of one "DUP," you hear a split sound: "T-DUP" (Fig. 20.23). During expiration, synchrony returns, and the aortic and pulmonic components fuse together. A split S_2 is heard only in the pulmonic valve area (the second left interspace).

SPLITTING OF THE SECOND HEART SOUND

EXPIRATION	INSPIRATION
S₁ S₂	S₁ S₂
A₂-P₂	A₂ P₂
lub — DUP	lub — T-DUP

20.23

Abnormal Findings

Causes of accentuated or diminished S_1 are listed in Table 20.3 (p. 526).

Both heart sounds are diminished with conditions in which the amount of tissue between the heart and your stethoscope is increased: emphysema (hyperinflated lungs), obesity, pericardial fluid.

Accentuated or diminished S_2 is described in Table 20.4 (p. 527).

Normal Range of Findings

Listen for Murmurs. A murmur is a blowing, swooshing sound that occurs with turbulent blood flow in the heart or great vessels. Except for the innocent murmurs described, murmurs are abnormal. If you hear a murmur, describe it by indicating the following characteristics.

Timing. It is crucial to define the murmur by its occurrence in systole or diastole. You must be able to identify S_1 and S_2 accurately to do this. Try to further describe the murmur as being in early, middle, or late systole or diastole; throughout the cardiac event (termed *pansystolic, holosystolic/pandiastolic,* or *holodiastolic*); and whether it obscures or muffles the heart sounds.

Normal heart tones[13]	**Lub** S_1	**Dup** S_2	**Lub** S_1	**Dup** S_2
Early systolic murmur	**LSHSHSH** S_1	**Dup** S_2	**LSHSHSH** S_1	**Dup** S_2
Midsystolic murmur	**LubSHSHDup** S_1　　S_2		**LubSHSHDup** S_1　　S_2	
Late systolic murmur	**Lub** S_1	**SHSHP** S_2	**Lub** S_1	**SHSHP** S_2
Late systolic murmur and click (C) of mitral valve prolapse	**Lub** S_1	**KSHSHP** C　S_2	**Lub** S_1	**KSHSHP** C　S_2
Holosystolic murmur	**SHSHSHSHSH** S_1　　S_2		**SHSHSHSHSH** S_1　　S_2	

Loudness. Describe the intensity in terms of six "grades." For example, record a grade 2 murmur as 2/6.

Grade 1: barely audible, heard only in a quiet room and then with difficulty

Grade 2: clearly audible, but faint

Grade 3: moderately loud, easy to hear

Grade 4: loud, associated with a thrill palpable on the chest wall

Grade 5: very loud, heard with one corner of the stethoscope lifted off the chest wall; associated thrill

Grade 6: loudest, still heard with entire stethoscope lifted just off the chest wall; associated thrill

Pitch. Describe the pitch as high, medium, or low. The pitch depends on the pressure and the rate of blood flow producing the murmur.

Pattern. The intensity may follow a pattern during the cardiac phase, growing louder (crescendo), tapering off (decrescendo), or increasing to a peak and then decreasing (crescendo–decrescendo, or diamond-shaped). Because the whole murmur is just milliseconds long, it takes practice to diagnose any pattern.

Quality. Describe the quality as musical, blowing, harsh, or rumbling.

Location. Describe the area of maximum intensity of the murmur (where it is best heard) by noting the valve area or intercostal spaces.

Radiation. The murmur may be transmitted downstream in the direction of blood flow and may be heard in another place on the precordium, on the neck, on the back, or on the axilla.

Abnormal Findings

Murmurs may be caused by congenital defects and acquired valvular defects. Study Tables 20.9 and 20.10, pp. 533–534, for a complete description.

A systolic murmur may occur with a normal heart or with heart disease; a diastolic murmur always indicates heart disease.

The murmur of mitral stenosis is rumbling, whereas that of aortic stenosis is harsh (see Table 20.10, p. 534).

Normal Range of Findings

Posture. Some murmurs disappear or are enhanced by a change in position. Some murmurs are common in healthy children or adolescents and are termed *innocent* or *functional*. **Innocent murmurs** have no valvular or other pathological cause; **functional murmurs** are caused by increased blood flow in the heart (e.g., in anemia, fever, pregnancy, hyperthyroidism). The contractile force of the heart is greater in children; this increases blood flow velocity. Because of the increased velocity and a smaller chest measurement, a murmur is audible.

The innocent murmur is soft (grade 2), midsystolic, short, crescendo–decrescendo, and with a vibratory or musical quality "vooot" sound (like fiddle strings). It is heard between the second and third intercostal space and disappears with sitting, and the young person has no other associated signs of cardiac dysfunction. It is important to distinguish innocent murmurs from pathological ones. Diagnostic tests such as ECG and echocardiography will establish an accurate diagnosis.

Change Position. After auscultating in the supine position, roll the patient toward his, her, or their left side. Listen with the bell at the apex for the presence of any diastolic filling sounds (i.e., the S_3 or S_4).

Ask the patient to sit up, lean forward slightly, and exhale. Listen with the diaphragm firmly pressed at the base, right, and left sides. Check for the soft, high-pitched, early diastolic murmur of aortic or pulmonic regurgitation (Fig. 20.24).

20.24

 DEVELOPMENTAL CONSIDERATIONS

Infants

The transition from fetal to pulmonic circulation occurs in the immediate neonatal period. Fetal shunts normally close within 10 to 15 hours after birth but may take up to 48 hours. Thus you should assess the CV system during the first 24 hours and again in 2 to 3 days.

Abnormal Findings

The innocent murmur is generally soft (grade 2), midsystolic, short, crescendo-decrescendo, and with a vibratory or musical quality (like fiddle strings). Also, the innocent murmur is heard at the second or third left intercostal space and disappears with sitting, and the young person has no associated signs of cardiac dysfunction.

S_3 and S_4, and the murmur of mitral stenosis are sometimes heard only when on the left side.

Murmur of aortic regurgitation sometimes may be heard only when the patient is leaning forward in the sitting position.

Failure of shunts to close (e.g., patent ductus arteriosus, atrial septal defect); see Table 20.9, p. 533.

Normal Range of Findings

Note any extracardiac signs that may reflect heart status (particularly in the skin), liver size, and respiratory status. The skin colour should be pink to pinkish brown, depending on the infant's genetic heritage. If cyanosis is present, determine its first appearance: at or shortly after birth versus after the neonatal period. Normally, the liver is not enlarged, and the respirations are not laboured. Also, note the expected parameters of weight gain throughout infancy.

Palpate the apical impulse to determine the size and position of the heart. Because the infant's heart has a more horizontal placement, expect to palpate the apical impulse at the fourth intercostal space just lateral to the midclavicular line. It may or may not be visible.

The heart rate is best auscultated because radial pulses are hard to count accurately. Use the small (pediatric size) diaphragm and bell (Fig. 20.25). The heart rate may range from 100 to 180 per minute immediately after birth and then stabilize to an average of 120 to 140 per minute. Infants normally have wide fluctuations with activity, from 170 per minute or more during crying or other activity to 70 to 90 per minute during sleep. Variations are greatest at birth and are even more so with premature babies.

20.25

Expect the heart rhythm to have sinus arrhythmia, the phasic speeding up or slowing down with the respiratory cycle.

Rapid rates make it more challenging to evaluate heart sounds. Expect heart sounds to be louder in infants than in adults because of the infant's thinner chest wall. Also, S_2 has a higher pitch and is sharper than S_1. Splitting of S_2 just after the height of inspiration is common, not at birth, but beginning a few hours after birth.

Abnormal Findings

Cyanosis at or just after birth signals oxygen desaturation of congenital heart disease (Table 20.9, p. 533).

The most important signs of heart failure in an infant are persistent tachycardia, tachypnea, and liver enlargement. Engorged veins, gallop rhythm, and pulsus alternans are additional signs. Respiratory crackles (rales) is an important sign in adults but not in infants.

Failure to thrive occurs with cardiac disease.

The apex is displaced in certain conditions:

- Cardiac enlargement: shifts to the left
- Pneumothorax: shifts away from affected side
- Diaphragmatic hernia: shifts usually to right because this hernia occurs more often on the left
- Dextrocardia: a rare anomaly in which the heart is located on right side of chest

Persistent tachycardia is a heart rate of more than 200 per minute in newborns and more than 150 per minute in older infants.

Bradycardia is a heart rate of less than 90 per minute in newborns and less than 60 in older infants or children. This causes a serious drop in cardiac output because the small muscle mass of their hearts cannot increase stroke volume significantly.

Investigate any irregularity except sinus arrhythmia.

Fixed split S_2 indicates atrial septal defect (see Table 20.5, p. 528).

Objective Data

Normal Range of Findings

Murmurs in the immediate neonatal period do not necessarily indicate congenital heart disease. Murmurs are relatively common in the first 2 to 3 days because of fetal shunt closure. These murmurs are usually grade 1 or 2, are systolic, accompany no other signs of cardiac disease, and disappear in 2 to 3 days. The murmur of patent ductus arteriosus is a continuous machinery-like murmur, which disappears by 2 to 3 days. On the other hand, absence of a murmur in the immediate neonatal period does not ensure that the heart is perfect; congenital defects can be present but not signalled by an early murmur. It is best to listen frequently and to note and describe any murmur according to the characteristics listed on p. 517.

Children

Note any extracardiac or cardiac signs that may indicate heart disease: poor weight gain, developmental delay, persistent tachycardia, tachypnea, DOE, cyanosis, and clubbing. Note that clubbing of fingers and toes usually does not appear until late in the first year, even with severe cyanotic defects.

The apical impulse is sometimes visible in children with thin chest walls. Note any obvious bulge or any heave; these are **not** normal.

Palpate the apical impulse: in the fourth intercostal space to the left of the midclavicular line until age 4 years; at the fourth interspace at the midclavicular line from ages 4 to 6 years; and in the fifth interspace to the right of the midclavicular line at age 7 years (Fig. 20.26).

20.26

The average heart rate slows as the child grows older, although it still varies with rest and activity (see Table 10.2, p. 165).

The heart rhythm remains characterized by sinus arrhythmia. Physiological S_3 is common in children (see Table 20.7, p. 530). It occurs in early diastole, just after S_2, and is a dull, soft sound that is best heard at the apex.

A **venous hum**—which represents turbulence of blood flow in the jugular venous system—is common in healthy children and has no pathological significance. It is a continuous, low-pitched, soft hum that is heard throughout the cycle, although it is loudest in diastole. Listen with the bell over the supraclavicular fossa at the medial third of the clavicle, especially on the right or over the upper anterior chest.

Abnormal Findings

Persistent murmur after 2 to 3 days, holosystolic murmurs or those that last into diastole, and those that are loud all warrant further evaluation.

A precordial bulge to the left of the sternum with a hyperdynamic precordium signals cardiac enlargement. The bulge occurs because the cartilaginous rib cage is more compliant.

A substernal heave occurs with right ventricular enlargement, and an apical heave occurs with left ventricular hypertrophy.

The apical impulse moves laterally with cardiac enlargement.

Thrill (palpable vibration) is abnormal.

Normal Range of Findings

The venous hum is usually not affected by respiration, may sound louder when the child stands, and is easily obliterated by occluding the jugular veins in the neck with your fingers.

Heart murmurs that are innocent (or functional) in origin are very common throughout childhood (often called *Still's murmur*). Results of some studies indicate that they have a 30% occurrence, and others indicate that nearly all children may demonstrate a murmur at some time. Most innocent murmurs have these characteristics: soft, relatively short systolic ejection murmur; medium pitch; vibratory; and best heard at the left lower sternal or midsternal border, with no radiation to the apex, base, or back.

For a child whose murmur has been shown to be innocent, it is very important that the parents understand this completely. They need to believe that this murmur is just a "noise" and has no pathological significance. Otherwise, the parents may become overprotective and limit activity for the child, which may cause the child to develop a negative self-concept.

Pregnant Women

The vital signs usually reveal that the resting pulse rate is increased by 10 to 15 beats per minute and that blood pressure is lower than the normal prepregnancy level. The blood pressure decreases to its lowest point during the second trimester and then slowly rises during the third trimester. The blood pressure varies with position. Usually lowest in left lateral recumbent position, a bit higher in the supine position, and highest in the sitting. Inspection of the skin often reveals a mild hyperemia in light-skinned women because the increased cutaneous blood flow is an attempt to eliminate the excess heat generated by the increased metabolism. Palpation of the apical impulse is higher and lateral than when the heart is in the normal position because the enlarging uterus elevates the diaphragm and displaces the heart up and to the left and rotates it on its long axis.

Auscultation of the heart sounds reveals changes caused by the increased blood volume and workload:
* Heart sounds
  Exaggerated splitting of S^1 and increased loudness of S^1
  A loud, easily heard S^3
* Heart murmurs
  A systolic murmur in 90%, which disappears soon after delivery

A continuous murmur from breast vasculature is termed a **mammary souffle** (pronounced *soof´f'l*). Mammary souffle occurs in 10% of women near term or when the mother is lactating; it is caused by increased blood flow through the internal mammary artery. The murmur is heard in the second, third, or fourth intercostal space; it is continuous, although it is accented in systole. You can obliterate it by pressure with the stethoscope or one finger lateral to the murmur.

The ECG shows no changes except for a slight left axis deviation as a result of the change in the heart's position.

Older Adults

A gradual rise in systolic blood pressure is common in older patients; the diastolic blood pressure stays fairly constant, with a resulting widening of pulse pressure. Some older adults experience **orthostatic hypotension**, a sudden drop in blood pressure when rising to sit or stand.

Use caution in palpating and auscultating the carotid artery. Avoid pressure in the carotid sinus area, which could cause a reflex slowing of the heart rate. Also, pressure on the carotid artery could compromise circulation if the artery is already narrowed by atherosclerosis.

Abnormal Findings

This latter manoeuvre helps differentiate the venous hum from other cardiac murmurs (e.g., that of patent ductus arteriosus).

Distinguish innocent murmurs from pathological ones. This may involve referral to another examiner or the performance of diagnostic tests such as electrocardiography or ultrasonography.

Suspect pregnancy-induced hypertension with a sustained rise of 30 mm Hg systolic or 15 mm Hg diastolic under basal conditions.

Murmurs of aortic valve disease cannot be obliterated.

Objective Data

Normal Range of Findings

The chest often increases in anteroposterior diameter in older patients. This makes it more difficult to palpate the apical impulse and to hear the splitting of S_2. The S_4 often occurs in older people with no known cardiac disease. Systolic murmurs are common, occurring in more than 50% of older adults.

Occasional premature ectopic beats are common and do not necessarily indicate underlying heart disease. When in doubt, obtain an ECG. However, consider that the ECG is a recording of only 1 isolated minute in time and may need to be supplemented by a test of 24-hour ambulatory heart monitoring.

Abnormal Findings

The S_3 is associated with heart failure and is always abnormal when present after 40 years of age (see Table 20.7, p. 530).

SPECIAL CONSIDERATIONS FOR ADVANCED PRACTICE

Normal Range of Findings

Estimate the Jugular Venous Pressure

Think of the jugular veins as a central venous pressure (CVP) manometer attached directly to the right atrium. You can "read" the CVP at the highest level of pulsations. Use the angle of Louis (sternal angle) as an arbitrary reference point, and compare it with the highest level of venous pulsation.

Abnormal Findings

This evaluation is considered by many authorities to be an advanced skill for practitioners in the cardiopulmonary environments in particular.

Elevated pressure is a level of pulsation that is more than 3 cm above the sternal angle while at 45 degrees (see Fig. 20.27, *B*). This occurs with heart failure.

A

Angle of Louis
(sternal angle)

5 cm

RA

2 cm

45 degrees

B   External jugular

20.27   **B**, © Pat Thomas, 2014.

Objective Data

Special Considerations for Advanced Practice

Normal Range of Findings	**Abnormal Findings**

Hold a vertical ruler on the sternal angle. Align a straight edge on the ruler like a T-square, and adjust the level of the horizontal straight edge to the level of pulsation (Fig. 20.27, A). Read the level of intersection on the vertical ruler; normal jugular venous pulsation is 2 cm or less above the sternal angle. Also state the patient's position: for example, "internal jugular vein pulsations 3 cm above sternal angle when elevated 30 degrees."

If you cannot find the internal jugular veins, use the external jugular veins and note the point where they look collapsed. Be aware that the technique of estimating venous pressure is difficult and is not always a reliable predictor of CVP. Consistency in grading among examiners is difficult to achieve.

If venous pressure is elevated, or if you suspect heart failure, perform the **abdominojugular test** (formerly *hepatojugular reflux*) (Fig. 20.28). Position the patient comfortably supine and instruct the patient to breathe quietly through an open mouth. Hold your right hand on the right upper quadrant of the patient's abdomen just below the rib cage. Watch the level of jugular pulsation as you push in with your hand. Exert firm sustained pressure for 30 seconds. This empties venous blood out of the liver sinusoids and adds its volume to the venous system. If the heart is able to pump this additional volume (i.e., if CVP is not elevated), the jugular veins will rise for a few seconds and then recede back to the previous level.

> If heart failure is present, the jugular veins will stay elevated as long as you push.

20.28 Abdominojugular test.

Splitting of S$_2$

When you first hear the split S$_2$, do *not* be tempted to ask the patient to hold the breath so that you can concentrate on the sounds. Breath-holding will only equalize ejection times in the right and left sides of the heart and cause the split to go away. Instead, concentrate on the split as you watch the patient's chest rise up and down with breathing. The split S$_2$ occurs about every fourth heartbeat, fading in with inhalation and fading out with exhalation.

> A **fixed split** is unaffected by respiration; the split is always there.
>
> A **paradoxical split** is the opposite of what you would expect; the sounds fuse on inspiration and split on expiration (see Table 20.5, p. 528).

Focus on Systole, Then on Diastole, and Listen for Any Extra Heart Sounds

Listen with the diaphragm, and then switch to the bell, covering all auscultatory areas (Fig. 20.29). Usually, these are silent periods. When you do detect an extra heart sound, listen carefully to note its timing and characteristics. During systole, the **midsystolic click** (which is associated with mitral valve prolapse) is the most common extra sound (see Table 20.6, p. 528). The third and fourth heart sounds occur in diastole; either may be normal or abnormal (see Table 20.7, pp. 530–531).

> A pathological S$_3$ (ventricular gallop) occurs with heart failure and volume overload; a pathological S$_4$ (atrial gallop) occurs with CAD (see Table 20.7, pp. 530–531, for a full description).

Normal Range of Findings	Abnormal Findings

20.29

DOCUMENTATION AND CRITICAL THINKING

Sample Charting

SUBJECTIVE

No chest pain, dyspnea, orthopnea, cough, fatigue, or edema. No personal history of hypertension, abnormal blood tests, heart murmur, or rheumatic fever. Last ECG 2 years PTA [prior to arrival], result normal. No stress ECG or other heart tests.

Family history: Father with obesity, smoking, and hypertension, treated with diuretic medication. No other family history significant for CVD.

Personal habits: Diet balanced in 4 food groups, 2 to 3 regular coffees/day; no smoking; alcohol, 1 to 2 beers occasionally on weekend; exercise, runs 5 km, 3 to 4 ×/week; no prescription or OTC [over-the-counter] medications or street drugs.

OBJECTIVE

Neck: Carotids 2+ and = bilaterally. Internal jugular vein pulsations present when supine, and disappear when elevated to a 45-degree position.

Precordium: Inspection. No visible pulsations, no heave or lift.

Palpation: Apical impulse in fifth ICS [intercostal space] at left midclavicular line, no thrill.

Auscultation: Rate 68 bpm [beats per minute], rhythm regular, S_1–S_2 are normal, not diminished or accentuated, no S_3, no S_4 or other extra sounds, no murmurs.

ASSESSMENT

Neck vessels healthy by inspection and auscultation
Heart sounds normal

Focused Assessment: Clinical Case Study

Mr. Norm Vernon (N.V.) is a 53-year-old Euro-Canadian male woodcutter admitted to the critical care unit at Toronto General Hospital (TGH) with chest pain.

SUBJECTIVE

1 year PTA: N.V. admitted to TGH with crushing substernal chest pain, radiating to L shoulder, accompanied by nausea, vomiting, diaphoresis.

Diagnosis: MI [myocardial infarction]; hospitalized 7 days, discharged with nitroglycerine prn [as needed] for anginal pain. Did not return to work. Activity included walking 2 km/day, hunting. Had occasional episodes of chest pain with exercise, relieved by rest.

1 day PTA: Had increasing frequency of chest pain, about every 2 hours, lasting few minutes, saw pain as warning to go to doctor.

Day of admission: Severe substernal chest pain ("like someone sitting on my chest") unrelieved by rest. Saw personal doctor; while in office had episode of chest pain same as last year's, accompanied by diaphoresis, no N & V [nausea and vomiting] or shortness of breath, relieved by 1 nitroglycerine. Transferred to TGH by paramedics. No further pain since admission 2 hours ago.

Family hx [history]: Mother died of MI at age 57.

Personal habits: Smokes 1½ pack cigarettes daily × 34 years, no alcohol; diet—trying to limit fat and fried food, still high in added salt.

OBJECTIVE

Extremities: Skin pink, no cyanosis. Upper extrem.: capillary refill sluggish, no clubbing. Lower extrem.: no edema, no hair growth 10 cm below knee bilaterally.

Pulses:

Carotid: 2+

Brachial: 2+

Radial: 2+

Femoral: 2+

Popliteal: 0

P.T. [posterior tibial]: 0

D.P. [dorsalis pedis]: 1+

BP [blood pressure] R [right] arm, 104/66 mm Hg

Neck: External jugular veins flat. Internal jugular pulsations present when supine and absent when elevated to 45 degrees.

Precordium: Inspection. Apical impulse visible fifth ICS, 7 cm left of midsternal line, no heave.

Palpation: Apical impulse palpable in fifth and sixth ICSs. No thrill.

Auscultation: Apical rate, 92 regular; S_1–S_2 are normal, not diminished or accentuated; no S_3 or S_4; grade 3/6 systolic murmur present at left lower sternal border.

ASSESSMENT

Substernal chest pain

Systolic murmur

Ineffective tissue perfusion R/T [related to] interruption in flow

Decreased cardiac output R/T reduction in stroke volume

Documentation and Critical Thinking

ABNORMAL FINDINGS

TABLE 20.2	Clinical Portrait of Heart Failure

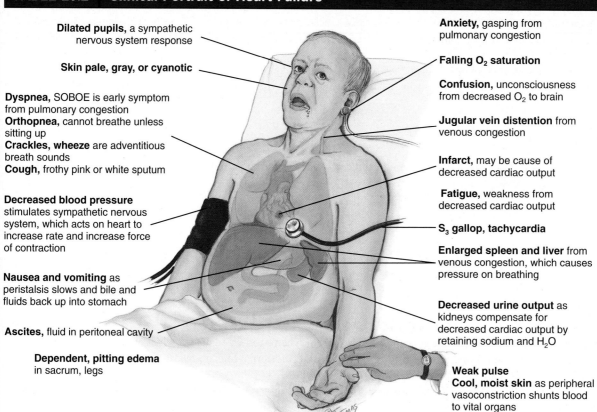

Dilated pupils, a sympathetic nervous system response

Skin pale, gray, or cyanotic

Dyspnea, SOBOE is early symptom from pulmonary congestion
Orthopnea, cannot breathe unless sitting up
Crackles, wheeze are adventitious breath sounds
Cough, frothy pink or white sputum

Decreased blood pressure stimulates sympathetic nervous system, which acts on heart to increase rate and increase force of contraction

Nausea and vomiting as peristalsis slows and bile and fluids back up into stomach

Ascites, fluid in peritoneal cavity

Dependent, pitting edema in sacrum, legs

Anxiety, gasping from pulmonary congestion

Falling O$_2$ saturation

Confusion, unconsciousness from decreased O$_2$ to brain

Jugular vein distention from venous congestion

Infarct, may be cause of decreased cardiac output

Fatigue, weakness from decreased cardiac output

S$_3$ gallop, tachycardia

Enlarged spleen and liver from venous congestion, which causes pressure on breathing

Decreased urine output as kidneys compensate for decreased cardiac output by retaining sodium and H$_2$O

Weak pulse
Cool, moist skin as peripheral vasoconstriction shunts blood to vital organs

Decreased cardiac output occurs when the heart fails as a pump and the circulation becomes backed up and congested.

Signs and symptoms of heart failure come from two basic mechanisms: (a) the heart's inability to pump enough blood to meet the metabolic demands of the body and (b) the kidney's compensatory mechanisms of abnormal retention of sodium and water to compensate for the decreased cardiac output. This increases blood volume and venous return, which causes further congestion.

Onset of heart failure may be (a) *acute*, as after a myocardial infarction, when direct damage to the heart's contracting ability has occurred, or (b) *chronic*, as with hypertension, when the ventricles must pump against chronically increased pressure.

In illustration: *CO,* Cardiac output; *SOBOE,* shortness of breath on exertion.

TABLE 20.3	Variations in S$_1$

The intensity of S$_1$ depends on three factors: (a) position of AV valve at the start of systole, (b) structure of the valve leaflets, and (c) how quickly pressure rises in the ventricle.

Variation	Factor	Examples
Loud (Accentuated) S$_1$ S$_1$ S$_2$	1. Position of AV valve at start of systole: wide open and no time for leaflets to drift together. 2. Change in valve structure: calcification of valve, increasing ventricular pressure needed to close the valve against increased atrial pressure.	Hyperkinetic states in which blood velocity is increased: exercise, fever, anemia, hyperthyroidism Mitral stenosis with leaflets still mobile

TABLE 20.3	Variations in S₁—cont'd	

Faint (Diminished) S₁

S₁   S₂

1. Position of AV valve: delayed conduction from atria to ventricles. Mitral valve drifts shut before ventricular contraction closes it.
2. Change in valve structure: extreme calcification, which limits mobility.
3. More forceful atrial contraction into noncompliant ventricle; delays or diminishes ventricular contraction.

First-degree heart block (prolonged PR interval)

Mitral insufficiency

Severe hypertension: systemic or pulmonary

Varying Intensity of S₁

S₁   S₂   S₁   S₂

1. Position of AV valve varies before closing from beat to beat.
2. Atria and ventricles beat independently.

Atrial fibrillation: irregularly irregular rhythm

Complete heart block with changing PR interval

Split S₁

S₁   S₂

T
M

Mitral and tricuspid components are heard separately.

Normal but uncommon

AV, Atrioventricular.

TABLE 20.4	Variations in S₂	
	Condition	**Example**
Accentuated S₂ S₁ S₂	1. Higher closing pressure 2. Increased pressure in aorta 3. Pulmonary hypertension 4. Semilunar valves calcified but still mobile	Systemic hypertension, ringing or booming S₂ Exercise and excitement Mitral stenosis, heart failure Aortic or pulmonic stenosis
Diminished S₂ S₁ S₂	1. Decrease in valve strength, caused by a fall in systemic blood pressure 2. Semilunar valves thickened and calcified, with decreased mobility	Shock Aortic or pulmonic stenosis

TABLE 20.5   Variations in Split S₂

Variation	Condition	Example
Normal Splitting		
Fixed Split	A fixed split is unaffected by respiration; the split is always there.	Atrial septal defect Right ventricular failure
Paradoxical Split	Conditions that delay aortic valve closure cause the opposite of a normal split. In inspiration, P₂ is normally delayed, so with a paradoxical split, the sounds fuse. In expiration you hear the split, in the order of P₂A₂.	Aortic stenosis Left bundle branch block Patent ductus arteriosus
Wide Split	When the right ventricle has delayed electrical activation, the split is very wide on inspiration and is still there on expiration.	Right bundle branch block (which delays P₂)

Normal Splitting

EXPIRATION — S₁   S₂   A₂-P₂

INSPIRATION — S₁   S₂   A₂ P₂

Fixed Split

EXPIRATION — S₁   S₂   A₂ P₂

INSPIRATION — S₁   S₂   A₂ P₂

Paradoxical Split

EXPIRATION — S₁   S₂   P₂ A₂

INSPIRATION — S₁   S₂

Wide Split

EXPIRATION — S₁   S₂   M T   A₂ P₂

INSPIRATION — S₁   S₂   A₂ P₂

TABLE 20.6   Systolic Extra Sounds

Early systolic:
  Ejection click
  Aortic prosthetic valve sounds

Mid-/late systolic:
  Midsystolic (mitral) click

Early Systolic

Aortic ejection click
(apex and base)

EXPIRATION — S₁   S₂   Eⱼ

INSPIRATION — S₁   S₂   Eⱼ

TABLE 20.6   Systolic Extra Sounds—cont'd

Pulmonic ejection click (base only)

Ejection Click

The ejection click occurs early in systole at the start of ejection because it results from opening of the semilunar valves. Normally, the semilunar valves open silently, but in the presence of stenosis (e.g., aortic stenosis, pulmonic stenosis), their opening makes a sound. It is short and high pitched, with a click quality, and is heard better with the diaphragm of the stethoscope.

The aortic ejection click is heard at the second right interspace and apex and may be loudest at the apex. Its intensity does not change with respiration. The pulmonic ejection click is best heard in the second left interspace and often grows softer with inspiration.

"Ball-in-cage"
AO = aortic opens
AC = aortic closes

Aortic Prosthetic Valve Sounds*

As a sequela of modern technological intervention for heart problems, some people now have *iatrogenically* induced heart sounds. The opening of an aortic ball-in-cage prosthesis (e.g., Starr–Edwards prosthesis) produces an early systolic sound. This sound is less intense with a tilting disc prosthesis (e.g., Bjork–Shiley prosthesis) and is absent with a tissue prosthesis (e.g., porcine).

Mid-/Late Systolic

Apex
C = click

Midsystolic (Mitral) Click

Although it is systolic, this is not an ejection click. It is associated with *mitral valve prolapse*, in which the mitral valve leaflets not only close with contraction but balloon back up into the left atrium. During ballooning, the sudden tensing of the valve leaflets and the chordae tendineae creates the click.

The sound occurs in mid- to late systole and is short and high pitched, with a click quality. It is best heard with the diaphragm of the stethoscope at the apex, but it also may be heard at the left lower sternal border. The click usually is followed by a systolic murmur. The click and murmur move with postural change; when the patient assumes a squatting position, the click may sound sooner after S_2, and the murmur may sound louder and delayed. The Valsalva manoeuvre also moves the click sooner after S_2.

*In illustration: *SEM,* Soft ejection murmur.

TABLE 20.7 Diastolic Extra Sounds

Early diastole:	Mid-diastole:	Late diastole:
Opening snap	Third heart sound	Fourth heart sound
Mitral prosthetic valve sound	Summation sound ($S_3 + S_4$)	Pacemaker-induced sound

Early Diastole

Opening Snap

Normally the opening of the AV valves is silent. In the presence of stenosis, increasingly higher atrial pressure is needed to open the valve. The deformed valve opens with a noise: the opening snap. It is sharp and high pitched, with a snapping quality. It sounds after S_2 and is best heard with the diaphragm of the stethoscope at the third or fourth left interspace at the sternal border; it is less well heard at the apex.

The OS usually is not an isolated sound. As a sign of mitral stenosis, the opening snap usually ushers in the low-pitched diastolic rumbling murmur of that condition.

Mitral Prosthetic Valve Sound*

An iatrogenic sound, the opening of a ball-in-cage mitral prosthesis produces an early diastolic sound: an opening click just after S_2. It is loud, is heard over the whole precordium, and is loudest at the apex and left lower sternal border.

Mid-Diastole

Third Heart Sound

The S_3 is a ventricular filling sound. It occurs in early diastole during the rapid filling phase. Your hearing quickly accommodates to the S_3, so it is best heard when you listen initially. It sounds after S_2 but later than an opening snap would be. It is a dull, soft sound, and it is low pitched, like "distant thunder." It is heard best in a quiet room, at the apex, with the bell of the stethoscope held lightly (just enough to form a seal), and with the patient in the left lateral position.

The S_3 can be confused with a split S_2. Use these guidelines to distinguish the S_3:

- *Location:* The S_3 is heard at the apex or left lower sternal border; the split S_2 is heard at the base.
- *Respiratory variation:* The S_3 does not vary in timing with respirations; the split S_2 does.
- *Pitch:* The S_3 is lower pitched; the pitch of the split S_2 stays the same.

The S_3 may be normal (physiological) or abnormal (pathological). The *physiological* S_3 is heard frequently in children and young adults; it occasionally persists after age 40 years, especially in women. The normal S_3 usually disappears when the patient sits up.

In adults, the S_3 is usually abnormal. The *pathological* S_3 is also called a *ventricular gallop* or an S_3 *gallop*, and it persists when the patient is sitting up. The S_3 indicates decreased compliance of the ventricles, as in heart failure. The S_3 may be the earliest sign of heart failure. The S_3 may originate from either the left or the right ventricle; a left-sided S_3 is heard at the apex in the left lateral position, and a right-sided S_3 is heard at the left lower sternal border with the patient supine and is louder on inspiration.

TABLE 20.7	Diastolic Extra Sounds—cont'd

The S₃ occurs also with conditions of volume overload, such as mitral regurgitation and aortic or tricuspid regurgitation. The S₃ is also found in states of high cardiac output in the absence of heart disease, such as hyperthyroidism, anemia, and pregnancy. When the primary condition is corrected, the gallop disappears.

Summation Sound (S₃ + S₄)

When both the pathological S₃ and S₄ are present, a quadruple rhythm is heard. Often, in cases of cardiac stress, one response is tachycardia. During rapid rates, the diastolic filling time shortens, and the S₃ and S₄ move closer together. They sound superimposed in mid-diastole, and you hear one loud, prolonged, summated sound, often louder than either S₁ or S₂.

Late Diastole

Fourth Heart Sound

The S₄ is a ventricular filling sound. It occurs when the atria contract late in diastole. It is heard immediately before S₁. This is a very soft sound, of very low pitch. You need a good bell, and you must listen for it. It is heard best at the apex, with the patient in left lateral position.

A *physiological* S₄ may occur in adults older than 40 or 50 years of age with no evidence of cardiovascular disease, especially after exercise.

A *pathological* S₄ is termed an atrial gallop or an S₄ *gallop*. It occurs with decreased compliance of the ventricle (e.g., coronary artery disease, cardiomyopathy) and with systolic overload (afterload), including outflow obstruction to the ventricle (aortic stenosis) and systemic hypertension. A left-sided S₄ occurs with these conditions. It is heard best at the apex, in the left lateral position.

A right-sided S₄ is less common. It is heard at the left lower sternal border and may increase with inspiration. It occurs with pulmonary stenosis or pulmonary hypertension.

Extracardiac Sounds

Pericardial Friction Rub

Inflammation of the precordium gives rise to a friction rub. The sound is high pitched and scratchy, like sandpaper being rubbed. It is best heard with the diaphragm of the stethoscope, with the patient sitting up and leaning forward, and with the breath held in expiration.

A friction rub can be heard any place on the precordium but usually is best heard at the apex and left lower sternal border, places where the pericardium comes in close contact with the chest wall. Timing may be systolic and diastolic. The friction rub of pericarditis is common during the first week after a myocardial infarction and may last only a few hours.

AV, Atrioventricular.
*In illustrations: *OS,* Opening snap; *SEM,* Soft ejection murmur.

TABLE 20.8   Abnormal Pulsations on the Precordium

Base

A *thrill* in the second and third right interspaces occurs with severe aortic stenosis and systemic hypertension.

A *thrill* in the second and third left interspaces occurs with pulmonic stenosis and pulmonic hypertension.

Left Sternal Border

A *lift (heave)* occurs with right ventricular hypertrophy, as found in pulmonic valve disease, pulmonic hypertension, and chronic lung disease. You feel a diffuse lifting impulse during systole at the left lower sternal border. It may be associated with retraction at the apex because the left ventricle is rotated posteriorly by the enlarged right ventricle.

Apex

Cardiac enlargement displaces the apical impulse laterally and over a wider area when left ventricular hypertrophy and dilatation are present. This is *volume overload*, which occurs in mitral regurgitation, aortic regurgitation, and left-to-right shunts.

Apex

The apical impulse is increased in force and duration but is not necessarily displaced to the left when left ventricular hypertrophy occurs alone without dilatation. This is *pressure overload*, which occurs in aortic stenosis or systemic hypertension.

Images © Pat Thomas, 2006.

TABLE 20.9 Congenital Heart Defects

Condition	Description	Clinical Data

Patent Ductus Arteriosus (PDA)

Persistence of the channel joining left pulmonary artery to aorta. This is normal in the fetus and usually closes spontaneously within hours of birth.

S: Usually no symptoms in early childhood; growth and development are normal.

O: Blood pressure has wide pulse pressure and bounding peripheral pulses from rapid runoff of blood into low-resistance pulmonary bed during diastole. Thrill often palpable at left upper sternal border. The continuous murmur heard in systole and diastole is called a *machinery murmur*.

Atrial Septal Defect (ASD)

Abnormal opening in the atrial septum, resulting usually in left-to-right shunting of blood and causing a large increase in pulmonary blood flow.

S: Defect is remarkably well tolerated. Symptoms in infants are rare; growth and development are normal. Affected children and young adults have mild fatigue and DOE.

O: Sternal lift often present. S_2 has fixed split, with P_2 often louder than A_2. Murmur is systolic ejection, medium pitch, best heard at base in second left interspace. Murmur caused not by shunting itself but by increased blood flow through pulmonic valve.

Ventricular Septal Defect (VSD)

Abnormal opening in septum between the ventricles, usually in subaortic area. The size and exact position vary considerably.

S: Small defects are asymptomatic. Infants with large defects have poor growth, slow weight gain; later look pale, thin, and delicate. Affected infants may have feeding problems; DOE; frequent respiratory infections; and, when the condition is severe, heart failure.

O: Loud, harsh holosystolic murmur, best heard at left lower sternal border, may be accompanied by thrill. Large defects also produce soft diastolic murmur at apex (mitral flow murmur) as a result of increased blood flow through mitral valve.

Continued

TABLE 20.9	Congenital Heart Defects—cont'd	
Condition	Description	Clinical Data
Tetralogy of Fallot 	Four components: (a) right ventricular outflow stenosis, (b) VSD, (c) right ventricular hypertrophy, and (d) overriding aorta. The result is a large amount of venous blood shunted directly into aorta away from pulmonary system, so that blood is never oxygenated.	S: Severe cyanosis, not in first months of life but developing as infant grows and RV outflow (i.e., pulmonic) stenosis gets worse. Cyanosis initially with crying and exertion, then at rest. Affected child uses squatting posture after starts walking. DOE common. Growth and development are slowed. O: Thrill is palpable at left lower sternal border. S_1 is normal; in S_2, A_2 is loud and P_2 is diminished or absent. Murmur is systolic, loud, crescendo–decrescendo.
Coarctation of the Aorta 	Severe narrowing of descending aorta, usually at the junction of the ductus arteriosus and the aortic arch, just distal to the origin of the left subclavian artery. Results in increased workload on left ventricle. Associated with defects of aortic valve in most cases, as well as associated patent ductus arteriosus and associated VSD.	S: In infants with associated lesions or symptoms, diagnosis occurs in first few months as symptoms of heart failure develop. For affected children and adolescents without symptoms, growth and development are normal. Diagnosis is usually incidental, as a result of blood pressure findings. Adolescents may complain of vague lower extremity cramping that is worse with exercise. O: Upper extremity hypertension, with readings 20 mm Hg higher than those of lower extremity, is a hallmark of coarctation. Another important sign is absence of or greatly diminished femoral pulses. A systolic murmur is heard best at the left sternal border, radiating to the back.

DOE, Dyspnea on exertion; *O,* objective data; *RV,* right ventricular; *S,* subjective data.
Images © Pat Thomas, 2006.

TABLE 20.10	Murmurs Caused by Valvular Defects

Midsystolic Ejection Murmurs

Caused by forward flow through semilunar valves. Examples below have the murmur pictured here:

SYSTOLE   DIASTOLE

S1   S2   S1   S2   S1   S2

TABLE 20.10	Murmurs Caused by Valvular Defects—cont'd	
Type of Defect	**Description**	**Clinical Data**
Aortic Stenosis	Calcification of aortic valve cusps restricts forward flow of blood during systole; hypertrophy of LV develops.	S: Fatigue, DOE, palpitation, dizziness, fainting, and anginal pain are present. O: Pallor, slow diminished radial pulse, low blood pressure, and auscultatory gap are common. Apical impulse is sustained and displaced to left. Thrill occurs in systole over second and third right interspaces and right side of neck. S_1 is normal; ejection click is often present, paradoxical split S_2 is often present, and S_4 is present with hypertrophy of LV. Murmur is loud, harsh, midsystolic, crescendo–decrescendo, and loudest at second right interspace; it radiates widely to side of neck, down left sternal border, or to apex.
Pulmonic Stenosis	Calcification of pulmonic valve restricts forward flow of blood.	O: Thrill occurs in systole at second and third left interspace, ejection click is often present after S_1, S_2 is diminished and usually with wide split, and S_4 is common with hypertrophy of RV. Murmur is systolic, medium pitch, coarse, crescendo–decrescendo (diamond shape), and best heard at second left interspace, and it radiates to left and neck.

Pansystolic Regurgitant Murmurs

Caused by backward flow from area of higher pressure to one of lower pressure. Examples below have the murmur pictured here:

SYSTOLE DIASTOLE

S1 S2   S1 S2   S1 S2

Type of Defect	**Description**	**Clinical Data**
Mitral Regurgitation	Stream of blood regurgitates back into LA during systole through incompetent mitral valve. In diastole, blood passes back into LV again along with new flow; results in dilatation and hypertrophy of LV.	S: Fatigue, palpitation, orthopnea, and PND are common. O: Thrill occurs in systole at apex. Lift occurs at apex. Apical impulse is displaced down and to left. S_1 is diminished, S_2 is accentuated, S_3 at apex is often present. Murmur is pansystolic, often loud, blowing, and best heard at apex, and it radiates well to left axilla.

Continued

TABLE 20.10   Murmurs Caused by Valvular Defects—cont'd

Tricuspid Regurgitation

Backflow of blood through incompetent tricuspid valve into RA.

O: Neck veins are engorged and pulsating; liver is enlarged. Lift occurs at sternum if RV is hypertrophied; a thrill is often present at left lower sternal border.

Murmur is soft, blowing, pansystolic, and best heard at left lower sternal border, and it increases with inspiration.

Diastolic Rumbles of AV Valves

Filling murmurs at low pressures, best heard with bell of stethoscope lightly touching skin. Examples below have the murmur pictured here:

SYSTOLE   DIASTOLE

OS   OS   OS

S1   S2   S1   S2   S1   S2

Type of Defect	Description	Clinical Data
Mitral Stenosis	Calcified mitral valve does not open properly, impedes forward flow of blood into LV during diastole. Results in enlargement of LA and increasing pressure in LA.	S: Fatigue, palpitations, DOE, orthopnea are common; PND or pulmonary edema occasionally occur. O: Arterial pulse is diminished and often irregular. Lift occurs at apex; diastolic thrill is common at apex. S_1 is accentuated; opening snap after S_2 is heard over wide area of precordium, followed by murmur. Murmur is a low-pitched diastolic rumble, best heard at apex with patient in left lateral position; it does not radiate.
Tricuspid Stenosis	Calcification of tricuspid valve impedes forward flow into RV during diastole.	O: Arterial pulse is diminished; jugular venous pulse is prominent. Murmur is a diastolic rumble; it is best heard at left lower sternal border and is louder in inspiration.

TABLE 20.10 Murmurs Caused by Valvular Defects—cont'd

Early Diastolic Murmurs

Caused by semilunar valve incompetence. Examples below have the murmur pictured here:

SYSTOLE   DIASTOLE

S1   S2   S1   S2   S1   S2

Type of Defect	Description	Clinical Data
Aortic Regurgitation	Stream of blood regurgitates back through incompetent aortic valve into LV during diastole. Dilatation and hypertrophy of LV are caused by increased stroke volume of LV. Large stroke volume is ejected rapidly into poorly filled aorta; then rapid runoff occurs in diastole as part of blood is pushed back into LV.	S: Affected patients have only minor symptoms for many years and then rapid deterioration: DOE, PND, angina, dizziness. O: Bounding "water-hammer" pulse is present in carotid, brachial, and femoral arteries. Blood pressure has wide pulse pressure. Pulsations are palpable in cervical and suprasternal areas; apical impulse is displaced to left and down and feels brief. Murmur starts almost simultaneously with S_2: It is soft, high-pitched, blowing diastolic, and decrescendo, best heard at third left interspace at base; as patient sits up and leans forward, murmur radiates down.
Pulmonic Regurgitation	Blood flows backward through incompetent pulmonic valve, from pulmonary artery to RV.	Murmur has same timing and characteristics as that of aortic regurgitation, and the two are hard to distinguish on physical examination.

AV, Atrioventricular; *DOE,* dyspnea on exertion; *LA,* left atrium; *LV,* left ventricle; *O,* objective data; *PND,* paroxysmal nocturnal dyspnea; *RA,* right atrium; *RV,* right ventricle; *S,* subjective data.
Images © Pat Thomas, 2006.

Abnormal Findings

Summary Checklist: Heart and Neck Vessels Examination

Neck
1. **Carotid pulse:** observe and palpate
2. **Jugular venous pulse:** observe
3. **Jugular venous pressure:** estimate

Precordium
1. **Inspect and palpate:**
   Describe location of apical impulse; note any heave (lift) or thrill
2. **Auscultate:**
   Identify anatomical areas where you listen

Note rate and rhythm of heartbeat

Identify S_1 and S_2, and note any variation

Listen in systole and diastole for any extra heart sounds

Listen in systole and diastole for any murmurs

Repeat sequence with bell of stethoscope

Listen at apex with patient in left lateral position

Listen at base with patient in sitting position

3. **Engage in teaching and health promotion**

REFERENCES

1. Simmons, A., & Steffen, K. (2011). Peripheral arterial disease in women. *Reviews in Cardiovascular Medicine, 12*(3), 123–131.
2. Mann, D., Zipes, D., Libby, P., et al. (2014). *Braunwald's heart disease: A textbook of cardiovascular medicine* (10th ed.). Philadelphia: Saunders.
3. Statistics Canada. (2015). *High blood pressure, 2014.* Retrieved from http://www.statcan.gc.ca/pub/82-625-x/2015001/article/14184-eng.htm.
4. Public Health Agency of Canada. (2016). *Health status of Canadians 2016.* Ottawa: Her Majesty the Queen in Right of Canada as represented by the Minister of Health. Retrieved from http://healthycanadians.gc.ca/publications/department-ministere/state-public-health-status-2016-etat-sante-publique-statut/alt/pdf-eng.pdf.
5. Public Health Agency of Canada. (2016). *Chronic disease and injury indicator framework. 2016 edition.* Retrieved from http://www.phac-aspc.gc.ca/publicat/hpcdp-pspmc/36-8/assets/pdf/ar-04-eng.pdf.
6. First Nations Information Governance Centre. (2012). *First Nations Regional Health Survey (RHS) 2008/10: National report on adults, youth and children living in First Nations communities.* Ottawa: Author.
7. Government of Canada. (2017). *Heart disease in Canada: Highlights from the Canadian Chronic Disease Surveillance System.* Retrieved from https://www.canada.ca/en/public-health/services/publications/diseases-conditions/heart-disease-canada-fact-sheet.html.
8. Heart and Stroke Foundation of Canada. (2017). *Ms. Understood.* Retrieved from http://www.heartandstroke.ca/-/media/pdf-files/canada/2018-heart-month/hs_2018-heart-report_en.ashx?la=en&hash=3BBC7F1DD1DA3EDC6B2B0E9BB31E855268C051EB.
9. Government of Canada. (2018). *Surveillance of heart diseases and conditions.* Retrieved from https://www.canada.ca/en/public-health/services/diseases/heart-health/heart-diseases-conditions/surveillance-heart-diseases-conditions.html.
10. Statistics Canada. (2018). *Leading causes of death, by sex.* Retrieved from http://www.statcan.gc.ca/tables-tableaux/sum-som/l01/cst01/hlth36a-eng.htm.
11. Fairholm, J. (1999). *Urban agriculture and food security initiatives in Canada: A survey of Canadian non-governmental organizations.* Ottawa: International Development Research Centre.
12. Public Health Agency of Canada. (2010). *Prevalence: Report from the Canadian Chronic Disease Surveillance System: Hypertension in Canada, 2010.* Retrieved from https://www.canada.ca/en/public-health/services/chronic-diseases/cardiovascular-disease/report-canadian-chronic-disease-surveillance-system-hypertension-canada-2010/adults-with-diagnosed-hypertension.html.
13. Statistics Canada. (2016). *High blood pressure, by sex, and by province and territory.* http://www.statcan.gc.ca/tables-tableaux/sum-som/l01/cst01/health70a-eng.htm.
14. Government of Canada. (2015). *Canadian Tobacco Use Monitoring Survey (CTUMS) 2012.* Retrieved from https://www.canada.ca/en/health-canada/services/publications/healthy-living/canadian-tobacco-use-monitoring-survey-ctums-2012.html.
15. Statistics Canada. (2016). *Smoking, 2016.* Retrieved from https://www150.statcan.gc.ca/n1/pub/82-625-x/2017001/article/54864-eng.htm.
16. Statistics Canada. (2015). *Overweight and obese adults (self-reported), 2014.* Retrieved from https://www.statcan.gc.ca/pub/82-625-x/2015001/article/14185-eng.htm.
17. Government of Canada. (n.d.). *Curbing childhood obesity: A federal, provincial and territorial framework for action to promote healthy weights.* Retrieved from https://www.canada.ca/content/dam/phac-aspc/migration/phac-aspc/hp-ps/hl-mvs/framework-cadre/pdf/ccofw-eng.pdf.
18. Doucet, G., & Beatty, M. (2010). The cost of diabetes in Canada: The economic tsunami. *Canadian Journal of Diabetes, 34*(1), 27–29.
19. Diabetes Canada. (2018). *Diabetes statistics in Canada.* Retrieved from http://www.diabetes.ca/how-you-can-help/advocate/why-federal-leadership-is-essential/diabetes-statistics-in-canada.
20. Rosella, I. C., Lebenbaum, M., Fitzpatrick, T., et al. (2015). Impact of diabetes on healthcare costs in a population-based cohort: A cost analysis. *Diabetic Medicine: A Journal of the British Diabetic Association, 33*(3), 395–403. doi:10.1111/dme.12858.

CHAPTER 21

Peripheral Vascular System and Lymphatic System

Written by Carolyn Jarvis, PhD, APN, CNP
Adapted by June MacDonald-Jenkins, RN, BScN, MSc

http://evolve.elsevier.com/Canada/Jarvis/examination/

STRUCTURE AND FUNCTION

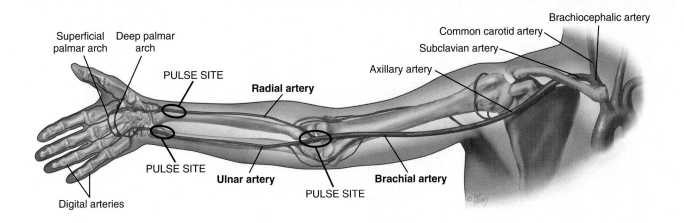

21.1 Arteries in the arm. (© Pat Thomas, 2010.)

The vascular system consists of the vessels of the body. Vessels are tubes for transporting fluid, such as the blood or lymph. Any disease in the vascular system creates problems with delivery of oxygen and nutrients to the tissues or with elimination of waste products from cellular metabolism.

ARTERIES

The heart pumps freshly oxygenated blood through the arteries to all body tissues (Fig. 21.1). The pumping of the heart makes this a high-pressure system. The artery walls are strong, tough, and tense to withstand pressure demands. Arteries contain elastic fibres, which allow their walls to stretch with systole and recoil with diastole. Arteries also contain muscle fibres (vascular smooth muscle), which control the amount of blood delivered to the tissues. The vascular smooth muscle contracts and dilates, which changes the diameter of the arteries to control the rate of blood flow.

Each heartbeat creates a pressure wave, which makes the arteries expand and then recoil. It is the recoil that propels blood through like a wave. All arteries have this pressure

wave, or **pulse**, throughout their length, but you can feel it only at body sites where the artery lies close to the skin and over a bone. The arteries described in the following sections are accessible to examination.

Temporal Artery

The temporal artery is palpated in front of the ear, as discussed in Chapter 14.

Carotid Artery

The carotid artery is palpated in the groove between the sternomastoid muscle and the trachea and is discussed in Chapter 20 in the section on great vessels.

Arteries in the Arm

The major artery supplying the arm is the **brachial artery**, which runs in the biceps–triceps furrow of the upper arm and surfaces at the antecubital fossa in the elbow medial to the biceps tendon (see Fig. 21.1). Immediately below the elbow, the brachial artery bifurcates into the **ulnar** and **radial arteries**. These run distally and form two arches

539

supplying the hand; these are called the *superficial* and *deep palmar arches*. The radial pulse can be palpated just medial to the radius at the wrist; the ulnar artery is located in the same relation to the ulna, but it is deeper and often difficult to feel.

Arteries in the Leg

The major artery in the leg is the **femoral artery**, which passes under the inguinal ligament (Fig. 21.2). The femoral artery travels down the thigh. At the lower thigh, it courses posteriorly; then it is termed the **popliteal artery**. Below the knee, the popliteal artery divides. The anterior tibial artery travels down the front of the leg on to the dorsum of the foot, where it becomes the **dorsalis pedis**. In back of the leg, the **posterior tibial artery** travels down behind the medial malleolus and forms the **plantar arteries** in the foot.

21.2 Arteries in the leg. (© Pat Thomas, 2010.)

The function of the arteries is to supply oxygen and essential nutrients to the tissues. **Ischemia** is a deficient supply of oxygenated arterial blood to a tissue, caused by obstruction of a blood vessel. A complete blockage leads to death of the distal tissue. A partial blockage causes the supply to be insufficient, and the ischemia may be apparent only during exercise, when oxygen needs increase. **Peripheral artery disease (PAD)** affects noncoronary arteries and usually refers to arteries supplying the limbs. It usually is caused by atherosclerosis, and less commonly by embolism, hypercoagulable states, or arterial dissection.

VEINS

The course of veins parallels that of arteries, but the body has more veins, and they lie closer to the skin surface. The following veins are accessible to examination.

Jugular Veins

Assessment of the jugular veins is described in Chapter 20.

Veins in the Arm

Each arm has two sets of veins: superficial and deep. The superficial veins are in the subcutaneous tissue and are responsible for most of the venous return.

Veins in the Leg

The legs have three types of veins (Fig. 21.3):
1. The **deep veins** run alongside the deep arteries and conduct most of the venous return from the legs. These are the **femoral** and **popliteal veins**. As long as these veins remain intact, the superficial veins can be excised without harming the circulation.
2. The **superficial veins** are the **great** and **small saphenous veins**. The great saphenous vein, inside the leg, starts at the medial side of the dorsum of the foot. You can see it ascend in front of the medial malleolus; then it crosses the tibia obliquely and ascends along the medial side of the thigh. The small saphenous vein, in the outer portion of the leg, starts on the lateral side of the dorsum of the foot and ascends behind the lateral malleolus and up the back of the leg, where it joins the popliteal vein. Blood flows from the superficial veins into the deep leg veins.
3. **Perforators** (not illustrated) are connecting veins that join the two sets. They also have one-way valves that route blood from the superficial veins into the deep veins and prevent reflux into the superficial veins.

VENOUS FLOW

Veins drain the deoxygenated blood and its waste products from the tissues and return it to the heart. Unlike the arteries, veins are a low-pressure system. Because veins do not have a pump to generate their blood flow, the veins need a mechanism to keep blood moving (Fig. 21.4). This movement is accomplished by (a) the contracting skeletal muscles that milk the blood proximally, back toward the heart; (b)

Inferior vena cava

Common iliac vein

External iliac vein

Great saphenous vein

Femoral vein

Popliteal vein

Small saphenous vein

Anterior tibial vein

Great saphenous vein

Dorsal venous arch

21.3 Veins in the leg. (© Pat Thomas, 2010.)

the pressure gradient caused by breathing, in which inspiration makes the thoracic pressure decrease and the abdominal pressure increase; and (c) the intraluminal valves, which ensure unidirectional flow. Each valve is a paired semilunar pocket that opens toward the heart and closes tightly when filled to prevent backflow of blood.

In the legs, this mechanism is called the *calf pump*, or "peripheral heart." During walking, the calf muscles alternately contract (systole) and relax (diastole). In the contraction phase, the gastrocnemius and soleus muscles squeeze the veins and direct the blood flow proximally. Because of the valves, venous blood flows just one way: toward the heart.

Besides the presence of intraluminal valves, venous structure differs from arterial structure. Because venous pressure is lower, walls of the veins are thinner than those of the arteries. Veins have a larger diameter and are more distensible; they can expand and hold more blood when blood

volume increases. This is a compensatory mechanism to reduce stress on the heart. Because of this ability to stretch, veins are called **capacitance vessels**.

Efficient venous return is dependent on contracting skeletal muscles, competent valves in the veins, and a patent lumen. Problems with any of these three elements lead to venous stasis. The risk for venous disease is increased by prolonged standing, sitting, or bed rest because of the absence of the milking action that walking accomplishes. Hypercoagulable states and vein wall trauma are other factors that increase risk for venous disease. Also, dilated and tortuous (varicose) veins have **incompetent valves**, wherein the lumen is so wide the valve cusps cannot approximate. This condition increases venous pressure, which further dilates the vein. Some people have a genetic predisposition to varicose veins, but venous pooling also occurs in obesity and following multiple pregnancies.

LYMPHATICS

The lymphatics form a completely separate vessel system, which retrieves excess fluid from the tissue spaces and returns it to the bloodstream (Fig. 21.5). During circulation of the blood, somewhat more fluid leaves the capillaries than the veins can absorb. Without lymphatic drainage, fluid would build up in the interstitial spaces and produce edema.

The lymphatic vessels converge and drain into two main trunks, which empty into the venous system at the subclavian veins (see Fig. 21.5):

1. The **right lymphatic duct** empties into the right subclavian vein. It drains the right side of the head and neck, right arm, right side of thorax, right lung and pleura, right side of the heart, and right upper section of the liver.

2. The **thoracic duct** drains the rest of the body. It empties into the left subclavian vein.

The functions of the lymphatic system are (a) to conserve fluid and plasma proteins that leak out of the capillaries, (b) to form a major part of the immune system that defends the body against disease, and (c) to absorb lipids from the intestinal tract.

The immune system is a complicated network of organs and cells that work together to protect the body. It detects and eliminates foreign pathogens, both those that come in from the environment and those arising from inside (abnormal or mutant cells). It accomplishes this by phagocytosis (digestion) of the substances by neutrophils and by monocytes or macrophages, as well as by production of specific antibodies or specific immune responses by the lymphocytes.

The lymphatic vessels have a unique structure. Lymphatic capillaries start as microscopic open-ended tubes, which siphon interstitial fluid. The capillaries converge to form small vessels. The small vessels, like veins, drain into larger ones. The vessels have valves, and so flow is in one direction from the tissue spaces into the bloodstream. The many valves make the vessels look beaded. The flow of lymph is slower than that of the blood. Lymph flow is propelled by

② Inspiration: ⬇Thoracic pressure ⬆Abdominal pressure

① Skeletal muscle pressure

③ Intraluminal valves

Open   Closed

MECHANISMS OF VENOUS FLOW

21.4   © Pat Thomas, 2006.

contracting skeletal muscles, by pressure changes secondary to breathing, and by contraction of the vessel walls themselves.

Lymph nodes are small oval clumps of lymphatic tissue located at intervals along the vessels. Most nodes are arranged in groups, both deep and superficial, in the body. Nodes filter the fluid before it is returned to the bloodstream and filter out micro-organisms that could be harmful to the body. The pathogens are exposed to lymphocytes in the lymph nodes. The lymphocytes mount an antigen-specific response to eliminate the pathogens. When local inflammation occurs, the nodes in that area become swollen and tender.

The superficial groups of nodes are accessible to inspection and palpation and give clues to the status of the lymphatic system:

- **Cervical nodes** drain the head and neck. They are described in Chapter 14.
- **Axillary nodes** drain the breast and upper arm. They are described in Chapter 18.
- The **epitrochlear node** is in the antecubital fossa and drains the hand and lower arm.
- The **inguinal nodes** in the groin drain most of the lymph of the lower extremity, the external genitalia, and the anterior abdominal wall.

Related Organs

The spleen, tonsils, and thymus gland aid the lymphatic system (Fig. 21.6). The **spleen** is located in the left upper quadrant of the abdomen. It has four functions: (a) to destroy old red blood cells, (b) to produce antibodies, (c) to

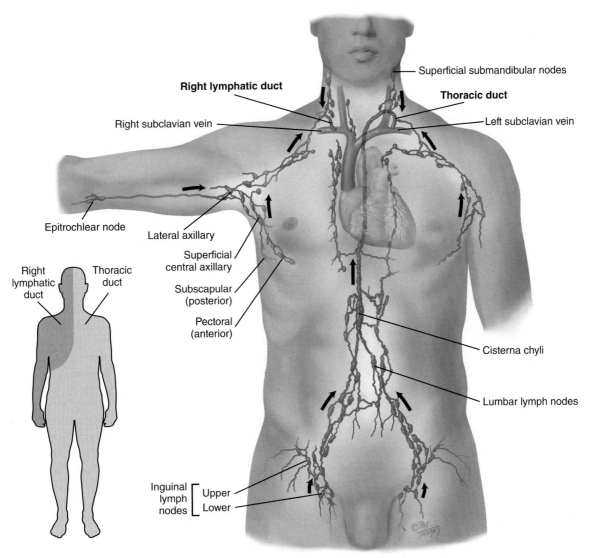

LYMPHATIC DUCTS AND DRAINAGE PATTERNS

21.5 © Pat Thomas, 2010.

store red blood cells, and (d) to filter micro-organisms from the blood.

The **tonsils** (palatine, pharyngeal, and lingual) are located at the entrance to the respiratory and gastro-intestinal tracts and respond to local inflammation.

The **thymus gland** is flat, pink-grey, and located in the superior mediastinum behind the sternum and in front of the aorta. It is relatively large in the fetus and young child and atrophies after puberty. It is important in developing the T lymphocytes of the immune system in children, but it serves no function in adults. The T and B lymphocytes originate in the bone marrow and mature in the lymphoid tissue.

 DEVELOPMENTAL CONSIDERATIONS

Infants and Children

The lymphatic system has the same function in children as in adults. Lymphoid tissue has a unique growth pattern in

comparison with other body systems. It is well developed at birth and grows rapidly until age 10 or 11 years. By age 6 years, the lymphoid tissue reaches adult size; it surpasses adult size by puberty, and then it slowly atrophies. It is possible that the excessive antigen stimulation in children causes the early rapid growth.

Lymph nodes are relatively large in children, and the superficial ones are often palpable even in healthy children. With infection, excessive swelling and hyperplasia occur. Enlargement of the tonsils is a familiar sign in respiratory infections. The excessive lymphoid response also may account for the common childhood symptom of abdominal pain with seemingly unrelated problems such as upper respiratory infections. Possibly, the inflammation of mesenteric lymph nodes produces the abdominal pain.

Pregnant Women

Hormonal changes cause vasodilatation and the resulting drop in blood pressure in the first and second trimesters

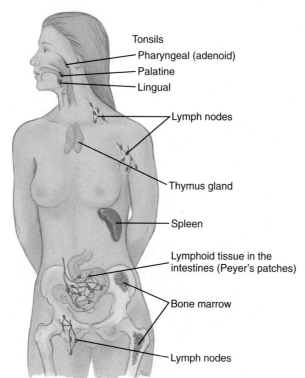

Tonsils
— Pharyngeal (adenoid)
— Palatine
— Lingual

Lymph nodes

Thymus gland

Spleen

Lymphoid tissue in the
intestines (Peyer's patches)

Bone marrow

Lymph nodes

RELATED ORGANS IN IMMUNE SYSTEM

21.6   © Pat Thomas, 2006.

of the pregnancy, as described in Chapter 20. The growing uterus obstructs drainage of the iliac veins and the inferior vena cava. This condition lowers blood flow and increases venous pressure. These developments, in turn, cause dependent edema, varicosities in the legs and vulva, and hemorrhoids.

Older Adults

Peripheral blood vessels grow more rigid with age, which results in **arteriosclerosis** (once called *hardening of the arteries*). This condition produces the rise in systolic blood pressure discussed in Chapter 10. Do not confuse this process

with another one, **atherosclerosis**, which is the deposition of fatty plaques on the intima of the arteries. Both processes are present with PAD in aging adults. PAD is underdiagnosed and undertreated, yet it is a large cause of morbidity (painful walking, poor wound healing) and mortality in Canada (see Table 21.6, p. 564).

PAD is a common, serious disease that is underdiagnosed, misdiagnosed, and undertreated. PAD is a condition characterized by atherosclerotic occlusive disease of the lower extremities and is a major risk factor for lower extremity amputation. PAD affects approximately 800 000 Canadians and is widespread within the population; it is frequently a **silent** cardiovascular disease. Therefore, many people remain at risk for preventable heart attacks and strokes. The incidence of PAD rises with age. It is suggested that approximately 4.3% of those over age 40 may have PAD, increasing to 14.5% in those older than 70 years of age.[1]

In people over 85 years of age, the prevalence of PAD is higher in women (39%) than it is in men (27%). It is not clear why women develop PAD a decade later than men do. When women do develop PAD, they also may have arthritis or peripheral neuropathy that masks their symptoms and delays diagnosis.[2] (If you are elderly, disabled, and cannot walk, you will not show leg pain.) Despite its prevalence and the risk for coronary artery disease (CAD), only 70 to 80% of those diagnosed with PAD are treated with antiplatelet or lipid-lowering medications; the rest are untreated. Many more are undiagnosed.

Aging produces a progressive enlargement of the intramuscular calf veins. Prolonged bed rest, prolonged immobilization, and heart failure increase the risk for deep vein thrombosis (DVT) and subsequent pulmonary embolism. These conditions are common in aging and also with malignancy and myocardial infarction (MI). Low-dose anticoagulant medication reduces the risk for venous thromboembolism.

Loss of lymphatic tissue leads to fewer numbers of lymph nodes in older people and to a decrease in the size of remaining nodes.

SUBJECTIVE DATA

1. Leg pain or cramps
2. Skin changes on arms or legs
3. Swelling in arms or legs
4. Lymph node enlargement
5. Medications

HEALTH HISTORY QUESTIONS

Examiner Asks	Rationale
1. Leg pain or cramps. Any leg **pain (cramps)**? Where? • Describe the type of pain: Is it burning, aching, cramping, stabbing? Did this come on gradually or suddenly? • Is it aggravated by activity, walking?	Such pain and cramps are signs of peripheral vascular disease; see Table 21.3, p. 561.

Examiner Asks	Rationale
• How many blocks (stairs) does it take to produce this pain?	**Claudication distance** is the number of blocks walked or stairs climbed that produces pain.
• Has this amount changed recently? • Is the pain worse with elevation? Worse with cool temperatures? • Does the pain wake you up at night?	Note sudden decrease in claudication distance or pain not relieved by rest. Night leg pain is common in older adults. It may indicate the ischemic rest pain of peripheral vascular disease, severe night muscle cramping (usually the calf), or restless leg syndrome.
• Tell me about your exercise pattern: Any recent change in exercise, a new exercise, increasing exercise? • Do you have a foot care routine? • Tell me about your job: Are you on your feet during the day or sitting at a desk?	Determine whether pain is of musculoskeletal origin rather than vascular. Chronic venous insufficiency, musculoskeletal pain of the lower back and feet, preterm birth, and spontaneous abortions are health risks associated with working conditions that required prolonged standing.
• What relieves this pain: dangling, walking, rubbing? Is the leg pain associated with any skin changes? • Is it associated with any change in sexual function (in men)?	Aortoiliac occlusion is associated with impotence (Leriche's syndrome).
• Any history of vascular problems, heart problems, diabetes, obesity, pregnancy, smoking, trauma, prolonged standing, or prolonged bed rest?	
2. Skin changes on arms or legs. Any **skin changes** in arms or legs? What colour: redness, pallor, blueness, brown discolorations? • Any change in temperature: excess warmth or coolness?	Coolness is associated with arterial disease.
• Do your leg veins look enlarged or crooked? Are these areas painful? • How have you treated these? Do you use support hose?	**Varicose veins** are swollen, twisted, and sometimes painful veins that have filled with an abnormal collection of blood.
• Any leg sores or ulcers? Where on the leg? Any pain with the leg ulcer?	Leg ulcers occur with chronic arterial and chronic venous disease (see Table 21.4, p. 562).
3. Swelling in arms or legs. Do you have **swelling** in one or both legs? When did this swelling start? • What time of day is the swelling at its worst: morning, or after you have been up most of day? • Does the swelling come and go, or is it constant? • What seems to trigger it: trauma, standing all day, sitting? • What relieves swelling: elevation, support hose? • Is swelling associated with pain, heat, redness, ulceration, hardened skin?	**Edema** is bilateral when caused by a systemic problem such as heart failure or unilateral when it is the result of a local obstruction or inflammation.
4. Lymph node enlargement. Any **"swollen glands"** (lumps, kernels)? Where in body? How long have you had them? • Any recent change? • How do they feel to you: hard, soft? • Are the swollen glands associated with pain, or local infection?	Lymph nodes enlarge with infection, malignancies, and immunological diseases.
5. Medications. What **medications** are you taking (e.g., oral contraceptives, hormone replacement, Aspirin)?	

OBJECTIVE DATA

PREPARATION

During a complete physical examination, examine the arms at the very beginning when you are checking the vital signs and the patient is sitting. Examine the legs directly after the abdominal examination while the patient is still supine. Then have the patient stand up to evaluate the leg veins.

Examination of the arms and legs includes peripheral vascular characteristics (described in this chapter), the skin (see Chapter 13), musculo-skeletal findings (see Chapter 24), and neurological findings (see Chapter 25). A method of integrating these steps is discussed in Chapter 28.

Room temperature should be approximately 22°C (72°F) and draft-free to prevent vasodilatation or vasoconstriction.

Use inspection and palpation. Compare your findings in one extremity with those in the opposite extremity.

EQUIPMENT NEEDED

Occasionally needed:
Paper tape measure
Tourniquet or blood pressure cuff
Stethoscope
Doppler ultrasonic stethoscope

Normal Range of Findings	Abnormal Findings

Inspect and Palpate the Arms

Lift both the patient's hands in your hands. Inspect, then turn the patient's hands over, noting colour of skin and nail beds; temperature, texture, and turgor of skin; and the presence of any lesions, edema, or clubbing. Use the **profile sign** (viewing the finger from the side) to detect early clubbing. The normal nail bed angle is 160 degrees. (See Chapter 13 for a full discussion of skin colour, lesions, and clubbing.)

With the patient's hands near the level of his, her, or their heart, check **capillary refill**. This is an index of peripheral perfusion and cardiac output. Depress and blanch the nail beds; release and note how long it takes for colour to return. Usually, the vessels refill within a fraction of a second. Consider it normal if the colour returns in less than 1 or 2 seconds. Note conditions that can skew your findings: a cool room, decreased body temperature, cigarette smoking, peripheral edema, and anemia.

The two arms should be symmetrical in size.

Note the presence of any scars on hands and arms. Many occur normally with usual childhood abrasions or with occupations involving hand tools.

Palpate radial pulses bilaterally, noting rate, rhythm, elasticity of vessel wall, and equal force (Fig. 21.7). Grade the force (amplitude) on a four-point scale:

   3+: increased, full, bounding
   2+: **normal**
   1+: weak
   0: absent

Abnormal Findings

Flattening of nail bed angle and clubbing (diffuse enlargement of terminal phalanges) occur with congenital cyanotic heart disease and cor pulmonale.

Refill time of more than 1 or 2 seconds signifies vasoconstriction or decreased cardiac output (hypovolemia, heart failure, shock). The hands are cold, clammy, and pale.

Edema of upper extremities occurs when lymphatic drainage is obstructed, which may occur after breast surgery (see Table 21.2, p. 560).

Needle tracks in antecubital fossae occur with intravenous drug use; linear scars in wrists may signify past self-inflicted injury.

The pulse is full and bounding (3+) in hyperkinetic states (exercise, anxiety, fever), anemia, and hyperthyroidism.

The pulse is weak and "thready" in shock and peripheral arterial disease. See Table 21.1, p. 559 for illustrations of these and irregular pulse rhythms.

Normal Range of Findings	Abnormal Findings

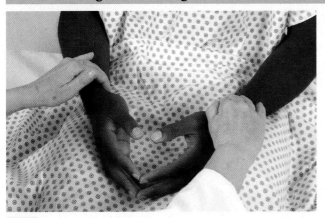

21.7

It usually is not necessary to palpate the ulnar pulses. If doing so is indicated, palpate along the medial side of the inner forearm (Fig. 21.8), although the ulnar pulses often are not palpable in normal people.

21.8

Palpate the brachial pulses; their force should be equal bilaterally (Fig. 21.9).

21.9

Objective Data

Normal Range of Findings

Check the epitrochlear lymph node in the depression above and behind the medial condyle of the humerus. Do this by "shaking hands" with the patient and reaching your other hand under the patient's elbow to the groove between the biceps and triceps muscles, above the medial epicondyle (Fig. 21.10). This node is normally not palpable.

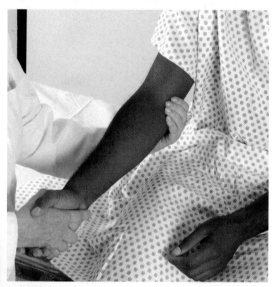

21.10

Inspect and Palpate the Legs

Uncover the patient's legs while keeping the genitalia draped. Inspect both legs together, noting skin colour, hair distribution, venous pattern, size (swelling or atrophy), and any skin lesions or ulcers.

Normally, hair covers the legs. Even if leg hair is shaved, you will still note hair on the dorsa of the toes.

The venous pattern normally is flat and barely visible. Note obvious varicosities, although these are best assessed while the patient is standing.

Both legs should be symmetrical in size without any swelling or atrophy. If the lower legs look asymmetrical or if DVT is suspected, measure the calf circumference with a nonstretchable tape measure (Fig. 21.11). Measure at the widest point, taking care to measure the other leg in exactly the same place: the same number of centimetres down from the patella or other landmark. If lymphedema is suspected, measure also at the ankle, distal calf, knee, and thigh. Record your findings in centimetres.

Abnormal Findings

The epitrochlear node becomes enlarged in infection of the hand or forearm.

Epitrochlear nodes are palpable in conditions of generalized lymphadenopathy: lymphoma, chronic lymphocytic leukemia, sarcoidosis, infections, mononucleosis.

Abnormalities include pallor with vasoconstriction, erythema with vasodilatation, and cyanosis.

In malnutrition, skin is thin, shiny, and atrophic; nails have thick ridges; hair loss occurs; and ulcers and gangrene may be present. Malnutrition, pallor, and coolness occur with arterial insufficiency.

Diffuse bilateral edema occurs with systemic illnesses.

Acute, unilateral, painful swelling and asymmetry of calves of 1 cm or more is abnormal; refer the patient to determine whether DVT is present.

Asymmetry of 1 to 3 cm occurs with mild lymphedema; 3 to 5 cm with moderate lymphedema; and more than 5 cm with severe lymphedema (see Table 21.2, p. 560).

Normal Range of Findings	**Abnormal Findings**

21.11

In the presence of skin discoloration, skin ulcers, or gangrene, note the size and the exact location.

Palpate for temperature (using the dorsa of your hand) along the patient's legs down to the feet, comparing symmetrical spots (Fig. 21.12). The skin should be warm and of equal warmth bilaterally. Both feet may be cool because of environmental factors such as cool room temperature, apprehension, and cigarette smoking. If temperature is increased higher up the leg, note whether this increase is gradual or abrupt.

21.12

Abnormal Findings

Brown discoloration occurs with chronic venous stasis as a result of hemosiderin deposits from red blood cell degradation.

Venous ulcers occur usually at the medial malleolus because of bacterial invasion of poorly drained tissues (see Table 21.4, p. 562).

With arterial deficit, ulcers occur on tips of toes, metatarsal heads, and lateral malleoli.

With arterial deficit, one foot or leg may be cool or the temperature may drop suddenly as you move down the leg.

Normal Range of Findings

Abnormal Findings

Flex the patient's knee, then gently compress the gastrocnemius (calf) muscle anteriorly against the tibia; no tenderness should be present.

CRITICAL FINDINGS

Calf pain with this manoeuvre is a positive **Homan's sign**, which also can occur when you sharply dorsiflex the foot toward the tibia. This test was once considered important but has lost its significance because of its **low sensitivity** in predicting the actual presence of a clot. As well, there is research to suggest that it can result in the dislodgement of an existing clot and increasing the risk for a pulmonary embolus.[3] Venous ultrasonography is considered the **highly sensitive** diagnostic test to determine the presence or absence of a clot. Approximately half of all patients with DVT have no clinically detectable signs or symptoms.

Palpate the inguinal lymph nodes. It is not unusual to find palpable nodes that are small (1 cm or less), movable, and nontender.

Palpate the peripheral arteries in both legs: femoral, popliteal, dorsalis pedis, and posterior tibial. Grade the force on the four-point scale. Locate the **femoral arteries** just below the inguinal ligament, halfway between the pubis and anterior superior iliac spines (Fig. 21.13). To help expose the femoral area, particularly in obese patients, ask the patient to bend the knees to the side in a froglike position. Press firmly and then slowly release, noting the pulse tap under your fingertips. Should this pulse be weak or diminished, auscultate the site for a bruit.

The **popliteal pulse** is a more diffuse pulse and can be difficult to localize. With the leg extended but relaxed, anchor your thumbs on the knee, and curl your fingers around into the popliteal fossa (Fig. 21.14). Press your fingers forward hard to compress the artery against the bone (the lower edge of the femur or the upper edge of the tibia). Often the pulse is just lateral to the medial tendon.

If you have difficulty with this manoeuvre, turn the patient prone and lift up the lower leg (Fig. 21.15). Let the leg relax against your arm, and press in deeply with your two thumbs. Often a normal popliteal pulse is impossible to palpate.

Nodes are not normally enlarged, tender, or fixed in area.

A bruit occurs with turbulent blood flow, indicating partial occlusion (see Table 21.6, p. 564).

21.13

21.14

Normal Range of Findings	Abnormal Findings

21.15

For the **posterior tibial pulse**, curve your fingers around the medial malleolus (Fig. 21.16). You will feel the tapping right behind it in the groove between the malleolus and the Achilles tendon. If you cannot feel it, try passive dorsiflexion of the foot to make the pulse more accessible.

The **dorsalis pedis pulse** requires a very light touch. Normally the pulse is just lateral to and parallel with the extensor tendon of the big toe (Fig. 21.17). Do not mistake the pulse in your own fingertips for that of the patient.

In adults older than 45 years of age, occasionally either the dorsalis pedis or the posterior tibial pulse may be hard to find, but not both on the same foot.

21.16   Posterior tibial pulse.

21.17   Dorsalis pedis pulse.

Check for pretibial edema. Firmly depress the skin over the tibia or the medial malleolus for 5 seconds and then release (Fig. 21.18, *A*). Normally, your finger should leave no indentation, although a pit commonly is seen if the patient has been standing all day or during pregnancy.

Bilateral, dependent, pitting edema occurs with heart failure, diabetic neuropathy, and hepatic cirrhosis (see Fig. 21.18, *B*).

Objective Data

Normal Range of Findings	Abnormal Findings

21.18 **A,** Checking for pretibial edema. **B,** Pitting edema.

If pitting edema is present, grade it on the following scale:

1+: Mild pitting, slight indentation, no perceptible swelling of the leg

2+: Moderate pitting, indentation subsides rapidly

3+: Deep pitting, indentation remains for a short time, swelling of leg

4+: Very deep pitting, indentation lasts a long time, gross swelling and distortion of leg

This classical method of capturing pit depth and recovery time is commonly used. Interestingly, is has been thought to be an arbitrary measure and not very reliable, but a recent study by Kogo and colleagues found there was a significant relationship between the depth of the surface imprint and the thickness of the subcutaneous soft tissue as measured on an ultrasonogram.[4] Ankle circumference is more reliable using a nonstretchable tape at a point 7 cm proximal to the midpoint of the medial malleolus. Because peripheral edema is a common clinical sign in a great number of conditions, it is important to detect true changes in the most accurate way available. Check with your own institution to conform to a consistently used scale.

Ask the patient to stand so that you can assess the venous system. Note any visible, dilated, and tortuous veins. If varicose veins are present, ask if they cause pain, swelling, fatigue, or cramping.

Unilateral edema occurs with occlusion of a deep vein. Unilateral or bilateral edema occurs with lymphatic obstruction. With these factors, it is "brawny" or nonpitting and feels hard to the touch.

Obtaining daily weights on the same scale is a useful method for standardizing data about water retention in the form of edema in the legs or other parts of the body (see the Critical Findings box).

CRITICAL FINDINGS

An increase in weight of >2.5 kg in a single day is cause for immediate concern. A complete head-to-toe evaluation is necessary to determine the cause of such significant fluid accumulation. Daily weights are a much better indicator of fluid status than intake and output measurements in individuals with compromised cardiovascular or peripheral vascular status.

Varicosities occur in the saphenous veins (see Table 21.5, p. 563). Examination techniques to assess valve incompetency within varicose veins are not reliable because varicosities occur below or between even competent valves.[5] Imaging by Doppler ultrasound is an objective, noninvasive measure of valvular incompetency.

Normal Range of Findings	**Abnormal Findings**

Colour Changes

If you suspect an arterial deficit, raise the legs approximately 30 cm off the table and ask the patient to wag the feet for approximately 30 seconds to drain off venous blood (Fig. 21.19). The skin colour now reflects only the contribution of arterial blood. A light-skinned person's feet normally look a little pale but still should be pink. A dark-skinned person's feet are more difficult to evaluate, but the soles should reveal extreme colour change.

Elevational pallor (marked) indicates arterial insufficiency.

21.19

Now have the patient sit up with the legs over the side of the table (Fig. 21.20, *A*). Compare the colour of both feet. Note the time it takes for colour to return to the feet. Normally, this is 10 seconds or less. Note also the time it takes for the superficial veins around the feet to fill; the normal time is approximately 15 seconds. This test is unreliable if the patient has concomitant venous disease with incompetent valves. (See the Promoting Health: Foot Care box, p. 555.)

Dependent rubor (deep blue-red colour) occurs with severe arterial insufficiency (see Fig. 21.20, *B*). Chronic hypoxia produces a loss of vasomotor tone and causes blood to pool in the veins.

Venous filling is delayed with arterial insufficiency (see Table 21.5, p. 563).

21.20 **A,** Checking for colour by having the patient sit with legs dangling over the examination table. **B,** Dependent rubor.

Test the lower legs for strength (see Chapter 24). Test the lower legs for sensation (see Chapter 25).

Motor loss occurs with severe arterial deficit.

Sensory loss occurs with arterial deficit, especially diabetes.

Objective Data

Normal Range of Findings	Abnormal Findings

Normal Range of Findings

The Doppler Ultrasonic Stethoscope

Use this device to detect a weak peripheral pulse, to monitor blood pressure in infants or children, or to measure a low blood pressure or blood pressure in a lower extremity (Fig. 21.21). The Doppler ultrasonic stethoscope magnifies pulsatile sounds from the heart and blood vessels. Position the patient supine, with the legs externally rotated so that the medial ankles are accessible. Place a drop of coupling gel on the end of the handheld transducer. Place the transducer over a pulse site, swivelled at a 45-degree angle. Apply very light pressure; locate the pulse site by the swishing, whooshing sound.

21.21

❖ DEVELOPMENTAL CONSIDERATIONS

Infants and Children

Transient acrocyanosis and skin mottling at birth are discussed in Chapter 13. Pulse force should be normal and symmetrical. Pulse force also should be the same in the upper and lower extremities.

Lymph nodes are often palpable in healthy infants and children. They are small, firm (shotty), mobile, and nontender. Their palpability may be the sequelae of past infection, such as a diaper rash (inguinal nodes) or a respiratory infection (cervical nodes). Vaccinations also can produce local lymphadenopathy. Note characteristics of any palpable nodes and whether they are local or generalized.

Pregnant Women

Expect diffuse bilateral pitting edema in the lower extremities, especially at the end of the day and into the third trimester. Varicose veins in the legs also are common in the third trimester.

Older Adults

The dorsalis pedis and posterior tibial pulses may become more difficult to find. Trophic changes associated with arterial insufficiency (thin, shiny skin, thick-ridged nails, loss of hair on lower legs) also occur normally with aging.

Abnormal Findings

Pulses are weak with vasoconstriction or diminished cardiac output.

Pulses are full and with patent ductus arteriosus as a result of the large left-to-right shunt.

Diminished or absence of femoral pulses in the presence of normal upper extremity pulses are suggestive of coarctation of aorta.

Enlarged, warm, tender nodes indicate current infection. Look for source of infection.

Remain alert for generalized edema in addition to hypertension, which are suggestive of pre-eclampsia, a dangerous obstetric condition.

PROMOTING HEALTH: FOOT CARE

Take Care of Your Feet

Foot problems are often the first sign of more serious health conditions such as arthritis, diabetes, and nerve or circulatory disorders. Health care providers not only should remember to examine the feet for common foot problems but also should be prepared to explain what "good foot care" really means. Too often health care providers advise "good foot care" but do not take the time to explain what it entails.

Foot problems are a major cause of morbidity and mortality in people with diabetes and contribute to increased health care costs. Management of foot ulceration requires an interdisciplinary approach that addresses glycemic control, infection, lower extremity vascular status, and local wound care.*

Good foot care entails the following:

1. Checking your feet every day:
   - If patients are unable to see the bottoms of their feet, they need to be instructed to use a mirror or to ask someone to help them.
   - Each foot should be examined for red spots or sensitive areas, discoloration of skin or nails, ingrown nails, pain, cuts, swelling, or blisters. A good time to examine feet is after a shower or bath. Patients should not soak their feet because this can cause skin to become dry. Feet should be dried carefully, especially between the toes.
   - Toenails should be kept trimmed, straight across, and filed at the edges with an emery board or nail file.
   - Although freshly applied nail polish does not increase the number of bacteria, chipped nail polish may support the growth of larger numbers of organisms on nails. This is especially important for individuals who already are at risk for infection.

2. Keeping the blood flowing to your feet:
   - It is important to keep blood circulating to the feet. This is accomplished by increasing activity. Walking is one of the best exercises for overall circulation.
   - When unable to walk, individuals should put their feet up when sitting or lying down, stretch the feet, wiggle the toes, and have a gentle foot massage.
   - Patients should not cross their legs for long periods of time.
   - Patients should not smoke.

3. Wearing shoes that fit and are comfortable:
   - Patients should wear comfortable shoes that fit well. The size of the feet changes with age, and so it is important to be measured each time a person buys new shoes. The best time to measure feet is toward the end of the day, when feet tend to be the largest.
   - In most individuals, one foot is larger than the other. It is recommended that shoes are fit to the larger foot. Furthermore, just as people have different body shapes, the feet have different shapes, too.
   - It is important to select shoes that are shaped like one's feet. The ball of the foot should fit comfortably into the widest part of the shoe, and toes should not be crowded.
   - For women, low-heeled shoes are safer and less damaging than high-heeled shoes.

4. Keeping skin soft and smooth:
   - A thin coat of skin lotion over the tops and bottoms of the feet helps keep skin soft and smooth. However, this extra moisture should not go between toes.
   - Patients should use mild soap to clean the feet.
   - Patients should be careful about adding oils to bath water. They can make the feet and the bathtub both very slippery.

For more information on foot care, consult the following:

- Diabetes Canada. (2018). Foot care: A step toward good health. Retrieved from http://guidelines.diabetes.ca/docs/patient-resources/foot-care.pdf.
- Canadian Podiatric Medical Association: https://www.podiatrycanada.org.

References

*Canadian Diabetes Association. (2013). Clinical practice guidelines: Screening for type 1 and type 2 diabetes. *Canadian Journal of Diabetes*, *37*, S12–S15.

Objective Data

SPECIAL CONSIDERATIONS FOR ADVANCED PRACTICE

Normal Range of Findings	Abnormal Findings

Modified Allen Test

The **modified Allen test** is used to evaluate the adequacy of collateral circulation before the radial artery is cannulated: (a) Firmly occlude both the ulnar and radial arteries of one hand while the patient makes a fist several times. This causes the hand to blanch (Fig. 21.22, *A*). (b) Ask the patient to open the hand without hyperextending it; then release pressure on the ulnar artery while maintaining pressure on the radial artery. If circulation is adequate, the hand's normal colour returns in approximately 2 to 5 seconds (Fig. 21.22, *B*). Although this test is simple and useful, it is relatively crude and subject to error; that is, you must occlude both arteries uniformly with 5 kg (11 lb) of pressure for the test result to be accurate.

Persistent pallor or a sluggish return to colour is suggestive of occlusion of the collateral arterial flow (Fig. 21.22, *C*). Avoid radial artery cannulation until adequate circulation is shown. This test is not considered part of a basic health assessment.

If Not Now, When?

This test is specifically a precannulation evaluation of a radial artery. It is commonly performed by respiratory therapists before blood gases are measured, to determine arterial competence. Advanced practitioners and health care practitioners in the critical care environment use this test as a means of determining arterial competence.

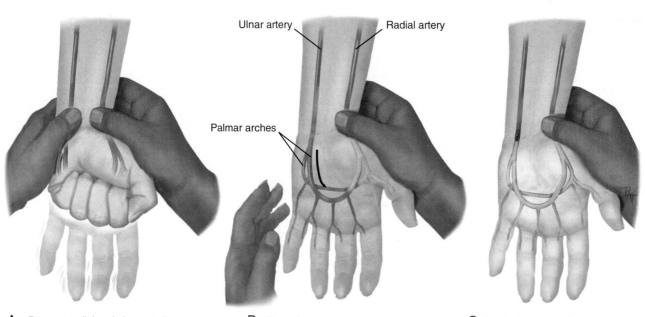

Ulnar artery   Radial artery

Palmar arches

A Depress radial and ulnar arteries— person opens and closes fist

B Normal— blood returns via ulnar artery

C Occluded ulnar artery— no blood return

21.22

The Wells Score for Leg Deep Vein Thrombosis[6]

Many of the assessment findings for DVT are unreliable and also occur with other conditions. Wells and others have combined findings into a simple scoring system. These criteria separate patients into groups of low, moderate, or high probability of DVT.[7]

| **Normal Range of Findings** | **Abnormal Findings** |

Clinical Model for Predicting Pretest Probability of Deep Vein Thrombosis*

Clinical Characteristic	Score
Active cancer (treatment ongoing, administered within previous 6 months or palliative)	1
Paralysis, paresis, or recent plaster immobilization of the lower extremities	1
Recently bedridden >3 days or major surgery within previous 12 weeks requiring general or regional anaesthesia	1
Localized tenderness along the distribution of the deep venous system	1
Swelling of entire leg	1
Calf swelling >3 cm larger than asymptomatic side (measured 10 cm below tibial tuberosity)	1
Pitting edema confined to the symptomatic leg	1
Collateral superficial veins (nonvaricose)	1
Previously documented DVT	1
Alternative diagnosis at least as likely as DVT	-2

*A score of 0 or less = low probability of DVT.
From Scarvelis, D., & Wells, P. S. (2006). Diagnosis and treatment of deep-vein thrombosis. *Canadian Medical Association Journal, 175*(9), 1087–1092.

Score of 1 or 2 = moderate probability of DVT; score of 3 points or more = high probability.

The Ankle–Brachial Index

Use of the Doppler stethoscope is a highly specific, noninvasive, and readily available way to determine the extent of PAD. Have the patient lie flat, with the head and heels fully supported.[8] Confirm no smoking within 2 hours of the measurement and allow a 5- to 10-minute rest period supine before measurement. Choose the correct cuff width for the arm and the ankle; width should be 40% of limb circumference. Position the ankle cuff just above the malleoli with straight wrapping.

Use the Doppler probe for both brachial and ankle measurements. In all sites, locate the pulse by Doppler and inflate the cuff 20 mm Hg above disappearance of flow signal; then deflate slowly to detect reappearance of flow signal. Moving counterclockwise, measure the following: right arm, right posterior tibial (PT), right dorsalis pedis (DP), left PT, left DP, and left arm. Calculate both ankle–brachial index (ABI) using this formula:

$$\text{Right ABI} = \frac{\text{Highest right ankle pressure (DP or PT)}}{\text{Highest arm pressure (right or left)}}$$

$$\text{Example:} \frac{132 \text{ ankle systolic}}{124 \text{ arm systolic}} = \frac{1.06 \text{ or } 106\%, \text{indicating}}{\text{no flow reduction}}$$

$$\text{Left ABI} = \frac{\text{Highest left ankle pressure (DP or PT)}}{\text{Highest arm pressure (right or left)}}$$

People with diabetes mellitus or renal failure may have calcified arteries that occasionally are noncompressible and give a falsely high ankle pressure. Thus the presence or severity of PAD may be underestimated.[9]

An ABI between 0.91 and 1 indicates borderline cardiovascular risk.

An ABI of 0.90 or less indicates PAD:
- 0.90 to 0.71: mild PAD
- 0.70 to 0.41: moderate PAD
- 0.40 to 0.30: severe PAD, usually with rest pain, except in the presence of diabetic neuropathy
- <0.30: ischemia, with impending loss of tissue

Special Considerations for Advanced Practice

DOCUMENTATION AND CRITICAL THINKING

Sample Charting

SUBJECTIVE

No leg pain, no skin changes, no swelling or lymph node enlargement. No history of heart or vascular problems, diabetes, or obesity. Does not smoke. On no medications.

OBJECTIVE

Inspection: Extremities have pink-tan colour without redness, cyanosis, or any skin lesions. Extremity size is symmetrical without swelling or atrophy.

Palpation: Temperature is warm and = bilaterally. All pulses present, 2+ and = bilaterally. No lymphadenopathy.

ASSESSMENT

Healthy tissue integrity
Effective tissue perfusion

Focused Assessment: Clinical Case Study

James Knowles (J.K.) is a 43-year-old, married male city sanitation worker, admitted to Queen Elizabeth II Medical Centre today for "bypass surgery tomorrow to fix my aorta and these black toes."

SUBJECTIVE

6 years PTA [prior to arrival]: Motorcycle accident with handle bars jammed into groin. J.K. treated and released at local hospital. No apparent injury, although M.D. now thinks accident may have precipitated current stenosis of aorta.

1 year PTA: Radiating pain in right calf on walking 1.5 km. Pain relieved by stopping walking.

3 months PTA: Problems with sex, unable to maintain erection during intercourse.

1 month PTA: Leg pain present after walking two blocks. Numbness and tingling in right foot and calf. Tips of three toes on right foot look black. Saw MD. Diagnostic studies showed stenosis of aorta "below vessels that go to my kidneys."

Today: Leg pain at rest, constant and severe, worse at night, partially relieved by dangling leg over side of bed.

History: No history of heart or vessel disease, no hypertension, no diabetes, no obesity.

Personal habits: Smokes cigarettes three ppd [packs of cigarettes per day] × 23 years. Now cut down to one ppd. Walking is part of occupation, although has been driving city truck past 3 months because of leg pain. On no medications.

OBJECTIVE

Inspection: Lower extremity size = bilaterally with no swelling or atrophy. No varicosities. Colour L [left] leg pink, R [right] leg pink when supine, but marked pallor in R foot on elevation. Black gangrene at tips of R second, third, fourth toes. Leg hair present but absent on involved toes.

Palpation: R foot cool and temperature gradually warms as proceed to palpate up R leg.

Pulses: Femoral pulses, both 1+; popliteal pulses, both 0; posterior tibial pulses, both 0 but present with Doppler stethoscope; dorsalis pedis pulses 0, but L dorsalis pedis pulse is present with Doppler stethoscope, and R is not present with Doppler stethoscope.

ASSESSMENT

Ischemic rest pain R leg
Ineffective tissue perfusion R/T [related to] interruption of flow
Impaired tissue integrity R/T altered circulation
Activity intolerance R/T leg pain
Sexual dysfunction R/T effects of disease

ABNORMAL FINDINGS

TABLE 21.1   Variations in Arterial Pulse

Description	Associated With

Weak, "Thready" Pulse: 1+

Hard to palpate, hard to find, may fade in and out, easily obliterated by pressure

Decreased cardiac output; peripheral arterial disease; aortic valve stenosis

Full, Bounding Pulse: 3+

Easily palpable, pounds under examiner's fingertips

Hyperkinetic states (exercise, anxiety, fever), anemia, hyperthyroidism

Water–Hammer (Corrigan's) Pulse: 3+

Greater than normal force, then sudden collapse

Aortic valve regurgitation; patent ductus arteriosus

Pulsus Bigeminus

Coupled rhythm, wherein every other beat comes early or normal beat is followed by premature beat; force of premature beat is decreased because of shortened cardiac filling time

Conduction disturbance (e.g., premature ventricular contraction, premature atrial contraction)

Pulsus Alternans

Regular rhythm, but force varying with alternating beats of large and small amplitude

When heart rate is normal: pulsus alternans occurs with severe left ventricular failure, which in turn is caused by ischemic heart disease, valvular heart disease, chronic hypertension, or cardiomyopathy

Pulsus Paradoxus

Amplitude of beats: weaker with inspiration, stronger with expiration; rhythm best determined during blood pressure measurement; pressure decreases (>10 mm Hg) during inspiration and increases with expiration

A common finding in cardiac tamponade (pericardial effusion in which high pressure compresses the heart and blocks cardiac output); also in severe bronchospasm of acute asthma

Pulsus Bisferiens

Two strong systolic peaks, with a dip in between, in each pulse; best assessed at the carotid artery

Aortic valve stenosis plus regurgitation

TABLE 21.2   Peripheral Vascular Disease in the Arms

◀ Raynaud's Phenomenon

This condition is characterized by episodes of abrupt progressive tricolour change of the fingers in response to cold, vibration, or stress: (a) white (pallor; in top photo) from arteriospasm and resulting deficit in supply; (b) blue (cyanosis; in lower photo) from slight relaxation of the spasm that allows a slow trickle of blood through the capillaries and increased oxygen extraction of hemoglobin; (c) and red (rubor) in heel of hand because of return of blood into the dilated capillary bed or reactive hyperemia.

Cold, numbness, or pain may accompany the pallor or cyanosis stage; then burning, throbbing pain, and swelling occur with rubor. Lasts minutes to hours; occurs bilaterally. Several medications predispose episodes, and smoking can increase the symptoms.

◀ Lymphedema

Lymphedema is high-protein swelling of the limb, most commonly caused by breast cancer treatment. Surgical removal of lymph nodes with breast surgery or damage to lymph nodes and vessels with radiation therapy for breast cancer can impede drainage of lymph. Protein-rich lymph builds up in the interstitial spaces, which further raises local colloid oncotic pressure and promotes more fluid leakage. Stagnation of lymphatic fluid can lead to infection, delayed wound healing, chronic inflammation, and fibrosis of surrounding tissue.

Lymphedema after breast cancer is common but usually mild. Obesity increases risk. Early symptoms include self-reported sensations of "tired," thick, heavy arm; tightness of jewellery; swelling; and tingling sensation. Objective data include a unilateral swelling and nonpitting brawny edema, with induration of overlying skin. Early recognition is important because evidence supports effectiveness of interventions, such as complete decongestive physiotherapy, exercise, nonelastic wrapping, compression garments, and skin care. Without treatment, lymphedema is chronic and progressive, which is psychologically demoralizing as a threat to body image and as a constant reminder of the cancer.

See Illustration Credits for source information.

TABLE 21.3	**Pain Profiles of Peripheral Vascular Disease**	
Symptom Analysis	Chronic Arterial Symptoms	Acute Arterial Symptoms

Arterial Disease Causes Symptoms and Signs of Oxygen Deficit

Location	Deep muscle pain, usually in calf, but may be lower leg or dorsum of foot	Varies, distal to occlusion, may involve entire leg
Character	Intermittent claudication, feels like "cramp," "numbness and tingling," "feeling of cold"	Throbbing
Onset and duration	Chronic pain, onset gradual after exertion	Sudden onset (within 1 hr)
Aggravating factors	Activity (walking, stairs); "claudication distance" is specific number of blocks or stairs it takes to produce pain Elevation (rest pain indicates severe involvement)	
Relieving factors	Rest (usually within 2 min [e.g., standing]) Dangling (severe involvement)	
Associated symptoms	Cool, pale skin	Six Ps: *pain, pallor, pulselessness, paresthesia, poikilothermia* (coldness), *paralysis* (indicates severe)
Those at risk	Older adults; more middle-age males than females, more older age females than males; history of hypertension, smoking, diabetes, hypercholesterolemia, obesity, vascular disease	History of vascular surgery; arterial invasive procedure; abdominal aneurysm (emboli); trauma, including injured arteries; chronic atrial fibrillation
	Chronic Venous Symptoms	Acute Venous Symptoms

Venous Disease Causes Symptoms and Signs of Metabolic Waste Buildup

Location	Calf, lower leg	Calf
Character	Aching, tiredness, feeling of fullness	Intense, sharp; deep muscle tender to touch
Onset and duration	Chronic pain, increases at end of day	Sudden onset (within 1 hr)
Aggravating factors	Prolonged standing, sitting	Pain may increase with sharp dorsiflexion of foot
Relieving factors	Elevation, lying, walking	
Associated symptoms	Edema, varicosities, weeping ulcers at ankles	Red, warm, swollen leg
Those at risk	Job with prolonged standing or sitting; obesity; pregnancy; prolonged bed rest; history of heart failure, varicosities, or thrombophlebitis; veins crushed by trauma or surgery	

TABLE 21.4	Leg Ulcerations: Arterial, Venous, or Diabetic
Chronic Arterial Insufficiency	Chronic Venous Insufficiency

Arterial (Ischemic) Ulceration

Arterial ulcers result from the buildup of fatty plaques on intima (atherosclerosis) plus hardening and calcification of the arterial wall (arteriosclerosis).

S: Deep muscle pain in calf or foot, claudication (pain with walking), pain at rest (indicative of worsening of condition).

O: Coolness, pallor, elevational pallor, and dependent rubor; diminished pulses; systolic bruits; trophic skin; signs of malnutrition (thin, shiny skin, thick-ridged nails, absence of hair, atrophy of muscles); xanthoma formation; distal gangrene.

Ulcers occur at toes, metatarsal heads, heels, and lateral ankle and are characterized by pale ischemic base, well-defined edges, and no bleeding.

Venous (Stasis) Ulceration

Venous ulcers occur after acute DVT or with chronic incompetent valves in deep veins.

S: Aching pain in calf or lower leg, worse at end of the day, worse with prolonged standing or sitting.

O: Firm, brawny edema; coarse, thickened skin; normal pulses; brown pigment discoloration; petechiae; dermatitis.

Venous stasis causes increased venous pressure, which then causes RBCs to leak out of veins and into the skin. The RBCs break down and leave hemosiderin (iron deposits) behind, which are the brown pigment deposits. A weepy, pruritic stasis dermatitis may be present.

Ulcers occur at medial malleolus and are characterized by bleeding and uneven edges.

◀ **Diabetes** hastens changes described with ischemic ulcer, with generalized dysfunction in all arterial areas: peripheral, coronary, cerebral, retinal, and renal. Peripheral involvement is associated with diabetic neuropathy and local infection. Without careful vigilance of pressure points on the feet, an ulcer may go unnoticed. Pain and other sensation are decreased, and surrounding skin is callused.

DVT, Deep venous thrombosis; *O*, objective data; *RBCs*, red blood cells; *S*, subjective data.
See Illustration Credits for source information.

TABLE 21.5	Peripheral Vascular Disease in the Legs
Chronic Venous Disease	Acute Venous Disease

Superficial Varicose Veins

Incompetent valves allow reflux of blood, which causes veins to become dilated and tortuous. Unremitting hydrostatic pressure causes distal valves to be incompetent and causes worsening of the varicosity.

After age 45 years, occurrence is three times more common in women than in men.

S: Aching, heaviness in calf, easy fatigability, night leg or foot cramps.

O: Dilated, tortuous veins.

Deep Venous Thrombophlebitis

A deep vein is occluded by a thrombus, which causes inflammation, blockage of venous return, cyanosis, and edema. Virchow's triad consists of the classical three factors that promote thrombogenesis: (a) stasis, (b) hypercoagulability, and (c) endothelial dysfunction. Cause may be prolonged bed rest; history of varicose veins; trauma; infection; cancer; and, in younger women, the use of oral estrogenic contraceptives.

Note that upper extremity deep venous thrombophlebitis is increasingly common because of the frequent use of invasive lines such as central venous catheters.[3]

S: Sudden onset of intense, sharp, deep muscle pain; may increase with sharp dorsiflexion of foot.

O: Increased warmth; swelling (to compare swelling, observe the usual shoe size); redness; possibly mild dependent cyanosis; tenderness to palpation; Homan's sign, only in a few cases (but a poor diagnostic measure).

O, objective data; *S*, subjective data.
See Illustration Credits for source information.

TABLE 21.6   Peripheral Artery Disease

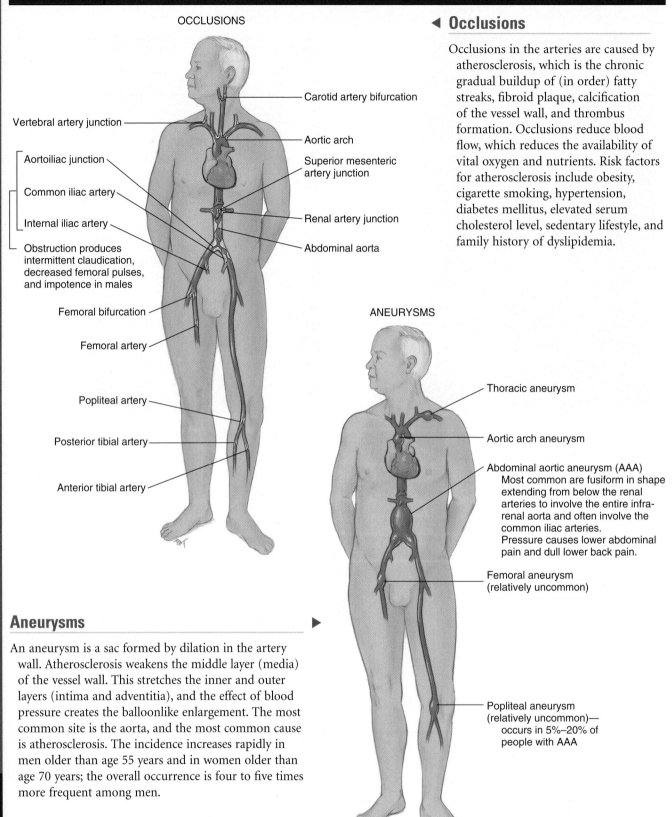

OCCLUSIONS

- Carotid artery bifurcation
- Vertebral artery junction
- Aortic arch
- Aortoiliac junction
- Superior mesenteric artery junction
- Common iliac artery
- Internal iliac artery
- Renal artery junction
- Obstruction produces intermittent claudication, decreased femoral pulses, and impotence in males
- Abdominal aorta
- Femoral bifurcation
- Femoral artery
- Popliteal artery
- Posterior tibial artery
- Anterior tibial artery

ANEURYSMS

- Thoracic aneurysm
- Aortic arch aneurysm
- Abdominal aortic aneurysm (AAA) Most common are fusiform in shape extending from below the renal arteries to involve the entire infra-renal aorta and often involve the common iliac arteries. Pressure causes lower abdominal pain and dull lower back pain.
- Femoral aneurysm (relatively uncommon)
- Popliteal aneurysm (relatively uncommon)— occurs in 5%–20% of people with AAA

◀ Occlusions

Occlusions in the arteries are caused by atherosclerosis, which is the chronic gradual buildup of (in order) fatty streaks, fibroid plaque, calcification of the vessel wall, and thrombus formation. Occlusions reduce blood flow, which reduces the availability of vital oxygen and nutrients. Risk factors for atherosclerosis include obesity, cigarette smoking, hypertension, diabetes mellitus, elevated serum cholesterol level, sedentary lifestyle, and family history of dyslipidemia.

Aneurysms   ▶

An aneurysm is a sac formed by dilation in the artery wall. Atherosclerosis weakens the middle layer (media) of the vessel wall. This stretches the inner and outer layers (intima and adventitia), and the effect of blood pressure creates the balloonlike enlargement. The most common site is the aorta, and the most common cause is atherosclerosis. The incidence increases rapidly in men older than age 55 years and in women older than age 70 years; the overall occurrence is four to five times more frequent among men.

Summary Checklist: Peripheral Vascular Examination

1. **Inspect arms** for colour, size, any lesions
2. **Palpate pulses:** radial, brachial
3. **Check epitrochlear node**
4. **Inspect legs** for colour, size, any lesions, trophic skin changes
5. **Palpate the skin for temperature** of feet and legs
6. **Palpate inguinal nodes**
7. **Palpate pulses in lower extremities:** femoral, popliteal, posterior tibial, dorsalis pedis
8. **Engage in teaching and health promotion**

CRITICAL FINDINGS

Deep venous thrombophlebitis necessitates emergency referral because of the risk for pulmonary embolism.

REFERENCES

1. Lovell, M., Dickson, C., & Lindsay, T. F. (2015). Peripheral artery disease: The unknown cardiovascular risk. *Diabetic Foot Canada, 3*(2), 6–9.
2. Harvard Women's Health Watch. (2012, April 12). Peripheral arterial disease. Cambridge, MA: Harvard Health Publishing. Retrieved from https://www.health.harvard.edu/heart-health/peripheral-artery-disease.
3. Lancaster, S., Owens, A., Bryant, A. S., et al. (2010). Upper-extremity deep vein thrombosis. *American Journal of Nursing, 110*(5), 48–52.
4. Kogo, H., Murata, J., Murata, S., et al. (2017). Validity of a new quantitative evaluation method that uses the depth of the surface imprint as an indicator for pitting edema. *PLoS ONE, 12*(1), e0170810. doi:https://doi.org/10.1371/journal.pone.0170810.
5. Oklu, R., Habito, R., Mayr, M., et al. (2012). Pathogenesis of varicose veins. *Journal of Vascular and Interventional Radiology, 23*(1), 33–39.
6. Scarvelis, D., & Wells, P. S. (2006). Diagnosis and treatment of deep-vein thrombosis. *Canadian Medical Association Journal, 175*(9), 1087–1092.
7. McGee, S. (2018). *Evidence-based physical diagnosis* (4th ed.). Philadelphia: Saunders.
8. American Heart Association. (2012). Measurement and interpretation of the ankle-brachial index. *Circulation, 126*(24), 2890–2909.
9. Aronow, W. S. (2012). Peripheral arterial disease of the lower extremities. *Archives of Medical Science, 8*(2), 375–388.

22 CHAPTER

The Abdomen

Written by Carolyn Jarvis, PhD, APN, CNP
Adapted by Marian Luctkar-Flude, RN, PhD

(e) http://evolve.elsevier.com/Canada/Jarvis/examination/

STRUCTURE AND FUNCTION

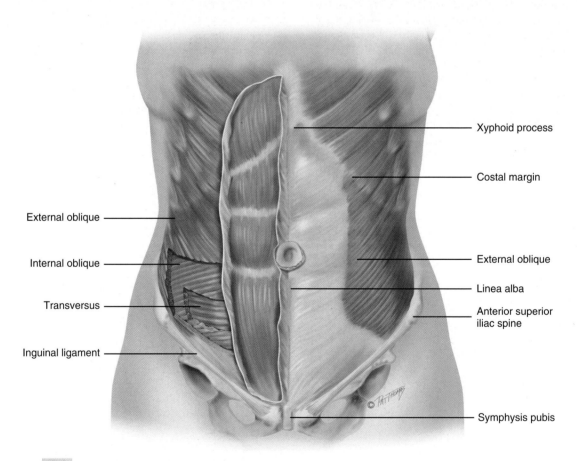

- Xyphoid process
- Costal margin
- External oblique
- Linea alba
- Anterior superior iliac spine
- External oblique
- Internal oblique
- Transversus
- Inguinal ligament
- Symphysis pubis

22.1 © Pat Thomas, 2006.

SURFACE LANDMARKS

The **abdomen** is a large oval cavity extending from the diaphragm down to the top of the pelvis. It is bordered in back by the vertebral column and paravertebral muscles and at the sides and front by the lower rib cage and abdominal muscles

(Fig. 22.1). Four layers of large, flat muscles form the ventral abdominal wall. These are joined at the midline by a tendinous seam, the **linea alba**. One muscle, the **rectus abdominis**, forms a strip extending the length of the midline, and its edge is often palpable. The muscles protect and hold the organs in place, and flex the vertebral column.

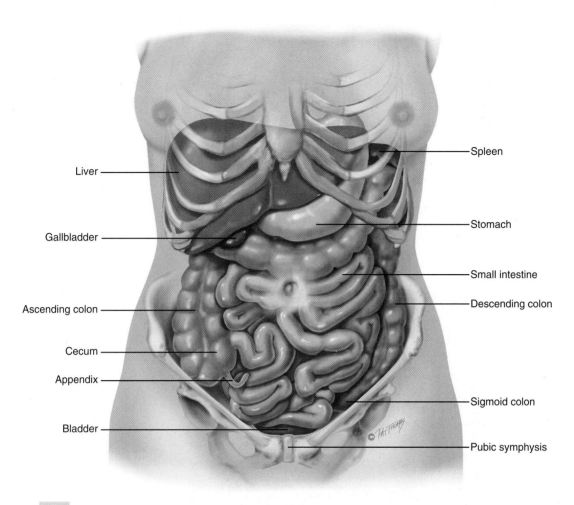

Liver

Gallbladder

Ascending colon

Cecum

Appendix

Bladder

Spleen

Stomach

Small intestine

Descending colon

Sigmoid colon

Pubic symphysis

22.2 © Pat Thomas, 2006.

INTERNAL ANATOMY

Inside the abdominal cavity, all the internal organs are called the **viscera**. It is important to know the location of these organs (Fig. 22.2) in order to visualize each organ as you auscultate or palpate through the abdominal wall.

The **solid viscera** are those that maintain a characteristic shape (liver, pancreas, spleen, adrenal glands, kidneys, ovaries, and uterus). The **liver** fills most of the right upper quadrant (RUQ) and extends over to the left midclavicular line. The lower edge of the liver and the right kidney may normally be palpable. The ovaries normally are palpable only on bimanual assessment during the pelvic examination.

The shape of the **hollow viscera** (stomach, gallbladder, small intestine, colon, and bladder) depends on the contents. They are usually not palpable, although you may feel a colon distended with feces or a bladder distended with urine. The stomach is just below the diaphragm, between the liver and spleen. The gallbladder rests under the posterior surface of the liver, just lateral to the right midclavicular line. The small intestine is located in all four quadrants, extending from the stomach's pyloric valve to the ileocecal valve in the right lower quadrant (RLQ), where it joins the colon.

The **spleen** is a soft mass of lymphatic tissue on the posterolateral wall of the abdominal cavity, immediately under the diaphragm (see illustration, Fig. 22.3). It lies obliquely with its long axis behind and parallel to the tenth rib, lateral to the midaxillary line. Its width extends approximately 7 cm from the ninth to the eleventh ribs. It is normally not palpable. If it becomes enlarged (see photo, Fig. 22.3), its lower edge moves downward and toward the midline.

The **aorta** is just left of midline in the upper part of the abdomen (Fig. 22.4). It descends behind the peritoneum and bifurcates 2 cm below the umbilicus into the right and left common iliac arteries opposite the fourth lumbar vertebra. Aortic pulsations can be palpated easily in the upper anterior abdominal wall. The right and left iliac arteries become the femoral arteries in the groin area. Their pulsations are also easily palpated, at a point halfway between the anterior superior iliac spine and the symphysis pubis.

The **pancreas** is a soft, lobulated gland located behind the stomach. It stretches obliquely across the posterior abdominal wall to the left upper quadrant (LUQ).

The bean-shaped **kidneys** are retroperitoneal, or posterior to the abdominal contents (Fig. 22.5). They are well protected by the posterior ribs and musculature. The twelfth rib forms an angle, the **costovertebral angle**, with the vertebral column. The left kidney lies at that point, at the eleventh and twelfth ribs. Because of the placement of the liver, the

22.3 © Pat Thomas, 2006.

right kidney rests 1 to 2 cm lower than the left kidney and is sometimes palpable.

For convenience in description, the abdominal wall is divided into **four quadrants** by a vertical and a horizontal line bisecting the umbilicus (Fig. 22.6). (According to an older, more complicated scheme, the abdomen was divided into nine regions. Although the old system is generally not used, some regional names persist, such as **epigastric** for the area between the costal margins, **umbilical** for the area around the umbilicus, and **hypogastric** or **suprapubic** for the area above the pubic bone.)

The anatomical location of each organ by quadrants is as follows:

Right Upper Quadrant (RUQ)
Liver
Gallbladder
Duodenum
Head of pancreas
Right kidney and adrenal gland
Hepatic flexure of colon
Parts of ascending and transverse colon

Left Upper Quadrant (LUQ)
Stomach
Spleen
Left lobe of liver
Body of pancreas
Left kidney and adrenal gland
Splenic flexure of colon
Parts of transverse and descending colon

Right Lower Quadrant (RLQ)
Cecum
Appendix
Right ovary and fallopian tube
Right ureter
Right spermatic cord

Midline
Aorta
Uterus (if enlarged)
Bladder (if distended)

Left Lower Quadrant (LLQ)
Part of descending colon
Sigmoid colon
Left ovary and fallopian tube
Left ureter
Left spermatic cord

❖ DEVELOPMENTAL CONSIDERATIONS

Infants and Children

In newborns, the umbilical cord shows prominently on the abdomen. It contains two arteries and one vein. The liver takes up proportionately more space in the abdomen at birth than in later life. In healthy full-term newborns, the lower edge may be palpated 0.5 to 2.5 cm below the right costal margin. (Age-related values of expected liver size are listed in the Objective Data section.) The urinary bladder is

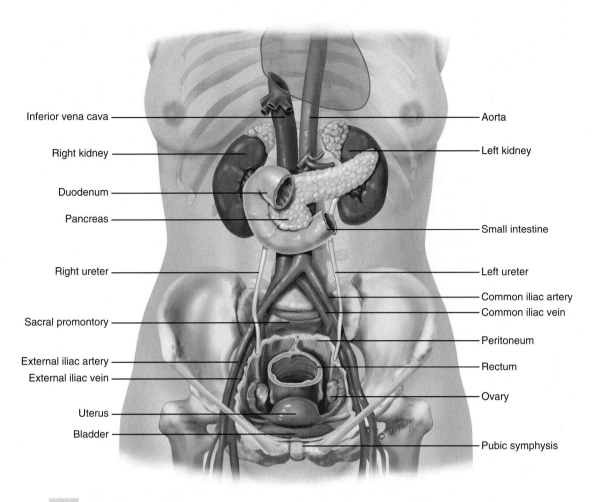

Inferior vena cava

Right kidney

Duodenum

Pancreas

Right ureter

Sacral promontory

External iliac artery

External iliac vein

Uterus

Bladder

Aorta

Left kidney

Small intestine

Left ureter

Common iliac artery

Common iliac vein

Peritoneum

Rectum

Ovary

Pubic symphysis

22.4 © Pat Thomas, 2006.

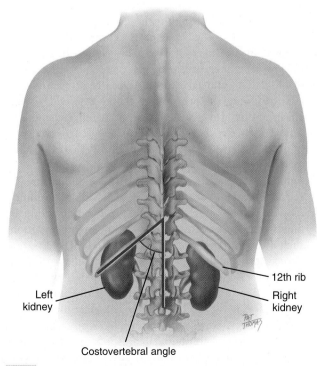

Left kidney

12th rib

Right kidney

Costovertebral angle

22.5 © Pat Thomas, 2006.

located higher in the abdomen in newborns than in adults. It lies between the symphysis and the umbilicus. During early childhood, the abdominal wall is less muscular, which may make the organs easier to palpate.

Children with gastroenteritis, particularly those younger than 1 year of age, are at increased risk for dehydration because of their relatively small body weights and high turnover of water and electrolytes. Signs of clinical dehydration that indicate increased risk for progression to shock include altered responsiveness (irritability, lethargy), sunken eyes, tachycardia, tachypnea, and reduced skin turgor.[1]

Pregnant Women

Nausea and vomiting, or "morning sickness," is an early sign of pregnancy in many pregnant women, starting between the first and second missed periods. The cause is unknown but may be related to hormone changes, such as the production of human chorionic gonadotropin. Another symptom is "acid indigestion," or heartburn, caused by esophageal reflux. Elevated levels of progesterone relax all smooth muscle, which leads to a decrease in gastro-intestinal motility and prolongation of gastric emptying time. As a result of decreased motility, more water is reabsorbed from the colon, which leads to constipation. Constipation, as well as

Four quadrants

22.6

increased venous pressure in the lower pelvis, may lead to formation of hemorrhoids.

The enlarging uterus displaces the intestines upward and posteriorly. Bowel sounds are diminished. Although the appendix may move during pregnancy, causing appendicitis-related pain in an atypical location, most pregnant women with appendicitis experience RLQ pain.[2] Skin changes on the abdomen, such as striae and linea nigra, are discussed later in this chapter and in Chapter 13.

Older Adults

Aging alters the appearance of the abdominal wall. During and after middle age, some fat accumulates in the suprapubic area in women as a result of decreased estrogen levels. Men also show some fat deposits in the abdominal area, resulting in the "big belly." This development is accentuated in adults with a sedentary lifestyle. With further aging, adipose tissue is redistributed away from the face and extremities to the abdomen and hips, and the abdominal musculature relaxes. Changes of aging occur in the gastro-intestinal system but do not significantly affect function as long as no disease is present.

- Salivation decreases, causing dryness of the mouth and a decrease in the sense of taste. Further changes are discussed in Chapter 17.
- Esophageal emptying is delayed. Feeding an older adult in the supine position increases the risk for aspiration.
- Gastric acid secretion decreases with aging. As a result, the absorption of orally administered medications may be impaired or delayed. This may cause pernicious anemia (as a result of impaired vitamin B_{12} absorption), iron deficiency anemia, and malabsorption of calcium.

- Older adults are more susceptible to dehydration because the ability to conserve water is reduced, as are the ability to respond to changes in temperature and the acuteness of thirst.
- Liver size decreases with age, particularly after 80 years, although most liver function remains normal. Age-related reductions in liver blood flow and medication-metabolizing enzyme content influences medication metabolism and the variability in response to beneficial and adverse medication effects seen in older adults.[3]
- Renal function decreases with age, contributing to the increased risk for adverse or toxic medication effects, as most medications are eventually cleared through the kidneys after metabolism in the liver. Older adults who drink alcohol and take medications are at even greater risk, including exacerbation of therapeutic and adverse effects and interference with medication effectiveness.[4]
- The incidence of gallstones increases with age, occurring in up to 20% of Canadian women and 10% of Canadian men by age 60.[5]
- Age-related changes alone do not account for the frequent reports of constipation by older adults. Common risk factors in older adults include functional impairments such as decreased mobility, pathological conditions such as hypothyroidism, adverse medication effects, and poor dietary habits, including inadequate intake of fluids and fibre.[6] Additional lifestyle factors that contribute to constipation include prolonged use and overuse of laxatives; ignoring the defecation urge; sedentary lifestyle; and polypharmacy.[7] Medications associated with constipation include opioids, nonsteroidal anti-inflammatory drugs (NSAIDs), antacids containing aluminum or calcium,

anticholinergics (e.g., anticonvulsants, antidepressants, antiparkinson agents) diuretics, calcium channel blockers, and calcium or iron supplements.

- The risk for colorectal cancer increases with age. See Chapter 23 for screening recommendations.

 ## SOCIAL DETERMINANTS OF HEALTH CONSIDERATIONS

Although the prevalence of obesity has increased significantly in all Canadian provinces over the past decade, prevalence rates among women in lower-income households continues to be 1.5 times higher than among women in higher-income households (20% versus 13%).[8] Obesity increases the risk for health problems including diabetes, certain types of cancer including esophageal cancer, and digestive problems including gallstones, fatty liver, cirrhosis of the liver, and **gastroesophageal reflux disease (GERD)**. On average, 5 million Canadians experience troublesome symptoms of heartburn and/or acid regurgitation associated with GERD at least once each week.[9] Risk factors for GERD include increasing age, obesity, hiatus hernia, smoking, pregnancy, food choices, and family history of GERD.

According to the Canadian Digestive Health Foundation (CDHF), **lactose intolerance** affects more than 7 million Canadians.[10] These individuals have lower levels of lactase, the intestinal enzyme that digests lactose found in milk, and experience cramps, bloating, abdominal pain, and diarrhea when dairy products are consumed in large amounts. However, avoidance of milk products can compromise calcium and vitamin D intakes, and research has found that lactose-intolerant individuals can consume moderate amounts of lactose without perceptible symptoms.[11]

Celiac disease is an inherited autoimmune condition in which intestinal tissue is damaged in response to eating gluten, which prevents nutrients from being properly absorbed. It is estimated that as many as 330 000 Canadians are living with celiac disease, with only about 110 000 having been diagnosed.[12] Untreated celiac disease can lead to medical problems such as lactose intolerance, malnutrition, osteoporosis, colon cancer, and lymphoma.

Canada has the highest incidence of **gastro-intestinal ulcers** in the world. Peptic ulcer disease increases with age and occurs with frequent use of NSAIDS, alcohol, smoking, and infection with *Helicobacter pylori*. Eight to 10 million Canadians have *H. pylori* infection, which is also associated with development of stomach cancer; approximately 75% of First Nations people are infected with *H. pylori*.[13]

Canada also has among the highest prevalence and incidence rates of **inflammatory bowel disease (IBD)** and **irritable bowel syndrome (IBS)** in the world. Approximately 233 000 Canadians are living with IBD: 129 000 people have Crohn's disease, 104 000 have ulcerative colitis.[14] In addition, approximately 5 million Canadians are living with IBS.[15] IBD can be diagnosed at any age, but usual onset is in the 20s for Crohn's disease and throughout adulthood for ulcerative colitis; incidence for both diseases peaks by age 30 and does not decline until age 80. A diagnosis of IBD is associated with a higher risk for colorectal cancer.

Infectious diseases such as hepatitis A and gastro-intestinal illnesses are often related to socioeconomic factors such as inadequate housing, sewage, and water-treatment facilities (see the box Promoting Health: Hepatitis Risk). These conditions are often present in Indigenous communities.[16] The most common gastro-intestinal and parasitic infections in refugee populations are *Giardia*, worm infections (e.g., roundworm [*Ascaris*], whipworm [*Trichuris*], and hookworm), and parasites of the *Strongyloides* and *Schistosoma* species.[17] Screening for *Strongyloides* with serological tests is recommended for immigrants and refugees newly arrived from Southeast Asia and Africa; screening for *Schistosoma* is recommended for individuals newly arrived from Africa.[18]

PROMOTING HEALTH: HEPATITIS RISK

How Is Your Liver Doing?

The liver is the largest organ in the body. It has an immense capacity to heal and regenerate, but that capacity is not infinite. Unfortunately, signs of severe liver damage or disease usually do not become apparent until the liver has been significantly harmed. The best protection for the liver is to prevent damage *before* it occurs!

Many self-management measures can be taken to protect the liver:

- *Practise safer sex.* Do not have unprotected sex with a man or woman.
- *Do not share items that may have bodily fluids on them.* This means needles, razors, nail clippers, cuticle scissors, and toothbrushes. When getting a tattoo, make sure that a new bottle of ink is opened and used only for you. Access clean needle exchange programs if you use injected drugs.
- *Be aware of your environment.* Be careful with aerosol cleaners. Make sure rooms are well ventilated. Wear a

mask, a hat, or protective clothing when you use insecticides, fungicides, paint, or other toxic chemicals. The liver can be damaged by what you breathe or absorb through your skin.

- *Monitor your diet and weight.* Obesity can cause a condition called *nonalcoholic fatty liver disease*, which may include cirrhosis.
- *Travel wisely.* Visit a travel medicine clinic before travelling. If you travel to an area with an increased rate of hepatitis A, such as Mexico, Central America, and the Caribbean, get vaccinated; avoid eating uncooked food, including raw vegetables; avoid drinking unboiled or unbottled water (including ice cubes); and brush your teeth with boiled or bottled water.
- *Use medications wisely.* Use prescription and over-the-counter medications only when needed. Be sure to take only the recommended doses.

Continued

Structure and Function

Subjective Data

PROMOTING HEALTH: HEPATITIS RISK—cont'd

How Is Your Liver Doing?

- *Do not mix medications without consulting a health care provider.* Mixing certain medications can form toxic compounds that can cause liver damage. Be certain that all medications, including over-the-counter and herbal preparations, are approved by a health care provider.
- *Drink alcohol in moderation.* More than one drink a day for women or two drinks a day for men over many years may be enough to lead to cirrhosis. A cirrhotic liver shrinks to a fraction of its former size and ability.
- *Do not mix medications and alcohol.* Acetaminophen (Tylenol) can be toxic to the liver even if a person drinks alcohol in moderation.
- *Do not use illegal drugs.* Cocaine is one of many illegal drugs known to cause liver damage.
- *Get vaccinated.* A vaccine is available for both hepatitis A and hepatitis B. Universal immunization of children and adolescents against hepatitis B is now part of the publicly funded vaccine programs offered in all Canadian provinces and territories.
- *Be aware of your risk for hepatitis.* Six hepatitis viruses have been identified, but three—hepatitis A (HAV), hepatitis B (HBV), and hepatitis C (HCV)—cause approximately 90% of acute hepatitis cases in Canada. The annual incidence of HAV illness has been estimated at 2.9 cases per 100 000 persons in Canada; the annual incidence of HBV illness is higher, at approximately 4.9 cases per 100 000 persons; and the annual incidence of HCV illness is highest, at between 10 and 20 cases per 100 000 persons.

HAV is spread primarily through food or water contaminated by feces from an infected patient. Risk factors for HAV infection include the following:

- Eating food prepared by someone who has HAV infection and poor hygiene
- Eating raw or undercooked shellfish (such as oysters or clams)
- Eating uncooked food, including unpeeled fruits and vegetables

- Travelling to HAV-endemic areas
- Having homosexual relations
- Sharing a household with an HAV-infected patient

HBV is spread primarily through contact with infected blood or bodily fluids. Risk factors for HBV infection include the following:

- Having unprotected sex, especially with someone with HBV infection or whose sexual history is unknown
- Sharing needles or other drug use equipment, including spoons, water, and cotton, to inject illegal drugs
- Handling blood or bodily fluids as a routine part of your job (e.g. nurses and other health care providers; morticians and embalmers)
- Getting body piercings or tattoos from a site in which infection control practices are poor
- Travelling to HBV-endemic areas
- Sharing a household with an HBV-infected patient
- Receiving dialysis treatment

HCV is spread primarily through contact with infected blood. Risk factors for HCV infection include the following:

- Having received a transfusion before 1992 or clotting factors before 1987
- Using illegal intravenous drugs or intranasal cocaine
- Handling blood or bodily fluids as a routine part of a job
- Receiving dialysis treatment
- Getting body piercings or tattoos from a site in which infection control practices are poor
- Sharing a household with an HCV-infected patient

References

Canadian Liver Foundation. (2016). *Viral hepatitis A, B, C*. Retrieved from http://www.liver.ca/liver-disease/types/viral-hepatitis-a-b-c.aspx.

Health Canada. (2013). *Hepatitis*. Retrieved from http://www.hc-sc.gc.ca/hc-ps/dc-ma/hep-eng.php.

SUBJECTIVE DATA

1. Appetite
2. Dysphagia
3. Food intolerance
4. Abdominal pain
5. Nausea/vomiting
6. Bowel habits
7. Past abdominal history
8. Medications
9. Alcohol and tobacco
10. Nutritional assessment

HEALTH HISTORY QUESTIONS

Examiner Asks	Rationale
1. Appetite. Any change in **appetite**? Is it increased or decreased? • Any change in weight? How much weight gained or lost? Over what time period? Due to change in diet?	**Anorexia** is a loss of appetite that occurs with gastro-intestinal disease, is an adverse effect of some medications, occurs with pregnancy, or occurs with psychological disorders. Loss of appetite and unexplained weight loss may be a sign of gastro-intestinal cancers such as stomach, esophageal, and pancreatic cancer.
2. Dysphagia. Any **difficulty swallowing**? When did you first notice this?	**Dysphagia** occurs with disorders of the throat or esophagus (e.g. later stages of esophageal cancer).
3. Food intolerance. Are there any foods you **cannot eat**? • What happens if you do eat them: allergic reaction, heartburn, belching, bloating, indigestion? • Do you use antacids? How often?	Examples of food intolerance are lactase deficiency (resulting in bloating, excessive gas, or diarrhea after ingesting milk products) and wheat allergy or gluten intolerance (resulting in abdominal pain, distension, or diarrhea). **Pyrosis** (heartburn) is a burning sensation in esophagus and stomach, caused by reflux of gastric acid. **Excessive belching** may occur with food intolerance or hiatal hernia (stomach bulges up into the chest through the hiatal opening).
4. Abdominal pain. Do you have any **abdominal pain**? Please point to it. • Is the pain in one spot, or does it move around? • How did it start? How long have you had it? • Is the pain constant, or does it come and go? Does it occur before or after meals? Does it peak? When? • How would you describe the character: cramping (colic type), burning in pit of stomach, dull, stabbing, aching? • Is the pain relieved by food, or is it worse after eating? • Is the pain associated with menstruation or menstrual irregularities, stress, dietary indiscretion, fatigue, nausea and vomiting, gas, fever, rectal bleeding, frequent urination, vaginal or penile discharge? • What makes the pain worse: food, position, stress, medication, activity? • What have you tried to relieve pain: rest, heating pad, change in position, medication?	Abdominal pain may be *visceral*, from an internal organ (dull, general, poorly localized); *parietal*, from inflammation of overlying peritoneum (sharp, precisely localized, aggravated by movement); or *referred*, from a disorder in another site (see Table 22.3, p. 600). Acute pain that necessitates urgent diagnosis occurs with appendicitis, cholecystitis, bowel obstruction, or perforation of an organ. Pain in the upper abdomen is a symptom that may occur in the later stages of gastro-intestinal neoplasms (e.g. liver or pancreatic cancer). Chronic pain of gastric ulcers usually occurs on an empty stomach; pain of duodenal ulcers occurs 2 to 3 hours after a meal and is relieved by more food.
5. Nausea/vomiting. Any **nausea** or **vomiting**? • How often? How much comes up? What is the colour? Does it have an odour?	Nausea/vomiting is a common adverse effect of many medications, with gastro-intestinal disease, and in early pregnancy.

Examiner Asks	Rationale

Nausea/vomiting may occur in later stages of gastro-intestinal neoplasms, such as stomach, liver, or pancreatic cancer.

Hematemesis (blood in vomit) occurs with stomach or duodenal ulcers and esophageal varices.

- Is it bloody?

- Are the nausea and vomiting associated with colicky pain, diarrhea, fever, chills?
- What foods did you eat in the past 24 hours? Where: at home, school, a restaurant? Has anyone else in the family had the same symptoms in the past 24 hours?

Consider food poisoning.

- Any recent travel? Where to? Did you drink the local water or eat fruit? Did you swim in public beaches or pools?

Nausea, vomiting and diarrhea occur when exposed to new local pathogens in developing countries. Water supply may be contaminated.

6. **Bowel habits**. How often do you have a **bowel movement**?
   - What is the colour? Consistency?
   - Any diarrhea or constipation? How long?
   - Any recent change in bowel habits?
   - Do you use laxatives? Which ones? How often do you use them?

Assess usual **bowel habits**.

Stools may be black and tarry because of occult blood (melena) from gastro-intestinal bleeding, or they may be black but nontarry because of iron medications. Grey stools occur with hepatitis.

Red blood in stools occurs with gastro-intestinal bleeding or localized bleeding around the anus. A change in bowel habits, stools that are narrower than usual, blood in the stool, diarrhea, and constipation are possible symptoms of colorectal cancer and necessitate further investigations.

7. **Past abdominal history**. Any **history** of gastro-intestinal problems: ulcer, gallbladder disease, hepatitis/jaundice, appendicitis, colitis, hernia?
   - Any **family history** of inflammatory bowel disease (IBD), colorectal cancer, or **familial adenomatous polyposis (FAP)**?
   - Ever had any operations in the abdomen? Please describe.
   - Any problems after surgery?
   - Any abdominal X-ray studies? How were the results?

FAP is caused by a genetic mutation that can be inherited. In individuals with FAP, the risk for colon cancer is 87% by age 45.

Abdominal adhesions (scar tissue in the abdomen) from previous abdominal surgery or infections can cause pain, nausea, vomiting, cramping, constipation, bloating or a complete bowel obstruction.

8. **Medications**. What **medications** are you currently taking?
   - Do you take over-the-counter remedies?
   - Do you take natural or herbal supplements?
   - Do you use probiotics or prebiotics?

Many prescription and over-the-counter medications, such as acetaminophen and salicylates, can have toxic effects on the liver. Peptic ulcer disease occurs with frequent use of NSAIDs, alcohol, smoking, and *H. pylori* infection.

Herbal supplements such as ginkgo biloba may cause gastro-intestinal upset, nausea and vomiting, or prolonged bleeding.

Preliminary evidence exists for several uses for probiotics, including ulcerative colitis.[19] However, patients often rely on nonclinical information sources; therefore, nurses should offer evidence-informed advice.[20]

Examiner Asks	Rationale

9. Alcohol and tobacco. How much **alcohol** would you say you drink each day? Each week? When was your most recent alcoholic drink?
- Do you **smoke**? How many packs per day? How long have you smoked?

Heavy alcohol drinking is a risk factor for esophageal cancer, liver cancer, and cirrhosis of the liver. Alcohol can also increase the toxic effects of medications such as acetaminophen, resulting in damage to the liver and kidneys.

Smoking is a risk factor for esophageal, stomach, and pancreatic cancers.

10. Nutritional assessment. Now I would like to ask you about your **diet**. Please tell me all the food you ate yesterday, starting with breakfast.
- Does the diet follow *Eating Well with Canada's Food Guide*?[21] Does the diet include adequate fluids and fibre?
- Which fresh-food markets are located in your neighbourhood?

Nutritional assessment is based on a 24-hour recall (see Chapter 12 for a complete discussion).

Eating high-fibre foods and drinking plenty of fluids helps keep the bowels regular, helps with weight control, and may protect against colon cancer.[22]

Many inner-city neighbourhoods are fresh-food deserts, lacking produce markets but full of fast-food restaurants.

Additional History for Infants and Children

1. Feeding infants. Are you breastfeeding or formula feeding the baby? If formula feeding, how does the baby tolerate the formula?

2. Table foods. What table foods have you introduced? How does the infant tolerate the food?

Consider a new food as a possible allergen. Adding only one new food at a time to the infant's diet helps identify allergies.

3. Eating patterns. How often does your child eat? Does your child eat regular meals?
- Does the child's diet follow Canada's Food Guide?
- How do you feel about your child's eating problems?
- Please describe all that your child had to eat yesterday, starting with breakfast. What foods does the child eat for snacks?
- Does the child ever eat nonfoods (grass, dirt, paint chips)?

Irregular eating patterns are common among children and a source of parental anxiety. As long as a child shows normal growth and development and only nutritious foods are offered, parents may be reassured. Refer to *Eating Well with Canada's Food Guide* in Chapter 12.

Although children may attempt to eat nonfoods (**pica**) at some time, they should recognize which materials are edible by age 2 years.

4. Constipation. Does your child have constipation: How long?
- What are the number of stools per day? Stools per week?
- How much water or juice is in the diet?
- Does the constipation seem to be associated with toilet training?
- What have you tried to treat the constipation?

5. Abdominal pain. Does the child have abdominal pain? Please describe what you have noticed and when it started.

Pain is hard to assess with young children. Many conditions of unrelated organ systems (e.g., otitis media) are associated with vague abdominal pain. Children cannot articulate specific symptoms and often focus on "the tummy." Abdominal pain accompanies inflammation of the bowel, constipation, urinary tract infection, and anxiety.

Subjective Data

Examiner Asks	Rationale
6. Overweight children. How long has weight been a problem? • At what age did the child first seem overweight? Did any change in diet pattern occur then? Is Canada's Food Guide being followed? • Describe the diet pattern now. • Describe the child's physical activity pattern. Are the *Canadian 24-Hour Movement Guidelines for Children and Youth*[23] being followed? • Do any other family members have a similar problem? • How does child feel about his, her, or their weight?	Poor food choices and reduced physical activity contribute to obesity. Children and youth should limit sedentary behaviours (especially screen time), and participate in a range of physical activities in a variety of environments (e.g., indoors, outdoors) and contexts (e.g., play, sport, hobbies, chores). Assess for family history of obesity. Assess body image and social adjustment.

Additional History for Adolescents

Examiner Asks	Rationale
1. Schedule and content. What do you eat at regular meals? Do you eat breakfast? What do you eat for snacks? • How many calories do you figure you consume?	Adolescents take control of eating and may reject family values (e.g., skipping breakfast; consuming junk foods, soft drinks). The only control parents have is over what food is in the home. You probably cannot change an adolescent's eating pattern, but you can supply nutritional facts.
2. Exercise. What is your exercise pattern?	Boys need, on average, 4 000 calories/day to maintain weight and more calories if they participate in sports. Girls need 20% fewer calories and the same nutrients as boys. Fast food is high in fat, calories, and salt, and has no fibre.
3. Underweight. If weight is less than body requirements: How much have you lost? By diet, exercise, or how? • How do you feel? Tired, hungry? How do you think your body looks? • What is your activity pattern? • Is the weight loss associated with any other body change, such as menstrual irregularity? • What do your parents say about your eating? Your friends?	Screen any extremely thin adolescent for **anorexia nervosa**, a serious psychosocial disorder that includes loss of appetite, voluntary starvation, and grave weight loss. Such patients may augment weight loss by purging (self-induced vomiting) and using laxatives. Denial of hunger and tiredness is common in anorexia. Although thin, such patients insist that they look fat and "disgusting." Body image is distorted. Patients with anorexia may have healthy activity and exercise, but many are hyperactive. Amenorrhea is common with anorexia nervosa. This is a family problem involving control issues. Anyone at risk requires immediate referral to a physician or psychologist.

Additional History for Older Adults

Examiner Asks	Rationale
1. Food access. How do you acquire your groceries and prepare your meals?	Assess risk for nutritional deficit: limited access to grocery store, limited income, or limited cooking facilities; physical disability (impaired vision, decreased mobility, decreased strength, neurological deficit).

Examiner Asks	Rationale
2. Emotional characteristics. Do you eat alone or share meals with others?	Assess risk for nutritional deficit if the patient is living alone; the patient may not bother to prepare all meals. Assess for social isolation and depression.
3. Recall. Please tell me all that you had to eat yesterday, starting with breakfast.	Note: 24-hour recall may not be sufficient because daily pattern may vary. The patient should attempt a week-long diary of intake. Food pattern may be different during a month if monthly income (e.g., Old Age Security pension cheque) runs out.
• Do you have any trouble swallowing these foods? • What do you do right after eating: walk, take a nap?	
4. Bowel movements. How often do your bowels move? • If the patient reports constipation: What do you mean by "constipation"? How much liquid is in your diet? How much bulk or fibre? • Have you had fecal incontinence or soiling? • Do you take anything for constipation, such as laxatives? Which ones? How often? • What medications do you take?	To prevent constipation, fluid intake should be between 1 500 and 2 000 mL/day; dietary fibre intake should be from 21 to 25 g/day.[7] Fecal incontinence and constipation often occur together. Consider gastro-intestinal adverse effects (e.g., nausea, upset stomach, anorexia, dry mouth).

OBJECTIVE DATA

PREPARATION

Expose the patient's abdomen so that it is fully visible. Drape the genitalia and female breasts.

The following measures will enhance abdominal wall relaxation:

- Instruct the patient to empty the bladder, saving a urine specimen if needed.
- Keep the room warm to avoid chilling and tensing of muscles.
- Position the patient supine, with the head on a pillow, the knees bent or on pillow, and the arms at the sides or across the chest. (Note: Discourage the patient from placing arms over the head, because this tenses abdominal musculature.)
- To avoid abdominal tensing, warm the stethoscope endpiece and your hands, and keep your fingernails very short.
- Inquire about any painful areas. Examine such an area last to avoid any muscle guarding.

Finally, learn to use distraction: enhance muscle relaxation through breathing exercises and/or emotive imagery; keep your voice low and soothing; and encourage the patient to relate any personal abdominal history while you palpate.

EQUIPMENT NEEDED

Strong overhead light
Secondary stand light
Stethoscope
Small centimetre ruler
Skin-marking pen
Alcohol wipe (to clean endpiece)
Drape

Objective Data

Normal Range of Findings	Abnormal Findings

Inspect the Abdomen

Contour

Stand on the patient's right side and look down on the abdomen. Then stoop or sit to gaze across the abdomen. Your head should be slightly higher than the abdomen. Determine the profile from the rib margin to the pubic bone. The contour describes the nutritional state and normally ranges from flat to rounded (Fig. 22.7 and Fig. 22.8).

A scaphoid abdomen caves in. Protuberant abdomen and abdominal distension (see Table 22.1, p. 597) are abnormal.

Flat

Scaphoid

Rounded

Protuberant

22.7

22.8

Symmetry

Shine a light across the abdomen toward you or lengthwise across the patient. The abdomen should be symmetrical bilaterally. Note any localized bulging, visible mass, or asymmetrical shape. Even small bulges are highlighted by shadow. Step to the foot of the examination table to recheck symmetry.

Ask the patient to take a deep breath to further highlight any change. The abdomen should stay smooth and symmetrical. You can also ask the patient to perform a sit-up without using the hands to push up.

Bulges, masses.

Hernia: protrusion of abdominal viscera through abnormal opening in muscle wall (see Table 22.4, p. 601).

Note any localized bulging.

Hernia, enlarged liver, or spleen may show.

Umbilicus

Normally the umbilicus is midline and inverted, with no sign of discoloration, inflammation, or hernia. It becomes everted and pushed upward during pregnancy.

The umbilicus is a common site for piercings in young women. The site should not be red or crusted.

Everted: with ascites or underlying mass (see Table 22.1, p. 598).

Deeply sunken: with obesity.

Enlarged and everted: with umbilical hernia.

Bluish periumbilical colour: with intra-abdominal bleeding (Cullen's sign), although rare.

Normal Range of Findings

Skin

The surface is smooth and even, with homogeneous colour. This area is helpful for judging pigment because it is often protected from sun.

One common pigment change is **striae** (lineae albicantes), which are silvery white, linear, jagged marks approximately 1 to 6 cm long (Fig. 22.9). They occur when elastic fibres in the reticular layer of the skin are broken after rapid or prolonged stretching, as in pregnancy or excessive weight gain. Recent striae are pink or blue; then they turn silvery white.

22.9   Striae.

Pigmented nevi (moles), which are circumscribed brown macular or papular areas, are common on the abdomen.

Normally, no lesions are present. If a scar is present, ask about it and draw its location in the patient's record, indicating the length in centimetres (Fig. 22.10). A surgical scar alerts you to the possible presence of underlying adhesions and excess fibrous tissue.

6 cm

11 cm

22.10

Abnormal Findings

Redness: with localized inflammation.

Jaundice (shows best in natural daylight).

Glistening and tautness of skin: with ascites.

Striae also occur with ascites.

Striae look purple-blue in patients with Cushing's syndrome (because excess adrenocortical hormone causes the skin to be fragile and easily broken from normal stretching).

Unusual colour or change in shape of mole (see Chapter 13).

Petechiae.

Cutaneous angiomas (spider nevi) occur with portal hypertension or liver disease.

Lesions and rashes warrant investigation (see Chapter 13).

Underlying adhesions are inflammatory bands that connect opposite sides of serous surfaces after trauma or surgery.

Normal Range of Findings

Veins usually are not seen, but a fine venous network may be visible in thin patients.

Good skin turgor reflects healthy nutrition. Gently pinch up a fold of skin; then release to note the skin's immediate return to original position.

Pulsation or Movement

Normally, you may see the pulsations from the aorta beneath the skin in the epigastric area, particularly in thin patients with good muscle wall relaxation. Respiratory movement also shows in the abdomen, particularly in men. Waves of peristalsis are sometimes visible in very thin patients. They ripple slowly and obliquely across the abdomen.

Hair Distribution

The pattern of pubic hair growth normally has a diamond shape in men and an inverted triangle shape in women (see Chapters 26 and 27).

Demeanour

A comfortable patient is quietly relaxed on the examining table, has a benign facial expression, and has slow, even respirations.

Auscultate Bowel Sounds and Vascular Sounds

Departing from the usual examination sequence, auscultation is done next because percussion and palpation can increase peristalsis, which would give a false interpretation of bowel sounds. If you hear a bruit during auscultation, you should avoid percussion and palpation. Use the diaphragm endpiece because bowel sounds are relatively high pitched. Hold the stethoscope lightly against the skin; pushing too hard may stimulate more bowel sounds (Fig. 22.11). Listen in all four quadrants, beginning in the RLQ at the ileocecal valve area because bowel sounds are normally always present here.

22.11

Abnormal Findings

Veins may become prominent and dilated with portal hypertension, cirrhosis, ascites, or vena caval obstruction. Veins are more visible with malnutrition as a result of thinned adipose tissue.

Turgor is poor with dehydration, which often accompanies gastro-intestinal disease.

Pulsation of the aorta is marked with widened pulse pressure (e.g., hypertension, aortic insufficiency, thyrotoxicosis) and with aortic aneurysm.

Markedly visible peristalsis, together with abdominal distension, indicates intestinal obstruction.

Patterns alter with endocrine or hormone abnormalities or chronic liver disease.

Restlessness and constant turning to find comfort occur with the colicky pain of gastroenteritis or bowel obstruction (see Table 22.2, p. 599, and Table 22.3, p. 601).

Absolute stillness, resisting any movement, occurs with the pain of peritonitis.

Upward flexing of the knees, facial grimacing, and rapid, uneven respirations also indicate pain.

Normal Range of Findings

Bowel Sounds

Note the character and frequency of bowel sounds. Bowel sounds originate from the movement of air and fluid through the small intestine. Depending on the time elapsed since eating, normal sounds range widely. Bowel sounds are high-pitched, gurgling, cascading sounds, occurring irregularly anywhere from 5 to 30 times per minute. Do not bother to count them. Judge whether they are normal, hyperactive, or hypoactive.

One type of hyperactive bowel sounds is fairly common: the hyperperistalsis when you feel your "stomach growling," termed **borborygmus**. A perfectly "silent abdomen" is uncommon; you must listen for 5 minutes by your watch before deciding that bowel sounds are completely absent.

Vascular Sounds

Using firmer pressure, listen with the bell of the stethoscope to check over the aorta and the renal, iliac, and femoral arteries, especially in patients with hypertension (Fig. 22.12). Note the presence of any vascular sounds or **bruits**. Usually, no such sound is present.

Aorta

Left renal artery

Iliac artery

Femoral artery

22.12

Percuss General Tympany

Percuss to assess the relative density of abdominal contents, to locate organs, and to screen for abnormal fluid or masses.

General Tympany

First, percuss lightly in all four quadrants to determine the prevailing amount of tympany and dullness (Fig. 22.13). Move clockwise. Tympany should predominate because air in the intestines rises to the surface when the patient is supine.

Abnormal Findings

Abnormal bowel sounds have two distinct patterns:
1. **Hyperactive sounds** are loud, high-pitched, rushing, tinkling sounds that signal increased motility and may indicate bowel obstruction.
2. Sounds may be **hypoactive** or **absent** after abdominal surgery or with inflammation of the peritoneum (see Table 22.5, p. 603).

Note location, pitch, and timing of a vascular sound.

A systolic bruit is a pulsatile blowing sound and occurs with stenosis or occlusion of an artery.

Venous hum and peritoneal friction rub are rare (see Table 22.6, p. 603 and the following Critical Findings box).

CRITICAL FINDINGS

If a bruit is heard over the aorta, you should *not* palpate the area, to avoid rupturing a possible aortic aneurysm. Report findings immediately.

Dullness is heard over solid structures (e.g., liver), a distended bladder, adipose tissue, fluid, or a mass.

Hyper-resonance is heard with gaseous distension.

Objective Data

Normal Range of Findings	Abnormal Findings

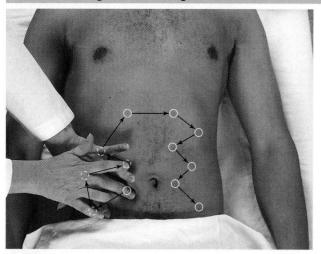

22.13

Palpate Surface Areas

Perform **light palpation** to assess surface characteristics such as texture, temperature, moisture, swelling, rigidity, pulsation, and presence of tenderness or pain. Review comfort measures under Preparation on p. 577. Because most people are naturally inclined to protect their abdomen, use additional measures to enhance complete muscle relaxation:

1. Bend the patient's knees.
2. Keep your palpating hand low and parallel to the abdomen. Holding the hand high and pointing down would make anyone tense up.
3. Coach the patient to breathe slowly (in through the nose, and out through the mouth).
4. Keep your own voice low and soothing. Conversation may relax the patient.
5. Try "emotive imagery." For example, you might say, "Imagine you are dozing on the beach, with the sun warming your muscles and the sound of the waves lulling you to sleep. Let yourself relax."
6. With a very ticklish patient, keep the patient's hand under your own with your fingers curled over the patient's fingers. Move both hands around as you palpate; people are not ticklish to themselves.
7. Alternatively, perform palpation just after auscultation. Keep the stethoscope in place and curl your fingers around it, palpating as you pretend to auscultate. People generally do not perceive a stethoscope as a ticklish object. You can slide the stethoscope out when the patient is used to being touched.

Light Palpation

With the first four fingers close together, depress the skin approximately 1 cm (Fig. 22.14). Make a gentle rotary motion, sliding the fingers and skin together. Then lift the fingers (do not drag them) and move clockwise to the next location around the abdomen. The objective here is not to search for organs but to form an overall impression of the skin surface and superficial musculature. Save the examination of any identified tender areas until last. This avoids causing pain and the resulting muscle rigidity that would obscure deep palpation later in the examination (if applicable).

Muscle guarding.
Rigidity.
Large masses.
Tenderness (see the following Critical Findings box).

Normal Range of Findings

22.14

As you circle the abdomen, discriminate between voluntary muscle guarding and involuntary rigidity. **Voluntary guarding** occurs when the patient is cold, tense, or ticklish. It is bilateral, and you will feel the muscles relax slightly during exhalation. Use the relaxation measures described previously to try to eliminate this type of guarding. If rigidity persists, it is probably involuntary.

❖ DEVELOPMENTAL CONSIDERATIONS

Infants

Inspection. The contour of the abdomen is protuberant because of the immature abdominal musculature. The skin exhibits a fine, superficial venous pattern that may be visible in lightly pigmented children until puberty.

Inspect the umbilical cord throughout the neonatal period. At birth, it is white and contains two umbilical arteries and one vein surrounded by mucoid connective tissue, called *Wharton's jelly.* The umbilical stump dries within a week, hardens, and falls off by 10 to 14 days after birth. Skin covers the area by 3 to 4 weeks.

The abdomen should be symmetrical, although two bulges are common. You may note an **umbilical hernia**. It appears 2 to 3 weeks after birth and is especially prominent when the infant cries. The hernia reaches maximum size at 1 month of age (up to 2.5 cm) and usually disappears by 1 year of age. Another common variation is **diastasis recti**, a separation of the rectus muscles with a visible bulge along the midline (see Table 22.4, p. 602). The condition is more common in infants of African descent, and it usually disappears by early childhood.

The abdomen shows respiratory movement. The only other abdominal movement you should note is occasional peristalsis, which may be visible because of thin musculature.

Auscultation. Auscultation yields only bowel sounds—the metallic tinkling of peristalsis. No vascular sounds should be heard.

Abnormal Findings

CRITICAL FINDINGS

RLQ tenderness on palpation in a patient with acute abdominal pain migrating from the umbilicus to the RLQ is indicative of acute appendicitis, which can progress to perforation and peritonitis.[24]

Immediate referral to a surgeon is required. Associated symptoms include nausea, vomiting, fever, and loss of appetite. Additional signs include guarding, rigidity, rebound tenderness, and iliopsoas (see p. 594).

RLQ, Right lower quadrant.

Involuntary rigidity is a constant board-like hardness of the muscles. It is a protective mechanism accompanying peritonitis, an acute inflammation of the peritoneum. It may be unilateral, and the same area usually becomes painful when the patient increases intra-abdominal pressure by attempting a sit-up.

Scaphoid shape: occurs with dehydration.

Dilated veins.

The presence of only one artery signals the possibility of congenital defects.

Inflammation should be investigated.

Drainage after cord stump falls off is abnormal and should be investigated.

Refer for investigation any umbilical hernia that is larger than 2.5 cm (see Table 22.4, p. 601); continues to grow after 1 month; or lasts more than 2 years in a child of European descent or for more than 7 years in a child of African descent.

Refer for investigation diastasis recti that lasts more than 6 years.

Marked peristalsis with pyloric stenosis (see Table 22.5, p. 602).

Bruit.
Venous hum.

Normal Range of Findings	Abnormal Findings

Percussion. Percussion reveals tympany over the stomach (the infant swallows some air with feeding) and dullness over the liver. The spleen is not percussed in infants. The abdomen sounds tympanitic, although it is normal to percuss dullness over the bladder. This dullness may extend up to the umbilicus.

Palpation. Aid palpation by flexing the baby's knees with one hand while palpating with the other (Fig. 22.15). Alternatively, hold the upper back and flex the neck slightly with one hand. Offer a pacifier to a crying baby. The liver fills the RUQ. It is normal to feel the liver edge at the right costal margin or 1 to 2 cm below. Normally, you may palpate the spleen tip, both kidneys, and the bladder. Also easily palpated are the cecum in the RLQ and the sigmoid colon, which feels like a sausage in the left inguinal area.

Make note of the newborn's first stool, a sticky, greenish black meconium stool within 24 hours of birth. By the fourth day, stools of breastfed babies are golden yellow, pasty, and smell like sour milk, whereas those of formula-fed babies are brown-yellow, firmer, and more fecal smelling.

22.15

Children

At ages younger than 4 years, the abdomen looks protuberant when the child is both supine and standing. After age 4 years, the potbelly remains when the child stands because of lumbar lordosis, but the abdomen looks flat when the child is supine. Normal movement on the abdomen includes respirations, which remain abdominal until 7 years of age.

To palpate the abdomen, position a young child on the parent's lap as you sit knee to knee with the parent (Fig. 22.16). Flex the child's knees up, and elevate the head slightly. You can ask the child to "pant like a dog" to further relax abdominal muscles. Hold your entire palm flat on the abdominal surface for a moment before starting palpation. This accustoms the child to being touched. If the child is very ticklish, hold the child's hand under your own as you palpate, or apply the stethoscope and palpate around it.

A scaphoid abdomen is associated with dehydration or malnutrition.

Before age 7 years of age, abdominal respirations are absent with inflammation of the peritoneum.

Normal Range of Findings	**Abnormal Findings**

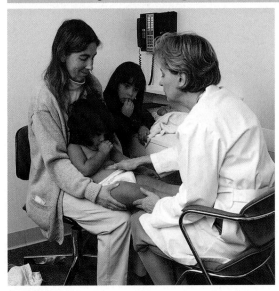

22.16

The liver remains easily palpable 1 to 2 cm below the right costal margin. The edge is soft and sharp and moves easily. On the left, the spleen also is easily palpable as a soft, sharp, movable edge. Usually you can feel 1 to 2 cm of the right kidney and the tip of the left kidney. Percussion of the liver span reveals measurements of approximately 3.5 cm at age 2 years, 5 cm at age 6 years, and 6 to 7 cm during adolescence.

When asking young children about abdominal tenderness, remember they often answer this question affirmatively no matter how the abdomen actually feels. Use objective signs to aid assessment, such as a cry changing in pitch as you palpate, facial grimacing, movement away from you, and guarding.

The school-age child has a slim abdominal shape once the potbelly is lost. This slimming trend continues into adolescence. Many adolescents are easily embarrassed by exposure of the abdomen, and adequate draping is necessary. The physical findings are the same as those listed for adults.

Older Adults

On inspection, you may note increased deposits of subcutaneous fat on the abdomen and hips because it is redistributed away from the extremities. Abdominal musculature is thinner and has less tone than that of younger adults; therefore, in the absence of obesity, you may note peristalsis.

Because the abdominal wall is thinner and softer, organs may be easier to palpate (in the absence of obesity). The liver is easier to palpate. Normally, you can feel the liver edge at or just below the costal margin. When the lungs are distended and the diaphragm is depressed, the liver is palpated lower, descending 1 to 2 cm below the costal margin with inhalation. The kidneys are easier to palpate.

Abdominal rigidity with acute abdominal conditions is less common in older adults.

Older adults with conditions that cause severe abdominal pain ("acute abdomen") often complain of less pain than do younger patients.

Objective Data

SPECIAL CONSIDERATIONS FOR ADVANCED PRACTICE

Normal Range of Findings	Abnormal Findings

Percuss Liver Span and Splenic Dullness

Liver Span

Percuss to map out boundaries of certain organs. Measure height of the liver in the right midclavicular line. (For a consistent placement of the midclavicular line landmark, remember to palpate the acromioclavicular and the sternoclavicular joints, and judge the line at a point midway between the two.)

Begin in the area of lung resonance, and percuss down the intercostal spaces until the sound changes to a dull quality (Fig. 22.17). Mark the spot on the patient's body, usually in the fifth intercostal space. Then find abdominal tympany and percuss up in the midclavicular line. Mark the spot on the patient's body where the sound changes from tympany to a dull sound, normally at the right costal margin.

22.17

Normal Range of Findings

Measure the distance between the two marks; the normal liver span in adults ranges from 6 to 12 cm (Fig. 22.18). The height of the liver span is correlated with the height of the patient; taller people have longer livers. Also, men have a longer liver span than women of the same height. Overall, the mean liver span is 10.5 cm in men and 7 cm in women.

22.18

One variation occurs in people with chronic emphysema, in which the liver is displaced downward by the hyperinflated lungs. Although you hear a dull percussion note well below the right costal margin, the overall span is still within normal limits.

Clinical estimation of liver span is important in screening for hepatomegaly and in monitoring changes in liver size. However, this measurement is a gross estimate; the liver span may be underestimated because of inaccurate detection of the upper border.

Scratch Test. Another assessment technique is the *scratch test*, which may help define the liver border when the abdomen is distended or the abdominal muscles are tense. Place your stethoscope over the liver. With one fingernail, scratch short strokes over the abdomen, starting in the RLQ and moving progressively up toward the liver (Fig. 22.19). When the scratching sound in your stethoscope becomes magnified, you will have crossed the border from over a hollow organ to over a solid one.

22.19

Abnormal Findings

Elongation of the liver span indicates liver enlargement (hepatomegaly).

Detection of liver borders is rendered inaccurate by dullness above the fifth intercostal space, which occurs with lung disease (e.g., pleural effusion or consolidation). Detection at the lower border is rendered inaccurate when dullness is pushed up with ascites or pregnancy or with gas distension in the colon, which obscures the lower border.

Normal Range of Findings	Abnormal Findings

Splenic Dullness

Often the spleen is obscured by stomach contents, but you may locate it by percussing for a dull note from the ninth to eleventh intercostal spaces just behind the left midaxillary line (Fig. 22.20). The area of splenic dullness normally is not wider than 7 cm in the adult and should not encroach on the normal tympany over the gastric air bubble.

A dull note forward of the midaxillary line indicates enlargement of the spleen, as occurs with mononucleosis, trauma, and infection.

22.20

Now percuss in the lowest intercostal space in the left *anterior* axillary line. You should hear tympany. Ask the patient to take a deep breath. Normally, tympany remains through full inspiration.

In the anterior axillary line, a change in percussion from tympany to a dull sound with full inspiration is a positive spleen percussion sign, indicating splenomegaly. This method helps detect mild to moderate splenomegaly before the spleen becomes palpable, as in mononucleosis, malaria, or hepatic cirrhosis.

Costovertebral Angle Tenderness

Indirect fist percussion causes the tissues to vibrate instead of producing a sound. To assess the kidney, place one hand over the twelfth rib at the costovertebral angle on the back (Fig. 22.21). Thump that hand with the ulnar edge of your other fist. The patient normally feels a thud but no pain. Perform the assessment bilaterally. (Although this step is explained here with percussion techniques, its usual sequence in a complete examination is with thoracic assessment, when the patient is sitting up and you are standing behind the patient.)

Sharp pain occurs with inflammation of the kidney or paranephric area.

Normal Range of Findings	Abnormal Findings

22.21

Palpate Deep Areas

If appropriate, perform **deep palpation** following light palpation to judge the size, location, and consistency of certain organs and to screen for an abnormal mass or tenderness.

Perform deep palpation using the same technique described earlier for light palpation, but push down approximately 5 to 8 cm (Fig. 22.22). Moving clockwise, palpate the entire abdomen.

22.22

To overcome the resistance of a very large or obese abdomen, use a bimanual technique. Place your two hands on top of each other (Fig. 22.23). The top hand does the pushing; the bottom hand is relaxed and can concentrate on the sense of palpation. With either a single-handed or bimanual technique, note the location, size, consistency, and mobility of any palpable organs and the presence of any abnormal enlargement, tenderness, or masses.

Normal Range of Findings	Abnormal Findings

22.23

Making sense of what you are palpating is more difficult than it seems. Inexperienced examiners complain that the abdomen "all feels the same," as if they are pushing their hand into a soft sofa cushion. It helps to memorize the anatomy and visualize what is under each quadrant as you palpate. Also remember that some structures are normally palpable, as illustrated in Fig. 22.24.

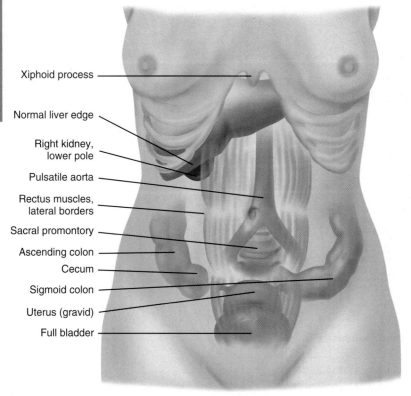

Xiphoid process

Normal liver edge

Right kidney, lower pole

Pulsatile aorta

Rectus muscles, lateral borders

Sacral promontory

Ascending colon

Cecum

Sigmoid colon

Uterus (gravid)

Full bladder

NORMALLY PALPABLE STRUCTURES

22.24

Normal Range of Findings

Mild tenderness normally is present when the sigmoid colon is palpated. Any other tenderness should be investigated.

If you identify a mass, first distinguish it from a normally palpable structure or an enlarged organ. Then note the following:
1. Location
2. Size
3. Shape
4. Consistency (soft, firm, hard)
5. Surface (smooth, nodular)
6. Mobility (including movement with respirations)
7. Pulsatility
8. Tenderness

Liver

Next, palpate for specific organs, beginning with the liver in the RUQ (Fig. 22.25). Place your left hand under the patient's back, parallel to the eleventh and twelfth ribs, and lift up to support the abdominal contents. Place your right hand on the RUQ, with fingers parallel to the midline. Push deeply down and under the right costal margin. Ask the patient to take a deep breath. It is normal to feel the edge of the liver bump your fingertips as the diaphragm pushes it down during inhalation. It feels like a firm, regular ridge. However, the liver is often not palpable, and you feel nothing firm.

22.25

Hooking Technique. An alternative method of palpating the liver is to stand at the patient's right shoulder and swivel your body to the right so that you face the patient's feet (Fig. 22.26). Hook your fingers over the costal margin from above. Ask the patient to take a deep breath. Try to feel the liver edge bump your fingertips.

22.26

Abnormal Findings

Tenderness occurs with local inflammation, with inflammation of the peritoneum or underlying organ, and with an enlarged organ whose capsule is stretched.

Except with a depressed diaphragm, a liver palpated more than 1 to 2 cm below the right costal margin is enlarged. Record the number of centimetres it descends, and note its consistency (hard, nodular) and tenderness (see Table 22.7, p. 604).

Normal Range of Findings	Abnormal Findings

Spleen

Normally, the spleen is not palpable and must be enlarged to three times its normal size to be felt. To search for it, reach over the abdomen with your left hand and behind the left side at the eleventh and twelfth ribs (Fig. 22.27, *A*). Lift up for support. Place your right hand obliquely on the LUQ with the fingers pointing toward the left axilla and just inferior to the rib margin. Push your hand deeply down and under the left costal margin, and ask the patient to take a deep breath. You should feel nothing firm.

When enlarged, the spleen slides out and bumps your fingertips (see the Critical Findings box to the right). It can grow so large that it extends into the lower quadrants. When this condition is suspected, start low on the abdomen so that you will not miss it. An alternative position is to roll the patient onto the right side to displace the spleen more forward and downward (Fig. 22.27, *B*). Then palpate as described earlier.

CRITICAL FINDINGS

The spleen becomes enlarged with mononucleosis and trauma (see Table 22.7, p. 605). If you feel enlargement of the spleen, refer the patient, but do *not* continue to palpate it. An enlarged spleen is friable and can rupture easily with overpalpation.

Describe the number of centimetres that the spleen extends below the left costal margin.

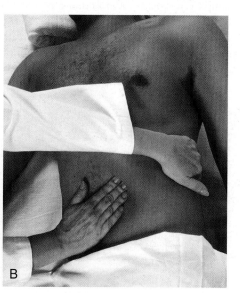

22.27

Kidneys

Search for the right kidney by placing your hands together in a "duck bill" position at the patient's right flank (Fig. 22.28, *A*). Press your two hands together firmly (you need deeper palpation than that used with the liver or spleen), and ask the patient to take a deep breath. In most people, you will feel no change. On occasion, you may feel the lower pole of the right kidney slide between your fingers as a round, smooth mass. Either condition is normal.

The left kidney sits 1 cm higher than the right kidney and is normally not palpable. Search for it by reaching your left hand across the abdomen and behind the left flank for support (see Fig. 22.28, *B*). Push your right hand deep into the abdomen, and ask the patient to breathe deeply. You should feel no change with the inhalation.

Enlarged kidney.
Kidney mass.

Normal Range of Findings	Abnormal Findings

22.28

Aorta

Using your opposing thumb and fingers, palpate the aortic pulsation in the upper abdomen slightly to the left of midline (Fig. 22.29). In adults, it is normally 2.5 to 4 cm wide and pulsates in an anterior direction.

22.29

Additional Special Procedures

Rebound Tenderness (Blumberg's Sign). Assess rebound tenderness when the patient reports abdominal pain or when you elicit tenderness during palpation. Choose a site away from the painful area. Hold your hand 90 degrees, or perpendicular, to the abdomen. Push down slowly and deeply (Fig. 22.30, *A*); then lift up quickly (Fig. 22.30, *B*). This makes structures that are indented by palpation rebound suddenly. A normal, or negative, response is no pain on release of pressure. Perform this test at the end of the examination, because it can cause severe pain and muscle rigidity.

Widened pulsation with abdominal aortic aneurysm (see Tables 22.6 and 22.7, pp. 603 and 605).

Prominent lateral pulsation with abdominal aortic aneurysm (see the following Critical Findings box).

CRITICAL FINDINGS

If a bruit was heard on auscultation, you should *not* palpate the area, to avoid rupturing an abdominal aortic aneurysm. Report findings immediately.

Pain on release of pressure confirms rebound tenderness, which is a reliable sign of peritoneal inflammation. Peritoneal inflammation accompanies appendicitis.

Cough tenderness that is localized to a specific spot also signals peritoneal irritation. Refer the patient with suspected appendicitis for computed tomographic (CT) scanning.

Special Considerations
for Advanced Practice

Normal Range of Findings	Abnormal Findings

22.30   Rebound tenderness.

Inspiratory Arrest (Murphy's Sign). Normally, palpating the liver causes no pain. In a patient with inflammation of the gallbladder, or cholecystitis, pain occurs. Hold your fingers under the liver border. Ask the patient to take a deep breath. A normal response is to complete the deep breath without pain.

Iliopsoas Muscle Test. Perform the iliopsoas muscle test when the acute abdominal pain is suspect for appendicitis. With the patient supine, lift the right leg straight up, flexing at the hip (Fig. 22.31); then push down over the lower part of the right thigh as the patient tries to hold the leg up. When the test result is negative, the patient feels no change.

22.31   Iliopsoas muscle test.

When the test result is positive, as the descending liver pushes the inflamed gallbladder onto the examining hand, the patient feels sharp pain and abruptly stops inspiration midway. (Note: This sign is less accurate in patients older than 60 years of age, who may not have any abdominal tenderness.)

When the iliopsoas muscle is inflamed (which occurs with an inflamed or perforated appendix), pain is felt in the RLQ.

Normal Range of Findings

The Alvarado Score. This scoring system combines findings to assist evaluation in patients with RLQ pain. It is also called the **MANTRELS score**, from the mnemonic in the following list.[25]

Finding	Points
Symptoms:	
Migration to right iliac fossa	1
Anorexia*	1
Nausea and vomiting	1
Signs:	
Tenderness, RLQ	2
Rebound tenderness	1
Elevation of temperature (oral ≥37.3°C)	1
Laboratory Findings:	
Leukocytosis (white blood cell count >10 000/μL)	2
Shift to the left (>75% neutrophils)	1
Total Possible Points	10

*For *anorexia*, may substitute *acetone in urine*.

Abnormal Findings

An Alvarado cut-off score of 4 or less is sufficiently sensitive to rule out appendicitis; The Alvarado Score is not sufficiently specific in diagnosing acute appendicitis; however, a score of 7 or more indicates an increased probability of appendicitis.[24,26]

DOCUMENTATION AND CRITICAL THINKING

Sample Charting

SUBJECTIVE

States appetite is good with no recent change, no dysphagia, no food intolerance, no pain, no nausea/vomiting. Has one formed BM [bowel movement]/day. Takes vitamins, no other prescribed or over-the-counter medication. No history of abdominal disease, injury, or surgery. Diet recall of past 24 hours listed at end of history.

OBJECTIVE

Inspection: Abdomen flat, symmetrical, with no apparent masses. Skin smooth with no striae, scars, or lesions.
Auscultation: Bowel sounds present, no bruits.
Percussion: Tympany predominates in all four quadrants; liver span is 8 cm in right midclavicular line. Splenic dullness located at tenth intercostal space in left midaxillary line.
Palpation: Abdomen soft; no organomegaly, no masses, no tenderness.

ASSESSMENT

Healthy abdomen, bowel sounds present

Focused Assessment: Clinical Case Study 1

George Eng (G.E.) is a 58-year-old unemployed, divorced man with chronic alcoholism who enters the chemical dependency treatment centre.

SUBJECTIVE

States past 6 months has been drinking 500 mL whisky/day. Last alcohol use 1 week PTA [prior to arrival], with "5 or 6" drinks that episode. Estranged from family, lives alone. Makes a few meals on hot plate. States never has appetite. Has fatigue and weakness.

OBJECTIVE

Inspection: G.E. appears older than stated age. Oriented, although verbal response time slowed. Weight loss of 5.5 kg in last 3 months. Abdomen protuberant, symmetrical, no visible masses. Poor skin turgor. Dilated venous pattern over abdominal wall. Hair sparse in axillary, pubic areas.

Auscultation: Bowel sounds present. No vascular sounds.

Percussion: Tympany predominates over abdomen. Liver span is 16 cm in right midclavicular line.

Palpation: Soft. Liver palpable 10 cm below right costal margin, smooth and nontender. No other organomegaly or masses.

ASSESSMENT

Alcohol dependence, severe, with physiological dependence
Imbalanced nutrition: less than body requirements R/T [related to] impaired absorption
Ineffective coping R/T effects of chronic alcoholism
Social isolation

Focused Assessment: Clinical Case Study 2

Edith Jules (E.J.) is a 63-year-old female, retired homemaker who has a history of lung cancer with metastasis to the liver.

SUBJECTIVE

Feeling "puffy and bloated" for the past week. States unable to get comfortable. Also short of breath "all the time now." Difficulty sleeping. "I feel like crying all the time now."

OBJECTIVE

Inspection: Weight increase of 3.7 kg in 1 week. E.J.'s abdomen is distended with everted umbilicus and bulging flanks. Girth at umbilicus is 85 cm. Prominent dilated venous pattern present over abdomen.

Auscultation: Bowel sounds present, no vascular sounds.

Percussion: When supine, tympany present at dome of abdomen, dullness over flanks. Liver span is 12 cm in right midclavicular line.

Palpation: Abdominal wall firm, able to feel liver with deep palpation at 6 cm below right costal margin. Liver feels firm, nodular, nontender. 4+ pitting edema in both ankles.

ASSESSMENT

Ascites
Grieving
Ineffective breathing pattern R/T increased intra-abdominal pressure
Pain R/T distended abdomen
Risk for impaired skin integrity: R/T ascites, edema, and faulty metabolism
Insomnia

Focused Assessment: Clinical Case Study 3

Dan Grieg (D.G.) is a 17-year-old male high school student who enters the emergency department with abdominal pain of 2 days' duration.

SUBJECTIVE

2 days PTA: D.G. noted general abdominal pain in umbilical region. Now pain is sharp and severe, and D.G. points to location in RLQ. No BM for 2 days. Nausea and vomiting off and on 1 day.

OBJECTIVE

Inspection: BP 112/70 mm Hg, temp 38°C (100.4°F), pulse 116 bpm [beats per minute], resp 18/min.

Lying on side with knees drawn up under chin. Resists any movement. Face tight and occasionally grimacing. Cries out with any sudden movement.

Auscultation: No bowel sounds present. No vascular sounds.

Percussion: Tympany. Percussion over RLQ leads to tenderness.

Palpation: Abdominal wall is rigid and boardlike. Extreme tenderness to palpation in RLQ. Rebound tenderness is present in RLQ.

ASSESSMENT

Acute abdominal pain in RLQ

Nausea

ABNORMAL FINDINGS

TABLE 22.1	Abdominal Distension[a]

Tympany
scattered dullness

Tympany

Obesity

Inspection: Uniformly rounded; umbilicus sunken (it adheres to peritoneum, and layers of fat are superficial to it)

Auscultation: Normal bowel sounds

Percussion: Tympany; scattered dullness over adipose tissue

Palpation: Normal; may be hard to feel through thick abdominal wall

Air or Gas

Inspection: Single round curve

Auscultation: Depends on cause of gas (e.g., decreased or absent bowel sounds with ileus); hyperactive with early intestinal obstruction

Percussion: Tympany over large area

Palpation: May have muscle spasm of abdominal wall

Continued

TABLE 22.1 Abdominal Distension—cont'd

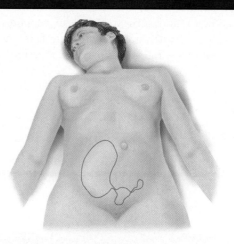

Ascites[b]

Inspection: Single curve; everted umbilicus; bulging flanks in supine position; taut, glistening skin; recent weight gain; increase in abdominal girth
Auscultation: Normal bowel sounds over intestines; diminished over ascitic fluid
Percussion: Tympany at top where intestines float; dull over fluid
Palpation: Limited by taut skin and increased intra-abdominal pressure

Ovarian Cyst (Large)

Inspection: Curve in lower half of abdomen, midline; everted umbilicus
Auscultation: Normal bowel sounds over upper abdomen where intestines are pushed superiorly
Percussion: Top dull over fluid; intestines pushed superiorly
Palpation: Aortic pulsation present (in ascites, it is not)

Pregnancy[c]

Inspection: Single curve; umbilicus protruding; breasts engorged
Auscultation: Fetal heart tones; diminished bowel sounds
Percussion: Tympany over intestines; dull over enlarging uterus
Palpation: Fetal parts; fetal movements

Feces

Inspection: Localized distension
Auscultation: Normal bowel sounds
Percussion: Tympany predominates; scattered dullness over fecal mass
Palpation: Plasticlike or ropelike mass with feces in intestines

TABLE 22.1   Abdominal Distension—cont'd

◀ **Tumour**

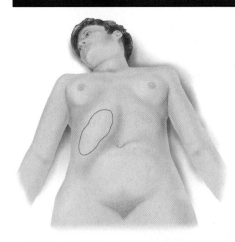

Inspection: Localized distension
Auscultation: Normal bowel sounds
Percussion: Dull over mass if mass reaches up to skin surface
Palpation: Used to define borders and distinguish from enlarged organ or normally palpable structure

[a]A mnemonic device to recall the common causes of abdominal distension is the seven *F*s: fat, flatus, fluid, fetus, feces, fetal growth, and fibroid.
[b]Ultrasonography study is the definitive tool for detecting ascites.
[c]Obviously a normal finding, pregnancy is included for comparison of conditions causing abdominal distension.

TABLE 22.2   Clinical Portrait of Intestinal Obstruction

- History of previous abdominal surgery with adhesions

- Vomiting

- Absence of stool or gas passage

- Distended abdomen (after 2nd day)

- Radiograph shows dilated air-filled loops of small bowel with multiple air-fluid levels

- Hyperactive bowel sounds in early obstruction; hypoactive or silent in late obstruction

- Dehydration and loss of electrolytes

- Accumulation of fluid and gas in bowel proximal (above) to obstruction

- Colicky pain from strong peristalsis above the obstruction

- Fever

- Pressure from excess fluid and gas may ➡leaking fluid into peritoneum

- Hypovolemic shock
  (⬇ BP, ⬆ pulse, cool skin if left untreated)

© Pat Thomas, 2014.

BP, Blood pressure.

TABLE 22.3 Common Sites of Referred Abdominal Pain

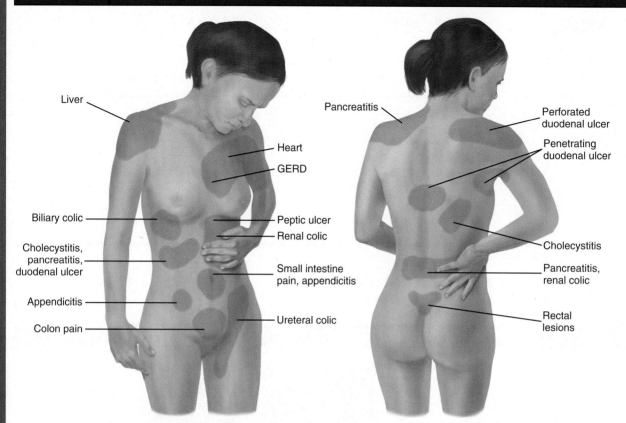

When a patient gives a history of abdominal pain, the location of the pain may not necessarily be directly over the involved organ. That is because the human brain has no felt image for internal organs. Rather, pain is referred to a site where the organ was located in fetal development. Although the organ migrates during fetal development, its nerves persist in referring sensations from the former location. The following are examples, not a complete list.

Liver

Hepatitis may produce mild to moderate dull pain in RUQ or epigastrium, along with anorexia, nausea, malaise, and low-grade fever.

Esophagus

Gastroesophageal reflux disease (GERD) is a complex of symptoms of esophagitis, including burning pain in midepigastrium or behind lower sternum that radiates upward, or "heartburn." The pain occurs 30–60 minutes after eating; it is aggravated by lying down or bending over.

Gallbladder

Cholecystitis is biliary colic, sudden pain in RUQ that may radiate to the right or left scapula and that builds over time, lasts 2 to 4 hours, and occurs after ingestion of fatty foods, alcohol, or caffeine. It is associated with nausea and vomiting and a positive Murphy's sign (sudden stop in inspiration with RUQ palpation).

Stomach

Gastric ulcer pain is dull, aching, gnawing epigastric pain, usually brought on by eating; it radiates to the back or substernal area. Perforated ulcer produces burning epigastric pain of sudden onset that is referred to one or both shoulders.

Appendix

Appendicitis typically starts as dull, diffuse pain in periumbilical region that later shifts to severe, sharp, chronic pain and tenderness localized in RLQ (McBurney's point). Pain is aggravated by movement, coughing, and deep breathing; it is associated first with anorexia, then with nausea and vomiting, and later with fever.

Kidney

Kidney stones prompt a sudden onset of severe, colicky flank or lower abdominal pain.

TABLE 22.3	Common Sites of Referred Abdominal Pain—cont'd

Pancreas

Pancreatitis produces acute, boring midepigastric pain radiating to the back and sometimes to the left scapula or flank, severe nausea, and vomiting.

Duodenum

Duodenal ulcer typically produces dull, aching, gnawing pain; it does not radiate, may be relieved by food, and may awaken the patient from sleep.

Small Intestine

Gastroenteritis produces diffuse, generalized abdominal pain, with nausea and diarrhea.

Colon

Large bowel obstruction produces moderate, colicky pain of gradual onset in lower abdomen, with bloating. IBS is accompanied by sharp or burning, cramping pain over a wide area; the pain, which does not radiate, is triggered by meals and relieved by bowel movement.

IBS, Irritable bowel syndrome; *RLQ*, right lower quadrant; *RUQ*, right upper quadrant.
Image © Pat Thomas, 2006.

TABLE 22.4	Abnormalities on Inspection

Epigastric Hernia

A protrusion of abdominal structures that presents as a small, fatty nodule at the epigastrium in the midline, through the linea alba. Usually it can be palpated rather than observed. It may be palpable only when the patient is standing.

Umbilical Hernia

A soft, skin-covered mass, which is the protrusion of the omentum or intestine through a weakness or incomplete closure in the umbilical ring. It is accentuated by increased intra-abdominal pressure, which occurs with crying, coughing, vomiting, or straining, but the bowel rarely becomes incarcerated or strangulated. It is more common in infants of African or Asian descent and in premature infants. Most umbilical hernias resolve spontaneously by age 1 year; parents should avoid affixing a belt or coin at the hernia because this will not speed closure and may cause contact dermatitis.

In an adult, it occurs with pregnancy and chronic ascites, or it may result from chronic intrathoracic pressure (e.g., asthma, chronic bronchitis).

Continued

TABLE 22.4	**Abnormalities on Inspection—cont'd**

Incisional Hernia

A bulge near an old operative scar that may not show when patient is supine but is apparent when the patient increases intra-abdominal pressure by a sit-up, by standing, or by performing the Valsalva manoeuvre.

Diastasis Recti

A midline longitudinal ridge that is a separation of the abdominal rectus muscles revealed when intra-abdominal pressure is increased by raising the head while in the supine position. It occurs congenitally and as a result of pregnancy or marked obesity in which distension is prolonged or muscle tone has decreased. It is not clinically significant.

See Illustration Credits for source information.

TABLE 22.5	**Abnormal Bowel Sounds**

◀ Succussion Splash

Unrelated to peristalsis, this is a very loud splash auscultated over the upper abdomen when the infant is rocked side to side. It indicates increased air and fluid in the stomach, as occurs with pyloric obstruction or large hiatus hernia.

Marked peristalsis, together with projectile vomiting in the newborn, is suggestive of **pyloric stenosis**, an obstruction of the stomach's pyloric valve. Pyloric stenosis is a congenital defect and appears in the second or third week after birth. After feeding, pronounced peristaltic waves cross from left to right, leading to projectile vomiting. Then, the examiner can palpate an olive-sized mass in the RUQ midway between the right costal margin and umbilicus. Affected infants must be referred promptly because of the risk for weight loss.

TABLE 22.5	Abnormal Bowel Sounds—cont'd

Hypoactive Bowel Sounds

Diminished or absence of bowel sounds signal decreased motility that results from inflammation, as with peritonitis; from paralytic ileus, as after abdominal surgery; or from late bowel obstruction. It also occurs with pneumonia.

Hyperactive Bowel Sounds

Loud, gurgling sounds (borborygmi) signal increased motility. They occur with early mechanical bowel obstruction (high-pitched), gastroenteritis, brisk diarrhea, laxative use, and subsiding paralytic ileus.

RUQ, Right upper quadrant.

TABLE 22.6	Abdominal Friction Rubs and Vascular Sounds

◀ **Peritoneal Friction Rub**

A rough, grating sound, like two pieces of leather rubbed together, indicates peritoneal inflammation. Occurs rarely. Usually occurs over organs with a large surface area in contact with the peritoneum.

Liver

Friction rub over lower right rib cage, caused by abscess or metastatic tumour.

Spleen

Friction rub over lower left rib cage in left anterior axillary line, caused by abscess, infection, or tumour.

Vascular Sounds

Arterial

A *bruit* indicates turbulent blood flow, as found in constricted, abnormally dilated, or tortuous vessels. Listen with the bell. Occurs with the following three conditions:
- *Abdominal aortic aneurysm:* Murmur is harsh, systolic, or continuous and accentuated with systole. Note in patient with hypertension.
- *Renal artery stenosis:* Murmur is midline or toward flank; soft, low-to-medium pitch.
- *Partial occlusion of femoral arteries:* Murmur is heard in the inguinal region (groin).

Peritoneal friction rub

Vascular sounds

Continued

TABLE 22.6	**Abdominal Friction Rubs and Vascular Sounds—cont'd**

Venous Hum

Occurs rarely. Heard in periumbilical region. Originates from inferior vena cava. Medium pitch, continuous sound; pressure on bell may obliterate it. A palpable thrill may be present. Occurs with portal hypertension and cirrhotic liver.

TABLE 22.7	**Abnormalities Detected on Palpation of Organs**

Enlarged Liver

The liver becomes enlarged, smooth, and nontender with fatty infiltration, portal obstruction or cirrhosis, obstruction high in the inferior vena cava, and lymphocytic leukemia. The liver feels enlarged and smooth but is tender to palpation with early heart failure, acute hepatitis, and hepatic abscess.

Enlarged Nodular Liver

The liver becomes enlarged and nodular with late portal cirrhosis, metastatic cancer, and tertiary syphilis.

TABLE 22.7 **Abnormalities Detected on Palpation of Organs—cont'd**

Enlarged Gallbladder

An enlarged, tender gallbladder is suggestive of acute cholecystitis. It is palpated behind the liver border as a smooth and firm mass like a sausage, although it may be difficult to palpate because of involuntary rigidity of abdominal muscles. The area is exquisitely painful to fist percussion, and inspiratory arrest (Murphy's sign) is present.

An enlarged, nontender gallbladder also feels like a smooth, sausagelike mass. This condition occurs when the gallbladder is filled with stones, as with obstruction of the common bile duct.

Enlarged Spleen

Because any enlargement superiorly is stopped by the diaphragm, the spleen enlarges downward and toward the midline. When enlargement is extreme, the spleen can extend down to the left aspect of the pelvis. It retains the splenic notch on the medial edge. When splenomegaly occurs with acute infections (mononucleosis), the spleen is moderately enlarged and soft, with rounded edges. When it is the result of a chronic cause, the enlargement is firm or hard, with sharp edges. An enlarged spleen is usually not tender to palpation; it is tender only if the peritoneum is also inflamed.

Enlarged Kidney

A kidney may become enlarged with hydronephrosis, cyst, or neoplasm. It may be difficult to distinguish an enlarged kidney from an enlarged spleen because they have a similar shape. Both extend forward and downward. However, the spleen may have a sharp edge, whereas the kidneys never do. The spleen retains the splenic notch, whereas the kidneys have no palpable notch. Percussion over the spleen yields dullness, whereas over the kidneys the sound is tympanitic because of the overriding bowel.

Abdominal Aortic Aneurysm

Most aortic aneurysms (more than 95%) are located in the abdomen below the renal arteries and extending to the umbilicus, and are referred to as abdominal aortic aneurysms (*AAA*, or *triple A*). Approximately 80% of these are detectable during routine physical examination. You will hear a bruit. Femoral pulses are present but decreased. An AAA has a high risk for rupture. If you hear a bruit, you should *not* palpate the area, to avoid rupturing the aneurysm.

Additional information on AAA appears in Table 22.6.

Abnormal Findings

Summary Checklist: Abdomen Examination

1. **Inspect:**
   Contour
   Symmetry
   Umbilicus
   Skin
   Pulsation or movement
   Hair distribution
   Demeanour

2. **Auscultate:**
   Bowel sounds
   Any vascular sounds

3. **Percuss:**
   All four quadrants
   Borders of liver, spleen

4. **Palpate:**
   Light palpation in all four quadrants
   Deeper palpation in all four quadrants
   Palpation for liver, spleen, and kidneys

5. **Engage in teaching and health promotion**

REFERENCES

1. Khanna, R., Lakhanpaul, M., Burman-Roy, S., et al. (2009). Diarrhoea and vomiting caused by gastroenteritis in children under 5 years: Summary of NICE guidelines. *British Medical Journal, 338*, 1009–1012. doi:10.1136/bmj.b1350.

2. Diegelmann, L. (2012). Nonobstetric abdominal pain and surgical emergencies in pregnancy. *Emergency Medicine Clinics of North America, 30*, 885–901. doi:10.1016/j.emc.2012.08.012.

3. McLachlan, A. J., & Pont, L. G. (2012). Drug metabolism in older people—A key consideration in achieving optimal outcomes with medicines. *The Journals of Gerontology. Series A, Biological Sciences and Medical Sciences, 67A*(2), 175–180. doi: https://doi.org/10.1093/gerona/glr118.

4. Mohanty, M., & Slattum, P. (2011). Alcohol, medications, and older adults. *Age in Action, 26*(3), 1–5.

5. Canadian Liver Foundation. (2011). *Gallstones*. Retrieved from http://www.liver.ca/Liver_Disease/Adult_Liver_Diseases/Gallstones.aspx.

6. Miller, C. A. (2012). *Nursing for wellness in older adults* (6th ed.). Philadelphia: Lippincott Williams & Wilkins.

7. Registered Nurses' Association of Ontario. (2011). *Prevention of constipation in the older adult population: Guideline supplement.* Retrieved from http://rnao.ca/sites/rnao-ca/files/Constipation_supplement_2011.pdf.

8. Canadian Institute for Health Information. (2015). *Trends in income-related health inequalities in Canada: Summary Report.* Ottawa: CIHI. Retrieved from https://www.cihi.ca/en/summary_report_inequalities_2015_en.pdf.

9. Canadian Digestive Health Foundation. (2017). *Understanding gastroesophageal reflux disease (GERD).* Retrieved from http://cdhf.ca/bank/document_en/12understanding-gerd-.pdf#zoom=100.

10. Canadian Digestive Health Foundation. (2017). *Understanding lactose intolerance.* Retrieved from http://cdhf.ca/bank/document_en/16understanding-lactose-intolerance-.pdf#zoom=100.

11. Suchy, F. J., Brannon, P. M., Carpenter, T. O., et al. (2010). NIH Consensus Development Conference: Lactose intolerance and health. *NIH Consensus and State-of-the-Science Statements, 27*(2), 1–27. Retrieved from https://consensus.nih.gov/2010/docs/LI_CDC_2010_Final%20Statement.pdf.

12. Canadian Digestive Health Foundation. (2017). *Understanding celiac disease.* Retrieved from http://cdhf.ca/bank/document_en/4understanding-celiac-disease-.pdf#zoom=100.

13. Canadian Digestive Health Foundation. (2017). *Understanding peptic ulcers.* Retrieved from http://cdhf.ca/bank/document_en/18understanding-peptic-ulcers-.pdf#zoom=100.

14. Crohn's and Colitis Foundation of Canada. (2012). *The impact of inflammatory bowel disease in Canada: 2012 final report and recommendations.* Toronto: Author. Retrieved from http://www.isupportibd.ca/pdf/ccfc-ibd-impact-report-2012.pdf.

15. Canadian Digestive Health Foundation. (2017). *Understanding irritable bowel syndrome (IBS).* Retrieved from http://cdhf.ca/bank/document_en/15understanding-irritable-bowel-syndrome-ibs-.pdf#zoom=100.

16. Reading, C., & Wien, F. (2013). *Health inequalities and social determinants of Aboriginal peoples' health.* Retrieved from http://www.nccah-ccnsa.ca/Publications/Lists/Publications/Attachments/46/health_inequalities_EN_web.pdf.

17. Canadian Paediatric Society. (2017). *Gastrointestinal parasitic infections in immigrant and refugee children.* Retrieved from http://www.kidsnewtocanada.ca/conditions/gastrointestinal-parasitic-infections.

18. Pottie, K., Greenaway, C., Feightner, J., et al. (2011). Evidence-based clinical guidelines for immigrants and refugees. *Canadian Medical Association Journal, 183*(12), E824–E925. doi:10.1503/cmaj.090313.

19. Derikx, L. A., Dieleman, L. A., & Hoentjen, F. (2016). Probiotics and prebiotics in ulcerative colitis. *Best Practice & Research. Clinical Gastroenterology, 30*, 55–71. doi:10.1016/j.bpg.2016.02.00.

20. Guarner, F., Khan, A. G., Garisch, J., et al. (2011). World Gastroenterology Organisation global guidelines: Probiotics and prebiotics. *Journal of Clinical Gastroenterology, 46*(6), 468–481.

21. Health Canada. (2016). *Eating well with Canada's food guide.* Retrieved from http://www.hc-sc.gc.ca/fn-an/food-guide-aliment/index-eng.php.

22. Dietitians of Canada. (2016). *Food sources of fibre.* Retrieved from http://www.dietitians.ca/Your-Health/Nutrition-A-Z/Fibre/Food-Sources-of-Fibre.aspx.

23. *Canadian 24-hour movement guidelines for children and youth.* (2016). Retrieved from http://www.csep.ca/CMFiles/Guidelines/24hrGlines/Canadian24HourMovementGuidelines2016.pdf.

24. Di Saverio, S., Birindelli, A., Kelly, M. D., et al. (2016). WSES Jerusalem guidelines for diagnosis and treatment of acute appendicitis. *World Journal of Emergency Surgery, 11*, 34. doi:10.1186/s13017-016-0090-5.

25. McGee, S. (2018). *Evidence-based physical diagnosis* (4th ed.). Philadelphia: Elsevier.

26. Ohle, R., O'Reilly, F., O'Brien, K. K., et al. (2011). The Alvarado score for predicting acute appendicitis: A systematic review. *BMC Medicine, 9*, 139. Retrieved from http://www.biomedcentral.com/1741-7015/9/139.

CHAPTER 23

Anus, Rectum, and Prostate

Written by Carolyn Jarvis, PhD, APN, CNP
Adapted by Marian Luctkar-Flude, RN, PhD

℮ http://evolve.elsevier.com/Canada/Jarvis/examination/

STRUCTURE AND FUNCTION

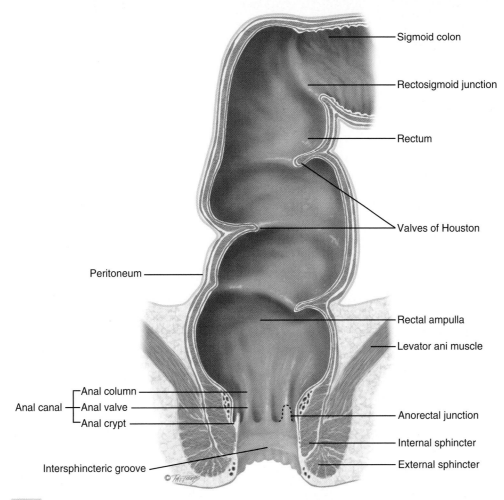

Sigmoid colon

Rectosigmoid junction

Rectum

Valves of Houston

Peritoneum

Rectal ampulla

Levator ani muscle

Anal canal — Anal column — Anal valve — Anal crypt

Anorectal junction

Internal sphincter

External sphincter

Intersphincteric groove

23.1 Anatomy of the anal sphincters. (© Pat Thomas, 2010.)

ANUS AND RECTUM

The **anal canal** is the outlet of the gastro-intestinal tract, and it is about 3.8 cm long in adults. It is lined with modified skin (which has no hair or sebaceous glands) that merges with rectal mucosa at the anorectal junction. The canal slants forward toward the umbilicus, forming a distinct right angle with the rectum, which rests back in the hollow of the sacrum. Although the rectum contains only autonomic nerves, numerous somatic sensory nerves are present in the

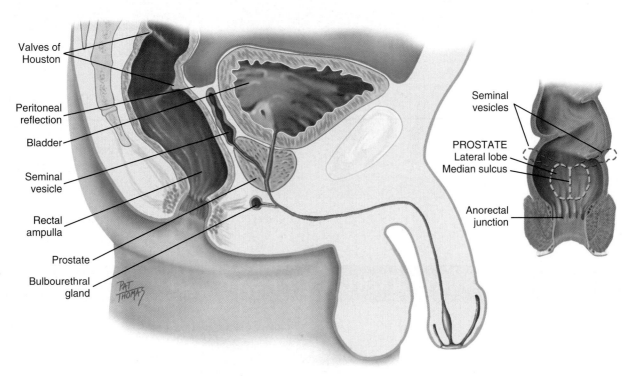

Valves of
Houston

Peritoneal
reflection

Bladder

Seminal
vesicle

Rectal
ampulla

Prostate

Bulbourethral
gland

PAT THOMAS

Seminal
vesicles

PROSTATE
Lateral lobe
Median sulcus

Anorectal
junction

23.2

anal canal and external skin, so any trauma to the anal area will cause sharp pain.

The anal canal is surrounded by two concentric layers of muscle called **sphincters** (Fig. 23.1). The internal sphincter is under involuntary control by the autonomic nervous system. The external sphincter surrounds the internal sphincter and has a small section overriding the tip of the internal sphincter at the opening. It is under voluntary control. Except for the passing of feces and gas, the sphincters keep the anal canal tightly closed. The **intersphincteric groove** separates the internal and external sphincters and is palpable.

The **anal columns** (or columns of Morgagni) are folds of mucosa. These extend vertically down from the rectum and end in the **anorectal junction** (also called the *mucocutaneous junction*, *pectinate line*, or *dentate line*). This junction is not palpable, but it is visible on proctoscopy. Each anal column contains an artery and a vein. Under conditions of chronic increased venous pressure, the vein may enlarge, forming a hemorrhoid. At the lower end of each column is a small crescent fold of mucous membrane called the **anal valve**. The space above the anal valve (between the columns) is a small recess called the **anal crypt**.

The **rectum**, which is 12 cm long, is the distal portion of the large intestine. It extends from the sigmoid colon, at the level of the third sacral vertebra, and ends at the anal canal. Just above the anal canal, the rectum dilates and turns posteriorly, forming the rectal ampulla. The rectal interior has three semilunar transverse folds called the **valves of Houston**. These cross half the circumference of the rectal lumen. Their function is unclear, but they may serve to hold feces as the flatus passes. The lowest is within reach of

palpation, usually on the left side, and must not be mistaken for an intrarectal mass.

Peritoneal Reflection. The peritoneum covers only the upper two-thirds of the rectum. In males, the anterior part of the peritoneum reflects down to within 7.5 cm of the anal opening, forming the **rectovesical pouch** (Fig. 23.2), and then covers the bladder. In females, this area is termed the **rectouterine pouch**, and it extends down to within 5.5 cm of the anal opening.

PROSTATE

In males, the **prostate gland** lies in front of the anterior wall of the rectum and 2 cm behind the symphysis pubis. It surrounds the bladder neck and the urethra and has 15 to 30 ducts opening into the urethra. The prostate secretes a thin, milky alkaline fluid that helps sperm viability. It is a bilobed structure that is round or heart-shaped. It measures 2.5 cm long and 4 cm in diameter. The two lateral lobes are separated by a shallow groove called the **median sulcus.**

The two **seminal vesicles** project like rabbit ears above the prostate. The seminal vesicles secrete a fluid that is rich in fructose, which nourishes the sperm, and contains prostaglandins. The two **bulbourethral glands** (also called *Cowper's glands*) are pea-sized and located inferior to the prostate on either side of the urethra (see Fig. 23.5, p. 616). They secrete a clear, viscid mucus.

REGIONAL STRUCTURES

In females, the uterine cervix lies in front of the anterior rectal wall and may be palpated through the wall.

The combined length of the anal canal and rectum is about 16 cm in adults. The average examining finger is 6 to 10 cm long; thus, many rectal structures are within reach.

The sigmoid colon is named for its S-shaped course in the pelvic cavity. It extends from the iliac flexure of the descending colon, ending at the rectum. It is 40 cm long and accessible to examination only through the colonoscope, which provides a view of the entire mucosal surface of the sigmoid colon and the colon itself.

 ## DEVELOPMENTAL CONSIDERATIONS

The first stool passed by the newborn is dark green meconium; its occurrence, within 24 to 48 hours of birth, indicates anal patency. From that time on, the infant usually has a stool after each feeding. This response to eating is a wave of peristalsis called the *gastrocolic reflex*. It continues throughout life, although children and adults usually produce no more than one or two stools per day.

The infant passes stools by reflex. Voluntary control of the external anal sphincter cannot occur until nerves supplying the area have become fully myelinated, usually around $1\frac{1}{2}$ to 2 years of age. Toilet training usually starts after age 2 years.

At male puberty, the prostate gland undergoes a very rapid increase to more than twice its prepubertal size. During early adulthood, its size remains fairly constant.

The prostate gland commonly starts to enlarge during the middle adult years. This enlargement, benign prostatic hypertrophy (BPH), is present in 10% of men by 40 years of age and increases with age. Hypertrophy is thought to be caused by a hormonal imbalance leading to proliferation of benign adenomas. These gradually impede urine output by obstructing the urethra. The risk of developing prostate cancer also increases with age (see the Promoting Heath: Screening for Prostate Cancer box, p. 614).

 ## SOCIAL DETERMINANTS OF HEALTH CONSIDERATIONS

Colorectal cancer (CRC) is the second most common cancer, accounting for 13% of all cancers in Canada.[1] It is expected that CRC will be diagnosed in 1 in 14 Canadian men and 1 in 16 Canadian women during their lifetime. Although more than half of Canadians were up to date with CRC screening in 2012, there were large differences among provinces, and individuals in lower-income groups were less likely to be screened than those in the highest income group, even in provinces with well-established population-based screening programs.[2] Risk factors for developing CRC are being of older age, particularly >50 years; having polyps; having a family history of CRC, especially a parent, sibling, or child who developed it before the age of 45; having familial adenomatous polyposis or hereditary nonpolyposis colon cancer; having inflammatory bowel disease; eating a diet high in red and processed meats; consuming alcohol; smoking; being physically inactive; being obese; and having Ashkenazi (Eastern European) Jewish ancestry. However, CRC develops in some people who have none of these risk factors. A diet high in vegetables and fruit is known to lower the risk. Research also suggests that a diet high in fibre and low in animal fats may also decrease the risk.

Prostate cancer is the most common cancer in men, and is more common in North America and northwestern Europe. A Canadian man has a 1 in 7 chance of receiving a diagnosis of prostate cancer during his lifetime.[1] The Canadian Cancer Society estimated that 21 300 Canadian men would be diagnosed with prostate cancer in 2017, which would account for 21% of all new male cancer cases. Risk factors for developing prostate cancer are being of older age, particularly >65 years; a family history of prostate cancer; a low-fibre, high-fat diet; and African ancestry. Obesity, physical inactivity, and exposure to cadmium are being studied as possible risk factors. Some men develop prostate cancer without any of these risk factors.

Cancer Risk and Indigenous Communities

Although limited data are available on Indigenous peoples in Canada and cancer rates, studies suggest that CRC incidence is increasing at a higher rate in the Indigenous population than in the general population.[3] Moreover, Indigenous people are more likely to be diagnosed at a later stage of disease, which lowers survival.[4] One in four Indigenous Canadians is obese, a risk factor for many cancers, including colorectal and prostate cancers. However, many rural and remote Indigenous communities face challenges changing unhealthy behaviours that contribute to obesity. Fresh, healthy foods are expensive and in limited supply, and it is often too cold to be active outside. Resources are available to support First Nations people in being active and eating healthy.[5]

SUBJECTIVE DATA

1. Usual bowel routine
2. Change in bowel habits
3. Rectal bleeding, blood in the stool

4. Medications
5. Rectal conditions
6. Family history

7. Self-care behaviours

HEALTH HISTORY QUESTIONS

Examiner Asks	Rationale

1. **Usual bowel routine.** Do you **defecate regularly**? How often? What is the usual colour? Is it usually hard or soft?
   - Do you have any **straining at stool**, incomplete evacuation, or urge to have bowel movement but nothing comes?
   - Do you eat breakfast? Drink coffee or tea?

   - Do you have pain while passing a bowel movement?

A visual aid such as the **Bristol stool chart** that follows can be used to assess stool quality.

Assess usual bowel routine. Constipation is defined as three or fewer stools per week and is a common concern among older adults.

Eating breakfast or drinking coffee or tea increases colon motility and prompts a bowel movement in many people.

Pain with defecation (**dyschezia**) may be caused by a local condition (hemorrhoid, fissure) or constipation.

Classification of the type of stool passed is a useful guide to intestinal transit time.[6]

Bristol Stool Chart

Type 1	Separate hard lumps, like nuts (hard to pass)	Severe Constipation
Type 2	Sausage-shaped but lumpy	Mild Constipation
Type 3	Like a sausage but with cracks on the surface	Normal
Type 4	Like a sausage or snake smooth and soft	Normal
Type 5	Soft blobs with clear-cut edges	Lacking Fiber
Type 6	Fluffy pieces with ragged edges, a mushy stool	Mild Diarrhea
Type 7	Watery, no solid pieces. **Entirely Liquid**	Severe Diarrhea

© The Rome Foundation.

2. **Change in bowel habits.** Any **change** in usual **bowel habits**? Do you have loose stools or diarrhea? When did this start? Is the diarrhea associated with nausea, vomiting, abdominal pain, something you ate recently?
   - Have you eaten at a restaurant recently? Anyone else in your group or family have similar symptoms?
   - Have you travelled to a foreign country during the past 6 months?
   - Do your stools have a hard consistency? When did this start?

Diarrhea occurs with gastroenteritis, colitis, and irritable bowel syndrome.

Consider food poisoning.

Consider parasitic infection.
Constipation is characterized by stool hardness.

3. **Rectal bleeding, blood in the stool.** Have you ever had **rectal bleeding** or **blood in the stool**?
   - When did you first notice blood in the stool? What is the colour: bright red or dark red-black? How much blood: spotting on the toilet paper or outright passing of blood with the stool? Does the bloody stool have a particular smell?

Black or bloody stools (**melena**) should be investigated.

Black stools may be tarry as a result of occult blood (melena) from gastro-intestinal bleeding, or they may be nontarry as a result of ingestion of iron medications.

Examiner Asks	Rationale

| | Red blood in stools occurs with gastro-intestinal bleeding or localized bleeding around the anus and also with colon and rectal cancer. |

- Have you ever had clay-coloured stool?

Clay colour indicates absence of bile pigment.

- Have you ever had mucus or pus in stool?

Excessive mucus or pus may indicate an infection, inflammatory bowel disease, or cancer.

- Is your stool frothy?

Steatorrhea is excessive fat in the stool, as occurs in malabsorption of fat.

- Do you need to pass gas frequently?

Excessive passing of gas (flatulence) should be investigated.

4. **Medications.** What **medications** do you take: prescription and over-the-counter? Laxatives or stool softeners? Which ones? How often? Iron pills? Do you ever use enemas to move your bowels? How often?

5. **Rectal conditions.** Do you have any **problems in rectal area**: itching, pain or burning sensation, hemorrhoids? How do you treat these? Do you use any hemorrhoid preparations? Ever had a fissure or fistula? How was this treated?

Pruritus (itching) can be caused by hemorrhoids.

- Have you ever had a **problem controlling your bowels**?

Such a problem is known as *fecal incontinence.*

Mucoid discharge and soiling of underwear occur with prolapsed hemorrhoids.

6. **Family history.** Any **family history** of polyps or cancer in the colon or rectum, inflammatory bowel disease, prostate cancer?

Assess risk factors for colon cancer, rectal cancer, prostate cancer.

7. **Self-care behaviours.** What is the usual amount of **high-fibre foods** in your daily diet: cereals, apples or other fruits, vegetables, whole-grain breads?
   - How many glasses of water do you drink each day?
   - How often do you exercise?

High-fibre foods of the soluble type (beans, prunes, barley, carrots, broccoli, cabbage) have been shown to lower cholesterol, and insoluble-fibre foods (cereals, wheat germ) reduce the risk for colon cancer. Also, high-fibre foods fight obesity, stabilize blood glucose levels, and help alleviate certain gastro-intestinal disorders. Exercise helps prevent constipation.

- When was your most recent colon or prostate screening test? Stool test, blood test or flexible sigmoidoscopy?

For colon and prostate cancer screening guidelines for the early detection of cancer, refer to Table 23.1, p. 612, and the Promoting Health boxes on p. 614.

Additional History for Infants and Children

1. **Skin problems.** Have you noticed any irritation in your child's anal area: redness, raised skin, frequent itching?

In children, pinworms are a common cause of intense itching and irritation of the anal skin.

2. **Bowel movements.** How are your child's bowel movements (BMs)? Frequency? Any problems? Any pain or straining with BM?

Constipation is a decrease in BM frequency, with difficult passing of very hard, dry stools. **Encopresis** is persistent passing of stools into clothing by a child older than age 4 years, at which age continence would be expected.

TABLE 23.1	Colorectal Cancer Screening Guidelines
AGE	RECOMMENDATIONS FOR ADULTS WHO ARE NOT AT HIGH RISK FOR COLORECTAL CANCER[a]
50–59 years	FOBT (either gFOBT or FIT) every 2 years OR flexible sigmoidoscopy every 10 years (*weak recommendation, moderate quality evidence*)[b]
60–74 years	FOBT (either gFOBT or FIT) every 2 years OR flexible sigmoidoscopy every 10 years (*strong recommendation; moderate quality evidence*)[c]
75 years and over	No screening recommended

[a]Recommendations do not apply to those with previous colorectal cancer (CRC) or polyps, inflammatory bowel disease, signs or symptoms of CRC, hereditary syndromes predisposing to CRC (e.g., familial adenomatous polyposis, Lynch syndrome), or history of CRC in one or more first-degree relative(s).
[b]Potential harms and benefits of screening should be discussed with the patient.
[c]Most individuals will be best served by screening.
FIT, Fecal immunochemical test; *FOBT*, fecal occult blood test; gFOBT, guaiac fecal occult blood test.
Modified from Canadian Task Force on Preventive Health Care. (2016). *Colorectal cancer (2016)*. Retrieved from https://canadiantaskforce.ca/guidelines/published-guidelines/colorectal-cancer/#documents.

OBJECTIVE DATA

PREPARATION

To perform a rectal examination on an adult, ask the patient to assume one of the positions shown in Fig. 23.3.

Examine the male patient in the left lateral decubitus or standing position. Instruct the standing male patient to point his toes together; this relaxes the regional muscles, making it easier to spread the buttocks.

Place the female patient in the lithotomy position if you are examining genitalia as well; use the left lateral decubitus position for examination of the rectal area alone. Place the transgender woman in a gender-affirming lithotomy position.

These positions leave many patients feeling vulnerable and embarrassed. Help the patient relax and retain a sense of control by using these measures:

- Ensure privacy.
- Explain each step in the examination before you perform it.
- Use a gentle, firm touch and gradual movements.
- Communicate throughout the examination. Maintain a dialogue to share information.

EQUIPMENT NEEDED

Penlight
Lubricating jelly
Glove
Guaiac test container

Left lateral decubitus

Lithotomy

Standing

23.3 Positions for rectal examination.

Normal Range of Findings	Abnormal Findings

Inspect the Perianal Area

Spread the buttocks wide apart, and observe the perianal region. The anus normally looks moist and hairless, with coarse folded skin that is more pigmented than the perianal skin. The anal opening is tightly closed. No lesions are present.

Inflammation; lesions or scars.
Linear split: fissure.
Flabby skin sac: hemorrhoid.

Normal Range of Findings	Abnormal Findings
	Shiny blue skin sac: thrombosed hemorrhoid.
	Small round opening in anal area: fistula (Table 23.2, p. 619).
Inspect the sacrococcygeal area. Normally, it appears smooth and even.	Inflammation or tenderness, swelling, tuft of hair, or dimple at tip of coccyx may indicate pilonidal cyst (see Table 23.2, p. 619).
	Appearance of fissure or hemorrhoids.
Instruct the patient to hold the breath and bear down (i.e., perform a Valsalva manoeuvre). No break in skin integrity or protrusion through the anal opening should be present. Describe any abnormality in clock face terms, with "12:00 position" as the anterior point toward the symphysis pubis and "6:00 position" toward the coccyx.	Circular red "doughnut" of tissue: rectal prolapse.

 DEVELOPMENTAL CONSIDERATIONS

Infants and Children

To examine a newborn, hold the feet with one hand and flex the knees up onto the abdomen. Note the presence of the anus. Confirm patency of the rectum and anus by noting the first meconium stool passed within 24 to 48 hours of birth. To assess sphincter tone, check the *anal reflex:* Gently stroke the anal area and note a quick contraction of the sphincter.

In an infant or child, note that the buttocks are firm and rounded with no masses or lesions. Recall that the *mongolian spot* is a common variation of hyperpigmentation in newborns of African, Asian, Mediterranean, or Indigenous descent (see Chapter 13).

Abnormal Findings (continued):

Imperforate anus.

Flattened buttocks, as in cystic fibrosis or celiac syndrome.
Coccygeal mass.
Meningocele (sac containing meninges that protrude through a defect in the bony spine).
Tuft of hair or pilonidal dimple.
Pustules indicate secondary infection of diaper rash.
Signs of physical or sexual abuse include anal abrasions and perianal tears.
Fissure is a common cause of constipation or rectal bleeding in children. (Because it is painful, the child does not defecate.)

The perianal skin is free of lesions. However, diaper rash is common in infants and manifests as a generalized reddened area with papules or vesicles.

Omit palpation unless the history or symptoms warrant. When internal palpation is needed, position the infant or child on the back with the legs flexed, and gently insert a gloved, well-lubricated finger into the rectum. Your fifth finger usually is long enough, and its smaller size is more comfortable for an infant or child. However, you may need to use the index finger because of its better control and increased tactile sensitivity. On withdrawing the finger, scant bleeding or protruding rectal mucosa may be evident.

Inspect the perianal region of a school-age child or adolescent during examination of the genitalia. Internal palpation is not performed routinely in patients of these ages.

Older Adults

As an older patient performs the Valsalva manoeuvre, you may note relaxation of the perianal musculature and decreased sphincter control. Otherwise, the full examination proceeds as described earlier for younger adults.

Objective Data

PROMOTING HEALTH: SCREENING FOR COLORECTAL CANCER

Screening for Life

Colorectal cancer (CRC) may not cause any symptoms in its early stages. Symptoms often appear once the tumour causes bleeding or blocks the bowel. Possible symptoms include a change in bowel habits, such as diarrhea or constipation; general abdominal discomfort (bloating, sensation of fullness, cramps); bloody stools (bright red or very dark); stools that are narrower than usual; a strong urge to defecate; a feeling that the bowel has not completely emptied; nausea or vomiting; fatigue; and weight loss.

Currently in Canada, screening for CRC with stool tests every 2 years or flexible sigmoidoscopy every 10 years is recommended for people aged 50 to 74 years (see Table 23.1, p. 612).* Two types of fecal occult blood tests (FOBTs) are used in Canada. The guaiac fecal occult blood test (gFOBT) is the most common and uses a chemical reaction on a paper card to find traces of blood in the stool from adenomatous polyps or tumours. The fecal immunochemical test (FIT) is a newer, more sensitive test that uses specific antibodies for human blood to find traces of blood in the stool. A positive FOBT or

FIT result may be followed up with a colonoscopy, flexible sigmoidoscopy, or double-contrast barium enema.*

Resources, test availability, and patient preferences should be considered when selecting a screening test. FIT is a more expensive test being used by some, but not all, CRC screening programs in Canada. Individuals who prefer less frequent testing or are averse to stool testing may choose flexible sigmoidoscopy for screening. However, access may be limited in some regions. Individuals who are at a higher-than-average risk of developing CRC may need testing more often and at an earlier age than people with average risk. They should talk to their doctor about a personal plan for testing.[†]

References

*Canadian Cancer Society. (2016). *Colorectal cancer: Understanding your diagnosis*. Retrieved from http://www.cancer.ca/en/support-and-services/resources/publications/?region=on.
†Canadian Task Force on Preventive Health Care. (2016). Recommendations on screening for colorectal cancer in primary care. *Canadian Medical Association Journal*, 188(5), 340–348. doi:10.1503/cmaj.151125.

PROMOTING HEALTH: SCREENING FOR PROSTATE CANCER

"To Screen or Not to Screen"

Throughout much of a man's life, the prostate gland is typically the size of a walnut. However, by the time a man is age 40, it may grow slightly larger, to the size of an apricot. By age 60, it may be lemon-sized. Although size varies between individuals, this gradual enlargement is considered to be a normal part of aging, and is termed **benign prostatic hypertrophy (BPH)**. It does not increase an individual's risk for prostate cancer, but symptoms for BPH are very similar to those of prostate cancer. Prostate cancer may not cause signs or symptoms, especially in the early stages. Symptoms may appear if the tumour enlarges the prostate and starts to press on the urethra, making the passage of urine difficult or painful, or increasing frequency of urination. Only a small proportion of men with prostate cancer have symptoms or die from the disease, as most prostate cancers are slowly progressive and not life-threatening.

The **digital rectal examination (DRE)** and the **prostate-specific antigen (PSA)** blood test can help detect prostate cancer early, but they can also yield false-positive results or miss prostate cancer that is present (false-negative results). In some cases, these tests can detect prostate cancer that may not pose a serious threat to a man's health. A biopsy performed during transrectal ultrasonography is usually necessary to make a definitive diagnosis of cancer.

There is no evidence that PSA screening reduces overall mortality for men of any age, and there is conflicting evidence that it leads to a small and very uncertain potential reduction in prostate cancer mortality in men aged 55 to 69 years. However, there is consistent evidence that screening and active treatment lead to potential significant harms such as bleeding, infection, urinary incontinence, erectile dysfunction, false positives, and overdiagnosis. Thus, screening with the PSA test is not recommended for men of any age, regardless

of whether DRE is performed. There is no evidence that DRE reduces prostate cancer mortality on its own or when used with the PSA test. There is also no evidence that high-risk groups such as men of African ancestry or those with a family history of prostate cancer (one or more first-degree relatives) should be screened differently.

If a patient raises the issue of PSA screening, it is important to discuss the benefits and harms associated with screening, ideally using decision aids to facilitate comprehension (see https://canadiantaskforce.ca/prostate-cancer-tools/).

In the DRE, the examiner inserts a gloved, lubricated finger into the patient's rectum. The prostate gland is located just in front of the rectum, thus it is possible to palpate the surface of the gland manually for bumps or hard areas that may represent developing cancer. The PSA blood test detects PSA, a substance made by the normal prostate gland. When prostate cancer develops, the PSA level increases. However, benign or noncancerous enlargement of the prostate (e.g., BPH), age, and prostatitis can also cause PSA levels to increase. Ejaculation causes a temporary increase in PSA levels, and men need to be instructed to abstain from ejaculation for 2 days before PSA level testing. In addition, some medications, such as finasteride (Proscar) or dutasteride (Avodart), artificially lower PSA levels. If the PSA level is elevated, further laboratory work or transrectal ultrasonography and biopsy may be recommended.

References

Canadian Cancer Society. (2016). *Prostate cancer: Understanding your diagnosis*. Retrieved from http://www.cancer.ca/en/support-and-services/resources/publications/?region=on.
Canadian Task Force on Preventive Health Care. (2014). Recommendations on screening for prostate cancer with the prostate-specific antigen test. *Canadian Medical Association Journal*, 186(16), 1225–1234. doi:10.1503/cmaj.140703.

SPECIAL CONSIDERATIONS FOR ADVANCED PRACTICE

Normal Range of Findings	Abnormal Findings

Palpate the Anus and Rectum

Drop lubricating jelly onto your gloved index finger. Inform the patient that palpation is not painful, but they may feel the need to move the bowels. Place the pad of your index finger gently against the anal verge (Fig. 23.4). You will feel the sphincter tighten and then relax. As it relaxes, flex the tip of your finger and slowly insert it into the anal canal in a direction toward the umbilicus. *Never* approach the anus at right angles with your index finger extended. Such a jabbing motion does not promote sphincter relaxation and is painful.

23.4 Palpating the anus and rectum.

Rotate your examining finger to palpate the entire muscular ring. The canal should feel smooth and even. Note the intersphincteric groove circling the canal wall. To assess tone, ask the patient to tighten the muscle. The sphincter should tighten evenly around your finger without causing pain for the patient.

Use a bidigital palpation technique, with your thumb against the perianal tissue (Fig. 23.5). Press your examining finger toward it. This manoeuvre helps detect any swelling or tenderness and helps you assess the bulbourethral glands.

Decreased tone should be investigated. Increased tone occurs with inflammation and anxiety.

Tenderness should be investigated.

Normal Range of Findings	Abnormal Findings

Bulbourethral gland

23.5 Examiner's thumb against perianal tissue.

Above the anal canal, the rectum turns posteriorly, following the curve of the coccyx and sacrum. Insert your finger farther, and explore all around the rectal wall. It normally feels smooth with no nodularity. Promptly report any mass you discover for further examination.

An internal hemorrhoid above the ano-rectal junction is not palpable unless it is thrombosed.

A soft, slightly movable mass may be a polyp.

A firm or hard mass with irregular shape or rolled edges may signify carcinoma (Table 23.3, p. 622).

Prostate Gland. On the anterior wall in a male patient, note the elastic, bulging prostate gland (Fig. 23.6). Palpate the entire prostate in a systematic manner, but note that only the superior surface and part of the lateral surface are accessible to examination. Press *into* the gland at each location, because when a nodule is present, it does not project into the rectal lumen. The surface should feel smooth and muscular; search for any distinct nodule or diffuse firmness.

Normal Range of Findings

Abnormal Findings

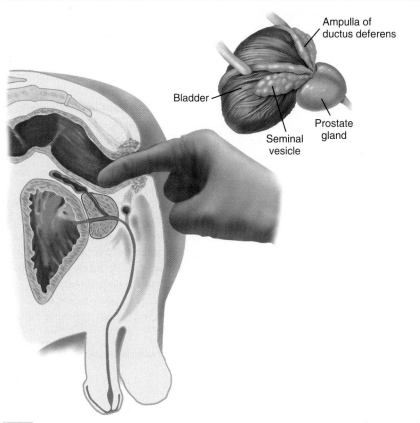

Ampulla of ductus deferens

Bladder

Prostate gland

Seminal vesicle

23.6 Palpating the prostate gland.

Note these characteristics:
Size: 2.5 cm long by 4 cm wide; should not protrude more than 1 cm into the rectum
Shape: heart shape, with palpable central groove
Surface: smooth
Consistency: elastic, rubbery
Mobility: slightly movable
Sensitivity: nontender to palpation

In a transgender woman who has undergone vaginoplasty, the prostate remains in situ and may be palpated anteriorly via digital vaginal examination in a gender-affirming lithotomy position.[7]

In a female patient, palpate the cervix through the anterior rectal wall. It normally feels like a small round mass. You also may palpate a retroverted uterus or a tampon in the vagina. Do not mistake the cervix or a tampon for a tumour.

Withdraw your examining finger; normally, no mucus or bright red blood is on the glove. To complete the examination, offer the patient tissues to remove the lubricant, and help the patient to a more comfortable position.

Enlargement or atrophy.

Flatness with no groove.
Nodularity.
Hardness or boggy, soft, fluctuant texture.
Fixed position.
Tenderness.
Enlargement, firmness, and smoothness with central groove obliterated: suggestive of BPH.
Swelling and exquisite tenderness accompanies prostatitis.
Any stone-hard, irregular, fixed nodule indicates carcinoma (Table 23.4, p. 623).

Special Considerations for Advanced Practice

Normal Range of Findings	Abnormal Findings
Examination of Stool. Inspect any feces remaining on the glove. Normally, the colour is brown, and the consistency is soft.	Jellylike shreds of mucus mixed in stool indicate inflammation. Bright red blood on stool surface indicates rectal bleeding. Bright red blood mixed with feces indicates possible colonic bleeding.
Test any stool on the glove for **occult blood**; use the specimen container that your agency directs. A negative response is normal. A positive *Hematest* result indicates occult blood. However, a false-positive finding may occur if the patient has ingested significant amounts of red meat within 3 days of the test.	Black tarry stool with distinct malodour indicates upper gastro-intestinal bleeding with blood partially digested. (More than 50 mL of blood from upper gastro-intestinal tract must be lost for this stool to be considered melena.) Black stool also occurs with ingesting iron or bismuth preparations. Grey, tan stool indicates the absence of bile pigment, as in obstructive jaundice. Pale yellow, greasy stool is indicative of increased fat content (steatorrhea), as occurs with malabsorption syndrome. Occult bleeding usually indicates cancer of the colon.

DOCUMENTATION AND CRITICAL THINKING

Sample Charting

SUBJECTIVE

Has one BM daily, soft, brown; no pain, no change in bowel routine. Taking no medications. Has no history of pruritus, hemorrhoids, fissure, or fistula. Diet includes one to two servings daily each of fresh fruits and vegetables but no whole-grain cereals or breads.

OBJECTIVE

No fissure, hemorrhoids, fistula, or skin lesions in perianal area. Sphincter tone good, no prolapse. Rectal walls smooth, no masses or tenderness. Prostate not enlarged, no masses or tenderness. Stool brown, Hematest result negative.

ASSESSMENT

Rectal structures intact, no palpable lesions

Focused Assessment: Clinical Case Study

Chand Mehta (C.M.) is a 62-year-old male with chronic obstructive pulmonary disease for 15 years, who today describes having had "diarrhea for 3 days."

SUBJECTIVE

7 days PTA [prior to arrival]: C.M. seen at this agency for acute respiratory infection that was diagnosed as acute bronchitis and treated with oral ampicillin. Took medication as directed.

3 days PTA: Symptoms of respiratory infection improved. Ingesting usual diet. Onset of four to five loose, unformed, brown stools a day. No abdominal pain or cramping. No nausea.

Now: Diarrhea continues. No blood or mucus noticed in stool. No new foods or restaurant food in past 3 days. Wife not ill.

OBJECTIVE

Vital signs: Temp 37°C (98.6°F), pulse 88 bpm, resp 18/min, BP 142/82 mm Hg.

Respiratory: Respirations unlaboured. Barrel chest. Hyper-resonant to percussion. Lung sounds clear but diminished. No crackles or rhonchi today.

Abdomen: Flat. Bowel sounds present. No organomegaly or tenderness to palpation.

Rectal: No lesions in perianal area. Sphincter tone good. Rectal walls smooth, no mass or tenderness. Prostate smooth and firm, no median sulcus palpable, no masses or tenderness. Stool brown, Hematest result negative.

ASSESSMENT

Diarrhea R/T [related to] effects of antibiotic medication

ABNORMAL FINDINGS

TABLE 23.2	Abnormalities of the Anal Region

Sinus tract

Fistula

Indurated cord

Pilonidal Cyst or Sinus

A hair-containing cyst or sinus located in the midline over the coccyx or lower sacrum. Often opens as a dimple with visible tuft of hair and, possibly, an erythematous halo, or may appear as a palpable cyst. When advanced, has a palpable sinus tract. Although congenital, the lesion is first diagnosed between the ages of 15 and 30 years.

Anorectal Fistula

A chronically inflamed gastro-intestinal tract creates an abnormal passage from inner anus or rectum out to skin surrounding anus. Usually originates from a local abscess. The red, raised tract opening may drain serosanguineous or purulent matter when pressure is applied. Bidigital palpation may reveal an indurated cord.

Continued

TABLE 23.2	Abnormalities of the Anal Region—cont'd

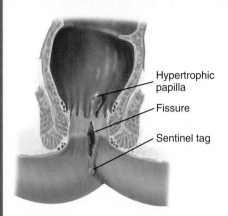

Hypertrophic papilla

Fissure

Sentinel tag

Internal hemorrhoid

Thrombosed external hemorrhoid

Fissure

A painful longitudinal tear in the superficial mucosa at the anal margin. Most fissures (>90%) occur in the posterior midline area. They are frequently accompanied by a papule of hyperplastic skin, called a *sentinel tag*, on the anal margin below. Fissures often result from trauma: for example, from passing a large, hard stool or from irritant diarrheal stools. Fissures cause itching, bleeding, and exquisite pain. A resulting spasm in the sphincters makes the area painful to examine; local anaesthesia may be indicated.

Hemorrhoids

These painless, flabby papules are caused by a varicose vein. An *external hemorrhoid* originates below the anorectal junction and is covered by anal skin. When *thrombosed*, it contains clotted blood and becomes a painful, swollen, shiny blue mass that itches and bleeds with defecation. When it resolves, it leaves a painless, flabby skin sac around the anal orifice. An *internal hemorrhoid* originates above the anorectal junction and is covered by mucous membrane. When the patient performs a Valsalva manoeuvre, it may appear as a red mucosal mass. Hemorrhoids result from increased portal venous pressure, as occurs with straining at stool, chronic constipation, pregnancy, obesity, chronic liver disease, or the low-fibre diet common in Western society.

TABLE 23.2   Abnormalities of the Anal Region—cont'd

Rectal Prolapse

The rectal mucous membrane protrudes through the anus, appearing as a moist red doughnut with radiating lines. When prolapse is incomplete, only the mucosa bulges. When complete, the anal sphincters also bulge. Occurs after a Valsalva manoeuvre, such as straining at stool, or with exercise. Caused by weakened pelvic support muscles and requires surgery.

Pruritus Ani

Intense perianal itching and burning is manifested by red, raised, thickened, excoriated skin around the anus. Common causes are pinworms in children and fungal infections in adults. The area is swollen and moist, and with a fungal infection, it appears dull greyish pink. The skin is dry and brittle with psychosomatic itching. Other causes include irritants (e.g., fecal soiling, soaps and detergents, medications and topical creams), anorectal disorders (e.g., hemorrhoids, fissures, colorectal cancer), dermatological disorders (e.g., psoriasis, dermatitis), psychological factors (e.g., stress, anxiety, depression) systemic disease (e.g., diabetes, liver or renal disease), or idiopathic causes.[8]

TABLE 23.3   Abnormalities of the Rectum

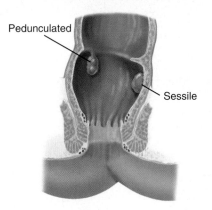

Abscess

A localized cavity of pus from infection in a pararectal space. Infection usually extends from an anal crypt. Characterized by persistent throbbing rectal pain. Termed according to the space it occupies (e.g., a perianal abscess is superficial around the anal skin) and appears red, hot, swollen, indurated, and tender. An ischiorectal abscess (lateral, between the anus and ischial tuberosity) is deep and tender to bidigital palpation and is rare. It must be drained before it worsens or develops sepsis.

Rectal Polyp

A growth protruding from the rectal mucous membrane that is fairly common. The polyp may be *pedunculated* (on a stalk) or *sessile* (a mound on the surface, close to the mucosal wall). The soft nodule is difficult to palpate. Sigmoidoscopy and biopsy are needed to screen for malignancy.

Fecal Impaction

A complete colon blockage by hard, desiccated immovable stool in the rectum, which presents as constipation or overflow incontinence. Abdominal palpation or DRE reveals mass. Results from decreased bowel motility as in hospitalized older adults and people with spinal cord injuries; also with low-fibre diet, hypothyroidism, opiate use, and retained barium after X-ray examination.[9] Community-dwelling older adults are at risk, especially those with dementia who cannot communicate.

Carcinoma

A malignant neoplasm in the rectum is asymptomatic; thus, the importance of routine DRE. An early lesion may be a single firm nodule. You may palpate an ulcerated centre with rolled edges. As the lesion grows, its shape is irregular, like cauliflower, and is fixed and stone hard. Refer a person with any rectal lesion for cancer screening.

DRE, Digital rectal examination.

TABLE 23.4 Abnormalities of the Prostate Gland

Benign Prostatic Hypertrophy

S: Urinary frequency, urgency, hesitancy, straining to urinate, weak stream, intermittent stream, sensation of incomplete emptying, nocturia.

O: A symmetrical, nontender enlargement commonly occurs in men beginning in middle age. The prostate surface feels smooth, rubbery, or firm (like the consistency of the nose), with the median sulcus obliterated.

Prostatitis

S: Fever, chills, malaise, urinary frequency and urgency, dysuria, urethral discharge; dull, aching pain in perineal and rectal area.

O: *Acute* inflammation: extremely tender, slightly asymmetric, swollen enlargement of the gland; *Chronic* inflammation: signs can vary from tender enlargement with a boggy texture to isolated firm areas caused by fibrosis, or the gland may feel normal.

◄ Carcinoma

S: Frequency, nocturia, hematuria, weak stream, hesitancy, pain or burning sensation on urination, continuous pain in lower back, pelvis, thighs.

O: A malignant neoplasm often starts as a single hard nodule on the posterior surface (see diagram *A*), producing asymmetry and a change in consistency. As it invades normal tissue, multiple hard nodules appear, or the entire gland feels stone hard and fixed (see diagram *B*), with the median sulcus obliterated.

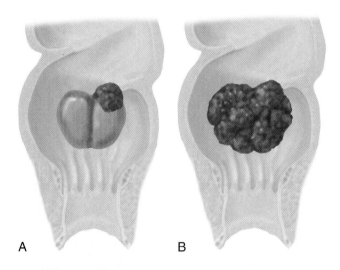

A   B

O, Objective data; *S*, subjective data.

Summary Checklist: Anus, Rectum, and Prostate Examination

1. **Inspect anus** and **perianal area**
2. **Inspect** during **Valsalva manoeuvre**
3. **Palpate anal canal** and **rectum** in all adults
4. **Test stool** for occult blood
5. **Engage in teaching and health promotion**

REFERENCES

1. Canadian Cancer Society Advisory Committee on Cancer Statistics. (2017). *Canadian cancer statistics 2017*. Toronto: Canadian Cancer Society. Retrieved from http://www.cancer.ca/~/media/cancer.ca/CW/cancer%20information/cancer%20101/Canadian%20cancer%20statistics/Canadian-Cancer-Statistics-2017-EN.pdf?la=en.

2. Singh, H., Bernstein, C. D., Samadder, J. N., et al. (2015). Screening rates for colorectal cancer in Canada: A cross-sectional study. *CMAJ Open, 3*(2), E149–E157. doi:10.9778/cmajo.20140073.

3. Young, S. W., Nishri, E. D., Candido, E., et al. (2015). *Colorectal cancer incidence in the Aboriginal population of Ontario, 1998 to 2009*. Retrieved from http://www.statcan.gc.ca/pub/82-003-x/2015004/article/14157-eng.htm.

4. Cyca, M. (2014). *Cancer risk and Aboriginal communities*. Retrieved from https://cancerprevent.ca/blog/cancer-risk-and-aboriginal-communities.

5. First Nations Health Authority. (2017). *Wellness for First Nations*. Retrieved from http://www.fnha.ca/wellness/wellness-for-first-nations.

6. Lewis, S. J., & Heaton, K. W. (1997). Stool form scale as a useful guide to intestinal transit time. *Scandinavian Journal of Gastroenterology, 32*(9), 920–924. doi:10.3109/00365529709011203.

7. Bournes, A. (2015). *Guidelines and protocols for hormone therapy and primary health care for trans clients*. Retrieved from http://sherbourne.on.ca/lgbt-health/guidelines-protocols-for-trans-care/.

8. Asgeirsson, T., Nunoo, R., & Luchtefeld, M. A. (2011). Hidradenitis suppurativa and pruritus ani. *Clinics in Colon and Rectal Surgery, 24*(1), 71–80. doi:10.1055/s-0031-1272826.

9. Fargo, M. V., & Latimer, K. M.(2012). Evaluation and management of common anorectal conditions. *American Family Physician, 85*(6), 624–630.

CHAPTER 24

Musculo-Skeletal System

Written by Carolyn Jarvis, PhD, APN, CNP
Adapted by Marian Luctkar-Flude, RN, PhD

ⓔ http://evolve.elsevier.com/Canada/Jarvis/examination/

STRUCTURE AND FUNCTION

24.1 Synovial joints.

The musculo-skeletal system consists of the body's bones, joints, and muscles. Humans need this system for *support* to stand erect and for *movement*. The musculo-skeletal system also functions to encase and *protect* the inner vital organs (e.g., brain, spinal cord, heart), to *produce* the red blood cells in the bone marrow (hematopoiesis), and as a *reservoir* for storage of essential minerals such as calcium and phosphorus in the bones.

COMPONENTS OF THE MUSCULO-SKELETAL SYSTEM

The skeleton has 206 bones that provide the framework of the body. Bone and cartilage are specialized forms of connective tissue. **Bone** is hard, rigid, and very dense. Its cells are continually turning over and remodelling. The **joint** (or articulation) is the place of union of two or more bones. Joints are the functional units of the musculo-skeletal system because they enable the mobility needed for activities of daily living (ADLs).

Nonsynovial or Synovial Joints

In **nonsynovial joints**, the bones are united by fibrous tissue or cartilage and are immovable (e.g., the sutures in the skull) or only slightly movable (e.g., the vertebrae). **Synovial joints** are freely movable because the bones are separated from each other and enclosed in a joint cavity (Fig. 24.1). This cavity is filled with a lubricant: synovial fluid that allows sliding of opposing surfaces, which enables movement.

625

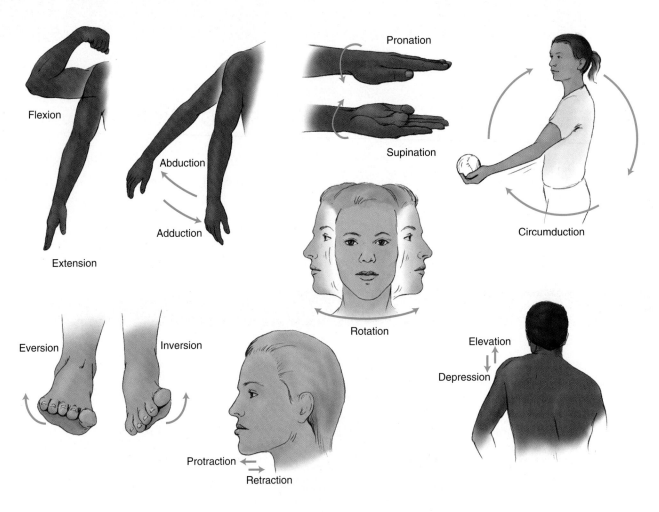

SKELETAL MUSCLE MOVEMENTS

24.2   © Pat Thomas, 2006.

In synovial joints, a layer of resilient **cartilage** covers the surface of opposing bones. Cartilage is avascular, receiving nourishment from synovial fluid that circulates during joint movement. It is a very stable connective tissue with a slow cell turnover. It has a tough, firm consistency, yet is flexible. Cartilage cushions the bones and provides a smooth surface to facilitate movement.

Each joint is surrounded by a fibrous capsule and is supported by ligaments. **Ligaments** are fibrous bands running directly from one bone to another that strengthen the joint and help prevent movement in undesirable directions. A **bursa** is an enclosed sac filled with viscous synovial fluid, much like a joint. Bursae are located in areas of potential friction (e.g., subacromial bursa of the shoulder, prepatellar bursa of the knee) and help muscles and tendons glide smoothly over bone.

Muscles

Muscles account for 40% to 50% of the body's weight. When they contract, they produce movement. Muscles are of three types: (a) skeletal, (b) smooth, and (c) cardiac. This chapter is concerned with skeletal, or voluntary, muscles, which are under conscious control.

Each **skeletal muscle** is composed of bundles of muscle fibres (**fasciculi**). Skeletal muscle is attached to bone by a **tendon**, a strong fibrous cord. Skeletal muscles produce the following movements (Fig. 24.2):

1. Flexion: bending a limb at a joint
2. Extension: straightening a limb at a joint
3. Abduction: moving a limb away from the midline of the body
4. Adduction: moving a limb toward the midline of the body
5. Pronation: turning the forearm so that the palm is down
6. Supination: turning the forearm so that the palm is up
7. Circumduction: moving the arm in a circle around the shoulder
8. Inversion: moving the sole of the foot inward at the ankle
9. Eversion: moving the sole of the foot outward at the ankle
10. Rotation: moving the head around a central axis

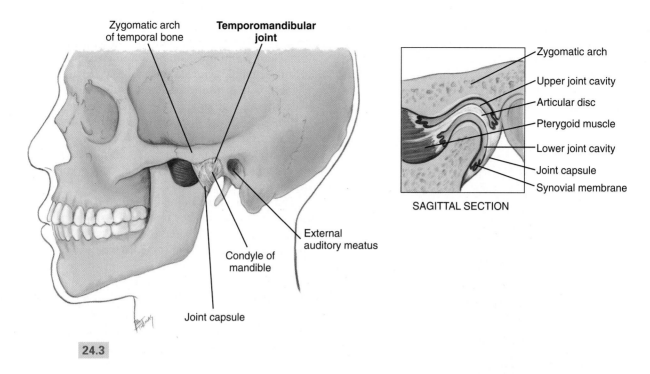

Zygomatic arch
of temporal bone

**Temporomandibular
joint**

Zygomatic arch

Upper joint cavity

Articular disc

Pterygoid muscle

Lower joint cavity

Joint capsule

Synovial membrane

SAGITTAL SECTION

External
auditory meatus

Condyle of
mandible

Joint capsule

24.3

11. Protraction: moving a body part forward and parallel to the ground
12. Retraction: moving a body part backward and parallel to the ground
13. Elevation: raising a body part
14. Depression: lowering a body part

Temporomandibular Joint

The temporomandibular joint is the articulation of the mandible and the temporal bone (Fig. 24.3). You can feel it in the depression anterior to the tragus of the ear. The temporomandibular joint enables jaw function for speaking and chewing. The joint allows three motions: (a) hinge action to open and close the jaws, (b) gliding action for protrusion and retraction, and (c) gliding action for side-to-side movement of the lower jaw.

Spine

The **vertebrae** are 33 connecting bones stacked in a vertical column (Fig. 24.4). You can feel their spinous processes in a furrow down the midline of the back. The furrow has paravertebral muscles mounded on either side down to the sacrum, where it flattens. Humans have 7 cervical, 12 thoracic, 5 lumbar, 5 sacral, and 3 to 4 coccygeal vertebrae. The following surface landmarks will orient you to their levels:

- The spinous processes of C7 and T1 are prominent at the base of the neck.
- The inferior angle of the scapula normally is at the level of the interspace between T7 and T8.
- An imaginary line connecting the highest point on each iliac crest crosses L4.
- An imaginary line joining the two symmetrical dimples that overlie the posterior superior iliac spines crosses the sacrum.

T1

C7

T7

Scapula

T8

T12

L1

Iliac crest

L4

Posterior
superior
iliac spine

S2

Coccyx

LANDMARKS OF THE SPINE

24.4

A lateral view (Fig. 24.5) shows that the vertebral column has four curves (a double S-shape). The cervical and lumbar curves are concave (inward or anterior), and the thoracic and sacrococcygeal curves are convex. The balanced or compensatory nature of these curves, together with the resilient intervertebral discs, allows the spine to absorb a great deal of shock.

24.5

The **intervertebral discs** are elastic fibrocartilaginous plates that constitute one-fourth of the length of the column (Fig. 24.6). Each disc centre has a **nucleus pulposus**, made of soft, semifluid, mucoid material that has the consistency of toothpaste in young adults. The discs cushion the spine like a shock absorber and help it move. As the spine moves, the elasticity of the discs allows compression on one side, with compensatory expansion on the other. If compression is too great, a disc can rupture, and the nucleus pulposus can herniate out of the vertebral column, compressing the spinal nerves and causing pain.

The unique structure of the spine enables both upright posture and flexibility for motion. The motions of the vertebral column are flexion (bending forward), extension (bending back), abduction (to either side), and rotation.

Shoulder

The **glenohumeral joint** is the articulation of the humerus with the glenoid fossa of the scapula (Fig. 24.7). Its ball-and-socket action allows great mobility of the arm in many axes. The joint is enclosed by a group of four powerful muscles and tendons that support and stabilize it. Together, these muscles and tendons are called the **rotator cuff** of the shoulder. The large **subacromial bursa** helps during abduction of the arm so that the greater tubercle of the humerus moves easily under the acromion process of the scapula.

The bones of the shoulder have palpable landmarks to guide examination (Fig. 24.8). The scapula and clavicle connect to form the shoulder girdle. You can feel the bump of the scapula's **acromion process** at the very top of the

24.6 The vertebrae.

SHOULDER JOINT

24.7

SHOULDER WITH ARM ELEVATED – SUPERIOR VIEW

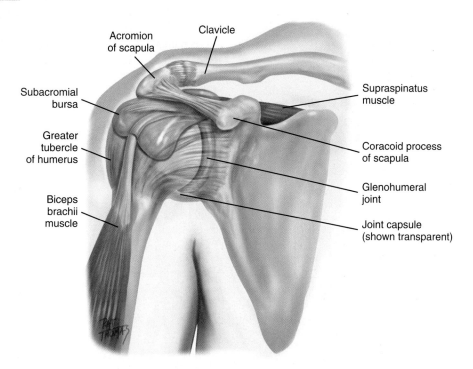

BONY LANDMARKS OF THE SHOULDER – ANTERIOR VIEW

24.8

shoulder. Move your fingers in a small circle outward, down, and around. The next bump is the **greater tubercle** of the humerus a few centimetres down and laterally, and from that the **coracoid process** of the scapula is a few centimetres medially. These surround the deeply situated joint.

Elbow

The elbow joint contains three bony articulations of the (a) humerus, (b) radius, and (c) ulna of the forearm (Fig. 24.9). Its hinge action moves the forearm (radius and ulna) on one plane, allowing flexion and extension. The olecranon bursa lies between the olecranon process and the skin.

Palpable landmarks are the **medial** and **lateral epicondyles** of the humerus and the large **olecranon process** of the ulna in between them. The sensitive ulnar nerve runs between the olecranon process and the medial epicondyle.

The radius and ulna articulate with each other at two radioulnar joints, one at the elbow and one at the wrist. These move together, enabling pronation and supination of the hand and forearm.

Wrist and Carpal Joints

Of the body's 206 bones, more than half are in the hands and feet. The wrist, or **radiocarpal joint**, is the articulation of the radius (on the thumb side) and a row of carpal bones (Fig. 24.10). Its condyloid action enables movement in two planes at right angles: (a) flexion and extension and (b)

side-to-side deviation. You can feel the groove of this joint on the dorsum of the wrist.

The **midcarpal joint** is the articulation between two parallel rows of carpal bones. It allows flexion, extension, and some rotation. The **metacarpophalangeal** and the **interphalangeal joints** enable finger flexion and extension. The flexor tendons of the wrist and hand are enclosed in synovial sheaths.

Hip

The hip joint is the articulation between the acetabulum and the head of the femur (Fig. 24.11). As in the shoulder, ball-and-socket action enables a wide range of motion (ROM) on many axes. The hip has somewhat less ROM than the shoulder, but it has more stability, which befits its weight-bearing function. Hip stability is enabled by powerful muscles that spread over the joint, a strong fibrous articular capsule, and the very deep insertion of the head of the femur. Three bursae facilitate movement.

Palpation of bony landmarks will guide your examination: you can feel the entire iliac crest, from the **anterior superior iliac spine** to the posterior superior iliac spine. The **ischial tuberosity** lies under the gluteus maximus muscle and is palpable when the hip is flexed. The **greater trochanter** of the femur is normally the width of the person's palm below the iliac crest and halfway between the anterior superior iliac spine and the ischial tuberosity. You can palpate it, when the person is standing, in a flat depression on the upper lateral side of the thigh.

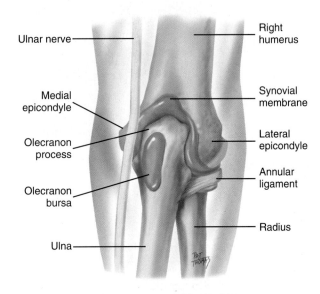

Ulnar nerve

Medial epicondyle

Olecranon process

Olecranon bursa

Ulna

Right humerus

Synovial membrane

Lateral epicondyle

Annular ligament

Radius

RIGHT ELBOW – POSTERIOR VIEW

24.9

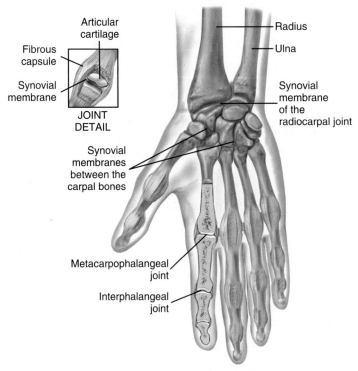

Articular cartilage

Fibrous capsule

Synovial membrane

JOINT DETAIL

Synovial membranes between the carpal bones

Radius

Ulna

Synovial membrane of the radiocarpal joint

Metacarpophalangeal joint

Interphalangeal joint

BONES OF THE HAND – PALMAR VIEW

24.10

HIP JOINT

24.11

LEFT KNEE – MEDIAL VIEW

24.12

SAGITTAL SECTION

Knee

The knee joint is the articulation of three bones—(a) the femur, (b) the tibia, and (c) the patella (kneecap)—in one common articular cavity (Fig. 24.12). It is the largest joint in the body and is complex. It is a hinge joint, enabling flexion and extension of the lower leg on a single plane.

The knee's synovial membrane is the largest in the body. At the superior border of the patella, it forms a sac, the **suprapatellar pouch**, that extends up as much as 6 cm behind the quadriceps muscle. Two wedge-shaped cartilages, the **medial** and **lateral menisci**, cushion the tibia and femur.

The joint is stabilized by two sets of ligaments. The **cruciate ligaments** (not shown in Fig. 24.12) criss-cross within the knee, providing anterior and posterior stability and helping control rotation. The **collateral ligaments** connect the joint at both sides, providing medial and lateral stability and preventing dislocation. Numerous bursae prevent friction. One, the **prepatellar bursa**, lies between the patella and the skin. The **infrapatellar fat pad** is a small, triangular fat pad below the patella and behind the patellar ligament.

Landmarks of the knee joint start with the large **quadriceps muscle**, which you can feel on your anterior and lateral thigh (Fig. 24.13). The muscle's four heads merge into a common tendon that continues down to enclose the round bony patella. Then the tendon inserts down on the **tibial tuberosity**, which you can palpate as a bony prominence in the midline. Move to the sides and a bit superiorly, and note the lateral and medial condyles of the tibia. Superior to these on either side of the patella are the medial and lateral epicondyles of the femur.

Ankle and Foot

The ankle, or **tibiotalar joint**, is the articulation of the tibia, fibula, and talus (Fig. 24.14). It is a hinge joint, limited to flexion (dorsiflexion) and extension (plantar flexion) in one plane. Landmarks are two bony prominences on either side: (a) the **medial malleolus** and (b) the **lateral malleolus**. Strong, tight medial and lateral ligaments extend from each malleolus onto the foot. They promote lateral stability of the

ankle joint, although they may be torn in eversion or inversion sprains of the ankle.

Joints distal to the ankle provide additional mobility in the foot. The subtalar joint enables inversion and eversion of the foot. The foot has a longitudinal arch, so that weight bearing is distributed between the parts that touch the ground: the heads of the metatarsals and the calcaneus (heel).

❖ DEVELOPMENTAL CONSIDERATIONS

Infants and Children

By 3 months' gestation, a "scale model" of the skeleton that is made up of cartilage has formed. During succeeding months in utero, the cartilage ossifies into true bone and starts to grow. Bone growth continues after birth—rapidly during infancy and then steadily during childhood—and during adolescence.

Long bones grow in two dimensions. They increase in width or diameter by deposition of new bony tissue around the shafts. Lengthening occurs at the **epiphyses** (growth plates). These specialized growth centres are transverse discs located at the ends of long bones. Trauma or infection at this location puts the growing child at risk for bone deformity. Longitudinal growth continues until closure of the epiphyses; the last closure occurs at about age 20 years.

Skeletal contour changes are apparent at the vertebral column. At birth the spine has a single C-shaped curve. At 3 to 4 months, when the baby can raise the head from the prone position, the anterior curve in the cervical neck region develops. From ages 1 year to 18 months, standing erect causes the development of the anterior curve in the lumbar region.

Although the skeleton contributes to linear growth, muscles and fat are significant for weight increase. Individual muscle fibres grow through childhood, but growth is marked during the **adolescent growth spurt**. At this time, muscles respond to increased secretion of growth hormone,

LANDMARKS OF THE RIGHT KNEE JOINT

24.13

ANKLE JOINT IN SECTION

24.14

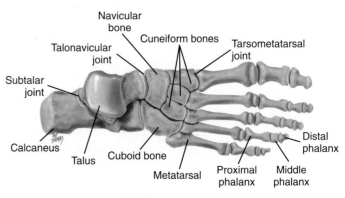

DORSAL VIEW (TOP OF FOOT)

to adrenal androgens, and, in boys, to further stimulation by testosterone. Muscles vary in size and strength in different people. This variation is attributable to genetic programming, nutrition, and exercise. All through life, muscles increase with use and atrophy with disuse. Obesity and osteoporosis have their beginnings in childhood. The following factors help prevent obesity and promote peak bone mass accrual: regular exercise; a diet rich in dark green and deep yellow vegetables, and dairy products; and a diet low in fried foods and carbonated beverages.[1] Routine growth monitoring is recommended for all children and youth to identify those who are not following a healthy body mass index (BMI) trajectory according to the World Health Organization (WHO) Growth Charts for Canada.[2]

The term *developmental dysplasia of the hip* (DDH) refers to a number of congenital abnormalities of the hip joint, including dislocated hip and subluxation of the hip. The Canadian Task Force on Preventive Health Care recommends clinical examination of the hips by a trained clinician in the periodic health examination of all infants until they are walking independently.[3] Potential risk factors for DDH include having a first-degree relative with DDH, breech delivery, and clinical evidence of joint instability. Girls are more predisposed than boys to DDH, and Indigenous people in Canada have a high risk for DDH.

The most common cause of childhood musculo-skeletal pain is termed "growing pains," a noninflammatory pain syndrome affecting children mainly between the ages of 3 and 12 years. The pain is usually nonarticular, bilateral, and located in the lower extremities; it occurs late in the day or is nocturnal, often awakening the child, and frequently occurs on days of increased physical activity. The pain can be mild or very severe, lasting minutes to hours; is generally episodic but may occur daily; and usually resolves by late childhood. Other causes should be considered when a child is younger than 3 years of age, is limping, or interrupts play or exercise due to the pain.

Pregnant Women

Increased levels of circulating hormones (estrogen, relaxin from the corpus luteum, and corticosteroids) cause increased mobility in the joints. Increased mobility in the sacroiliac, sacrococcygeal, and symphysis pubis joints in the pelvis contributes to the noticeable changes in maternal posture. The most characteristic change is progressive **lordosis**, which compensates for the enlarging fetus; otherwise, the centre of balance would shift forward. Lordosis compensates by shifting the weight farther back on the lower extremities. This shift in balance, in turn, creates strain on the low back muscles, which in some women is felt as low back pain during late pregnancy.

Anterior flexion of the neck and slumping of the shoulder girdle are other postural changes that compensate for the lordosis. These upper back changes may put pressure on the ulnar and median nerves during the third trimester. Nerve pressure creates aching, numbness, and weakness in the upper extremities in some women.

Older Adults

Bone remodelling is a cyclical process of loss of bone matrix (bone resorption) and new bone growth (deposition). Deposition predominates until skeletal maturity at 25 to 35 years, when bone mass reaches its peak.[4] After age 40, resorption occurs more rapidly than deposition. The net effect is a loss of bone density (**osteoporosis**). Although some degree of osteoporosis is nearly universal, women are more affected than men because lack of estrogen after menopause causes bone loss to accelerate. Risk factors for fracture associated with osteoporosis are listed in Table 24.1.

Postural changes are evident with aging, and decreased height is the most noticeable. Long bones do not shorten with age; decrease in height results from shortening of the vertebral column caused by loss of water content and thinning of the intervertebral discs, which occurs more in

TABLE 24.1 **Indications for Measuring Bone Mineral Density to Assess for Osteoporosis**	
OLDER ADULTS (AGE ≥50 YEARS)	**YOUNGER ADULTS (AGE <50 YEARS)**
Age ≥65 years (both women and men)	Fragility fracture
Clinical risk factors for fracture in men aged 50–64 years and in menopausal women:	Prolonged use of glucocorticoids[a]
• Fragility fracture after age 40 years	Use of other high-risk medication[b]
• Prolonged use of glucocorticoids[a]	Hypogonadism or premature
• Use of other high-risk medications[b]	menopause (age <45 years)
• Parental hip fracture	Malabsorption syndrome
• Vertebral fracture or osteopenia identified on radiography	Primary hyperparathyroidism
• Current smoking	Other disorders strongly associated with
• High alcohol intake	rapid bone loss and/or fracture
• Low body weight (<60 kg) or major weight loss (>10% of body weight at age 25 years)	
• Rheumatoid arthritis	
• Other disorders strongly associated with osteoporosis	

[a]At least 3 months of cumulative therapy in the previous year at a prednisone-equivalent dose of ≥7.5 mg daily.
[b]For example, aromatase inhibitors or androgen deprivation therapy.
From Papaioannou, A., Morin, S., Cheung, A. M., et al. (2010). 2010 Clinical practice guidelines for the diagnosis and management of osteoporosis in Canada: Summary. *Canadian Medical Association Journal, 182*(17), 1864–1873. doi:10.1503/cmaj.100771.

middle age. Both men and women can expect a progressive decrease in height beginning in the 40s, although this is not significant until age 60 years. A greater decrease occurs in the 70s and 80s as a result of osteoporotic collapse of the vertebrae, which results in shortening of the trunk and the appearance of comparatively long extremities. Other postural changes are kyphosis, a backward head tilt to compensate for the kyphosis, and a slight flexion of hips and knees.

The distribution of subcutaneous fat changes through life. Usually, men and women gain weight in their 40s and 50s. The body contour is different, even if the weight is the same as when they were younger. They begin to lose fat in the face and deposit it in the abdomen and hips. In the 80s and 90s, fat further decreases in the periphery, noticeably in the forearms and over the abdomen and hips.

Loss of subcutaneous fat leaves bony prominences more marked (e.g., tips of vertebrae, ribs, iliac crests) and body hollows deeper (e.g., cheeks, axillae). An absolute loss in muscle mass occurs; some muscles decrease in size, and some atrophy, which causes weakness. Muscle contours become more prominent, and muscle bundles and tendons feel more distinct.

Lifestyle affects musculo-skeletal changes; a sedentary lifestyle hastens the musculo-skeletal changes of aging. However, physical exercise increases skeletal mass, helping prevent or delay osteoporosis in postmenopausal women[5] and older men.[6] (See the box Promoting Health: Preventing Osteoporosis). In 2014, only 54% of Canadians were at least moderately active during their leisure time, equivalent to walking at least 30 minutes a day or taking an hour-long exercise class at least three times a week.[7]

PROMOTING HEALTH: PREVENTING OSTEOPOROSIS

Do Not Overlook Osteoporosis

Bone is a living tissue that continually grows and changes. Every day old bone dissolves and is replaced with new, stronger bone. Until a person is 30 years old, new bone appears at a faster rate than the bone disappears. As people age, however, the opposite begins to occur. When this happens, bones can become "spongy," weak, and more likely to break with even the slightest of twists or bumps. This condition is called *osteoporosis*. The bones of the wrist, hip, and spine are most often affected.

Osteoporosis is more common in women, slender people, and individuals of European descent. An estimated 2 million Canadians are affected by osteoporosis and at least one in three women and one in five men will break a bone due to osteoporosis in their lifetime.* Postmenopausal women are especially vulnerable because of hormonal changes. Osteoporosis tends to run in families, but lifestyle choices can increase the risk even in individuals without a family history. A person whose calcium intake is low or who lacks exercise, smokes, or consumes large quantities of alcohol is at a higher risk of developing osteoporosis. Although long-term use of proton pump inhibitor (PPI) medications to treat acid-related conditions such as stomach ulcers has been associated with an increased risk for bone fractures, recent randomized trials show no impact of PPI therapy on either calcium absorption or risk for osteoporosis.†

Osteoporosis Canada recommends that all women and men older than age 50 be assessed for risk factors for osteoporosis and fracture. Bone mineral density (BMD) testing is used to diagnose osteoporosis and predict fracture risk.‡ BMD testing is recommended for all women aged 65 and older and for those with clinical risk factors for fracture such as fragility fracture after age 40, prolonged use of glucocorticoids, or parental hip fracture (see Table 24.1, p. 633).

Prevention of osteoporosis is important because there is no cure, only treatment, for osteoporosis. The gold standard for treatment of osteoporosis has traditionally been hormone replacement therapy (HRT), which has been shown to prevent bone loss and improve bone mineralization. However, new research indicates that HRT may carry an increased risk for breast cancer and myocardial infarction in women. Alternative therapies that include exercise and diet provide similar, if not equal, benefits for women at risk for osteoporosis.

Recommendations for Bone Health
1. **Diet.** Adequate intake of calcium and vitamin D are necessary to maintain bone health.
   a. **Dine on dairy.** Low-fat milk, yogourt, and cheese are healthy sources of calcium. Fortified milk products also contain vitamin D, which is needed to absorb calcium.
   b. **Go fish.** Salmon and sardines, which are canned with their bones, are rich in calcium, and oily fish such as mackerel are rich in vitamin D.
   c. **Eat your greens.** Leafy green vegetables have a lot of calcium. Fill up on broccoli, kale, Swiss chard, turnip greens, and bok choy. These foods also contain potassium and vitamin K, which help block calcium loss from bones.
   d. **Try soy.** Soy contains calcium and plant estrogens. Try substituting soy flour for regular flour in recipes, nibbling on soybean "nuts," or drinking soy milk.
   e. **Limit caffeine.** Caffeine causes the body to excrete calcium more readily. Caffeine is present in coffee, tea, hot chocolate, and many carbonated drinks (e.g., cola).
   f. **Eat onions.** Although onions are not known to have any nutritive value, they appear to reduce the bone breakdown process that can lead to osteoporosis.
2. **Exercise.** Bones and muscles must work against gravity to have a bone-building effect. A regular program of weight-bearing exercise for at least 30 minutes three times a week is recommended as the minimum. Try walking, low-impact aerobics, dancing, or stationary cycling. Resistance training with light weights or resistance bands is also recommended, and exercises that focus on posture and balance, such as tai chi, can help reduce the risk for falls.

PROMOTING HEALTH: PREVENTING OSTEOPOROSIS—cont'd

Do Not Overlook Osteoporosis

Sunshine also helps the body produce vitamin D. About 15 minutes of exposure to sunshine a day is all that is needed to maintain a good vitamin D supply.

3. **Lifestyle.** Avoid smoking and excessive alcohol, and seek help for depression. People who smoke have twice the risk for spinal and hip fractures. Furthermore, fractures heal more slowly in people who smoke and are more apt to heal improperly. Too much alcohol prevents the body from absorbing calcium. In addition, seek help for depression. Research has shown that women with clinical depression have lower bone densities.

4. **Medical options.** Talk to a health care provider about bone health. Although many people consider osteoporosis prevention to be important, fewer than half discuss the topic with health care providers or undergo BMD screening. Ask that your height be measured on an annual basis. A loss of 2 to 5 cm is an early sign of undiagnosed vertebral fractures and osteoporosis. Seek treatment for conditions that can jeopardize BMD, including thyroid disease, certain intestinal and kidney diseases, and some cancers. Also, remember that some medications may contribute to bone loss: for example, corticosteroids, anticoagulants, thyroid supplements, and certain anticonvulsants.

5. **Supplements.** Most people do not get enough calcium in their diets, and supplements may help achieve the minimum dosage. The total daily intake of elemental calcium (through diet and supplements) is 1 200 mg for adults over age 50 years. It is impossible for adults to get sufficient vitamin D from diet alone. The recommended daily dose of vitamin D is 400 to 1 000 IU for healthy adults between 19 and 50 years of age and 800 to 2 000 IU for adults over 50 years of age or younger adults at high risk (with osteoporosis, multiple fractures, or vitamin D malabsorption).

References

*Osteoporosis Canada. (2018). *About the disease*. Retrieved from https://osteoporosis.ca/about-the-disease/.

†Leontiadis, G. I., & Moayyedi, P. (2014). Proton pump inhibitors and risk of bone fractures. *Current Treatment Options in Gastroenterology*, 12(4), 414–423. doi:10.1007/s11938-014-0030-y.

‡Papaioannou, A., Morin, S., Cheung, A. M., et al. (2010). 2010 Clinical practice guidelines for the diagnosis and management of osteoporosis in Canada: Summary. *Canadian Medical Association Journal*, 182(17), 1864–1873. doi:10.1503/cmaj.100771.

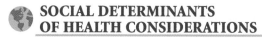

SOCIAL DETERMINANTS OF HEALTH CONSIDERATIONS

Arthritis is one of the most prevalent chronic health conditions and a leading cause of pain, physical disability, and health care system use in Canada. In 2016, about 6.1 million Canadians (20.4%) aged 15 and older reported that they had arthritis.[8] In that year, arthritis was prevalent among 23.9% of females and 17.3% of males. The prevalence of arthritis increases with age, and the highest number of people affected are age 75 years and older.[9] For individuals with arthritis who are under age 65, this condition frequently results in loss of work and productivity. Prevalence of arthritis is higher in women and in individuals living in rural areas, but lower among immigrants, particularly recent immigrants (less than 15 years since immigration). Prevalence of arthritis is also higher among people with a lower education and income level, and 1.3 to 1.6 times higher among First Nations and Métis adults.

Osteoarthritis is the most prevalent type of arthritis, affecting more than 3 million Canadians.[10] Risk factors for osteoarthritis include increasing age, family history, excess weight, and joint injury. Low educational attainment and nonprofessional occupations are also associated with poorer arthritis outcomes.[11] About 300 000 Canadians have rheumatoid arthritis, with three times more women affected than men.[10] The cause of rheumatoid arthritis is; it can occur at any age, but usually appears between the ages of 40 and 60.

About 4.27 million Canadians aged 12 or older suffered an injury severe enough to limit their usual activities in 2009–10.[12] The most common types of injury were sprains and strains (51%), followed by fractures and broken bones (17%). Most adolescent patients were injured playing sports (66%), younger and middle-aged adults were injured playing sports or at work (47%), and more than half of older adults' injuries occurred while they were walking or performing household chores. (See the box Promoting Health: Preventing Workplace Pains and Strains.) Falls were the leading cause of injury among older adults (63%), adolescents (50%), and younger and middle-aged adults (35%).

Hip fractures are a serious consequence of falls in older adults. It is estimated that about 30 000 hip fractures occur in Canada each year.[13] Women are twice as likely as men to fracture a hip. Hip fractures can result in loss of mobility and independence, financial difficulties, and increased use of health care services. In a large Canadian study, adults aged 50 years and older with hip or vertebral fractures were more likely to die during the 5-year follow-up than were those without fractures.[14] Similarly, adults aged 65 or older accounted for the majority of joint replacements—63% of hip replacements and 64% of knee replacements—in Canada during 2006–07.[15] A high proportion of patients undergoing hip and knee replacement were obese, according to BMI. Across the country, efforts have been made to reduce wait times for hip and joint replacement surgeries.

PROMOTING HEALTH: PREVENTING WORKPLACE PAINS AND STRAINS

Protecting Your Spine on the Job

Musculo-skeletal disorders in the workplace often result from repetitive, forceful, or awkward movements on bones, joints, ligaments, and other tissues resulting in pain, numbness, tingling, weakness, or restricted movements. Workplace pains and strains, also referred to as *repetitive strain* or *repetitive motion injuries*, include back pain, shoulder pain, tennis elbow, rotator cuff syndrome, carpal tunnel syndrome, muscle strain, and tendinitis. Low back injuries are among the most common occupational injuries, often resulting from prolonged sitting, standing, or lifting. Most people experience back pain at least once in their lifetime, and the lower back is the primary site of chronic pain among Canadians.* Low back pain is more common among men, and increases in prevalence until age 65 years. Common risk factors include low educational status, sedentary lifestyle, obesity, stress, anxiety, depression, job dissatisfaction, low levels of workplace social support, and whole-body vibration.[†] Research studies have documented a higher prevalence of low back pain in nurses.[‡] Chronic pain such as back pain can contribute to activity restriction, psychological distress, and decreased mental health.[§]

Recommendations for Back Health

1. **Sitting.** Limit the amount of uninterrupted time sitting and take breaks every 30 minutes for 1 to 2 minutes. Stand, stretch, or take a short walk.
2. **Standing.** When standing for long periods, rest one foot on a low stool to relieve pressure on the lower back. Switch feet every 5 to 15 minutes, change position frequently, and move around as much as possible. Wear flat shoes or low heels (2.5 cm or lower) and maintain good posture.
3. **Lifting.** Learn and use appropriate body mechanics to reduce lower back stress: lift loads close to the body, lift smoothly without jerking, and avoid twisting and side

bending when lifting. Use mechanical aids to eliminate heavy lifting.
4. **Lifestyle.** Extra abdominal weight creates stress on the lower back, and sedentary lifestyle leads to muscle weakening, stiffness, and degeneration of spinal discs. Get regular physical activity, including stretching, strengthening, and low-impact aerobic activities, to help prevent occurrence and recurrence of low back pain. Exercises that strengthen the back and abdominal muscles provide better support for the spine.

References

*Schopflocher, D., Taenzer, P., & Jovey, R. (2011). The prevalence of chronic pain in Canada. *Pain Research & Management*, 16(6), 445–450.

[†]Hoy, D., Brooks, P., Blyth, F., et al. (2010). The epidemiology of low back pain. *Best Practice & Research. Clinical Rheumatology*, 24, 769–781. doi:10.1016/j.berh.2010.10.002.

[‡]Yassi, A., & Lockhart, K. (2013). Work-relatedness of low back pain in nursing personnel: A systematic review. *International Journal of Occupational and Environmental Health*, 19(3), 223–244. doi:10.1179/2049396713Y.0000000027.

[§]Gilmour, H. (2015). Chronic pain, activity restriction and flourishing mental health. *Health Reports*, 26(1), 15–22.

Additional Resources

Canadian Centre for Occupational Health and Safety. (2017). *Back injury prevention.* Retrieved from https://www.ccohs.ca/oshanswers/ergonomics/inj_prev.html.

The College of Family Physicians of Canada. (2012). *Low back pain: Tips on pain relief and prevention.* Retrieved from http://www.cfpc.ca/uploadedFiles/Resources/Resource_Items/Patients/LowerBackPain_EN.pdf.

Ontario Ministry of Labour. (2009). *Prevent workplace pains and strains! It's time to take action!* Retrieved from https://www.labour.gov.on.ca/english/hs/pubs/ergonomics/is_ergonomics.php.

Statistics Canada. (2014). *Work injuries.* Retrieved from http://www.statcan.gc.ca/pub/82-003-x/2006007/article/injuries-blessures/4149017-eng.htm.

SUBJECTIVE DATA

1. Joints:
   Pain
   Stiffness
   Swelling, heat, redness
   Limitation of movement
2. Knee joint (if injured)

3. Muscles:
   Pain (cramps)
   Weakness
4. Bones:
   Pain
   Deformity

   Trauma (fractures, sprains, dislocations)
5. Functional assessment (ADLs)
6. Self-care behaviours

HEALTH HISTORY QUESTIONS

Examiner Asks	Rationale
1. Joints. Any problems with your joints? Any **pain**?	**Joint pain** and loss of function are the most common musculo-skeletal concerns.

Examiner Asks	Rationale
• Location: Which joints? On one side or both sides?	Rheumatoid arthritis is symmetrical, involving the same joints on both sides; other musculo-skeletal illnesses involve isolated or unilateral joints. Exquisite tenderness occurs with acute inflammation.
• Quality: What does the pain feel like: aching, stiff, sharp or dull, shooting? • Severity: How strong is the pain? • Onset: When did this pain start? • Timing: What time of day does the pain occur? How long does it last? • How often does it occur?	Rheumatoid arthritis pain is worse in the morning on arising; osteoarthritis is worse later in the day; tendinitis is worse in the morning and improves during the day.
• Is the pain aggravated by movement, rest, position, weather? Is the pain relieved by rest, medications, application of heat or ice?	Movement increases most joint pain except in rheumatoid arthritis, in which movement decreases pain.
• Is the pain associated with chills, fever, recent sore throat, trauma, repetitive activity?	Joint pain 10 to 14 days after an untreated streptococcal infection ("strep throat") is suggestive of rheumatic fever. Joint injury is caused by trauma and repetitive motion.
• Any **stiffness** in your joints?	Rheumatoid arthritis stiffness occurs in morning and after rest periods.
• Any **swelling, heat, redness** in the joints?	These signs are suggestive of acute inflammation.
• Any **limitation of movement** in any joint? Which joint? • Which activities give you problems? (See Functional Assessment [ADLs].)	Decrease in ROM may be caused by joint injury to cartilage or the capsule, or it may result from muscle contracture.
2. **Knee joint (if injured).** How did you **injure** your knee? Hit inside of knee? Outside? Twisting or pivoting? Overuse such as jumping or kneeling?	Inside knee injury can strain or rupture medial ligament; outside injury can strain or rupture lateral ligament; abrupt twisting can injure anterior cruciate ligament.[16]
• Hear a "pop" at injury? Can you stand on that leg? Can you flex the knee? Point to where it hurts the most.	Pop may mean tear in ligament or fracture. With direct knee trauma, obtain radiograph if the patient is unable to flex knee to 90 degrees or unable to bear weight, if pain is experienced at fibula head or patella, or if patient is over age 55 years (Ottawa Knee Rules).
3. **Muscles.** Any problems in the muscles, such as any **pain** or **cramping**? Which muscles? • If pain is widespread: How long have you had this pain? Is the pain associated with fatigue?	**Myalgia** is usually felt as cramping or aching. Widespread musculo-skeletal pain lasting 3 months or longer and associated with fatigue is suggestive of fibromyalgia.[17]
• If pain is in calf muscles: Does the pain occur with walking? Does it go away with rest? • Are your muscle aches associated with fever, chills, the "flu"?	Calf pain may represent intermittent claudication (see Chapter 21). Symptoms of viral illness often include myalgia.
• Any **weakness** in muscles? • Location: Where is the weakness? How long have you noticed weakness? • Do the muscles look smaller there?	Weakness may involve musculo-skeletal or neurological systems (see Chapter 25). Decrease in muscle size is indicative of atrophy.

Examiner Asks	Rationale

4. Bones. Any **bone pain**? Is the pain affected by movement?
- Any **deformity** of any bone or joint? Caused by injury or trauma? Does the deformity affect ROM?
- Have any **accidents** or **trauma** ever affected the bones or joints: fractures, joint strain, sprain, dislocation? Which ones?
- When did this occur? What treatment was given? Any problems or limitations now as a result?
- Any back pain? In which part of your back? Is pain felt anywhere else, such as shooting down your leg?
- Any numbness and tingling? Any limping?

CRITICAL FINDINGS

Fracture causes sharp pain that increases with movement (other bone pain usually feels "dull" and "deep" and is unrelated to movement). A fractured bone may also be misaligned. Report findings immediately. Never attempt to realign broken bones. Monitor vital signs and peripheral vascular circulation distal to the injury until the patient's care is transferred.

5. Functional assessment (ADLs). Do problems with your joints (muscle, bone) impose any limits on your usual **ADLs**? Which ones? (Note: Ask about each category; if the patient answers "yes," ask specifically about each activity in category.)
- Bathing: getting in and out of the tub, turning faucets
- Toileting: urinating, defecating, ability to get self on and off toilet, wiping self
- Dressing: manipulating buttons and zippers, fastening openings behind the neck, pulling dress or sweater over head, pulling up pants, tying shoes, wearing shoes that fit
- Grooming: shaving, brushing teeth, brushing or fixing hair, applying makeup
- Eating: preparing meals, pouring liquids, cutting up foods, bringing food to mouth, drinking
- Mobility: walking, walking up or down stairs, getting in and out of bed, getting out of the home
- Communicating: talking, using phone, writing

Functional assessment is used to assess the safety of independent living, the need for home health care services, and quality of life (see Chapter 31).
Assess any self-care deficit.

Assess for impairment in physical mobility.
Assess for impairment in verbal communication.

6. Self-care behaviours. Any occupational hazards that could affect the muscles and joints? Does your work involve heavy lifting? Or any repetitive motion or chronic stress to joints? Any efforts to alleviate these?
- Tell me about your exercise program: type of exercise, frequency, warm-up program?
- Any pain during exercise? How do you treat it?
- Have you had any recent weight gain? Please describe your usual daily diet. (Note the patient's usual caloric intake, all four food groups, daily amount of protein, calcium.)
- Are you taking any medications for musculo-skeletal system: Aspirin, anti-inflammatory, muscle relaxant, pain reliever?
- If patient has chronic disability or crippling illness: How has your illness affected the following:
  Your interaction with family?
  Your interaction with friends?
  The way you view yourself?

Assess risk for back pain or carpal tunnel syndrome.

Assess **self-care behaviours**.

Assess for the following:
- Self-esteem disturbance
- Loss of independence
- Body image disturbance
- Role performance disturbance
- Social isolation

Examiner Asks	Rationale

Additional History for Infants and Children

1. **Birth trauma.** Were you told about any trauma to the infant during labour and delivery? Did the baby come out head first? Were forceps needed?

Traumatic delivery increases risk for fractures (e.g., humerus, clavicle).

2. **Anoxia.** Did the baby need resuscitation?

A period of anoxia may result in hypotonia of muscles.

3. **Milestones.** Were the baby's motor milestones achieved at about the same time as those of siblings or other children the same age?

4. **Bone injuries.** Has your child ever broken any bones? Any dislocations? How were these treated?

5. **Bone deformities.** Have you ever noticed any bone deformity in your child? Spinal curvature? Unusual shape of toes or feet? At what age? Have you ever sought treatment for any of these?

Additional History for Adolescents

1. **Athletics.** Are you involved in any sports at school or after school? How frequently (times per week)?

Assess safety of sport for the child. Note whether the child's height and weight are adequate for the particular sport (e.g., football).

2. **Sports equipment.** Do you use safety equipment? Does any training program exist for your sport?

Use of safety equipment and presence of adult supervision decrease the risk for sports injuries.

3. **Warming up.** What is the nature of your daily warm-up?

Lack of adequate warm-up increases the risk for sports injury.

4. **Injury.** What do you do if you get hurt?

Students may not report injury or pain for fear that their participation in the sport will be restricted.

5. **Time management.** How does your sport fit in with other school demands and other activities?

Additional History for Older Adults

Use the functional assessment history questions in Chapter 5 (pp. 70–71) to elicit any loss of function, self-care deficit, or safety risk that may occur as a process of aging or musculo-skeletal illness. (Review the complete functional assessment in Chapter 31.)

Age-related changes in the musculo-skeletal, neurological, and sensory systems increase the probability of falls and fractures in older adults.

1. **Weakness.** Any change in weakness over the past months or years?

2. **Injury.** Any increase in falls or stumbling over the past months or years?

3. **Mobility.** Do you use any mobility aids to help you get around: cane, walker?

OBJECTIVE DATA

PREPARATION

The purpose of the musculo-skeletal examination is to assess function for ADLs and to screen for any abnormalities. By documenting the history, you will already have considerable data regarding ADLs. Note additional ADL data as the patient goes through the motions necessary for an examination: gait, posture, how the patient sits in a chair, raises from a chair, takes off a jacket, manipulates a small object such as a pen, raises from a supine position.

A **screening musculo-skeletal examination** suffices for most patients:

- Inspection and palpation of joints, integrated with inspection of each body region
- Observation of ROM as patient proceeds through motions described earlier
- Age-specific screening measures, such as the Ortolani manoeuvre for infants or scoliosis screening for adolescents

A **complete musculo-skeletal examination**, as described in this chapter, is appropriate for patients with articular disease, a history of musculo-skeletal symptoms, or any problems with ADLs. Nurses may work in collaboration with other health care providers (e.g., physiotherapists or occupational therapists) when performing these assessments in acute, rehabilitative, long-term, and home care settings.

Make the patient comfortable before and throughout the examination. Drape for full visualization of the body part you are examining without needlessly exposing the rest of the patient's body.

Use an orderly approach: head to toe, proximal to distal. The approach may need to be modified for patients with limitations in mobility, pain, or fatigue. Provide analgesics, rest periods, or both, as required.

Support each joint at rest. Muscles must be soft and relaxed for you to assess the joints under them accurately. Take care when examining any inflamed area, where rough manipulation could cause pain and muscle spasm. To avoid pain and spasm, use firm support, gentle movement, and gentle return to a relaxed state. Compare corresponding paired joints. Expect symmetry of structure and function, and normal parameters for each joint.

EQUIPMENT NEEDED

Tape measure
Skin marking pen

Normal Range of Findings

Order of the Examination

Inspection

Note the *size* and *contour* of the joint. Inspect the skin and tissues over the joint for *colour*, *swelling*, and any *masses* or *deformity*. The presence of swelling is significant and signals joint irritation.

Abnormal Findings

Swelling may be caused by excess joint fluid (effusion), thickening of the synovial lining, inflammation of surrounding soft tissue (bursae, tendons), or bony enlargement.

Deformities include **dislocation** (one or more bones in a joint being out of position), **subluxation** (partial dislocation of a joint), **contracture** (shortening of a muscle leading to limited ROM of joint), or **ankylosis** (stiffness or fixation of a joint).

Normal Range of Findings	**Abnormal Findings**

Palpation

Palpate each joint, including its skin, for temperature, its muscles, its bony articulations, and the area of the joint capsule. Note any heat, tenderness, swelling, or masses. Normally, joints are not tender to palpation. If any tenderness does occur, try to localize it to specific anatomical structures (e.g., skin, muscles, bursae, ligaments, tendons, fat pads, or joint capsule).

Normally, the synovial membrane is not palpable. When thickened, it feels doughy or boggy. A small amount of fluid is present in the normal joint, but it is not palpable.

Warmth and tenderness signal inflammation.

Palpable fluid is abnormal. Fluid is contained in an enclosed sac; therefore, if you push on one side of the sac, the fluid will shift and cause a visible bulging on another side.

Range of Motion

Ask for **active (voluntary) ROM** while modelling the movements yourself as appropriate; you can use your own movements as a control. You may stabilize the body area proximal to that being moved. Familiarize yourself with each joint type and its normal ROM so you can recognize limitations. If you see a limitation, gently attempt **passive motion** with the person's muscles relaxed while you move the body part. Anchor the joint with one hand while your other hand slowly moves it to its limit. The normal ranges of active and passive motion should be the same.

Joint motion normally causes no tenderness, pain, or crepitation. Do not confuse crepitation with the normal discrete "crack" heard as a tendon or ligament slips over bone during motion, such as a knee bend.

Limitation in ROM is the most sensitive sign of joint disease.[18] The amount of limitation may alert you to the cause of disease. **Articular** disease (inside the joint capsule, such as arthritis) produces swelling and tenderness around the whole joint, and it limits both active and passive ROM in all planes. **Extra-articular** disease (injury to a specific tendon, ligament, nerve) produces swelling and tenderness to that one spot in the joint and affects ROM in only certain planes, especially during active (voluntary) motion.

Crepitation is an audible and palpable crunching or grating that accompanies movement. It occurs when articular surfaces in the joints are roughened, as in rheumatoid arthritis (see Table 24.2, p. 673).

Muscle Testing

Test the strength of the prime mover muscle groups for each joint. Instruct the patient to repeat the motions you tested for active ROM. Now ask the patient to flex (tighten or contract) the muscle and hold as you apply opposing force. Muscle strength should be equal bilaterally and should fully resist your opposing force. (Note: Muscle status and joint status are interdependent and should be interpreted together. Chapter 25 discusses the examination of muscles for size, strength, tone, and involuntary movements.)

Strength varies widely among people. You may wish to use a system of grading from "no voluntary movement" to "full strength," such as the following:

Grade	Description	% Normal	Assessment
5	Full ROM against gravity, full resistance	100	Normal
4	Full ROM against gravity, some resistance	75	Good
3	Full ROM with gravity	50	Fair
2	Full ROM with gravity eliminated (passive motion)	25	Poor
1	Slight contraction	10	Trace
0	No contraction	0	Zero

Objective Data

Normal Range of Findings		**Abnormal Findings**

Note: Although certain movements are assessed during both ROM and muscle testing, some movements are assessed in ROM testing only. The following table summarizes which movements are assessed in each type of test:

Joint	ROM and Muscle Testing Movements	Additional Movements for ROM Testing Only
Temporomandibular joints	Vertical motion Lateral motion Protrusion	
Cervical spine	Flexion Extension Lateral bend Rotation	Hyperextension
Shoulder	Flexion Extension Abduction Adduction	Internal rotation External rotation
Elbow	Flexion Extension	Supination Pronation
Wrist and hands	Flexion Extension	Ulnar deviation Radial deviation Abduction
Hip	Flexion Extension Internal rotation External rotation Abduction Adduction	
Knee	Flexion Extension	Hyperextension
Ankle	Flexion Extension Inversion Eversion	
Spine	Flexion Extension	Hyperextension Rotation Lateral bending

Temporomandibular Joint

With the patient seated, *inspect* the area just anterior to the ear. Place the tips of your first two fingers in front of each ear, and ask the patient to open and close the mouth. Drop your fingers into the depressed area over the joint, and note smooth motion of the mandible. An audible and palpable snap or click occurs in many healthy people as the mouth opens (Fig. 24.15).

Test ROM as follows:

Instructions to Patient	Motion and Expected Range
• Open mouth maximally.	Vertical motion. You can measure the space between the upper and lower incisors. Normal space is 3 to 6 cm, or three fingers inserted sideways.
• Partially open mouth, thrust lower jaw, and move it side to side.	Lateral motion. Normal extent is 1 to 2 cm (Fig. 24.16).
• Stick out lower jaw.	Protrusion without deviation.

Instruct the patient to clench the teeth, and palpate the patient's contracted temporalis and masseter muscles. Compare right and left sides for size, firmness, and strength. Ask the patient to move the jaw forward and laterally against your resistance, and to open mouth against your resistance. This also tests the integrity of cranial nerve V (trigeminal nerve).

Abnormal Findings

Swelling looks like a round bulge over the joint, although it must be moderate or marked to be visible.

Crepitus and pain occur with temporomandibular joint dysfunction.

Lateral motion may be lost earlier and more significantly than vertical motion.

Normal Range of Findings	Abnormal Findings

24.15

24.16

Cervical Spine

Inspect the alignment of the head and neck. The spine should be straight and the head erect. *Palpate* the spinous processes and the sternomastoid, trapezius, and paravertebral muscles. They should feel firm, with no muscle spasm or tenderness.

Test ROM as follows (Fig. 24.17)*:

Head tilted to one side.
Asymmetry of muscles.
Tenderness and hard muscles with muscle spasm.

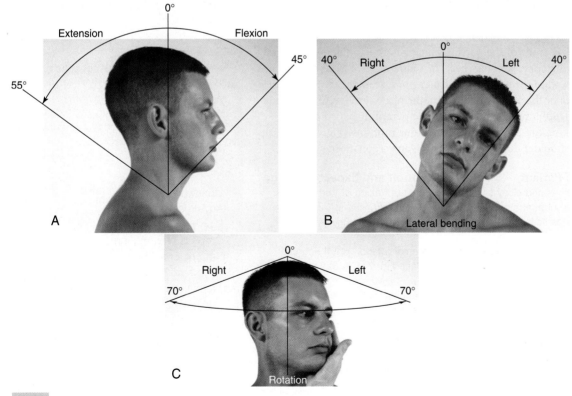

24.17

*Do not attempt if you suspect neck trauma.

Objective Data

Normal Range of Findings	Abnormal Findings

Normal Range of Findings

Instructions to Patient	Motion and Expected Range
• Touch chin to chest.	Flexion of 45 degrees (see Fig. 24.17, *A*).
• Lift the chin toward the ceiling.	Hyperextension of 55 degrees.
• Move each ear toward the corresponding shoulder. Do not lift up the shoulder.	Lateral bending of 40 degrees (see Fig. 24.17, *B*).
• Turn the chin toward each shoulder.	Rotation of 70 degrees (see Fig. 24.17, *C*).

Ask the patient to repeat the motions while you apply opposing force. The patient normally can maintain flexion against your full resistance. This is also a test of the integrity of cranial nerve XI (spinal nerve).

Upper Extremity

Shoulders

Inspect and compare both shoulders posteriorly and anteriorly, checking the size and contour of the joint, and the equality of bony landmarks. Normally, no redness, muscular atrophy, deformity, or swelling is present. Check the anterior aspect of the joint capsule and the subacromial bursa for abnormal swelling.

If the patient reports any shoulder pain, ask the patient to point to the spot with the hand of the unaffected side. Be aware that shoulder pain may have local causes, or it may be referred pain from a hiatal hernia or a cardiac or pleural condition, which is potentially serious. Pain from a local cause is reproducible during the examination by palpation or motion.

While you stand in front of the patient, *palpate* both shoulders, noting any muscular spasm or atrophy, swelling, heat, or tenderness. Start at the clavicle and methodically explore the acromioclavicular joint, scapula, greater tubercle of the humerus, area of the subacromial bursa, the biceps groove, and the anterior aspect of the glenohumeral joint. Palpate the pyramid-shaped axilla.

Test ROM by asking the patient to perform four motions (Fig. 24.18). Cup one hand over the shoulder during ROM to note any crepitation.

Instructions to Patient	Motion and Expected Range
• With arms at sides and elbows extended, move both arms forward and up in wide vertical arcs, and then move them back.	Forward flexion of 180 degrees; hyperextension of up to 50 degrees (see Fig. 24.18, *A*).
• Rotate arms internally behind back, and place back of hands as high as possible toward the scapulae.	Internal rotation of 90 degrees (see Fig. 24.18, *B*).
• With arms at sides and elbows extended, raise both arms in wide arcs in the coronal plane. Touch palms together above head.	Abduction of 180 degrees. Adduction of 50 degrees (see Fig. 24.18, *C*).
• Touch both hands behind the head with elbows flexed and rotated posteriorly.	External rotation of 90 degrees (see Fig. 24.18, *D*).

Test the shoulder muscle strength by asking the patient to shrug the shoulders, flex them forward and up, and abduct them against your resistance. The shoulder shrug also tests the integrity of cranial nerve XI (spinal nerve).

Abnormal Findings

Limited ROM.
Pain with movement.

The patient cannot maintain flexion.

Redness.
Inequality of bony landmarks.
Atrophy, manifesting as lack of fullness.
Dislocated shoulder: loses the normal rounded shape and looks flattened laterally.
Swelling from excess fluid: best seen anteriorly; considerable fluid must be present to cause a visible distension because the capsule is normally loose (see Table 24.3, p. 674).
Swelling of subacromial bursa is localized under the deltoid muscle and may be accentuated when the patient tries to abduct the arm.

Swelling.
Hard muscles with muscle spasm.
Tenderness or pain.
Adenopathy or masses.

Limited ROM.
Asymmetry.
Pain with motion.
Crepitus with motion.
Rotator cuff lesions may cause limited ROM, pain, and muscle spasm during abduction, whereas forward flexion stays fairly normal.

Normal Range of Findings   **Abnormal Findings**

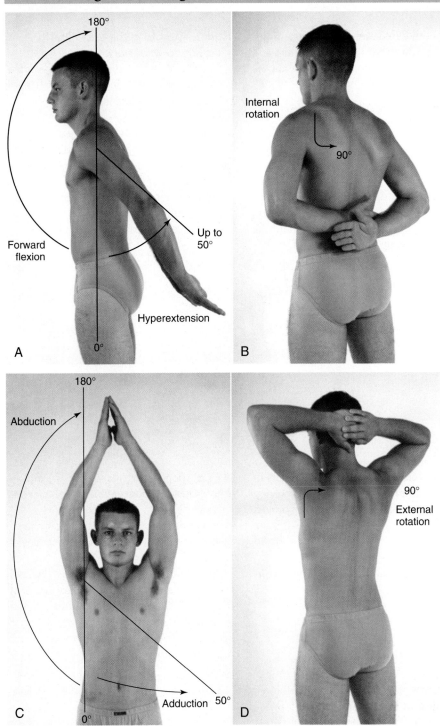

180°

Forward
flexion

Up to
50°

Hyperextension

0°

A

Internal
rotation

90°

B

180°

Abduction

Adduction   50°

0°

C

90°

External
rotation

D

24.18

Normal Range of Findings	Abnormal Findings

Normal Range of Findings

Elbow

Inspect the size and contour of the elbow in both flexed and extended positions. Look for any deformity, redness, or swelling. Check the olecranon bursa and the normally present hollows on either side of the olecranon process for abnormal swelling.

Palpate with the patient's elbow flexed about 70 degrees and as relaxed as possible (Fig. 24.19). Use your left hand to support the patient's left forearm, and palpate the extensor surface of the elbow—the olecranon process and the medial and lateral epicondyles of humerus—with your right thumb and fingers.

24.19

With your thumb in the lateral groove and your index and middle fingers in the medial groove, palpate either side of the olecranon process, using varying pressure. Normally, tissues and fat pads feel fairly solid. Check for any synovial thickening, swelling, nodules, or tenderness.

Palpate the area of the olecranon bursa for heat, swelling, tenderness, consistency, or nodules.

Test ROM as follows:

Instructions to Patient	**Motion and Expected Range**
• Bend and then straighten the elbow.	Flexion of 150 to 160 degrees; extension at 0 (see Fig. 24.20).
	Some healthy people lack 5 to 10 degrees of full extension, and others have 5 to 10 degrees of hyperextension.
• Hold the hand midway; then touch the front and back sides of the hand to the table.	Movement of 90 degrees in pronation and supination (see Fig. 24.21).

Abnormal Findings

In subluxation of the elbow, the forearm is dislocated posteriorly.

Swelling and redness of olecranon bursa are localized and easy to observe because of the nearness of the bursa to skin.

Effusion or synovial thickening manifests first as a bulge or fullness in groove on either side of the olecranon process, and occurs with gouty arthritis.

Epicondyles, head of radius, and tendons are common sites of inflammation and local tenderness, or "tennis elbow."

Soft, boggy, or fluctuant swelling in both grooves occurs with synovial thickening or effusion.

Local heat or redness (signs of inflammation) can extend beyond the synovial membrane.

Subcutaneous nodules are raised, firm, and nontender, and overlying skin moves freely. Common sites are in the olecranon bursa and along the extensor surface of the ulna. These nodules occur with rheumatoid arthritis (see Table 24.4, p. 676).

Normal Range of Findings	Abnormal Findings

24.20   **24.21**

While you test *muscle strength*, stabilize the patient's arm with one hand (Fig. 24.22). Apply resistance just proximal to the wrist, and instruct the patient to flex the elbow against your resistance and then extend the elbow against your resistance.

24.22

Wrist and Hand

Inspect the hands and wrists on the dorsal and palmar sides, noting position, contour, and shape. In the normal functional position of the hand, the wrist is in slight extension. This way, the fingers can flex efficiently, and the thumb can oppose them for grip and manipulation. The fingers lie straight in the same axis as the forearm. Normally, no swelling or redness, deformity, or nodules are present.

The skin looks smooth, with knuckle wrinkles present and no swelling or lesions. Muscles are full, with the palm showing a rounded mound proximal to the thumb (the thenar eminence) and a smaller rounded mound proximal to the little finger.

Subluxation of wrist.
Ulnar deviation; fingers list to ulnar side.
Ankylosis; wrist in extreme flexion.
Dupuytren's contracture: flexion contracture of one or more fingers (see Table 24.5, p. 677).
Swan-neck or boutonnière deformity in fingers.
Atrophy of the thenar eminence (see Table 24.5, p. 676).

Objective Data

Normal Range of Findings

Palpate each joint in the wrist and hands. Face the patient, support the patient's hand with your fingers under it, and palpate the wrist firmly with both your thumbs on its dorsum (Fig. 24.23). Make sure the patient's wrist is relaxed and in straight alignment. Move your palpating thumbs side to side to identify the normal depressed areas that overlie the joint space. Use gentle but firm pressure. Normally, the joint surfaces feel smooth, with no swelling, bogginess, nodules, or tenderness.

24.23

Palpate the metacarpophalangeal joints with your thumbs, just distal to and on either side of the knuckle (Fig. 24.24).

24.24

Abnormal Findings

Ganglion cyst in wrist (see Table 24.5, p. 676).
Synovial swelling on dorsum.
Generalized swelling.
Tenderness.

Normal Range of Findings

Use your thumb and index finger in a pinching motion to palpate the sides of the interphalangeal joints (Fig. 24.25). Normally, no synovial thickening, tenderness, warmth, or nodules are present.

24.25

Test ROM as follows (Fig. 24.26):

Instructions to Patient
- Bend the hand up at the wrist.

- Bend the hand down at the wrist.
- Bend the fingers up and down at metacarpophalangeal joints.

- With palms flat on table, turn them outward and in.

- Spread fingers apart; then, make a fist.

- Touch the thumb to each finger and to the base of the little finger.

Motion and Expected Range
Hyperextension of 70 degrees (see Fig. 24.26, *A*).
Palmar flexion of 90 degrees.
Flexion of 90 degrees; hyperextension of 30 degrees (see Fig. 24.26, *B*).
Ulnar deviation of 50 to 60 degrees; radial deviation of 20 degrees (see Fig. 24.26, *C*).
Abduction of 20 degrees; tight fist; equal bilateral responses (see Fig. 24.26, *D, E*).
Ability to perform this manoeuvre, and equal bilateral responses (see Fig. 24.26, *F*).

Abnormal Findings

Heberden's and Bouchard's nodes are hard and nontender and occur with osteoarthritis (see Table 24.5, p. 677).

Loss of ROM (in this location, the most common and most significant functional loss in the wrist).
Limited motion.
Pain on movement.

Normal Range of Findings

Abnormal Findings

A

B

C

D

E

F

24.26

For *muscle testing*, position the patient's forearm supinated (palm up) and resting on a table (Fig. 24.27). Stabilize the patient's arm by holding your hand at the mid-forearm. Ask the patient to flex the wrist against your resistance at the palm.

24.27

SPECIAL CONSIDERATIONS FOR ADVANCED PRACTICE: WRIST AND HAND

Normal Range of Findings	Abnormal Findings

Phalen Test

Ask the patient to hold both hands back to back while flexing the wrists 90 degrees. Acute flexion of the wrist for 60 seconds produces no symptoms in the normal hand (Fig. 24.28).

Positive Phalen test: numbness and burning sensation occurs with **carpal tunnel syndrome** (see Table 24.5, p. 676).

24.28 Phalen test.

Tinel's Sign

Direct percussion of the location of the median nerve at the wrist produces no symptoms in the normal hand (Fig. 24.29).

Positive Tinel's sign: burning and tingling sensations along its distribution occurs with carpal tunnel syndrome.

24.29 Tinel's sign.

Normal Range of Findings	Abnormal Findings

Lower Extremity

Hip

Inspect the hip joint together with the spine a bit later in the examination as the patient stands. At that time, note symmetrical levels of iliac crests, gluteal folds, and equal-sized buttocks. A smooth, even gait reflects equal leg lengths and functional hip motion.

Help the patient into the supine position, and *palpate* the hip joints. The joints should feel stable and symmetrical, with no tenderness or crepitation.

Test ROM as follows (Fig. 24.30):

Pain with palpation.
Crepitation.

24.30

Normal Range of Findings

Abnormal Findings

Instructions to Patient
- Raise each leg with knee extended.

- Bend each knee up to the chest while keeping the other leg straight.

- Flex knee and hip to 90 degrees. (Examiner stabilizes by holding the thigh with one hand and the ankle with the other hand.) Swing the foot outward. Swing the foot inward. (Foot and thigh move in opposite directions.)
- Swing leg laterally, then medially, with knee straight. Stabilize pelvis by pushing down on the opposite anterior superior iliac spine.
- When standing (later in examination), swing straight leg back behind body. (Examiner stabilizes pelvis to eliminate exaggerated lumbar lordosis. The most efficient way is to ask patient to bend over the table and support the trunk on the table, or lie prone on the table.)

Motion and Expected Range
Hip flexion of 90 degrees (see Fig. 24.30, *A*).
Hip flexion of 120 degrees; the opposite thigh should remain on the table (see Fig. 24.30, *B*).
Internal rotation of 40 degrees.
External rotation of 45 degrees (see Fig. 24.30, *C*).

Abduction of 40 to 45 degrees.
Adduction of 20 to 30 degrees (see Fig. 24.30, *D*).
Hyperextension of 15 degrees when stabilized.

Limited motion.
Pain with motion.
Flexion flattens the lumbar spine; if this reveals a flexion deformity in the opposite hip, it represents a positive sign of the *Thomas test*.
Limited internal rotation of hip is an early and reliable sign of hip disease.
Limitation of abduction of the hip in the supine position is the most common motion dysfunction in hip disease.

Knee

The patient should remain supine with legs extended, although some examiners prefer the knees to be flexed and dangling for *inspection*. The skin normally looks smooth, with even colouring and no lesions.

Inspect lower leg alignment. The lower leg should extend in the same axis as the thigh.

Inspect the knee's shape and contour. Normally, distinct concavities (hollows) are present on either side of the patella. Check them for any sign of fullness or swelling. Check other locations, such as the prepatellar bursa and the suprapatellar pouch, for any abnormal swelling.

Check the quadriceps muscle in the anterior thigh for any atrophy. Because it is the prime mover of knee extension, this muscle is important for joint stability during weight bearing.

Shiny and atrophic skin.
Swelling or inflammation (see Table 24.6, p. 679).
Lesions (e.g., psoriasis).
Angulation deformity:
- Genu varum (bowlegs; see p. 666)
- Genu valgum (knock knees)
  Flexion contracture.
  With synovial thickening or effusion, hollows disappear; then they may bulge.

Atrophy occurs with disuse or chronic disorders. It first appears in the medial part of the muscle, although it is difficult to note because the vastus medialis is relatively small.

Objective Data

Normal Range of Findings

Palpate the patient's knee in the supine position with complete relaxation of the quadriceps muscle. Start high on the anterior thigh, about 10 cm above the patella. Palpate with your left thumb and fingers in a grasping manner (Fig. 24.31). Proceed down toward the knee, exploring the region of the suprapatellar pouch. Note the consistency of the tissues. The muscles and soft tissues should feel solid, and the joint should feel smooth, with no warmth, tenderness, thickening, or nodularity.

24.31

When swelling is present, distinguish whether it represents soft tissue swelling or increased fluid in the joint by testing for the bulge sign and ballottement of the patella.

Abnormal Findings

Fluctuant or boggy texture with synovitis of suprapatellar pouch.

SPECIAL CONSIDERATIONS FOR ADVANCED PRACTICE: KNEE

Normal Range of Findings

Bulge Sign

The bulge sign confirms presence of small amounts of fluid in the suprapatellar pouch as you try to move the fluid from one side of the joint to the other. Firmly stroke up on the medial aspect of the knee two or three times to displace any fluid (see Fig. 24.32, *A*). Tap the lateral aspect (see Fig. 24.32, *B*). Watch the medial side in the hollow for a distinct bulge from a fluid wave. Normally, none is present.

Abnormal Findings

The bulge sign occurs with very small amounts (4 to 8 mL) of fluid flowing across the joint (see Fig. 24.32, *C*).

Normal Range of Findings	Abnormal Findings

24.32

Ballottement of the Patella

This test is reliable when larger amounts of fluid are present. Use your left hand to compress the suprapatellar pouch to move any fluid into the knee joint. With your right hand, push the patella sharply against the femur. If no fluid is present, the patella is already snug against the femur (see Fig. 24.33, *A*).

If fluid has collected, your tap on the patella moves it through the fluid, and you will hear a tap as the patella bumps up on the femoral condyles (see Fig. 24.33, *B*).

24.33

Continue assessment with palpation of the tibiofemoral joint (Fig. 24.34). Note smooth joint margins and absence of pain. Palpate the infrapatellar fat pad and the patella. Check for crepitus by holding your hand on the patella as the knee is flexed and extended. Some crepitus in an otherwise symptom-free knee is not uncommon.

Irregular bony margins (present with osteoarthritis).

Pain at joint line.

Pronounced crepitus (a significant finding, which occurs with degenerative diseases of the knee).

Normal Range of Findings	Abnormal Findings

24.34

Test ROM as follows (Fig. 24.35):

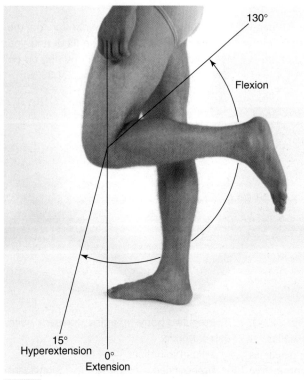

130°

Flexion

15°
Hyperextension

0°
Extension

24.35

Special Considerations for Advanced Practice

Instructions to Patient
- Bend each knee.
- Extend each knee.

- Ambulate. (Examiner checks knee ROM during ambulation.)

Motion and Expected Range
Flexion of 130 to 150 degrees.
A straight line of 0 degrees in some persons; a hyperextension of 15 degrees in others.

Limited ROM.
Contracture.
Pain with motion.
Limpness.
In sudden locking, the patient is unable to extend the knee fully. This usually occurs with a painful and audible "pop" or "click." Sudden buckling, or "giving way," occurs with ligament injury, which causes weakness and instability.

Normal Range of Findings	**Abnormal Findings**

Check muscle strength by asking the patient to maintain knee flexion while you oppose by trying to pull the leg forward. The patient demonstrates muscle extension by successfully rising from a seated position in a low chair or rising from a squat without using the hands for support.

Special Test for Meniscal Tears

McMurray Test. Perform this test when a patient has reported a history of trauma followed by locking, giving way, or local pain in the knee. Position the patient supine as you stand next to the affected side. Hold the heel, and flex the knee and hip. Place your other hand on the knee with fingers on the medial side. Rotate the leg in and out to loosen the joint. Externally rotate the leg and push a valgus (inward) stress on the knee. Then slowly extend the knee. Normally, the leg extends smoothly with no pain (Fig. 24.36).

A "click" is a positive result of the *McMurray test* that signifies a torn meniscus.

24.36

Normal Range of Findings	**Abnormal Findings**

Ankle and Foot

Inspect with the patient in a sitting, non–weight-bearing position, as well as when standing and walking. Compare both feet, noting position of feet and toes, contour of joints, and skin characteristics. The foot should align with the long axis of the lower leg; an imaginary line would fall from mid-patella to between the first and second toes.

Weight bearing should be borne on the middle of the foot, from the heel, along the midfoot, to between the second and third toes. Most feet have a longitudinal arch, although the arch can vary normally from "flatfeet" to a high instep.

Special Considerations for Advanced Practice

Objective Data

Normal Range of Findings	Abnormal Findings

The toes point straight forward and lie flat. The ankles (malleoli) are smooth bony prominences. Normally, the skin is smooth, with even colouring and no lesions. Note the locations of any calluses or bursal reactions because they reveal areas of abnormal friction. Examining well-worn shoes helps assess areas of wear and accommodation.

In **hallux valgus**, the distal part of the great toe is directed *away* from the body midline (Fig. 24.37).

24.37

Hammertoes; claw toes.
Swelling or inflammation.
Calluses; ulcers (see Table 24.7, p. 682).
Swelling or inflammation.
Tenderness.

Support the ankle by grasping the heel with your fingers while palpating with your thumbs (Fig. 24.38). Explore the joint spaces. They should feel smooth and depressed, with no fullness, swelling, or tenderness.

24.38

Palpate the metatarsophalangeal joints between your thumb on the dorsum and your fingers on the plantar surface (Fig. 24.39).

Using a pinching motion of your thumb and forefinger, palpate the interphalangeal joints on the medial and lateral sides of the toes.

Swelling or inflammation; tenderness.

Normal Range of Findings	Abnormal Findings

24.39

Test ROM as follows (Fig. 24.40):

24.40

Instructions to Patient
- Point toes toward the floor.
- Point toes toward your nose.

- Turn soles of feet out, then in. (Examiner stabilizes the ankle with one hand and holds heel with the other to test the subtalar joint.)
- Flex and straighten toes.

Motion and Expected Range
Plantar flexion of 45 degrees.
Dorsiflexion of 20 degrees (see Fig. 24.40, *A*).
Eversion of 20 degrees.
Inversion of 30 degrees (see Fig. 24.40, *B*).

Limited ROM.
Pain with motion.

Assess muscle strength by asking the patient to maintain dorsiflexion and plantar flexion against your resistance.

The patient cannot maintain flexion.

Normal Range of Findings	Abnormal Findings

Spine

The patient should be standing, draped in a gown open at the back. Place yourself far enough behind the patient so that you can see the entire back. *Inspect* and note whether the spine is straight by following an imaginary vertical line from the head through the spinous processes and down through the gluteal cleft; by noting equal horizontal positions for the shoulders, scapulae, iliac crests, and gluteal folds; and by noting equal spaces between the arm and lateral thorax on the two sides (see Fig. 24.41, *A*). The patient's knees and feet should be aligned with the trunk and should be pointing forward.

A difference in shoulder elevation and in the level of scapulae and iliac crests occur with scoliosis (see Table 24.8, p. 683).

A   B

24.41

From the side, note the normal convex thoracic curve and concave lumbar curve (see Fig. 24.41, *B*). An enhanced thoracic curve, or kyphosis, is common in older adults. A pronounced lumbar curve, or lordosis, is common in obese people.

Palpate the spinous processes. Normally, they are straight and not tender. Palpate the paravertebral muscles; they should feel firm with no tenderness or spasm.

Lateral tilting and forward bending occur with a herniated nucleus pulposus (see Table 24.8, p. 684).

Spinal curvature.
Tenderness; spasm of paravertebral muscles.
Chronic axial skeletal pain occurs with fibromyalgia syndrome.

Objective Data

Normal Range of Findings	**Abnormal Findings**

Test ROM of the spine by asking the patient to bend forward and touch the toes (Fig. 24.42). Look for flexion of 75 to 90 degrees and smoothness and symmetry of movement. Note that the concave lumbar curve should disappear with this motion, and the back should have a single convex C-shaped curve.

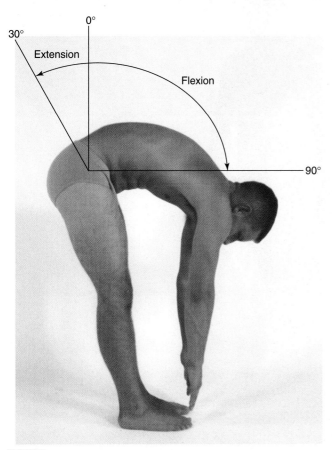

24.42

If you suspect a spinal curvature during inspection, this may be more clearly seen when the patient touches the toes. While the patient is bending over, mark a dot on each spinous process. When the patient resumes standing, the dots should form a straight vertical line.

Stabilize the pelvis with your hands. *Test ROM* as follows (Fig. 24.43):

Instructions to Patient	**Motion and Expected Range**
• Bend sideways.	Lateral bending of 35 degrees (see Fig. 24.43, *A*).
• Bend backward.	Hyperextension of 30 degrees.
• Twist shoulders to one side, then the other.	Rotation of 30 degrees, bilaterally (see Fig. 24.43, *B*).

Abnormal Findings:

If the dots form a slight S-shape when the patient stands, a spinal curve is present.

Limited ROM.
Pain with motion.

Objective Data

Normal Range of Findings	Abnormal Findings

A   B

24.43

These manoeuvres reveal only gross restriction. Movement is still possible even if some spinal fusion has occurred. Finally, ask the patient to walk on the toes for a few steps and then to walk on the heels.

SPECIAL CONSIDERATIONS FOR ADVANCED PRACTICE: SPINE

Normal Range of Findings	Abnormal Findings

Straight Leg Raising: Lasègue Test

These manoeuvres reproduce back and leg pain and help confirm the presence of a herniated nucleus pulposus. Straight leg raising while keeping the knee extended normally produces no pain. Raise the affected leg just short of the point where it produces pain. Then dorsiflex the foot (Fig. 24.44).

Positive Lasègue test: lifting the affected leg reproduces sciatic pain, confirming the presence of a herniated nucleus pulposus.

Normal Range of Findings	Abnormal Findings

24.44

Raise the unaffected leg while leaving the other leg flat. Inquire about the involved side.

If lifting the unaffected leg reproduces sciatic pain, it strongly suggests a herniated nucleus pulposus.

Measure Leg Length Discrepancy

Perform this measurement if you need to determine whether one leg is shorter than the other. For *true leg length*, measure between fixed points, from the anterior superior iliac spine to the medial malleolus, crossing the medial side of the knee (Fig. 24.45). Normally, these measurements are equal or within 1 cm, indicating no true bone discrepancy.

Unequal leg lengths.
True leg lengths are equal, but leg lengths may appear unequal as a result of pelvic obliquity or adduction or flexion deformity in the hip.

24.45

Sometimes the true leg length is equal, but the legs still look unequal. For apparent leg length, measure from a nonfixed point (the umbilicus) to a fixed point (medial malleolus) on each leg.

Evaluate Back Pain

Consider using a back pain screening tool such as the **Clinically Organized Relevant Exam (CORE) Back Tool** to evaluate individuals with back pain.[19]

Screening tools help the advanced practice nurse recognize common mechanical pain syndromes and screen for other conditions contributing to back pain.

Special Considerations
for Advanced Practice

Normal Range of Findings	Abnormal Findings

 DEVELOPMENTAL CONSIDERATIONS

Review the developmental milestones discussed on the Evolve website. Keep handy a concise chart of the usual sequence of motor development so you can refer to expected findings for the age of each child you are examining. Use the Denver II test to identify fine and gross motor skills expected for the child's age. Because some aspects of musculo-skeletal and neurological examinations overlap, assessment of muscle tone, resting posture, and motor activity are discussed in the next chapter.

Infants

Examine the infant with the infant fully undressed and lying on the back. Take care to place the newborn on a warming table to maintain body temperature.

Feet and Legs. Start with the feet and work your way up the extremities. Note any *positional deformities*, a residual of fetal positioning. Often the newborn's feet are not held straight but in a varus (apart) or valgus (together) position. It is important to distinguish whether this position is flexible (and thus usually self-correctable) or fixed. Scratch the outside of the bottom of the foot. If the deformity is self-correctable, the foot assumes a normal right angle to the lower leg. Alternatively, immobilize the heel with one hand and gently push the forefoot to the neutral position with the other hand. If you can move it to neutral position, it is flexible.

Note the relationship of the forefoot to the hindfoot. Commonly, the hindfoot is in alignment with the lower leg and just the forefoot angles inward. This forefoot adduction is *metatarsus adductus*. It is usually present at birth and usually resolves spontaneously by age 3 years.

Check for *tibial torsion*, a twisting of the tibia. Place the child's feet flat on the table, and push to flex up the knees. With the patella and the tibial tubercle in a straight line, place your fingers on the malleoli. In an infant, note whether an imaginary line connecting the four malleoli is parallel to the table.

Tibial torsion may originate from intrauterine positioning and then may be exacerbated at a later age by continuous sitting in a reverse tailor position, the "W" sitting position (sitting with the buttocks on the floor and the lower legs splayed back and out on either side).

Hips. Check the hips for *congenital dislocation* by performing the **Ortolani manoeuvre** at every professional visit until the infant is 1 year old. With the infant supine, flex the knees by holding your thumbs on the inner mid-thighs and with your fingers outside on the hips, touching the greater trochanters. Adduct the legs until your thumbs touch (see Fig. 24.46, *A*). Then gently lift and *abduct* the legs, moving the knees apart and down so their lateral aspects touch the table (see Fig. 24.46, *B*). This normally feels smooth and produces no sound.

A true deformity is fixed and assumes a right angle only with forced manipulation or not at all.

Metatarsus varus: adduction and inversion of forefoot.

Talipes equinovarus (clubfoot): inversion and adduction of forefoot, with downward pointing of foot (see Table 24.9, p. 685).

Tibial torsion: more than 20 degrees of deviation or location of lateral malleolus anterior to medial malleolus.

With a dislocated hip, the head of the femur is not cupped in the acetabulum but rests posterior to it.

Hip instability feels like a clunk as the head of the femur pops back into place. This is a *positive Ortolani sign* and warrants referral.

24.46 Ortolani manoeuvre.

Normal Range of Findings	Abnormal Findings

The **Allis test** is also used to check for hip dislocation by comparing leg lengths (Fig. 24.47). Place the baby's feet flat on the table, and flex the knees up. Scan the tops of the knees; normally, they are at the same elevation.

Positive Allis sign: one knee is significantly lower than the other, which suggests hip dislocation.

24.47 Allis test.

Note the gluteal folds. Normally, they are equal on both sides. However, some asymmetry may be present in healthy children.

Hands and Arms. Inspect the hands, noting shape, number, and position of fingers and palmar creases. The palm usually has three strong horizontal lines (palmar flexion creases). A simian crease (single palmar crease) is often a normal finding, occurring in about 1 out of 30 people and twice as often in males.[20]

Palpate the length of the clavicles because the clavicle is the bone most frequently fractured during birth. The clavicles should feel smooth, regular, and without crepitus. Also note equal ROM of arms during the Moro reflex (see Chapter 25, p. 724 for description).

Back. Lift up the infant and examine the back. Note the normal single C-shaped curve of the newborn's spine (Fig. 24.48). By 2 months of age, the infant can lift the head while prone. This builds the concave cervical spinal curve and indicates normal forearm strength. Inspect the length of the spine for any tuft of hair, dimple in midline, cyst, or mass. Normally, none are present. A sacral dimple is often normal.

Unequal gluteal folds may accompany hip dislocation after 2 to 3 months of age.

Polydactyly is the presence of extra fingers or toes. *Syndactyly* is webbing between adjacent fingers or toes (see Table 24.5, p. 678).

A simian crease frequently occurs with other conditions (e.g., Down syndrome or fetal alcohol spectrum disorder) and is accompanied by short broad fingers, incurving of little fingers, and low-set thumbs.

Fractured clavicle: Note irregularity at the fracture site, crepitus, and angulation. The site has rapid callus formation with a palpable lump within a few weeks. Observe limited arm ROM and unilateral response in the Moro reflex.

A small dimple in the midline—anywhere from the head to the coccyx—suggests dermoid sinus.

A tuft of hair, birthmark, or skin tag over a sacral dimple in the midline may indicate spina bifida.

Mass, such as meningocele, necessitates referral.

24.48

Objective Data

Normal Range of Findings

Observe ROM through spontaneous movement of extremities. Test muscle strength by lifting up the infant with your hands under the axillae (Fig. 24.49). A baby with normal muscle strength wedges securely between your hands.

24.49

Preschool-Age and School-Age Children

Once the infant learns to crawl and then to walk, the waking hours are spent seemingly in perpetual motion. Observe the muscles and joints during spontaneous play before a table-top examination. Most young children enjoy showing off their physical accomplishments. For specific motions, coax the toddler: "Show me how you can walk to Mom"; "Climb the step stool." Ask the preschooler to hop on one foot or to jump.

Back. While the child is standing, note posture. From behind, note the plumb line from the back of the head, along the spine, to the middle of the sacrum. Shoulders are level within 1 cm, and scapulae are symmetrical. From the side, lordosis is common throughout childhood, appearing more pronounced in children with a protuberant abdomen.

Legs and Feet. Anteriorly, note the leg position. A bowlegged stance (*genu varum*) is a lateral bowing of the legs (see Fig. 24.50, *A*). It is characterized by a persistent space of more than 2.5 cm between the knees when the medial malleoli are together. Genu varum is normal for 1 year after the child begins to walk. The child may walk with a waddling gait. Genu varum resolves with growth; no treatment is indicated.

Knock knees (*genu valgum*) are characterized by a span of more than 2.5 cm between the medial malleoli when the knees are together (see Fig. 24.50, *B*). It occurs normally between 2 and 3½ years of age. Treatment is not indicated for genu valgum.

Flatfoot (*pes planus*) is pronation, or turning in, of the medial side of the foot. The young child may look flatfooted because the normal longitudinal arch is concealed by a fat pad until age 3 years. When standing begins, the child takes a broad-based stance, which causes pronation. Thus, pronation is common between 12 and 30 months. You can see it best from behind the child, where the medial side of the foot drops down and in.

Pigeon toes, or toeing in, are demonstrated when the child tends to walk on the lateral side of the foot, and the longitudinal arch looks higher than normal. It often starts as a forefoot adduction, which usually resolves spontaneously by age 3 years, as long as the foot is flexible.

Abnormal Findings

A baby who starts to "slip" between your hands shows weakness of the shoulder muscles.

Lordosis is marked in muscular dystrophy and rickets.

Severe bowing or unilateral bowing also occurs with rickets.

Genu valgum also occurs in rickets, poliomyelitis, and syphilis.

Pronation beyond 30 months.

Toeing in from forefoot adduction that is fixed or lasts beyond age 3 years.
Toeing in from tibial torsion.

Normal Range of Findings   **Abnormal Findings**

24.50   Leg position. **A**, Genu varum. **B**, Genu valgum.

Check the child's gait while the child walks away from and toward you. Let the child wear socks because a cold tile floor will distort the usual gait. In children 1 to 2 years of age, expect a broad-based gait, with arms out for balance. Weight bearing is borne on the inside of the foot. From 3 years of age, the base narrows, and arms are kept closer to the sides. Inspect shoes for spots of greatest wear to aid judgement of the gait. Normally, shoes show the most wear on the outside of the heel and inside of the toe.

Check for the **Trendelenburg sign** to screen for progressive subluxation of the hip (see Fig. 24.51, *A*). As you watch from behind, ask the child to stand on one leg, then the other. Note the iliac crests; they should stay level when weight is shifted.

The child may sit for the remainder of the examination. Start with the feet and hands of the child from 2 to 6 years of age because the child is happy to show these off, and proceed through the examination as described earlier.

In particular, check the arm for full ROM and presence of pain. Look for subluxation of the elbow (head of the radius). This occurs most often between 2 and 4 years of age as a result of forceful removal of clothing or dangling while adults suspend the child by the hands.

Palpate the bones, joints, and muscles of the extremities as described for the adult examination.

Limp, usually caused by trauma, fatigue, or hip disease.

Abnormal gait patterns (see Chapter 25).

Positive Trendelenburg sign: occurs with severe subluxation of one hip. When the child stands on the "good" leg, the pelvis looks level. When the child stands on the affected leg, the pelvis drops toward the "good" side. The hip abductors on the standing side are too weak to hold the pelvis level (see Fig. 24.51, *B*).

Inability to supinate the hand while the arm is flexed, together with pain in elbow, indicates subluxation of the head of the radius.

Pain or tenderness in extremities is usually caused by trauma or infection.

Fractures usually result from trauma and are exhibited as an inability to use the area, a deformity, or an excess motion in the involved bone with pain and crepitation.

Enlargement of the tibial tubercles with tenderness is suggestive of Osgood-Schlatter disease (see Table 24.6, p. 680).

Normal Range of Findings	Abnormal Findings

Normal hip abductors

Level iliac crests

A

B

24.51

Adolescents

Proceed with the musculo-skeletal examination as for adults, with special attention to spinal posture. Kyphosis is common during adolescence because of chronic poor posture. Be aware of the risk for sports-related injuries because sports participation and competition often peak in this age group.

The Canadian Task Force on Preventive Health Care recommends routine screening of symptom-free adolescents for idiopathic scoliosis;[21] however, periodic visual inspection of the backs of adolescents seen for other reasons is reasonable.

Normal Range of Findings

Inspect for scoliosis with the *forward bend test* (Fig. 24.52, *A, B*). Seat yourself behind the standing child, and ask the child to stand with feet shoulder-width apart and to bend forward slowly to touch the toes. Expect a straight vertical spine while the child is both standing and bending forward. The posterior ribs should be symmetrical, with equal elevation of shoulders, scapulae, and iliac crests. You may wish to mark each spinous process with a felt marker. The lineup of ink dots highlights even a subtle curve.

A   B

24.52

Abnormal Findings

Scoliosis is most apparent during the preadolescent growth spurt. Asymmetry is suggestive of scoliosis: The ribs "hump up" on one side as the child bends forward, and landmark elevation is unequal (see Table 24.8, p. 683).

Normal Range of Findings	Abnormal Findings

Pregnant Women

Proceed through the examination described for adults. Expected postural changes in pregnancy include progressive lordosis and, toward the third trimester, anterior cervical flexion, kyphosis, and slumped shoulders (see Fig. 24.53, A). At full term, the protuberant abdomen and relaxed mobility in the joints create the characteristic waddling gait (see Fig. 24.53, B).

A   B

24.53

Older Adults

Postural changes include a decrease in height, which is more apparent in the eighth and ninth decades (Fig. 24.54). "Lengthening of the arm–trunk axis" describes this shortening of the trunk with the appearance of comparatively long extremities. Kyphosis is common, with a backward head tilt to compensate. This creates the outline of a figure 3, as in the older adult pictured, viewed from the left side. Slight flexion of hips and knees is also common.

Contour changes include a decrease of fat in the body periphery and fat deposition over the abdomen and hips. Bony prominences become more marked.

ROM and muscle strength are much the same as in younger adults, provided no musculo-skeletal illnesses or arthritic changes are present.

Functional Assessment for ADLs. For patients with changes caused by advanced aging or arthritis and those with musculo-skeletal disability, perform a **functional assessment for ADLs**. ROM and muscle strength are tested with regard to accomplishment of specific activities. You need to determine adequate and safe performance of functions essential for independent home life. See Chapter 31 for further assessments.

Normal Range of Findings

Abnormal Findings

24.54

Instructions to Patient	**Common Adaptation for Aging Changes**
1. Walk (with shoes on).	Shuffling pattern; swaying; arms out to help balance; broader base of support; watching own feet.
2. Climb up stairs.	Holds tightly onto hand rail; may haul body up with arm; may lead with favoured (stronger) leg.
3. Walk down stairs.	Holds hand rail tightly, sometimes with both hands.
	With weakness, descending sideways, lowering the weaker leg first; with unsteadiness, watching the feet.
4. Pick up object from floor.	Often bends at the waist instead of at the knees; holds onto furniture for support while bending or straightening.
5. Rise up from sitting in chair.	Uses arms to push off chair arms, upper trunk leans forward before body straightens, feet are planted wide in broad base of support.
6. Rise up from lying in bed.	May roll to one side, pushes with arms to lift up torso; grabs bedside table to increase leverage.

Objective Data

DOCUMENTATION AND CRITICAL THINKING

Sample Charting

SUBJECTIVE

Reports no joint pain, stiffness, swelling, or limitation. No muscle pain or weakness. No history of bone trauma or deformity. Able to manage all usual daily activities with no physical limitations. No occupational risk factors. Exercise pattern is brisk walk 2 km 5×/week.

OBJECTIVE

Joints and muscles symmetrical; no swelling, masses, deformity; normal spinal curvature. No tenderness to palpation of joints; no heat, swelling, or masses. Full ROM; movement smooth, no crepitation, no tenderness. Muscle strength: able to maintain flexion against resistance and without tenderness.

ASSESSMENT

Muscles and joints: healthy and functional

Focused Assessment: Clinical Case Study

Margaret Tan (M.T.) is a 45-year-old female salesperson with rheumatoid arthritis, diagnosed 3 years ago, who seeks care now for "swelling and burning pain in my hands" for 1 day.

SUBJECTIVE

M.T. received a diagnosis of rheumatoid arthritis at age 41 years, with flare-ups occurring every 6 to 8 months. Acute episodes involve hand joints and are treated with naproxen, which gives relief; she feels better in a few days and decreases dose herself. Typically experiences morning stiffness, lasting $\frac{1}{2}$ to 1 hour. Joints feel warm, swollen, tender. Has had weight loss of 7 kg (15 lb) over past 4 years and feels fatigued much of the time. States should rest more, but "I can't take the time." Daily exercises have been prescribed, but M.T. does not do them regularly.

OBJECTIVE

Body joints within normal limits except joints of wrist and hands. Radiocarpal, metacarpophalangeal, and proximal interphalangeal joints are red, swollen, tender to palpation. Spindle-shaped swelling of proximal interphalangeal joints of third digit right hand and second digit left hand; ulnar deviation of metacarpophalangeal joints.

ASSESSMENT

Acute pain R/T [related to] inflammation
Impaired physical mobility R/T inflammation
Deficient knowledge about naproxen treatment R/T lack of exposure
Nonadherence with exercise program R/T lack of perceived benefits of treatment
Nonadherence with advised rest periods R/T lack of perceived benefits of treatment

ABNORMAL FINDINGS

TABLE 24.2 Abnormalities Affecting Multiple Joints

Articular cartilage — Joint capsule — Synovial membrane

NORMAL JOINT
(joint space enlarged for clarity)

Inflamed synovial membrane

Cyst

Erosion

Fibrous formation

Swelling of soft tissue

◀ **Inflammatory Conditions**

Rheumatoid Arthritis

Chronic, systemic inflammatory disease of the joints and surrounding connective tissue. Inflammation of the synovial membrane leads to thickening; then to fibrosis, which limits motion; and finally to bony ankylosis. The disorder is symmetrical and bilateral and is characterized by heat, redness, swelling, and painful motion of the affected joints. Rheumatoid arthritis is associated with fatigue, weakness, anorexia, weight loss, low-grade fever, and lymphadenopathy. Associated signs are described in the following tables, especially Table 24.5, p. 677.

Ankylosing Spondylitis (Not Illustrated)

Chronic progressive inflammation of spine, sacroiliac, and larger joints of the extremities, leading to bony ankylosis and deformity. A form of rheumatoid arthritis, this affects primarily men by a 10:1 ratio, starting in late adolescence or early adulthood. Spasm of paraspinal muscles pulls the spine into forward flexion, obliterating cervical and lumbar curves. The thoracic curve is exaggerated into a single kyphotic rounding. Manifestations also include flexion deformities of the hips and knees.

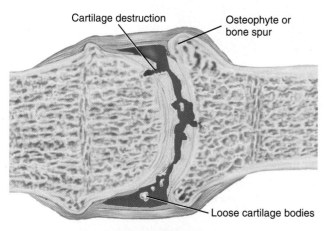

Cartilage destruction

Osteophyte or bone spur

Loose cartilage bodies

◀ **Degenerative Conditions**

Osteoarthritis (Degenerative Joint Disease)

Noninflammatory, localized, progressive disorder involving deterioration of articular cartilages and subchondral bone, and formation of new bone (osteophytes) at joint surfaces. Aging increases incidence; nearly all adults older than age 60 years show some signs of osteoarthritis on radiographs. Asymmetrical joint involvement commonly affects hands, knees, hips, and lumbar and cervical spine. Affected joints have stiffness; swelling with hard, bony protuberances; pain with motion; and limitation of motion (see Table 24.5, p. 678).

Bone resorption

◀ **Osteoporosis**

Decrease in skeletal bone mass occurring when rate of bone resorption is greater than that of bone formation. The weakened bone state increases risk for stress fractures, especially at wrist, hip, and vertebrae. Occurs primarily in postmenopausal women of European descent. Osteoporosis risk is also associated with smaller height and weight, younger age at menopause, lack of physical activity, and lack of estrogen replacement therapy.

TABLE 24.3   Abnormalities of the Shoulder

Atrophy

Loss of muscle mass is exhibited as a lack of fullness
surrounding the deltoid muscle. In the case pictured (on
the patient's left side), atrophy is caused by axillary nerve
palsy. Atrophy also results from disuse, muscle tissue
damage, or motor nerve damage.

Dislocated Shoulder

Anterior dislocation (95%) is exhibited when the shoulder
is hunched forward and the tip of the clavicle dislocates.
It occurs with trauma involving abduction, extension, and
rotation (e.g., falling on an outstretched arm or diving
into a pool).

Joint Effusion

Swelling is caused by excess fluid in the joint capsule:
in the case pictured, from rheumatoid arthritis. It is
best observed anteriorly and is fluctuant on palpation.
Considerable fluid must be present to cause a visible
distension because the capsule is normally loose.

Tear of Rotator Cuff

Characteristics are a hunched position and limited
abduction of arm (in the case pictured, on the patient's
right side). Such tears are caused by traumatic adduction
while the arm is held in abduction; by a fall on shoulder;
by throwing; or by heavy lifting. In the *drop arm test*, the
arm is passively abducted at the shoulder; a positive result
is the patient's inability to sustain the position, and the
arm falls to the side.

TABLE 24.3 Abnormalities of the Shoulder—cont'd

◀ Frozen Shoulder: Adhesive Capsulitis

Fibrous tissues form in the joint capsule, causing stiffness, progressive limitation of motion, and pain. Abduction and external rotation are limited; affected patients cannot reach overhead. It may lead to atrophy of shoulder girdle muscles. Onset is gradual, and the cause is unknown. It is associated with prolonged bedrest or shoulder immobility and may resolve spontaneously. It is a frequent adverse effect of breast cancer treatment.

Subacromial Bursitis (Not Illustrated)

Inflammation and swelling of the subacromial bursa over the shoulder cause both limitation in ROM and pain with motion. Localized swelling under the deltoid muscle may increase with partial passive abduction of the arm. This condition is caused by direct trauma, strain during sports, local or systemic inflammatory process, or repetitive motion injury.

ROM, Range of motion.

TABLE 24.4 Abnormalities of the Elbow

Olecranon Bursitis

Large soft knob, or "goose egg," and redness from inflammation of olecranon bursa. Localized and easy to see because bursa lies just under skin.

Gouty Arthritis

Joint effusion or synovial thickening, seen first as bulge or fullness in grooves on either side of olecranon process. Redness and heat can extend beyond area of synovial membrane. Soft, boggy, or fluctuant fullness to palpation. Limited extension of elbow.

Continued

TABLE 24.4	Abnormalities of the Elbow—cont'd

Subcutaneous Nodules

Raised, firm, nontender nodules that occur with rheumatoid arthritis. Common sites are in the olecranon bursa and along extensor surface of arm. The skin slides freely over the nodules.

Epicondylitis: Tennis Elbow

Chronic, disabling pain at lateral epicondyle of humerus, radiates down extensor surface of forearm. Pain can be located by touching with one finger (as in illustration). Resisting extension of the hand will increase pain. Occurs with activities combining excessive pronation and supination of forearm with an extended wrist (e.g., racket sports or using a screwdriver).

Medial epicondylitis is rarer and is caused by activity of forced palmar flexion of the wrist against resistance.

TABLE 24.5	Abnormalities of the Wrist and Hand

(Reprinted from the *Clinical Slide Collection on the Rheumatic Diseases*, © 1991, 1995, 1997. Used by permission of the American College of Rheumatology.)

Carpal Tunnel Syndrome With Atrophy of Thenar Eminence

Atrophy (pictured) is caused by interference with motor function as a result of compression of the median nerve inside the carpal tunnel. Caused by chronic repetitive motion; occurs between 30 and 60 years of age and is five times more common in women than men. Symptoms of carpal tunnel syndrome include pain, burning sensation and numbness, positive findings on Phalen test, positive Tinel's sign, and often atrophy of thenar muscles.

Ganglion Cyst

Round, cystic, nontender nodule overlying a tendon sheath or joint capsule, usually on dorsum of wrist. Flexion makes it more prominent. A common benign tumour; it does not become malignant.

TABLE 24.5	**Abnormalities of the Wrist and Hand—cont'd**

Ankylosis

Wrist in extreme flexion, as a result of severe rheumatoid arthritis. The affected hand is functionally useless because when the wrist is palmar flexed, a good deal of power is lost from the fingers, and the thumb cannot oppose the fingers.

Colles' Fracture (Not Illustrated)

Nonarticular fracture of distal radius, with or without fracture of ulna at styloid process. Usually results from a fall on an outstretched hand; occurs most often in older women. Wrist looks puffy, with "silver fork" deformity, a characteristic hump when viewed from the side.

Dupuytren's Contracture

Chronic hyperplasia of the palmar fascia causes flexion contractures of the digits, first in the fourth digit, then the fifth digit, and then the third digit. Note the bands that extend from the mid-palm to the digits and the puckering of palmar skin. The condition occurs commonly in men older than 40 years of age and is usually bilateral. It occurs with diabetes, epilepsy, and alcoholic liver disease and as an inherited trait. The contracture is painless but impairs hand function.

Conditions Caused by Chronic Rheumatoid Arthritis

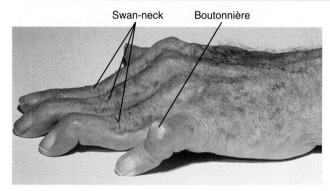

(Reprinted from the *Clinical Slide Collection on the Rheumatic Diseases*, © 1991, 1995, 1997. Used by permission of the American College of Rheumatology.)

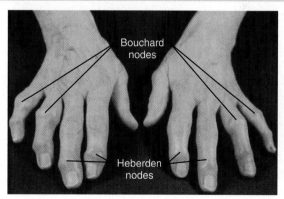

Swan-Neck and Boutonnière Deformity

In **swan-neck deformity**, the flexion contracture resembles the curve of a swan's neck. Note flexion contracture of metacarpophalangeal joint, hyperextension of the proximal interphalangeal joint, and flexion of the distal interphalangeal joint. It occurs with chronic rheumatoid arthritis and is often accompanied by ulnar drift of the fingers.

Ulnar Deviation or Drift

Fingers drift to the ulnar side because of stretching of the articular capsule and muscle imbalance (right hand in illustration). Also note subluxation and swelling in the joints and muscle atrophy on the dorsa of the hands. These are caused by chronic rheumatoid arthritis.

Continued

TABLE 24.5 Abnormalities of the Wrist and Hand—cont'd

In **boutonnière deformity**, the knuckle looks as if it is being pushed through a buttonhole. It is a relatively common deformity and includes flexion of proximal interphalangeal joint with compensatory hyperextension of distal interphalangeal joint.

Degenerative Joint Disease or Osteoarthritis

Osteoarthritis is characterized by hard, nontender nodules (osteophytes, or bony overgrowths), 2 to 3 mm or more in diameter. The osteophytes of the distal interphalangeal joints are called **Heberden's nodes**, and those of the proximal interphalangeal joints are called **Bouchard's nodes**.

Syndactyly

Webbed fingers are a congenital deformity, usually necessitating surgical separation. The metacarpals and phalanges of the webbed fingers are different lengths, and the joints do not line up. Not correcting fused fingers would limit their flexion and extension.

Acute Rheumatoid Arthritis

Painful swelling and stiffness of joints, with fusiform or spindle-shaped swelling of the soft tissue of proximal interphalangeal joints. Fusiform swelling is usually symmetrical, the hands are warm, and the veins are engorged. The inflamed joints have limited ROM.

Polydactyly

Extra digits are a congenital deformity, usually occurring at the fifth finger or the thumb. Surgical removal is considered for cosmetic reasons. The sixth finger shown here was not removed because it had full ROM and sensation and a normal appearance.

TABLE 24.5   Abnormalities of the Wrist and Hand—cont'd

◀ **Gout in the Thumb**

See explanation of gout in Table 24.7, p. 681.

ROM, Range of motion.

TABLE 24.6   Abnormalities of the Knee

Mild Synovitis

Loss of normal hollows on either side of the patella, which are replaced by mild distension. Occurs with synovial thickening or effusion (excess fluid). Also note mild distension of the suprapatellar pouch.

Prepatellar Bursitis

Localized swelling on anterior knee between patella and skin. A tender fluctuant mass indicates swelling; in some cases, infection spreads to surrounding soft tissue. The condition is limited to the bursa, and the knee joint itself is not involved. Overlying skin may be red, shiny, and either atrophic or coarse and thickened.

Continued

TABLE 24.6 Abnormalities of the Knee—cont'd

Swelling of Menisci

Localized soft swelling from cyst in lateral meniscus shows at the midpoint of the anterolateral joint line (right leg in illustration). Semiflexion of the knee makes swelling more prominent.

Osgood-Schlatter Disease

Painful swelling of the tibial tubercle just below the knee, probably from repeated stress on the patellar tendon. Occurs mostly in puberty during rapid growth and most often in boys. Pain increases with kicking, running, bicycling, stair climbing, or kneeling. The condition is usually self-limited, and symptoms resolve with rest.

Postpolio Muscle Atrophy

Leg and foot muscle atrophy as a result of childhood polio (in illustration, the patient's right leg and foot). Poliomyelitis epidemics peaked in North America in the 1940s and 1950s. The development of the oral polio vaccine (1962) has almost eradicated the disease. However, thousands of polio survivors have this muscle atrophy.

Chondromalacia Patellae (Not Illustrated)

Degeneration of articular surface of patellae. Occurs most often in females, adolescents and young adults. Cause is unknown, but condition is associated with overuse and injury. May produce mild effusion. Joint motion is painless, but crepitus may be present. Kneeling causes onset of pain.

TABLE 24.7	Abnormalities of the Ankle and Foot

Achilles Tenosynovitis

Inflammation of a tendon sheath near the ankle (in illustration, the Achilles tendon) produces a superficial linear swelling and a localized tenderness along the route of the sheath. Movement of the involved tendon usually causes pain.

Tophi With Chronic Gout

In illustration, a hard, painless nodule (tophus) over the metatarsophalangeal joint of the first toe. Tophi are collections of sodium urate crystals that develop in and around the joint with chronic gout; they cause extreme swelling and joint deformity. They sometimes burst with a chalky discharge.

Continued

TABLE 24.7	Abnormalities of the Ankle and Foot—cont'd

Acute Gout

Acute episode of gout usually involves the first metatarsophalangeal joint. Clinical findings consist of redness, swelling, heat, and extreme tenderness. Gout is a metabolic disorder of disturbed purine metabolism, associated with elevated serum levels of uric acid. It occurs primarily in men older than 40 years of age.

Hallux Valgus With Bunion and Hammertoes

Hallux valgus is a common deformity caused by rheumatoid arthritis. It is a lateral or outward deviation of the great toe with medial prominence of the head of the first metatarsal. The **bunion** is the inflamed bursa that forms at the pressure point. The great toe loses power to push off while walking; this stresses the second and third metatarsal heads, and they develop calluses and pain. Chronic sequelae include corns, calluses, hammertoes, and joint subluxation.

Note the **hammertoe** deformities in the second, third, fourth, and fifth toes. Often associated with hallux valgus, hammertoe includes hyperextension of the metatarsophalangeal joint and flexion of the proximal interphalangeal joint.

Corns (thickening of soft tissue) develop on the dorsum over the bony prominence as a result of prolonged pressure from shoes.

Callus

Hypertrophy of the epithelium develops because of prolonged pressure, commonly on the plantar surface of the first metatarsal head in the hallux valgus deformity. The condition is not painful.

Ingrown Toenail

"Ingrown toenail" is a misnomer; the nail does not grow in, but the soft tissue grows over the nail and obliterates the groove. It occurs almost always on the great toe on the medial or lateral side. It is caused by trimming the nail too short or crowding of toes in tight shoes. The area becomes infected when the nail grows and its corner penetrates the soft tissue.

TABLE 24.7	Abnormalities of the Ankle and Foot—cont'd

◀ Plantar Wart

Verrucae plantaris (plantar warts) are common lesions occurring on the sole of the foot, caused by the human papillomavirus (HPV). They may cause pain or tenderness when walking or standing.

TABLE 24.8	Abnormalities of the Spine

◀ Scoliosis

Lateral curvature of thoracic and lumbar segments of the spine, usually with some rotation of involved vertebral bodies.

Functional scoliosis is flexible, apparent on standing, and disappears on forward bending. It may be compensatory for other abnormalities such as leg length discrepancy.

Structural scoliosis is fixed; the curvature shows both on standing and on bending forward. In illustration, note rib hump with forward flexion. With the patient standing, note unequal shoulder elevation, unequal scapulae, obvious curvature, and unequal hip level. At greatest risk are girls aged 10 years through adolescence, during the peak of the growth spurt.

TABLE 24.8   Abnormalities of the Spine—cont'd

◄ **Herniated Nucleus Pulposus**

The nucleus pulposus (at the centre of the intervertebral disc) ruptures into the spinal canal and puts pressure on the local spinal nerve root. It is usually caused by stress, such as lifting, twisting, continuous flexion with lifting, or a fall onto the buttocks. It occurs mostly in men 20 to 45 years of age. Lumbar herniations occur mainly in interspaces L4–L5 and L5–S1. Note sciatic pain, numbness, and paraesthesia of involved dermatome; listing away from affected side; decreased mobility; low back tenderness; and decreased motor and sensory function in leg. Straight leg raising tests reproduce sciatic pain.

TABLE 24.9   Common Congenital or Pediatric Abnormalities

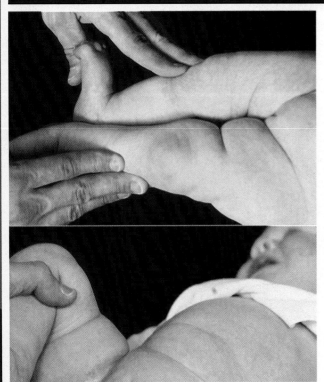

◄ **Congenital Dislocated Hip**

Head of the femur is displaced out of the cup-shaped acetabulum.

The degree of the condition varies; subluxation may occur as stretched ligaments allow partial displacement of the femoral head, and acetabular dysplasia may develop because of excessive laxity of the hip joint capsule.

Occurrence is 1:500 to 1:1 000 births; more common in girls (7:1 ratio). Signs include limited abduction of flexed thigh; positive findings of Ortolani manoeuvre and positive Barlow's sign; asymmetrical skin creases or gluteal folds; limb length discrepancy; and positive indication of the Trendelenburg sign in older children.

TABLE 24.9	Common Congenital or Pediatric Abnormalities—cont'd

Talipes Equinovarus (Clubfoot)

Congenital, rigid, and fixed malposition of foot, including (a) inversion, (b) forefoot adduction, and (c) foot pointing downward (equinus). A common birth defect, with an incidence of 1:1000 to 3:1000 live births. Boys are affected twice as frequently as girls.

Spina Bifida

Incomplete closure of posterior part of vertebrae results in a neural tube defect. Seriousness varies from skin defect along the spine to protrusion of the sac containing meninges, spinal fluid, or malformed spinal cord. The most serious type is myelomeningocele (shown in illustration), in which the meninges and neural tissue protrude. Most children with myelomeningocele are paralyzed below the level of the lesion.

Coxa Plana (Legg-Calvé-Perthes Syndrome) (Not Illustrated)

Avascular necrosis of the femoral head, occurring primarily in boys between 3 and 12 years of age, peaking at age 6 years. In the initial inflammatory stage, interruption of blood supply to femoral epiphysis occurs, halting growth. Revascularization and healing occur later, but significant residual deformity and dysfunction may be present.

Summary Checklist: Musculo skeletal Examination

For each joint to be examined:
1. **Inspect:**
   Size and contour of joint
   Skin colour and characteristics
2. **Palpate joint area:**
   Skin
   Muscles

Bony articulations
Joint capsule
3. **Test range of motion (ROM):**
   Active
   Passive (if active ROM is limited)
4. **Test muscles**

5. **Engage in teaching and health promotion**

REFERENCES

1. Weaver, C. M., Gordon, C. M., Janz, K. F., et al. (2016). The National Osteoporosis Foundation's position statement on peak bone mass development and lifestyle factors: A systematic review and implementation recommendations. *Osteoporosis International, 27,* 1281–1386. doi:10.1007/s00198-015-3440-3.

2. Canadian Task Force on Preventive Health. (2015). Recommendations for growth monitoring, and prevention and management of overweight and obesity in children and youth in primary care. *Canadian Medical Association Journal, 187*(6), 411–421. doi:10.1503/cmaj.141285.

3. Canadian Task Force on Preventive Health Care. (2001). *Screening and management of developmental dysplasia of the hip in newborns.* Retrieved from http://canadiantaskforce.ca/other-guidelines-1979-2006/screening-and-management-of-developmental-dysplasia-of-the-hip-in-newborns-2001/.

4. Pigozzi, E., Rizzo, M., Giombinin, A., et al. (2009). Bone mineral density and sport: Effect of physical activity. *Journal of Sports Medicine and Physical Fitness, 49*(2), 177–183.

5. Schmitt, N. M., Schmitt, J., & Doren, M. (2009). The role of physical activity in the prevention of osteoporosis in postmenopausal women—An update. *Maturitas, 63*(1), 34–38. doi:10.1016/j.maturitas.2009.03.002.

6. Cousins, J. M., Petit, M. A., Paudel, M. L., et al. (2010). Muscle power and physical activity are associated with bone strength in older men: The osteoporotic fractures in men study. *Bone, 47*(2), 205–211. doi:10.1016/j.bone.2010.05.003.

7. Statistics Canada. (2015). *Physical activity during leisure time, 2014.* Retrieved from http://www.statcan.gc.ca/pub/82-625-x/2015001/article/14189-eng.htm.

8. Statistics Canada. (2017). *Health fact sheet: Chronic conditions.* Ottawa: Minister of Industry. Retrieved from http://www.statcan.gc.ca/pub/82-625-x/2017001/article/54858-eng.pdf.

9. Public Health Agency of Canada. (2011). *Chapter 1: Life with arthritis in Canada: A personal and public health challenge—What is arthritis and how common is it?* Retrieved from https://www.canada.ca/en/public-health/services/chronic-diseases/arthritis/life-arthritis-canada-a-personal-public-health-challenge/chapter-one-what-is-arthritis-and-how-common-is-it.html.

10. Arthritis Society. (2015). *Types of arthritis.* Retrieved from http://arthritis.ca/understand-arthritis/types-of-arthritis.

11. Luong, M. N., Cleveland, R. J., Nyrop, K. A., et al. (2012). Social determinants and osteoarthritis outcomes. *Aging Health, 8*(4), 413–437. doi:10.2217/ahe.12.43.

12. Statistics Canada. (2015). *Injuries in Canada: Insights from the Canadian Community Health Survey.* Retrieved from http://www.statcan.gc.ca/pub/82-624-x/2011001/article/11506-eng.htm.

13. Osteoporosis Canada. (2017). *#Betterbonehealth: 2015–2016 Annual Report, Osteoporosis Canada.* Retrieved from https://osteoporosis.ca/wp-content/uploads/Osteo-Annual-Report-2015-2016-Web-Version.pdf.

14. Ioannidis, G., Papaioannou, A., Hopman, W. M., et al. (2009). Relation between fractures and mortality: Results from the Canadian Multicentre Osteoporosis Study. *Canadian Medical Association Journal, 181*(5), 265–271.

15. Canadian Institute for Health Information. (2009). *Hip and knee replacements in Canada—Canadian Joint Replacement Registry (CJRR) 2008–2009 annual report.* Retrieved from https://secure.cihi.ca/free_products/2008_cjrr_annual_report_en.pdf.

16. Schraeder, T. L., Terek, R. M., & Smith, C. C. (2010). Clinical evaluation of the knee. *New England Journal of Medicine, 363*(4), e5.

17. Wolfe, F., & Hauser, W. (2011). Fibromyalgia diagnosis and diagnostic criteria. *Annals of Medicine, 43*(7), 495–502. doi:10.3109/07853890.2011.595734.

18. McGee, S. (2012). *Evidence-based physical diagnosis* (3rd ed.). St. Louis: Saunders.

19. Centre for Effective Practice. (2016). *Clinically Organized Relevant Exam (CORE) Back Tool.* Retrieved from https://thewellhealth.ca/low-back-pain/.

20. Kaneshiro, N. K. (2011). *Simian crease.* Retrieved from http://www.nlm.nih.gov/medlineplus/ency/article/003290.htm.

21. Goldbloom, R. B. (1994). Screening for idiopathic adolescent scoliosis. In Canadian Task Force on the Periodic Health Examination (Ed.), *Canadian guide to clinical preventive health care* (pp. 346–354). Ottawa: Health Canada.

CHAPTER 25

Neurological System

Written by Carolyn Jarvis, PhD, APN, CNP
Adapted by Annette J. Browne, PhD, RN

http://evolve.elsevier.com/Canada/Jarvis/examination/

STRUCTURE AND FUNCTION

Precentral gyrus—
primary motor area

Central sulcus

Postcentral gyrus—
primary sensory area

trunk

hand

PARIETAL LOBE—
sensation

fingers

Wernicke's area—
speech comprehension

face

lips

OCCIPITAL LOBE—
visual reception

tongue

FRONTAL LOBE—
personality
behaviour
emotion
intellectual functions

Broca's area—
motor speech

Lateral sulcus

TEMPORAL LOBE—
hearing
taste
smell

CEREBELLUM—
motor coordination
equilibrium
balance

CEREBRAL CORTEX
Left Lateral View

25.1 (© Pat Thomas, 2006.)

The nervous system can be divided into two parts: (a) central and (b) peripheral. The **central nervous system (CNS)** includes the brain and spinal cord. The **peripheral nervous system (PNS)** includes the 12 pairs of cranial nerves, the 31 pairs of spinal nerves, and all their branches. The PNS carries sensory (*a*fferent) messages *to* the CNS from sensory receptors, motor (*e*fferent) messages *from* the CNS out to muscles and glands, and autonomic messages that govern the internal organs and blood vessels.

The meninges (dura, arachnoid, and pia mater) are the layers of membranes that envelope the CNS. The primary function of the meninges and of the cerebrospinal fluid is to protect the CNS.

THE CENTRAL NERVOUS SYSTEM

Cerebral Cortex

The cerebral cortex is the cerebrum's outer layer of nerve cell bodies; this layer looks like "grey matter" because it

COMPONENTS OF THE CENTRAL NERVOUS SYSTEM

25.2 (© Pat Thomas, 2006.)

lacks myelin. Myelin is the white insulation on the axon that increases the conduction velocity of nerve impulses.

The cerebral cortex (cerebrum) is the centre for humans' highest functions, governing thought, memory, reasoning, sensation, and voluntary movement (Fig. 25.1). Each half of the cerebrum is a **hemisphere**; the left hemisphere is dominant in about 95% of right-handed people, and in many who are left-handed.

Each hemisphere is divided into four **lobes**: (a) frontal, (b) parietal, (c) occipital, and (d) temporal. The lobes have certain areas that mediate specific functions:

- The **frontal** lobe has areas concerned with personality, behaviour, emotions, and intellectual function.
- The precentral gyrus of the frontal lobe initiates voluntary movement.
- The **parietal** lobe contains the postcentral gyrus, which is the primary centre for sensation.
- The **occipital** lobe is the primary visual receptor centre.
- The portion of the **temporal** lobe behind the ear contains the primary auditory reception centre.
- **Wernicke's area** in the temporal lobe is associated with language comprehension. When it is damaged in a person's dominant hemisphere, receptive aphasia results. The person hears sound, but it has no meaning, like hearing a foreign language.
- **Broca's area** in the frontal lobe mediates motor speech. When it is injured in the dominant hemisphere, expressive aphasia results; the person cannot talk. The person

can understand language and knows what he, she, or they would like to say, but can produce only a garbled sound.

Damage to any of these specific cortical areas produces a corresponding loss of function: motor weakness, paralysis, loss of sensation, or impairment of the ability to understand and process language. Damage occurs when the highly specialized neurological cells are deprived of their blood supply, such as when a cerebral artery becomes occluded or when vascular bleeding or vasospasm occurs.

Basal Ganglia

The basal ganglia are additional bands of grey matter buried deep within the two cerebral hemispheres that form the subcortical associated motor system (the extrapyramidal system; Fig. 25.2). They control automatic associated movements of the body, such as the arm swing that alternates with the leg movement during walking.

Thalamus

The thalamus is the main relay station for the nervous system. Sensory pathways of the spinal cord and brain stem form **synapses** (sites of contact between two neurons) on their way to the cerebral cortex.

Hypothalamus

The hypothalamus is a major control centre with many vital functions: controlling temperature, heart rate, and blood pressure; regulating sleep and the anterior and posterior pituitary gland; and coordinating autonomic nervous system activity and emotional status.

Cerebellum

The cerebellum is a coiled structure located under the occipital lobe that is concerned with motor coordination of voluntary movements, equilibrium (i.e., the postural balance of the body), and muscle tone. It does not initiate movement but coordinates and smoothes it, such as the complex and quick coordination of the many different muscles needed in playing the piano, swimming, or juggling. It is like the automatic pilot on an airplane in that it adjusts and corrects the voluntary movements but operates entirely below the conscious level.

Brain Stem

The brain stem is the central core of the brain consisting of mostly nerve fibres. It has three areas:

1. **Midbrain:** the most anterior part of the brain stem that still has the basic tubular structure of the spinal cord. It merges into the thalamus and hypothalamus. It contains many motor neurons and tracts.
2. **Pons:** the enlarged area containing ascending and descending fibre tracts.
3. **Medulla:** the continuation of the spinal cord in the brain that contains all ascending and descending fibre tracts connecting the brain and spinal cord. It has vital autonomic centres (respiratory, cardiac, gastro-intestinal functions), as well as nuclei for cranial nerves VIII through XII. Pyramidal decussation (crossing of the motor fibres) occurs here (see under Corticospinal or Pyramidal Tract).

Spinal Cord

The spinal cord is the long cylindrical structure of nervous tissue approximately as big around as the little finger. It occupies the upper two-thirds of the vertebral canal from the medulla to lumbar vertebrae L1 and L2. It is the main pathway for ascending and descending fibre tracts that connect the brain to the spinal nerves, and it mediates reflexes. Its grey matter is arranged in a butterfly shape with anterior and posterior "horns" and contains the nerve cell bodies.

Pathways of the Central Nervous System

Crossed representation is a notable feature of the nerve tracts. The *left* cerebral cortex receives sensory information from, and controls motor function to, the *right* side of the body, whereas the *right* cerebral cortex interacts with the *left* side of the body. Knowledge of where the fibres cross the midline helps you interpret clinical findings.

Sensory Pathways

Millions of sensory receptors are embroidered into the skin, mucous membranes, muscles, tendons, and viscera. They monitor conscious sensations, internal organ functions, body positions, and reflexes. Sensation travels in the afferent fibres in the peripheral nerve, then through the posterior (dorsal) root, and then into the spinal cord. In the spinal cord, it may take one of two routes: the spinothalamic tract or the posterior (dorsal) columns (see Fig. 25.3, *B*).

Spinothalamic Tract. The spinothalamic tract contains sensory fibres that transmit the sensations of pain, temperature, and crude or light touch (i.e., touch not precisely localized). The fibres enter the dorsal root of the spinal cord and synapse with a second sensory neuron. The second-order neuron fibres cross to the opposite side and ascend the spinothalamic tract to the thalamus. Fibres carrying pain and temperature sensations ascend the *lateral* spinothalamic tract, whereas those carrying sensations of crude touch form the *anterior* spinothalamic tract. At the thalamus, the fibres synapse with a third sensory neuron, which carries the message to the sensory cortex for full interpretation.

Posterior (Dorsal) Columns. These fibres conduct the sensations of position, vibration, and finely localized touch:

- **Position (proprioception):** the sense of where your body parts are in space and in relation to each other, without your looking at them.
- **Vibration:** the ability to feel vibrating objects.
- **Finely localized touch (stereognosis):** the ability to identify familiar objects by touch, without looking.

These fibres enter the dorsal root and proceed immediately up the same side of the spinal cord to the brain stem. At the medulla, they synapse with a second sensory neuron and then cross. They travel to the **thalamus**, synapse again, and proceed to the sensory cortex, which localizes the sensation and makes full discrimination.

The sensory cortex is arranged in a specific pattern forming a corresponding "map" of the body (see Fig. 25.3, *A*: The *homunculus* [Latin for "little man"] is an illustration representing the proportion of the brain that is responsible for sensations in particular body parts). Pain in the right hand is perceived at its specific spot on the left cortex map. Some organs—such as the heart, liver, and spleen—are not represented in the brain map. You know you have such organs, but you have no "felt image" of them. Pain originating in these organs is referred: that is, it is felt "by proxy" by another body part that does have a felt image. For example, pain in the heart is referred to the chest, shoulder, and left arm, which were its neighbours during fetal development. Pain originating in the spleen is felt on the top of the left shoulder.

Motor Pathways

Corticospinal or Pyramidal Tract. This area has been named *pyramidal* because it originates in pyramid-shaped cells in the motor cortex (Fig. 25.4). Motor nerve fibres originate in the motor cortex and travel to the brain stem, where they cross to the opposite or contralateral side (*pyramidal decussation*) and then pass down in the lateral column of the spinal cord. At each cord level, they synapse with a lower motor neuron contained in the anterior horn of the spinal cord. Ten percent of corticospinal fibres do not cross, and these descend in the anterior column of the spinal cord. Corticospinal fibres mediate voluntary movement, particularly very skilled, discrete, purposeful movements such as writing.

Major Sensory Pathways

—Lateral spinothalamic tract—
  pain, temperature

—Anterior spinothalamic tract—
  crude touch

—Posterior (dorsal) columns—
  fine touch

25.3 Sensory pathways. (© Pat Thomas, 2006.)

The corticospinal tract is a newer, "higher" motor system in humans that enables very skilled and purposeful movements. The origin of this tract in the motor cortex is arranged in a specific pattern called *somatotopic organization.* Another type of body map, a cortical *homunculus* (see Fig. 25.3, *A*) shows the portion of the human brain directly responsible for the movement and exchange of sensory and motor information of the body; that is, body parts whose movements are relatively more important to humans (e.g., the hand) occupy proportionally more space on the brain map.

Extrapyramidal Tracts. The extrapyramidal tracts include all the motor nerve fibres originating in the motor cortex, basal ganglia, brain stem, and spinal cord that are *outside* the pyramidal tract. They constitute a phylogenetically older, more primitive motor system. These subcortical motor fibres maintain muscle tone and control body movements, especially gross automatic movements such as walking.

Cerebellar System. This complex motor system coordinates movement, maintains equilibrium, and helps maintain posture. The cerebellum receives information about the position of muscles and joints—the body's equilibrium—and

the kind of motor messages that are being sent from the cortex to the muscles. The information is integrated, and the cerebellum uses feedback pathways to exert its control back on the cortex or down to lower motor neurons in the spinal cord. This entire process occurs on a subconscious level.

Upper and Lower Motor Neurons

Upper motor neurons are a complex of all the descending motor fibres that can influence or modify the lower motor neurons. Upper motor neurons are located completely within the CNS. The neurons convey impulses from the motor areas of the cerebral cortex to the lower motor neurons in the anterior horn cells of the spinal cord (Fig. 25.5).

Examples of upper motor neurons are the corticospinal, corticobulbar, and extrapyramidal tracts. Examples of upper motor neuron diseases are cerebrovascular accident, cerebral palsy, and multiple sclerosis.

Lower motor neurons are located mostly in the PNS. The cell body of the lower motor neuron is located in the anterior grey column of the spinal cord, but the nerve fibre extends from there to the muscle. The lower motor neuron is the "final common pathway" because it funnels many

25.4 Motor pathways. (© Pat Thomas, 2010.)

neural signals and it provides the final direct contact with the muscles. Any movement must be translated into action by lower motor neuron fibres. Examples of lower motor neurons are the cranial nerves and spinal nerves of the PNS. Examples of lower motor neuron diseases are spinal cord lesions, poliomyelitis, and amyotrophic lateral sclerosis.

THE PERIPHERAL NERVOUS SYSTEM

A **nerve** is a bundle of fibres *outside* the CNS. The peripheral nerves carry input to the CNS via their sensory afferent fibres and deliver output from the CNS via the efferent fibres.

Reflex Arc

Reflexes are basic defence mechanisms of the nervous system. They are involuntary, operating below the level of conscious control and enabling a quick reaction to potentially painful or damaging events. Reflexes also help the body maintain balance and appropriate muscle tone. There are four types of reflexes: (a) **deep tendon reflexes** (myotatic), such as patellar or knee jerk; (b) **superficial**, such as corneal reflex or abdominal reflex; (c) **visceral** (organic), such as pupillary response to light and accommodation; and (d) **pathological** (abnormal), such as the Babinski (extensor plantar) reflex.

The fibres that mediate the reflex are carried by a specific spinal nerve. In the most simple reflex, tapping the tendon stretches the muscle spindles in the muscle, which activates the sensory afferent nerve. The sensory afferent fibres carry the message from the receptor and travel through the dorsal root into the spinal cord (Fig. 25.6). They synapse directly in the cord with the motor neuron in the anterior horn. Motor efferent fibres leave via the ventral root and travel to the muscle, stimulating a sudden contraction.

The deep tendon (myotatic or stretch) reflex (DTR) has five components: (a) an intact sensory nerve (afferent); (b) a functional synapse in the cord; (c) an intact motor nerve fibre (efferent); (d) the neuromuscular junction; and (e) a competent muscle.

Cranial Nerves

Cranial nerves enter and exit the brain rather than the spinal cord (Fig. 25.7). Cranial nerves I and II extend from the cerebrum; cranial nerves III to XII extend from the

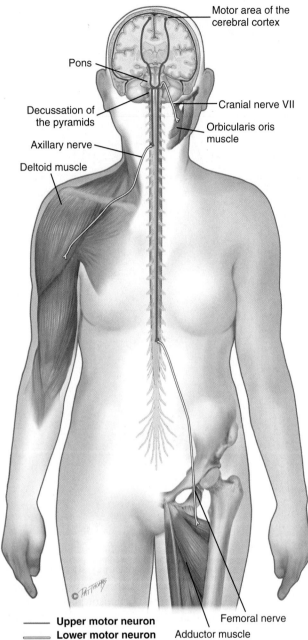

25.5 (© Pat Thomas, 2006.)

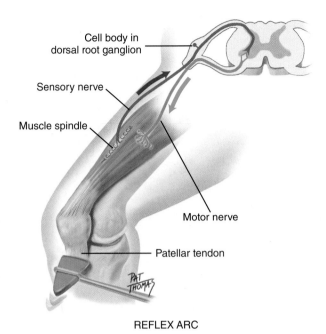

REFLEX ARC

25.6

through roots: sensory afferent fibres through the posterior (dorsal) roots, and motor efferent fibres through the anterior (ventral) roots.

The nerves exit the spinal cord in an orderly ladder shape. Each nerve innervates a particular segment of the body. **Dermal segmentation** is the cutaneous distribution of the various spinal nerves.

A **dermatome** is a circumscribed skin area that is supplied mainly from one spinal cord segment through a particular spinal nerve (Fig. 25.8). The dermatomes overlap, which is a form of biological insurance; that is, if one nerve is severed, most of the sensations will continue to be transmitted by the nerve above and the nerve below. Do not attempt to memorize all dermatome segments; focus on just the following as useful landmarks:

- The thumb, middle finger, and fifth finger are each in the dermatomes of C6, C7, and C8.
- The axilla is at the level of T1.
- The nipple is at the level of T4.
- The umbilicus is at the level of T10.
- The groin is in the region of L1.
- The knee is at the level of L4.

Somatic and Autonomic Nerve Fibres

The PNS is composed of cranial nerves and spinal nerves. These nerves carry fibres that can be divided functionally into two parts: (a) somatic and (b) autonomic. The somatic fibres innervate the skeletal (voluntary) muscles; the autonomic fibres innervate smooth (involuntary) muscles, cardiac muscle, and glands. The autonomic nervous system mediates unconscious activity. A detailed description of the autonomic nervous system is beyond the scope of this book; its overall function is to maintain homeostasis of the body.

lower diencephalon and brain stem. The 12 pairs of cranial nerves supply primarily the head and neck, except the vagus nerve (from the Latin *vagus*, or wanderer, as in "vagabond"), which travels to the heart, respiratory muscles, stomach, and gallbladder.

Spinal Nerves

The 31 pairs of **spinal nerves** arise from the length of the spinal cord and supply the rest of the body. They are named for the region of the spine from which they exit: 8 cervical, 12 thoracic, 5 lumbar, 5 sacral, and 1 coccygeal. They are "mixed" nerves because they contain both sensory and motor fibres. The nerves enter and exit the spinal cord

CRANIAL NERVES

- **I** Olfactory
- **II** Optic
- **III** Oculomotor
- **IV** Trochlear
- **VI** Abducens
- **V** Trigeminal
- **VII** Facial
- **VIII** Acoustic
- **IX** Glossopharyngeal
- **X** Vagus
- **XI** Spinal Accessory
- **XII** Hypoglossal

——— SENSORY
——— MOTOR

Cranial Nerve	Type	Function
I: Olfactory	Sensory	Smell
II: Optic	Sensory	Vision
III: Oculomotor	Mixed*	Motor—most extraocular movement (EOM), opening of eyelids Parasympathetic—pupil constriction, lens shape
IV: Trochlear	Motor	Downward and inward movement of eye
V: Trigeminal	Mixed	Motor—muscles of mastication Sensory—sensation of face and scalp, cornea, mucous membranes of mouth and nose
VI: Abducens	Motor	Lateral movement of eye
VII: Facial	Mixed	Motor—facial muscles, closing of eyes, labial speech, closing of mouth Sensory—taste (sweet, salty, sour, bitter) on anterior two-thirds of tongue Parasympathetic—saliva and tear secretion
VIII: Acoustic	Sensory	Hearing and equilibrium
IX: Glossopharyngeal	Mixed	Motor—pharynx (phonation and swallowing) Sensory—taste on posterior one-third of tongue, pharynx (gag reflex) Parasympathetic—parotid gland, carotid reflex
X: Vagus	Mixed	Motor—pharynx and larynx (talking and swallowing) Sensory—general sensation from carotid body, carotid sinus, pharynx, viscera Parasympathetic—carotid reflex
XI: Spinal	Motor	Movement of trapezius and sternomastoid muscles
XII: Hypoglossal	Motor	Movement of tongue

Mixed refers to a nerve carrying a combination of fibres: motor + sensory; motor + parasympathetic; or motor + sensory + parasympathetic.

25.7 (© Pat Thomas, 2006.)

SPINAL NERVES

DERMATOMES

DEVELOPMENTAL CONSIDERATIONS

Infants

The neurological system is not completely developed at birth. Motor activity in newborns is under the control of the spinal cord and medulla. Very little cortical control exists, and the neurons are not yet myelinated. Movements are directed primarily by primitive reflexes. As the cerebral cortex develops during the first year, it inhibits these reflexes, and they disappear at predictable times. Persistence of the primitive reflexes is an indication of CNS dysfunction.

Infants' sensory and motor development proceeds along with the gradual acquisition of myelin because myelin is needed to conduct most impulses. The process of myelinization follows a cephalocaudal order and a proximal-to-distal order (head, neck, trunk, and extremities). This is the order observed in infants as they gain motor control (lifting head, lifting head and shoulders, rolling over, moving whole arm, using hands, walking). As the milestones are achieved, each movement is more complex and coordinated. Milestones occur in an orderly sequence, although the exact age at occurrence may vary.

Sensation is also rudimentary at birth. Newborns need a strong stimulus and then respond by crying and with whole body movements. As myelinization develops, infants are able to localize the stimulus more precisely and to make a more accurate motor response.

Older Adults

The aging process causes a general atrophy with a steady loss of neurons in the brain and spinal cord. This causes a decrease in weight and volume with a thinning of the cerebral cortex, reduced subcortical brain structures, and expansion of the ventricles.[1] Neuron loss leads many people over 65 years of age to show signs that would be considered abnormal in the younger adult, such as general loss of muscle bulk; loss of muscle tone in the face, in the neck, and around the spine; decreased muscle strength; impaired fine coordination and agility; loss of vibratory sense at the ankle; decreased or absent Achilles reflex; loss of position sense at the big toe; and pupillary miosis, irregular pupil shape, and decreased pupillary reflexes.

The velocity of nerve conduction decreases between 5% and 10% with aging, which slows the reaction time in some older adults. An increased delay at the synapse also occurs, so that the impulse takes longer to travel. As a result, touch and pain sensation, taste, and smell may be diminished.

The motor system may show a general slowing down of movement. Muscle strength and agility decrease. A generalized decrease occurs in muscle bulk, which is most apparent in the dorsal hand muscles. Muscle tremors may occur in the hands, head, and jaw, along with possible repetitive facial grimacing (dyskinesias).

Aging involves a progressive decrease in cerebral blood flow and oxygen consumption. In some people, this causes dizziness and a loss of balance with position change. Older adults need to get up slowly; otherwise, they are at increased risk for falls and resulting injuries. In addition, older adults may forget that they fell, which makes it hard to diagnose the cause of an injury.

When they are in good health, older adults walk about as well as they did during their middle and younger years, except more slowly and more deliberately. Some survey the ground for obstacles or uneven terrain. Some show hesitation and take a slightly wayward path. Importantly, because two-thirds of strokes occur among people over age 65 years, it is important for nurses to engage in health promotion activities that are tailored to the context of peoples' lives.[2]

SOCIAL DETERMINANTS OF HEALTH CONSIDERATIONS

As with all aspects of health, the social determinants of health have an impact on neurological health and related systems. For example, the latest evidence on socioeconomic status and stroke shows that stroke disproportionately affects socioeconomically disadvantaged populations in high-income countries such as Canada, and a similar trend exists in lower income nations.[3] These disparities are reflected not only in risk for stroke but also in short-term and long-term outcomes after stroke. Among stroke survivors, lower socioeconomic status is significantly associated with higher rates of disability following acute ischemic stroke.[4] Research has shown that people in low-income neighbourhoods are more likely to be hospitalized for stroke than those in higher income areas.[5] The underlying reasons are complex and relate to intersecting factors such as poor access to health care and preventive services, lack of opportunities for exercise, and low socioeconomic status (which is known to have a negative impact on health overall).

Research also indicates that in comparison with the general population, First Nations, Inuit, and Métis people experience higher rates of hypertension, Type 2 diabetes, and smoking, which combined contribute to a death rate due to stroke that is twice as high than in the general population.[6] Similarly, people of South Asian or African heritage are more likely to have hypertension and diabetes, and, thus, an elevated risk for heart disease and stroke.[7] Epidemiologists and others have shown that these health issues are strongly impacted by patients' experiences of racism and other forms of discrimination; they are not (as may have been previously assumed) clearly attributable to so-called lifestyle factors such as exercise and diet.[8] Recognizing the importance of early detection of stroke, the Heart and Stroke Foundation of Canada has translated and adapted selected health education resources into Ojibway, Oji-cree, Punjabi, Hindi, Mandarin, and Cantonese, among other languages, to help patients from diverse populations learn the risk factors and warning signs. (See the box Promoting Health: Stroke.)

PROMOTING HEALTH: STROKE

Stroke Prevention

Stroke is the third leading cause of death and the leading cause of disability in Canada. Each year, over 62 000 new cases of stroke occur in Canada,* with nearly 14 000 Canadians dying from stroke each year.[†] The prevalence of stroke increases with age and other risk factors, such as hypertension, smoking, and associated cardiac conditions such as atrial fibrillation. A stroke, or cerebrovascular accident, occurs when the blood flow is interrupted to a part of the brain, which is why it is often referred to as a "brain attack." The most common type is an ischemic stroke, in which a blood clot blocks a blood vessel in the brain. Less common is a hemorrhagic stroke, which occurs when a blood vessel in the brain ruptures and causes bleeding. The symptoms and aftereffects of a stroke depend on which area of the brain is affected and to what extent. This can make a stroke difficult to diagnose. However, early recognition of symptoms and prompt treatment are essential so that appropriate treatments and interventions can be initiated as soon as possible. Only approximately 5% of patients with stroke receive appropriate therapy in a timely manner.[‡]

Time from symptom onset is the most important piece of information in the initial assessment.[‡] Early assessment is particularly important because symptoms of stroke or transient ischemic attacks (TIAs) may be similar to those of other conditions, such as hypoglycemia, migraine, seizure, trauma, or medication overdose. The *most common* symptoms of stroke are as follows:

1. Sudden weakness or numbness in the face, arms, or legs, especially when it is on one side of the body
2. Sudden confusion, trouble speaking, or understanding speech
3. Sudden changes in vision, such as blurry vision or partial or complete loss of vision in one or both eyes
4. Sudden trouble walking, dizziness, or loss of balance or coordination
5. Sudden severe headache with no reason or explanation
   Less common symptoms of stroke are as follows:
1. Sudden nausea or vomiting
2. Brief loss of consciousness, including fainting

Continued

PROMOTING HEALTH: STROKE—cont'd

Stroke Prevention

Many Canadians continue to ignore, or fail to recognize, the symptoms of stroke. Stroke symptoms usually do not hurt, which is why many people ignore them or delay seeking medical attention. A "mini-stroke," or TIA, can also occur. In these cases, the stroke symptoms are only temporary and then disappear, often within an hour. Because the symptoms "go away," people too often do not report them or seek medical attention. However, a TIA is a warning sign that should not be ignored. Nearly one-third of people who survive a stroke or a TIA go on to have another stroke within the next five years.[†] When people experience chest pain, they usually know to seek medical attention to rule out a heart attack. Having a TIA should also prompt people to seek medical attention to rule out the possibility of a future TIA. One significant reason for delay is that patients consult with their physician or relatives at the onset of symptoms.[‡] Patients must be instructed to call an ambulance for immediate transportation to a hospital instead. To promote swift recognition of the symptoms of stroke among members of the public, the Heart and Stroke Foundation of Canada developed the following mnemonic:[§]

- **F**ACE—Is it drooping?
- **A**RMS—Can you raise both?
- **S**PEECH—Is it slurred or jumbled?
- **T**IME—To call 9-1-1 right away.

Most risk factors for stroke, such as high blood pressure, diabetes, smoking, inactivity, and high cholesterol, are equivalent for men and women and are potentially modifiable, depending on personal and social contexts. Gender, however, is an important risk factor. In Canada, the risk for stroke is higher for men than for women, but the mortality rate is 45% higher for women at all ages,[†] and the gap is widening. In part, this is because women live longer on average than do men, but new research suggests that there may exist some risk factors that are uniquely important for women. For example, women who have migraines with visual disturbances, such as flashing dots or blind spots, can be up to 10 times more likely to have a stroke than those without visual disturbances; women who develop pre-eclampsia in pregnancy may have a 60% greater risk for non–pregnancy-related ischemic stroke; and women who smoke and who are taking oral contraceptives or have high blood pressure, migraines, or blood clotting disorders have an increased risk for stroke.

The following modifiable risk factors for stroke have been well documented:

1. History of cardiovascular disease
   a. Coronary heart disease
   b. Cardiac failure
   c. Symptomatic peripheral artery disease (PAD)
2. Hypertension
3. Cigarette smoking or exposure to second-hand smoke
4. Diabetes
5. Atrial fibrillation
6. Other cardiac conditions
   a. Dilated cardiomyopathy
   b. Valvular heart disease (e.g., mitral valve prolapse, endocarditis, and prosthetic cardiac valves)
   c. Intracardiac congenital defects (e.g., patent foramen ovale, atrial septal defect, and atrial septal aneurysm)

7. Dyslipidemia
8. Asymptomatic carotid stenosis
9. Sickle cell disease
10. Postmenopausal hormone therapy
11. Diet and nutrition
12. Physical inactivity
13. Obesity and fat distribution
14. History of TIA

Nonmodifiable risk factors for stroke may still help identify people who, in conjunction with well-documented modifiable risks, are at highest risk for stroke and who may benefit from more rigorous treatment of modifiable risk factors. Nonmodifiable risk factors for stroke include the following:

1. Age
2. Gender: Strokes are generally more prevalent in men than in women. However, the mortality rate for women is higher.
3. Low birth weight
4. Ethnocultural background: Indigenous people and people of African or South Asian descent are more likely to have high blood pressure and diabetes and are therefore at greater risk for heart disease and stroke than is the general population.
5. Genetic factors and genetic disorders such as Marfan's syndrome, Fabry's disease, and cerebral autosomal dominant arteriopathy with subcortical infarcts and leukoencephalopathy (CADASIL)

The *Canadian Stroke Best Practice Recommendations*[‖] recommend that patients at risk for stroke and who have had a stroke focus on the following areas for prevention: eating a healthy balanced diet; adhering to the recommended daily limit of sodium intake, known as the Adequate Intake; undertaking moderate exercise; maintaining a healthy weight; participating in smoking cessation or reduction; limiting alcohol intake; and managing underlying medical conditions, including hypertension, dyslipidemia, previous stroke or TIA, atrial fibrillation and stroke, and carotid stenosis. These areas of prevention have important implications for the range of health assessments conducted by nurses working in a range of settings.

References

*Blacquiere, D., Lindsay, P., Foley, N., et al. (2017). Canadian stroke best practice recommendations: Telestroke best practice guidelines update 2017. *International Journal of Stroke*, 12(8), 886–895. doi:10.1177/1747493017706239.

†Ontario Stroke Network. (2016). *Stroke stats & facts.* Retrieved from http://ontariostrokenetwork.ca/information-about-stroke/stroke-stats-and-facts/.

‡Bergman, D. (2011). Preventing recurrent cerebrovascular events in patients with stroke or transient ischemic attack: The current data. *Journal of the American Academy of Nurse Practitioners*, 23(12), 659–666. doi:10.1111/j.1745-7599.2011.00650.x.

§Heart and Stroke Foundation of Canada. (2017). *Signs of stroke.* Retrieved from http://www.heartandstroke.ca/stroke/signs-of-stroke.

‖Coutts, S. B., Wein, T. H., Lindsay, M. P., et al. (2015). Canadian stroke best practice recommendations: Secondary prevention of stroke guidelines, update 2014. *International Journal of Stroke*, 10(3), 282–291. doi:10.1111/ijs.12439.

SUBJECTIVE DATA

1. Headache
2. Head injury
3. Dizziness or vertigo
4. Seizures
5. Tremors

6. Weakness
7. Incoordination
8. Numbness or tingling sensation
9. Difficulty swallowing
10. Difficulty speaking

11. Significant past history
12. Environmental and occupational hazards

HEALTH HISTORY QUESTIONS

Examiner Asks	Rationale
1. Headache. Do you have any unusually frequent or severe **headaches**? • When did this start? How often does it occur? • Where in your head do you feel the headaches? Do the headaches seem to be associated with anything? (Headache history is fully discussed in Chapter 14.)	
2. Head injury. Have you ever had any **head injury**? Please describe. • What part of your head was hit? • Did you experience loss of consciousness? For how long? • Do you use a helmet consistently to prevent head injuries (e.g., helmet use with sports such as biking, skating, skiing, snowboarding)?	
3. Dizziness or vertigo. Do you ever feel lightheaded or a swimming sensation, like feeling faint? • When have you noticed this? How often does it occur? Does it occur with activity, change in position? • Do you ever feel a rotational spinning sensation? (Note: Distinguish **vertigo** from **dizziness**.) Do you feel as if the room spins (objective vertigo)? Or do you feel that you are spinning (subjective vertigo)? Did this come on suddenly or gradually?	**Syncope** is a sudden loss of strength and a temporary loss of consciousness (fainting) caused by lack of cerebral blood flow, as occurs with low blood pressure. True **vertigo** is the sensation of rotational spinning, caused by neurological disease in the vestibular apparatus in the ear or in the vestibular nuclei in the brain stem.
4. Seizures. Have you ever had any **seizures**? When did they start? How often do they occur? • Course and duration: When a seizure starts, do you have any warning sign? What type of sign? • Motor activity: Where in your body do the seizures begin? Do the seizures travel through your body? On one side or both? Does your muscle tone seem tense or limp? • Any associated signs, such as colour change in face or lips, loss of consciousness (for how long), automatisms (eyelid-fluttering, eye-rolling, lip smacking), incontinence? • Postictal phase: After the seizure, are you told that you spend time sleeping, or do you have any confusion, weakness, headache, or muscle ache? • Precipitating factors: Does anything seem to bring on the seizures: activity, discontinuing medication, fatigue, stress? • Are you taking any medication? • Coping strategies: How have the seizures affected daily life, your occupation?	**Seizures** occur with epilepsy, a paroxysmal disease characterized by altered or loss of consciousness, involuntary muscle movements, and sensory disturbances. *Aura* is a subjective sensation that precedes a seizure; it could be auditory, visual, or motor.

Subjective Data

Examiner Asks	Rationale
5. Tremors. Do you have any shakes or **tremors** in the hands or face? When did these start? • Do they seem to grow worse with anxiety, intention (purposeful movement), or rest? • Are they relieved with rest, activity, alcohol? Do they affect daily activities?	Tremor is an involuntary shaking, vibrating, or trembling.
6. Weakness. Do you have any **weakness** in, or problem moving, any body part? Is this generalized or local? Does weakness occur with any particular movement, such as difficulty getting up out of a chair or reaching for an object (proximal or large muscle weakness) or difficulty opening a jar, writing, using scissors, or walking without tripping (distal or small muscle weakness)?	*Paresis* refers to weakness of voluntary movements or impaired movement. *Paralysis* is a loss of motor function as a result of a lesion in the neurological or muscular system or loss of sensory innervation.
7. Incoordination. Do you have any problem with **coordination**? Any problem with balance when walking? Do you list to one side? Any falling? Which way? Do your legs seem to give way? Any clumsy movement?	*Dysmetria* is the inability to control the range of motion (ROM) of muscles.
8. Numbness or tingling sensation. Do you have any **numbness** or **tingling sensation** in any body part? Does it feel like pins and needles? When did this start? Where do you feel it? Does it occur with activity?	*Paraesthesia* is an abnormal sensation, such as burning or tingling.
9. Difficulty swallowing. Do you have any problem **swallowing**? Does it occur with solids or liquids? Have you experienced excessive salivation, drooling?	Dysphagia refers to difficulty swallowing.
10. Difficulty speaking. Do you have any problem **speaking**: with forming words or with saying what you intended to say? When did you first notice this? How long did it last?	*Dysarthria* is difficulty forming words; aphasia is difficulty with language comprehension or expression (see Table 25.12, p. 745).
11. Significant past history. Have you ever had a stroke (cerebrovascular accident), spinal cord injury, meningitis or encephalitis, congenital defect, or alcoholism?	
12. Environmental and occupational hazards. Are you exposed to any **environmental or occupational hazards**: insecticides, organic solvents, lead? • Are you taking any medications now? • How much alcohol do you drink? Each week? Each day? • Do you take other mood-altering drugs, such as marijuana, cocaine, barbiturates, tranquilizers?	Review the patient's anticonvulsant, anti-tremor, antivertigo, and pain medications.

Additional History for Infants and Children

1. Maternal health. Did you (the mother) have any health problems during the pregnancy: any infections or illnesses, toxemia, hypertension, alcohol or drug use, diabetes? Medications taken?	Prenatal history may affect an infant's neurological development.
2. Neonatal period. Please tell me about this baby's birth. Was the baby full term or premature? What was the birth weight? • Any birth trauma? Did the baby breathe immediately? • Were you told the baby's Apgar scores? • Any congenital defects?	

Examiner Asks	Rationale

3. Reflexes. What have you noticed about the baby's behaviour? Do the baby's sucking and swallowing seem coordinated? When you touch the cheek, does the baby turn the head toward the touch? Is the baby startled by a loud noise or shake of the crib? Does the baby grasp your finger?

4. Weakness and balance. Does the child seem to have any problem with balance? Have you noted any unexplained falling, clumsy or unsteady gait, progressive muscular weakness, problem with going up or down stairs, problem with getting up from a lying position?

> If any of these signs occurs, it may not be noticed until child starts to walk (in late infancy).
> Screen for muscular dystrophy.

5. Seizures. Has this child had any seizures? Please describe. Did the seizure occur with a high fever? Did any loss of consciousness occur? For how long? How many seizures occurred with this same illness (if occurred with high fever)?

> In infants and toddlers, seizures may occur with high fever. Seizures may also be a sign of neurological disease.

6. Physical development. Did this child's motor or developmental milestones seem to occur at approximately the right age? Does this child seem to be growing and maturing normally to you? How does this child's development compare with that of siblings or other children the same age?

7. Environmental hazards. Do you know whether your child has had any environmental exposure to lead?

> Chronically elevated lead levels may cause developmental delay or loss of a newly acquired skill, or no clinical signs may be present.

8. Cognitive development. Have you been told about any learning problems in school: whether the child has problems with attention span, cannot concentrate, is hyperactive?

9. Family history. Any family history of seizure disorder, cerebral palsy, muscular dystrophy?

Additional History for Older Adults

1. Risk for falls. Any problem with dizziness? Does this occur when you first sit or stand up, when you move your head, when you get up and walk just after eating? Does this occur with any of your medications?

> Diminished cerebral blood flow and diminished vestibular response may produce staggering with position change, which increases the risk for falls.
> Micturition syncope.

- (For men) Do you ever get up at night and then feel faint while standing to urinate?
- How does dizziness affect your daily activities? Are you able to drive safely and to manoeuvre within your house safely?
- What safety modifications have you applied at home?

2. Cognitive function. Have you noticed any decrease in memory, changes in mental function? Have you felt any confusion? Did this seem to come on suddenly or gradually?

3. Tremor. Have you ever noticed any tremor? Is this in your hands or face? Is this worse with anxiety, activity, rest? Does the tremor seem to be relieved with alcohol, activity, rest? Does the tremor interfere with daily or social activities?

> Senile tremor is relieved by alcohol, although this is not a recommended treatment. Assess whether the patient is using alcohol in an effort to relieve tremor.

4. Vision. Have you ever had any sudden vision change, fleeting blindness? Did this occur along with weakness? Did you have any loss of consciousness?

> Screen for symptoms of stroke. (See the Critical Findings box.)

Subjective Data

Examiner Asks	Rationale

CRITICAL FINDINGS

Critical findings that necessitate immediate medical intervention or immediate transport to a hospital include the following signs and symptoms:
- Sudden decline in alertness (loss of consciousness)
- Sudden change in speech or a new onset of speech difficulties
- Signs of stroke or transient ischemic attack (TIA)
- Sudden onset of severe headache
- Signs of raised intracranial pressure
- Sudden onset of weakness, numbness, eye movement problems, and double vision
- Seizures
- Lethargy that persists beyond appropriate times and circumstances

OBJECTIVE DATA

PREPARATION

Perform a **screening neurological examination** (items identified in the following sections) of seemingly healthy patients whose histories reveal no significant subjective findings.

Perform a **complete neurological examination** of patients who have neurological concerns (e.g., headache, weakness, loss of coordination) or who have shown signs of neurological dysfunction.

Perform a **neurological recheck examination** of patients with demonstrated neurological deficits who require periodic assessments (e.g., hospitalized patients or those in extended care), using the examination sequence beginning on p. 727.

Integrate the steps of the neurological examination with the examination of each particular part of the body, as much as you are able: for example, test cranial nerves while you assess the head and neck (recall Chapters 14 through 17) and superficial abdominal reflexes while you assess the abdomen (recall Chapter 22). When you record your findings, however, consider all neurological data as a functional unit, and record them all together.

Use the following sequence for the complete neurological examination:
1. Mental health (see Chapter 6)
2. Cranial nerves
3. Motor system
4. Sensory system
5. Reflexes

Ask the patient to sit up with the head at your eye level.

EQUIPMENT NEEDED

Penlight
Tongue blade
Cotton swab
Cotton ball
Tuning fork (128 Hz or 256 Hz)
Percussion hammer
(Possibly) familiar aromatic substances, such as peppermint, coffee, vanilla

Normal Range of Findings	Abnormal Findings

Test Cranial Nerves

Cranial Nerve I: Olfactory Nerve

Do not test routinely. Test the sense of smell in patients who report loss of smell, those with head trauma, and those with abnormal mental status and when the presence of an intracranial lesion is suspected. First, assess patency by occluding one nostril at a time and asking the patient to sniff. Then, with the patient's eyes closed, occlude one nostril and present an aromatic substance. Use familiar, conveniently obtainable, and non-noxious smells, such as coffee, toothpaste, orange, vanilla, soap, or peppermint. Alcohol wipes smell familiar and are easy to find but are irritating.

Anosmia (decrease or loss of smell) occurs bilaterally with tobacco smoking, allergic rhinitis, and cocaine use.

Normally, a person can identify an odour through each side of the nose. The sense of smell normally decreases bilaterally with aging. Any asymmetry in the sense of smell is important.

Unilateral loss of smell in the absence of nasal disease is *neurogenic anosmia* (see Table 25.2, p. 735).

> Smell cannot be tested when air passages are occluded, as in upper respiratory infection or sinusitis.

Cranial Nerve II: Optic Nerve

Test visual acuity, and test visual fields by confrontation (see Chapter 15).

Using the ophthalmoscope, examine the ocular fundus to determine the colour, size, and shape of the optic disc (see Chapter 15).

> Visual field loss (see Table 15.5, p. 342). Papilledema with increased intracranial pressure; optic atrophy (see Table 15.9, p. 346).

Cranial Nerves III, IV, and VI: Oculomotor, Trochlear, and Abducens Nerves

Palpebral fissures are usually equal, or nearly so, in width.

> Ptosis (drooping) occurs with myasthenia gravis, dysfunction of cranial nerve III, or Horner's syndrome (see Table 15.2, p. 337).

Check pupils for size, regularity, equality, direct and consensual light reactions, and accommodation (see Chapter 15).

> Increasing intracranial pressure causes sudden, unilateral dilation and nonreactivity of a pupil.

Assess extraocular movements with the cardinal positions of gaze (see Chapter 15).

Nystagmus is a back-and-forth oscillation of the eyes. Endpoint nystagmus—a few beats of horizontal nystagmus at extreme lateral gaze—is normal.

Assess any other nystagmus carefully, noting the following:

- Presence of nystagmus: Document whether it is in one or both eyes.
- Pendular movement (oscillations move equally left to right) or *jerk* (a quick phase in one direction, then a slow phase in the other): Classify the jerk nystagmus in the direction of the quick phase.
- Amplitude: Judge whether the degree of movement is fine, medium, or coarse.
- Frequency: Note whether the nystagmus is constant or whether it fades after a few beats.
- Plane of movement: Note whether the nystagmus is horizontal, vertical, rotary, or a combination.

> Strabismus (deviated gaze) or limited movement (see Table 15.1, p. 335).
>
> Nystagmus occurs with disease of the vestibular system, cerebellum, or brain stem.

Objective Data

Normal Range of Findings	Abnormal Findings

Cranial Nerve V: Trigeminal Nerve

Motor Function. Assess the muscles of mastication by palpating the temporal and masseter muscles as the patient clenches the teeth (Fig. 25.9). Muscles should feel equally strong on both sides. Next, try to separate the jaws by pushing down on the chin; normally, you cannot.

Decreased strength on one or both sides.
Asymmetry in jaw movement.
Pain with clenching of teeth.

25.9

Sensory Function. With the patient's eyes closed, test light touch sensation by brushing a cotton wisp on designated areas of the patient's face: forehead, cheeks, and chin (Fig. 25.10). Ask the patient to say "Now" whenever the touch is felt. This tests all three divisions of the nerve: (a) ophthalmic, (b) maxillary, and (c) mandibular.

Decreased or unequal sensation.

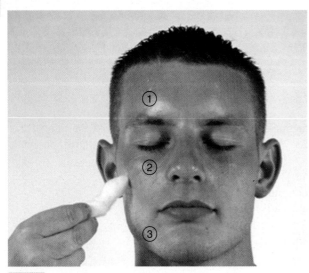

25.10

Normal Range of Findings

Corneal Reflex. (Omit this test, unless the patient has abnormal facial sensation or abnormalities of facial movement.) Ask the patient to remove any contact lenses. With the patient looking forward, bring a wisp of cotton in from the side (to minimize defensive blinking) and lightly touch the cornea, not the conjunctiva (Fig. 25.11). Normally, a person will blink bilaterally. The corneal reflex may be decreased or absent in people who have worn contact lenses. This procedure tests the sensory afferent fibres in cranial nerve V and the motor efferent fibres in cranial nerve VII (muscles that close the eye).

25.11

Cranial Nerve VII: Facial Nerve

Motor Function. Note mobility and facial symmetry as the patient responds to your requests to smile (Fig. 25.12), frown, close eyes tightly (against your attempt to open them), lift eyebrows, show teeth, and puff cheeks (Fig. 25.13). Then, press the patient's puffed cheeks in, and note whether the air escapes equally from both sides.

Sensory Function. Do not test routinely. Test only when you suspect facial nerve injury. When it is indicated, test sense of taste by applying to the tongue a cotton applicator soaked in a solution of sugar, salt, or lemon juice (sour). Ask the patient to identify the taste.

25.12

25.13

Abnormal Findings

No blink occurs with a lesion of cranial nerve V or with cranial nerve VII paralysis.

Muscle weakness is demonstrated by flattening of the nasolabial fold, drooping of one side of the face, lower eyelid sagging, and escape of air from only one cheek that is pressed in.

Loss of movement and asymmetry of movement occur both with CNS lesions (e.g., cerebrovascular accident that affects the lower face on one side) and with lesions of the PNS (e.g., cases of Bell's palsy that affect the upper *and* lower portions of one side of the face).

Normal Range of Findings	Abnormal Findings

Cranial Nerve VIII: Acoustic (Vestibulocochlear) Nerve

Test hearing acuity by determining the patient's ability to hear normal conversation, using the whispered voice test (see Chapter 16).

Cranial Nerves IX and X: Glossopharyngeal and Vagus Nerves

Motor Function. Depress the tongue with a tongue blade, and note pharyngeal movement as the patient says "ahhh" or yawns; the uvula and soft palate should rise in the midline, and the tonsillar pillars should move medially.

Touch the posterior pharyngeal wall with a tongue blade, and note the gag reflex. Also note that the voice sounds smooth and not strained.

Sensory Function. Cranial nerve IX does mediate taste on the posterior one-third of the tongue, but technically this sensation is too difficult to test.

Absence or asymmetry of soft palate movement.
Deviation of uvula to side.
Asymmetry of tonsillar pillar movement.
Hoarseness or brassy quality of the voice occurs with vocal cord dysfunction; nasal twang occurs with weakness of soft palate.

Cranial Nerve XI: Spinal Accessory Nerve

Examine the sternomastoid and trapezius muscles for equal size. Check equal strength by asking the patient to rotate the head forcibly against resistance applied to the side of the chin (Fig. 25.14). Then ask the patient to shrug the shoulders against resistance (Fig. 25.15). These movements should feel equally strong on both sides.

Atrophy.
Muscle weakness or paralysis.

25.14

25.15

Cranial Nerve XII: Hypoglossal Nerve

Inspect the tongue. No wasting or tremors should be present. Note the forward thrust in the midline as the patient sticks out the tongue. Also ask the patient to say "light, tight, dynamite," and note that lingual speech (sounds of letters *l, t, d, n*) is clear and distinct.

Atrophy; fasciculations.
Tongue deviates to side with lesions of the hypoglossal nerve. (When this occurs, deviation is toward the paralyzed side.)

Normal Range of Findings	Abnormal Findings

Inspect and Palpate the Motor System

Muscles

Size. As you proceed through the examination, inspect all muscle groups for size. Compare the right side with the left. Muscle groups should be within the normal size limits for age and should be symmetricical bilaterally. When muscles in the extremities look asymmetrical, measure each in centimetres, and record the difference. A difference of 1 cm or less is not significant. Note that it is difficult to assess muscle mass in very obese patients.

Strength. (See Chapter 24.) Test the power of homologous muscles simultaneously. Test muscle groups of the extremities, neck, and trunk.

Tone. Tone is the normal degree of tension (contraction) in voluntarily relaxed muscles. It is demonstrated as mild resistance to passive stretch. To test muscle tone, move the extremities through a passive ROM. First, persuade the patient to relax completely—to "go limp like a rag doll." Move each extremity smoothly through a full ROM. Support the arm at the elbow and the leg at the knee (Fig. 25.16). Normally, you will note a mild, even resistance to movement.

Atrophy: abnormally small muscle with a wasted appearance; occurs with disuse, injury, lower motor neuron disease such as polio, diabetic neuropathy.

Hypertrophy: increased size and strength; occurs with isometric exercise.

Paresis (weakness) is diminished strength; paralysis (plegia) is absence of strength.

Limited ROM.

Pain with motion.

Flaccidity: decreased resistance, hypotonicity.

Spasticity and rigidity: types of increased resistance (see Table 25.3, p. 736).

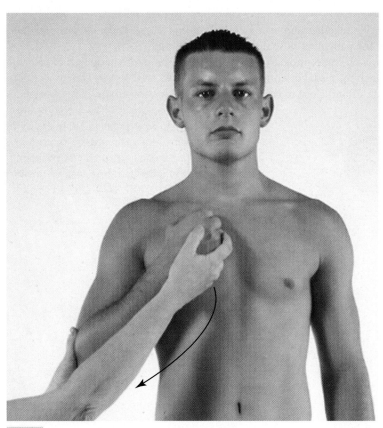

25.16

Involuntary Movements. Normally, no involuntary movements occur. If they are present, note their location, frequency, rate, and amplitude. Note whether the movements can be controlled at will.

Tic, tremor, fasciculation, myoclonus, chorea, and athetosis (see Table 25.4, p. 737).

Normal Range of Findings	Abnormal Findings

Cerebellar Function

Balance Tests

Gait. Observe as the patient walks 3 to 6 m, turns, and returns to the starting point. Normally, a person moves with a sense of freedom. The gait is smooth, rhythmic, and effortless; the opposing arm swing is coordinated; the turns are smooth. The step length is approximately 30 cm from heel to heel.

Ask the patient to walk a straight line in a heel-to-toe manner (tandem walking; Fig. 25.17). This decreases the base of support and accentuates any problem with coordination. Normally, a person can walk straight and stay balanced.

You may also test for balance by asking the patient to walk on the toes and then on the heels for a few steps.

The Romberg Test. Ask the patient to stand up with feet together and arms at the sides. Once the patient is in a stable position, ask the patient to close the eyes and to hold the position (Fig. 25.18). Wait approximately 20 seconds. Normally, a person can maintain posture and balance even with the visual orienting information blocked, although slight swaying may occur. (Stand close to catch the patient in case the patient falls.)

Stiff, immobile posture; staggering or reeling; wide base of support.

Lack of arm swing or rigid arms.

Unequal rhythm of steps; slapping of foot; scraping of toe of shoe.

Ataxia: uncoordinated or unsteady gait (see Table 25.5, p. 739).

Crooked line of walk.

Widening of base to maintain balance.

Staggering, reeling, loss of balance.

An ataxia that did not appear with regular gait may appear now. Inability to tandem walk is indicative of an upper motor neuron lesion, such as multiple sclerosis, or acute cerebellar dysfunction, as with alcohol intoxication.

Muscle weakness in the legs makes toe and heel walking difficult.

Swaying, falling, widening base of feet to avoid falling.

Positive Romberg sign is loss of balance that occurs when the eyes are closed. You eliminate the advantage of orientation with the eyes, which had compensated for sensory loss. A positive Romberg sign occurs with cerebellar ataxia (caused by multiple sclerosis, alcohol intoxication), loss of proprioception, and loss of vestibular function.

25.17   Tandem walking.   **25.18**   Romberg test.

Normal Range of Findings

Ask the patient to perform a shallow knee bend or to hop in place, first on one leg, then the other (Fig. 25.19). This demonstrates normal position sense, muscle strength, and cerebellar function. Note that some individuals cannot hop because of aging or obesity.

25.19

Coordination and Skilled Movements

Rapid Alternating Movements. Ask the patient to pat the knees with both hands, lift up and turn over the hands, and pat the knees with the backs of the hands (Fig. 25.20). Then ask the patient to do this faster. Normally, this is done with equal turning and a quick rhythmic pace.

Alternatively, ask the patient to touch the thumb to each finger on the same hand, starting with the index finger, then reverse direction (Fig. 25.21). Normally, this can be done quickly and accurately.

25.20

25.21

Abnormal Findings

Inability to perform knee bend because of weakness in quadriceps muscle or hip extensors.

Lack of coordination.
Slow, clumsy, and sloppy response is termed *dysdiadochokinesia* and occurs with cerebellar disease.
Lack of coordination.

Normal Range of Findings	Abnormal Findings

Normal Range of Findings

Finger-to-Finger Test. With the patient's eyes open, ask that the patient use the index finger to touch your finger and then his, her, or their own nose (Fig. 25.22). After a few times, move your finger to a different spot. The patient's movement should be smooth and accurate.

25.22

Finger-to-Nose Test. Ask the patient to close the eyes and to stretch out the arms. Ask the patient to touch the nose with each index finger, alternating hands and increasing speed. Normally, this movement is accurate and smooth.

Heel-to-Shin Test. Test lower extremity coordination by asking the patient to assume a supine position, to place the heel on the opposite knee, and run it down the shin from the knee to the ankle (Fig. 25.23). Normally, a person moves the heel in a straight line down the shin.

25.23

Abnormal Findings

Dysmetria is clumsy movement with overshooting of the mark; it occurs with cerebellar disorders and acute alcohol intoxication.

Past-pointing is a constant deviation to one side.

The patient's finger misses the nose.

Worsening of coordination when the eyes are closed occurs with cerebellar disease or alcohol intoxication.

Lack of coordination (heel falls off shin) occurs with cerebellar disease.

Normal Range of Findings	Abnormal Findings

Assess the Sensory System

To test the intactness of the peripheral nerve fibres, the sensory tracts, and higher cortical discrimination, ask the patient to identify various sensory stimuli.

Ensure the validity of sensory system testing by making sure the patient is alert, cooperative, and comfortable and has an adequate attention span; otherwise, you may get misleading and invalid results. Testing of the sensory system can be fatiguing. You may need to repeat the examination later or to conduct only parts of it when the patient is tired.

You do not need to test the entire skin surface for every sensation. Routine screening procedures include testing superficial pain, light touch, and vibration in a few distal locations, and testing stereognosis. This will suffice for all patients who have not demonstrated any neurological symptoms or signs. Complete testing of the sensory system is warranted in patients with neurological symptoms (e.g., localized pain, numbness, and tingling sensation) or when you discover abnormalities (e.g., motor deficit). In those cases, test all sensory modalities, and cover most dermatomes of the body.

Compare sensations on symmetrical parts of the body. When you find a definite decrease in sensation, map it out by systematic testing in that area. Proceed from the point of decreased sensation toward the sensitive area. By asking the patient to tell you where the sensation changes, you can map the exact borders of the deficient area. Note your results on a diagram.

Avoid asking leading questions, such as "Can you feel this pinprick?" This creates an expectation of how the patient should feel the sensation, which is called *suggestion*. Instead, use unbiased directions.

Note whether the topographical pattern of sensory loss is distal—that is, over the hands and feet in a "glove-and-stocking" distribution—or whether it is over a specific dermatome.

The patient's eyes should be closed during each of the tests. Take time to explain what will be happening and exactly how you expect the patient to respond.

Spinothalamic Tract

Pain. Pain is tested by the patient's ability to perceive a pinprick. Break a tongue blade lengthwise, forming a sharp point at the fractured end and a dull spot at the rounded end. Lightly apply the sharp point or the dull end to the patient's body in a random, unpredictable order (Fig. 25.24). Ask the patient to say "sharp" or "dull," depending on the sensation felt. (Note that the sharp edge is used to test for pain (see Fig. 25.24, *A*); the dull edge is used as a general test of the patient's responses (see Fig. 25.24, *B*).)

Let at least 2 seconds elapse after each stimulus, to avoid *summation*. With summation, frequent consecutive stimuli are perceived as one strong stimulus. When you are done, discard the tongue blade.

Hypoalgesia: decreased pain sensation.
Analgesia: absence of pain sensation.
Hyperalgesia: increased pain sensation.

25.24

Normal Range of Findings	Abnormal Findings

Normal Range of Findings

Temperature. Test temperature sensation only when pain sensation is abnormal; otherwise, you may omit it because the fibre tracts are much the same. Fill two test tubes, one with hot water and one with cold water, and apply the bottom ends to the patient's skin in a random order. Ask the patient to say which temperature is felt. Alternatively, you could place the flat side of a tuning fork on the skin; its metal always feels cool.

Light Touch. Apply a wisp of cotton to the skin. Stretch a cotton ball to lengthen it, and brush it over the skin in a random order of sites and at irregular intervals (Fig. 25.25). This prevents the patient from responding just from repetition. Include the arms, forearms, hands, chest, thighs, and legs. Ask the patient to say "now" or "yes" when touch is felt. Compare symmetrical points.

25.25

Posterior Column Tract

Vibration. Test the patient's ability to feel vibrations of a tuning fork over bony prominences. Use a low-pitch tuning fork (128 Hz or 256 Hz) because its vibration has a slower decay. Strike the tuning fork on the heel of your hand, and hold the base on a bony surface of the patient's fingers and great toe (Fig. 25.26). Ask the patient to indicate when the vibration starts and stops. If the patient feels the normal vibration or buzzing sensation on these distal areas, you may assume that the proximal spots are normal, too, and proceed no further. If no vibrations are felt, move proximally and test ulnar processes, ankles, patellae, and iliac crests. Compare responses on the right side with those on the left side. If you find a deficit, note whether it is gradual or abrupt.

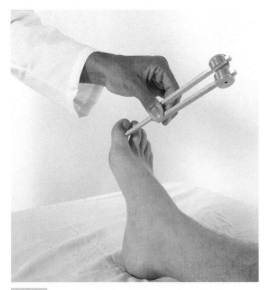

25.26

Abnormal Findings

Hypoaesthesia: decreased touch sensation.

Anaesthesia: absent touch sensation.

Hyperaesthesia: increased touch sensation.

Inability to feel vibration: Loss of vibration sense occurs in peripheral neuropathy such as diabetes and alcoholism. Often, this is the first sensation lost.

Peripheral neuropathy is worst at the feet, and sensation gradually improves up the leg, whereas a specific nerve lesion produces a clear zone of deficit for its dermatome.

Normal Range of Findings	Abnormal Findings

Normal Range of Findings

Position (Kinaesthesia). Test the patient's ability to perceive passive movements of the extremities. Move a finger or the big toe up and down, and ask the patient to tell you which way it is moved (Fig. 25.27). The test is done with the patient's eyes closed, but to be sure it is understood, have the patient watch a few trials first. Vary the order of movement up or down. Hold the digit by the sides because upward or downward pressure on the skin may provide a clue as to how it has been moved. Normally, a person can detect movement of a few millimetres.

25.27

Tactile Discrimination (Fine Touch). The following tests also measure the discrimination ability of the sensory cortex. As a prerequisite, the patient needs a normal or near-normal sense of touch and a normal position sense.

Stereognosis. Test the patient's ability to recognize objects by feeling their forms, sizes, and weights, with the eyes closed. Place a familiar object (paper clip, key, coin, cotton ball, or pencil) in the patient's hand, and ask the patient to identify it (Fig. 25.28). Normally, a person's fingers explore the object, and then the person correctly names it. Test a different object in each hand; testing the left hand helps you assess functioning of the right parietal lobe.

25.28

Abnormal Findings

Loss of position sense.

Problems with tactile discrimination occur with lesions of the sensory cortex or posterior column.

Astereognosis (inability to identify objects correctly) occurs with sensory cortex lesions such as cerebrovascular accident (stroke).

Normal Range of Findings

Graphaesthesia. Graphaesthesia is the ability to "read" a number by having it traced on the skin. Ask the patient to close the eyes, and use a blunt instrument to trace a single-digit number or a letter on the patient's palm (Fig. 25.29). Ask the patient to tell you what the character is. Graphaesthesia is a good measure of sensory loss if the patient cannot make the hand movements needed for stereognosis, as occurs in arthritis.

25.29 Testing for graphaesthesia.

Two-Point Discrimination. Test the patient's ability to distinguish the separation of two simultaneous pinpoints on the skin. Apply the two points of an opened paper clip lightly to the skin in ever-closing distances. Note the distance at which the patient no longer perceives two separate points. The level of perception varies considerably with the region tested; it is most sensitive in the fingertips (2 to 8 mm) and least sensitive on the upper arms, thighs, and back (40 to 75 mm).

Extinction. Simultaneously touch both sides of the body at the same point. Ask the patient to state how many sensations are felt and where they are. Normally, both sensations are felt.

Point Location. Touch the skin, and withdraw the stimulus promptly. Tell the patient, "Put your finger where I touched you." You can perform this test simultaneously with light touch sensation.

Test the Reflexes

Stretch (Deep Tendon) Reflexes

Measurement of the stretch reflexes reveals the intactness of the reflex arc at specific spinal levels, as well as the normal override on the reflex of the higher cortical levels.

For an adequate response, the limb should be relaxed and the muscle partially stretched. Stimulate the reflex by directing a short, snappy blow of the reflex hammer onto the muscle's insertion tendon. Use a relaxed hold on the hammer. As with the percussion technique, the action takes place at the wrist. Strike a brief, well-aimed blow, and bounce up promptly; do not let the hammer rest on the tendon. Use the pointed end of the reflex hammer when aiming at a smaller target, such as your thumb, on the tendon site; use the flat end when the target is wider or to diffuse the impact and prevent pain.

Abnormal Findings

Inability to distinguish the number or letter occurs with lesions of the sensory cortex.

The distance it normally takes to identify two separate points is increased with sensory cortex lesions.

The ability to recognize only one of the stimuli occurs with sensory cortex lesion; the stimulus is extinguished on the side *opposite* the cortex lesion.

With a sensory cortex lesion, the sensation cannot be localized accurately, even though light touch sensation may be retained.

Normal Range of Findings

Use just enough force to get a response. Compare responses on the right and left sides; they should be equal. The reflex response is graded on a five-point scale:

4+: Very brisk, hyperactive with clonus, indicative of disease
3+: Brisker than average, may indicate disease
2+: Average, normal
1+: Diminished, low normal
0: No response

This is a subjective scale, and its use requires some clinical practice. Even then the scale is not completely reliable because no standard exists to say *how* brisk a reflex should be to warrant a grade of 3+. Also, normality in reflex responses has a wide range. Healthy people may have diminished or brisk reflexes. Your best plan is to interpret the DTRs *only* within the context of the other results of the neurological examination.

Sometimes the reflex response fails to appear. Try further encouragement of relaxation, varying the patient's position, or increasing the strength of the blow. **Reinforcement** is another technique to relax the muscles and enhance the response (Fig. 25.30). Ask the patient to perform an isometric exercise in a muscle group somewhat distant from the one being tested. For example, to enhance a patellar reflex, ask the patient to lock the fingers together and "pull." Then strike the tendon. To enhance a biceps response, ask the patient to clench the teeth or to grasp the thigh with the opposite hand.

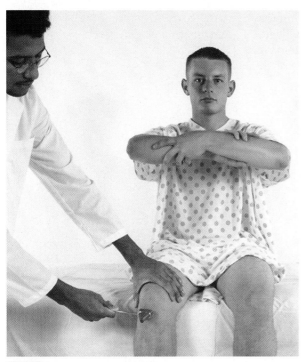

25.30   Reinforcement.

Abnormal Findings

Clonus is a set of rapid, rhythmic contractions of the same muscle.

Hyper-reflexia is the exaggerated reflex that occurs when the monosynaptic reflex arc is released from the usually inhibiting influence of higher cortical levels. This occurs with upper motor neuron lesions, such as a cerebrovascular accident.

Hyporeflexia is the reduced functioning of a reflex. In some cases, the reflex may be absent. Hyporeflexia is a lower motor neuron problem. It results from interruption of sensory afferent pathways or destruction of motor efferent fibres and anterior horn cells, as in spinal cord injury.

Objective Data

Normal Range of Findings	Abnormal Findings

Biceps Reflex (C5 to C6). Support the patient's forearm on yours; this position relaxes, as well as partially flexes, the patient's arm. Place your thumb on the biceps tendon, and strike a blow on your thumb. You can feel as well as see the normal response, which is contraction of the biceps muscle and flexion of the forearm (Fig. 25.31).

25.31   Biceps reflex.

Triceps Reflex (C7 to C8). Tell the patient to let the arm "just go limp" as you suspend it by holding the upper arm. Strike the triceps tendon directly just above the elbow (Fig. 25.32). The normal response is extension of the forearm. Alternatively, hold the patient's wrist across the chest to flex the arm at the elbow, and tap the tendon.

25.32   Triceps reflex.

Normal Range of Findings	Abnormal Findings

Normal Range of Findings

Brachioradialis Reflex (C5 to C6). Hold the patient's thumbs to suspend the forearms in relaxation. Strike the forearm directly, approximately 2 to 3 cm above the radial styloid process (Fig. 25.33). The normal response is flexion and supination of the forearm.

25.33   Brachioradialis reflex.

Quadriceps or Patellar ("Knee Jerk") Reflex (L2 to L4). Let the patient's lower legs dangle freely to flex the knee and stretch the tendons. Strike the tendon directly just below the patella (Fig. 25.34). Extension of the lower leg is the expected response. Contraction of the quadriceps will also be palpable.

25.34   Quadriceps reflex.

To test this reflex with the patient in the supine position, use your own arm as a lever to support the weight of one of the patient's legs against the other leg (Fig. 25.35). This manoeuvre also flexes the knee.

Abnormal Findings

Objective Data

Normal Range of Findings	Abnormal Findings

25.35 Supine quadriceps reflex.

Achilles ("Ankle Jerk") Reflex (L5 to S2). Position the patient with the knee flexed and the hip externally rotated. Hold the patient's foot in dorsiflexion, and strike the Achilles tendon directly (Fig. 25.36). Feel the normal response as the foot plantar flexes against your hand.

25.36 Achilles reflex.

To test this reflex with the patient in the supine position, flex one of the patient's knees and support that lower leg against the other leg so that it falls "open." Dorsiflex the foot, and tap the tendon (Fig. 25.37).

25.37 Supine Achilles reflex.

Normal Range of Findings

Clonus. Test for clonus, particularly when the reflexes are hyperactive. Support one of the patient's lower legs in one of your hands. With your other hand, move the foot up and down a few times to relax the muscle. Then stretch the muscle by briskly dorsiflexing the foot. Hold the stretch (Fig. 25.38). A normal response is no further movement. When clonus is present, rapid rhythmic contractions of the calf muscle and movement of the foot are visible and palpable.

25.38

Superficial (Cutaneous) Reflexes

For cutaneous reflexes, the sensory receptors are in the skin rather than in the muscles. The motor response is a localized muscle contraction.

Abdominal Reflexes: Upper (T8 to T10) and Lower (T10 to T12). Have the patient assume a supine position, with the knees slightly bent. Use the handle end of the reflex hammer, a wood applicator tip, or the end of a split tongue blade to stroke the skin. Move from the side of the abdomen toward the midline at both the upper and lower abdominal levels (Fig. 25.39). The normal response is ipsilateral contraction of the abdominal muscle, with an observed deviation of the umbilicus toward the stroke. When the abdominal wall is very thick, pull the skin to the opposite side; the muscle palpably contracts toward the stimulus.

Abdominal reflex

Cremasteric reflex

25.39

Abnormal Findings

Clonus is repeated reflex muscular movements. A hyperactive reflex with sustained clonus (lasting as long as the stretch is held) occurs with upper motor neuron disease.

Superficial reflexes are absent with diseases of the pyramidal tract (e.g., they are absent on the contralateral side with cerebrovascular accident).

Normal Range of Findings

Cremasteric Reflex (L1 to L2). This reflex is not routinely tested. On a male patient, lightly stroke the inner aspect of the thigh with the reflex hammer or tongue blade (see Fig. 25.39). Note the elevation of the ipsilateral testicle.

Plantar Reflex (L4 to S2). Position the thigh in slight external rotation. With the reflex hammer, stroke lightly up the lateral side of the sole of the foot and inward across the ball of the foot, in an upside-down J shape (see Fig. 25.40, *A*). The normal response is plantar flexion of the toes and inversion and flexion of the forefoot.

Abnormal Findings

This reflex is absent in both upper and lower motor neuron lesions.

Except in infancy, the abnormal response is dorsiflexion of the big toe and fanning of all toes, which is a positive Babinski sign, also called *upgoing toes* (see Fig. 25.40, *B*). This occurs with upper motor neuron disease of the corticospinal (or pyramidal) tract.

25.40   **A**, Plantar reflex. **B**, Babinski sign.

❖ DEVELOPMENTAL CONSIDERATIONS

Infants (Birth to Age 12 Months)

The neurological system undergoes dramatic growth and development during the first year of life. Assessment includes noting that milestones you normally would expect for each month have indeed been achieved and that the early, more primitive reflexes are eliminated from the baby's repertory when they are supposed to be.

At birth, the newborn is very alert, with the eyes open, and demonstrates strong, urgent sucking. The normal cry is loud and lusty and may even sound angry. The next 2 or 3 days may be spent mostly sleeping as the baby recovers from the birth process. After that, the pattern of sleep and waking activity is highly variable; it depends on the baby's individual body rhythm, as well as external stimuli.

The behavioural assessment should include your observations of the infant's spontaneous waking activity, responses to environmental stimuli, and social interaction with the parents and others.

By 2 months of age, the baby smiles responsively and recognizes the parent's face. Babbling begins at 4 months, and one or two words (mama, dada) are used nonspecifically after 9 months.

The cranial nerves cannot be tested directly, but you can infer their proper functioning by the manoeuvres shown in Table 25.1.

Failure to attain a skill by expected time. Persistence of reflex behaviour beyond the normal time.

With CNS damage, the cry may be high-pitched or shrill or sound like a feline screech.

With respiratory distress, the cry may be weak or groaning, or an expiratory grunt occurs.

Lethargy, hyporeactivity, hyperirritability, and parent's report of significant change in behaviour all warrant referral.

Normal Range of Findings

TABLE 25.1	Testing Cranial Nerve Function of Infants
CRANIAL NERVE	**RESPONSE**
II, III, IV, VI	Optical blink reflex: shine light in open eyes, note rapid closure
	Size, shape, equal-sized pupils
	Looking at face or close object
	Eyes follow movement
V	Rooting reflex, sucking reflex
VII	Facial movements (e.g., wrinkling forehead and nasolabial folds) symmetrical when crying or smiling
VIII	Moro reflex (until age 4 months): elicited by loud noise
	Acoustic blink reflex: infant blinks in response to a loud hand clap 30 cm (12 in) from head (avoid creating air current)
	Eyes follow direction of sound
IX, X	Swallowing, gag reflex
	Coordinated sucking and swallowing
XII	In response to pinching of nose, infant's mouth opens and tongue rises in midline

The Motor System

Observe spontaneous motor activity for smoothness and symmetry. Smoothness of movement suggests proper cerebellar function, as does the coordination involved in sucking and swallowing. To screen gross and fine motor coordination, use the Nipissing District Developmental Screen (NDDS), or other parent-report screening tool (as discussed in Chapter 2), with its age-specific developmental milestones. You also can assess movement by testing the reflexes listed in the following section. Note their smoothness of response and symmetry. Also, note whether their presence or absence is appropriate for the infant's age.

Assess muscle tone by first observing resting posture. The newborn favours a flexed position; extremities are symmetrically folded inward, the hips are slightly abducted, and the fists are tightly flexed (Fig. 25.41). Infants born by breech delivery, however, will not immediately demonstrate flexion in the lower extremities.

25.41

Motor activity is delayed with brain damage, intellectual disability, peripheral neuromuscular damage, prolonged illness, and parental neglect.

Frog position: hips abducted and almost flat against the table, externally rotated (normal only after breech delivery).

Opisthotonos: head arched back, stiffness of neck, and extension of arms and legs; occurs with meningeal or brain stem irritation and kernicterus (see Table 25.9, p. 744).

Extension of limbs may occur with intracranial hemorrhage.

Continual asymmetry of any type (e.g., asymmetry of upper limbs) occurs with brachial plexus palsy.

Normal Range of Findings

After 2 months of age, flexion gives way to gradual extension, beginning with the head and continuing in a cephalocaudal direction. Now is the time to check for spasticity; none should be present. Test for spasticity by flexing the infant's knees onto the abdomen and then quickly releasing them. They will unfold but not too quickly. Also, gently push the head forward; the baby should comply.

The fists normally are held in tight flexion for the first 3 months. Then the fists open for part of the time. A purposeful reach for an object with both hands occurs at approximately 4 months of age; a transfer of an object from one hand to the other hand, at 7 months of age; a grasp with fingers and opposing thumb, at 9 months of age; and a purposeful release, at 10 months of age. Babies are normally ambidextrous for the first 18 months.

Head control is an important milestone in motor development. You can incorporate the following two movements into every infant assessment to check the muscle tone necessary for head control.

First, with the baby supine, hold the wrists and pull the baby up to a sitting position, and note head control (Fig. 25.42). The newborn will hold the head almost in the same plane as the body; the head will balance briefly when the baby reaches the sitting position and then flop forward. (Even premature infants demonstrate this.) At 4 months of age, the head stays in line with the body and does not flop.

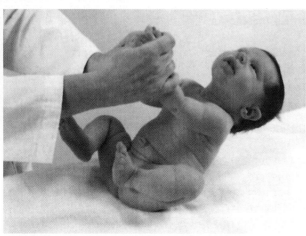

25.42

Second, lift up the baby in a prone position, with one of your hands supporting the baby's chest (Fig. 25.43). The full-term newborn holds the head at an angle of 45 degrees or less from horizontal, the back is straight or slightly arched, and the elbows and knees are partly flexed.

25.43

Abnormal Findings

Spasticity is an early sign of cerebral palsy. In affected infants, after you release the flexed knees, the legs quickly extend and adduct, even to a "scissoring" motion. Also, affected infants often resist head flexion and extend back against your hand.

Note persistent one-hand preference in babies younger than 18 months of age, which may indicate a motor deficit on the opposite side.

Because development progresses in a cephalocaudal direction, a lag in head control is an early sign of brain damage.

Any baby who cannot hold the head in midline when sitting after 6 months of age should be referred for neurological evaluation.

Normal Range of Findings	Abnormal Findings

At 3 months of age, the baby raises the head and arches the back, as in a swan dive. This is the *Landau reflex*, which persists until 1½ years of age (Fig. 25.44).

25.44

Assess muscle strength by noting the strength of sucking and of spontaneous motor activity. Normally, no tremors are present, and in a baby aged 4 months or older, no continual overshooting of the mark occurs when the baby reaches for an object.

The Sensory System

You will perform very little sensory testing with infants and toddlers. The newborn normally has hypoaesthesia, and a stimulus must be strong to elicit a response. The baby responds to pain by crying and a general reflex withdrawal of all limbs. By 7 to 9 months of age, the infant can localize the stimulus and shows more specific signs of withdrawal. Other sensory modalities are not tested.

Reflexes

Infantile automatisms are reflexes that have a predictable timetable of appearance and disappearance. The reflexes most commonly tested are listed in the following section. For the screening examination, you need check only the rooting, grasp (palmar and plantar), tonic neck, and Moro reflexes.

Rooting Reflex. Brush the infant's cheek near the mouth. Note whether the infant turns the head toward that side and opens the mouth (Fig. 25.45). This reflex is present at birth and disappears at ages 3 to 4 months.

Sucking Reflex. Touch the lips and offer your gloved little finger to suck. Note strong sucking reflex. This reflex is present at birth and disappears at ages 10 to 12 months.

Abnormal Findings (right column):

Head lag, a limp floppy trunk, and dangling arms and legs are abnormal signs.

Absence of the Landau reflex indicates motor weakness, upper motor neuron disease, or intellectual disability.

Unusually rapid withdrawal is *hyperaesthesia*, which occurs with spinal cord lesions, CNS infections, increased intracranial pressure, and peritonitis.

No withdrawal is indicative of decreased sensation, which occurs with decreased consciousness, mental disability, and lesions of the spinal cord or peripheral nerves.

Normal Range of Findings	**Abnormal Findings**

Objective Data

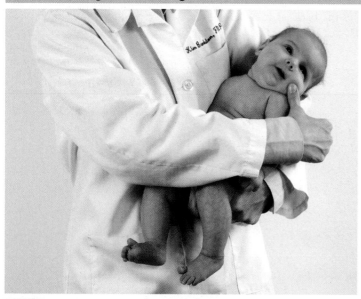

25.45

Palmar Grasp. Place the baby's head midline to ensure symmetrical response. Offer your finger from the baby's ulnar side, away from the thumb. Note tight grasp of all the baby's fingers (Fig. 25.46). Sucking enhances grasp. Often, you can pull the baby to a sit with the palmar grasp. This reflex is present at birth, is strongest at ages 1 to 2 months, and disappears at ages 3 to 4 months.

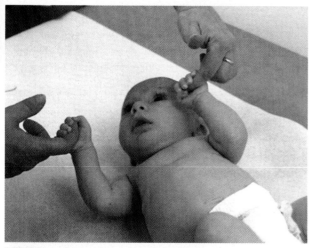

25.46

Plantar Grasp. Touch your thumb at the ball of the baby's foot. Note that the toes curl down tightly (Fig. 25.47). This reflex is present at birth and disappears at ages 8 to 10 months.

The palmar grasp reflex is absent at birth with brain damage and with local muscle or nerve injury.

The palmar grasp reflex persists after 4 months of age with frontal lobe lesion.

Normal Range of Findings	Abnormal Findings

25.47

Babinski Reflex. Stroke your finger up the lateral edge and across the ball of the infant's foot. Note fanning of toes (positive Babinski reflex; Fig. 25.48). The reflex is present at birth and disappears (changes to the adult response) by approximately 24 months of age (variable).

The Babinski reflex persists after 2 or 2½ years of age with pyramidal tract disease.

25.48

Tonic Neck Reflex. With the baby supine, relaxed, or sleeping, turn the head to one side with the chin over the shoulder. Note ipsilateral extension of the arm and leg, and flexion of the opposite arm and leg; this is the "fencing" position (Fig. 25.49). If you turn the infant's head to the opposite side, arm and leg positions will switch sides. This reflex appears by ages 2 to 3 months, decreases at ages 3 to 4 months, and disappears by ages 4 to 6 months.

This reflex persists in later infancy with brain damage.

Normal Range of Findings

Abnormal Findings

25.49 Tonic neck reflex.

Moro Reflex. Startle the infant by jarring the crib, making a loud noise, or supporting the head and back in a semisitting position and quickly lowering the infant to 30 degrees. The baby looks as if to be hugging a tree; that is, symmetrical abduction and extension of the arms and legs, fanning of fingers, and curling of the index finger and thumb to a C-shape position occur (Fig. 25.50). The infant then brings in both arms and legs. This reflex is present at birth and disappears at ages 1 to 4 months.

Absence of the Moro reflex in the newborn or its persistence after 5 months of age indicates severe CNS injury.

Absence of movement in just one arm occurs with fracture of the humerus or clavicle and with brachial nerve palsy.

Absence of movement in one leg occurs with a lower spinal cord problem or a dislocated hip.

The Moro reflex appears hyperactive with tetany or CNS infection.

25.50 Moro reflex.

Placing Reflex. Hold the infant upright under the arms, close to a table. Let the dorsal aspect (top) of the foot touch the underside of table. Note flexing of hip and knee, followed by extension at the hip, to place foot on table (Fig. 25.51). This reflex appears 4 days after birth.

Normal Range of Findings	Abnormal Findings

Normal Range of Findings

Stepping Reflex. Hold the infant upright under the arms, with the feet on a flat surface. Note regular alternating steps (Fig. 25.52). This reflex disappears before voluntary walking begins.

 25.51   Placing reflex.

25.52   Stepping reflex.

Preschool- and School-Age Children

Use the same sequence of neurological assessment as with adults, except for the omissions and modifications mentioned in this section.

Assess the child's general behaviour during play activities, reaction to parent, and cooperation with parent and with you.

Smell and taste are almost never tested, but if you need to test the child's sense of smell (cranial nerve I), use a scent familiar to the child, such as an orange peel. When testing visual fields (cranial nerve II) and cardinal positions of gaze (cranial nerves III, IV, VI), you often need to gently immobilize the head, or else the child will track with the whole head. Make a game out of asking the child to imitate your "funny faces" (cranial nerve VII); thus, the child has fun, and you have the child's friendship.

Much of the motor assessment can be derived from watching the child undress and dress and manipulate buttons. This indicates muscle strength, symmetry, joint ROM, and fine motor skills. Use the NDDS or other parent-report screening tool to screen gross and fine motor skills that are appropriate for the child's specific age. Be familiar with developmental milestones (examples are provided on the Evolve website).

Note the child's gait during both walking and running. A wide-based gate is normal in toddlers, and a knock-kneed walk is normal in preschoolers. Normally, children can balance on one foot for approximately 5 seconds by 4 years of age, can balance for 8 to 10 seconds at 5 years of age, and can hop at 4 years of age. Children enjoy participating in these tests (Fig. 25.53).

Abnormal Findings

Extensor thrust, or "scissoring"; crossing of lower extremities.

Muscle hypertrophy or atrophy occurs with muscular dystrophy.

Muscle weakness should be investigated.

Incoordination should be investigated.

Causes of motor delay are listed earlier in the Infants (Birth to Age 12 Months) section.

Staggering and falling should be investigated.

Normal Range of Findings

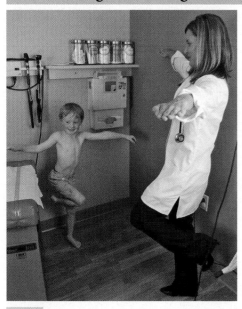

25.53

Observe as the child rises from the supine position on the floor to the sitting position and then to the standing position. Note the child's muscles of the neck, abdomen, arms, and legs. Normally, the child curls up in the midline to sit up and then pushes off with both hands against the floor to stand (see Fig. 25.54, *A*).

A

25.54

Assess fine coordination by using the finger-to-nose test if you can be sure the young child understands your directions. Demonstrate the procedure first, then ask the child to do the test with the eyes open, then with the eyes closed. Fine coordination is not fully developed until the child has reached 4 or 6 years of age. If a younger child can bring the finger to within 2 to 5 cm of the nose, consider the result normal.

Testing sensation is very unreliable in toddlers and preschoolers. You may test the sense of light touch by asking the child to close the eyes and then to point to the spot where you touch or tickle. Senses of vibration, position, stereognosis, graphaesthesia, and two-point discrimination are usually not tested in children younger than 6 years of age. Also, do not test for perception of superficial pain. In children older than 6 years of age, you may perform sensory testing as with adults. Use a broken tongue blade if you need to test superficial pain.

Abnormal Findings

Weakness climbing up or down stairs occurs with muscular dystrophy.

Broad-based gait beyond toddlerhood and scissor gait should be investigated (see Table 25.5, p. 739).

Failure to hop after 5 years of age indicates incoordination of gross motor skill.

Weak pelvic muscles are a sign of muscular dystrophy; from the supine position, affected children roll to one side, bend forward to all four extremities, plant hands on legs, and literally "climb" up themselves. This is *Gower's sign* (see Fig. 25.54, *B*).

B

Failure of the finger-to-nose test with the eyes open indicates gross incoordination; failure of the test with the eyes closed indicates minor incoordination or lack of position sense.

Sensory loss occurs with decreased consciousness, mental deficiency, or spinal cord or peripheral nerve dysfunction.

Normal Range of Findings

The DTRs usually are not tested in children younger than 5 years of age because they cannot be relied upon to cooperate in relaxation. When you need to test DTRs in a young child, use your finger to percuss the tendon. Use a reflex hammer only with older children. Coax the child to relax, or distract and percuss discreetly when the child is not paying attention. The knee jerk is present at birth, then the ankle jerk and brachial reflex appear, and the triceps reflex is present at 6 months.

Older Adults

Use the same examination as used with younger adults. Be aware that some older adults show a slower response to your requests, especially to those involving coordination of movements. The conditions discussed in this section are normal variants related to aging.

Although the cranial nerves mediating taste and smell are not usually tested, they may show some decline in function.

Any decrease in muscle bulk is most apparent in the hand, as seen by guttering between the metacarpals. These dorsal hand muscles often look wasted, even with no apparent arthropathy. The grip strength remains relatively good.

Senile tremors occasionally occur. These benign tremors include an intention tremor of the hands, head nodding (as if saying yes or no), and tongue protrusion. *Dyskinesias* are the repetitive stereotyped movements in the jaw, lips, or tongue that may accompany senile tremors. No associated rigidity is present.

The gait may be slower and more deliberate than that in younger adults, and it may deviate slightly from a midline path.

Rapid alternating movements, such as pronating and supinating the hands on the thigh, may be more difficult to perform by an older adult.

After 65 years of age, loss of the sensation of vibration at the ankle malleolus is common and is usually accompanied by loss of the ankle jerk reflex. Position sense in the big toe may be lost, although this is less common than vibration loss. Tactile sensation may be impaired. Older adults may need stronger stimuli for light touch and especially for pain.

The DTRs are less brisk. Those in the upper extremities are usually present, but the ankle jerk reflex is commonly lost. The knee jerk reflex may be lost, but this occurs less often. Because older adults find it difficult to relax their limbs, always encourage relaxation when eliciting the DTRs.

The plantar reflex may be absent or difficult to interpret. A definite normal flexor response is often not apparent.

The superficial abdominal reflexes may be absent, probably because of stretching of the musculature through pregnancy or obesity.

Neurological Recheck

Some hospitalized patients have a neurological deficit caused by head trauma or a systemic disease process. These patients must be monitored closely for any improvement or deterioration in neurological status and for any indication of increasing intracranial pressure. Signs of increasing intracranial pressure signal impending cerebral disaster and death and necessitate early and prompt intervention.

Conduct an abbreviated neurological examination in the following sequence:
1. Level of consciousness
2. Motor function
3. Pupillary response
4. Vital signs

Abnormal Findings

Hyperactivity of DTRs occurs with upper motor neuron lesion, hypocalcemia, and hyperthyroidism, and with muscle spasm associated with early poliomyelitis.

Reflexes are decreased or absent with a lower motor neuron lesion, muscular dystrophy, and flaccidity or flaccid paralysis.

Clonus may occur with fatigue, but it usually indicates hyper-reflexia.

Hand muscle atrophy is worsened with disuse and degenerative arthropathy.

Distinguish senile tremors from tremors of parkinsonism. The latter include rigidity, slowness, and weakness of voluntary movement.

The rhythmic reciprocal gait pattern may be absent in parkinsonism and hemiparesis (see Table 25.5, p. 739).

Note any difference in sensation between right and left sides, which may indicate a neurological deficit.

A definite extensor response should be considered abnormal.

Objective Data

Normal Range of Findings

Level of Consciousness. A *change* in the level of consciousness is the most important factor in this examination. It is the earliest and most sensitive index of change in neurological status. Note the ease of *arousal* and the state of awareness, or *orientation*. Assess orientation by asking questions about the following:

- Person: own name, occupation, names of workers around person, their occupations
- Place: where person is, nature of building, city, province
- Time: day of week, month, year

Vary the questions during repeat assessments to ensure that the patient is not merely memorizing and recalling answers. Note the quality and the content of the verbal response; articulation, fluency, manner of thinking; and any deficit in language comprehension or production (see Chapter 6).

When a patient is intubated and cannot speak, you will have to ask questions that require a nod or shake of the head: "Is this a hospital?" "Are you at home?" "Are we in Alberta?"

A patient is fully alert when the eyes open at your approach or spontaneously; when the patient is oriented to person, place, and time; and when the patient is able to follow verbal commands appropriately.

If the patient is not fully alert, increase the amount of stimulus used in this order:

1. Calling of name
2. Light touch on patient's arm
3. Vigorous shake of patient's shoulder
4. Pain applied (pinch the patient's nail bed, pinch the patient's trapezius muscle, rub your knuckles on the patient's sternum)

Record the stimulus used, as well as the patient's response to it.

Motor Function. Check the voluntary movement of each extremity by giving the patient specific commands. (With this procedure, you also test level of consciousness by noting the patient's ability to follow commands.)

Ask the patient to lift the eyebrows, frown, and bare teeth. Note symmetrical facial movements and bilateral nasolabial folds (cranial nerve VII).

You can check upper arm strength by testing hand grasps. Ask the patient to squeeze your fingers. Offer your two fingers, one on top of the other, so that a strong hand grasp does not hurt your knuckles (Fig. 25.55). Be judicious about asking the patient to squeeze your hands; in some patients with diffuse brain damage, especially frontal lobe injury, the grasp is a reflex only.

25.55

Abnormal Findings

A change in consciousness may be subtle. Note any decreasing level of consciousness, disorientation, memory loss, uncooperative behaviour, or even complacency in a previously combative patient.

Review Table 6.2: Levels of Consciousness, p. 99.

Normal Range of Findings	Abnormal Findings

Normal Range of Findings

Alternatively, ask the patient to lift each hand or to hold up one finger. You also can check upper extremity strength by palmar drift. Ask the patient to extend both arms forward or halfway up, palms up, eyes closed, and hold for 10 to 20 seconds (Fig. 25.56). Normally, the arms stay steady with no downward drift.

25.56

Check lower extremities by asking the patient to perform straight leg raises, in which the supine patient lifts one leg at a time straight up off the bed (Fig. 25.57). Full strength enables the patient to lift the leg 90 degrees. If multiple trauma, pain, or equipment preclude this motion, ask the patient to push one foot at a time against your hand's resistance, "like putting your foot on the gas pedal of your car" (Fig. 25.58).

25.57

25.58

In a patient with decreased level of consciousness, note whether movement occurs spontaneously and as a result of noxious stimuli such as pain or suctioning. An attempt to push away your hand after such stimuli is called *localizing* and is characterized as purposeful movement.

Abnormal Findings

Any abnormal posturing, decorticate rigidity, or decerebrate rigidity indicates diffuse brain injury (see Table 25.9, p. 744).

Normal Range of Findings

Pupillary Response. Note the size, shape, and symmetry of both pupils. Shine a light into each pupil and note the direct and consensual light reflex. Both pupils should constrict briskly. (Allow for the effects of any medication that could affect pupil size and reactivity.) When you record pupil size, express the value in millimetres. Tape a millimetre scale onto a tongue blade and hold it next to the patient's eyes for the most accurate measurement (Fig. 25.59).

25.59

Vital Signs. Measure the temperature, pulse, respiration, and blood pressure as often as the patient's condition warrants. Although they are vital to the overall assessment of the critically ill patient, pulse and blood pressure are notoriously unreliable parameters of CNS deficit. Any changes are late consequences of rising intracranial pressure.

Assessment of Unconscious and Brain-Damaged Patients

The Glasgow Coma Scale. The assessment of *comatose* patients is an important aspect of critical care. The Glasgow Coma Scale (Fig. 25.60) was originally designed for patients with head trauma and has become the most widely used scoring system for patients with an altered level of consciousness in the critical care unit.[9] The Glasgow Coma Scale is used to assess the functional state of the brain as a whole, not of any particular site in the brain, and it is a standardized assessment that defines the level of consciousness by giving it a numerical value.

The scale is divided into three areas: (a) eye opening, (b) verbal response, and (c) motor response. Each area is rated separately, and the patient's best response is scored numerically. The three numbers are added; the total score reflects the brain's functional level. A fully alert, normal patient has a score of 15, whereas a score of 7 or less reflects coma. Serial assessments can be plotted on a graph to illustrate visually whether the patient is stable, improving, or deteriorating.

Abnormal Findings

In a brain-injured patient, sudden, unilateral dilation and nonreactivity of a pupil is an ominous sign. Cranial nerve III runs parallel to the brain stem. When increasing intracranial pressure pushes the brain stem down (uncal herniation), it puts pressure on cranial nerve III, causing pupil dilation.

The Cushing reflex consists of signs of increasing intracranial pressure: sudden elevation of blood pressure with widening pulse pressure and decreased pulse rate or slow and bounding pulse.

Objective Data

Normal Range of Findings **Abnormal Findings**

GLASGOW COMA SCALE									
EYE OPENING RESPONSE		**MOTOR RESPONSE**		**VERBAL RESPONSE**			
Spontaneous	4	Obeys verbal command *wiggle your fingers*	6	Oriented X3 -appropriate *what year is it?* [correct response]	5	Normal total 15
To speech *open your eyes*	3	Localizes pain	5	Conversation confused *what year is it?* 1962	4	
		Flexion - withdrawal	4	Speech inappropriate *what year is it?* after lunch	3	
To pain	2	Flexion - abnormal	3	Speech incomprehensible *what year is it?* aawagga	2	
		Extension - abnormal	2			
No response	1	No response	1	No response	1	
	SUB-TOTAL	– – – → plus	SUB-TOTAL	– – – → plus	SUB-TOTAL	**TOTAL SCORE**

25.60   (Images © Pat Thomas, 2014.)

Limitations of the Glasgow Coma Scale include inconsistent interrater reliability and the impossibility of assessing the verbal score in intubated or aphasic patients.[9,10] Since 2000, alternative scoring systems have been developed, including new coma scales that are not reliant on verbal responses, such as the Full Outline of UnResponsiveness (FOUR).[11]

The Canadian Neurological Scale. The Canadian Neurological Scale is a valid, reliable, standardized neurological assessment tool that is used to evaluate and monitor both mentation (level of consciousness, orientation, and speech) and motor function (face, arm, and leg) in patients with *stroke*.[12-15] An advantage is that it is a short, simple assessment that does not need to be administered by a neurologist. The Canadian Neurological Scale can be used to monitor change and predict patient outcomes, such as length of stay, death, and dependency. The Canadian Neurological Scale Reference Card is shown in Fig. 25.61.

Objective Data

Normal Range of Findings	Abnormal Findings

Objective Data (side tab)

SECTION A	MENTATION			*SCORE*
	Level of Consciousness		Alert Drowsy	3.0 1.5
	Orientation Place: city or hospital Time: month and year Patient can speak, write, or gesture a response.	*Score:* If patient is oriented (can correctly state both place and correct month and year), score 1.0. If patient cannot state both (disoriented), score 0.0.	Oriented Disoriented/NA	1.0 0.0
	Speech *Receptive:* Ask patient the following separately (do not prompt by gesturing): 1. Close your eyes 2. Point to the ceiling *Expressive:* 1. Show patient 3 items separately, and ask patient to name each object. 2. Ask patient what each object is used for, while holding each one up again.	*Score:* If patient is unable to do both (Receptive Deficit), score 0.0 and go to Section A2. If patient obeys commands, leave blank and assess expressive speech. *Score:* If patient is able to state the name and use of all 3 objects (Normal Speech), score 1.0. If patient is not able to state the name and use of all 3 objects (Expressive Deficit), score 0.5.	Normal Expressive Deficit Receptive Deficit	1.0 0.5 0.0
			TOTAL:	

SECTION A1 NO COMPREHENSION DEFICIT	MOTOR FUNCTIONS: WEAKNESS		WEAKNESS	
	Face Ask patient to smile/grin, note weakness in mouth or nasal/labial folds.	*Score:* None (no weakness) = 0.5; Present (weakness) = 0.0	None Present	0.5 0.0
	Arm: Proximal Ask patient to lift arm 45-90 degrees; apply resistance between shoulder and elbow.	*Score:* None (no weakness present) = 1.5; Mild (mild weakness, full ROM, cannot withstand resistance) = 1.0; Significant (moderate weakness, some movement, not full ROM) = 0.5; Total (complete loss of movement; total weakness) = 0	None Mild Significant Total	1.5 1.0 0.5 0
	Arm: Distal Ask patient to make a fist and flex wrist backwards; apply resistance between wrist and knuckles.	*Score:* None (no weakness present) = 1.5; Mild (mild weakness, full ROM, cannot withstand resistance) = 1.0; Significant (moderate weakness, some movement, not full ROM) = 0.5; Total (complete loss of movement; total weakness) = 0	None Mild Significant Total	1.5 1.0 0.5 0
	Leg: Proximal With patient in supine position, ask patient to flex hip to 90 degrees; apply pressure to mid-thigh.	*Score:* None (no weakness present) = 1.5; Mild (mild weakness, full ROM, cannot withstand resistance) = 1.0; Significant (moderate weakness, some movement, not full ROM) = 0.5; Total (complete loss of movement; total weakness) = 0	None Mild Significant Total	1.5 1.0 0.5 0
	Leg: Distal Ask patient to dorsiflex foot; apply resistance to top of foot.	*Score:* None (no weakness present) = 1.5; Mild (mild weakness, full ROM, cannot withstand resistance) = 1.0; Significant (moderate weakness, some movement, not full ROM) = 0.5; Total (complete loss of movement; total weakness) = 0	None Mild Significant Total	1.5 1.0 0.5 0
			TOTAL:	

SECTION A2 COMPREHENSION DEFICIT	MOTOR FUNCTIONS: MOTOR RESPONSE			
	Face Have patient mimic your smile. If patient is unable, note facial expression while applying sternal pressure.		Symmetrical Asymmetrical	0.5 0.0
	Arms Demonstrate or lift patient's arms to 90 degrees; score ability to maintain raised arms; apply nail bed pressure to assess reflex response.		Equal Unequal	1.5 0.0
	Legs Lift patient's hip to 90 degrees; score ability to maintain equal levels (>5 seconds). If patient is unable to maintain raised position, apply nail bed pressure to assess reflex response.		Equal Unequal	1.5 0.0
			TOTAL:	

25.61   The Canadian Neurological Scale Reference Card. *NA,* Not applicable; *ROM,* range of motion.

DOCUMENTATION AND CRITICAL THINKING

Sample Charting

SUBJECTIVE

No unusually frequent or severe headaches; no head injury, dizziness or vertigo, seizures, or tremors. No weakness, numbness, or tingling; no difficulty swallowing or speaking. Has no past history of stroke, spinal cord injury, meningitis, or alcoholism.

OBJECTIVE

Mental status: Appearance, behaviour, and speech appropriate; alert and oriented to person, place, and time; recent and remote memory intact.

Cranial nerves:

I: Identifies coffee and peppermint.

II: Vision 20/20 O.S. [left eye], 20/20 O.D. [right eye], peripheral fields intact by confrontation, fundi normal.

III, IV, VI: EOMs intact, no ptosis or nystagmus; PERRLA [*p*upils *e*qual, *r*ound, *r*eact to *l*ight and *a*ccommodation].

V: Sensation intact and equal bilaterally, jaw strength equal bilaterally.

VII: Facial muscles intact and symmetrical.

VIII: Hearing: whispered words heard bilaterally.

IX, X: Swallowing intact, gag reflex present, uvula rises in midline on phonation.

XI: Shoulder shrug, head movement intact and equal bilaterally.

XII: Tongue protrudes midline, no tremors.

Motor: No atrophy, weakness, or tremors. Gait smooth and coordinated, able to tandem walk, negative Romberg reflex. Rapid alternating movements: finger-to-nose smoothly intact.

Sensory: Pinprick, light touch, vibration intact. Stereognosis: able to identify key.

Reflexes: Normal abdominal, no Babinski sign, DTRs 2+ and = bilaterally with downgoing toes; see the following drawing:

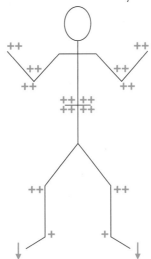

ASSESSMENT

Neurological system intact, normal function

Focused Assessment: Clinical Case Study

Jack Tibeaud (J.T.) is a 61-year-old male carpenter at a large building firm; he is admitted to the Rehabilitation Institute with a diagnosis of right hemiplegia and aphasia after a cerebrovascular accident (CVA) 4 weeks PTA (prior to arrival).

SUBJECTIVE

Because of J.T.'s speech dysfunction, history was provided by wife.

4 weeks PTA: J.T. complained of severe headache, then had sudden onset of collapse and loss of consciousness while at work. Did not strike head as fell. Transported by ambulance to Memorial Hospital where admitting physician said J.T. "probably had a stroke." Right arm and leg were limp, and he remained unconscious. Admitted to CCU [critical care unit]. Regained consciousness day 3 after admission, unable to move right side, unable to speak clearly or write. Remained in CCU 4 more days until "doctors were sure heart and breathing were steady."

3 weeks PTA: Transferred to medical floor where care included physical therapy 2×/day and passive ROM 4×/day.

Now: Some improvement in right motor function. Bowel control achieved with use of commode same time each day (after breakfast). Bladder control improved. Some occasional incontinence, usually when unable to tell people he needs to urinate.

OBJECTIVE

Mental status: Dressed in jogging suit, sitting in wheelchair, appears alert with appropriate eye contact, listening intently to history. Speech is slow, requires great effort, able to give one-word answers that are appropriate but lack normal tone. Seems to understand all language spoken to him. Follows requests appropriately, within limits of motor weakness.

Cranial nerves:

II: Acuity normal, fields by confrontation: right homonymous hemianopsia, fundi normal.

III, IV, VI: EOMs intact, no ptosis or nystagmus, PERRLA.

V: Sensation intact to pinprick and light touch. Jaw strength weak on right.

VII: Flat nasolabial fold on right, motor weakness on right lower face. Able to wrinkle forehead bilaterally, but unable to smile or bare teeth on right.

VIII: Hearing intact.

IX, X: Swallowing intact, gag reflex present, uvula rises midline on phonation.

XI: Shoulder shrug, head movement weaker on right.

XII: Tongue protrudes midline, no tremors.

Motor: Right hand grip weak, right arm drifts, right leg weak, unable to support weight. Spasticity in right arm and leg muscles, limited ROM on passive motion. Unable to stand up and walk unassisted. Unable to perform finger-to-nose or heel-to-shin on right side; left side smoothly intact.

Sensory: Pinprick and light touch present but diminished on right arm and leg. Vibration intact. Position sense impaired on right side. Stereognosis intact.

Reflexes: Hyperactive 4+ with clonus, and upgoing toes in right leg. Abdominal and cremasteric reflexes absent on right; see the following drawing:

ASSESSMENT

Impaired verbal communication R/T [related to] effects of CVA

Impaired physical mobility R/T neuromuscular impairment

Disturbed body image R/T effects of loss of body function

Self-care deficits: feeding, bathing, toileting, dressing/grooming R/T muscular weakness

Disturbed sensory perception (absent right visual fields) R/T neurological impairment

Risk for injury R/T visual field deficit

ABNORMAL FINDINGS

TABLE 25.2	Abnormalities in Cranial Nerves		
Nerve	**Test**	**Abnormal Findings**	**Possible Causes**
I: Olfactory	Identifying familiar odours	Neurogenic anosmia	Upper respiratory infection (temporary); tobacco or cocaine use; fracture of cribriform plate or ethmoid area; frontal lobe lesion; tumour in olfactory bulb or tract
II: Optic	Visual acuity Visual fields Shining light in eye	Defect in or absence of central vision Defect in peripheral vision, hemianopsia Absence of light reflex	Congenital blindness, refractive error, acquired vision loss as result of numerous diseases (e.g., cerebrovascular accident, diabetes), trauma to globe or orbit (see discussion of cranial nerve III)
	Direct inspection	Papilledema Optic atrophy Retinal lesions	Increased intracranial pressure Glaucoma Diabetes
III: Oculomotor	Inspection	Dilated pupil, ptosis, eye turns out and slightly down	Paralysis in cranial nerve III from internal carotid aneurysm, tumour, inflammatory lesions, uncal herniation with increased intracranial pressure
	Extraocular muscle movement	Failure to move eye up, in, down	Ptosis from myasthenia gravis, oculomotor nerve palsy, Horner's syndrome
	Shining light in eye	Absence of light reflex	Blindness, medication influence, increased intracranial pressure, CNS injury, circulatory arrest, CNS sequelae of syphilis
IV: Trochlear	Extraocular muscle movement	Failure to turn eye down or out	Fracture of orbit, brain stem tumour
V: Trigeminal	Superficial touch: three divisions Corneal reflex Clenching teeth	Absence of sense of touch and pain, paraesthesias No blink Weakness of masseter or temporalis muscles	Trauma, tumour, pressure from aneurysm, inflammation, sequelae of alcohol injection for trigeminal neuralgia Unilateral weakness with cranial nerve V lesion; bilateral weakness with upper or lower motor neuron disorder
VI: Abducens	Extraocular muscle movement to right and left sides	Failure to move laterally, diplopia on lateral gaze	Brain stem tumour or trauma, fracture of orbit

Continued

TABLE 25.2	Abnormalities in Cranial Nerves—cont'd		
Nerve	Test	Abnormal Findings	Possible Causes
VII: Facial	Wrinkling forehead, closing eyes tightly	Absence of or asymmetrical facial movement	Bell's palsy (lower motor neuron lesion), which causes paralysis of entire half of face
	Smiling, puffing cheeks Identifying tastes	Loss of taste	Upper motor neuron lesions (cerebrovascular accident, tumour, inflammation), which cause paralysis of lower half of face, leaving forehead intact; lower motor neuron lesions that cause paralysis: swelling from ear or meningeal infections
VIII: Acoustic	Hearing acuity	Decrease or loss of hearing	Inflammation, occluded ear canal, otosclerosis, presbycusis, medication toxicity, tumour
IX: Glossopharyngeal	Gag reflex	See cranial nerve X	
X: Vagus	Phonating "ahhh"	Deviation of uvula to side	Brain stem tumour, neck injury, cranial nerve X lesion
	Gag reflex	No gag reflex	Vocal cord weakness
	Voice quality	Hoarse or brassy voice	Soft palate weakness
		Nasal twang Husky voice	Unilateral cranial nerve X lesion
	Swallowing	Dysphagia, regurgitation of fluids through nose	Bilateral cranial nerve X lesion
XI: Spinal Accessory	Turning head, shrugging shoulders against resistance	Absence of movement of sternomastoid or trapezius muscles	Neck injury, torticollis
XII: Hypoglossal	Protruding tongue	Deviation to side	Lower motor neuron lesion
	Wiggling tongue from side to side	Slowed rate of movement	Bilateral upper motor neuron lesion

CNS, Central nervous system.

TABLE 25.3	Abnormalities in Muscle Tone	
Condition	Description	Associated With
Flaccidity	Decreased muscle tone (*hypotonia*); muscle feels limp, soft, and flabby; muscle is weak and easily fatigued	Lower motor neuron injury anywhere from the anterior horn cell in the spinal cord to the peripheral nerve (peripheral neuritis, poliomyelitis, Guillain-Barré syndrome) Early cerebrovascular accident and spinal cord injury: flaccidity at first
Spasticity	Increased tone (*hypertonia*); increased resistance to passive lengthening and then suddenly giving way (clasp-knife phenomenon)	Upper motor neuron injury to corticospinal motor tract, such as paralysis with cerebrovascular accident (chronic stage)
Rigidity	Constant state of resistance (lead-pipe rigidity); resistance to passive movement in any direction; dystonia	Injury to extrapyramidal motor tracts: for example, basal ganglia with parkinsonism
Cogwheel rigidity	Type of rigidity in which the increased tone lessens by degrees during passive ROM so that it feels like small, regular jerks	Parkinsonism

ROM, Range of motion.

TABLE 25.4   Abnormalities in Muscle Movement

Paralysis

Decrease in or loss of motor power caused by problem with motor nerve or muscle fibres. Acute causes: trauma, spinal cord injury, cerebrovascular accident, poliomyelitis, polyneuritis, Bell's palsy; chronic causes: muscular dystrophy, diabetic neuropathy, multiple sclerosis; episodic causes: myasthenia gravis

Patterns of paralysis: *hemiplegia* (spastic or flaccid paralysis of one [right or left] side of body and extremities); *paraplegia* (symmetrical paralysis of both lower extremities); *quadriplegia* (paralysis in all four extremities); *paresis* (weakness of muscles rather than paralysis)

Fasciculation

Rapid, continuous twitching of resting muscle or part of muscle, without movement of limb, which can be seen or palpated. Types: fine (occurs with lower motor neuron disease, associated with atrophy and weakness) and coarse (occurs with cold exposure or fatigue and is not significant).

Tic

Involuntary, compulsive, repetitive twitching of a muscle group, such as wink, grimace, head movement, shoulder shrug; has a neurological cause, such as tardive dyskinesias and Tourette's syndrome, or a psychogenic cause (habit tic).

Myoclonus

Rapid, sudden jerk or a short series of jerks at fairly regular intervals. A hiccup is a myoclonus of the diaphragm. Single myoclonic arm or leg jerk is normal when a person is falling asleep; myoclonic jerks are severe with tonic–clonic seizures.

Tremor (Not Illustrated)

Involuntary contraction of opposing muscle groups. Results in rhythmic, back-and-forth movement of one or more joints. May occur at rest or with voluntary movement. All tremors disappear during sleep. Tremors may be slow (3 to 6 per second) or rapid (10 to 20 per second).

Continued

Abnormal Findings

TABLE 25.4   Abnormalities in Muscle Movement—cont'd

Rest Tremor

Coarse and slow (3 to 6 per second); partly or completely disappears with voluntary movement (e.g., "pill rolling" tremor of parkinsonism, with thumb and opposing fingers).

Intention Tremor

Rate varies; worse with voluntary movement. Occurs with cerebellar disease and multiple sclerosis.

Essential tremor (familial): a type of intention tremor; most common tremor in older adults. Benign (no associated disease) but causes emotional stress in work or social situations. Improves with the administration of sedatives, propranolol, and alcohol, but use of alcohol is discouraged because of the risk for addiction.

Chorea

Sudden, rapid, jerky, purposeless movement involving limbs, trunk, or face.

Occurs at irregular intervals, not rhythmic or repetitive, more convulsive than a tic. Some are spontaneous, and some are initiated; all are accentuated by voluntary acts. Disappears with sleep. Common with Sydenham's chorea and Huntington's disease.

Athetosis

Slow, twisting, writhing, continuous movement, resembling a snake or worm. Involves distal part of limb more than the proximal part. Occurs with cerebral palsy. Disappears with sleep. "Athetoid" hand: some fingers are flexed and some are extended.

TABLE 25.5 Abnormal Gaits

Type	Characteristic Appearance	Possible Causes
Spastic Hemiparesis	Arm is immobile against the body, with flexion of the shoulder, elbow, wrist, and fingers and adduction of shoulder. The leg is stiff and extended and circumducts with each step (patient drags toe in a semicircle).	Upper motor neuron lesion of the corticospinal tract, such as those caused by cerebrovascular accident, trauma
Cerebellar Ataxia	Patient has staggering, wide-based gait; difficulty with turns; uncoordinated movement with positive Romberg sign.	Alcohol or barbiturate effect on cerebellum; cerebellar tumour; multiple sclerosis
Parkinsonian (Festinating)	Posture is stooped; trunk is pitched forward; elbows, hips, and knees are flexed. Steps are short and shuffling. Patient hesitates to begin walking and has difficulty stopping suddenly. Patient holds the body rigid, walks and turns body as one fixed unit, and has difficulty with any change in direction.	Parkinsonism
Scissors	Knees cross or are in contact, like holding an orange between the thighs. The patient uses short steps, and walking requires effort.	Paraparesis of legs, multiple sclerosis
Steppage or Footdrop	Slapping quality: Gait looks as if patient is walking up stairs and finding no stair there. Patient lifts knee and foot high and slaps it down hard and flat to compensate for footdrop.	Weakness of peroneal and anterior tibial muscles; caused by lower motor neuron lesion at the spinal cord, such as poliomyelitis, Charcot-Marie-Tooth disease (an inherited peripheral neuropathy)

Continued

Abnormal Findings

TABLE 25.5	Abnormal Gaits—cont'd	
Type	Characteristic Appearance	Possible Causes
Waddling	Weak hip muscles: When the patient takes a step, the opposite hip drops, which allows compensatory lateral movement of pelvis. Often, the patient also has marked lumbar lordosis and a protruding abdomen.	Hip girdle muscle weakness, caused by muscular dystrophy, dislocation of hips
Short Leg	Leg length discrepancy >2.5 cm. Vertical telescoping of affected side, which dips as the patient walks. Appearance of gait varies, depending on amount of accompanying muscle dysfunction.	Congenital dislocated hip; acquired shortening as a result of disease, trauma

TABLE 25.6	Characteristics of Upper and Lower Motor Neuron Lesions	
Characteristic	Upper Motor Neuron Lesion	Lower Motor Neuron Lesion
Weakness or paralysis	In muscles that correspond to distribution of damage in pyramidal tract lesion; usually in hand grip, arm extensors, leg flexors	In specific muscles served by damaged spinal segment, ventral root, or peripheral nerve
Location	Descending motor pathways that originate in the motor areas of cerebral cortex and carry impulses to the anterior horn cells of the spinal cord	Nerve cells that originate in the anterior horn of spinal cord or in brain stem and carry impulses by the spinal nerves or cranial nerves to the muscles, the "final common pathway"
Examples	Cerebrovascular accident	Poliomyelitis; herniated intervertebral disc
Muscle tone	Increased tone; spasticity	Loss of tone, flaccidity
Bulk	Some atrophy from disuse; otherwise normal	Atrophy (wasting), may be marked
Abnormal movements	None	Fasciculations
Reflexes	Hyper-reflexia, ankle clonus; diminished or absent superficial abdominal reflexes; positive Babinski sign	Hyporeflexia or areflexia; no Babinski sign, no pathological reflexes
Possible nursing diagnoses	Risk for contractures; impairment in physical mobility	Impairment in physical mobility

TABLE 25.7 Patterns of Motor System Dysfunction

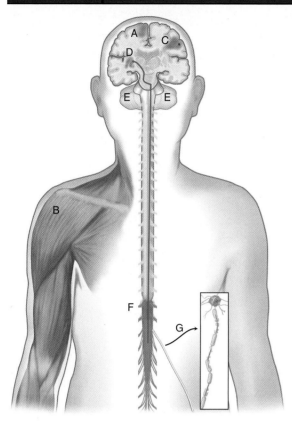

A: Cerebral Palsy

Mixed group of paralytic neuromotor disorders of infancy and childhood; results from damage to cerebral cortex caused by a developmental defect, intrauterine meningitis or encephalitis, birth trauma, anoxia, or kernicterus.

B: Muscular Dystrophy

Chronic, progressive wasting of skeletal musculature, which produces weakness, contractures, and in severe cases, respiratory dysfunction and death. Onset of symptoms occurs in childhood. Many types exist; the most severe is Duchenne's muscular dystrophy, characterized by the waddling gait described in Table 25.5 (p. 740).

C: Hemiplegia

Damage to corticospinal tract (e.g., cerebrovascular accident). Upper motor neuron damage occurs above the pyramidal decussation crossover; thus, motor impairment is on contralateral (opposite) side. Affected muscles are initially flaccid when the lesion is acute; later, the muscles become spastic, and abnormal reflexes appear. Characteristic posture of arm: shoulder adducted, elbow flexed, wrist pronated, leg extended; characteristic facies: weakness only in lower muscles. Hyper-reflexia and sometimes clonus occur on the involved side; loss of corneal, abdominal, and cremasteric reflexes; positive Babinski and Hoffman reflexes.

D: Parkinsonism

Defect of extrapyramidal tracts, in the region of the basal ganglia, with loss of the neurotransmitter dopamine. Classic triad of symptoms: tremor, rigidity, akinesia. Also slower monotonous speech and diminutive writing. Body tends to stay immobile; facial expression is flat, staring, expressionless; excessive salivation occurs; eye blinking is reduced. Posture is stooped; equilibrium is impaired; balance is easily lost; gait is as described in Table 25.5 (p. 739). Parkinsonian tremor; cogwheel rigidity on passive ROM.

E: Cerebellar

A lesion in one hemisphere produces motor abnormalities on the ipsilateral side. Characterized by ataxia, lurching forward of affected side during walking, rapid alternating movements that are slow and arrhythmic; finger-to-nose test reveals ataxia and tremor with overshoot or undershoot, and eyes display coarse nystagmus.

F: Paraplegia

Lower motor neuron damage caused by spinal cord injury. A severe injury or complete transection initially produces "spinal shock" (no movement or reflex activity below the level of the lesion). Gradually, deep tendon reflexes reappear and become increased, flexor spasms of legs occur, and then extensor spasms of legs occur; these spasms lead to prevailing extensor tone.

G: Multiple Sclerosis

Chronic, progressive, immune-mediated disease in which axons undergo inflammation, demyelination, degeneration, and sclerosis.[a] Structures most frequently involved are the optic nerve, oculomotor nerve, corticospinal tract, posterior column tract, and cerebellum. Thus symptoms are varied but include blurred vision, diplopia, extreme fatigue, weakness, spasticity, numbness and tingling sensation, and loss of balance.

[a]Courtney, A. M., Treadaway, K., Remington, G., et al. (2009). Multiple sclerosis. *Medical Clinics of North America, 93*(2), 451–476. doi:10.1016/j.mcna.2008.09.014.
Image © Pat Thomas, 2010.
ROM, Range of motion.

TABLE 25.8   Common Patterns of Sensory Loss

Type	Characteristics	Possible Causes
Peripheral Neuropathy 	Loss of sensation involves *all* modalities. Loss is most severe distally (feet and hands); response improves as stimulus is moved proximally (glove-and-stocking anaesthesia). Zone of anaesthesia gradually merges into a hypoaesthesia zone, then gradually becomes normal.	Diabetes, chronic alcoholism, nutritional deficiency
Individual Nerves or Roots 	Decrease in or loss of *all* sensory modalities. Area of sensory loss corresponds to distribution of the involved nerve.	Trauma, vascular occlusion
Spinal Cord Hemisection (Brown-Séquard Syndrome)	Loss of pain and temperature sensation on the contralateral side, starting one to two segments below the level of the lesion. Loss of vibration sensation and position discrimination on the ipsilateral side, below the level of the lesion.	Meningioma, neurofibroma, cervical spondylosis, multiple sclerosis

TABLE 25.8	Common Patterns of Sensory Loss—cont'd	
Type	Characteristics	Possible Causes
Complete Transection of the Spinal Cord 	Complete loss of *all* sensory modalities below the level of the lesion. Condition is associated with motor paralysis and loss of sphincter control.	Spinal cord trauma, demyelinating disorders, tumour
Thalamus 	Loss of *all* sensory modalities on the face, arm, and leg on the side contralateral to the lesion.	Vascular occlusion
Cortex 	Because pain, vibration sensation, and crude touch sensation are mediated by the thalamus, little loss of these sensory functions occurs with a cortex lesion. Loss of discrimination occurs on the contralateral side. Loss of graphaesthesia, stereognosis, recognition of shapes and weights, finger finding.	Cerebral cortex, parietal lobe lesion (e.g., cerebrovascular accident)

TABLE 25.9 Abnormal Postures

Decorticate Rigidity

Upper extremities: flexion of arm, wrist, and fingers; adduction of arm (i.e., tight against thorax). Lower extremities: extension, internal rotation, plantar flexion. This type of rigidity indicates hemispheric lesion of cerebral cortex.

Decerebrate Rigidity

Upper extremities: stiffly extended, adducted, and internally rotated; palms pronated. Lower extremities: stiffly extended; plantar flexion. Other areas: teeth clenched; back hyperextended. More ominous than decorticate rigidity; indicates lesion in brain stem at midbrain or upper pons.

Flaccid Quadriplegia

Complete loss of muscle tone and paralysis of all four extremities, indicating completely nonfunctional brain stem.

Opisthotonos

Prolonged arching of the back, with head and heels bent backward. This indicates meningeal irritation.

Images © Pat Thomas, 2006.

TABLE 25.10 Pathological Reflexes

Reflex	Method of Testing	Abnormal Response (Reflex Is Present)	Indications
Babinski	Stroke lateral aspect and across ball of foot.	Extension of great toe, fanning of toes	Corticospinal (pyramidal) tract disease (e.g., stroke, trauma)
Oppenheim	Using heavy pressure with your thumb and index finger, stroke anterior medial tibial muscle.	Same as for Babinski reflex	Same as for Babinski reflex
Gordon	Firmly squeeze calf muscles.	Same as for Babinski reflex	Same as for Babinski reflex
Hoffman	With patient's hand relaxed, wrist dorsiflexed, and fingers slightly flexed, sharply flick nail of distal phalanx of middle or index finger.	Clawing of fingers and thumb	Same as for Babinski reflex
Kernig	With patient in flat-lying supine position, raise leg straight or flex thigh on abdomen, then extend knee.	Resistance to straightening (because of hamstring spasm), pain down posterior thigh	Meningeal irritation (e.g., meningitis, infections)
Brudzinski	With one hand under patient's neck and other hand on patient's chest, sharply flex chin on chest, and watch hips and knees.	Resistance and pain in neck with flexion of hips and knees	Meningeal irritation (e.g., meningitis, infections)

TABLE 25.11	Frontal Release Signs			
Reflex		Method of Testing	Abnormal Response (Reflex Is Present)	Indications
Snout Snout		Gently percuss patient's oral region	Puckering of lips	Frontal lobe disease, cerebral degenerative disease (Alzheimer's disease), amyotrophic sclerosis, corticobulbar lesions
Sucking Sucking		Touch patient's oral region	Sucking movement of lips, tongue, and jaw; swallowing	Same as for snout reflex
Grasp Grasp		Touch patient's palm with your finger	Uncontrolled, forced grasping (grasp is usually last of these signs to appear, so its presence indicates severe disease)	When grasping is unilateral: frontal lobe lesion on contralateral side When grasping is bilateral: diffuse bifrontal lobe disease

Images © Pat Thomas, 2006.

TABLE 25.12	Speech Disorders	
Condition	Function Affected	Description
Dysphonia	Voice	Difficulty or discomfort in talking, with abnormal pitch or volume, caused by laryngeal disease. Voice sounds hoarse or whispered, but articulation and language are intact.
Dysarthria	Articulation	Distorted speech sounds; speech may sound unintelligible; basic language (word choice, grammar, comprehension) is intact.
Aphasia	Language comprehension and production	True language disturbance, defect in word choice and grammar or defect in comprehension; defect is in *higher* integrative language processing and is secondary to brain damage.
Types of Aphasia[a]		
	Speech production	An earlier dichotomy classified aphasias as expressive (difficulty producing language) or receptive (difficulty understanding language). Because all people with aphasia have some difficulty with expression, beginning examiners tend to classify all types as expressive. The following system is more descriptive.

Continued

TABLE 25.12	Speech Disorders—cont'd	
Condition	Function Affected	Description
• Global aphasia		The most common and severe form. Spontaneous speech is absent or reduced to a few stereotyped words or sounds. Comprehension is absent or reduced to only the patient's own name and a few select words. Repetition, reading, and writing are severely impaired. Prognosis for language recovery is poor. Caused by a large lesion that damages most of combined anterior and posterior language areas.
• Broca's aphasia		Expressive aphasia. The patient can understand language but cannot express himself or herself with language. This is characterized by nonfluent, dysarthric, and effortful speech. The speech is mostly nouns and verbs (high-content words) with few grammatical fillers ("agrammatic" or "telegraphic" speech). Repetition and reading aloud are severely impaired. Auditory and reading comprehensions are surprisingly intact. Lesion is in anterior language area called the *motor speech cortex* or *Broca's area.*
• Wernicke's aphasia		Receptive aphasia. The linguistic opposite of Broca's aphasia. The person can hear sounds and words but cannot relate them to previous experiences. Speech is fluent, effortless, and well-articulated but has many paraphasias (word substitutions that are malformed or wrong) and neologisms (made-up words) and often lacks substantive words. Speech can be totally incomprehensible. Often, there is a great urge to speak. Repetition, reading, and writing also are impaired. Lesion is in posterior language area called the *association auditory cortex* or *Wernicke's area.*

ᵃFor a discussion of other types of aphasia (e.g., conduction, anomic, transcortical), please consult a neurology text.

Summary Checklist: Neurological Examination

Screening Neurological Examination
1. **Mental status**
2. **Cranial nerves:**
   II: Optic
   III, IV, VI: Extraocular muscles
   V: Trigeminal
   VII: Facial mobility
3. **Motor function:**
   Gait and balance
   Knee flexion: hop or shallow knee bend
4. **Sensory function:**
   Superficial pain and light touch: arms and legs
   Vibration: arms and legs

5. **Reflexes:**
   Biceps
   Triceps
   Patellar
   Achilles
Complete Neurological Examination
1. **Mental status**
2. **Cranial nerves II through XII**
3. **Motor system:**
   Muscle size, strength, tone
   Gait and balance
   Rapid alternating movements
4. **Sensory function:**
   Superficial pain and light touch
   Vibration

Position sense
Stereognosis, graphaesthesia, two-point discrimination
5. **Reflexes:**
   Deep tendon: biceps, triceps, brachioradialis, patellar, Achilles
   Superficial: abdominal, plantar

REFERENCES

1. Fjell, A. M., Walhovd, K. B., & Fennema-Notestine, C. (2009). One-year brain atrophy evident in healthy aging. *Journal of Neuroscience, 29*(48), 1523–1531. doi:10.1523/JNEUROSCI.3252-09.2009.

2. Ontario Stroke Network. (2016). *Stroke stats & facts.* Retrieved from http://ontariostrokenetwork.ca/information-about-stroke/stroke-stats-and-facts/.

3. Marshall, I. J., Wang, Y., Crichton, S., et al. (2015). The effects of socioeconomic status on stroke risk and outcomes. *The Lancet. Neurology, 14*(12), 1206–1218. doi:10.1016/S1474-4422(15)00200-8.

4. Bettger, J. P., Zhao, X., Bushnell, C., et al. (2014). The association between socioeconomic status and disability after stroke: Findings from the Adherence eValuation After Ischemic stroke Longitudinal (AVAIL) registry. *BMC Public Health, 14*(1), 281. doi:10.1186/1471-2458-14-281.

5. Menec, V. H., Shooshtari, S., Nowicki, S., et al. (2010). Does the relationship between neighborhood socioeconomic status and health outcomes persist into very old age? A population-based study. *Journal of Aging and Health, 22*(1), 27–47. doi:10.1177/0898264309349029.

6. Heart and Stroke Foundation of Canada. (2017). *Taking control: Lower your risk of heart disease and stroke: A guide for Aboriginal Peoples.* Retrieved from http://www.heartandstroke.ca/-/media/pdf-files/canada/other/aboriginal_takingcontrol.ashx.

7. Heart and Stroke Foundation of Canada. (2017). *Risk factors you cannot change.* Retrieved from http://www.heartandstroke.ca/stroke/risk-and-prevention/risk-factors-you-cannot-change.

8. Krieger, N. (2014). Discrimination and health inequities. *International Journal of Health Services, 44*(4), 643–710. doi:10.2190/HS.44.4.b.

9. Fischer, M., Rüegg, S., Czaplinski, A., et al. (2010). Inter-rater reliability of the Full Outline of UnResponsiveness score and the Glasgow Coma Scale in critically ill patients: A prospective observational study. *Critical Care, 14*(2), R64. Retrieved from http://ccforum.com/content/14/2/R64.

10. Kornbluth, J., & Bhardwaj, A. (2011). Evaluation of coma: A critical appraisal of popular scoring systems. *Neurocritical Care, 14*(1), 134–143. doi:10.1007/s12028-010-9409-3.

11. Wijdicks, E., Bamlet, W., Maramattom, B., et al. (2005). Validation of a new coma scale: The FOUR score. *Annals of Neurology, 58*(4), 585–593. doi:10.1002/ana.20611.

12. Côté, R., Battista, R. N., Wolfson, C., et al. (1989). The Canadian Neurological Scale: Validation and reliability assessment. *Neurology, 39*, 638–643.

13. Côté, R., David, M., Deveber, G., et al. (2007). *Stroke prevention: The Thrombosis Interest Group of Canada.* Retrieved from http://www.tigc.org/eguidelines/previschemstroke05.htm.

14. Côté, R., Hachinski, V. C., Shurvell, B. L., et al. (1986). The Canadian Neurological Scale: A preliminary study in acute stroke. *Stroke, 17*, 731–737. doi:10.1161/01.STR.17.4.731.

15. O'Farrell, B., & Zou, G. Y. (2008). Implementation of the Canadian Neurological Scale on an acute care neuroscience unit: A program evaluation. *Journal of Neuroscience Nursing, 40*(4), 201–211.

Male Genitourinary System

Written by Carolyn Jarvis, PhD, APN, CNP
Adapted by Marian Luctkar-Flude, RN, PhD

http://evolve.elsevier.com/Canada/Jarvis/examination/

STRUCTURE AND FUNCTION

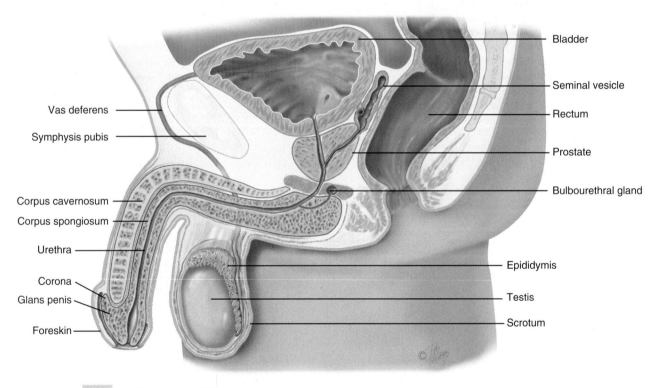

26.1 (© Pat Thomas, 2010.)

THE MALE GENITALIA

The male genital structures include the penis and scrotum externally and the testis, epididymis, and vas deferens internally. Glandular structures accessory to the genital organs (the prostate, seminal vesicles, and bulbourethral glands) are discussed in Chapter 23.

Penis

The **penis** is composed of three cylindrical columns of erectile tissue: the two corpora cavernosa on the dorsal side and the corpus spongiosum ventrally (Fig. 26.1). At the distal end of the shaft, the corpus spongiosum expands into a cone of erectile tissue, the **glans**. The area where the glans joins

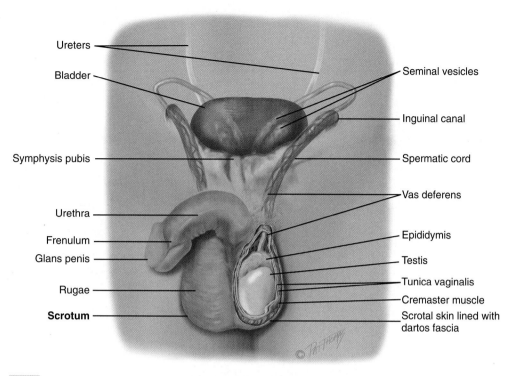

26.2   Male genital structures. (© Pat Thomas, 2010.)

the shaft is the **corona**. The **urethra** transverses the corpus spongiosum, and its meatus forms a slit at the glans tip. Over the glans, the skin folds in and back on itself, forming a hood or flap. This is the **foreskin**, or **prepuce**. Sometimes, it is surgically removed shortly after birth by circumcision. The **frenulum** is a fold of the foreskin extending from the urethral meatus ventrally.

Scrotum

The **scrotum** is a loose protective sac that is a continuation of the abdominal wall (Fig. 26.2). After adolescence, the scrotal skin is deeply pigmented and has large sebaceous follicles. The scrotal wall consists of thin skin lying in folds, or **rugae**, and the underlying cremaster muscle. The **cremaster** and **dartos muscles** control the size of the scrotum by responding to ambient temperature. This is to keep the testes at the best temperature for producing sperm: 3°C below abdominal temperature. When it is cold, the cremaster muscle contracts, raising the sac and bringing the testes closer to the body to absorb heat necessary for sperm viability. The dartos muscle, located within the dartos fascia, also contracts, causing the scrotal skin to wrinkle. When it is warmer, these muscles relax, the scrotum lowers, and the skin looks smoother.

Inside, a septum separates the sac into two halves. In each scrotal half is a **testis**, which produces sperm. Each testis is a solid oval structure that is compressed laterally and measures 4 to 5 cm long by 3 cm wide in adults. The testis is suspended vertically by the spermatic cord (see Fig. 26.2). The left testis is lower than the right because the left spermatic cord is longer. Each testis is covered by a double-layered

membrane, the tunica vaginalis, which separates it from the scrotal wall. The two layers are lubricated by fluid so that the testis can slide a little within the scrotum; this helps prevent injury.

Sperm are transported along a series of ducts. First, the testis is capped by the **epididymis**, which is a markedly coiled duct system and the main storage site of sperm. It is a comma-shaped structure, curved over the top and the posterior surface of the testis. In 6% to 7% of males, the epididymis is anterior to the testis.

The lower part of the epididymis is continuous with a muscular duct, the **vas deferens**. This duct approximates with other vessels (arteries and veins, lymphatic vessels, nerves) to form the **spermatic cord**. The spermatic cord ascends along the posterior border of the testis and runs through the tunnel of the inguinal canal into the abdomen. At that point, the vas deferens continues back and down behind the bladder, where it joins the duct of the seminal vesicle to form the **ejaculatory duct**. This duct empties into the urethra.

The **lymphatic vessels** of the penis and scrotal surface drain into the inguinal lymph nodes, whereas those of the testes drain into the abdomen. Abdominal lymph nodes are not accessible to clinical examination.

Inguinal Area

The **inguinal area**, or groin, is the juncture of the lower abdominal wall and the thigh (Fig. 26.3). Its diagonal borders are the anterior superior iliac spine and the symphysis pubis. Between these landmarks lies the **inguinal ligament** (Poupart's ligament). Superior to the ligament lies the

Anterior superior iliac spine

Inguinal ligament

Inguinal lymph node

Inguinal canal

External ring

Fascia over symphysis pubis

External oblique muscle

Internal oblique muscle

Transverse abdominis muscle

Internal ring

Cremaster muscle

Spermatic cord

Femoral canal

Femoral vein

Femoral artery

STRUCTURES OF INGUINAL AREA

26.3   (© Pat Thomas, 2010.)

inguinal canal, a narrow tunnel passing obliquely between layers of abdominal muscle. It is 4 to 6 cm long in the adult. Its openings are an internal ring, located 1 to 2 cm above the midpoint of the inguinal ligament, and an external ring, located just above and lateral to the pubis.

Inferior to the inguinal ligament is the **femoral canal**. It is a potential space located 3 cm medial to and parallel with the femoral artery. You can use the artery as a landmark to find this space.

Knowledge of these anatomical areas in the groin is useful because they are potential sites for a hernia, which is a loop of bowel protruding through a weak spot in the musculature.

 DEVELOPMENTAL CONSIDERATIONS

Infants

During gestation, the testes develop in the abdominal cavity near the kidneys. During the later months of gestation, the testes migrate, pushing the abdominal wall in front of them and dragging the vas deferens, the blood vessels, and nerves behind. The testes descend along the inguinal canal into the scrotum before birth. At birth, each testis measures 1.5 to 2 cm long and 1 cm wide. Their size increases only slightly during the prepubertal years.

Adolescents

Puberty begins sometime between the ages of 9½ and 13½. The first sign is enlargement of the testes. Next, pubic hair

appears, and then penis size increases. The developmental stages are documented in Tanner's sexual maturity rating (see Table 26.1, p. 751).

The complete change from a preadolescent to an adult takes approximately 3 years; the normal range is 2 to 5 years (Fig. 26.4). The chart shown in Fig. 26.4 is useful in teaching a boy the expected sequence of events and in reassuring him about the wide range of ages when these events normally occur.

Adults and Older Adults

The level of sexual development at the end of puberty remains constant through early and middle adulthood, with no further genital growth and no change in circulating sex hormone.

Men do not experience a definite end to fertility, as women do. At approximately age 40 years, the production of sperm begins to decrease, although production continues into the 80s and 90s. After age 55 to 60 years, testosterone production declines very gradually so that resulting physical changes are not evident until later in life. Aging changes also result from decreased muscle tone, decreased subcutaneous fat, and decreased cellular metabolism.

In older men, the amount of pubic hair decreases, and the remaining hair turns grey. Penis size decreases. Because of decreased tone of the dartos muscle, the scrotal contents hang lower, the rugae decrease, and the scrotum looks pendulous. The testes decrease in size and are less firm to palpation. Increased connective tissue is present in

TABLE 26.1   Sexual Maturity Ratings in Boys

DEVELOPMENTAL STAGE	PUBIC HAIR	PENIS	SCROTUM
1	No pubic hair; fine body hair on abdomen (vellus hair) continues over pubic area	Preadolescent; size and proportion are the same as during childhood	Preadolescent; size and proportion are the same as during childhood
2	Few straight, slightly darker hairs at base of penis are long and downy	Little or no enlargement	Enlargement of testes and scrotum; scrotal skin reddens and changes in texture
3	Sparse growth over entire pubis; hair is darker, coarser, and curly	Enlargement, especially in length	Further enlargement
4	Thick growth over pubic area but not on thighs; hair coarse and curly, as in adult	Continued enlargement in length and diameter, with development of glans	Testes almost fully grown; scrotum darker
5	Growth spread over medial thighs, although not yet up toward umbilicus; after puberty, pubic hair growth continues until the mid-20s, extending up the abdomen toward the umbilicus	Adult size and shape	Adult size and shape

Adapted from Tanner, J. M. (1962). *Growth at adolescence.* Oxford, UK: Blackwell Scientific Publications.

Structure and Function

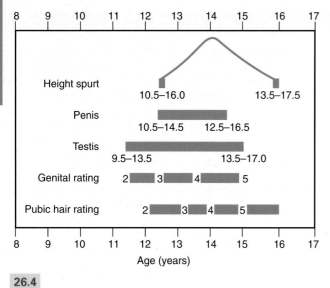

26.4

the tubules, and so these become thickened and produce less sperm.

In general, declining testosterone production leaves older men with a slower and less intense sexual response. Although a wide range of individual differences can occur, an older man may find that an erection takes longer to develop and that it is less full or firm. Once obtained, the erection may be maintained for longer periods without ejaculation. Ejaculation is shorter and less forceful, and the volume of seminal fluid is less than when the man was younger. After ejaculation, detumescence (return to the flaccid state) is rapid, especially after 60 years of age. This occurs in a few seconds, in comparison with minutes or hours in a younger man. The refractory state—when the man is physiologically unable to ejaculate—lasts longer (from 12 to 24 hours) than in a younger man (2 minutes).

Sexual Expression in Later Life

Chronological age by itself should not halt sexual activity. The aforementioned physical changes need not interfere with libido or pleasure from sexual intercourse. An older man is capable of sexual function as long as he is in reasonably good health and has an interested, willing partner. Even chronic illness does not put a complete end to sexual desire or activity.

An older man may misinterpret normal age changes as sexual failure. Once this idea occurs, it may demoralize the man and place undue emphasis on performance rather than on pleasure. In the absence of disease, older men may withdraw from sexual activity for various reasons: loss of spouse; depression; preoccupation with work; marital or family conflict; adverse effects of medications such as antihypertensives, psychotropics, antidepressants, antispasmodics, sedatives, tranquilizers or narcotics, and estrogens; heavy use of alcohol; lack of privacy (living with adult children or in a nursing home); economic or emotional stress; poor nutrition; or fatigue.

 ## SOCIAL DETERMINANTS OF HEALTH CONSIDERATIONS

Circumcision is an elective surgical procedure to remove all or part of the foreskin (prepuce) from the penis, usually performed on newborn males. Parents need an unbiased presentation of risks and benefits of this procedure so they can be weighed in the context of their own religious and cultural beliefs. Circumcision of newborn males in Canada has declined over the past few decades to the current Canadian average of 32%, in response to past recommendations from the Canadian Paediatric Society (CPS) affirming the procedure was not medically indicated.[1] While the CPS does not recommend routine circumcision of every newborn male, recent evidence indicates there are potential health benefits associated with male circumcision, particularly in populations at high risk for sexually transmitted infections (STIs). Infant circumcision reduces incidence of urinary tract infections (UTIs) and eliminates the need for medical circumcision in later childhood to treat recurrent balanoposthitis, paraphimosis, and phimosis. Circumcised men have a lower risk of developing penile cancer or contracting STIs, including human immunodeficiency virus (HIV), herpes simplex virus (HSV), and human papillomavirus (HPV), while their female sexual partners have a reduced incidence of trichomonas, bacterial vaginosis, and cervical cancer.

Circumcision carries a very small risk for complications. Most are minor and treatable: pain, bleeding, swelling, or inadequate skin removal. Serious complications are rare and include excess bleeding, wound infections, and urinary retention.[2] Neonates are capable of perceiving pain; therefore, parents need to be apprised of pain-relief measures for the circumcision procedure, including local anaesthetic given by a needle, topical anaesthetic creams, and oral pain medication, as well as comfort measures such as providing a sucrose pacifier, holding the infant, and nursing often.[3]

For an uncircumcised newborn, assess parental knowledge about care of the uncircumcised penis. The infant's penis should be cleansed with soap and water, but the foreskin should not be forcibly retracted. When the foreskin retracts easily, the area under the foreskin should be cleansed occasionally. By the age of 3 or 4 years, a boy can be taught to clean under his foreskin. When a boy reaches puberty, he needs to clean under his foreskin daily.

Infection with HPV is common in boys and men, causes most cases of genital warts, and is associated with cancers of the penis, anus, and head and neck. The quadrivalent HPV vaccine previously approved for prevention of cervical cancer in girls and women (see p. 757) has demonstrated efficacy in preventing HPV infection and diseases in boys and men.[4] In Canada, the vaccine is recommended for prevention of penile and anal cancers and anogenital warts in males aged 9 to 26, and in males who have sex with males aged 9 and over.[5]

When conducting a physical examination of a transgender person, examination of the genitalia should be relevant to the anatomy that is present and must be done with sensitivity. Sex organs and secondary sex characteristics will vary depending on history of gender-affirming surgery (GAS), hormone therapy, or both. Nurses should use a gender-affirming approach by using general terminology for body parts or asking patients if they have a preferred term to be used. Routine cancer screening for transgender patients should be conducted in accordance with current guidelines if they have the particular body part or organ and otherwise meet criteria for screening based on risk factors or symptoms, regardless of hormone use.[6] Transgender women who have not undergone GAS may practise "tucking" to provide a female-appearing genital contour by manually displacing their testes up into the inguinal canal and positioning the penis and scrotal skin back between the legs with tape or tight underwear. Prolonged tucking may result in pain, urinary reflux, prostatitis, or cystitis.

SUBJECTIVE DATA

1. Frequency, urgency, and nocturia
2. Dysuria
3. Hesitancy and straining
4. Urine colour
5. Past genitourinary history
6. Penis: pain, lesion, discharge
7. Scrotum: self-care behaviours, lump
8. Sexual activity and contraceptive use
9. STI contact
10. STI risk reduction

HEALTH HISTORY QUESTIONS

Examiner Asks	Rationale
1. **Frequency, urgency, and nocturia.** Are you urinating more often than usual?	The average adult voids five to six times per day; this amount varies with fluid intake, individual habits. Polyuria: excessive quantity. Oliguria: diminished quantity, <400 mL/24 hr.
• When you need to urinate, do you feel as if you cannot wait?	Urgency may be indicative of infection or conditions causing irritation or obstruction.
• Do you awaken during the night because you need to urinate? How often? Is this a recent change?	Nocturia occurs together with frequency and urgency in urinary tract disorders. Other origins: cardiovascular, diabetes, habitual, diuretic medication.
2. **Dysuria.** Any pain or burning sensation with urinating?	Dysuria is a burning sensation that is common with acute cystitis, prostatitis, and urethritis.
3. **Hesitancy and straining.** Any trouble starting the urine stream?	Hesitancy may be indicative of prostate enlargement.
• Do you need to strain to start or maintain the stream?	Straining may be indicative of prostate enlargement.
• Any change in force of stream: narrowing, becoming weaker?	Loss of force and decreased calibre should be investigated.
• Do you experience dribbling, so that you must stand closer to the toilet?	Terminal dribbling should be investigated.
• Afterwards, do you still feel you need to urinate?	Sense of residual urine should be investigated.

Examiner Asks	Rationale
• Have you ever had any urinary tract infections (UTIs)?	Recurrent episodes of acute cystitis should be investigated. Aforementioned symptoms (i.e., hesitancy and so on) suggest progressive prostatic obstruction.
4. Urine colour. What colour is your urine? Is urine usually clear or discoloured, cloudy, foul-smelling, bloody (Table 26.2, p. 768)?	Dark yellow, strong-smelling urine is a sign of dehydration. Urine is cloudy in UTI. Some colour changes are temporary or harmless. However, for blood in urine or for a colour change lasting more than 1 day, the patient should seek health care (see Critical Findings box below). For a complete description, see Table 26.2, p. 768.

CRITICAL FINDINGS

Hematuria (blood in the urine)—a danger sign that warrants further workup—is the most common symptom of cancers of the bladder and kidney. Hematuria is also associated with disease, inflammation, infection, or trauma within the urinary tract.

Examiner Asks	Rationale
5. Past genitourinary history. Do you have any difficulty controlling your urine?	True incontinence: loss of urine without warning. Urge incontinence: involuntary urine loss from overactive detrusor muscle in bladder; bladder contracts, causing urgent need to void. Stress incontinence: involuntary loss of urine with physical strain, sneezing, or coughing; caused by weakness in pelvic floor.
• Do you accidentally urinate when you sneeze, laugh, cough, or bear down? • Any history of kidney disease, kidney stones, flank pain, UTIs, prostate trouble? • Are you using any medications? Prescription, over-the-counter or natural therapies? Which ones?	
6. Penis: pain, lesion, discharge. Any problem with your penis: pain, lesions? • Any discharge? How much? Has that increased or decreased since it started? • What colour is it? Any odour? Is the discharge associated with pain or with urination?	Urethral discharge occurs with infection (see Table 26.3, p. 769).
7. Scrotum: self-care behaviours, lump. Any problem with the scrotum or testicles? • Do you perform testicular self-examination (TSE)? • Have you noticed any lump or swelling on your testes? • Have you noted any change in size of the scrotum? • Have you noted any bulge or swelling in the scrotum? For how long? Have you ever been told you have a hernia? Any dragging, heavy feeling in scrotum?	Assess self-care behaviours (see Self-Care: Knowing Your Testicles, p. 764). Concern about any self-discovered mass (spermatocele, hydrocele, varicocele, rarely testicular cancer) alerts you to careful exploration during examination. Assess for possible hernia.

Examiner Asks	Rationale

8. Sexual activity and contraceptive use. Have you been engaged in sexual activity in the last 6 months?
- Do you have a regular sexual partner?
- Are aspects of sex satisfactory to you and your partner/s?
- Are you satisfied with the way you and your partner/s communicate about sex?

- Occasionally a man notices a change in ability to have an erection when aroused. Have you noticed any changes?* Have you used any medications or natural therapies for erectile dysfunction? Which ones?

- How many sexual partners have you had in the past 6 months?

- What is your sexual preference: sexual activity with a woman, a man, both?
- Do you or your partner/s use a contraceptive? Which method? Is this satisfactory? Any questions about this method? Other methods?

9. STI contact. Any sexual contact with a partner who has an STI, such as gonorrhea, herpes, HIV, *Chlamydia* infection, genital warts, syphilis? When? How was this treated? Were there any complications? Any questions or concerns about any of these infections?

10. STI risk reduction. Do you take any precautions to reduce risk for STIs? Do you use condoms every time you have sexual intercourse? Other methods?

Rationale

Questions about sexual activity should be routine in review of body systems for these reasons:

- This question communicates your acceptance of the patient's sexual activity and belief it is important.
- Your comfort with discussion prompts patient's interest and possibly relief that topic has been introduced and gives the patient permission to talk about sexual health.
  - Erectile dysfunction (ED) is the inability to get and keep an erection firm enough for sex, and may be a warning sign of current or future heart disease or type 2 diabetes.
- This question helps you establish a database for comparisons with any future sexual activities.
- It also provides an opportunity to screen for sexual problems.
  Your questions should be objective and matter-of-fact.
  Gay and bisexual men need to feel acceptance to discuss their health concerns.

An STI is any condition that can be transmitted during intercourse or intimate sexual contact with an infected partner.

Male and female condoms help protect both partners from STIs, including HIV. Dental dams or condoms cut open help prevent STI transmission during oral sex.

Additional History for Infants and Children

1. Urination. Does your child have any problem urinating? Does the urine stream look straight?
- Any pain, crying, or holding the genitals when your child urinates?
- Has your child had any urinary tract infection (UTI)?

2. Toilet training. (If child is older than 2½ years of age.) Has toilet training started? How is it progressing?
- (If child is 5 years or older.) Does the child wet the bed at night? Is this a problem for the child or for you (parents)? What have you done? How does the child feel about it?

Nocturnal enuresis: involuntary passing of urine after an age at which continence is expected.

*Phrase your questions so that the patient is comfortable acknowledging a problem.

Examiner Asks	Rationale

3. **Abnormalities.** Any problem with child's penis or scrotum: sores, swelling, discoloration?
   - Have you been told whether the child's testes are descended or undescended?
   - Has the child ever had a hernia or hydrocele?
   - Have you seen swelling in the child's scrotum during crying or coughing?

4. **Molestation.** (Ask directly of preschooler or young school-age child.) "Has anyone ever touched your penis or in between your legs and you did not want them to? Sometimes that happens to children, and it's not okay."

Screen for sexual abuse (see Chapter 8). Service providers, including nurses, have an ethical and legal obligation to report suspected child abuse. For prevention, teach the child that it is not "okay" for someone to look at or touch his private parts while telling him it is a secret. The patient who has been abused should be told that he has not been "bad" and that he should try to tell an adult about it: "Can you tell me three different big people you trust who you could talk to?" Being asked to name three trusted adults will help the child include someone outside the family; this is important because molestation is often performed by a parent.

Additional History for Preadolescents and Adolescents

Use the following questions, as appropriate, to assess sexual growth and development and sexual behaviour:
- Ask questions appropriate for a child's age, but be aware that norms vary widely. When in doubt, it is better to ask too many questions than to omit something. Children obtain information, often misinformation, from the media and from peers at surprisingly early ages. Your information will be more thoughtful and accurate.
- Ask direct, matter-of-fact questions. Avoid sounding judgemental.
- Start with a *permission statement*. "Often boys your age experience … ." This conveys that it is normal and all right to think or feel a certain way.
- Try the *ubiquity approach*. "When did you … ?" rather than "Do you … ?" This method is less threatening because it implies that the topic is normal and unexceptional.
- Do not be concerned if an adolescent will not discuss sexuality with you or respond to offers for information. Adolescents may not feel comfortable letting on that they need or want more information. You should convey your willingness to talk when the adolescent is ready. The adolescent may come back at a future time.

1. **Puberty.** At approximately 12 to 13 years old, but sometimes earlier, boys start to change and grow around the penis and scrotum. What changes have you noticed? Have you ever seen charts and pictures of normal growth patterns for boys? Let's go over these now.
   - Whom can you talk to about your body changes and about sex information? How do these talks go? Do you think you get enough information? What about sex education classes at school? How about your parents? Is there a favourite teacher, nurse, doctor, minister, or counsellor to whom you can talk?

Examiner Asks	Rationale
2. Nocturnal emission. Boys approximately 12 to 13 years old (sexual maturity rating 3) have a normal experience of fluid coming out of the penis at night, called a *nocturnal emission*, or "wet dream." Have you had this?	On occasion, a boy confuses this with a sign of STI or feels guilty.
3. Erotic feelings. Teenage boys have other normal experiences and wonder if they are the only ones who ever had them, like having an erection at embarrassing times, having sexual fantasies, or masturbating. Also, a boy might have a thought about touching another boy's genitals and wonder whether this means he might be homosexual. Would you like to talk about any of these things?	A boy may feel guilty about experiencing these feelings if he is not informed that they are normal.
4. Sexual activity. Often boys your age have questions about sexual activity. What questions do you have? How about things such as birth control, or STIs such as gonorrhea or herpes? Any questions about these? • Are you dating? Someone steady? Male or female? Have you had sexual intercourse? Oral sex? Are you using birth control? What kind? • What kind of birth control did you use the *last* time you had intercourse?	Assess level of knowledge. Many boys do not admit that they need more knowledge. Teach STI risk reduction. Avoid the term "having sex." It is ambiguous, and teenagers can take it to mean anything from foreplay to intercourse. Use behaviour-specific words. This particular question often elicits the information that the teenager is not using any method of birth control.
5. Immunization. Have you and your parents discussed the HPV vaccine (Gardasil)? It is recommended before boys become sexually active.	HPV vaccines are approved for males aged 9 to 26 for prevention of anal cancers and anogenital warts.
6. Self-examination. Has a nurse or doctor ever taught you how to examine your testicles to make sure they are healthy?	Assess knowledge of testicular self-examination (see Self-Care: Knowing Your Testicles, p. 764).
7. Molestation. Has anyone ever touched your genitals when you did not want them to? Another boy, or an adult, even a relative? Sometimes that happens to teenagers.	Patients should understand that it is not their fault. They should tell another adult they trust. Service providers, including nurses, have an ethical and legal obligation to report suspected child abuse.

Additional History for Older Adults

1. Prostate enlargement. Do you have any difficulty urinating? Any hesitancy and straining? Is the force of stream weaker? Any dribbling? Or any incomplete emptying?	Early symptoms of enlarging prostate may be tolerated or ignored. Later symptoms are more dramatic: hematuria, UTI.
2. Incontinence. Do you ever leak water/urine when you do not want to? Do you use pads or tissue to catch urine in your underwear?	*Incontinence* is any involuntary leaking of urine.
3. Nocturia. Do you need to get up at night to urinate? What medications are you taking? What fluids do you drink in the evening?	Nocturia may be habitual, or it may be caused by diuretic medication or fluid ingestion 3 hours before bedtime; coffee and alcohol in particular have a diuretic effect. Also, fluid retention from mild heart failure or varicose veins produces nocturia because recumbency at night mobilizes fluid.

Subjective Data

Examiner Asks	Rationale
4. Sexual function. A man in his 70s or older may experience changes in his sexual relationship or his sexual response; have you noticed this? Have you wondered whether it is normal? For example, it is normal for an erection to develop slowly at this age. This is not a sign of impotence, but a man might wonder if it is. Except in cases of physical illness, older men are fully capable of sexual function.	Some older men assume that normal changes mean they are "old men" and withdraw from sexual activity. Older men are not usually reluctant to discuss sexual activity, and most welcome the opportunity. Substances that depress sexual desire and function include antihypertensives, sedatives, tranquilizers, estrogens, and alcohol. Alcohol decreases the sexual response even more dramatically in older men.

OBJECTIVE DATA

PREPARATION

Position the male patient standing, with underwear down. Appropriate draping protects the modesty of the patient. This is important for male patients of all ethnocultural backgrounds. The examiner should be sitting. Alternatively, the patient may be supine for the first part of the examination and stand to be checked for a hernia.

It is normal for a male patient to feel apprehensive about having his genitalia examined, especially by a female examiner. Younger adolescents usually have more anxiety than do older adolescents. However, any male patient may have difficulty dissociating a necessary, matter-of-fact step in the physical examination from the feeling that this is an invasion of his privacy. His concerns are similar to those experienced by the female patient during the examination of the genitalia: modesty, fear of pain, cold hands, negative judgement, or memory of previously uncomfortable examinations. In addition, he may fear comparison with other male patients, or he may fear having an erection during the examination and that this would be misinterpreted by the examiner.

This normal apprehension becomes manifested in different behaviours. Many patients act resigned and embarrassed and avoid eye contact. Some will laugh and make jokes to cover embarrassment. Also, a man may refuse examination by a female and insist on a male examiner.

Take time to consider these feelings, and explore your own. It is normal for you to feel embarrassed and apprehensive, too. You may worry about your age, lack of clinical experience, causing pain, or even that your movements might "cause" an erection. Some examiners feel guilty when this occurs. You need to accept these feelings and work through them so you can examine the male patient in a professional way. Discuss these concerns with an experienced examiner. Your unresolved discomfort magnifies any discomfort the patient may have.

Your demeanour should be confident and relaxed, unhurried and yet businesslike. Do not discuss genitourinary history or sexual practices while you are performing the examination; this may be perceived as judgemental. Use a firm, deliberate touch, not a soft, stroking one. If an erection does occur, do *not* stop the examination or leave the room. This only focuses more attention on the erection and increases embarrassment. Reassure the male patient that this is only a normal physiological response to touch, just as when the pupil constricts in response to bright light. Proceed with the rest of the examination.

EQUIPMENT NEEDED

Gloves: wear gloves during every examination of male genitalia
Occasionally: glass slide for urethral specimen
Materials for cytological study
Flashlight

Normal Range of Findings

Inspect and Palpate The Penis

The skin normally looks wrinkled, hairless, and without lesions (Fig. 26.5). The dorsal vein may be apparent.

26.5

The glans looks smooth and lesion-free. Ask the uncircumcised male patient to retract the foreskin, or you retract it. It should move easily. Some cheesy smegma may have collected under the foreskin. After inspection, slide the foreskin back to the original position.

The urethral meatus is positioned just about centrally.

At the base of the penis, pubic hair distribution is consistent with age. Hair is without infestations.

Abnormal Findings

Inflammation.
Lesions: nodules, solitary ulcer (chancre), grouped vesicles or superficial ulcers, wartlike papules (see Table 26.4, p. 770).

Inflammation; lesions on glans or corona.
Phimosis: inability to retract the foreskin.
Paraphimosis: inability to return foreskin to original position.
Hypospadias: ventral location of meatus.
Epispadias: dorsal location of meatus (see Table 26.5, p. 773).
Pubic lice or nits can be seen with the unaided eye. Excoriated skin usually accompanies their presence.

Objective Data

Normal Range of Findings

Compress the glans anteroposteriorly between your thumb and forefinger (Fig. 26.6). The meatus edge should appear pink, smooth, and without discharge.

26.6

If you note urethral discharge, collect a smear for microscopic examination and a culture. If no discharge shows but the person gives a history of it, ask him to milk the shaft of the penis. This should produce a drop of discharge.

Palpate the shaft of the penis between your thumb and first two fingers. Normally, the penis feels smooth, semifirm, and nontender.

Inspect and Palpate The Scrotum

Inspect the scrotum as the patient holds the penis out of the way. Alternatively, you hold the penis out of the way with the back of your hand (Fig. 26.7). Scrotal size varies with ambient room temperature. Asymmetry is normal; the left scrotal half is usually lower than the right half.

26.7

Abnormal Findings

Stricture: narrowed opening.

Edges that are red, everted, and edematous, along with purulent discharge, are suggestive of urethritis (see Table 26.3, p. 769).

Urethral discharge occurs with infection.

Nodule or induration.
Tenderness.

Scrotal swelling (edema) may be taut and pitting. This occurs with heart failure, renal failure, and local inflammation.

Lesions should be investigated.

Normal Range of Findings

Spread rugae out between your fingers. Lift the sac to inspect the posterior surface. Normally, no scrotal lesions are present, except for sebaceous cysts, which are commonly found. These are yellowish, 1-cm nodules and are firm, nontender, and often multiple.

Palpate each scrotal half gently between your thumb and first two fingers (Fig. 26.8). The scrotal contents should slide easily. Testes normally feel oval, firm and rubbery, smooth, and equal bilaterally, and they are freely movable and slightly tender to moderate pressure. Each epididymis normally feels discrete, softer than the testis, smooth, and nontender.

26.8

Palpate each spermatic cord between your thumb and forefinger, along its length from the epididymis up to the external inguinal ring (Fig. 26.9, *A*). You should feel a smooth, nontender cord.

26.9   **A,** Palpating each spermatic cord. **B,** Varicocele.

Abnormal Findings

Inflammation.

Absence of testis: may be a temporary migration or true cryptorchidism (see Table 26.6, p. 769).
Atrophied testes: small and soft.
Fixed testes.
Nodules on testes or epididymides.
Marked tenderness.
An indurated, swollen, and tender epididymis: indicative of epididymitis.

Thickened cord.
Soft, swollen, and tortuous cord: see the varicocele in Fig. 26.9, *B*.

Normal Range of Findings

Normally, no other scrotal contents are present. If you do find a mass, note the following:

- Is there any tenderness?
- Is the mass distal or proximal to testis?
- Can you place your fingers over it?
- Is it reduced when the patient lies down?
- Can you auscultate bowel sounds over it?

Transillumination. Perform this manoeuvre only if you note a swelling or mass. Darken the room. Shine a strong flashlight from behind the scrotal contents. Normal scrotal contents cannot be transilluminated.

Inspect and Palpate for Hernia

Inspect the inguinal region for a bulge as the patient stands and as the patient strains down. Normally, none is present.

Palpate the inguinal canal (Fig. 26.10). For the right side, ask the patient to shift his weight onto the left (unexamined) leg. Place your right index finger low on the right scrotal half. Palpate up the length of the spermatic cord, invaginating the scrotal skin as you go, to the external inguinal ring. It feels like a triangular slitlike opening, and it may or may not admit your finger. If it will admit your finger, gently insert it into the canal and ask the person to "bear down."* Normally, you feel no change. Repeat the procedure on the left side.

Palpate the femoral area for a bulge. Normally, you feel none.

External inguinal ring

26.10

Abnormal Findings

Abnormalities in the scrotum: hernia, tumour, orchitis, epididymitis, hydrocele, spermatocele, varicocele (see Table 26.6, p. 774).

Serous fluid (e.g., hydrocele or spermatocele) can be transilluminated and glows red. Solid tissue (e.g., hernia, epididymitis, or tumour) and blood cannot be transilluminated (see Table 26.6, p. 774).

Bulge at external inguinal ring or at femoral canal should be investigated. (A hernia may be present but is easily reduced and may appear only intermittently with an increase in intra-abdominal pressure.)

A palpable herniating mass bumps your fingertip or pushes against the side of your finger (see Table 26.7, p. 777).

*Avoid the old instruction to "turn your head and cough." For one thing, a brief cough does not produce the steady, increased intra-abdominal pressure you need. For another, the patient might cough in your face.

Objective Data

Normal Range of Findings

Palpate the Inguinal Lymph Nodes

Palpate the horizontal chain along the groin inferior to the inguinal ligament and the vertical chain along the upper inner thigh.

It is normal to palpate an isolated node on occasion; it then feels small (<1 cm), soft, discrete, and movable (Fig. 26.11).

Enlarged, hard, matted, fixed nodes.

26.11

Assessment of Urine Output

Normal adult urine output is 1 500 mL per day, and most people urinate five to six times during the day and occasionally at night; however, the amount and frequency of urination varies with food and fluid intake, and bladder capacity, which normally ranges from 600 to 1 000 mL. On average, 200 to 250 mL of urine in the bladder causes moderate distension and the urge to urinate; whereas 400 to 600 mL or more causes discomfort.[7]

> ### CRITICAL FINDINGS
>
> **Acute urinary retention** is an inability to pass urine, characterized by lower abdominal pain and bladder distension. It may be confirmed by bladder scan. Report acute urinary retention immediately; management involves bladder decompression by intermittent or indwelling urinary catheter.

Assessment of Patient With Indwelling Urinary Catheter

Monitor catheterized patients for signs and symptoms of catheter-acquired UTI, the most common infection in acute and long-term care settings. Risk factors include prolonged catheterization (>6 days), female gender, diabetes, malnutrition, old age, and impaired immunity.

Catheter should be properly anchored; tubing should be free from kinking; collecting bag should be below bladder level (Fig. 26.12); urethral meatus is pink, smooth, and without discharge.

Assess urine output.

Urgency, suprapubic tenderness, costovertebral angle pain or tenderness, fever >38°C (100.4°F), change in character of urine (bloody, foul smell, increased sediment), positive dipstick for leukocytes, worsening of mental or functional status.

Drainage or excoriation of urethral orifice.

Normal Range of Findings	Abnormal Findings

26.12 Indwelling urinary catheter.

Self-Care: Knowing Your Testicles

The overall incidence is rare, but testicular cancer occurs most commonly in men aged 15 to 29. Other risk factors include delayed descent of the testicles (if not corrected early), family or personal history of testicular cancer, and abnormal development of the testicle. Some men develop testicular cancer without having any of these risk factors. If detected early by palpation and treated, the cure rate is almost 100%; therefore, all men aged 15 years and older should be aware of how their testicles normally look and feel.

A good time to examine the testicles is just after a warm bath or shower. The heat from the water relaxes the scrotum and makes the testicles descend. Carefully feel each testicle for any changes such as a lump or tenderness. The testicle is egg-shaped and movable. It feels rubbery with a smooth surface, like a peeled hard-boiled egg. Compare the two sides and note any differences; it is normal for one testicle to be larger than the other one. The epididymis is a tube on top and behind each testicle and feels like a soft cord or small bump. Report any changes to a doctor as soon as possible.[9]

❖ DEVELOPMENTAL CONSIDERATIONS

Infants and Children

For an infant or toddler, perform this procedure right after the abdominal examination. In preschool-age and young school-age children (3 to 8 years of age), leave underwear on until just before the examination. In an older school-age child or adolescent, offer an extra drape, as with an adult. Reassure the child and parents of normal findings.

CRITICAL FINDINGS

Decreased urine output may be a sign of renal or systemic problems such as dehydration, renal failure, or hypovolemic shock. In an adult, urine output of less than 30 mL/hour can indicate decreased renal perfusion and should be reported.[8]

Normal Range of Findings

Inspect the penis and scrotum. Penis size is usually small in infants (2 to 3 cm; Fig. 26.13) and in young boys until puberty. In obese boys, the penis looks even smaller because of folds of skin covering the base.

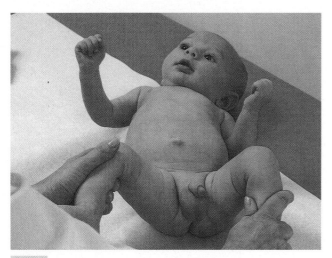

26.13

In the circumcised infant, the glans looks smooth with the meatus centred at the tip. During the diaper-wearing stage, the meatus may become ulcerated from ammonia irritation. This is more common in circumcised infants.

If possible, observe the newborn's first voiding to assess strength and direction of stream.

If the infant is uncircumcised, the foreskin is normally tight during the first 3 months and should *not* be retracted because of the risk of tearing the membrane attaching the foreskin to the shaft. This leads to scarring and, possibly, adhesions later in life. In infants older than 3 months of age, retract the foreskin gently to check the glans and meatus. It should return to its original position easily.

The scrotum looks pink in light-skinned infants and dark brown in dark-skinned infants. Rugae are well formed in full-term infants. Size varies with ambient temperature, but overall, the infant's scrotum looks large in relation to the penis. No bulges, either constant or intermittent, are present.

Palpate the scrotum and testes. The cremasteric reflex is strong in the infant, pulling the testes up into the inguinal canal and abdomen from exposure to cold, touch, exercise, or emotion. Take care not to elicit the reflex; to prevent it, keep your hands warm and palpate from the external inguinal ring down, and block the inguinal canals with the thumb and forefinger of your other hand to prevent the testes from retracting (Fig. 26.14).

Abnormal Findings

In rare cases, a very small penis may be an enlarged clitoris in a genetically female infant.

Enlarged penis is indicative of precocious puberty.

Redness, swelling, and lesions should be investigated.

Urethral discharge occurs with infection.

Hypospadias, epispadias (see Table 26.5, p. 773) should be corrected.

Stricture is a narrowed opening.

On occasion, ulceration may produce a stricture, evidenced by a pinpoint meatus and a narrow stream. This increases the risk for urine obstruction.

Poor stream is significant because it may indicate a stricture or neurogenic bladder.

In phimosis, the foreskin is tight and cannot be retracted.

In paraphimosis, the foreskin cannot be slipped forward once it is retracted.

Dirt and smegma may collect under the foreskin.

Objective Data

Normal Range of Findings	Abnormal Findings

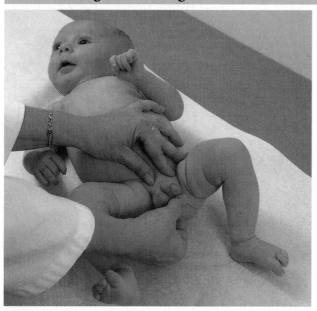

26.14

Normally, the testes are descended and equal in size bilaterally (1.5 to 2 cm until puberty). It is important to document that you have palpated the testes. Once palpated, they are considered descended, even if they have retracted momentarily at the next visit.

If the scrotal half feels empty, search for the testes along the inguinal canal and try to milk them down. Ask the toddler or child to squat with the knees flexed up; this pressure may force the testes down. Another manoeuvre is have the young child sit cross-legged to relax the reflex (Fig. 26.15).

Cryptorchidism: undescended testes (those that have never descended). Undescended testes are common in premature infants. They occur in 3% to 4% of full-term infants, although in most cases, they have descended by 3 months of age. Physicians have different opinions concerning the age at which an affected child should be referred (see Table 26.6, p. 774).

26.15

Migratory testes (physiological cryptorchidism) are common because of the strength of the cremasteric reflex and the small mass of the prepubertal testes. Note that the affected side has a normally developed scrotum (with true cryptorchidism, the scrotum is atrophic) and the testis can be milked down. These testes descend at puberty and are normal.

Normal Range of Findings	Abnormal Findings
Palpate the epididymis and spermatic cord as described for adults. A common scrotal finding in the boy younger than 2 years is a hydrocele (fluid in the scrotum). It appears as enlargement of the scrotum and glows faint pink under transillumination. It usually disappears spontaneously. Inspect the inguinal area for a bulge. If you do not see a bulge but the parent gives a positive history of one, try to elicit it by increasing intra-abdominal pressure. Ask the boy to hold his breath and strain down, or have him blow up a balloon. If a hernia is suspected, palpate the inguinal area. Use your little finger to reach the external inguinal ring.	A hydrocele is a cystic collection of serous fluid in the tunica vaginalis, surrounding the testis (see Table 26.6, p. 776).

Adolescents

Adolescents show wide variation in normal development of the genitals. Using the sexual maturity rating charts, note (a) enlargement of the testes and scrotum; (b) pubic hair growth; (c) darkening of scrotal colour; (d) roughening of scrotal skin; (e) increase in penis length and width; and (f) axillary hair growth.

Be familiar with the normal sequence of growth.

Older Adults

In older men, you may note thinner, greying pubic hair and decreased size of the penis. Testes may decrease in size and feel less firm. The scrotal sac is pendulous, with fewer rugae. The scrotal skin may become excoriated if the man continually sits on it.

DOCUMENTATION AND CRITICAL THINKING

Sample Charting

SUBJECTIVE

Urinates four to five times per day; urine clear, straw-coloured. No nocturia, dysuria, or hesitancy. No pain, lesions, or discharge from penis. Does not perform TSE. No history of genitourinary disease. Sexually active in a monogamous relationship. Sexual life satisfactory to self and partner. Uses birth control via barrier method (partner uses diaphragm). No known STI contact.

OBJECTIVE

No lesions, inflammation, or discharge from penis. Scrotum: testes descended, symmetrical, no masses. No inguinal hernia.

ASSESSMENT

Genital structures normal.

Focused Assessment: Clinical Case Study

Riku Tanaka (R.T.) is a 19-year-old student who noted acute onset of painful urination, frequency, and urgency 2 days ago. Noted some thick penile discharge.

SUBJECTIVE

States has no side pain, no abdominal pain, no fever, no genital skin rash. R.T. is concerned he has an STI because of episode of unprotected intercourse with a new partner 6 days ago. Has no known allergies.

OBJECTIVE

Vital signs: Temp 37°C (98.6°F), pulse 72 bpm [beats per minute], resp 16/min. No lesions or inflammation around penis or scrotum. Urethral meatus has mild edema with purulent urethral discharge. No pain on palpation of genitalia. Testes symmetrical with no masses. No lymphadenopathy.

ASSESSMENT

Urethral discharge
Deficient knowledge about STI prevention R/T [related to] lack of information recall

ABNORMAL FINDINGS

TABLE 26.2   Urine Colour and Discolorations

- Medication side effect: amitriptyline, indomethacin (Indocin)
- Foods: asparagus
- Dye after prostate surgery

Blue

- Urine contains melanin, melaninuria

Dark Grey

- Liver disease, especially with pale stools, jaundice
- Myoglobinuria
- Some medications or food dyes
- Blood in urine

Tea

- UTI
- Kidney stones

Cloudy

- Clear, watery with excess liquids
- Acute viral hepatitis, cirrhosis

Pale Yellow

- Some foods: beets, berries, food dyes
- Some laxatives
- Kidney stones
- UTI

Pink

- Natural yellow is urochrome excretion, a pigment in blood
- Bright neon yellow with vitamin supplements

Yellow

- Blood in urine
- Nephritis, cystitis
- Cancer
- Following prostate surgery

Red

Amber

- Gold coloured or concentrated with dehydration
- Some laxatives
- Food or supplements with B-complex vitamins

Orange

- Medication side effect: rifampin for meningitis, phenazopyridine (Pyridium), warfarin (Coumadin)
- Some foods, food dyes, laxatives
- Dehydration
- Jaundice (bilirubinemia)

UTI, Urinary tract infection.
See illustration Credits for source information.

TABLE 26.3   Urinary Problems

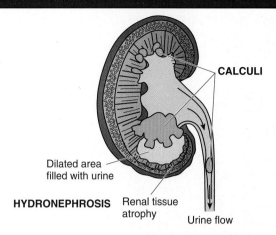

CALCULI

Dilated area
filled with urine

HYDRONEPHROSIS   Renal tissue
atrophy

Urine flow

Urethritis (Urethral Discharge and Dysuria)

Infection of urethra causes painful burning urination or
pruritus. Meatus edges are reddened, everted, and swollen
with purulent discharge. Urine is cloudy with discharge
and mucous shreds. Cause determined by culture: in
gonococcal urethritis, discharge is thick, profuse, and
yellow or grey-brown; in nonspecific urethritis, discharge
may be similar but often is scanty and mucoid. Of these
infections, about 50% are caused by *Chlamydia* organisms.
This is important to differentiate because antibiotic
treatment is different.

Renal Calculi

Renal stones (crystals of calcium oxalate or uric acid)
form in kidney tubules and then migrate. Their presence
becomes an emergency when they pass into the ureter,
become lodged, and obstruct urine flow. They cause
abrupt, severe flank pain, which radiates to the groin or
abdomen; nausea and vomiting; restlessness; and gross or
microscopic hematuria.

Acute Urinary Retention (Not Illustrated)

Affected patients experience abrupt inability to pass urine,
with bladder distension and lower abdominal pain.
This is much more common in men than in women
because of bladder outlet obstruction, such as benign
prostatic hypertrophy (see Chapter 23). Catheterization
must be performed to relieve acute discomfort; then the
underlying problem must be managed.

See illustration Credits for source information.

TABLE 26.4 Male Genital Lesions

Tinea Cruris

A fungal infection in the crural fold, not extending to scrotum, occurring in postpubertal males ("jock itch") after sweating or wearing layers of occlusive clothing. It forms a red-brown half-moon shape with well-defined borders.

Genital Herpes: HSV-2 Infection

Clusters of small vesicles with surrounding erythema, which are often painful, erupt on the glans or foreskin. These rupture to form superficial ulcers. Genital herpes is a sexually transmitted infection (STI); the initial manifestation lasts 7–10 days. The virus remains dormant indefinitely; recurrent manifestations last 3–10 days with milder symptoms.

◀ Syphilitic Chancre

Manifests within 2–4 weeks of infection as a small, solitary, silvery papule that erodes to a red, round or oval, superficial ulcer with a yellowish serous discharge. Palpation reveals a nontender, indurated base that can be lifted like a button between thumb and finger. Lymph nodes enlarge early but are nontender. Syphilis, an STI, is easily treated with penicillin G; if untreated, leads to cardiac problems, neurological problems, and blindness.

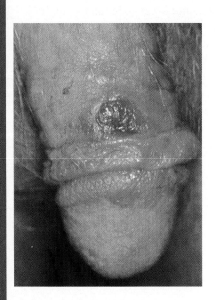

TABLE 26.4	Male Genital Lesions—cont'd

Genital Warts

Soft, pointed, moist, fleshy, painless papules may be single or multiple in a cauliflowerlike patch. Colour may be grey, pale yellow, or pink in Euro-Canadian men and black or translucent grey-black in men of African descent. They occur on the shaft of the penis, behind the corona, or around the anus, where they may grow into large grapelike clusters.

These are caused by the human papillomavirus (HPV), which is one of the most common STIs. The HPV infection is correlated with early onset of sexual activity, infrequent use of contraception, and multiple sexual partners.

Carcinoma

Begins as red, raised warty growth or as an ulcer, with watery discharge. As it grows, it may necrose and slough. It is usually painless. It almost always appears on the glans or inner lip of the foreskin and after chronic inflammation. Enlarged lymph nodes are common.

See illustration Credits for source information.

TABLE 26.5   Abnormalities of the Penis

Phimosis

Nonretractable foreskin forms a pointy tip with a tiny orifice. Foreskin is advanced and so tight that it is impossible to retract over glans. May be congenital or acquired from adhesions secondary to infection. Poor hygiene leads to retained dirt and smegma, which increases the risk for inflammation, calculus formation, and obstructive uropathy.

Paraphimosis

Foreskin is retracted and fixed. Once retracted behind glans, a tight or inflamed foreskin cannot return to its original position. Constriction impedes circulation, and so glans swells. A medical emergency; the constricting band prevents venous and lymphatic return from the glans and compromises arterial circulation.

TABLE 26.5	Abnormalities of the Penis—cont'd

Hypospadias

Urethral meatus opens on the ventral aspect (underside) of glans or shaft or at the penoscrotal junction. A groove extends from the meatus to the normal location at the tip. This congenital defect should be recognized at birth. Affected newborns should not be circumcised because surgical correction may entail use of foreskin tissue to extend urethral length.

Urethral Stricture (Not Illustrated)

Pinpoint, constricted opening at meatus or inside along urethra. Occurs congenitally or secondary to urethral injury. Gradual decrease in force and calibre of urine stream is the most common symptom. Shaft feels indurated along ventral aspect at the site of the stricture.

Priapism (Not Illustrated)

Prolonged, painful erection of penis without sexual stimulation and unrelieved by intercourse or masturbation; most common in men in their 30s and 40s. This condition is rare, but when it lasts 4 hours or longer, it can cause ischemia of penis, fibrosis of tissue, and erectile dysfunction. It can occur as an adverse effect of some medications and street drugs and with sickle cell trait or disease; with leukemia, when increased numbers of white blood cells produce engorgement; with malignancy; and as a result of local trauma or spinal cord injuries with autonomic nervous system dysfunction.

Epispadias

Meatus opens on the dorsal (upper) side of glans or shaft above a broad, spadelike penis. Rare; less common than hypospadias but more disabling because of associated urinary incontinence and separation of pubic bones. Corrective surgery is usually done in early childhood.

Peyronie's Disease

Hard, nontender, subcutaneous plaques palpated on dorsal or lateral surface of penis. May be single or multiple and asymmetrical. They are associated with painful bending of the penis during erection. Plaques are fibrosis of the covering of the corpora cavernosa. Usually occurs after age 45 years. Its cause is trauma to the erect penis, such as an unexpected change in angle during intercourse. More common in men with diabetes, gout, and Dupuytren's contracture of the palm.

TABLE 26.6 Abnormalities in the Scrotum

Disorder	Clinical Findings	Discussion
Absence of Testis (Cryptorchidism)	S: Empty scrotal half. O: Inspection: in true maldescent, atrophic scrotum on affected side. Palpation: no testis. A: Absence of testis.	True cryptorchidism: testes that have never descended. Incidence at birth is 3%–4%; in half these cases, the testes descend in first month. Incidence in premature infants is 30%; in adults, 0.7%–0.8%. True undescended testes undergo a histological change by 6 years, causing decreased spermatogenesis and infertility.
Small Testis	S: None. O: Palpation: small and soft (in rare cases, may be firm). A: Small testis.	Smallness with softness (<3.5 cm) indicates atrophy, as with cirrhosis, hypopituitarism, after estrogen therapy, or as a sequela of orchitis. Smallness with firmness (<2 cm) occurs with Klinefelter's syndrome (hypogonadism).

Testicular Torsion	S: Excruciating pain in testicle; of sudden onset, often during sleep or after trauma. May be accompanied by lower abdominal pain, nausea, and vomiting, but no fever.
	O:
	  • Inspection: red, swollen scrotum, one testis (usually left) higher as a result of rotation and shortening.
	  • Palpation: cord feels thick, swollen, tender; epididymis may be anterior; cremasteric reflex is absent on side of torsion.
	A: Acute, painful swelling of spermatic cord, with elevation of one testis.
		Sudden twisting of spermatic cord. Occurs in late childhood and early adolescence; rare after age 20 years. Torsion usually occurs on the left side. Faulty anchoring of testis on wall of scrotum allows testis to rotate. The anterior part of the testis rotates medially toward the other testis. Blood supply is cut off, which results in ischemia and engorgement. This is an emergency necessitating surgery; testis can become gangrenous in a few hours.

Epididymitis	S: Severe pain of sudden onset in scrotum, somewhat relieved by elevation (a positive Phren sign); also rapid swelling, fever.
	O:
	  • Inspection: enlarged scrotum; reddened.
	  • Palpation: exquisitely tender; epididymis enlarged, indurated; may be hard to distinguish from testis. Overlying scrotal skin may be thick and edematous.
	  • Laboratory: white blood cells and bacteria in urine.
	A: Tender swelling of epididymis.
		Acute infection of epididymis is commonly caused by prostatitis; occurs after prostatectomy because of trauma of urethral instrumentation; or is caused by *Chlamydia*, gonorrhea, or other bacterial infection. Distinguishing between epididymitis and testicular torsion is often difficult.

TABLE 26.6	Abnormalities in the Scrotum—cont'd	
Disorder	Clinical Findings	Discussion

Varicocele

S: Dull pain; constant pulling or dragging sensation; or may be asymptomatic.

O:

- Inspection: usually no sign. Bluish colour may show through light scrotal skin.
- Palpation: when patient is standing, a soft, irregular mass is palpable posterior to and above testis; collapses when patient is supine, refills when patient is upright. Feels distinctive, like a "bag of worms."
- The testis on the side of the varicocele may be smaller because of impaired circulation.

A: Soft mass on spermatic cord.

A varicocele is a collection of dilated, tortuous varicose veins in the spermatic cord as a result of incompetent valves within the vein, which enable reflux of blood. It occurs most often on left side, perhaps because left spermatic vein is longer and inserts at a right angle into left renal vein. Common in boys and young men. Screen at early adolescence; early treatment is important to prevent potential infertility in adulthood.

Spermatocele

S: Painless, usually found on examination.

O:

- Inspection: can be transilluminated higher in the scrotum than a hydrocele, and the sperm may be fluorescent.
- Palpation: round, freely movable mass lying above and behind testis. If large, feels like a third testis.

A: Free cystic mass on epididymis.

Retention cyst in epididymis. Cause unclear but may be obstruction of tubules. Filled with thin, milky fluid that contains sperm. Most spermatoceles are small (<1 cm); occasionally are larger and then may be mistaken for hydrocele.

Early Testicular Tumour

S: Painless, found on examination.

O: Palpation: firm nodule or harder than normal section of testicle.

A: Solitary nodule.

Most testicular tumours occur in men between the ages of 15 and 29. Practically all are malignant and occur most often in men of European descent. Biopsy is necessary to confirm malignancy. Most important risk factor is undescended testis, even those surgically corrected. Early detection is important in prognosis, but practice of testicular self-examination is currently low.

Diffuse Tumour

S: Enlarging testis (most common symptom). When enlarges, has feel of increased weight.

O:

- Inspection: enlarged, cannot be transilluminated.
- Palpation: enlarged, smooth, ovoid, firm.
- Important: firm palpation does *not* cause usual sickening discomfort as with normal testis.

A: Nontender swelling of testis.

Diffuse tumour maintains shape of testis.

Continued

TABLE 26.6	Abnormalities in the Scrotum—cont'd	
Disorder	Clinical Findings	Discussion
Hydrocele	S: Painless swelling, although affected patient may complain of weight and bulk in scrotum. O: • Inspection: enlargement; mass can be transilluminated, glows pink or red (in contrast to a hernia). • Palpation: nontender mass, fingers can reach above mass (in contrast to scrotal hernia). A: Nontender swelling of testis.	Cystic. Circumscribed collection of serous fluid in tunica vaginalis, surrounding testis. May occur after epididymitis, trauma, hernia, tumour of testis, or spontaneously in a newborn.
Scrotal Hernia	S: Swelling; pain may occur with straining. O: • Inspection: enlargement; may be reduced when patient is supine; cannot be transilluminated. • Palpation: soft mushy mass; palpating fingers cannot reach above mass; mass is distinct from testicle that is normal. A: Nontender swelling of scrotum.	Scrotal hernia is usually a result of indirect inguinal hernia (see Table 26.7, p. 777).
Orchitis	S: Acute or moderate pain of sudden onset, swollen testis, feeling of weight, fever. O: • Inspection: enlarged, edematous, reddened; cannot be transilluminated. • Palpation: swollen, congested, tense, and tender; hard to distinguish testis from epididymis. A: Tender swelling of testis.	Acute inflammation of testis. Most common cause is mumps; can occur with any infectious disease. May be associated with hydrocele, which can be transilluminated.
Scrotal Edema	S: Tenderness. O: • Inspection: enlarged, may be reddened (with local irritation). • Palpation: taut with pitting; scrotal contents probably cannot be palpated. A: Scrotal edema.	Accompanies marked edema in lower half of body (e.g., in heart failure, renal failure, and portal vein obstruction). Occurs with local inflammation: epididymitis, torsion of spermatic cord. Also, obstruction of inguinal lymphatic vessels produces lymphedema of scrotum.

A, Assessment; *O,* objective data; *S,* subjective data.
Images © Pat Thomas, 2006.

TABLE 26.7	Inguinal and Femoral Hernias

Characteristic	Indirect Inguinal	Direct Inguinal	Femoral
Course	Sac herniates through internal inguinal ring; can remain in canal or pass into scrotum	Directly behind and through external inguinal ring, above inguinal ligament; rarely enters scrotum	Through femoral ring and canal, below inguinal ligament, more often on right side
Clinical symptoms and signs	Pain with straining; soft swelling that increases with increased intra-abdominal pressure; swelling may decrease when patient is lying down	Usually painless; round swelling close to the pubis in area of internal inguinal ring; easily reduced when patient is supine*	Pain may be severe; hernia may become strangulated
Frequency	Most common; 60% of all hernias More common in infants <1 year old and in boys and men 16–20 years of age	Less common, occurs most often in men >40 years of age, rare in women	Least common; 4% of all hernias More common in women
Cause	Congenital or acquired	Acquired weakness; brought on by heavy lifting, muscle atrophy, obesity, chronic cough, or ascites	Acquired; caused by increased abdominal pressure, muscle weakness, or frequent stooping

*Reducible: contents return to abdominal cavity by gentle pressure or when patient is supine. Incarcerated: herniated bowel cannot be returned to abdominal cavity. Strangulated: blood supply to hernia is shut off; accompanied by nausea, vomiting, and tenderness.
Images © Pat Thomas, 2006.

Summary Checklist: Male Genitalia Examination

1. **Inspect** and **palpate** the **penis**
2. **Inspect** and **palpate** the **scrotum**
3. **If a mass exists**, transilluminate the scrotum
4. **Palpate** for an **inguinal hernia**
5. **Palpate** the **inguinal lymph nodes**
6. **Engage in teaching and health promotion**

REFERENCE

1. Sorokan, S. T., Finlay, J. C., & Jefferies, A. L. (2015). Canadian Paediatric Society position statement: Newborn male circumcision. *Paediatrics & Child Health, 20*(6), 311–315.

2. Weiss, H. A., Larke, N., Halperin, D., et al. (2010). Complications of circumcision in male neonates, infants and children: A systematic review. *BMC Urology, 10*, 2. doi:10.1186/1471-2490-10-2.

3. Canadian Paediatric Society. (2015). *Circumcision of baby boys: Information for parents.* Retrieved from http://www.caringforkids.cps.ca/handouts/circumcision.

4. Giuliano, A. R., Palefsky, J. M., Goldstone, S., 2011). Efficacy of quadrivalent HPV vaccine against HPV infection and diseases in males. *New England Journal of Medicine, 364*(5), 401–411. doi:10.1056/NEJMoa0909537.

5. Public Health Agency of Canada. (2012). *Update on human papillomavirus (HPV) vaccines.* Retrieved from http://www.phac-aspc.gc.ca/publicat/ccdr-rmtc/12vol38/acs-dcc-1/index-eng.php.

6. Deutsch, M. B. (2016). *Guidelines for the primary and gender-affirming care of transgender and gender nonbinary people* (2nd ed.). San Francisco: Center of Excellence for Transgender Health. Retrieved from http://transhealth.ucsf.edu/protocols.

7. Lewis, S. L., Heitkemper, M. M., Dirksen, S. R., et al. (Eds.) (2010). *Medical-surgical nursing in Canada* (2nd Can. ed.). Toronto: Elsevier.

8. Perry, A. G., & Potter, P. A. (2010). *Clinical nursing skills and techniques* (7th ed., p. 168). St. Louis: Elsevier.

9. Canadian Cancer Society. (2017). *Testicular cancer.* Retrieved from http://www.cancer.ca/en/cancer-information/cancer-type/testicular/testicular-cancer/?region=on.

CHAPTER 27

Female Genitourinary System

Written by Carolyn Jarvis, PhD, APN, CNP
Adapted by Marian Luctkar-Flude, RN, PhD

ⓔ http://evolve.elsevier.com/Canada/Jarvis/examination/

STRUCTURE AND FUNCTION

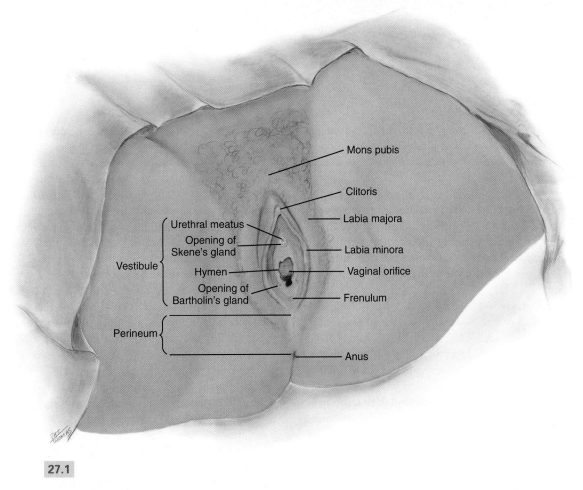

Mons pubis
Clitoris
Labia majora
Labia minora
Vaginal orifice
Frenulum

Urethral meatus
Opening of Skene's gland
Vestibule
Hymen
Opening of Bartholin's gland

Anus

Perineum

27.1

EXTERNAL GENITALIA

The external genitalia are called the **vulva**, or pudendum (Fig. 27.1). The **mons pubis** is a round, firm pad of adipose tissue covering the **symphysis pubis**, the cartilaginous joint between the two pubic bones. After puberty, it is covered with hair in an inverted triangle pattern. The **labia majora** are two rounded folds of adipose tissue extending from the mons pubis down and around to the perineum. After puberty, hair covers the outer surfaces of the labia, whereas the inner folds are smooth and moist, and contain sebaceous follicles.

Inside the labia majora are two smaller, darker folds of skin, the **labia minora**. These are joined anteriorly at the clitoris, where they form a hood (*prepuce*). The labia minora

779

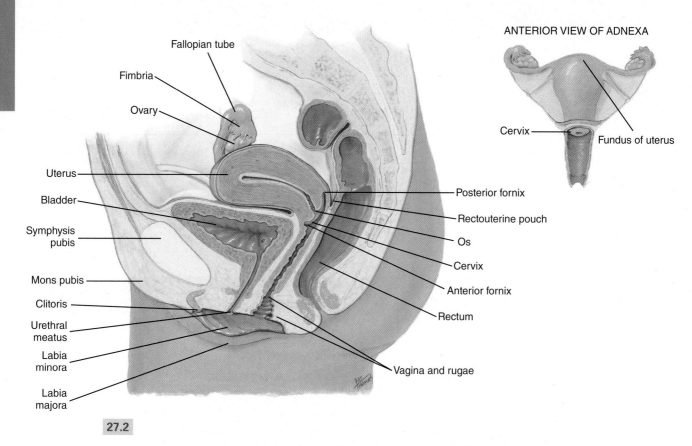

ANTERIOR VIEW OF ADNEXA

27.2

are joined posteriorly by a transverse fold, the **frenulum** (or *fourchette*). The **clitoris** is a small, pea-shaped erectile body, homologous with the male penis and highly sensitive to tactile stimulation.

The labial structures encircle a boat-shaped space, or cleft, termed the **vestibule**. Within it are numerous openings. The **urethral meatus** appears as a dimple 2.5 cm posterior to the clitoris. Surrounding the urethral meatus are multiple, tiny **paraurethral (Skene's) glands**. Their ducts are not visible but open posterior to the urethra at the 5:00 and 7:00 positions.

The **vaginal orifice** is posterior to the urethral meatus. It appears either as a thin median slit or as a large opening with irregular edges, depending on the presentation of the membranous hymen. The **hymen** is a thin, circular or crescent-shaped fold that may cover part of the vaginal orifice or may be absent completely. On either side posterior to the vaginal orifice are two **vestibular (Bartholin's) glands**, which secrete clear lubricating mucus during intercourse. Their ducts are not visible, but they open in the groove between the labia minora and the hymen.

INTERNAL GENITALIA

The internal genitalia include the **vagina**, a flattened, tubular canal extending from the orifice up and backward into the pelvis (Fig. 27.2). It is 9 cm long and sits between the rectum posteriorly and the bladder and urethra anteriorly. Its walls are in thick transverse folds, or **rugae**, which enable the vagina to dilate widely during childbirth.

At the end of the canal, the uterine **cervix** projects into the vagina. In nulliparous women, the cervix appears as a smooth, doughnut-shaped area with a small circular hole (the **os**). After childbirth, the os is slightly enlarged and irregular. The cervical epithelium is of two distinct types. The vagina and cervix are covered with smooth, pink, stratified squamous epithelium. Inside the os, the endocervical canal is lined with columnar epithelium that looks red and rough. The point where these two tissues meet is the **squamocolumnar junction** and is not visible.

A continuous recess is present around the cervix; the front part is the **anterior fornix**, and the rear aspect is the **posterior fornix**. Behind the posterior fornix, another deep recess is formed by the peritoneum. It dips down between the rectum and cervix to form the **rectouterine pouch**, or **cul-de-sac of Douglas**.

The **uterus** is a pear-shaped, thick-walled, muscular organ. It is flattened anteroposteriorly, measuring 5.5 to 8 cm long by 3.5 to 4 cm wide and 2 to 2.5 cm thick. It is freely movable and usually tilts forward and superior to the bladder (for an anteverted and anteflexed position, see Fig. 27.19, p. 802).

The **fallopian tubes** are two pliable, trumpet-shaped tubes, 10 cm in length, extending from the uterine fundus laterally to the brim of the pelvis. There they curve posteriorly, their fimbriated ends located near the **ovaries**. The two ovaries are located one on each side of the uterus at the level of the anterior superior iliac spine. Each is oval, 3 cm long by 2 cm wide by 1 cm thick, and serves to develop ova (eggs) and the female hormones.

TABLE 27.1   Sexual Maturity Ratings in Girls

Stage 1 (Not Illustrated)
Preadolescent. No pubic hair. Mons and labia covered with fine vellus hair, as on abdomen.

Stage 2
Hair growth sparse and mostly on labia. Long, downy hair, slightly pigmented, straight or only slightly curly.

Stage 3
Hair growth sparse but spreading over mons pubis. Hair is darker, coarser, curlier.

Stage 4
Hair is adult in type but over smaller area; none on medial thigh.

Stage 5
Hair is adult in type and pattern; inverse triangle. Also on medial thigh surface.

Adapted from Tanner, J. M. (1962). *Growth at adolescence.* Oxford, UK: Blackwell Scientific.

 ## DEVELOPMENTAL CONSIDERATIONS

Infants and Adolescents

At birth, the external genitalia are engorged because of presence of maternal estrogen. The structures recede in a few weeks, remaining small until puberty. The ovaries are located in the abdomen during childhood. The uterus is small with a straight axis and no anteflexion.

At puberty, estrogens stimulate cell growth in the reproductive tract and development of secondary sex characteristics. The first signs of puberty are breast and pubic hair development, beginning between the ages of 8½ and 13 years. These signs are usually concurrent, but it is not abnormal if they do not develop together, taking about 3 years to complete.

Menarche occurs during the latter half of this sequence, just after the peak of growth velocity. Irregularity of the menstrual cycle is common during adolescence because of occasional failure to ovulate. With menarche, the uterine body flexes on the cervix, and the ovaries have migrated to the pelvic cavity.

Tanner's sexual maturity rating scale is helpful in teaching girls the expected sequence of sexual development (Table 27.1).

Pregnant Women

Pregnancy is discussed in detail in Chapter 30. In summary, shortly after the first missed menstrual period, the genitalia show signs of pregnancy. The cervix softens (*Goodell's sign*) at 4 to 6 weeks, and the vaginal mucosa and cervix look cyanotic (*Chadwick's sign*) at 6 to 8 weeks. These changes occur because of increased vascularity and edema of the cervix and hypertrophy and hyperplasia of the cervical glands. The isthmus of the uterus softens (*Hegar's sign*) at 6 to 8 weeks.

The nonpregnant uterus has a flattened pear shape. In early pregnancy, its growth encroaches on the space occupied by the bladder, producing urinary frequency. By 10 to 12 weeks' gestation, the uterus becomes globular in shape and is too large to stay in the pelvis. At 20 to 24 weeks, the uterus has an oval shape. It rises almost to the liver, displacing the intestines superiorly and laterally.

A clot of thick, tenacious mucus (the mucous plug) forms in the spaces of the cervical canal, which protects the fetus from infection. This plug dislodges when labour begins at the end of term, producing a sign of labour called the "bloody show." Cervical and vaginal secretions increase during pregnancy and are thick, white, and more acidic. The acidity increases because of the action of *Lactobacillus acidophilus*, which changes glycogen into lactic acid. The acidic pH keeps pathogenic bacteria from multiplying in the vagina, but the increase in glycogen increases the risk for candidiasis (commonly called a *yeast infection*) during pregnancy.

Older Women

In contrast to the slowly declining levels of hormones in aging men, hormonal levels in women decrease rapidly. *Menopause* is cessation of the menses. It usually occurs between 48 to 51 years of age, although the variation in ages is wide (from 35 to 60 years of age). The stage of menopause includes the preceding 1 to 2 years of decline in ovarian function, shown by irregular menses that gradually become farther apart and whose flow is lighter. Ovaries stop producing progesterone and estrogen. Because cells in the reproductive tract are estrogen dependent, decreased estrogen levels during menopause bring dramatic physical changes.

The uterus shrinks in size because of decreased myometrium. The ovaries atrophy to 1 to 2 cm and are not palpable after menopause. Ovulation still may occur sporadically after menopause. The sacral ligaments relax and the pelvic musculature weakens, and so the uterus droops. Sometimes it may protrude, or prolapse, into the vagina. The cervix shrinks and looks paler, with a thick, glistening epithelium.

The vagina becomes shorter, narrower, and less elastic because of increased connective tissue. Without sexual activity, the vagina atrophies to one-half of its former length and width. The vaginal epithelium atrophies, becoming thinner, drier, and itchy. This results in a fragile mucosal surface that is at risk for bleeding and vaginitis. Decreased vaginal secretions leave the vagina dry and at risk for irritation and pain with intercourse (dyspareunia). The vaginal pH becomes more alkaline, and glycogen content decreases as a result of the decreased estrogen, resulting in conditions suitable for pathogens and increasing the risk for vaginitis.

Externally, the mons pubis looks smaller because the fat pad atrophies. The labia and clitoris gradually decrease in size. Pubic hair becomes thin and sparse.

Declining estrogen levels produce some physiological changes in the female sexual response cycle: reduced amount of vaginal secretion and lubrication during excitement; shorter duration of orgasm; and rapid resolution.

However, sexual desire and the need for full sexual expression continue. Like older men, older women are capable of sexual function if they are in reasonably good health and have an interested partner. The problem for many older heterosexual women is the availability of an acceptable sexual partner. Older women outnumber their male counterparts and are more likely to be single, whereas men of the same age are more likely to be married.

Urinary incontinence is prevalent among community-living older adults, with women most likely to be affected; it is associated with loss of independence and reduced social interaction, psychological well-being, and quality of life.[1] Urinary incontinence also impacts physical health by contributing to skin rashes, pressure sores, and urinary tract infections (UTIs). As well, it increases the financial burden of individuals as a result of the costs associated with personal care, care products, and medications.

SOCIAL DETERMINANTS OF HEALTH CONSIDERATIONS

Female genital cutting (FGC), also referred to as *female circumcision* or *female genital mutilation* (FGM), is the ritual removal of part or all of the external female genitalia, usually performed on prepubertal girls. The term FGC is preferred as it is considered medically correct, neutral, and culturally sensitive.[2] FGC is a cultural practice, most common in Africa, Asia, and the Middle East; it is estimated that more than 200 million girls and women alive today have undergone FGC. This practice is recognized internationally as harmful and a violation of human rights. The health implications include both (a) immediate effects, such as severe pain, hemorrhage, urinary retention, infection, sepsis, and death, and (b) long-term effects, such as urinary tract and genital tract dysfunction, painful menstruation, sexual and birth control difficulties, infertility, difficulties during pregnancy and childbirth, and psychological difficulties. FGC is illegal in Canada and most Western countries; however, an increasing number of immigrant women who have undergone these procedures are now living in Canada. Affected women may be reluctant to seek health care, and when they do, they may find it difficult and at times traumatic. Health care providers are in a position to educate immigrants from practising communities about the health considerations and legal consequences of FGC.

Sexually transmitted infections (STIs) are a major health concern, with the rates of chlamydia, gonorrhea, and infectious syphilis rising since the late 1990s. Chlamydia continues to be the most commonly reported STI in Canada; reported rates increased by 58% from 2003 to 2012.[3] Rates were highest in those aged 20 to 24 years, and women accounted for almost twice as many cases than did men. The highest rates were reported in the Northwest Territories, Manitoba, Saskatchewan, Yukon, and Alberta. The consequences of untreated chlamydia for women include pelvic inflammatory disease (PID), which can lead to chronic pelvic pain, ectopic pregnancy, and infertility. Some STIs are more common among lesbian and bisexual women, such as bacterial vaginosis, and are easily passed from woman to woman.

Women also represent an increasing proportion of Canadians living with human immunodeficiency virus (HIV) infection and acquired immune deficiency syndrome (AIDS), accounting for 25% of cases diagnosed in 2014.[4] HIV was also generally diagnosed at a younger age in females compared with males, with the majority diagnosed between the ages of 20 to 40 years. The two main risk factors for HIV infection in women are heterosexual contact and injection drug use; Indigenous women accounted for 31% of reported cases.

The incidence of cervical cancer and associated mortality rates have declined substantially in Canada as a result of cervical cancer screening programs;[5] however, rates remain higher among women living in less developed countries without screening programs.[6] Thus immigrant women from developing countries are at a higher risk, as most advanced cervical cancers occur among women who have not undergone regular screening.[7] Historically, Indigenous women have had lower cervical cancer screening rates and higher rates of invasive cervical cancer than non-Indigenous women in Canada. However, recent data have demonstrated an increase in screening among Indigenous women.[8]

UTI is one of the most common bacterial infections in women.[9] Women are more prone to developing UTIs than men because of the shortness of the female urethra, which makes it easier for bacteria to reach the bladder. Risk factors for development of UTI include abnormalities of the urinary tract, pregnancy, postmenopausal status, diabetes, and presence of an indwelling urinary catheter. Transgender women who have undergone vaginoplasty may experience urinary complications such as increased frequency of UTIs, stricture, and fistula.

When conducting a physical examination of a transgender person, examination of the genitalia should be relevant to the anatomy present, and must be done with sensitivity. Sex organs and secondary sex characteristics will vary depending on the person's history of gender assignment surgery (GAS), hormone therapy, or both. Nurses should follow a gender-affirming approach by using general terminology for body parts or asking patients if they have preferred terms that they would like used. Routine cancer screening for transgender patients should be conducted in accordance with current guidelines if they have the particular body part or organ and otherwise meet criteria for screening based on risk factors or symptoms, regardless of hormone use.[10] Transgender women, including those who have undergone vaginoplasty, do not have a cervix. Therefore, cervical cancer screening is not appropriate for them. However, transgender men are at risk for cervical cancer and less likely to be up-to-date on cervical cancer screening than nontransgender women.

SUBJECTIVE DATA

1. Menstrual history
2. Obstetrical history
3. Menopause
4. Self-care behaviours

5. Urinary symptoms
6. Vaginal discharge
7. Past history
8. Sexual activity

9. Contraceptive use
10. STI contact
11. STI risk reduction

HEALTH HISTORY QUESTIONS

Examiner Asks	Rationale
1. Menstrual history. Tell me about your menstrual periods:	Documentation of menstrual history is usually nonthreatening; thus, it is a good topic to use to start recording the history.
• What was the date of your last menstrual period (LMP)? • What was your age at the time of your first period?	Menarche: Mean age at onset is 12 to 13; delayed onset suggests endocrine or underweight problem.
• How often are your periods?	Cycle: normally every 18 to 45 days.
• How many days does your period last? • What is the usual amount of flow: light, medium, heavy? How many pads or tampons do you use each day or hour? • Have you noted any clotting?	Amenorrhea: absence of menses. Duration: average of 3 to 7 days. Menorrhagia: heavy menses. Clotting indicates heavy flow or vaginal pooling.
• Do you have any pain or cramps before or during your period? How do you treat it? Does it interfere with daily activities? Any other associated symptoms: bloating, breast tenderness, moodiness? Any spotting between periods?	Dysmenorrhea.
2. Obstetrical history. Have you ever been pregnant?	Record the obstetrical history (see Chapter 30, p. 856 for details).
• How many times? • How many babies have you had? • Any miscarriage or abortion?	Gravida (G): number of pregnancies. Para (P): number of births. Abortions (A): interrupted pregnancies, including elective abortions and spontaneous miscarriages.

Examiner Asks	Rationale

- For each pregnancy, describe the duration, any complication, labour and delivery, baby's sex, baby's birth weight, and baby's condition.
- Do you think you may be pregnant now? What symptoms have you noticed?

3. Menopause. Have your periods slowed down or stopped?

- Any associated symptoms of menopause (e.g., hot flash, numbness and tingling sensation, headache, palpitations, drenching sweats, mood swings, vaginal dryness, itching)? Any treatment?
- If you are taking hormone replacement, how much? How is it working? Any adverse effects?

- How do you feel about going through menopause?

4. Self-care behaviours. How often do you have a gynecological checkup?
- When was your most recent Papanicolaou (Pap) test? What were the results?
- Has your mother ever mentioned taking hormones while pregnant with you?

5. Urinary symptoms. Any problems urinating? Do you urinate frequently and in small amounts? When you feel the need to urinate, is it impossible to wait?
- Do you have any burning sensation or pain on urinating?
- Do you awaken during the night to urinate?
- Have you seen blood in the urine?
- Is urine dark, cloudy, foul smelling?
- Do you have any difficulty controlling urine or wetting yourself?

- Do you urinate when you sneeze, laugh, cough, or bear down?

6. Vaginal discharge. Have you noticed any unusual vaginal discharge? Has the amount increased?
- What is the character or colour: white, yellow-green, grey, curdlike, foul smelling?

- When did this begin?

Rationale

Menopause is the cessation of menstruation.

Perimenopausal period from ages 40 to 55 years is characterized by hormone shifts, which result in vasomotor instability.

Adverse effects of hormone replacement therapy include fluid retention, breast pain or enlargement, vaginal bleeding, possible breast cancer risk.

Although this is a normal life stage, reaction varies from acceptance to feelings of loss.

Assess self-care behaviours.

Maternal ingestion of diethylstilbestrol (DES) causes cervical and vaginal abnormalities in female offspring, which necessitates frequent follow-up.

Frequency.
Urgency.

Dysuria.
Nocturia.
Hematuria.
Bile in urine or UTI.
True incontinence: loss of urine without warning.
Urgency incontinence: sudden loss of urine, as with acute cystitis.
Functional incontinence: loss of urine associated with inability to access the toilet because of impairment in cognitive or physical functioning, or both, or because of an environmental barrier.
Stress incontinence: loss of urine with physical strain from muscle weakness.

Normal discharge is small, clear or cloudy, and always nonirritating.
With vaginal infection, character of discharge often suggests causative organism (see Table 27.5, pp. 813–814).
Determine whether problem is acute or chronic.

Examiner Asks	Rationale
• Is the discharge associated with vaginal itching, rash, pain with intercourse?	Itching or rash may occur as a result of irritation from discharge. Dyspareunia occurs with vaginitis of any cause.
• Are you taking any medications?	Factors that increase the risk for vaginitis: • Oral contraceptives increase glycogen content of vaginal epithelium, which renders epithelium conducive to the growth of some organisms. • Broad-spectrum antibiotics alter the balance of normal flora.
• Do you have a family history of diabetes? • What part of your menstrual cycle are you in now?	• Diabetes increases glycogen content. • Menses, postpartum status, and menopause cause vaginal pH to be more alkaline.
• Do you use a vaginal douche? How often? • Do you use feminine hygiene spray?	• Frequent douching alters vaginal pH. • Use of such sprays increases the risk for contact dermatitis.
• Do you use talcum powder in the genital area? Cornstarch powder?	• Talcum powder use is associated with a higher risk for ovarian cancer. Cornstarch powder is not.
• Do you wear nonventilating underwear, pantyhose? • Have you treated the discharge with anything? What was the result?	• Local irritation.
7. **Past history.** Any other problems in the genital area? Sores or lesions: now or in the past? How were these treated? • Any abdominal or pelvic pain? • Any past surgery on uterus, ovaries, vagina?	Assess the patient's feelings. Some women fear loss of sexual response after hysterectomy, which may cause problems in intimate relationships.
8. **Sexual activity.** Often women have questions about their sexual relationships and how it affects their health. Do you? • Have you engaged in sexual activity in the last 6 months? • Do you have a regular sexual partner? • Are aspects of your sexual relationship satisfactory to you and your partner/s? • Are you satisfied with the way you and your partner/s communicate about sex? • Are you satisfied with your ability to respond sexually? • Do you have more than one sexual partner?	Begin with open-ended question to assess individual needs. Include appropriate questions as a routine, for these reasons: • Such questions communicate your acceptance of the patient's sexual activity and your belief that it is important. • Your comfort with discussion prompts the patient's interest and possibly relief that the topic has been introduced. • This question helps establishes a database for comparison with any future sexual activities. • It also provides opportunity to screen for sexual problems.
• What is your sexual preference: relationship with a man, with a woman, both?	Lesbians and bisexual women need to feel acceptance to discuss their health concerns.

Subjective Data

Examiner Asks	Rationale

9. Contraceptive use. Are you currently planning a pregnancy or avoiding pregnancy?
- Do you use a **contraceptive**? Which method? Is this satisfactory? Do you have any questions about method?
- Which methods have you used in the past? Have you and your partner discussed having children?
- Have you ever had any problems becoming pregnant?

Assess smoking history. Oral contraceptives, together with cigarette smoking, increase the risk for vascular problems.

Infertility is considered after 1 year of engaging in unprotected sexual intercourse without conceiving.

10. STI contact. Any sexual contact with a partner who had an STI, such as gonorrhea, herpes, HIV, *Chlamydia* infection, genital warts, syphilis? When? How was this treated? Were there any complications? Any questions or concerns about any of these infections?

An STI is any condition that can be transmitted during intercourse or intimate sexual contact with an infected partner.

11. STI risk reduction. Do you take any precautions to reduce the risk for STIs? Do you use condoms every time you have sexual intercourse? Other methods?

Male and female condoms help protect both partners from STIs, including HIV. Dental dams or condoms cut open help prevent STI transmission during oral sex.

Additional History for Infants and Children

1. Urination problems. Does your child have any problem urinating? Does the child have pain with urinating? Does the child cry or hold the genitals while urinating? Has the child ever had a urinary tract infection (UTI)?
- (If the child is older than 2 to 2½ years of age.) Has toilet training started? How is it progressing?
- Does the child wet the bed at night? Is this a problem for the child or for you (parents)? What have you (parents) done?

2. Genital problems. Does the child have a problem with the genital area: itching, rash, vaginal discharge?

Such problems occur with poor perineal hygiene or insertion of a foreign body in the vagina.

3. Molestation. (To child) "Has anyone ever touched you in between your legs and you did not want them to? Sometimes that happens to children, and it's not okay."

Screen for sexual abuse (see Chapter 8). Service providers, including nurses, have an ethical and legal obligation to report suspected child abuse. For prevention, teach children that it is not "okay" for someone to look at or touch their private parts while telling them it is a secret. The patient who has been abused should be told that she has not been "bad" and that she should try to tell an adult about it: "Can you tell me three different big people you trust who you could talk to?" Being asked to name three trusted adults will help the child include someone outside the family; this is important because molestation is often performed by a parent.

Examiner Asks	Rationale

Additional History for Preadolescents and Adolescents

Use the following questions, as appropriate, to assess sexual growth and development and sexual behaviour:

- Ask questions that are appropriate for a child's age, but be aware that norms vary widely. When in doubt, it is better to ask too many questions than to omit something. Children obtain information, often misinformation, from the media and from peers at surprisingly early ages. You information will be more thoughtful and accurate.
- Ask direct, matter-of-fact questions. Avoid sounding judgemental.
- Start with a *permission statement*. "Often girls your age experience … ." This conveys that it is normal and all right to think or feel a certain way.
- Try the *ubiquity approach*. "When did you … ?" rather than "Do you … ?" This method is less threatening because it implies that the topic is normal and unexceptional.

1. **Puberty**. At approximately 9 or 10 years of age, girls start to develop breasts and pubic hair. Have you ever seen charts and pictures of normal growth patterns for girls? Let's go over these now.

2. **Menstruation**. Have your periods started? How did you feel? Were you prepared or surprised?

Assess the attitude of the girl and parents. Note inadequate preparation or attitude of distaste.

3. **Information**. Who in your family do you talk to about your body changes and about sex information? How do these talks go? Do you think you get enough information? What about sex education classes at school? Is there a teacher, a nurse or doctor, a minister, a counsellor to whom you can talk?
   - Often girls your age have questions about sexual activity. Do you have questions? Are you dating? Someone steady? Male or female?
   - Are you having sexual intercourse? Oral sex? Are you using condoms? Other protection?

Avoid the term "having sex." It is ambiguous, and teenagers can take it to mean anything from foreplay to intercourse. Use behaviour-specific words.

4. **Disease**. Has anyone ever talked to you about STIs, such as chlamydia, herpes, gonorrhea, or AIDS?

Teach STI risk reduction.

5. **Immunization**. Have you and your parents discussed the human papillomavirus (HPV) vaccine (Gardasil, Cervarix)? It is recommended before girls become sexually active.

HPV vaccines are approved for girls and women aged 9 to 45 for the prevention of cervical and other cancers. See the box Promoting Health: Cervical Cancer Prevention.

6. **Molestation**. Sometimes a person touches a girl in a way that she does not want to be touched. Has that ever happened to you?

Screen for sexual abuse. If abuse has occurred, patients should understand that it is not their fault and that they should tell another adult about it.

Additional History for Older Adults

1. **Bleeding**. Since menopause, have you noted any vaginal bleeding?

Postmenopausal bleeding warrants further workup and referral.

Subjective Data

Examiner Asks	Rationale
2. Vaginal problems. Any vaginal itching, dryness, discharge, pain with intercourse? Do you use a vaginal lubricant?	These problems are associated with atrophic vaginitis related to decreased estrogen levels. Lubricant may relieve vaginal dryness and decrease discomfort with intercourse.
3. Incontinence. Have you experienced any pressure in the genital area, back pain, constipation, or loss of urine when you cough or sneeze?	These problems occur with weakened pelvic musculature and uterine prolapse.
4. Sexuality. During and after menopause, a woman may notice changes in her sexual relationship or in her sexual response and wonder whether it is normal. Are you currently in a relationship involving intercourse? Are aspects of intercourse satisfactory to you and your partner? Is there adequate privacy for a sexual relationship?	Most older adults are not reluctant to discuss sexual activity and welcome the opportunity. A decline in libido and difficulty in maintaining arousal and achieving orgasm are normal changes that may occur with aging. In the absence of physical illness, an older woman is fully capable of sexual function.

PROMOTING HEALTH: CERVICAL CANCER PREVENTION

HPV Vaccine and Cervical Cancer Screening

HPV Vaccine

Human papillomavirus (HPV) is estimated to be the most prevalent sexually transmitted infection (STI) in Canada. HPV infection can lead to development of cancers of the cervix, vulva, and vagina in females, penile cancers in males, and anal and oropharyngeal cancers in both sexes. High-risk HPV types 16 and 18 cause about 70% of cervical cancers, with up to another 19% caused by HPV types 32, 33, 45, 52, and 58. Low-risk HPV types 6 and 11 cause over 90% of cases of anogenital warts (AGW).

In 2006, the first HPV vaccine, Gardasil (HPV4 vaccine), was approved for use in Canada for the prevention of HPV types 6- and 11-related AGWs, and HPV types 16- and 18-related cancers. In 2010, Cervarix (HPV2 vaccine) was approved for use in Canada for prevention of HPV types 16- and 18-related cervical cancers. In 2015, Gardasil 9 (HPV9 vaccine) was approved for use in Canada for prevention of infections, cancers, precancerous lesions, and AGWs caused by HPV types 6, 11, 16, 18, 31, 33, 45, 52, and 58. Most provinces have HPV immunization programs for girls and some also have them for boys.

The Canadian National Advisory Committee on Immunization recommends the following HPV vaccine immunization schedule:

- **Healthy females aged 9 to 14 years (immunocompetent, non-HIV infected):** a 2- or 3-dose schedule of Gardasil or Cervarix HPV vaccine.
- **Healthy females aged 15 years or older:** a 3-dose schedule of Gardasil or Cervarix HPV vaccine; if the first dose was administered between 9 to 14 years of age, a 2-dose schedule is sufficient.
- **Healthy males aged 9 to 14 years (immunocompetent, non-HIV infected):** a 2- or 3-dose schedule of Gardasil HPV4 vaccine.

- **Healthy males aged 15 years or older:** a 3-dose schedule of Gardasil HPV4 vaccine; if the first dose was administered between 9 to 14 years of age, a 2-dose schedule is sufficient.
- **Immunocompromised and immunocompetent HIV-infected females:** a 3-dose schedule of Gardasil or Cervarix HPV vaccine.
- **Immunocompromised and immunocompetent HIV-infected males:** a 3-dose schedule of Gardasil HPV4 vaccine.
  Infection with HPV is the most important risk factor for cervical cancer, and most cases occur in women younger than 50 years of age. Other known risk factors for HPV include smoking, lower socioeconomic status, giving birth many times, being sexually active, becoming sexually active at a young age, having many sexual partners, having a weakened immune system, using oral contraceptives for a long time, or prenatal exposure to diethylstilbestrol (DES). Reluctance to undergo screening may be attributed to lack of knowledge, lack of access, or failure of the clinician to offer screening.

Cervical Cancer Screening

Cervical cancer incidence and mortality rates have declined as a result of widespread Pap test screening. In 2013, the Canadian Task Force on Preventive Health Care released new recommendations on screening for cervical cancer for women with no symptoms of cervical cancer who are or who have been sexually active, regardless of sexual orientation:

- **Women under the age of 25 years:** routine Pap test screening is no longer recommended.
- **Women and transgender individuals with a cervix, aged 25 to 69 years:** screening every 3 years with cervical cytology is recommended.

PROMOTING HEALTH: CERVICAL CANCER PREVENTION—cont'd

HPV Vaccine and Cervical Cancer Screening

- **Women aged 70 years and older:** screening with cervical cytology every 3 years is recommended if previous screening was inadequate and until three negative results have been received; otherwise, screening may stop.

  More frequent testing may be considered for women at high risk. Women who have received the HPV vaccine should still take part in the currently recommended cervical cancer screening programs.

References

Canadian Cancer Society. (2016). *Cervical cancer: Understanding your diagnosis.* Retrieved from http://www.cancer.ca/~/media/cancer.ca/CW/publications/Cervical%20UYD/Cervical-UYD-2013-EN.pdf.

Canadian National Advisory Committee on Immunization. (2016). *Updated recommendations on human papillomavirus (HPV)* vaccines: *9-Valent HPV vaccine and clarification of minimum intervals between doses in the HPV immunization schedule.* Retrieved from https://www.canada.ca/en/public-health/services/publications/healthy-living/updated-recommendations-human-papillomavirus-immunization-schedule-immunocompromised-populations.html.

Canadian Task Force on Preventive Health Care. (2013). Recommendations on screening for cervical cancer. *Canadian Medical Association Journal,* 185(1), 35–45.

Public Health Agency of Canada. (2016). *Section 5-5: Canadian Guidelines on Sexually Transmitted Infections—Management and treatment of specific infections—Human papillomavirus (HPV) infections.* Retrieved from https://www.canada.ca/en/public-health/services/infectious-diseases/sexual-health-sexually-transmitted-infections/canadian-guidelines/sexually-transmitted-infections/canadian-guidelines-sexually-transmitted-infections-33.html.

OBJECTIVE DATA

PREPARATION

Examination of the internal genitalia is an advanced assessment; however, the generalist nurse may be asked to assist with the procedure, particularly if the physician or nurse practitioner performing the examination is male. Assemble the equipment before helping the patient into position. Arrange equipment within easy reach. Familiarize yourself with the vaginal speculum before the examination. Practise opening and closing the blades, locking them into position, and releasing them. Try both metal and plastic types. Note that the plastic speculum locks and unlocks with a resounding click that can be alarming to the uninformed patient.

EQUIPMENT NEEDED

Gloves
Goose-necked lamp with a strong light
Vaginal speculum of appropriate size (Fig. 27.3, *A* and *B*)
Graves speculum: useful for most women, available in varying lengths and widths
Pederson speculum: narrow blades, useful for young or postmenopausal women with narrowed introitus
Large cotton-tipped applicators (rectal swabs)
Materials for cytological study as specified within your region or facility:
- Glass slide with frosted end
- Specimen container for liquid-based cytological study
- Sterile endocervical brush (Cytobrush) or cotton-tipped applicator
- Ayre spatula
- Spray fixative
- Specimen container for gonorrhea/*Chlamydia* culture
- Small bottle of normal saline solution, potassium hydroxide (KOH), and acetic acid (white vinegar)
- Lubricant

27.3 Vaginal specula. *A,* side view. *B,* top view.

POSITION

Initially, the patient should be sitting up. An equal-status position is important for establishing trust and rapport before the vaginal examination. For the examination, help the patient into the lithotomy position, with the body supine, feet in stirrups, knees apart, and buttocks at edge of examining table (Fig. 27.4). Ask the patient to lift the hips as you guide the patient to the edge of the table. The examiner sits on a stool.

Place the patient's arms at the sides or across the chest and not over the head (because this position tightens the abdominal muscles). Appropriate draping protects the modesty of the patient. This is important for patients of all ethnocultural backgrounds. Drape the patient fully, covering the stomach and legs, exposing only the vulva to your view. Be sure to push down the drape between the legs, and elevate the head so you can see the patient's face.

The lithotomy position leaves many patients feeling helpless and vulnerable. Many women find it embarrassing and uncomfortable. Previous examinations may have been painful, or the previous examiner's attitude was hurried and patronizing.

Help the patient relax, decrease the patient's anxiety, and retain a sense of control by using these measures:

- Have the patient empty the bladder before the examination.
- Position the examination table so that the perineum is not exposed to an inadvertent open door.
- Ask whether the patient would like a friend, family member, or chaperone present. Position this person by the patient's head to maintain privacy.

- Elevate the patient's head and shoulders to a semi-sitting position to maintain eye contact.
- Place the stirrups so that the legs are not abducted too far.
- Explain each step in the examination before you do it.
- Assure the patient that you can stop the examination at any point if the patient feels any discomfort.
- Use a gentle, firm touch and gradual movements.
- Maintain a dialogue throughout the examination to share information, answer questions, and provide health teaching.
- Use the techniques of the *educational* or *mirror pelvic examination* (Fig. 27.5). This is a routine examination with some modifications in attitude, position, and communication. Patients are considered active participants interested in learning and sharing decisions about their own health care. They are propped up on one elbow, or the head of the table is raised. Their other hand holds a mirror between the legs, above the examiner's hands. Patients have a full view of their genitalia and can see all that the examiner is doing.

The mirror works well for teaching normal anatomy and its relation to sexual behaviour. Even those who are in a sexual relationship or who have had children may be surprisingly uninformed about their own anatomy. This is an ideal opportunity to provide teaching and to clarify any misconceptions. Most patients respond enthusiastically on seeing their own cervix.

The mirror pelvic examination also works well when abnormalities arise because the patient can see the rationale for treatment and can monitor progress at the next appointment. Patients are more willing to comply with treatment when they share in the decision.

27.4

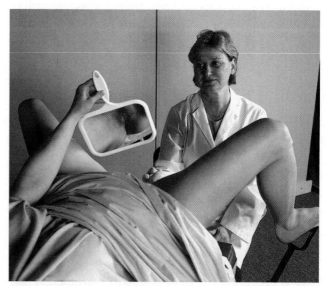

27.5

Normal Range of Findings	Abnormal Findings

External Genitalia

Inspection

Note the following characteristics:

- **Skin colour** (Fig. 27.6).

Refer any suspect pigmented lesion for biopsy.

27.6

- **Hair distribution.** The usual female pattern is an inverted triangle, although it may trail up the abdomen toward the umbilicus; this is normal.

Consider puberty delayed if no pubic hair or breast development has occurred by age 13 years.

Nits or lice at the base of pubic hair should be eradicated.

Swelling.

- **Labia majora.** Normally the labia are symmetrical, plump, and well formed. In nulliparous women, labia meet in the midline; after a vaginal delivery, the labia no longer meet in the midline, and appear slightly shrunken and less defined.
- **Skin texture.** No lesions should be present, except for occasional sebaceous cysts. These are yellowish, 1-cm nodules that are firm, nontender, and often multiple.

  With your gloved hand, separate the labia majora to inspect the following anatomical features:
- **Clitoris** (Fig. 27.7).

Excoriation, nodules, rash, or lesions (see Table 27.2, p. 809).

27.7

Normal Range of Findings	Abnormal Findings
• **Labia minora.** The labia minora are dark pink, moist, and usually symmetrical.	Inflammation or lesions.
• **Urethral opening.** This appears stellate or slitlike and is midline.	
• Vaginal opening, or introitus. This may appear as a narrow vertical slit or as a larger opening.	Polyp. Foul-smelling, irritating discharge.
• **Perineum.** The perineum is normally smooth. A well-healed episiotomy scar, midline or mediolateral, may be present after a vaginal birth.	
• **Anus.** The skin of the anus is coarse and has increased pigmentation (see Chapter 23 for assessment).	

SPECIAL CONSIDERATIONS FOR ADVANCED PRACTICE: EXTERNAL AND INTERNAL GENITALIA

Normal Range of Findings	Abnormal Findings

External Genitalia

Palpation

Assess the urethra and Skene's glands (Fig. 27.8). Dip your gloved finger in a bowl of warm water to lubricate. Then insert your index finger into the vagina, and gently milk the urethra by applying pressure up and out. This procedure should produce no pain. If any discharge appears, culture it.

Tenderness.
Induration along urethra.
Urethral discharge.

27.8

Assess Bartholin's glands. Palpate the posterior parts of the labia majora with your index finger in the vagina and your thumb outside (Fig. 27.9). Normally, the labia feel soft and homogeneous.

Swelling (see Table 27.2, p. 810).
Induration.
Pain with palpation.
Erythema around or discharge from duct opening.

Normal Range of Findings	Abnormal Findings

27.9

Assess the support of pelvic musculature by using these manoeuvres:

1. Palpate the perineum. Normally, it feels thick, smooth, and muscular in a nulliparous woman but thin and rigid in a multiparous woman.
2. Ask the patient to squeeze the vaginal opening around your fingers; it should feel tight in a nulliparous woman and should have less tone in a multiparous woman.
3. Using your index and middle fingers, separate the vaginal orifice and ask the patient to strain down. Normally, no bulging of vaginal walls or urinary incontinence occurs.

Tenderness.

Paper-thin perineum.

Absence or decrease of tone may diminish sexual satisfaction.

Bulging of the vaginal wall indicates cystocele, rectocele, or uterine prolapse (see Table 27.3, p. 811).

Urinary incontinence should be investigated.

Internal Genitalia

Speculum Examination

Select the proper-sized speculum. Warm and lubricate the speculum under warm running water. In many provinces, small amounts of carbomer-free water-soluble lubricants are allowable when performing speculum examinations for Pap tests, as research indicates there is no effect on cervical cytology results.[11]

A good technique is to dedicate one hand to the patient and the other hand to picking up equipment. For example, hold the speculum in your left hand (the equipment hand), with the index and the middle fingers surrounding the blades and your thumb under the thumbscrew. This prevents the blades from opening painfully during insertion. With your right index and middle fingers (the hand on the patient), push the introitus down and open to relax the pubococcygeal muscle (Fig. 27.10). Tilt the width of the blades obliquely and insert the speculum past your right fingers, applying any pressure *downward*. This avoids pressure on the sensitive urethra above it.

Normal Range of Findings	Abnormal Findings

27.10

Ease insertion by asking the patient to bear down. This method relaxes perineal muscles and opens the introitus. (With experience, you can combine speculum insertion with assessing support of the vaginal muscles.) As the blades pass your right fingers, withdraw your fingers. Now change the hand holding the speculum to your right hand, and turn the width of the blades horizontally. Continue to insert in a 45-degree angle *downward* toward the small of the woman's back, matching the natural slope of the vagina (Fig. 27.11).

27.11

Normal Range of Findings	Abnormal Findings

After the blades are fully inserted, open them by squeezing the handles together (Fig. 27.12). The cervix should be in full view. Sometimes this does not occur (especially for novice examiners), because the blades are angled above the location of the cervix. Try closing the blades, withdrawing about halfway, and reinserting in a more *downward* plane. Then slowly sweep upward. Once you have the cervix in full view, lock the blades open by tightening the thumbscrew.

27.12

Special Considerations for Vaginal Examination of Transgender Women

Physical examination should be relevant to the anatomy that is present. The transgender woman should be placed in a gender-affirming lithotomy position. The neovagina lacks surrounding fornices and may have a more posterior orientation; therefore, an anoscope may be more appropriate for a visual examination when indicated.[10] After insertion, the trocar is removed, and the vaginal walls can be visualized collapsing around the end of the anoscope as it is withdrawn. Transgender women who have undergone vaginoplasty do not have a cervix; therefore, cervical screening is not appropriate for them.

Granulation tissue, active hair follicles, warts, abnormal discharge, or malignancy of neovaginal wall.

Special Considerations for Pelvic Examination of Transgender Men

Physical examination should be relevant to the anatomy that is present. Administration of vaginal estrogens for 1 to 2 weeks prior to the pelvic examination may decrease vaginal atrophy in transgender men on testosterone therapy. Follow cervical cancer screening guidelines for nontransgender women if the cervix is present.

Inspect the Cervix and Its Os

Note the following characteristics:
- **Colour.** The cervical mucosa is normally pink and even. During the second month of pregnancy it looks blue (Chadwick's sign), and after menopause it is pale.

Redness, inflammation.
Pallor with anemia.
Cyanotic other than with pregnancy (see Table 27.4, p. 812).

- **Position.** The cervix is midline, either anterior or posterior. It projects 1 to 3 cm into the vagina.

Lateral position may result from adhesion or tumour. Projection of more than 3 cm may be a prolapse.

Normal Range of Findings	**Abnormal Findings**

Normal Range of Findings

- **Size.** Diameter is 2.5 cm (1 in).
- **Os.** This is small and round in nulliparous women. In parous women, it is a horizontal irregular slit, and healed lacerations may be visible on the sides (Fig. 27.13, *A* and *B*).

Abnormal Findings

Hypertrophy of more than 4 cm occurs with inflammation or tumour.

A

NORMAL VARIATIONS OF THE CERVIX

Nulliparous   Parous (after childbirth)

LACERATIONS

B   Unilateral transverse   Bilateral transverse   Stellate   Cervical eversion   Nabothian cysts

27.13   Cervix. **A,** View of os. **B,** Normal variations.

- **Surface.** This is normally smooth, but **cervical eversion**, or ectropion, may occur normally after vaginal deliveries. The endocervical canal is everted or "rolled out." It looks like a red, beefy halo inside the pink cervix surrounding the os. It is difficult to distinguish this normal variation from an abnormal condition (e.g., erosion or carcinoma), and biopsy may be needed.

Reddened, granular, and asymmetrical surface, particularly around os.

Friable, bleeding easily.

Any lesions: white patch on cervix; strawberry spot.

Refer any suspect red, white, or pigmented lesion for biopsy (see erosion and carcinoma, Table 27.4, pp. 812–813).

Normal Range of Findings

- **Nabothian cysts** are benign growths that commonly appear on the cervix after childbirth. They are small, smooth, yellow nodules that may be single or multiple and are less than 1 cm in diameter. They are retention cysts caused by obstruction of cervical glands.
- **Cervical secretions.** Depending on the day of the menstrual cycle, secretions may be clear and thin, or they may be thick, opaque, and stringy. They are always odourless and nonirritating.
  - If secretions are copious, swab the area with a thickly tipped rectal swab to get a better view of the structures.

Obtain Cervical Smears and Cultures

The Pap test is a screen for cervical cancer. Screening recommendations vary by province. Previously, guidelines recommended annual screening starting at early ages, but now all provinces have increased the starting age and intervals between screens.[12] See the box Promoting Health: Cervical Cancer Prevention (p. 788) for the latest screening guidelines. Do not obtain a Pap test during the woman's menses or if a heavy infectious discharge is present. Instruct the woman not to douche, have intercourse, or put anything into the vagina within 24 hours before the specimens are collected. Obtain the Pap test before other specimens so that you will not disrupt or remove cells.

Conventional **glass slide cytology** remains the most common screening test for cervical cancer available in Canada. A single slide is sufficient for the entire specimen.

Cervical Scrape. Insert the bifid end of the cervical spatula into the vagina with the more pointed bump into the cervical os. Rotate it 360 to 720 degrees, using firm pressure (Fig. 27.14, *A*). The rounded cervix fits snugly into the spatula's groove. The spatula scrapes the surface of the exocervix and the squamocolumnar junction (SCJ) or transformation zone (T-zone) as you turn the instrument. Failure to adequately sample the T-zone may result in a false negative test. The T-zone can be identified by a change in colour and texture: the mature squamous epithelium of the ectocervix appears pale pink, shiny, and smooth, whereas the columnar epithelium of the endocervix appears reddish with a granular surface. During child-bearing years, the T-zone can usually be visualized. However, in postmenopausal women, the SCJ often recedes into the endocervical canal and may not be easily visualized.

After withdrawing the spatula, spread the specimen from both sides of the spatula onto a glass slide. Use a single stroke to thin out the specimen, not a back-and-forth motion. Spray with a fixative (or not), according to your agency's procedures.

Abnormal Findings

Cervical polyp: bright red growth protruding from the os (see Table 27.4, p. 812).

Foul-smelling, irritating, with yellow, green, white, or grey discharge (see Table 27.5, p. 813).

A

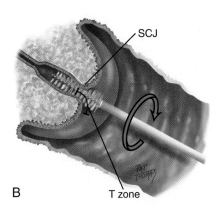

B

SCJ

T zone

27.14

Normal Range of Findings	Abnormal Findings

Normal Range of Findings

Endocervical Specimen. Insert an endocervical brush (instead of a cotton applicator) into the os (Fig. 27.14, *B*). With a brush, you obtain a higher yield of endocervical cells from the transformation zone, the area at greatest risk for development of cervical cancers. The patient may feel a slight pinch with the brush, and scant bleeding may occur. Collect the endocervical specimen last so that bleeding does not obscure cytological evaluation.

Rotate the brush 720 degrees in *one* direction in the endocervical canal, either clockwise or counter-clockwise. Then withdraw the brush and rotate it gently on a slide to deposit all the cells, rotating in the direction opposite to the one used to obtain the specimen. Avoid leaving a thick specimen, which would be hard to analyze under the microscope. For a patient after hysterectomy whose cervix has been removed, collect a scrape from the end of the vagina and a vaginal pool.

Immediately (within 2 seconds) spray the slide with fixative to avoid drying, if procedures require this step.

Label the frosted end of the slide with the patient's name. Send the slide to the laboratory with the following necessary data:

- Date of specimen
- Patient's date of birth
- Date of LMP
- Any hormone medication, including testosterone use in transgender men[13]
- If patient is pregnant, estimated date of delivery
- Known infections
- Prior surgery or radiation treatment
- Prior abnormal cytological findings
- Abnormal findings on physical examination

These data are important for accurate interpretation.

Liquid-based cytology (LBC), a newer method of cervical screening, offers advantages over conventional Pap testing. The sample is collected with a cervical spatula and an endocervical brush and placed in a jar containing a liquid preservative medium. LBC is now available in most provinces, but not within all regions across these provinces.[14]

In some regions, another screening tool, the **cervical broom** (Fig. 27.15), is used to simultaneously sample the exocervix and endocervix, including the T-zone.[15] The long central bristles of the broom are inserted into the cervical os until the lateral bristles bend against the exocervix. The broom is rotated three to five full rotations in one direction only.

The **HPV test** is available in some provinces and territories, and is only appropriate for women 30 years of age or older. It may be performed on the same sample of cells used for the Pap test, or as a follow-up test after an abnormal Pap test result to detect HPV DNA and determine whether the HPV type is high risk.

Abnormal Findings

Caution: The endocervical brush is contraindicated for pregnant women.

Normal Range of Findings	Abnormal Findings

27.15

To screen for STIs, and if you note any abnormal vaginal discharge, obtain the **gonorrhea/chlamydia culture**. Insert a sterile cotton applicator into the os, rotate it 360 degrees, and leave it in place 10 to 20 seconds for complete saturation. Withdraw the applicator, and insert it into a labelled specimen container.

On occasion, you need the following samples:

- **Saline mount, or "wet preparation."** Spread a sample of the discharge onto a glass slide, and add one drop of normal saline solution and a coverslip.
- **Potassium hydroxide preparation.** To a sample of the discharge on a glass slide, add one drop of KOH and a coverslip.
- **Anal culture.** Insert a sterile cotton swab into the anal canal about 1 cm. Rotate it, and move it side to side. Leave in place 10 to 20 seconds. If the swab collects feces, discard it and begin again. Withdraw the swab, and insert the culture sample into a labelled specimen container.

Inspect the Vaginal Wall

Loosen the thumbscrew but continue to hold the speculum blades open. Slowly withdraw the speculum, rotating it as you go, to fully inspect the vaginal wall. Normally, the wall looks pink, deeply rugated, moist, and smooth. Normal discharge is thin and clear, or opaque and stringy, but always odourless.

Inflammation or lesions should be investigated.

Leukoplakia appears as a spot of dried white paint.

Abnormal vaginal discharge has the following characteristics: thick, white, and curdlike (with candidiasis); profuse, watery, grey-green, and frothy (with trichomoniasis); or any grey, green-yellow, white, or foul-smelling discharge (see Table 27.5, p. 813).

When the blade ends of the speculum near the vaginal opening, let them close, being careful not to pinch the mucosa or catch any hairs. Turn the blades obliquely to avoid stretching the opening. Place a metal speculum in a basin to be cleaned later and soaked in a sterilizing and disinfecting solution; discard the plastic variety. Discard your gloves, and wash hands.

Special Considerations for Advanced Practice

| **Normal Range of Findings** | **Abnormal Findings** |

Bimanual Examination

Rise to a stand, and have the patient remain in lithotomy position. Drop lubricant onto the first two fingers of the gloved hand that will be inserted intravaginally (Fig. 27.16). Assume the "obstetrical" position with the first two fingers extended, the last two flexed onto the palm, and the thumb abducted. Insert your lubricated fingers into the vagina, with any pressure directed posteriorly. Wait until the vaginal walls relax, then insert your fingers fully.

27.16

Use both hands to palpate the internal genitalia; assess their location, size, and mobility, and screen for any tenderness or mass. One hand is on the abdomen (the "abdominal" hand), and the other (often the dominant, more sensitive hand) inserts two fingers into the vagina (the "intravaginal" hand; Fig. 27.17). It does not matter which hand you choose to be inserted intravaginally; try each way (on different patients), and settle on the method most comfortable for you.

27.17

Palpate the vaginal wall. Normally, it feels smooth and has no area of induration or tenderness.

Nodule.
Tenderness.

Normal Range of Findings	**Abnormal Findings**

Cervix. Locate the cervix in the midline, often near the anterior vaginal wall. The cervix points in the opposite direction of the fundus of the uterus. Palpate, using the palmar surface of your fingers. Note the following characteristics of a normal cervix:

- Consistency: smooth and firm, like the consistency of the tip of the nose. It softens and feels velvety at 5 to 6 weeks of pregnancy (Goodell's sign).
- Contour: evenly rounded.
- Mobility: With a finger on either side, move the cervix gently from side to side. Normally, this produces no pain (Fig. 27.18).

Hard with malignancy.
Nodular.
Irregular.
Immobile with malignancy.

27.18

Palpate all around the fornices; the wall should feel smooth.

Painful with inflammation or ectopic pregnancy.

Use your "abdominal" hand to push the pelvic organs closer for your intravaginal fingers to palpate. Place your "abdominal" hand midway between the umbilicus and the symphysis; push down in a slow, firm manner, fingers together and slightly flexed. Brace the elbow of your "intravaginal" arm against your hip, and keep it horizontal. The patient must be relaxed.

Normal Range of Findings	**Abnormal Findings**

Uterus. With your "intravaginal" fingers in the anterior fornix, assess the uterus. Determine the position, or *version,* of the uterus (Fig. 27.19). This compares the long axis of the uterus with the long axis of the body. In many women, the uterus is anteverted; you palpate it at the level of the pubis with the cervix pointing posteriorly. Two other positions are also normal (midposition and retroverted), as are two aspects of flexion, in which the long axis of the uterus is not straight but flexed.

Special Considerations for Advanced Practice

Anteverted

Midposition

Anteflexed

Retroflexed

Retroverted

27.19

Normal Range of Findings

Palpate the uterine wall with your fingers in the fornices. Normally, it feels firm and smooth, with the contour of the fundus rounded. It softens during pregnancy. Bounce the uterus gently between your abdominal and intravaginal hands. It should be freely movable and nontender.

Adnexa. Move both hands to the right to explore the adnexa. Place your abdominal hand on the lower quadrant just inside the anterior iliac spine and your "intravaginal" fingers in the lateral fornix (Fig. 27.20). Push the "abdominal" hand down, and try to palpate the ovary. In many patients, you cannot palpate the ovary. When you can, it normally feels smooth, firm, and almond-shaped and is highly movable, sliding through the fingers. It is slightly sensitive but not painful. The fallopian tube is normally not palpable. No other mass or pulsation should be felt.

27.20

A note of caution: Normal adnexal structures often are not palpable. Be careful not to mistake an abnormality for a normal structure. To be safe, consider abnormal any mass that you cannot *positively* identify, and refer the patient for further study.

Move to the left to palpate the other side. Then, withdraw your hand and check secretions on the gloved fingers before you discard the glove. Normal secretions are clear or cloudy and odourless.

Abnormal Findings

Enlarged uterus (see Table 27.6, p. 815).
Lateral displacement.
Nodular mass.
Irregular, asymmetrical uterus.
Fixed and immobile uterus.
Tenderness.
Enlarged adnexa; nodules or mass in adnexa.
Immobile adnexa.
Marked tenderness (see Table 27.7, p. 816).

CRITICAL FINDINGS

Pulsation or palpable fallopian tube suggests ectopic pregnancy; this warrants immediate referral (see Table 27.7, p. 816).

Special Considerations for Advanced Practice

Normal Range of Findings	**Abnormal Findings**

Rectovaginal Examination

Use this technique to assess the rectovaginal septum, posterior uterine wall, cul-de-sac, and rectum. Change gloves to avoid spreading any possible infection. Lubricate the first two fingers. Instruct the patient that this may feel uncomfortable and will mimic the feeling of moving the bowels. Ask the patient to bear down as you insert your index finger into the vagina and your middle finger gently into the rectum (Fig. 27.21).

Uterus retroflexed

RECTOVAGINAL PALPATION

27.21

While pushing with the "abdominal" hand, repeat the steps of the bimanual examination. Try to keep the "intravaginal" finger on the cervix so that the finger in the rectum does not mistake the cervix for a mass. Note the following characteristics:

- The rectovaginal septum should feel smooth, thin, firm, and pliable.
- The rectovaginal pouch, or cul-de-sac, is a potential space and usually not palpable.
- The uterine wall and fundus feel firm and smooth.

Rotate the "intrarectal" finger to check the rectal wall and anal sphincter tone. (See Chapter 23 for assessment of anus and rectum.) Check your gloved finger as you withdraw it; test any adherent stool for occult blood.

Give the patient tissues to wipe the area and help the patient up. Remind the patient to slide the hips back from the edge before sitting up in order to not fall.

Nodular or thickened.

Normal Range of Findings	Abnormal Findings

❖ DEVELOPMENTAL CONSIDERATIONS

Infants and Children
Preparation

- **Infant:** Place on examination table.
- **Toddler or preschooler:** Place on parent's lap in the frog-leg position: hips flexed and soles of feet together and touching the child's buttocks. A preschool-age child may want to separate her own labia. Do not use drapes; a young girl wants to see what you are doing.
- **School-age child:** place on examination table, frog-leg position, no drapes. During childhood, a routine screening is limited to inspection of the external genitalia to determine that (a) the structures are intact, (b) the vagina is present, and (c) the hymen is patent.

The newborn's genitalia are somewhat engorged. The labia majora are swollen; the labia minora are prominent and protrude beyond the labia majora; the clitoris looks relatively large; and the hymen appears thick. Because of transient engorgement, the vaginal opening is more difficult to see now than it will be later. Place your thumbs on the labia majora. Push laterally while pushing the perineum down, and try to note the vaginal opening above the hymenal ring. Do not palpate the clitoris because it is very sensitive.

A sanguineous vaginal discharge or leukorrhea (mucoid discharge) are normal during the first few weeks because of the maternal estrogen effect. (This also may cause transient breast engorgement and secretion.) During the early weeks, the genital engorgement resolves, and the labia minora atrophy and remain small until puberty (Fig. 27.22).

Ambiguous genitalia are rare but are suggested by the appearance of a markedly enlarged clitoris, fusion of the labia (resembling scrotum), and palpable mass in fused labia (resembling testes) (see Table 27.8, p. 817).

Imperforate hymen warrants referral.

Lesions, rash.

27.22

Between the ages of 2 months and 7 years, the labia majora are flat, the labia minora are thin, the clitoris is relatively small, and the hymen is tissue-paper thin. Normally, no irritation or foul-smelling discharge is present.

In young school-age girls (age 7 to 10 years), the mons pubis and labia majora thicken, and the labia minora become slightly rounded. Pubic hair begins to appear around age 11 years, although sparse pubic hair may appear as early as age 8 years. Normally, the hymen is perforate.

Poor perineal hygiene.

Pest inhabitants; excoriations.

During and after toddler age, foul-smelling discharge occurs with lodging of foreign body, pinworms, or infection.

Absence of pubic hair by age 13 years indicates delayed puberty.

Amenorrhea in an adolescent, together with bluish and bulging hymen, indicates imperforate hymen and warrants referral.

Normal Range of Findings	Abnormal Findings

Usually in these age groups, an external examination will suffice. An internal pelvic examination, if needed, is best performed by a pediatric gynecologist using specialized instruments.

Adolescents

Adolescents have special needs during the genitalia examination. Examine the patient alone, without the parent present. Assure the patient of privacy and confidentiality. Allow plenty of time for health education and discussion of pubertal progress. Assess the patient's growth velocity and menstrual history, and use sexual maturity rating charts to teach breast and pubic hair development. Assure the patient that increased vaginal fluid (physiological *leukorrhea*) is normal because of the estrogen effect.

Perform pelvic examination when contraception is desired, when sexual activity includes intercourse, or at age 18 years in virgins. Start periodic Pap tests at age 25 years. Use the examination techniques listed in the section for adults, but provide additional time and psychological support for adolescents undergoing their first pelvic examination.

The experience of the first pelvic examination determines how the adolescent will approach future care. Your accepting attitude and gentle, unhurried approach are important. Take the time to teach, using the patient's own body as illustration. Your frank discussion of anatomy and sexual behaviour communicates that these topics are not taboo and are acceptable to discuss with health care providers. This affirms the patient's self-concept and helps the patient understand that her or their body is normal.

During the bimanual examination, note that the adnexa are not palpable in an adolescent.

Pelvic or adnexal mass.

Pregnant Women

Depending on the week of the pregnancy, inspection reveals the enlarging abdomen (see Fig. 30.1, p. 851). The height of the fundus ascends gradually as the fetus grows. At 16 weeks, the fundus is palpable halfway between the symphysis and umbilicus; at 20 weeks, at the lower edge of the umbilicus; at 28 weeks, halfway between the umbilicus and the xiphoid process; and at 34 to 36 weeks, almost to the xiphoid process. Close to term, the fundus drops as the fetal head engages in the pelvis.

The external genitalia exhibit hyperemia of the perineum and vulva because of increased vascularity. Varicose veins may be visible in the labia or legs, and hemorrhoids may be visible around the anus. Both are caused by interruption in venous return from the pressure of the fetus.

Internally, the walls of the vagina appear violet or blue (Chadwick's sign) because of hyperemia. The vaginal walls are deeply rugated, and the vaginal mucosa thickens. The cervix looks blue, and feels velvety and softer than in the nonpregnant state; thus, it is a bit more difficult to differentiate from the vaginal walls.

During bimanual examination, the isthmus of the uterus feels softer and is more easily compressed between your two hands (Hegar's sign). The fundus balloons between your two hands; it feels connected to, but distinct from, the cervix because the isthmus is so soft.

Search the adnexal area carefully during early pregnancy. Normally, the adnexal structures are not palpable.

An ectopic pregnancy has serious consequences (see Table 27.7, p. 816).

Normal Range of Findings	Abnormal Findings

Older Women

Natural lubrication is decreased; to avoid a painful examination, lubricate instruments and the examining hand adequately. Use the Pederson speculum (rather than the Graves) because its narrower, flatter blades are more comfortable in women with vaginal stenosis or dryness.

Menopause and the resulting decrease in estrogen production cause numerous physical changes. Pubic hair gradually decreases, becoming thin and sparse in later years. The skin is thinner, and fat deposits decrease, leaving the mons pubis smaller and the labia flatter. Clitoris size also decreases after age 60 years.

Internally, the rugae of the vaginal walls decrease, and the walls look pale pink because of the thinned epithelium. The cervix shrinks and looks pale and glistening. It may retract, appearing to be flush with the vaginal wall. In some women, it is hard to distinguish the cervix from the surrounding vaginal mucosa. Alternately, the cervix may protrude into the vagina if the uterus has prolapsed.

With the bimanual examination, you may need to insert only one gloved finger if vaginal stenosis exists. The uterus feels smaller and firmer, and the ovaries are normally not palpable.

Older women may have special needs. For example, advise those with arthritis to take a mild analgesic or anti-inflammatory agent before the appointment to ease joint pain in positioning; schedule appointment times when joint pain or stiffness is at its least; allow extra time for positioning and "unpositioning" after the examination; and maintain dignity and privacy.

Refer any suspect red, white, or pigmented lesion for biopsy.

Vaginal atrophy increases the risk for infection and trauma.

Refer any mass for prompt evaluation.

DOCUMENTATION AND CRITICAL THINKING

Sample Charting

SUBJECTIVE

Menarche age 12 years, cycle usually q28 days, duration 5 days, flow moderate, no dysmenorrhea, LMP April 3. Grav 0/Para 0/Ab 0. Last Pap test 3 years ago, negative.

No urinary problems, no irritating or foul-smelling vaginal discharge, no sores or lesions, no history of pelvic surgery. Satisfied with sexual relationship with husband, uses vaginal diaphragm for birth control, no plans for pregnancy at this time. Not aware of any STI contact to herself or husband.

OBJECTIVE

External genitalia: No swelling, lesions, or discharge. No urethral swelling or discharge.
Internal: Vaginal walls have no bulging or lesions; cervix is pink with no lesions; scant clear mucoid discharge.
Bimanual: No pain on moving cervix; uterus anteflexed and anteverted; no enlargement or irregularity.
Adnexa: Ovaries not enlarged.
Rectal: No hemorrhoids, fissures, or lesions; no masses or tenderness; stool brown with guaiac test result negative.

ASSESSMENT

Genital structures intact and appear healthy

Focused Assessment: Clinical Case Study 1

Jan Keung (J.K.), 27-year-old, married newspaper journalist, Grav 0/Para 0/Ab 0. Presents at clinic with "urinary burning, vaginal itching, and discharge" × 4 days.

SUBJECTIVE

3 weeks ago: J.K. treated at clinic for bronchitis with erythromycin. J.K. improved within 5 days.

4 to 5 days ago: Noted burning sensation on urination; intense vaginal itching; thick, white, "smelly" discharge. Warm water douche; no relief.

No previous history of vaginal infection, UTI, or pelvic surgery. Monogamous sexual relationship, has used low-estrogen birth control pills for 3 years with no adverse effects.

OBJECTIVE

Vulva and vagina erythematous and edematous. Thick, white, curdlike discharge clinging to vaginal walls. Cervix pink, no lesions.

Bimanual examination: No pain on palpating cervix, uterus not enlarged, ovaries not enlarged.

Specimens: Pap smear, gonorrhea/chlamydia culture to laboratory. KOH preparation shows mycelia and spores of *Candida albicans*.

ASSESSMENT

Candida vaginitis
Pain R/T [related to] infectious process

Focused Assessment: Clinical Case Study 2

Brenda Dickson (B.D.), a 17-year-old high school student, comes to clinic for pelvic examination.

SUBJECTIVE

Menarche 12 years, cycle q30 days, duration 6 days, mild cramps relieved by acetaminophen. LMP March 10. No dysuria, vaginal discharge, vaginal itching. Relationship involving intercourse with one boyfriend for the past 8 months. For birth control, boyfriend uses condoms "sometimes." B.D. wants to start birth control pills. Never had pelvic examination. No knowledge of STIs except HIV. Smokes cigarettes, $\frac{1}{2}$ PPD, started age 11 years.

OBJECTIVE

Breasts: Symmetrical, no lesions or discharge, palpation reveals no mass or tenderness.
External genitalia: No redness, lesions, or discharge.
Internal: Vaginal walls and cervix pink with no lesions or discharge. Specimens obtained.
Bimanual examination: No tenderness to palpation, uterus anteverted with no enlargement, ovaries not enlarged.
Rectum: No masses, fissure, or tenderness. Stool brown, and guaiac test result negative.
Specimens: Gonorrhea/*Chlamydia* culture to laboratory.

ASSESSMENT

Breast and pelvic structures appear healthy
Deficient knowledge regarding birth control measures, STI prevention; cigarette smoking R/T lack of education

Documentation and Critical Thinking

ABNORMAL FINDINGS

TABLE 27.2	Abnormalities of the External Genitalia

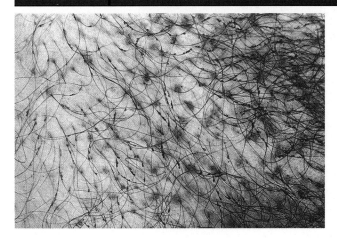

Pediculosis Pubis (Crab Lice)

S: Severe perineal itching.

O: Excoriations and erythematous areas. Little dark spots (lice are small); nits (eggs) adherent to pubic hair near roots may be visible. Usually localized in pubic hair, occasionally in eyebrows or eyelashes.

Herpes Simplex Virus Type 2 (Herpes Genitalis)

S: Episodes of local pain, dysuria, fever.

O: Clusters of small, shallow vesicles with surrounding erythema; erupt on genital areas and inner thigh. Also, inguinal adenopathy, edema. Vesicles on labia rupture in 1–3 days, leaving painful ulcers. Initial manifestation lasts 7–10 days. Virus remains dormant indefinitely; recurrent manifestations last 3–10 days with milder symptoms.

Syphilitic Chancre

O: Begins as a small, solitary silvery papule that erodes to a red, round or oval, superficial ulcer with a yellowish serous discharge. Palpation reveals a nontender indurated base that can be lifted like a button between thumb and finger. Nontender inguinal lymphadenopathy.

Red Rash: Contact Dermatitis

S: History of skin contact with allergenic substance in environment; intense pruritus.

O: Primary lesion: red, swollen vesicles, which may then weep; crusts, scales, thickening of skin, excoriations from scratching may be present. Rash may result from reaction to feminine hygiene spray or synthetic underwear.

Continued

TABLE 27.2 **Abnormalities of the External Genitalia—cont'd**

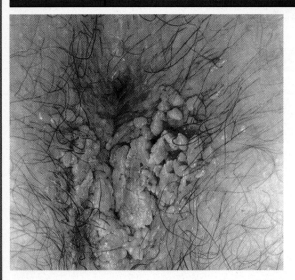

Human Papillomavirus (HPV) Genital Warts

S: Painless warty growths; may be unnoticed by woman.
O: Pink or flesh-coloured, soft, pointed, moist, warty papules. Single or multiple in a cauliflowerlike patch. Occur around vulva, introitus, anus, vagina, cervix.
HPV infection is common among sexually active women, especially adolescents, regardless of ethnicity or socioeconomic status. Risk factors include early age at menarche and multiple sexual partners. The long incubation period (6 weeks to 8 months) makes it difficult to establish history of exposure. HPV infection is strongly associated with abnormal cervical cytological findings.

Urethritis

Urethritis

S: Dysuria.
O: Palpation of anterior vaginal wall reveals erythema, tenderness, induration along urethra, purulent discharge from meatus. Caused by *Neisseria gonorrhoeae*, *Chlamydia*, or *Staphylococcus* infection.

Abscess of Bartholin's Gland

S: Local pain, can be severe.
O: Overlying skin red and hot. Posterior part of labia swollen; palpable fluctuant mass and tenderness. Red spot is visible on mucosa at site of duct opening; can express purulent discharge. Often secondary to gonococcal infection.

Urethral Caruncle

S: Tenderness, pain with urination, urinary frequency, hematuria, dyspareunia, or no symptoms.
O: Small, deep red mass protruding from meatus; usually secondary to urethritis or skenitis; lesion may bleed on contact.

O, Objective data; *S*, subjective data.
See Illustration Credits for source information.

TABLE 27.3 Abnormalities of the Pelvic Musculature

Cystocele (With Bladder Prolapse)

S: Sensation of pressure in vagina, stress incontinence.
O: With straining or standing, introitus widens, and a soft, round anterior bulge is evident. The bladder, covered by vaginal mucosa, prolapses into vagina; in the case illustrated, it is accompanied by an extreme uterine prolapse.

Rectocele

S: Sensation of pressure in vagina, possibly constipation.
O: With straining or standing, note introitus widening and the presence of a soft, round bulge from posterior. Here, part of the rectum, covered by vaginal mucosa, prolapses into vagina.

◀ Uterine Prolapse

O: With straining or standing, uterus protrudes into vagina. Prolapse is graded as follows:
- First degree: Cervix appears at introitus with straining.
- Second degree: Cervix bulges outside introitus with straining.
- Third degree (in illustration): Whole uterus protrudes even without straining; in essence, uterus is inside out.

O, Objective data; *S*, subjective data.
See Illustration Credits for source information.

TABLE 27.4   Abnormalities of the Cervix

Bluish Cervix: Cyanosis

O: Bluish discoloration of the mucosa is normal during pregnancy (Chadwick's sign at 6–8 weeks) and with any other condition causing hypoxia or venous congestion (e.g., heart failure, pelvic tumour).

Erosion

O: Cervical lips are inflamed and eroded. Reddened granular surface is superficial inflammation, with no ulceration (loss of tissue). It is usually secondary to purulent or mucopurulent cervical discharge. Biopsy is needed to distinguish erosion from carcinoma; clinician cannot rely on inspection.

Human Papillomavirus (HPV, Condylomata)

O: Virus can appear in various forms when affecting cervical epithelium. In illustration, warty growth appears as abnormal thickened white epithelium. Visibility of lesion is enhanced by acetic acid (vinegar) wash, which dissolves mucus and temporarily causes intracellular dehydration and coagulation of protein.

Polyp

S: Mucoid discharge or bleeding may occur.
O: Bright red, soft, pedunculated growth emerges from os. It is a benign lesion, but this must be determined through biopsy. It may be lined with squamous or columnar epithelium.

◀ Diethylstilbestrol (DES) Syndrome

S: Prenatal exposure to DES causes cervical and vaginal abnormalities.
O: Red, granular patches of columnar epithelium extend beyond normal squamocolumnar junction onto cervix and into fornices (vaginal adenosis). Cervical abnormalities may also be present: circular groove, transverse ridge, protuberant anterior lip, "cockscomb" formation. Frequent monitoring is warranted.

TABLE 27.4	Abnormalities of the Cervix—cont'd

◄ **Carcinoma**

S: Carcinoma may manifest as bleeding between menstrual periods or after menopause or as unusual vaginal discharge.

O: Chronic ulcer and induration are early signs of carcinoma, although the lesion may or may not show on the exocervix. (In illustration, lesion is mostly around the external os.) It is diagnosed through Pap smear and biopsy. Risk factors for cervical cancer are early age at first intercourse, multiple sex partners, cigarette smoking, and certain STIs.

O, Objective data; *S,* subjective data; *STI,* sexually transmitted infection.
See Illustration Credits for source information.

TABLE 27.5	Vulvovaginal Inflammations

Atrophic Vaginitis

S: Postmenopausal vaginal itching, dryness, burning sensation, dyspareunia, mucoid discharge (may be flecked with blood).

O: Mucosa is pale, with abraded areas that bleed easily; bloody discharge may be present.

This is an opportunistic infection related to chronic estrogen deficiency.

Candidiasis (Moniliasis)

S: Intense pruritus; thick, whitish discharge.

O: Vulva and vagina are erythematous and edematous. Discharge is usually thick, white, curdy, "like cottage cheese." Infection is diagnosed through microscopic examination of discharge on potassium hydroxide wet mount.

Predisposing causes include use of oral contraceptives or antibiotics, more alkaline vaginal pH (as with menstrual periods, postpartum, menopause), and pregnancy (because of increased glycogen and diabetes).

Continued

TABLE 27.5	Vulvovaginal Inflammations—cont'd

Trichomoniasis

S: Pruritus, watery and often malodorous vaginal discharge, urinary frequency, terminal dysuria. Symptoms are worse during menstruation, when the pH becomes optimal for the organism's growth.

O: Vulva may be erythematous. Vagina is diffusely red, granular, occasionally with red raised papules and petechiae ("strawberry" appearance). Discharge is frothy, yellow-green, and foul-smelling. Microscopic examination of saline wet mount specimen reveals characteristic flagellated cells.

Bacterial Vaginosis (*Gardnerella vaginalis, Haemophilus vaginalis,* or Nonspecific Vaginitis)

S: Profuse discharge, "constant wetness" with "foul, fishy, rotten" odour.

O: Discharge is thin, creamy, grey-white, and malodorous. No inflammation is present on vaginal wall or cervix because the pathogen is a surface parasite. Microscopic view of saline wet mount specimen reveals typical "clue cells."

Chlamydia

S: Mimics gonorrhea. Of infected women, 75% have no symptoms. Symptoms may include urinary frequency, dysuria, vaginal discharge, or postcoital bleeding.

O: Affected patients may have yellow or green mucopurulent discharge, friable cervix, or cervical motion tenderness. Signs are subtle, easily mistaken for gonorrhea. The two are important to distinguish because antibiotic treatment is different; if the wrong medication is given or if the condition is untreated, *Chlamydia* can ascend the reproductive tract to cause PID and result in infertility. This is the most common sexually transmitted infection in Canada; nearly 70% of all reported cases occur in the 15- to 24-year-old age cohort. Clinicians are urged to screen all sexually active girls and young women every 6 months, regardless of symptoms or risk.

Gonorrhea

S: Variable: vaginal discharge, dysuria, abnormal uterine bleeding, abscess in Bartholin's or Skene's glands; the majority of cases are asymptomatic.

O: Often no signs are apparent. Purulent vaginal discharge may be present. The disease is diagnosed through positive culture of organism. If the condition is untreated, it may progress to acute salpingitis, PID.

O, Objective data; *PID,* pelvic inflammatory disease; *S,* subjective data.
See Illustration Credits for source information.

TABLE 27.6 | Uterine Enlargement

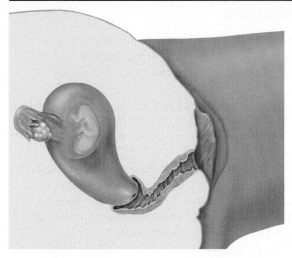

◀ Pregnancy

A normal condition; included here for comparison.

S: Amenorrhea, fatigue, breast engorgement, nausea, change in food tolerance, weight gain.

O: Early signs include cyanosis of vaginal mucosa and cervix (Chadwick's sign). Palpation reveals soft consistency of cervix, enlarging uterus with compressible fundus and isthmus (Hegar's sign) at 10–12 weeks.

◀ Myomas (Leiomyomas, Uterine Fibroids)

S: Varies, depending on size and location. Often no symptoms. Symptoms include vague discomfort, bloating, heaviness, pelvic pressure, dyspareunia, urinary frequency, backache, or hypermenorrhea if myoma disturbs endometrium. Heavy bleeding produces anemia.

O: Uterus irregularly enlarged, firm, mobile, and nodular with hard, painless nodules in the uterine wall.

Myomas are usually benign. Incidence is highest between the ages of 30 and 45 years and in women of African descent. Myomas are estrogen-dependent; after menopause, the lesions usually regress but do not disappear. Surgery may be indicated.

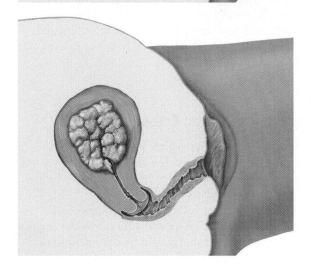

◀ Carcinoma of the Endometrium

S: Abnormal and intermenstrual bleeding before menopause; postmenopausal bleeding or mucosanguineous discharge. Pain and weight loss occur late in the disease.

O: Uterus may be enlarged.

The Pap test is rarely effective in detecting endometrial cancer. Women with abnormal vaginal bleeding or at high risk for endometrial cancer should undergo biopsy of an endometrial tissue sample. Risk factors for endometrial cancer are early menarche, late menopause, history of infertility, failure to ovulate, use of tamoxifen (Tamoxifene), unopposed estrogen therapy (which continually stimulates the endometrium, causing hyperplasia), and obesity (which increases endogenous estrogen).

Continued

TABLE 27.6	Uterine Enlargement—cont'd

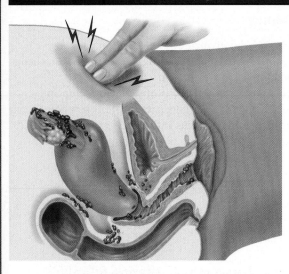

◄ Endometriosis

S: Cyclic or chronic pelvic pain, occurring as dysmenorrhea, dyspareunia, or low backache. It may include irregular uterine bleeding or hypermenorrhea, or it may be asymptomatic.

O: Uterus fixed, tender with movement. Small, firm nodular masses tender to palpation on posterior aspect of fundus, uterosacral ligaments, ovaries, sigmoid colon. Ovaries often enlarged.

Masses are aberrant growths of endometrial tissue scattered throughout pelvis as a result of transplantation of tissue by retrograde menstruation. Ectopic tissue responds to hormone stimulation: builds up between menstrual periods, sloughs during menstruation. May cause infertility through pelvic adhesions, tubal obstruction, decreased ovarian function.

O, Objective data; *S,* subjective data.

TABLE 27.7	Adnexal Enlargement

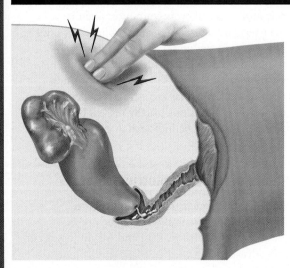

◄ Fallopian Tube Mass: Acute Salpingitis (PID)

S: Sudden fever >38°C (100.4°F), suprapubic pain and tenderness.

O:
- Acute: Rigid, boardlike lower abdominal musculature. Purulent discharge may emanate from cervix. Movement of uterus and cervix causes intense pain. Pain in lateral fornices and adnexa. Bilateral adnexal masses are difficult to palpate because of pain and muscle spasm.
- Chronic: Bilateral, tender, fixed adnexal masses.

Complications include ectopic pregnancy, infertility, and reinfection. PID is usually caused by *Neisseria gonorrhoeae* and *Chlamydia trachomatis.*

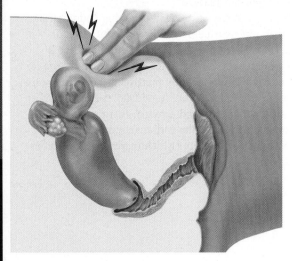

◄ Fallopian Tube Mass: Ectopic Pregnancy

S: Amenorrhea or irregular vaginal bleeding, pelvic pain.

O: Softening of cervix and fundus; movement of cervix and uterus causes pain; palpable, tender pelvic mass, which is solid, mobile, and unilateral.

This condition has potential for serious sequelae; seek gynecological consultation immediately before the mass ruptures or the patient shows signs of acute peritonitis.

TABLE 27.7	Adnexal Enlargement—cont'd

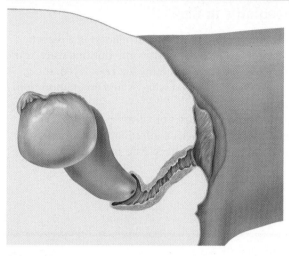

◀ Fluctuant Ovarian Mass: Ovarian Cyst

S: Usually asymptomatic.

O: Smooth, round, fluctuant, mobile, nontender mass on ovary. Some cysts resolve spontaneously within 60 days but must be monitored closely.

◀ Solid Ovarian Mass: Ovarian Cancer

S: Usually asymptomatic. Abdomen may enlarge from fluid accumulation.

O: Solid tumour palpated on ovary. Heavy, solid, fixed, poorly defined mass suggests malignancy; benign mass may feel mobile and solid.

Biopsy necessary to distinguish the two types of masses. The Pap test does not detect ovarian cancer. Women older than 40 years of age should have a thorough pelvic examination every year.

PID, Pelvic inflammatory disease; *O,* objective data; *S,* subjective data.

TABLE 27.8	Abnormalities in Pediatric Genitalia

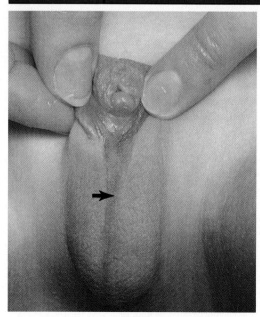

◀ Ambiguous Genitalia

Female pseudohermaphroditism is a congenital anomaly resulting from hyperplasia of the adrenal glands, which exposes the female fetus to excess amounts of androgens. This exposure causes masculinization of external genitalia, here shown as enlargement of the clitoris and fusion of the labia. *Ambiguous* means that the enlarged clitoris may look like a small penis with hypospadias, and the fused labia look like an incompletely formed scrotum with absent testes (*arrow* in illustration). Other forms of intersexual conditions occur, and the family must be referred for counselling and diagnostic evaluation of the child.

Continued

Abnormal Findings

TABLE 27.8 Abnormalities in Pediatric Genitalia—cont'd

◀ Vulvovaginitis in Child

This infection is caused by *Candida albicans* in a diabetic child. Symptoms include pruritus and burning when urine touches excoriated area. Examination reveals red, shiny, edematous vulva; vaginal discharge; and excoriation from scratching.

Other, more common causes of vulvovaginitis in prepubertal children include infection from a respiratory or bowel pathogen, STI, or presence of a foreign body.

STI, Sexually transmitted infection.
See Illustration Credits for source information.

Summary Checklist: Female Genitalia Examination

1. **Inspect external genitalia**
2. **Palpate labia, Skene's,** and **Bartholin's glands**
3. **Using vaginal speculum, inspect cervix and vagina**
4. **Obtain specimens** for cytological study
5. **Perform bimanual examination:** cervix, uterus, adnexa
6. **Perform rectovaginal examination**
7. **Test stool** for occult blood
8. **Engage in teaching and health promotion**

REFERENCES

1. Ramage-Morin, P. L., & Gilmour, H. (2013). *Urinary incontinence and loneliness in Canadian seniors.* Retrieved from http://www.statcan.gc.ca/pub/82-003-x/2013010/article/11872-eng.pdf.
2. Perron, L., Senikas, V., Burnett, M., et al. (2013). Female genital cutting: Clinical practice guidelines. *Journal of Obstetrics and Gynaecology Canada, 35*(11), e1–e18.
3. Public Health Agency of Canada. (2015). *Canadian guidelines on sexually transmitted infections: Primary care and sexually transmitted infections.* Retrieved from http://www.phac-aspc.gc.ca/std-mts/sti-its/cgsti-ldcits/section-2-eng.php#a2.
4. Public Health Agency of Canada. (2015). *HIV and AIDS in Canada: Surveillance report to December 31, 2014.* Retrieved from https://www.canada.ca/en/public-health/services/publications/diseases-conditions/hiv-aids-canada-surveillance-report-december-31-2014.html.
5. Dickinson, J. A., Stankiewicz, A., Popadiuk, C., et al. (2012). Reduced cervical cancer incidence and mortality in Canada: National data from 1932 to 2006. *BMC Public Health, 12,* 992. doi:10.1186/1471-2458-12-992.
6. Torre, L. A., Bray, F., Siegel, R. L., et al. (2015). Global cancer statistics, 2012. *CA: A Cancer Journal for Clinicians, 65*(2), 87–108. doi:10.3322/caac.21262.
7. Canadian Partnership Against Cancer. (2013). *Cervical cancer screening in Canada: Monitoring program performance 2009–2011.* Retrieved from http://www.cancerview.ca/preventionandscreening/cervicalcancercontrolincanada/.
8. Demers, A. A., Kliewer, E. V., Remes, O., et al. (2012). Cervical cancer among Aboriginal women in Canada. *Canadian Medical Association Journal, 184*(7), 743–744. doi:10.1503/cmaj.110523.
9. Epp, A., & Larochelle, A. (2010). SOGC clinical practice guideline: Recurrent urinary tract infection. *Journal of Obstetrics and Gynaecology Canada, 250,* 1082–1090.
10. Deutsch, M. B. (2016). *Guidelines for the primary and gender-affirming care of transgender and gender nonbinary people.* Retrieved from http://transhealth.ucsf.edu/protocols.
11. Lin, S. N., Taylor, J., Alperstein, S., et al. (2014). Does speculum lubricant affect liquid-based Papanicolaou test adequacy? *Cancer Cytopathology, 122,* 221–226. doi:10.1002/cncy.21369.
12. Canadian Task Force on Preventive Health Care. (2013). Recommendations on screening for cervical cancer. *Canadian Medical Association Journal, 185*(1), 35–45. doi:10.1503/cmaj.121505.
13. Bournes, A. (2015). *Guidelines and protocols for hormone therapy and primary health care for trans clients.* Retrieved from http://sherbourne.on.ca/lgbt-health/guidelines-protocols-for-trans-care/.
14. Canadian Partnership Against Cancer. (2016). *Cervical cancer screening in Canada: Environmental scan.* Retrieved from http://www.cancerview.ca/preventionandscreening/cervicalcancercontrolincanada/.
15. Cancer Care Nova Scotia. (2014). *Screening for cancer of the cervix: An office manual for health professionals.* Retrieved from http://www.cancercare.ns.ca/site-cc/media/cancercare/Office%20Manual%202014.pdf.

CHAPTER 28

The Complete Health Assessment: Putting It All Together

Written by Carolyn Jarvis, PhD, APN, CNP
Adapted by Marian Luctkar-Flude, RN, PhD

(e) http://evolve.elsevier.com/Canada/Jarvis/examination/

The choreography of the complete history and physical examination is the art of arranging the separate steps you have learned so far. For patients who do not speak English or another language spoken by the nurse, obtain a cultural interpreter whenever possible to ensure accuracy of communication. Your first examination may seem awkward; you may have to pause and think about what comes next. With repeated rehearsals, the procedure will flow naturally, and if you forget a step, you will be able to insert it gracefully at the next logical time. Continue to engage the patient in dialogue at appropriate moments during the physical examination to collect additional subjective data. Abnormal physical assessment findings will prompt you to explore further in a focused assessment. Remain attentive to physical signs suggestive of abuse. If abuse is suspected, ask the patient directly, in a nonjudgemental manner, about the presence of interpersonal violence. Although annual physical examinations are associated with improved delivery of some preventive health services and increased number of diagnoses, they do not reduce morbidity and mortality from cardiovascular disease or cancer.[1] Insurance coverage for annual physical examinations is not standardized across Canada, with each province having its own approach; however, a physical examination is generally conducted when medically necessary, and tailored to the patient's specific needs.[2]

A complete examination may be performed at a patient's initial outpatient visit or hospital admission. The following suggested examination sequence is intended to minimize the number of position changes for the patient and for you. With experience, you may rearrange this sequence in a way

that feels natural for you; you will learn which steps you must retain to be thorough and those you may safely omit when time is pressing. Individual organizations may have standardized documentation forms outlining which components of the complete health assessment are recommended for routine versus specialized encounters. The steps for the follow-up or shift assessment are described in Chapter 29.

Review Chapter 9 for preparing the setting, preparing patients, and your approach with regard to their age. Have all equipment prepared and accessible before the examination. Refer to the following list of equipment usually needed for a screening physical examination.

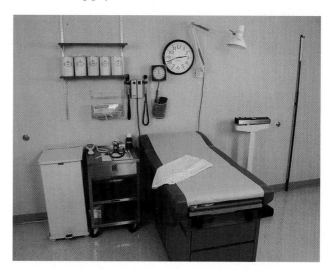

EQUIPMENT LIST

Platform scale with
    height attachment
Skinfold calipers (if
    indicated)
Flexible measuring tape
Sphygmomanometer
Stethoscope with bell
    and diaphragm
Thermometer
Pulse oximeter (if
    indicated)
Flashlight or penlight
Otoscope/
    ophthalmoscope
Tuning fork
Nasal speculum (if a
    short, broad speculum
    is not included with
    the otoscope)

Tongue depressor
Snellen eye chart
    or pocket vision
    screener
Skin-marking pen
Ruler marked in
    centimetres
Reflex hammer
Sharp object (split
    tongue blade)
Cotton balls
Bivalve vaginal speculum
Clean gloves
Materials for cytological
    study
Lubricant
Fecal occult blood test
    materials

SUBJECTIVE DATA

Sequence

Selected Photos

The patient walks into the room, sits; the examiner sits facing the patient; the patient remains in street clothes. (Note: Position changes are noted in *italics*.)

Health History

Collect the history, complete or limited as visit warrants (refer to Chapter 5):
1. Biographical data
2. Reason for seeking care
3. Present health or history of present illness
4. Past history
5. Family history
6. Review of systems
7. Functional assessment or activities of daily living (ADLs)

Throughout the history and examination, note data on the patient's general appearance.

OBJECTIVE DATA

Sequence	Selected Photos

General Survey

1. Whether patient appears stated age
2. Level of consciousness
3. Skin colour
4. Nutritional status
5. Posture and position; comfortably erect
6. Obvious physical deformities
7. Mobility:
   Gait
   Use of assistive devices
   Range of motion (ROM) of joints
   Involuntary movements
   Ability to rise from a seated position
8. Facial expression
9. Mood and affect
10. Speech: articulation, pattern; content appropriate; first language
11. Hearing
12. Personal hygiene

Measurement

1. Weight
2. Height
3. Body mass index (BMI)
4. Waist and hip measurements (not indicated for patients younger than age 18 years or for pregnant or lactating women)
5. Skinfold measurements (if indicated)
6. Vision with Snellen eye chart (if indicated)

Ask the patient to empty the bladder (save urine specimen, if needed), disrobe except for underwear, and put on a gown. The patient *sits with legs dangling* off side of the bed or table; you stand in front of the patient.

Vital Signs

1. Radial pulse
2. Respirations
3. Blood pressure in arms
4. Blood pressure in lower leg; compute ankle/brachial index (if indicated)
5. Temperature (if indicated)
6. Oxygen saturation (if indicated)
7. Patient's rating of pain level on a scale of 0 to 10; note location and quality of pain. If appropriate, use the Faces Pain Scale–Revised (see Fig. 11.5, p. 190).

Skin

1. Examine both hands and inspect nails.
2. For the rest of the examination, examine the skin of the corresponding region.

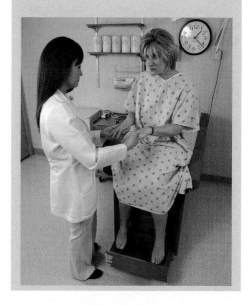

Sequence	**Selected Photos**

Head and Face

1. Inspect and palpate scalp, hair, and cranium.
2. Inspect face: expression, symmetry (cranial nerve VII).
3. Palpate the temporal artery and then the temporomandibular joint as the patient opens and closes the mouth.
4. Palpate the maxillary sinuses and frontal sinuses.

Eye

1. Test visual fields by confrontation (cranial nerve II).
2. Test extraocular muscles: corneal light reflex, six cardinal positions of gaze (cranial nerves III, IV, VI).
3. Inspect external eye structures.
4. Inspect conjunctivae, sclerae, corneas, irides.
5. Test pupil: size, response to light and accommodation.
6. Darken room. Using an ophthalmoscope, inspect ocular fundus: red reflex, disc, vessels, and retinal background (if indicated).

Ear

1. Inspect the external ear: position and alignment, skin condition, and auditory meatus.
2. Move auricle, and push tragus for tenderness.
3. With an otoscope, inspect the canal and then the tympanic membrane for colour, position, landmarks, and integrity.
4. Assess hearing with the whispered voice test.

Nose

1. Inspect the external nose: symmetry, lesions.
2. Inspect facial symmetry (cranial nerve VII).
3. Test the patency of each nostril.
4. With a speculum, inspect nares: nasal mucosa, septum, and turbinates.

Mouth and Throat

1. With a penlight, inspect the mouth: buccal mucosa, teeth, gums, tongue, floor of mouth, palate, and uvula.
2. Grade tonsils, if present.
3. Note mobility of uvula as the patient phonates "ahhh," and test gag reflex (cranial nerves IX, X).
4. Ask the patient to stick out the tongue (cranial nerve XII).
5. With a gloved hand, bimanually palpate the mouth (if indicated).

Objective Data

| **Sequence** | **Selected Photos** |

Neck

1. Inspect the neck: symmetry, lumps, and pulsations.
2. Palpate cervical lymph nodes.
3. Inspect and palpate carotid pulses, one side at a time. Listen for carotid bruits (if indicated).
4. Palpate trachea in midline.
5. Test ROM and muscle strength against your resistance: head forward and back, head turned to each side, and shoulder shrug (cranial nerve XI).

Step behind the patient, taking your stethoscope, ruler, and marking pen with you.

6. Palpate thyroid gland, posterior approach.
   Open the patient's gown to expose the back for examination of the thorax, but leave gown on shoulders and chest.

Chest, Posterior and Lateral

1. Inspect the posterior chest: configuration of the thoracic cage, skin characteristics, and symmetry of shoulders and muscles.
2. Palpate for symmetrical expansion; tactile fremitus; lumps or tenderness.
3. Palpate length of spinous processes.
4. Percuss over all lung fields; percuss diaphragmatic excursion.
5. Percuss costovertebral angle, noting tenderness.
6. Auscultate breath sounds, comparing side with side in upper and lateral lung fields; note any adventitious sounds. (Do *not* listen over the patient's gown.)

Move around to face the patient; the patient remains sitting. For a female breast examination, ask permission to lift gown to drape on the shoulders, exposing the chest; for a male patient, lower the gown to the lap.

Chest, Anterior

1. Inspect respirations and skin characteristics.
2. Palpate for tactile fremitus, lumps, or tenderness.
3. Percuss anterior lung fields.
4. Auscultate breath sounds, comparing side to side in upper and lower lung fields; note any adventitious sounds. (Do *not* listen over the patient's gown.)

Heart

1. Ask the patient to lean forward and exhale briefly; auscultate the cardiac base for any murmurs. (Do *not* listen over the patient's gown.)

Upper Extremities

1. Test ROM and muscle strength of hands, arms, and shoulders.
2. Palpate the epitrochlear nodes.
3. Palpate temperature, capillary refill.
4. Compare radial and brachial pulses.

Sequence	Selected Photos

Female Breasts

1. Inspect for symmetry, mobility, and dimpling as the patient lifts the arms over the head, pushes the hands on the hips, and leans forward.
2. Inspect supraclavicular and infraclavicular areas.
   Help the patient *lie supine with their head flat or up to a 30-degree angle.* Stand at the patient's right side. Drape the gown up across the patient's shoulders to expose the anterior chest, and place an extra sheet across the lower abdomen.
3. Palpate each breast, lifting the same-side arm up over the patient's head. As you palpate, include the tail of Spence and areola.
4. Palpate each nipple for discharge.
5. Support the patient's arm, and palpate the axilla and regional lymph nodes.
6. Teach breast self-examination, if the patient asks to learn it.

Male Breasts

1. Inspect and palpate the chest wall.
2. Supporting each arm, palpate the axillae and regional nodes.

Neck Vessels

1. Inspect each side of the patient's neck for a jugular venous pulse, turning the patient's head slightly to the other side.
2. Estimate jugular venous pressure (if indicated).

Heart

1. Inspect the precordium for any pulsations or heave (lift).
2. Palpate the apical impulse, and note location.
3. Palpate the precordium for any abnormal thrill.
4. Auscultate apical rate and rhythm.
5. Auscultate heart sounds with the diaphragm of the stethoscope, inching from the apex up to the base, or vice versa.
6. Auscultate heart sounds with the bell of the stethoscope, again inching through all locations.
7. Turn the patient to the left side while you auscultate the apex with the bell.

Abdomen

The patient should be *supine*, with the bed flat; arrange drapes to expose the abdomen from the chest to the pubis.

1. Inspect contour, symmetry, skin characteristics, umbilicus, and pulsations.
2. Auscultate bowel sounds.
3. Auscultate for vascular sounds over the aorta and renal arteries.
4. Percuss all quadrants.
5. Percuss height of the liver span at the right midclavicular line.
6. Percuss location of the spleen.
7. Palpate lightly in all quadrants; then palpate deeply in all quadrants.

Objective Data

Sequence	**Selected Photos**

8. Palpate for liver, spleen, kidneys, and aorta.
9. Test the abdominal reflexes (if indicated).

Inguinal Area

1. Palpate each side of the groin for the femoral pulse and inguinal nodes. Lift the drape to expose the legs.

Lower Extremities

1. Inspect symmetry, skin characteristics, and hair distribution.
2. Palpate pulses: popliteal, posterior tibial, dorsalis pedis.
3. Use Doppler technique to locate peripheral pulses (if indicated).
4. Palpate for temperature and pretibial edema.
5. Separate toes and inspect.
6. Test ROM and muscle strength of hips, knees, ankles, and feet.

Ask the patient to *sit up with the legs dangling* off the bed or table. Keep the gown on and the drape over the patient's lap.

Musculo-Skeletal

1. Note muscle strength as the patient sits up.

Neurological

1. Test sensation in selected areas on face, arms, hands, legs, and feet: superficial pain, light touch, and vibration.
2. Test position sense of finger, one hand.
3. Test stereognosis, using a familiar object.
4. Evaluate cerebellar function of upper extremities with the finger-to-nose test or test of rapid alternating movements.

Objective Data

Sequence	**Selected Photos**

5. Elicit deep tendon reflexes of upper extremities: biceps, triceps, and brachioradialis.

6. Test the cerebellar function of the lower extremities by asking the patient to run each heel down the opposite shin.
7. Elicit deep tendon reflexes of the lower extremities: patellar and Achilles.
8. Test for the Babinski reflex.

Ask the patient to *stand* with the gown on. Stand close to the patient.

Lower Extremities

1. Inspect the patient's legs for varicose veins.

Musculo-Skeletal

1. Ask the patient to *walk* across the room in regular gait, to turn, and to walk back toward you in heel-to-toe manner.
2. Ask the patient to walk on the toes for a few steps and then to walk on the heels for a few steps.
3. Stand close and check for the Romberg sign.

Objective Data

Sequence	**Selected Photos**

4. Ask the patient to hold the edge of the bed and to stand on one leg and perform a shallow knee bend, one for each leg.
5. Stand behind the patient, and check the spine as the patient touches the toes.
6. Stabilize the patient's pelvis and test ROM of the spine as the patient hyperextends, rotates, and laterally bends.

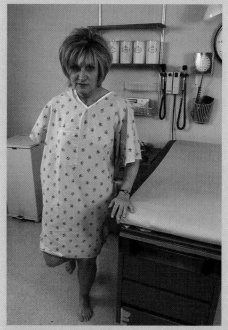

Male Genitalia

For a male patient, sit on a stool in front of him. The patient stands.
1. Inspect the penis and scrotum.
2. Palpate the scrotal contents. If a mass exists, transilluminate the scrotum.
3. Check for inguinal hernia.
4. Teach testicular self-examination.

Male Rectum

For a male patient, ask him to *bend over the examination table*, with his forearms on the table. Assist a bedridden man to a *left lateral position*, with his right leg drawn up.
1. Inspect the perianal area.
2. With a gloved lubricated finger, palpate rectal walls and prostate gland.
3. Save a stool specimen for an occult blood test.

Female Genitalia

Assist the female patient back to the examination table, and help them *assume the lithotomy position*. Drape the patient appropriately. For the speculum examination, sit on a stool at the foot of the table; for the bimanual examination, stand.

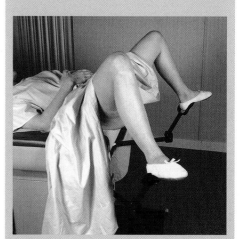

Objective Data

Sequence	Selected Photos

Sequence

1. Inspect the perineal and perianal areas.
2. With a vaginal speculum, inspect the cervix and vaginal walls.
3. Procure specimens.
4. Perform a bimanual examination; cervix, uterus, and adnexa.
5. Continue bimanual examination, checking the rectum and rectovaginal walls.
6. Save a stool specimen for an occult blood test.
7. Provide tissues for the patient to wipe the perineal area, and help the patient up to a *sitting position.*

Tell the patient that you are finished with the examination and that you will leave the room as the patient gets dressed. Return to discuss the examination and further plans and to answer any questions. Thank the patient for his, her, or their time.

For a hospitalized patient, return the bed and any room equipment to the way you found it. Make sure the call bell and telephone are within easy reach.

Newborns and Infants

Review Chapter 9 for the steps in preparation and positioning, and for developmental principles. The 1-minute and 5-minute Apgar results are important data about the newborn's immediate response to extrauterine life. The following sequence expands these data. You may reorder this sequence as the infant's sleep and wakefulness state or physical condition warrants.

The infant is *supine* on a warming table or examination table with an overhead heating element. The infant may be nude except for a diaper.

Vital Signs

Note pulse, respirations, and temperature.

Measurement

Measure and plot weight, length, and head circumference on growth curves for the infant's age.

General Survey

1. Body symmetry, spontaneous position, flexion of head and extremities, and spontaneous movement
2. Skin colour and characteristics; any obvious deformities
3. Symmetry and positioning of facial features
4. Alert, responsive affect
5. Strong, lusty cry

Chest and Heart

1. Inspect condition of the skin over the chest and abdomen; chest configuration; and nipples and breast tissue.
2. Note movement of the abdomen with respirations and any chest retraction.
3. Palpate the apical impulse and note its location; palpate the chest wall for thrills; assess tactile fremitus if infant is crying.
4. Auscultate breath sounds, heart sounds in all locations, and bowel sounds in the abdomen.

Sequence	Selected Photos

Abdomen

1. Inspect the shape of the abdomen and skin condition.
2. Inspect the umbilicus; count vessels; note the condition of the cord or stump and the presence of any hernia.
3. Palpate skin turgor.
4. Palpate lightly for muscle tone, liver, spleen tip, and bladder.
5. Palpate deeply for kidneys and any mass.
6. Palpate femoral pulses and inguinal lymph nodes.
7. Percuss all quadrants.

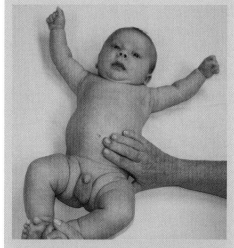

Head and Face

1. Note moulding of the cranium after delivery, any swelling on the cranium, and bulging of fontanelle with crying or at rest.
2. Palpate fontanelles, suture lines, and any swellings.
3. Inspect positioning and symmetry of facial features of infant at rest and during crying.

Eyes

To open a newborn's eyes, support the head and shoulders and gently lower the baby backward, or ask the parent to hold the baby over the shoulder while you stand behind the parent.

1. Inspect the eyelids (edematous in newborns), palpebral slant, conjunctivae, any nystagmus, and any discharge.
2. Use a penlight to elicit pupillary reflex, blink reflex, and corneal light reflex; assess tracking of a moving light.
3. Using an ophthalmoscope, elicit the red reflex.

Ears

(Defer otoscopic examination until the end of the complete examination.)

1. Inspect size, shape, alignment of auricles; patency of auditory canals; and any extra skin tags or pits.
2. Note the startle reflex in response to a loud noise.
3. Palpate flexible auricles.

Sequence	**Selected Photos**

Nose

1. Determine the patency of the nares.
2. Note nasal discharge, sneezing, and any flaring with respirations.

Mouth and Throat

1. Inspect the lips and gums, high-arched intact palate, buccal mucosa, tongue size, and frenulum of tongue; in a newborn, note absence of or minimal salivation.
2. Note the rooting reflex.
3. Insert a gloved little finger into the infant's mouth, note sucking reflex, and palpate palate.

Neck

1. Lift the infant's shoulders, and let the head lag to inspect the neck: Note midline trachea, any skinfolds, and any lumps.
2. Palpate the lymph nodes, the thyroid, and any masses.
3. While the infant is supine, elicit the tonic neck reflex; note suppleness of the neck with movement.

Upper Extremities

1. Inspect and manipulate, noting ROM, muscle tone, and absence of the scarf sign (elbow should not reach midline).
2. Count fingers, count palmar creases, and note colour of hands and nail beds.
3. Place your thumbs in the infant's palms to note the grasp reflex; wrap your hands around infant's hands to pull up, and note the head lag.

Lower Extremities

1. Inspect and manipulate the legs and feet, noting ROM, muscle tone, and skin condition.
2. Note alignment of feet and toes, look for flat soles, and count toes; note any syndactyly.
3. Perform the Ortolani manoeuvre to test for hip stability.

Objective Data

Sequence	**Selected Photos**

Genitalia

Girls: Inspect labia and clitoris (edematous in the newborn), vernix caseosa between labia, and patent vagina.

Boys:

1. Inspect position of urethral meatus (do not retract foreskin); strength of urine stream, if possible; and rugae on scrotum.
2. Palpate the testes in the scrotum.

Lift the infant under the axillae, and *hold the infant facing you* at eye level.

Neuromuscular

1. Note shoulder muscle tone and the infant's ability to stay in your hands without slipping.
2. Rotate the newborn slowly side to side; note the doll's eye reflex.
3. Turn the infant around so the back is to you; elicit the stepping reflex and the placing reflex against the edge of the examination table.

Spine and Rectum

Turn the infant over. Hold the infant prone in your hands or *place the infant prone* on the examination table.

1. Inspect the length of the spine, trunk incurvation reflex, and symmetry of gluteal folds.
2. Inspect the skin; note any sinus openings, protrusions, or tufts of hair.
3. Note patent anal opening. In a newborn, check for passage of meconium stool during the first 24 to 48 hours.

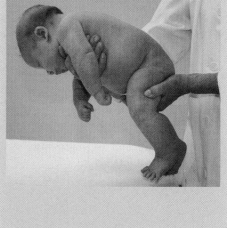

Sequence	Selected Photos

Objective Data

Final Procedures

1. With an otoscope, inspect the auditory canals and tympanic membranes.
2. Elicit the Moro reflex by letting the infant's head and trunk drop back a short way, by jarring crib sides or making a loud noise.

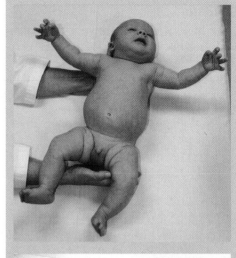

Young Children

Review the developmental considerations in preparing for an examination of a toddler and a young child in Chapter 9. The young child has a desire for independence, which conflicts with the child's basic dependence. Also, the child is fearful of a new environment, has a fear of invasive procedures, dislikes being restrained, and may be emotionally attached to a security object.

At the start of the examination, focus on the parent as the child plays with a toy.

The Health History

1. Collect the history, including developmental data. During the history, note data on general appearance.

General Survey

1. Note the child's ability to play independently while the parent speaks.
2. Note interactions between parent and child.
3. Note gross- and fine-motor skills as the child plays with a toy. Gradually involve the child, at first in a "play" period.
4. Evaluate developmental milestones by using an age-appropriate Nipissing District Developmental Screen (see Fig. 2.3, p. 24).
5. Evaluate posture while the child is sitting and standing. Evaluate alignment of legs and feet while the child is walking.
6. Evaluate speech acquisition.
7. Evaluate vision and hearing ability.
8. Evaluate social interaction.

Sequence	Selected Photos

Ask the parent to undress the child or help the child undress to the diaper or underwear. Position a child 6 months to 2 or 3 years of age in the *parent's lap*. Move your chair to sit knee-to-knee with the parent. Most 4- or 5-year-old children feel comfortable on the examination table.

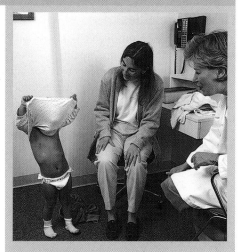

Measurement

Document the child's height, weight, and head circumference (you may need to defer measuring head circumference until later in the examination).

Chest and Heart

1. Auscultate breath sounds and heart sounds in all locations; count respiratory rate and heart rate; and auscultate bowel sounds.
2. Inspect size, shape, and configuration of the thoracic cage. Assess respiratory movement.
3. Inspect pulsations on the precordium. Note nipple and breast development.
4. Palpate apical impulse and note location; palpate chest wall for thrills and any tactile fremitus.

Abdomen

The child should be *sitting up in the parent's lap or on the examination table*, in diaper or underwear.
1. Inspect shape of the abdomen, skin condition, and periumbilical area.
2. Palpate skin turgor, muscle tone, liver edge, spleen, kidneys, and any masses.
3. Palpate femoral pulses. Compare strength with radial pulses.
4. Palpate inguinal lymph nodes.

Genitalia

1. Inspect the external genitalia.
2. On boys, palpate scrotum for testes. If masses are present, transilluminate the scrotum.

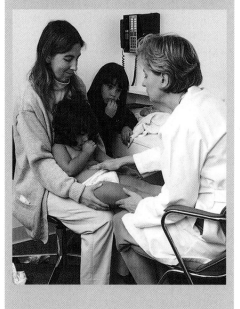

Objective Data

Sequence	Selected Photos

Lower Extremities

The child should be *sitting up in the parent's lap or lying supine on the examination table*, in diaper or underpants.

1. Perform the Ortolani manoeuvre for hip stability.
2. Note skin condition and alignment of legs.
3. Note alignment of feet. Inspect toes and longitudinal arch.
4. Palpate the dorsalis pedis pulse.
5. Obtain the child's cooperation for the reflex hammer test by allowing the child to play with the hammer. Elicit plantar, Achilles, and patellar reflexes.

Upper Extremities

The child should be *sitting up in the parent's lap or on the examination table*, in diaper or underwear.

1. Inspect the arms and hands for alignment and skin condition; inspect the fingers, and note palmar creases.
2. Palpate and count the radial pulse.
3. Test biceps and triceps reflexes with a reflex hammer.
4. Measure blood pressure.

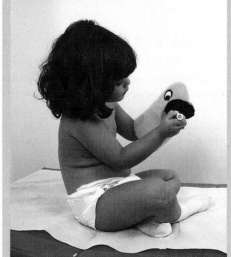

Head and Neck

1. Inspect the size and shape of the head and symmetry of facies.
2. Palpate the fontanels and cranium. Palpate cervical lymph nodes, trachea, and thyroid gland.
3. Measure the head circumference.

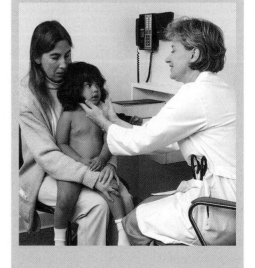

Eyes

1. Inspect the external structures. Note any palpebral slant.
2. With a penlight, test corneal and pupillary light reflexes.
3. Direct a moving penlight to test cardinal positions of gaze.
4. Perform the cover test (if indicated) by covering the child's eye with your thumb or with an index card.
5. Inspect conjunctivae and sclerae.
6. With an ophthalmoscope, check the red reflex. Inspect the fundus as much as possible.

Sequence	Selected Photos

Nose

1. Inspect the external nose and its skin condition.
2. With a penlight, inspect the nares for foreign body, mucosa, septum, and turbinates.

Mouth and Throat

1. Have the child stick out the tongue. (Use a tongue blade as the last resort.) With a penlight, inspect the mouth, buccal mucosa, teeth, gums, tongue, palate, and uvula in midline.

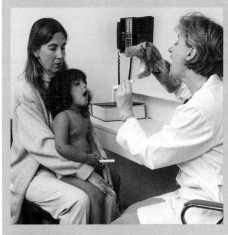

Ears

1. Inspect and palpate the auricles. Note any discharge from the auditory meatus. Check for any foreign body.
2. With an otoscope, inspect the ear canals and tympanic membranes. Obtain the child's cooperation by using a puppet, by encouraging the child to handle the equipment, or by having the child look in the parent's ear as you hold the otoscope. You may need the parent's help in restraining the child.

Objective Data

Sequence	Selected Photos

School-Age Children, Adolescents, and Older Adults

The sequence of the examination in these age groups is the head-to-toe format described for adults. However, review Chapter 9 for differences in approach and timing, and for special developmental considerations.

DOCUMENTATION AND CRITICAL THINKING

RECORDING THE DATA

Record the history and physical examination data as soon as possible. Memory fades over time, especially when you are responsible for the care of more than one patient.

It is difficult to strike a balance between recording too much and too little data; however, from a legal perspective, if a procedure is not documented, it was not performed. Data important for the diagnosis and treatment of the patient's health should be recorded, as should data that contribute to your decision-making process. This includes charting relevant normal or negative findings.

A listing of every assessment parameter described in this text will result in an unwieldy, unworkable record. One way to keep your record complete but succinct is to use short, clear phrases. Avoid redundant introductory phrases such as "The patient states that … ." Avoid redundant descriptions such as "No inguinal, femoral, or umbilical hernias." Just write "No hernias."

Use simple line drawings to describe your findings. Draw a simple sketch of a tympanic membrane, breast, abdomen, or cervix, and mark your findings on it.

Consider Ellen from Chapter 1, who is receiving care at a primary health care setting. Study the following complete history and physical examination for a sample write-up.

Focused Assessment: Clinical Case Study

HEALTH HISTORY

Biographical Data

Name: Ellen K.

Address: 123 Centre St.

Marital Status: Single

Birth date: 1/18/xxxx

Birthplace: Mt. Albert

Ethnocultural background: Euro-Canadian

Ellen K. is a 23-year-old, single female; was cashier in a large department store, currently unemployed for 6 months.

Objective Data

Documentation and Critical Thinking

Source: Ellen, seems reliable.

Reason for seeking care: "It's been over 5 years since I've had a checkup. I'm worried about my drinking."

History of present illness: Alcohol use started age 16. For past 2 years, has equivalent of 3–4 drinks per day × 4–5 days per week. Most recent alcohol intake was yesterday.

Past Health

Childhood illnesses: Chicken pox at age 6. No measles, mumps, croup, or pertussis. No rheumatic fever, scarlet fever, or polio.

Accidents: (a) Auto accident, age 12, father driving, Ellen thrown from car, R [right] leg crushed. Hospitalized at Memorial Hospital, surgery for leg pinning to repair multiple compound fracture. (b) Auto accident, age 21, head hit dashboard, no loss of consciousness, treated and released at Memorial Hospital ED. (c) Auto accident, age 23, "car hit median strip," no injuries, not seen at hospital.

Chronic illnesses: None.

Hospitalizations: Age 12, Memorial Hospital, surgery to repair R leg as described, Dr. M.J. Carlson, surgeon.

Obstetrical history: Grav 0/Para 0/Ab 0.

Immunizations: Childhood immunizations up to date. Last tetanus "probably high school." No TB [tuberculin] skin test.

Last examinations: Yearly pelvic examinations at the Public Health Sexual Health Clinic since age 18, told "normal." High-school-sports physical, age 16. Most recent dental examination, age 15; most recent vision test for driver's licence, age 16; has never had ECG [electrocardiography] or chest radiograph.

Allergies: No known allergies.

Current medications: Birth control pills, low-estrogen type, for 3 years. No other prescription or OTC [over-the-counter] medications.

Family History

Ellen is second and youngest child, parents divorced 8 years, father has chronic alcoholism. See the following family genogram:

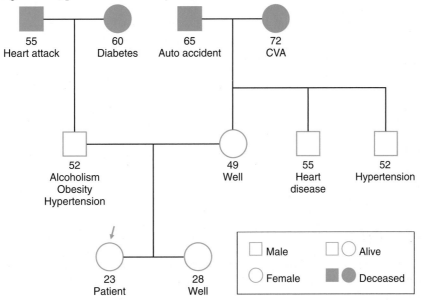

REVIEW OF SYSTEMS

General health: Reports usual health "OK." No recent weight change; no fatigue, weakness, fever, or sweats.

Skin: No change in skin colour, pigmentation, or nevi. No pruritus, rash, or lesions. Has bruise now over right eye, struck by boyfriend 1 week ago. No history of skin disease. Hair, no loss or change in texture. Nails, no change. Self-care: Stays in sun "as much as I can." No sunscreen use. Goes to tanning beds at hair salon twice/week during winter.

Head: No unusually frequent or severe headaches; no head injury, dizziness, syncope, or vertigo.

Eyes: No difficulty with vision or double vision. No eye pain, inflammation, discharge, or lesions. No history of glaucoma or cataracts. No corrective lenses.

Ears: No hearing loss or difficulty. No earaches, infections now or as child, no discharge, tinnitus, or vertigo. Self-care: No exposure to environmental noise; cleans ears with washcloth.

Nose: No discharge; has two to three colds per year; no sinus pain, nasal obstruction, epistaxis, or allergy.

Mouth and throat: No mouth pain, bleeding gums, toothache, sores or lesions in mouth, dysphagia, hoarseness, or sore throat. Has tonsils. Self-care: Brushes teeth twice/day, no flossing.

Documentation and Critical Thinking

Neck: No pain, limitation of motion, lumps, or swollen glands.

Breast: No pain, lump, nipple discharge, rash, swelling, or trauma. No history of breast disease in self, mother, or sister. No surgery.

Respiratory: No history of lung disease, no chest pain with breathing, no wheezing, no shortness of breath. Colds sometimes "go to my chest," treats with OTC cough medicine and acetaminophen. Occasional early morning cough, nonproductive. Smokes cigarettes ½ PPD [pack of cigarettes per day] × 2 years, prior use 1 PPD × 4 years. Never tried to quit. Boyfriend smokes.

Cardiovascular: No chest pain, palpitation, cyanosis, fatigue, dyspnea with exertion, orthopnea, paroxysmal nocturnal dyspnea, nocturia, or edema. No history of heart murmur, hypertension, coronary artery disease, or anemia.

Peripheral vascular: No pain, numbness or tingling, or swelling in legs. No coldness, discoloration, varicose veins, infections, or ulcers. Legs are unequal in length as sequela of accident age 12. Self-care: Usual work as cashier involves standing for 8-hour shifts, no support hose.

Gastro-intestinal: Appetite good with no recent change. No food intolerance, heartburn, indigestion, pain in abdomen, nausea, or vomiting. No history of ulcers, liver or gallbladder disease, jaundice, appendicitis, or colitis. Bowel movement 1/day, soft, brown; no rectal bleeding or pain. Self-care: No use of vitamins, antacids, laxatives. Diet recall: see Functional Assessment (below).

Urinary: No dysuria, frequency, urgency, nocturia, hesitancy, or straining. No pain in flank, groin, or suprapubic region. Urine colour yellow, no history of kidney disease.

Genitalia: Menarche age 11. LMP [last menstrual period] April 18. Cycle usually q28d, duration 4 to 5 days, flow moderate, no dysmenorrhea. No vaginal itching or discharge, sores or lesions.

Sexual health: In relationship that includes intercourse. This boyfriend has been her only sexual partner for 2 years; one other partner before that. Uses birth control pills to prevent pregnancy, partner uses no condoms. Concerned boyfriend may be having sex with other women but has not confronted him. Not aware of any STI [sexually transmitted infection] contact. Never tested for HIV [human immunodeficiency virus]. History of sexual abuse by father from ages 12 to 16 years, abuse did not include intercourse. Ellen unwilling to discuss further at this time.

Musculo-skeletal: No history of arthritis or gout. No joint pain, stiffness, swelling, deformity, or limitation of motion. No muscle pain or weakness. Bone trauma at age 12, has sequela of unequal leg lengths, R leg shorter, walks with limp. Self-care: No walking or running for sport or exercise "because of leg." Able to stand as cashier. Uses lift pad in right shoe to equalize leg length.

Neurological: No history of seizure disorder, stroke, fainting. Has had blackouts with alcohol use. No weakness, tremor, paralysis, problems with coordination, or difficulty speaking or swallowing. No numbness or tingling. Not aware of memory problem, nervousness or mood change, or depression. Had counselling for sexual abuse in the past. Denies any suicidal ideation or intent during adolescent years or now.

Hematological: No bleeding problems in skin or excessive bruising. Not aware of exposure to toxins; never had blood transfusion; never used needles to shoot drugs.

Endocrine: Paternal grandmother with diabetes. No increase in hunger, thirst, or urination; no problems with hot or cold environments; no change in skin, appetite, or nervousness.

FUNCTIONAL ASSESSMENT

Self-concept: Graduated from high school. Worked as a department store cashier. Unemployed now, on social assistance, does not perceive she has enough money for daily living. Lives with boyfriend of 2 years in a rented small basement suite. Raised as Presbyterian, believes in God, does not attend church. Believes self to be "honest, dependable." Believes limitations are "smoking, weight, drinking."

Activity and exercise: Typical day: arises 9 A.M., light chores or TV, spends day looking for work, running errands, with friends, bedtime at 11 P.M. No sustained physical exercise. Able to perform all ADLs; limp poses no problem in bathing, dressing, cooking, household tasks, mobility, driving a car, or work as cashier. No mobility aids. Hobbies are fishing, boating, and snowmobiling, although currently has no finances to engage in these.

Sleep and rest: Bedtime 11 P.M. Sleeps 8 to 9 hours. No sleep aids.

Nutrition: 24-Hour recall: breakfast, none; lunch, bologna sandwich, chips, diet pop; dinner, hamburger, French fries, coffee; snacks, peanuts, potato chips. This menu is typical of most days. Eats lunch at home alone. Most dinners at fast-food restaurants. Shares household grocery expenses and cooking with boyfriend. No food intolerances.

Alcohol: Alcohol use started age 16. For past 2 years, has equivalent of 3–4 drinks per day × 4–5 days per week. Most recent alcohol intake was yesterday. Denies use of street drugs.

Interpersonal relationships: Describes family life growing up as chaotic. Father physically abusive toward mother, and sexually abusive toward Ellen. Parents divorced because of father's continual drinking. Few support systems currently. Estranged from mother, "didn't believe me about my father." Father estranged from entire family. Gets along "OK" with sister. Relationship with boyfriend chaotic; he has hit her twice in the past. Ellen has never pressed legal charges. No close women friends. Most friends are "drinking buddies."

Coping and stress management: Believes housing adequate, adequate heat and utilities, and neighbourhood safe. Believes home has no safety hazards. Does not use seatbelts. No travel outside 100 km of hometown. Identifies current stresses to be drinking, unemployment, financial worries, and relationship with boyfriend. Considers her drinking to be problematic.

PERCEPTION OF HEALTH

Identifies alcohol as a health problem for herself, feels motivated for treatment. Never been interested in physical health and own body before; "Now I think it's time I learned." Expects health care providers to "help me with my drinking."

PHYSICAL EXAMINATION

Measurement

Height: 163 cm (5′4″); weight: 68.6 kg (151 lb)
BP [blood pressure]: 142/100 mm Hg right arm, sitting; 140/96 mm Hg right arm, lying; 138/98 mm Hg left arm, lying
Temp: 37°C (98.6°F); pulse: 76 bpm [beats per minute], regular; resp: 16/min, unlaboured
General survey: Ellen K. is a 23-year-old female, not currently under the influence of alcohol or other substances, articulates clearly, ambulates without difficulty, is in no distress, but is tearful when discussing her boyfriend or her drinking.

Head-to-Toe Examination

Skin: Uniformly tan-pink in colour, warm, dry, intact; turgor good. No lesions, birthmarks, or edema. Resolving 2-cm yellow-green hematoma present over R eye, no swelling, ocular structures not involved. Hair, normal distribution and texture, no visible infestations. Nails, no clubbing, biting, or discolorations. Nail beds pink and firm with prompt capillary refill.

Head: Normocephalic, no lesions, lumps, scaling, parasites, or tenderness. Face, symmetrical, no weakness, no involuntary movements.

Eyes: Acuity by Snellen chart 20/20 [right eye], 20/20 [left eye]. Visual fields full by confrontation. EOMs [extraocular movements] intact, no nystagmus. No ptosis, lid lag, discharge, or crusting. Corneal light reflex symmetrical, no strabismus. Conjunctivae clear. Sclera white, no lesion or redness. PERRLA [pupils equal, round, react to light, and accommodation]. Fundi: discs flat with sharp margins. Vessels present in all quadrants without crossing defects. Background has even colour, no hemorrhage or exudates.

Ears: Pinna has no mass, lesions, scaling, discharge, or tenderness to palpation. Canals clear. Tympanic membrane pearly grey, landmarks intact, no perforation. Whispered words heard bilaterally. Weber test: tone heard midline with lateralization. Rinne test: AC > BC and = bilaterally.

Nose: No deformities or tenderness to palpation. Nares patent. Mucosa pink, no lesions. Septum midline, no perforation. No sinus tenderness.

Mouth: Mucosa and gingivae pink, no lesions or bleeding. R lower first molar missing, multiple dark spots on most teeth, gums receding on lower incisors. Tongue symmetrical, protrudes midline, no tremor. Pharynx pink, no exudate. Uvula rises midline on phonation. Tonsils 1+. Gag reflex present.

Neck: Neck supple with full ROM. Symmetrical, no masses, tenderness, lymphadenopathy. Trachea midline. Thyroid nonpalpable, not tender. Jugular veins flat at 45 degrees. Carotid arteries 2+ and = bilaterally, no bruits.

Spine and back: Normal spinal profile, no scoliosis. No tenderness over spine, no CVA [costovertical angle] tenderness.

Thorax and lungs: AP [anteroposterior] < transverse diameter. Chest expansion symmetrical. Tactile fremitus equal bilaterally. Lung fields resonant. Diaphragmatic excursion 4 and 5 cm bilaterally. Breath sounds diminished. Expiratory wheeze in upper back at both bases, scattered rhonchi in upper back at both bases, do not clear with coughing.

Breasts: Symmetrical; no retraction, discharge, or lesions. Contour and consistency firm and homogeneous. No masses or tenderness, no lymphadenopathy.

Heart: Precordium, no abnormal pulsations, no heaves. Apical impulse at fifth ICS [intercostal space] in left MCL [midclavicular line], no thrills. S_1 and S_2 are not diminished or accentuated; no S_3 or S_4. Systolic murmur, grade II/VI, loudest at left lower sternal border, no radiation, present supine and sitting.

Abdomen: Flat, symmetrical. Skin smooth with no lesions, scars, or striae. Bowel sounds present, no bruits. Tympany predominates in all quadrants. Liver span 7 cm in right MCL. Abdomen soft, no organomegaly, no masses or tenderness, no inguinal lymphadenopathy.

Extremities: Colour tan-pink; no redness, cyanosis, or lesions other than surgical scar. Scar R lower leg, anterior, 28 cm × 2 cm wide, well healed. No edema or varicosities. No calf tenderness. All peripheral pulses present, 2+ and = bilaterally. Asymmetrical leg length, R leg 3 cm shorter than left.

Musculo-skeletal: Temporomandibular joint: no slipping or crepitation. Neck: full ROM, no pain. Vertebral column: no tenderness, no deformity or curvature; full extension, lateral bending, rotation. Arms symmetrical, legs measure as described, extremities have full ROM, no pain or crepitation. Muscle strength: able to maintain flexion against resistance and without tenderness.

Neurological: Mental status: Appearance, behaviour, speech appropriate. Alert and oriented to person, place, time. Thought coherent. Remote and recent memories intact. Cranial nerves II through XII intact. Sensory: pinprick, light touch, vibration intact. Stereognosis, able to identify key. Motor: no atrophy, weakness, or tremors. Gait has limp, able to tandem walk with shoes on. Negative Romberg sign. Cerebellar, finger-to-nose smoothly intact. DTRs [deep tendon reflexes]: see the following stick diagram:

Genitalia: External genitalia have no lesion or discharge. Internal: vaginal walls pink, no lesion. Cervix pink, nulliparous os, no lesions, small amount nonodorous clear discharge. Specimens for Pap test, gonorrhea/*Chlamydia*, trichomoniasis, and moniliasis obtained. Swabbing mucosa with acetic acid shows no acetowhitening.

Bimanual: no pain on moving cervix, uterus midline, no enlargement, masses, or tenderness. Adnexa, ovaries not enlarged, no tenderness. Anus, no hemorrhoids, fissures, or lesions. Rectal wall intact, no masses or tenderness. Stool soft, brown; Hematest negative.

ASSESSMENT

Alcohol dependence with physiological dependence
Nicotine dependence with physiological dependence
Right orbital contusion (resolving)
Systolic heart murmur
Elevated blood pressure
Ineffective airway clearance R/T [related to] tracheobronchial secretions and obstruction
Risk for trauma
Self-care deficit: oral hygiene R/T lack of motivation
Deficient knowledge about alcoholism disease process, treatment options, support systems R/T lack of exposure
Deficient knowledge about balanced diet R/T lack of exposure and substance abuse
Dysfunctional family processes: alcoholism
Chronic low self-esteem R/T effects of alcoholism, sexual abuse, and physical abuse

REFERENCES

1. Krogsbøll, L. T., Jørgensen, K. J., Grønhøj Larsen, C., et al. (2012). General health checks in adults for reducing morbidity and mortality from disease. *BMJ (Clinical Research Ed.), 345,* e7191.

2. College of Family Physicians of Canada. (2013). *Annual physical examination practices by province/territory in Canada.* Retrieved from http://www.cfpc.ca/uploadedFiles/Health_Policy/CFPC_Policy_Papers_and_Endorsements/CFPC_Policy_Papers/CFPC%20PT%20Annual%20Exam.pdf.

Documentation and Critical Thinking

CHAPTER 29

Bedside Assessment and Electronic Health Recording

Written by Ian M. Camera, MSN, ND, RN
Adapted by Marian Luctkar-Flude, RN, PhD

http://evolve.elsevier.com/Canada/Jarvis/examination/

In a hospital setting, patients do not require a complete head-to-toe physical examination during every 24-hour stay. Patients do require a consistent specialized examination that focuses on certain parameters at least every 8 hours. Some data, such as daily weights, abdominal girth, or the circumference of a limb, must be measured very carefully. The utility of such measurements depends entirely on consistency of procedure from nurse to nurse; for example, whether nurses use the same scale to measure the patient's daily weights at the same time of day. For patients who do not speak English, obtain a cultural interpreter whenever possible to ensure accuracy of communication. Documentation and communication of clinical findings are important aspects of assessment of a hospitalized adult. The *subjective, objective, assessment, plan* (SOAP) charting to organize findings related to a clinical problem facilitates clinical reasoning; the *situation, background, assessment, recommendation*

(SBAR) technique facilitates communication between health care providers (see p. 848).

Many assessments must be performed frequently throughout the course of a hospital shift. This chapter outlines the initial assessment that will allow you to get to know your patients. As you perform this sequence, take note of anything that necessitates continuous monitoring, such as a blood pressure (BP) or pulse oximetry reading that is not what you expect, or breath sounds that suggest a difficult respiratory effort. If no protocol is in place for a particular assessment situation, then decide for yourself how often you need to check on the patient's status. It is easy to be distracted by ringing bells and alarms as the shift progresses, but your own judgement about a patient's needs is just as important as any electronic alert or alarm.

The need for multiple assessments of each patient highlights the need for efficiency in the hospital setting. Assessments must be thorough and accurate, but you must be able to complete them rapidly without seeming hurried. The only solution to this paradox is practice. Remember that practising in a laboratory setting with simulated patients or with classmates may feel artificial, but it is the quickest route to feeling confident in the presence of hospitalized patients.

The basic reassessment applies to adults in medical-surgical and cardiac stepdown units. Each assessment must be customized to each patient, and findings must be integrated into your complete knowledge base regarding the patient. This knowledge base includes what you read in the chart, what you hear in report, and the results of any available laboratory tests and diagnostic imaging.

SUBJECTIVE AND OBJECTIVE DATA

Sequence	Selected Photos

Assist the patient into bed. During the examination, the patient is in a bed that is at a level comfortable for the examiner. Both subjective and objective data are collected simultaneously throughout the bedside assessment using a systems approach. Abnormal findings may prompt a more comprehensive assessment of the affected systems.

The Health History

On your way into the patient's room, verify that any necessary markers or flags are in place at the doorway with regard to such conditions as isolation precautions, latex allergies, or fall precautions. Once in the room, introduce yourself as the patient's nurse for the next 8 (or 12) hours.

Make direct eye contact, and do not allow yourself to be distracted by intravenous (IV) pumps or other equipment as you ask how the patient is feeling and how he, she, or they spent the previous shift. Assess for pain: "Are you currently having any pain or discomfort? Can you rate your pain on a scale from 0 to 10, with 0 being no pain and 10 being the worst pain you can imagine?" Or, if appropriate, use the Faces Pain Scale–Revised (see Fig. 11.5, p. 190). You should know when pain medication was most recently administered and what physician orders are written. Determine whether further dosing is needed or whether you need to contact the physician. With regard to written orders, confirm settings on the patient-controlled analgesia (PCA) pump or epidural setting if one of these is in place. Confirm that the IV solution hanging matches orders for rate and type.

Wash your hands in the patient's presence. Offer water as a courtesy if the patient is allowed water, and note the physical data this offer elicits: the patient's ability to hear, to follow directions, to cross the midline, and to swallow. Complete your initial overview by verifying that the correct name band has been applied to the patient's wrist. As you proceed with the examination, continue to question the patient to elicit both subjective and objective data related to each of the body systems. As you collect and document these data, note the following.

General Appearance

1. Facial expression: whether appropriate for the situation.
2. Body position: whether relaxed and comfortable or tense and in pain.
3. Level of consciousness: whether alert and oriented, attentive to your questions, and responding appropriately.
4. Skin colour: whether tone is even and consistent with ethnocultural heritage.
5. Nutritional status: whether weight appears in healthy range, fat distribution is even, and hydration appears healthy.
6. Speech: whether articulation is clear and understandable, pattern is fluent and even, and content is appropriate.

Sequence	Selected Photos

7. Hearing: whether responses and facial expression are consistent with what you have said.
8. Personal hygiene: ability to attend to hair, makeup, shaving.

Measurement

1. Measure baseline vital signs: temperature, pulse, respirations, BP. Note whether you must avoid an arm because of surgery, mastectomy, IV access, or dialysis shunt. Collect and document vital signs more frequently if patient is unstable or patient condition changes.
2. Measure oxygen saturation (pulse oximetry): maintain at 92% or higher, or as ordered (e.g., 88 to 92% for patients with chronic obstructive pulmonary disease [COPD]).
3. Ask the patient to rate pain level on a scale of 0 to 10, at rest and with activity; note location and quality of pain. If appropriate, use the Faces Pain Scale–Revised.
4. Assess pain intensity on a scale of 0 to 10 before and after administration of analgesics; note response according to known pharmacokinetics of the analgesic, approximately 15 minutes after IV administration and 1 hour after oral administration.

Neurological System

1. Note whether the patient's eyes open spontaneously to name.
2. Note whether the patient's verbal response makes sense and the speech is clear and articulate.
3. Measure right and left pupil sizes in millimetres, and assess reaction to light.
4. Note whether the patient's motor response in upper and lower extremities is strong and equal bilaterally.
5. Assess muscle strength of right and left upper extremities, with the use of hand grips.
6. Assess muscle strength of right and left lower extremities, pushing feet against your palms.
7. Note any ptosis or facial droop.
8. Evaluate sensation (omit unless indicated).
9. Assess the patient's ability to swallow.

Subjective and Objective Data

Subjective and Objective Data

Respiratory System

1. If the patient is receiving oxygen by mask or nasal prongs, check fitting and assess skin integrity of the nares and behind the ears.
2. Note fraction of inspired oxygen (FiO_2).
3. Assess respiratory effort.
4. Inquire whether the patient is short of breath at rest or on exertion.
5. Auscultate breath sounds (do *not* listen over the patient's gown), and compare sides:
   Anterior lobes: right upper, left upper, right middle and lower, left lower
   Posterior lobes: left upper, right upper, left lower, right lower (if the patient is not able to sit up, have another nurse hold patient to each side)
6. Instruct the patient to cough and breathe deeply. Check colour, consistency, and amount of any expectorant.
7. If an incentive spirometer is ordered, encourage the patient to use it every hour for 10 inspirations. If oxygen saturation or respiratory rate drops, encourage its use every 15 minutes.

Cardiovascular System

1. Auscultate rhythm at apex: Is it regular or irregular? (Do *not* listen over the patient's gown.)
2. Check apical pulse against radial pulse, noting perfusion of all beats.
3. Assess heart sounds in all auscultatory areas: first with the diaphragm of the stethoscope and then with the bell.
4. Check capillary refill for prompt return.
5. Check for pretibial edema.
6. Palpate the posterior tibial and dorsalis pedis pulses in both feet. (Assess pulses in the lower extremities by Doppler technique, if not palpable.)
7. Verify that the correct IV solution is hanging and flowing at the correct rate according to both the physician's orders and your own assessment of the patient's needs.

Sequence	Selected Photos

Skin

1. Note skin colour and whether it is consistent with the patient's ethnocultural heritage.
2. Palpate skin temperature; expect the skin to be warm and dry.
3. Pinch up a fold of skin under the clavicle or on the forearm to note mobility and turgor.
4. Note skin integrity, any lesions, and the condition of any dressings. Note any bleeding or infection, but do not change dressing until after physical examination.
5. Note the date on the IV site and the surrounding skin condition, observing for redness, edema, drainage, etc.
6. Complete any standardized scales used to quantify risk for skin breakdown (see the Braden Scale for Predicting Pressure Sore Risk, Table 13.1, p. 230).
7. Verify that any *air loss* or *alternating pressure* mattresses being used are properly applied and operating at the correct settings.

Abdomen

1. Assess contour of abdomen: flat, rounded, or protuberant.
2. Listen to bowel sounds in all four quadrants.
3. Perform light palpation in all four quadrants.
4. Inquire whether the patient is nauseated or has vomited.
5. Inquire whether the patient is passing flatus or stool, or experiencing constipation or diarrhea. Note date of most recent bowel movement.
6. Check any drainage tube placement for colour, consistency, odour, and amount of drainage, and evaluate the integrity of the insertion site. Assess all tubes from site to source for kinks, leaks, and disconnections.
7. Check any stoma for colour, moisture, excoriation, and bleeding, and evaluate the integrity of the stomal appliance. Check stomal drainage for colour, consistency, odour, and amount.
8. With regard to diet orders, determine whether the patient is tolerating ice chips, liquids, or solids. Order the correct diet as it is advanced. Note whether the patient is at high risk for nutrition deficit.

Genitourinary System

1. Inquire whether the patient is voiding regularly, or, if indicated, assess the indwelling urinary catheter and surrounding skin integrity.
2. Check urine for colour and clarity.
3. If catheter is in place, check colour, quantity, and clarity of urine with every check of vital signs.
4. If urine output is less than the expected amount, perform a bladder scan according to agency protocol. Determine whether the problem is associated with the production of urine or its retention.
5. Assess 24-hour fluid balance to identify hydration or dehydration, kidney function, and perfusion.

Subjective and Objective Data

Sequence	Selected Photos

Activity

1. With regard to activity orders, if the patient is on bed rest, the head of the bed should be angled at 15 degrees or higher. Note whether the patient is at high risk for skin breakdown.
2. If the patient is ambulatory, assist the patient to a sitting position. Assess for orthostatic hypotension and dizziness. If none, move the patient to a chair. Increase activity as tolerated.
3. Note any assistance needed, how the patient tolerates movement, distance walked to the chair, the patient's ability to turn, and whether the patient's gait is steady and symmetrical.
4. Note any need for ambulatory aid or equipment.
5. Complete any standardized scales used to quantify the patient's risk for falling and/or functional status, and assess need for referral to physiotherapy or occupational therapy.
6. If antiembolism compression (T.E.D.) stockings and sequential compression devices (SCDs) are ordered, the patient needs to use them for 22 of 24 hours. SCDs must be hooked up and turned on, except during ambulation.

Report Critical Findings

Note examination findings that necessitate immediate attention:
1. Altered level of consciousness, confusion
2. Systolic BP ≤90 or ≥160 mm Hg
3. Temperature ≥38°C (100.4°F)
4. Heart rate ≤60 or ≥100 bpm
5. Respiratory rate ≤10/min or ≥28/min
6. Oxygen saturation ≤92%
7. Urine output <30 mL/hour for 2 hours
8. Dark amber urine or bloody urine (except for urology patients)
9. Postoperative nausea or vomiting not relieved with medication
10. Surgical pain not controlled with medication; any other unusual pain, such as chest pain
11. Bleeding
12. Sudden restlessness or anxiety

DOCUMENTATION AND CRITICAL THINKING

ELECTRONIC HEALTH RECORDING

The use of health information and communications technology has the potential to improve the flow of information among health care providers to enhance the efficiency, quality, and safety of health care delivery.[1] Most hospitals or clinics now use a basic or comprehensive **electronic charting system** to replace paper medical records. **Electronic health records (EHRs)** are secure and private lifetime records that describe a person's health history and care, and are made up of information from a variety of sources, including hospitals, clinics, doctors, pharmacies, and laboratories.[2] They can be accessed by authorized health care providers and staff across more than one health care organization. The EHR can provide integrated clinical information to support the five *R*s of clinical decision-making: the *r*ight information, about the *r*ight patient, available to the *r*ight person, in the *r*ight place, and at the *r*ight time. Nurses use EHRs in day-to-day practice to review orders, diagnostic test results, dictated notes, and consults, and to document the nursing care provided, including the administration of medications.[3] An **electronic medical record (EMR)** is an electronic record of health information that is specific to a single health care organization or clinician's practice, and it is often integrated with scheduling and billing software.[4] The benefits of EHRs and EMRs include improved legibility and ability to find, search, and share patient records. The structure imposed by a computerized database can serve as a prompt to guide nurses through a complete assessment, and documentation time can be decreased through the use of check boxes and drop-down menus.

Nurses must understand how EHRs fit within the bigger picture of health care delivery.[3] When used to their full potential, interoperable EHRs provide data and functionalities that may contribute to quality improvement, improved health care access, effective surveillance and management of public health, and cost savings.[2] The Canadian Association of Schools of Nursing (CASN) publication *Nursing Informatics: Entry-to-Practice Competencies for Registered Nurses* focuses on the use of information and communication technologies (such as EHRs and EMRs) to support clinical decision-making and nursing-practice improvements and uses standardized nursing and other clinical terminology.[4]

Fig. 29.1 shows an example of what an EHR might look like.

Patient Safety

The meaningful use of EHRs and EMRs, which include physician order entry and clinical decision support, may increase patient safety and quality care. Within a single institution, EMRs allow all health care providers, regardless of geographical location, to access patient health information, place orders, and receive timely patient status updates. No longer does a provider have to be on the clinical unit to retrieve test results, vital signs, or the most recent nurse's or physician's note. Because of the recent adoption of EHRs, few research studies exist that identify their overall benefits.[5]

Canada Health Infoway is an independent, federally funded nonprofit organization that was tasked with establishing the key requirements and core components of an EHR, in consultation with the provinces, territories, and other stakeholders.[6] It also developed the **Electronic Health Record Solution Blueprint**, a technology framework for sharing health information securely and appropriately to guide the national development of EHRs. The Blueprint was released in 2003 and revised in 2006.[2]

EHRs support health care providers in meeting the safety competencies outlined by the Canadian Patient Safety Institute (CPSI), such as working as a team and communicating effectively.[7] EHRs also offer the possibility of automated chart audits to ensure complete documentation, compliance with standards, and a means to search for potentially dangerous practices.[8] The use of computerized physician order entry (CPOE) has decreased transcription and prescribing errors.[9] Well-designed EHR systems can notify providers of potential medication interactions, dosage adjustments for renal patients or advanced age, and additional required testing (e.g., laboratory tests). Nurses can benefit from EHR use in medication administration through the use of bar-code scanners, which identify both the patient and the medication. Checklists built into EHR systems can help clinicians identify health care–associated infections or patients at risk for these infections. Checklists have also been used successfully for depression and suicide screening.[10] Although no system is perfect, a well-designed EHR system can increase patient safety when successfully integrated into the

• Help	Patient Details		GP Details		
• Logout		**GME0000** **Smith,** **Caroline**	**Name:** Jones, Evans	**Phone:** 333-465-5545	**Address:** 11 Terrence Ave., Edmonton, AB T4Y 8U9

Patient Details

Sex: Female	**Phone:** 365-565-9090
DOB: 1940/01/01	**Address:** 19 Provincial Rd.
Next of kin: John Smith	Edmonton AB T6M 1R7

Other Healthcare Providers

Name	Disp.	Last Encounter	Next encounter	Right of Access
Diaz, Ellen	Cardiology	01/2006	07/2006	Y
Fournier, Janice	RN	08/2005		N
Cohen, Richard	Dermatology	07/2005		N

Patient Record
- Summary
- Lab Results
- Diagnostic
- Images
- Details
- Notes or
- Comments

Alerts

Allergies – Sulfa Drugs
- Pap smear due
- Td due
- A1C above target

Medications

Date	Medications	Prescriptions	Last Filled
11/1989	Hydrochlorothiazide 25 mg	One tab at breakfast	12/2005
03/1999	Glyburide 5 mg	One tab twice daily	12/2005
01/2001	Metformin 500 mg	Two tabs twice daily	12/2005
03/2001	Atorvastatin 20 mg	One tab at supper	12/2005
02/2002	Atenolol 50 mg	One tab at breakfast	12/2005
02/2002	ECASA 325 mg	One tab at breakfast	12/2005
02/2006	Ramipril 10mg	One tab at supper	02/2006
06/2005	Cloxacillin 500 mg	Discontinued	
05/2004	Beclomethasone Cream	Discontinued	

Encounter History

Date	Facility	Speciality	Clinician	Reason	Type
02/2006	GP			Hypertension	-
01/2006	Cardio Assoc	Cardiology	Diaz, E.	CAD	Outpatient
12/2005	GP			Diabetes	-
10/2005	General Hosp	Dietician	Johnson, H.	Diabetes teaching	Outpatient
08/2005	GP			Diabetes	-
08/2005	GP			Cellulitis	-
08/2005	Home Visit	RN	Fournier, J.	Cellulitis	-
08/2005	GP	-	-	Cellulitis	-
07/2005	Polyclinic	Dermatology	Cohen, R.	Stasis dermatitis	Outpatient

Diagnosis

Diagnosis	State	Status
Hypertension	11/1989	Ongoing
Diabetes	05/1996	Ongoing
Coronary Artery Disease	02/2002	Ongoing
Fasting lipids	12/2005	
Exercise stress test	1/2005	
Coronary angiogram / Cellulitis	02/2005	Resolved
Cholecystectomy	05/1981	Resolved
Cesarian section	01/1967	Resolved

Immunizations

Type	Most Recent	Number Received
Influenza	11/2005	7
Pneumovax	03/2005	1
Twinrix	08/2002	3
Td	04/1996	1

Diabetic Indices

Type	Value	Most Recent
A1C	0.071	12/2005
LDL	2.41	12/2005
BP	135/75	02/2006
Urine Microalb	0.02	08/2005
Eye Exam		05/2005
Home Gluc (average)	7.4	01/2006

29.1 Note: The individual is fictional. (© Minister of Public Works and Government Services Canada, 2010.)

workflow of a clinic or hospital. An EHR that is not carefully implemented with usability in mind can lead to unintended consequences, including risks to patient safety.[11] As EHR use becomes the standard of care, more research is needed to determine the specific factors that contribute to patient safety and increased quality of care when using EHRs.

USING THE SBAR TECHNIQUE FOR STAFF COMMUNICATION

Throughout this text, we have used the SOAP acronym (subjective, objective, assessment, plan) to organize assessment findings into written or charted communication. To organize assessment data for verbal communication (e.g., calls to physicians, nursing shift reports, patient transfers to other units), we use the SBAR framework: situation, background, assessment, recommendation.

The SBAR technique is a structured communication technique to standardize communication and prevent misunderstandings. Communication errors contribute to most patient safety incidents and medical errors in health care.[12] US Joint Commission data from 2010 to 2012 indicated that communication failures contributed to between 59 and 76% of sentinel events;[13] however, because reporting is voluntary, the data represent only a small proportion of actual events. With the incidence of patient safety incidents in Canada

as high as 7.5%, communication tools such as the SBAR technique are recommended to improve verbal communication and reduce medical errors.[14-16] The SBAR technique is a standardized framework to transmit important in-the-moment information. Using the SBAR technique will keep your message concise and focused on the immediate problem and yet give your colleagues enough information to understand the current situation and make a decision. To formulate your verbal message, use these four points:

Situation: What is happening right now? What are you calling about? State your name, your unit, patient's name, room number, patient's problem, when the problem happened or when it started, and how severe it is.

Background: Do not recite the patient's full history since admission. Do state the data pertinent to this moment's problem: admitting diagnosis, relevant comorbidities, time of admission, code status, and appropriate immediate assessment data (e.g., vital signs, pulse oximetry, change in mental status, allergies, current medications, IV fluids, laboratory results).

Assessment: What do *you* think is happening in regard to the current problem? If you do not know, at least state which body system you think is involved. How severe is the problem?

Recommendation: What do you want the physician to do to improve the patient's situation? Offer probable solutions:

Order more pain medication? Come and assess the patient?

Review the following examples of SBAR communication.

Situation 1

S: This is Bill on the Oncology Unit. I'm calling about Daniel Meyers in room 8417. He is refusing all oral medications as of now.

B: Daniel is a 59-year-old male with multiple myeloma. He was admitted for an autologous stem cell transplant and received chemotherapy 10 days ago. Now he is 5 days post transplantation. Vital signs are stable, he is alert and oriented, IV fluids are D$_5$W [5% dextrose in water]. As of 1 hour ago, he has been feeling extreme nausea and vomiting, refusing all food and oral meds.

A: I think the chemo he had before transplantation is hitting him now. His uncontrolled nausea isn't going away in the next few days.

R: I'm concerned that he cannot stay hydrated, and he needs his meds. I need you to please change the IV rate and change all scheduled oral meds to IV. I also think we need

to add an additional prn [as needed] antiemetic. If he continues to refuse food, we may have to consider starting him on TPN [total parenteral nutrition]/lipids.

Situation 2

S: This is Andrea. I'm the nurse taking care of Max Goodson in 6443. His condition has changed, and his most recent vital signs show a significant drop in BP.

B: Max is 40 years old with a history of alcoholism. He was admitted through the emergency department [ED] last night with abdominal pain and a suspected GI [gastro-intestinal] bleeding. His BPs have been running in the 130s/80s. He just produced a large amount of liquid maroon stool and reported feeling dizzy. I rechecked his vitals, and his BP is 88/50 and heart rate is 104.

A: I'm worried his GI bleed is getting worse.

R: Will you order a stat CBC [complete blood cell count] and place an order to transfuse RBCs [red blood cells] if his Hgb [hemoglobin] is below 8 g? Also, can you please come and assess? I think we may need to insert an NG [nasogastric] tube and do lavage.

REFERENCES

1. Registered Nurses' Association of Ontario. (2017). *Best practice guidelines: Adopting eHealth solutions: Implementation strategies.* Retrieved from http://rnao.ca/bpg/guidelines/ehealth-solutions.
2. Office of the Auditor General of Canada. (2010). *Electronic health records in Canada: An overview of federal and provincial audit reports.* Retrieved from http://www.oag-bvg.gc.ca/internet/English/parl_oag_201004_07_e_33720.html.
3. Furlong, K. E. (2015). Learning to use an EHR: Nurses' stories. *Canadian Nurse, 111*(5), 20–24.
4. Canadian Association of Schools of Nursing (2015). *Nursing informatics: Entry-to-practice competencies for registered nurses.* Ottawa: Author. Retrieved from https://www.casn.ca/wp-content/uploads/2014/12/Nursing-Informatics-Entry-to-Practice-Competencies-for-RNs_updated-June-4-2015.pdf.
5. Kelley, T. F., Brandon, D. H., & Docherty, S. L. (2011). Electronic nursing documentation as a strategy to improve quality of patient care. *Journal of Nursing Scholarship, 43*(2), 154–162. doi:10.1111/j.1547-5069.2011.01397.x.
6. Canadian Nurses Association. (2012). *New advances in patient safety through nursing assessments in electronic health records.* Retrieved from https://www.cna-aiic.ca/en/news-room/news-releases/2012/new-advances-in-patient-safety-through-nursing-assessments-in-electronic-health-records.
7. Canadian Patient Safety Institute. (2009). *The safety competencies: Enhancing patient safety across the health professions.* Retrieved from http://www.patientsafetyinstitute.ca/en/toolsResources/safetyCompetencies/Pages/default.aspx.
8. Joseph, A., & Kildea, J. (2014). *An analysis of the effectiveness of automated pre-, post- and intra-treatment auditing of electronic health records.* Retrieved from http://www.patientsafetyinstitute.ca/en/toolsResources/Research/studentships/Documents/2013-2014%20CPSI%20Studentships/Ackeem%20Joseph%20CPSI%20Final%20Report%202014.pdf.
9. Abramson, E. L., Barron, Y., Quaresimo, J., et al. (2011). Electronic prescribing within an electronic health record reduces ambulatory prescribing errors. *The Joint Commission Journal on Quality and Patient Safety, 37*(10), 470–478.
10. Radecki, R. P., & Sittig, D. F. (2011). Application of electronic health records to the Joint Commission's 2011 national patient safety goals. *JAMA: The Journal of the American Medical Association, 306,* 92–93.
11. Middleton, B., Bloomrosen, M., Dente, M. A., et al. (2013). Enhancing patient safety and quality of care by improving the usability of electronic health record systems. *Journal of the American Medical Informatics Association, 20,* e2–e8. doi:10.1136/amiajnl-2012-001458.
12. Leonard, M., Graham, S., & Bonacum, D. (2004). The human factor: The critical importance of effective teamwork and communication in providing safe care. *Quality and Safety in Health Care, 13*(Suppl. 1), i85–i90.
13. The Joint Commission. (2013). *Sentinel event data—Root causes by event type 2004–2012.* Retrieved from http://www.jointcommission.org/sentinel_event.aspx.
14. Canadian Patient Safety Institute (2011). *Canadian framework for teamwork and communication: Literature review, needs assessment, evaluation of training tools and expert consultations.* Edmonton: Author. Retrieved from http://www.patientsafetyinstitute.ca/en/toolsResources/teamworkCommunication/Documents/Canadian%20Framework%20for%20Teamwork%20and%20Communications.pdf.
15. Thomas, C. M., Bertram, E., & Johnson, D. (2009). The SBAR communication technique. *Nurse Educator, 34*(4), 176–180.
16. Trentham, B., Andreoli, A., Boaro, N., et al. (2010). *SBAR: A shared structure for effective team communication: An implementation toolkit* (2nd ed.). Toronto: Toronto Rehabilitation Institute.

Documentation and Critical Thinking

Pregnancy

Written by Deborah E. Swenson, MSN, ARNP, C-WHCNP
Adapted by Nancy Watts, RN, MN, PNC (C)

ⓔ http://evolve.elsevier.com/Canada/Jarvis/examination/

STRUCTURE AND FUNCTION

PREGNANCY AND THE ENDOCRINE PLACENTA

The first day of menses is day 1 of the menstrual cycle. For the first 14 days of the cycle, one or more follicles in the ovaries develop and mature. One follicle grows faster than the others, and on approximately day 14 of the menstrual cycle, this dominant follicle ruptures, and ovulation occurs. If the ovum meets viable sperm, fertilization occurs in the fallopian tube. The remaining cells in the follicle form the **corpus luteum**, or "yellow body," which produces various hormones. The most important hormone is progesterone, which prevents the sloughing of the endometrial wall, ensuring a rich vascular network into which the fertilized ovum, the blastocyst, will implant. The blastocyst or embryo, prior to implantation, includes an inner cell mass that will become the fetus, germ cells, and the trophectoderm that will become the placenta. The blastocyst is surrounded by the zona pellucida, which may be a barrier to viruses and bacteria within the uterus prior to implantation.[1]

The **blastocyst** continues to divide, differentiate, and grow rapidly. Specialized cells in the blastocyst produce human chorionic gonadotropin (hCG), stimulating the ongoing production of progesterone. Between days 20 and 24, the blastocyst becomes implanted into the uterine wall, which may cause a small amount of vaginal bleeding. The placenta starts to produce progesterone that supports the pregnancy at 7 weeks, and it takes over this function completely from the corpus luteum at approximately 10 weeks.

The **placenta** functions as an endocrine organ and produces several hormones. These hormones help fetal growth and development and direct changes in the woman's body in preparation for birth and lactation. The hCG stimulates the rise in progesterone levels during pregnancy. Progesterone maintains the endometrium around the fetus, increases the alveoli in the breast, and keeps the uterus in a quiescent state. Estrogen stimulates duct formation in the breast, increases

the weight of the uterus, and increases certain uterine receptors important to birth.

The average length of pregnancy is 280 days from the first day of the last menstrual period (LMP), which is equal to 40 weeks, 10 lunar months, or 9 calendar months. Note: this includes the 2 weeks when the follicle was maturing, before conception actually occurred. Pregnancy is divided into three trimesters: (a) the first 12 weeks, (b) weeks 13 to 27, and (c) week 28 to birth.

A woman (or trans or intersex person) who is pregnant for the first time is described as a **primigravida** (G), and with subsequent pregnancies is a **multigravida**. *Parity* (P) refers to a pregnancy that has led to birth at a minimum of 20 weeks' gestation (often referred to as the *age of viability*). A nulliparous woman is pregnant for the first time (notation: G1 P0), and becomes a **primipara** after giving birth once at 20 weeks' gestation or more (G1 P1). A **multipara** has given birth more than once (e.g., for a woman who has given birth twice, G2 P2). Preterm labour or preterm birth occurs at a minimum of 20 weeks' gestation but before 37 weeks' gestation. Pregnancy loss at less than 20 weeks is an abortion (A) that can be spontaneous (SA) (miscarriage) or a planned interruption of pregnancy (therapeutic [TA]). It is common to document pregnancy history with the notations G (gravida), T (term), P (preterm), A (abortion), and L (living children). If a woman is now pregnant for the fourth time, has given birth twice at 39 weeks gestation, has had one therapeutic abortion, and has two living children, the pregnancy history may be written "G4 T2 P0 TA1 L2" (or "G4 TPAL 2012").

CHANGES DURING NORMAL PREGNANCY

Pregnancy is diagnosed by three types of signs and symptoms. **Presumptive signs** are those the woman experiences, such as amenorrhea, breast tenderness, nausea, fatigue, and increased urinary frequency. **Probable signs** are those detected with examination, such as uterine enlargement. **Positive signs** are direct evidence of the fetus, such as auscultated fetal heart tones (FHTs) or positive cardiac activity on ultrasound.

First Trimester

The blastocyst becomes implanted in the uterus 6 to 10 days after conception. Serum hCG test results become positive after implantation, approximately 8 to 11 days after conception.

The following menstrual period is missed and hCG can now be detected in the urine. Tingling and breast tenderness begin as rising estrogen levels promote mammary growth and development of the ductal system; progesterone stimulates the alveolar system and mammary growth. Chorionic somatomammotropin (also called *human placental lactogen* [*hPL*]), produced by the placenta, stimulates breast growth and exerts lactogenic properties.[2] Up to 80% of all pregnant women experience nausea (and 50% also experience vomiting), which usually subsides by the sixteenth week but may continue throughout pregnancy in as many as 20% of women.[3] The cause is unclear but may involve the hormonal changes of pregnancy, hypoglycemia, gastric overloading, slowed peristalsis, enlargement of the uterus, and psychosocial factors. Up to one-quarter of women with severe nausea and vomiting consider interruption of pregnancy, and even women with mild nausea and vomiting report significant disruption in their lives related to child care, relationships, and work. Sleep disturbances including insomnia, frequent waking, and daytime sleepiness are common throughout pregnancy. They may be related to pain, restless leg syndrome, difficulty finding a comfortable position, and concerns about the pregnancy and infant.[4]

Estrogen, and possibly progesterone, causes hypertrophy of the uterine muscle cells, and uterine blood vessels and lymphatic vessels enlarge. The uterus becomes globular in shape, softens, and flexes easily over the cervix (**Hegar's sign**). This change causes compression of the bladder, which results in urinary frequency. Increased vascularity, congestion, and edema cause the cervix to soften (**Goodell's sign**) and become bluish purple in the primiparous woman (**Chadwick's sign**).

Early in the first trimester, blood pressure (BP) reflects prepregnancy values. BP, particularly diastolic pressure, decreases until approximately 24 to 32 weeks gestational age, mostly due to falling peripheral vascular resistance. BP gradually returns to the nonpregnant baseline value by term. Systemic vascular resistance decreases from the vasodilatory effect of progesterone and prostaglandins and vasodilatory effects of nitric oxide, which increases in pregnancy.[5]

At the end of 9 weeks, the embryonic period ends and the fetal period begins, at which time major structures are present.[5] FHTs can be heard through Doppler ultrasonography between 9 and 10 weeks.[5] The uterus may be palpated just above the symphysis pubis at approximately 12 weeks. Fig. 30.1 depicts uterine fundal growth during the first trimester.

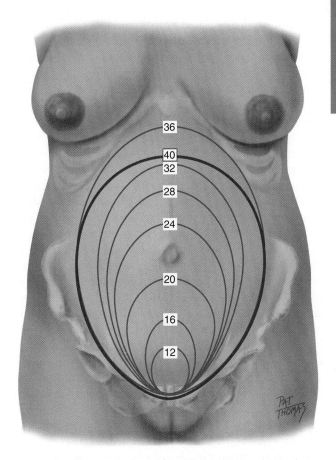

HEIGHT OF FUNDUS AT WEEKS OF GESTATION

30.1

Second Trimester

By weeks 12 to 16, the nausea, vomiting, and urinary frequency of the first trimester decrease. The woman recognizes fetal movement ("quickening") at approximately 18 to 20 weeks (earlier for the multigravida). As breast enlargement continues, the veins of the breast enlarge and are more visible through the skin. **Colostrum**, or first milk, is yellow and contains more minerals and protein but less carbohydrate and fat than mature milk, and is seen with spontaneous leaking by some women. Colostrum is rich in antibodies, which protect the newborn during the first weeks of life.[5]

The areolae and nipples darken because estrogen and progesterone have a melanocyte-stimulating effect that escalates from the second month of pregnancy until birth. For the same reason, the midline of the abdominal skin becomes pigmented; the dark area is called the **linea nigra**. **Striae gravidarum** ("stretch marks") may be seen on the breast, abdomen, and areas where enlargement has occurred.

During the second trimester, systolic BP may remain the same while diastolic BP drops 10 to 15 mm Hg lower than prepregnancy levels.[5] This drop is lowest at 24 to 32 weeks, causing dizziness and syncope, particularly with position changes. Enlargement of the uterus displaces the stomach, and progesterone causes alterations in esophageal sphincter and gastric tone, predisposing the woman to heartburn. The intestines are also displaced by the growing uterus, and tone and motility are decreased due to progesterone, often resulting in constipation. The gallbladder empties sluggishly and may become distended, possibly as a result of the action of progesterone on its smooth muscle. Bile stasis, together with the increased cholesterol saturation of pregnancy, predisposes some women to gallstone formation.

Progesterone and, to a lesser degree, estrogen cause increased respiratory effort during pregnancy by increasing tidal volume (amount of air entering the lungs with normal inhalation). Hemoglobin, and therefore oxygen-carrying capacity, also increases. Increased tidal volume causes a slight drop in partial pressure of arterial carbon dioxide, which in turn causes pregnant women to have occasional dyspnea.[6]

High levels of estrogen during pregnancy cause an increase in thyroxine-binding globulin, the major thyroxine transport protein. Several thyroid-stimulating factors of placental origin are produced. The thyroid gland enlarges as a result of hyperplasia and increased vascularity. Thyroid function plays a vital role in maternal–fetal morbidity and mortality, as 2.5% to 5% of pregnant women demonstrate some dysfunction. Maternal hypothyroidism increases the risk for miscarriage, hypertensive disorders, low birth weight, preterm birth, and placental abruption if not monitored and treated.[7] Even mild untreated maternal hypothyroidism adversely affects the fetus, leading to neurodevelopmental changes with potential to decrease mental function.

Cutaneous blood flow is augmented during pregnancy as a result of decreased vascular resistance. This may cause more frequent nosebleeds. Gums bleed more easily (**gingivitis of pregnancy**) as a result of growth of capillaries of the gums.[8] Pregnant women with periodontal disease, a chronic local oral infection, are at risk for pre-eclampsia and their fetuses for low birth weight.[9] Untreated, this condition may lead to a systemic infection affecting maternal levels of prostaglandin E_2, which may increase the risk for preterm birth.[8]

FHTs are audible with a fetoscope (as opposed to Doppler imaging) at approximately 17 to 19 weeks' gestation. The fetal outline is palpable through the abdominal wall at approximately 20 weeks. See Fig. 30.1 for the growth of the uterine fundus during the second trimester.

Third Trimester

Blood volume increases rapidly during the second trimester, peaking in the middle of the third trimester to approximately 30% to 45% higher than prepregnancy levels, and plateaus thereafter. This volume is greater with multiple gestations: up to 65% for twins, and even more for higher order multiple fetuses.[5] Erythrocyte mass increases by 20% to 30% (as a result of an increase in erythropoiesis, mediated by progesterone, estrogen, and placental chorionic somatomammotropin). However, plasma volume increases slightly more, causing a slight hemodilution and a small drop in hematocrit. BP slowly rises again to approximately prepregnancy levels.[5]

Uterine enlargement causes the diaphragm to rise and the shape of the rib cage to widen at the base. The decrease in space for lung expansion may cause a sense of dyspnea. The rising diaphragm displaces the heart up and to the left. Cardiac output, stroke volume, and force of contraction are increased. The pulse rate rises 15 to 20 beats per minute.[10] Due to increased blood volume, a functional systolic murmur, grade 2/6 or less, can be heard in more than 95% of pregnant women.[5]

Edema of the lower extremities may occur (a) because enlargement of the uterus impedes venous return and (b) because of lower colloid osmotic pressure. Edema worsens with dependency, such as that caused by prolonged standing. Varicosities, which have a familial tendency, may form or enlarge as a result of progesterone-induced vascular relaxation. Varicosities are also formed by the weight of the full uterus compressing the inferior vena cava and the vessels of the pelvic area, causing venous congestion in the legs, vulva, and rectum. Hemorrhoids are varicosities of the rectum worsened by constipation, and caused by relaxation of the large bowel by progesterone.

Progressive lordosis (an inward curvature of the lumbar spine) occurs to compensate for the shifting centre of balance caused by the anteriorly enlarging uterus, predisposing pregnant women to backaches. Slumping of shoulders and anterior flexion of the neck from increasing weight of the breasts causes compression of the median and ulnar nerves in the arm, which may result in aching and numbness of the arms and hands, a condition referred to as *carpal tunnel syndrome*.[11]

Approximately 2 weeks before going into labour, a primigravida experiences engagement (also called "lightening" or "dropping"), when the presenting part of the fetus, usually the head, moves down into the pelvis. The fundus appears to be lower, and its measurement is smaller; other symptoms include urinary frequency, increased vaginal secretions as a result of increased pelvic congestion, and increased lung capacity. In a multigravida, the fetus may move down any time in late pregnancy or, often, not until labour. The cervix, in preparation for labour, begins to thin (efface) and open (dilate). A thick **mucus plug**, formed in the cervix as a mechanical barrier during pregnancy, is expelled at variable times before or during labour. Between 37 and 40 to 41 weeks, the pregnancy is considered *full term*. After 41 completed weeks, the pregnancy is considered *post-term*. Placental function begins to decline after 41 completed weeks, so induction planning is usually done in collaboration with the woman.

Determining Gestational Age

The *expected date of birth* (EDB)—also known as the *due date*—occurs 266 days after conception or 280 days (40 weeks) after the first day of the LMP. The LMP is reliable to determine EDB if there is a history of spontaneous regular 28- to 30-day cycles with normal flow and duration. Implantation of the fertilized egg can cause some light bleeding and may be wrongly noted as the LMP. The EDB may be calculated according to **Nägele's rule**: by adding 7 days to the LMP and subtracting 3 months. Pregnancy wheels or calculators can also be used (Fig. 30.2); because Nägele's rule and the pregnancy wheels are based on regular 28-day cycles, adjustments must be considered for longer or shorter menstrual cycles. Accurate history of coitus, ovulation, and fertility treatments, combined with physical findings (pelvic and bimanual, auscultation of the fetal heart rate [FHR], β–human chorionic gonadotropin [β-hCG] levels, and perceived fetal movement), aid in estimating the EDB. The most reliable method of dating a pregnancy is first trimester ultrasonography (see Table 30.4, p. 886).

Weight Gain During Pregnancy

The amount of weight gained by term accounts for fetal weight, amniotic fluid, placenta, increased uterine size, increased blood volume, increased extravascular fluid, maternal fat stores, and increased breast size. Weight gain during pregnancy reflects gains in both the mother and the fetus and represents approximately 62% water gain, 30% fat gain, and 8% protein. Approximately 25% of the total gain is attributable to the fetus, 11% to the placenta and amniotic fluid, and the remainder to the mother.[5] A healthy outcome may be expected within a great range of weight gain and nutritional intake as well as prepregnant body mass index (BMI). These factors are important in the calculation of an appropriate weight gain,[12] as indicated in Table 30.1.

◈ DEVELOPMENTAL CONSIDERATIONS

The rate of adolescent pregnancy in Canada has been on the decline: it was 6.1% of all live births in 1993 and 3.1% of all live births in 2013.[13] In Canada, adolescents who become pregnant tend to live in rural areas, belong to lower socioeconomic groups, have little family support, and have limited access to prenatal care, or may be part of an Indigenous community.[14,15]

Pregnant adolescents face psychosocial stressors and medical as well as obstetrical risks. Young women who become pregnant may need to interrupt their education, which may lead to ongoing job and independence challenges. Nutritional risks are related to skeletal immaturity and the competition for nutrients between the fetus and the adolescent. An increased weight gain is suggested for the pregnant adolescent.[16] The risk factors for pregnant adolescents are generally related to poverty, inadequate nutrition, substance use, an increased rate of sexually transmitted infections (STIs), prepregnancy health challenges, and emotional and physical abuse from their partners (up to 35% reported by teenaged women).[15] Pregnant adolescents are also at risk for pre-eclampsia, a multi-system disease specific to pregnancy characterized by new-onset hypertension, proteinuria, or both, usually after 20 weeks' gestation.[17] Moreover, the infants of pregnant adolescents are at risk for low birth weight. Pregnant adolescents, for reasons such as denial, fear, and lack of knowledge, seek health care later in the pregnancy, even though early prenatal care has been shown to provide optimal management.

On the other hand, more women are delaying pregnancy. The average age of women who give birth in Canada is

30.2 Pregnancy wheel.

TABLE 30.1	Guidelines for Gestational Weight Gain Ranges			
PREPREGNANCY BMI CATEGORY	**MEAN RATE OF WEIGHT GAIN IN THE SECOND AND THIRD TRIMESTERS**		**RECOMMENDED RANGE OF TOTAL WEIGHT GAIN**	
	KILOGRAMS/WEEK	**POUNDS/WEEK**	**KILOGRAMS**	**POUNDS**
BMI <18.5 (underweight)	0.5	1.0	12.5–18	28–40
BMI 18.5–24.9 (normal weight)	0.4	1.0	11.5–16	25–35
BMI 25.0–29.9 (overweight)	0.3	0.6	7–11.5	15–25
BMI ≥30 (obese)	0.2	0.5	5–9	11–20

BMI, Body mass index.
Note: Values are rounded. Calculations assume a total weight gain of 0.5 to 2 kg in the first trimester. A narrower range of weight gain may be advised for women with a prepregnancy BMI of 35 or greater. Individualized advice is recommended for these women. In 2010, Health Canada adapted the US Institute of Medicine's 2009 guidelines.
From Health Canada. (2010). *Prenatal nutrition guidelines for health professionals: Gestational weight gain.* Ottawa: Minister of Health Canada. Retrieved from https://www.canada.ca/content/dam/hc-sc/migration/hc-sc/fn-an/alt_formats/pdf/nutrition/prenatal/ewba-mbsa-eng.pdf.

currently 30.2 years of age; 11% of first births are in women who are 35 years of age or older.[18,19] Fertility declines as women age, partly because of decreases both in viable eggs and in ovulation, and partly because of other conditions, including endometriosis, early-onset menopause, and an increase in pregnancy loss. Advanced paternal age is also a concern because quantity and quality of sperm may be decreased.[18] Pregnancy in women of advanced maternal age is related to an increase in congenital anomalies. The incidence of Down syndrome (trisomy 21) in an infant increases from 1 per 1 340 among mothers aged 25 years to 1 per 353 among mothers aged 35 years.[20] Older pregnant woman are at increased risk for multiple fetuses. In Canada, such pregnancies account for 3.0% of all births, and a large percentage occur as preterm births.

Women of advanced age are more likely than younger women to have coexisting medical conditions—such as hypertension, diabetes, and obesity—that further complicate pregnancy.[18,21] Hypertension and diabetes are associated with intrauterine growth restriction (IUGR) and pre-eclampsia, which, in turn, are associated with oligohydramnios, placental abruption, and preterm birth. Older women are more likely to experience complications in labour and birth, including the need for Caesarean birth as well as postpartum hemorrhaging.

SOCIAL DETERMINANTS OF HEALTH CONSIDERATIONS

Some complications of pregnancy occur more frequently in particular populations. In Canada, immigration has resulted in a complex mix of hereditary and genetic factors that may not always be discernible. Certain population groups have increased risks for particular genetic disorders.[12] For example, mutations for hemoglobinopathies (e.g., sickle cell anemia, β-thalassemia, α-thalassemia) are common among people whose ancestors were from areas where malaria is endemic, including Africa, the Mediterranean basin, the Middle East, the Indian subcontinent, Southeast Asia, and southern China. In practice, it has been recommended that everyone whose ancestors do not come from northern Europe should be considered at high risk for these genetically linked disorders. The carrier frequency for Tay-Sachs disease, another genetic disorder, is 1 per 30 among Ashkenazi Jews and 1 per 14 among French Canadians in Eastern Quebec. The frequency outside Eastern Quebec, however, is much lower (1 per 41 to 1 per 98).

While the overall Canadian teen pregnancy rate has declined, adolescent pregnancies in Indigenous communities are four times higher than the national average.[15] Rates of tobacco and marijuana use are increasing in this population, as is gestational diabetes mellitus. Pregnant Indigenous women in northern and remote communities also face potential separation from their community in terms of birthplace location. Supporting existing traditional practices (e.g., the inclusion of Elders in prenatal care, herbal medications, smudging, and retention of placental tissue) is key to the provision of culturally safe and competent care to all women within this cultural group.

Pregnancy and breastfeeding outcomes are significantly affected not only by maternal and fetal health but also by the social determinants of health, such as educational level, income, and social support systems. Many contributing factors, including knowledge and beliefs, can affect a woman's decision to seek prenatal care. Other factors can include work environment, transportation, caring for other family members, and support of a partner or friends.

All families, regardless of ethnocultural background, recognize the birth of a child as a significant psychological, social, and spiritual moment for women, families, and communities. Complex and important rituals, customs, and beliefs are integrated into this experience. Spiritual practices and beliefs that underlie women's lives are unique to each woman and her family. A relational approach to nursing (see Chapter 1) enables the provision of compassionate care in a culturally competent way as women deal with emotionally charged issues such as sexuality, relationships, contraception, maternal weight gain, and, in some cases, spontaneous or therapeutic abortion. Sensitivity and dialogue that communicates respect for preferences and care needs are essential components of developing rapport and enable the patient and her family to share concerns as they develop. Demonstrating sensitivity and openness to communication enhances the success of childbirth in its psychological and social dimensions and demonstrates value for the diversity of women and families.[22]

Safe Motherhood: Global Pregnancy Outcomes

The World Health Organization (WHO) defines **maternal death** as any death that occurs during pregnancy or within 42 days after termination of any pregnancy. It must be a direct or indirect result of the pregnancy or any condition aggravated by the pregnancy. It does not include deaths resulting from accidental or incidental causes. The **maternal mortality rate** is the number of maternal deaths per 100 000 live births. The maternal mortality rate represents the risk of dying that a pregnant woman faces with each pregnancy. In 2017, the WHO estimated that there were 216 per 100 000 maternal deaths in the world.[23] Developing nations account for the majority of these deaths, but mortality rates in developed countries are increasing. From 2009 to 2011, Canada had a maternal mortality rate of 6.1 per 100 000 births.[24] In contrast, women in developing nations have a lifetime risk of 1 per 180.[23] More than 80% of maternal deaths worldwide are caused by postpartum hemorrhage, sepsis, unsafe abortion, obstructed labour, and pre-eclampsia or eclampsia.[25]

SUBJECTIVE DATA

1. Menstrual history
2. Gynecological history
3. Obstetrical history
4. History of current pregnancy
5. Medical history
6. Family history
7. Review of systems
8. Nutritional history
9. Environment and hazards

HEALTH HISTORY QUESTIONS

Examiner Asks	Rationale
1. Menstrual history. When was the first day of your most recent menstrual period that was normal in timing?	Using Nägele's rule, calculate the EDB with the LMP. Using a pregnancy wheel, determine the current number of weeks of gestation.
• Did you have premenstrual symptoms? How long was your period? What was the amount of flow? Did you have cramping? • What is the usual number of days in a normal cycle for you? • What was your age at menarche?	Nägele's rule is less accurate if a woman's menstrual cycles are irregular and/or longer.
2. Gynecological history. Have you ever had surgery of the cervix or uterus?	Cervical surgery may affect integrity of the cervix during pregnancy and may impede cervical dilation during labour. Uterine surgery increases the risk for cervical insufficiency, uterine rupture, and abnormal placentation: for example, placenta accreta or placenta percreta, particularly with placenta previa.
• Any known history of or exposure to genital herpes?	Onset during pregnancy is potentially *teratogenic* (causing physical defects in the developing fetus) and can contribute to preterm birth. A lesion at time of birth precludes vaginal birth, so acyclovir is normally prescribed for the last 4 weeks.
• Papanicolaou (Pap) test: When was your most recent one? Any history of abnormality? If so, when? Have you ever had a colposcopy? Cervical biopsy?	Because more women delay childbearing, gynecological cancers may be increasingly diagnosed during pregnancy. Cervical cancer is the second most commonly diagnosed cancer in women 20 to 44 years of age, and has a mortality rate of 25%, so Pap screening is important in pregnancy.[26]
• Any history of infertility, fibroids, or uterine abnormalities?	These conditions may increase the risk for ectopic pregnancy, miscarriage, and preterm labour or preterm birth.
• Any history of gonorrhea, chlamydia, syphilis, trichomoniasis, bacterial vaginitis, or pelvic inflammatory disease (PID)?	STIs increase the risk for premature rupture of membranes, preterm labour or preterm birth, and postpartum maternal and fetal infections.
• Do you or your partner have more than one sexual partner?	Intercourse with multiple partners increases the risk for STIs, including human immunodeficiency virus (HIV) infection.
• Were you a preterm infant?	Women who were preterm infants are at increased risk for preterm birth.

Subjective Data

Examiner Asks	Rationale

- Have you had a mammogram, breast biopsy, breast implants, lumpectomy, or mastectomy?

Approximately 1 in 3 000 breast cancers are reported in pregnancy, particularly in women 32 to 38 years of age.[27] Breast surgery and/or implants may affect the woman's ability to breastfeed successfully.

3. **Obstetrical history.** In earlier pregnancies, did you experience hypertension, pre-eclampsia, eclampsia, HELLP (*h*emolysis, *e*levated *l*iver enzyme levels, *l*ow *p*latelet count) syndrome, diabetes, β-hemolytic *Streptococcus* infection, IUGR, congenital anomalies, preterm labour, postpartum hemorrhage, or postpartum depression?
  - How did you experience previous pregnancies and births?

A patient who has experienced complications in the past is at increased risk of developing them in subsequent pregnancies.

The subjective quality of previous experiences affects emotions and acceptance of the current pregnancy.

  - Have you ever had a Caesarean section? If so, what was the indication? At how many centimetres of dilation, if any, was surgery performed? What type of uterine incision was made? (Confirming records of this surgery must be obtained.) Have you ever had a vaginal birth after a Caesarean section?

A patient who has undergone uterine surgery is at risk for uterine rupture during labour and abnormal placentation. The vertical ("classic") incision increases the risk for rupture; in women with this incision, all subsequent births must be by Caesarean section. The pfannenstiel ("low transverse") horizontal incision carries a low risk, and subsequent births may be vaginal. Note that the direction of the scar does not indicate how the uterus was incised.

  - How many times have you been pregnant? How many full-term or preterm births have you delivered?
  - How many spontaneous miscarriages, elective abortions, or ectopic pregnancies have you experienced? Any fetal or neonatal deaths? Any losses?

Establishing an obstetrical history is beneficial in providing care during the current pregnancy. If a woman describes multiple early losses, it may be critical to assess her mental health status and ask about investigations into possible causes that may have been done (e.g., infectious disease assessment, bloodwork).

In the case of donor eggs, the age of the egg donor is used in calculating genetic testing.

  - Do you have any history of infertility? Have you used assisted reproductive technology?

  - Do you have any history of preterm labour or preterm rupture of membranes?

A patient with such a history requires close observation during the current pregnancy. Previous preterm birth is associated with recurrence.

  - Have you been told that you have cervical insufficiency or incompetence? Have you had a cervical cerclage placed in previous pregnancies?

A cervical cerclage is a stitch placed surgically to hold the cervix closed during pregnancy and is normally placed between weeks 12 and 18. This would indicate a high risk for previous preterm labour.

Examiner Asks	Rationale
• What were the gestational ages and weights of your babies at birth?	Small infant size may indicate prematurity or IUGR; these complications are repeatable. A large infant may indicate gestational diabetes (also repeatable). Birth weights of other children may indicate a "constitutional size" (e.g., tendency of a couple to conceive small but normal children). Also, a patient's pelvis has accommodated to the weight of the largest baby born vaginally; bear this number in mind as labour begins, estimating and comparing the weight of the baby about to be born.
• Have you breastfed before? How was that experience for you?	A patient's experience and knowledge base will shape your teaching and support.
• Do you have any history of mastitis?	A painful previous experience increases need for breastfeeding support after this pregnancy.
4. History of current pregnancy. (Having calculated the current number of weeks of gestation, reassess probable accuracy of that date when eliciting the following history.) • What method of contraceptive did you use most recently, and when did you discontinue it?	Recent use of birth control pills or other hormonal contraceptives may cause delays in ovulation and irregular menses; consider this when establishing the EDB. An intrauterine device that is still in place must be removed; it threatens the pregnancy. Also, presence of this device raises the question of whether pregnancy was planned.
• Was the pregnancy planned? How do you feel about it?	Even a planned pregnancy represents loss for a patient: perhaps a loss of freedom, compromise of goals, or loss of time with other children or a partner. Up to 50% of pregnancies are thought to be unplanned. Thus, the first trimester is known as the "trimester of ambivalence," and encouraging acceptance and expression of these feelings facilitates resolution.
• How does the baby's father or your support person feel about the pregnancy? How do other family members feel?	Women may need assistance in gathering support groups. Your patient may have a female partner, or the baby's father may not be involved. Inviting significant others to future office visits affirms their importance and supports involvement of whomever this woman wishes to include in her support group.
• Have you experienced any vaginal bleeding? When? How much? What colour? Accompanied by any pain? (Determine the patient's Rh status.)	Vaginal bleeding may indicate threatened abortion, cervicitis, or other complications and must be investigated. Rh-negative women should receive Rho(D) immune globulin within 72 hours of an episode of antepartum bleeding (prevents the formation of antibodies against Rh-positive blood cells possibly from the fetus if the partner is Rh positive).

Subjective Data

Examiner Asks	Rationale
• Are you experiencing any nausea, vomiting, or both? How are you coping?	Nausea and vomiting are symptoms of pregnancy that usually begin between weeks 4 and 5, peak between weeks 8 and 12, and resolve between weeks 14 and 16. Nausea and vomiting may lead to symptoms of depression or even wishing to interrupt the pregnancy. Persistent and severe nausea and vomiting lead to hyperemesis gravidarum in a small group of women that may continue throughout pregnancy (<3%).[28]
• Have you experienced abdominal pain? When? Where in your abdomen? Was it accompanied by vaginal bleeding?	The most common causes of abdominal pain in early pregnancy are spontaneous abortion (see Table 30.5, p. 888), ectopic pregnancy, urinary tract infection (UTI), and round ligament discomfort. Late in pregnancy, causes of pain are premature labour, placental abruption, and HELLP syndrome (see Table 30.3, p. 885). Consider other medical and surgical causes of abdominal pain.
• Have you experienced any contractions? How painful? How often? How long do they last?	Uterine contractions associated with true labour are painful, occur regularly at least every 5 minutes, last 30 to 60 seconds, and increase steadily in intensity and duration. *Braxton Hicks* contractions (false labour or prelabour) are generally painless, irregular, occur every 10 to 20 minutes, and last fewer than 30 seconds.
• Have you experienced any illnesses since being pregnant? Any recent fever, unexplained rash, or infections? Any travel in a country with Zika virus? • Since becoming pregnant, have you had any X-rays? Have you had regular dental care? Any bleeding when you brush your teeth?	Document any possible exposures to infectious agents.

CRITICAL FINDINGS

Good oral hygiene, including dental care for any dental problems, is important. Periodontal disease is a group of inflammatory diseases of periodontal tissues and has association with early pre-eclampsia.[9] Gingivitis has been associated with preterm birth and low weight for gestational age in infants. In addition, poor maternal oral health increases the risk for childhood caries, as the mother's saliva is the primary source of cariogenic bacteria in children's oral flora.

Examiner Asks	Rationale
• Are you experiencing any vision changes, such as new onset of blurred vision or seeing spots before your eyes?	In the third trimester, visual changes may be a sign of pre-eclampsia. Evaluate the patient for other signs and symptoms of pre-eclampsia (see Table 30.3, p. 885).
• Are you experiencing any edema? In what parts of your body, and under what circumstances?	In the third trimester, normal weight-dependent edema of pregnancy is common, particularly in the ankles and lower legs. Facial edema is more concerning.
• Are you experiencing any unusual frequency or burning sensation with urination? Any blood in your urine? Do you void in small amounts? Any history of UTIs, pyelonephritis, or kidney stones?	Differentiate the normal urinary frequency of the first and third trimesters from UTI, for which pregnant women are at increased risk. Confirm UTI by urinalysis. UTIs increase rates of preterm birth.
• Are you experiencing any vaginal burning sensation or itching? Any foul-smelling or coloured discharge?	Check for vaginal infection. If symptoms exist, obtain specimens for cultures or a wet mount during pelvic examination. Discuss partner treatment if necessary. Explain the normal increase in vaginal secretions during pregnancy.
• Do you have cats in the home? Do they go outside regularly? Do you live on a farm with other animals?	Explain toxoplasmosis, a teratogenic disease transmitted through cat feces. To avoid exposure, someone other than the pregnant patient should empty cat litter at frequent intervals, and the pregnant patient should wear gloves with outdoor gardening (outdoor cats, particularly those eating mice or other rodents). There is increased risk with farm animals.
• On what date did you first feel the baby move?	This sign is compared to the EDB to evaluate the accuracy of that date. Tell a patient who has not felt movement to note and report that event at the following prenatal visit.
• How does the baby move on a daily basis?	Fetal movement is an excellent indicator of fetal health. Clinicians encourage the patient to be aware daily of fetal movements starting at 26 to 28 weeks of pregnancy, and to count them if the patient is high risk.[29]
• Do you plan to breastfeed this baby?	Arrange for reading materials, classes, and other support for a patient who is breastfeeding for the first time or who had an unsuccessful earlier experience.
5. Medical history. Do you have allergies to medications or foods? If so, what type of reaction?	Document such allergies to prevent prescription errors. A "penicillin allergy" should be explored to understand the reaction (e.g., rash versus nausea and vomiting). Group B streptococcal infection is best treated with penicillin in patients without a true allergy.

Examiner Asks	Rationale

Subjective Data

- What is your blood group and type?

Rh-negative women should be identified early in pregnancy so that Rho(D) immune globulin can be given to prevent antibody stimulation in the event of an antepartum, intrapartum, or postpartum uptake of fetal blood.

- Any personal or family history of cancer?

Advanced maternal age increases the risk for breast, ovarian, uterine, and colon cancers.

- Do you have a history of asthma? If yes, have you ever been intubated?

Poor control and frequent exacerbations of asthma during pregnancy may result in maternal hypoxia and a decrease in fetal oxygenation.

- Have you ever had German measles (rubella)?

This disease, which has mild effects in children, is highly teratogenic in fetuses, especially during the first trimester. Instruct a patient who has not had rubella to avoid small children who are ill. Check immunity status in the serum prenatal panel. A nonimmune patient will be offered immunization after birth while in hospital.

- Have you ever had chicken pox?

In rare cases, varicella causes congenital anomalies. A nonimmune patient should avoid exposure. Offer postpartum immunization.

- Does anyone in your family have leukemia? Have you ever been tested for human T-lymphotropic virus (HTLV)?

HTLV-1 is the most clinically significant as it causes multiple disorders: leukemia, myelopathy, uveitis, infectious dermatitis, or another inflammatory disorder. HTLV-2 is associated with milder neurological disorders and chronic pulmonary infections.

Both can be transmitted via breast milk and sexual contact. The risk for HTLV-1 transmission reaches 20% with breastfeeding and is affected by duration of breastfeeding, the proviral load, and quantity of maternal antibodies. Intrauterine infection is only 5%.[30]

- Have you had any injury to the back or another weight-bearing part?

The localized and overall weight gain of pregnancy and the joint-softening effects of progesterone cause lordosis and aggravate such injuries with increasing gestational age.

- Have you been tested for HIV infection? When? What was the result? Have you ever had a blood transfusion? Used intravenous drugs? Had a sexual partner at risk for HIV infection? Are both you and your partner monogamous?

Address HIV status to promote patient's health and decrease the risk for transmission of the virus across the placenta to the fetus. Assess the viral load with serum testing throughout pregnancy to determine the risk at time of birth. Breastfeeding is contraindicated in HIV-positive mothers because the virus is present in breast milk. Provide information on "safer sex" to a patient who describes engaging in high-risk sexual behaviour, and consider retesting each trimester.

Examiner Asks	Rationale
• Do you smoke cigarettes? How many? For how many years? Have you ever tried to quit? Do you drink alcohol? How many times per week? Do you use any problematic substances or recreational drugs, for example, opioids that are not prescribed for you? Do you smoke or ingest marijuana?	Explain the danger of using these substances during pregnancy. Smoking increases the risk for ectopic pregnancy, spontaneous abortion, low birth weight, prematurity, preterm rupture of membranes, hypertensive disorders, placental abruption, and sudden unexpected infant death (SUID). Alcohol increases the risk for fetal alcohol spectrum disorder (see Table 14.2, p. 294). Cocaine use during pregnancy is associated with congenital anomalies, a fourfold increased risk for placental abruption, and the risk for withdrawal symptoms in newborns. Infants exposed to problematic substances during pregnancy may have developmental delays or behavioural disturbances.[6] Refer such patients to counselling or support programs and for periodic toxicology screening. Refer patients who smoke to a smoking cessation program. Discuss cannabis use with pregnant women, including the risks for long-term behavioural effects on the fetus and on parenting, particularly decision making. Breastfeeding is discouraged while continuing to use marijuana.[31]
• Do you take any prescribed, over-the-counter, or herbal medications?	Screen all medications to establish safety during pregnancy. Many women do not view herbal supplements as medications, so reviewing them for possible effects on the pregnancy is helpful.
• Do you participate in a regular exercise program? What type?	Regular exercise during pregnancy may reduce the risk for hypertension and helps control weight gain.
• How do you perceive your sleep at night? Do you take any medications to help you sleep? Is it hard for you to fall asleep? Do you nap in the daytime? Do you feel drowsy during the day?	Women may not identify medications to help them sleep, especially if they are taken occasionally. Talking about methods to help with sleep such as exercise and reading, rather than watching TV or computer screens just before bed, is helpful.
• Has your vitamin D level been checked?	Vitamin D is essential for maternal response to the calcium demands of the fetus for growth and bone development. Maternal anorexia and malaise are often associated with vitamin D deficiency,[32] and vitamin D intake should be evaluated when these symptoms occur.
6. Family history. Does anyone in your family have hypertension?	Hypertension increases the risk for chronic hypertension and for pre-eclampsia.

|

- Does anyone in your family have diabetes? Juvenile or adult onset? Insulin dependent? What about thyroid disease?

If a first-degree relative has type 2 diabetes, a pregnant patient is at higher risk for gestational diabetes. Complete the screening for gestational diabetes at 24 to 28 weeks and then counsel as needed.[33] If there is a family history of thyroid disease, ask about symptoms and consider screening early in pregnancy.[7]

- Has anyone in your family had a mental illness such as anxiety, depression, or schizophrenia?
- Do you have kidney disease?

Mental illness increases the risk for postpartum depression.[34]

Kidney disease increases the risk for renal disease, hypertension, and pre-eclampsia.

- Has anyone in your family had fraternal twins?

Tendency to ovulate twice in 1 month is familial, thus the incidence of twinning is increased in families of such women.

- Has anyone in your family, or in the family of the baby's father, had congenital anomalies?

Some anomalies, such as certain heart conditions, are familial. Offer genetic counselling if needed.

- Are you of Mediterranean descent?
- Are you of African descent?
- Are you of Ashkenazi Jewish descent?
- Are you of Irish descent?

Risk for β-thalassemia is increased.
Risk for sickle cell anemia is increased.
Risk for Tay-Sachs disease is increased.
Risk for spinal malformations is increased.

7. Review of systems. What was your weight before pregnancy?

Baseline weight is needed to evaluate changes. Calculating BMI with prepregnancy weight is helpful for determining the risk for gestational diabetes, large-for-gestational-age and small-for-gestational-age infants, and need for Caesarean birth.[35]

- Do you wear glasses?

A transient change in vision correction may occur during pregnancy.

- When did you most recently see the dentist? Do you need any dental work?

Gums may be puffy and bleed easily during pregnancy, predisposing to caries. Poor dental hygiene can lead to preterm birth, low birth weight, and neonatal death. Encourage dental hygiene. Suggest any dental work be performed during the second trimester and that the dentist be informed the patient is pregnant.

- Have you been exposed to tuberculosis or had a positive tuberculin test result or chest X-ray?
- Do you have any cardiovascular disease, such as coronary artery disease, heart failure, or disease of a heart valve?

Consider tuberculosis screening with the tuberculin skin test.

A patient with cardiac disease who becomes pregnant must be monitored carefully for signs of cardiac compromise. Blood volume increases by about 30% to 45%, and the demand on the heart is significantly increased.

Examiner Asks	Rationale
• Have you had anemia? What kind? When? Was it treated? How? Did it improve?	Pregnancy worsens any pre-existing anemia because iron in the mother's body is used by the fetus in growth and development. Identify the need for early supplementation and encourage ingestion of iron with a vitamin C source.[32] Sickle cell disease may worsen during pregnancy, whereas sickle cell carriers have more UTIs. Screen the latter regularly for bacteriuria.
• Have you had thrombophlebitis, pulmonary embolus, or deep venous thrombosis?	Pregnancy is a hypercoagulable state because of increases in coagulation factors I, VII, VIII, IX, and X. This increases the risk for phlebitis.[6]
• Have you had hypertension or kidney disease?	A pregnant patient with kidney disease or chronic hypertension is at increased risk for pre-eclampsia. Document baseline BP and renal function to evaluate any changes.
• Do you have any history of hepatitis B or C? Have you been immunized for hepatitis B prior to pregnancy?	Confirm hepatitis status with serum testing. Perinatal transmission of hepatitis B to the infant usually occurs through exposure to infected blood and genital secretions during birth and through cracked and bleeding nipples during breastfeeding. Immune globulin and hepatitis B vaccine are given to the newborn within the first 12 hours of life to prevent transmission of hepatitis B.[36] Hepatitis C-positive women can give birth vaginally and can breastfeed except when transmission can occur directly through blood, such as with cracked and bleeding nipples.
• Do you have any history of thyroid disease?	Uncontrolled hypothyroidism is associated with increased neonatal morbidity resulting from preterm birth and low birth weight. Uncontrolled hypothyroidism is related to delayed mental development in children.
• Do you have any history of seizures? Are you taking any medications for seizures?	Maternal seizure disorders are associated with increased incidences of stillbirths and IUGR. Medications given for seizure disorders need to be reviewed for safety with breastfeeding. Planning for safety at home postpartum is also important.
• Have you had a UTI?	The hormonal levels during pregnancy predispose women to UTIs; a history of UTIs before pregnancy is an indication for periodic screening. Pregnancy may also mask symptoms of UTI. Furthermore, a serious UTI may cause irritability of the uterus, posing a risk for preterm labour. Educate patients about measures to prevent UTI.

Subjective Data

Examiner Asks	Rationale
• Have you had a mental illness such as anxiety, depression, or schizophrenia? Were you treated? Are you still being treated?	Such a patient is at risk for prenatal and postpartum depression. Assist her to prepare a support network. Counselling may help her navigate the developmental challenges of becoming a mother. If a patient was taking antidepressants before pregnancy, it is important to establish whether she should continue taking them or be gradually weaned. If she has a condition such as schizophrenia, it is very important to continue with medication, and the patient should be encouraged to have regular care for this.
• Do you feel safe in your relationship or home environment?	Interpersonal violence during pregnancy is common. Questioning the safety of the patient privately is part of prenatal care.
• Are you in a relationship with someone who physically or emotionally abuses or threatens you?	Most abused patients do not freely offer this information. You must ask these questions at the appropriate time, privately, and without causing distress, by framing them as follows: "I ask everyone these questions because of my concern for all women."
• Has anyone forced you to perform sexual activities against your will?	Women who have been subjected to incest or other abuse are candidates for dysfunctional labour and subsequent Caesarean delivery.
• Do you have diabetes? Did you have diabetes during a previous pregnancy?	Diabetes is carefully managed during pregnancy to avoid serious complications, such as macrosomia in the infant, shoulder dystocia, and stillbirth. Consider early glucose screening (prior to the usual 26 to 28-week screening) and nutritional interventions. Plan for increased fetal assessments such as ultrasound and weekly nonstress test (NST) close to term, with a plan for induction prior to 40 weeks.[37]
8. Nutritional history. Are you taking a folic acid–fortified multivitamin every day?	A daily multivitamin with at least 0.4 to 1.0 mg of folic acid is recommended for all women who could become pregnant, for 3 months or longer before conception through the first 3 months of pregnancy, to prevent neural tube defects in the baby.

Subjective Data

Examiner Asks	Rationale

CRITICAL FINDINGS

For pregnant women with high medical risks, such as diabetic women taking insulin, women with epilepsy, women with a family history of neural tube defect, or women with a BMI exceeding 35 kg/m^2, a supplement of 4 mg of folic acid is encouraged 3 months before and up to 10 to 12 weeks of pregnancy.[32]

- Do you follow a special diet? Are you vegetarian?

A special diet may put the patient at nutritional risk. Help achieve optimal nutrition in collaboration with the woman and involve a dietitian if required.

- Any food intolerance? Do you have any gastro-intestinal conditions that make nutritional intake challenging, such as Crohn's disease, irritable bowel syndrome, celiac disease?

A food intolerance might affect the woman's and fetus's nutrition (e.g., lactose intolerance limits calcium intake). Explore dietary intake with the patient.

- Do you crave nonfoods such as ice, paint chips, dirt, or clay?

Craving for nonfood items is called *pica* and is associated with anemia.

9. **Environment and hazards.** What is your occupation? What are the physical demands of the work? Are you exposed to any strong odours, chemicals, radiation, or other harmful substances?

Environmental hazards represent possible teratogens. A patient who is not immune to rubella may be advised not to continue working in a day care centre. A patient whose job requires long hours of standing may need to stop work early in the pregnancy if signs of preterm labour occur.

- Do you consider your food and housing adequate?

If it is appropriate, refer the patient for provincial and federal programs to assist with food, housing, or other needs.

- How do you wear your seatbelt when driving?

For maternal and fetal safety, instruct the patient to place the lap belt below the abdomen.

- Do you have other questions or concerns?

Encourage the patient to write down questions that may come up between visits.

OBJECTIVE DATA

PREPARATION

The initial examination for pregnancy may be a patient's first pelvic examination, and many women become extremely anxious about it. Moreover, the patient may not know for certain whether she is pregnant and may be anxious about the findings. Before touching the patient, explain what will happen during the examination. Save the pelvic examination for last; by that time the patient will have become more comfortable with your gentle, informative approach. Communicate all findings as you proceed, to demonstrate respectful affirmation of the patient's control and responsibility in her own health and health care and that of her child's.

Ask the patient to empty the bladder before the examination; reserve a specimen for protein and glucose testing and, if necessary, for urinalysis. Before the examination, weigh the patient on the office scale. Provide the patient with a support person if desired. Some clinics require an additional person to be present during examinations.

Give the patient a gown and a drape, and time to undress and put on the gown. Begin the examination with the patient sitting on the examination table, wearing the gown and with the lap covered by the drape. Measure and record vital signs, including BP, pulse, temperature, and fetal heart rate. Before beginning the breast examination, help the patient lie down. She remains recumbent for the abdominal and extremity examination, but must be placed in the lithotomy position for the pelvic examination (see Chapter 27). Help the patient to the sitting position. Recheck after the examination if BP was previously elevated.

EQUIPMENT NEEDED

Stethoscope
BP cuff
Centimetre measuring tape
Fetoscope and Doppler sonometer
Reflex hammer
Urine collection containers
Urinalysis test strips to check urine for glucose and protein
Equipment needed for pelvic examination as noted in Chapter 27

Normal Range of Findings

General Survey

Observe the patient's state of nourishment, grooming, posture, mood, and affect, which reflect mental state. Throughout the examination, assess the patient's maturity and ability to pay attention and learn so that you can plan how to provide the information she needs to successfully complete a healthy pregnancy.

Abnormal Findings

Undernourished or obese.

Poor grooming, a slumped posture, and a flat affect may be signs of depression, risk for postpartum depression, or the influence of drugs. Poor grooming may reflect a lack of resources and need for a social service referral.

Lack of attention may indicate a preoccupation with some concern. The patient who has had learning difficulties may benefit from printed and oral information, special classes, and a support person to accompany her.

Normal Range of Findings	Abnormal Findings

Skin

Note any scars (particularly those of previous Caesarean delivery). Many pregnant women exhibit skin changes, such as acne or skin tags, that may resolve spontaneously after the pregnancy. Vascular spiders may be present on the upper body. Some women have **chloasma**, known as the "mask of pregnancy," which is a butterfly-shaped pigmentation of the face. Note the presence of the linea nigra, a hyperpigmented line that begins at the sternal notch and extends down the abdomen through the umbilicus to the pubis (Fig. 30.3). Also note striae, or stretch marks, in areas of enlargement, particularly on the abdomen and breasts of multiparous women. These marks are bright red when they first form, but shrink and lighten to a silvery colour (in light-skinned women) after the pregnancy. In dark-skinned women, the striae will appear lighter than the surrounding skin.

Multiple bruises may suggest physical abuse.

Tracks (scars along easily accessed veins) may indicate intravenous substance use.

Complaints of nasal irritation, crusting, or stuffiness, or recurrent nose bleeds, may indicate use of inhalants.

Palmar erythema in the first trimester may indicate hepatitis, but thereafter is not clinically significant.[38]

30.3

Mouth

Mucous membranes should be red and moist. Gum hypertrophy (surface looks smooth, and stippling disappears) may occur normally during pregnancy (pregnancy gingivitis). Gums may bleed as a result of estrogen stimulation, which increases vascularity and causes fragility.

Pale mucous membranes are indicative of anemia.

Poor dental hygiene during pregnancy may lead to preterm birth or low birth weight.

Neck

The thyroid may be palpable and feel full but smooth during the normal pregnancy of a euthyroid patient.

Solitary nodules indicate neoplasm; multiple nodules usually indicate inflammation or a multinodular goitre. Significant diffuse enlargement occurs with hyperthyroidism, thyroiditis, and hypothyroidism.

Objective Data

Normal Range of Findings	**Abnormal Findings**

Breasts

Breasts are enlarged (Fig. 30.4), perhaps with resulting striae, and may be very tender. Areolae and nipples enlarge and darken in pigmentation, nipples become more erect, and "secondary areolae" (mottling around the areolae) may develop. Blood vessels of the breast enlarge; the chest wall may seem more translucent than usual, with blue veins visible just below the skin. When you auscultate, you can hear blood flow through these blood vessels, and the sound may be mistaken for a cardiac murmur. This sound is called the *mammary souffle* (pronounced *soof' f'l*). Montgomery's tubercles, located around the areola and responsible for skin integrity of the areola, enlarge. Colostrum, a thick yellow fluid, may be expressed or leak from the nipples.

30.4

Breast tissue feels nodular as the mammary alveoli hypertrophy. The patient should expect changes in the breast tissue during pregnancy. Instruct her to palpate over her breasts in a circular motion to feel for any changes (e.g., hardened, hot, or reddened areas that are painful to the touch).

Recall that some women have an embryological remnant called a *supernumerary nipple*, which may or may not have breast tissue beneath it. These remnants, which may have been previously mistaken for moles, appear under the arm or in a line directly underneath each nipple on the abdominal wall (see Chapter 18). Such nipples and breast tissue may show the same changes of pregnancy.

For any unusual breast lump, refer the patient for further study. Ultrasonography of the breasts is used in lieu of mammography during pregnancy and lactation.

Heart

Many pregnant patients have a functional, soft, blowing, systolic murmur that occurs as a result of increased volume. The murmur necessitates no treatment and resolves after pregnancy.

If you note any other murmur, refer the patient for further evaluation. Valvular disease may necessitate use of prophylactic antibiotics at delivery. Pregnancy places a large hemodynamic burden on the heart, and a pregnant patient with cardiac disease must be managed closely.

Normal Range of Findings	Abnormal Findings

Lungs

Lungs are clear bilaterally to auscultation with no crackles or wheezing. Shortness of breath is common in the third trimester as a result of pressure on the diaphragm from the enlarged uterus.

Women with asthma exacerbations during pregnancy may have expiratory (and possibly inspiratory) wheeze.

Peripheral Vasculature

Diffuse, bilateral pitting edema may be observed on the legs, particularly during the third trimester and later in the day, when the patient has been on her feet. Varicose veins in the legs are common in the third trimester. Nondependent edema is no longer a criterion for diagnosing pre-eclampsia.

Pregnant patients are at risk for thrombophlebitis. Carefully evaluate any redness or red, hot, tender swelling to rule out phlebitis. Varicosities increase the risk for thrombophlebitis, and such patients should not wear restrictive clothing or sit for a long period without moving the legs. Varicosities worsen with the weight and volume of pregnancy, and support hose helps minimize them.

Neurological System

Using the reflex hammer, check the biceps, patellar, and ankle deep tendon reflexes (DTRs). Normally these are graded 1+ to 2+ and are equal bilaterally.

DTRs that are brisk or greater than grade 2+ and clonus may be associated with hypertension and cerebral edema in pre-eclamptic women.

Inspect and Palpate the Abdomen

Observe the shape and contours of the abdomen to discern signs of fetal position. Note the linea nigra and any bruises or cuts. As the patient lifts her head, you may see the **diastasis recti**, or separation of the abdominal muscles, which occurs during pregnancy. The muscles return together after pregnancy with abdominal exercise. When palpating, note the abdominal muscle tone, which grows more relaxed with each subsequent pregnancy. Note any tenderness; the uterus is normally nontender.

The fundus should be palpable abdominally after 12 weeks' gestation. Using the side of your hand, begin palpating centrally on the abdomen higher than you expect the uterus to be. Palpate down until you feel the fundus (the top of the uterus). Alternatively, stand at the patient's right side, facing her head (Fig. 30.5). Place the palm of your right hand on the curve of the uterus in the left lower quadrant and the palm of your left hand on the curve of the uterus in the right lower quadrant. Moving from hand to hand, allowing the curve of the uterus to guide you, move your hands to where they meet centrally at the fundus.

Suspect multiple gestation if uterine size is greater than expected for gestational age, if multiple fetal heart tones are auscultated, if multiple fetal parts are felt, or if the patient describes use of assisted reproductive technologies.[39]

Objective Data

Normal Range of Findings	Abnormal Findings

30.5

Note the fundal location by landmarks and fingerbreadths, as shown in Fig. 30.1 (p. 851). Because of individual women's variations in location of landmarks and examiners' variations in fingerbreadth, this measurement is inexact. From 20 weeks' gestation, measurement is more accurate using a centimetre measuring tape; measure the height of the fundus in centimetres from the superior border of the symphysis to the fundus (Fig. 30.6). After 20 weeks, the number of centimetres should approximate the number of weeks of gestation.

A lag in fundal height of more than 2 cm may indicate IUGR, transverse lie, oblique fetal presentation, oligohydramnios, or inaccurate calculation of gestational age.

An increase in fundal height of more than 2 cm may indicate multiple gestation, macrosomia, polyhydramnios, or inaccurate calculation of gestational age.

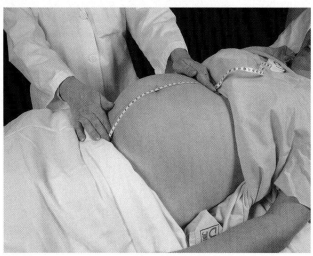

30.6

Normal Range of Findings	Abnormal Findings

Beginning at 20 weeks, you may feel fetal movement, and the fetus's head can be palpated with ballottement. A gentle, quick palpation with the fingertips can locate the head, which is hard not only when you push it away but also as it bobs or bounces back against your fingers.

If you suspect the patient to be in labour, palpate for uterine contractions. Palpate the uterus over its entire surface to familiarize yourself with its "indentability." Then rest your hand lightly on the uterine fundus with fingers opened. When the uterus contracts, it rises and pulls together, drawing your fingers closer together.

During the contraction, notice that the uterus is less "indentable." When the uterus relaxes, your fingers relax open again. In this way, contractions can be monitored for frequency (from the beginning of one contraction to the beginning of the next), length, and quality. Note that a mild contraction feels like the firmness of the tip of your nose; a moderate contraction feels like your chin; and a hard contraction feels like a forehead. (Make allowance for the amount of soft tissue between your fingers and the uterus.)

> An abnormal uterine contraction is dystonic in nature; the contraction begins in the lower uterine segment and may delay cervical dilation.
>
> An inadequate resting tone can indicate uterine irritability or tachysystole associated with placental abruption. Tenderness of the uterus may indicate chorioamnionitis or placental abruption.

True labour is characterized by painful, repetitive uterine contractions that increase steadily in intensity and duration and lead to progressive effacement and dilatation of the cervix.[40] True labour pains typically begin in the fundal region and upper abdomen and radiate into the pelvis and the lower back, whereas false labour is characterized by brief, irregular contractions, commonly called *Braxton Hicks contractions*, that are usually confined to the lower abdomen and do not lead to cervical changes.

Leopold's Manoeuvres

In the patient's third trimester, perform Leopold's manoeuvres to determine fetal lie, presentation, attitude, position, variety, and engagement. **Fetal lie** is the orientation of the fetal spine to the maternal spine and may be longitudinal, transverse, or oblique. **Presentation** describes the part of the fetus that is entering the pelvis first. **Attitude**, the position of fetal parts in relation to each other, may be flexed, military (straight), or extended. **Position** designates the location of a fetal part to the right or left of the maternal pelvis. **Variety** is the location of the fetal back to the anterior, lateral, or posterior part of the maternal pelvis. **Engagement** occurs when the widest diameter of the presenting part has passed through the pelvic inlet. In a full-term pregnancy, engagement usually occurs at the same time that the leading point of the presenting part reaches the level of the ischial spines.[38]

> Multiple gestational presentations (common) are illustrated in Table 30.6, p. 889. The most common presentation is vertex.

To perform **Leopold's first manoeuvre**, face the patient's head and place your fingertips around the top of the fundus (Fig. 30.7). Note its size, consistency, and shape. Imagine which fetal part is in the fundus. When a fetus is in the breech position, the fetal part at the top feels large and firm. Moving the fetal head between the thumb and fingers of the hand, because it is attached to the fetus at the waist, results in moving it slowly and with difficulty. The fetal head itself feels large, round, hard, and mobile. When the fetus is in a vertex position, the fetal parts in the pelvis feel more soft and the fetal head is in the pelvis. When it is in ballottement (not engaged and above the pelvis), the fetal head feels hard as you push it away and hard again as it bobs back against your fingers in response. Note that the bobbing movement occurs because the head is attached at the neck and moves easily. If you palpate no part in the fundus, the fetus is in the transverse lie.

Objective Data

Normal Range of Findings	Abnormal Findings

30.7   Leopold's first manoeuvre.

For **Leopold's second manoeuvre**, move your hands to the sides of the uterus (Fig. 30.8). Note whether small parts or a long, firm surface are palpable on the patient's left or right side. The long, firm surface is the fetal back. Note whether the back is anterior, lateral, or out of reach (posterior). The small parts, or limbs, indicate a posterior position when they are palpable all over the abdomen.

30.8   Leopold's second manoeuvre.

Leopold's third manoeuvre, also called *Pawlik's manoeuvre*, requires the patient to bend her knees up slightly (Fig. 30.9). Grasp the patient's lower abdomen just above the symphysis pubis between the thumb and fingers of one hand, as you did at the fundus during the first manoeuvre, to determine what part of the fetus is there. If the presenting part is beginning to engage, it will feel "fixed." With this manoeuvre alone, it may be difficult to differentiate the shoulder from the vertex.

By 36 weeks of gestation, the presenting part should be cephalic. If a breech or transverse presentation is detected, referral to an obstetrician is indicated. The patient should be offered external cephalic version in the absence of contraindications.

Normal Range of Findings	**Abnormal Findings**

30.9 Leopold's third manoeuvre.

Leopold's fourth manoeuvre assists in determining engagement and, in the vertex presentation, to differentiate shoulder from vertex (Fig. 30.10). The patient's knees are still bent. Face her feet, and place your palms, with fingers pointing toward the feet, on either side of the lower abdomen. Pressing your fingers firmly, move slowly down toward the pelvic inlet. If your fingers meet, the presenting part is not engaged. If your fingers diverge at the pelvic rim, meeting a hard prominence on one side, this prominence is the fetal occiput. This indicates vertex presentation with a deflexed head (the face presenting). If your fingers meet hard prominences on both sides, the vertex is engaged in either a military or a flexed position. If your fingers come to the pelvic brim diverged but with no prominences palpable, the vertex is "dipping" into the pelvis, or is engaged. In this case, the firm object felt above the symphysis pubis in the third manoeuvre is the fetal shoulder.

30.10 Leopold's fourth manoeuvre.

Objective Data

Normal Range of Findings	Abnormal Findings

Fig. 30.11 depicts various fetal positions and where to auscultate the FHTs for each. At the end of pregnancy, 96% of fetal presentations are vertex, 3.5% are breech, 0.3% are face, and 0.4% are shoulder.[6]

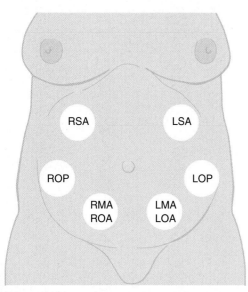

RSA and LSA = right and left sacral anterior (breech)
RMA and LMA = right and left mentum anterior (face)
ROA and LOA = right and left occiput anterior (vertex)
ROP and LOP = right and left occiput posterior (vertex)

30.11   Location of fetal heart tones (FHTs) for various fetal positions.

Auscultate Fetal Heart Tones

FHTs are a positive sign of pregnancy. A fetal heartbeat should be heard on Doppler ultrasonography by 12 to 13 weeks' gestation; it may be heard as early as 8 to 10 weeks in some women. Use of the fetoscope assists in dating the pregnancy. FHTs are auscultated best over the fetal back. After you identify the position of the fetus (see Fig. 30.11), use heart tones to confirm your findings. Count the FHTs for 15 seconds and multiply by 4 to obtain the rate (Fig. 30.12). The normal rate is between 110 and 160 beats per minute.[29] Spontaneous accelerations of FHTs indicate fetal well-being.

If no FHTs are heard, verify fetal cardiac activity with ultrasonography.

Further investigate any decelerations of FHTs because they can be an abnormal finding. Abrupt and brief decelerations are common in preterm fetuses. Decelerations cannot be classified by type unless the fetal heart is assessed by electronic fetal monitoring.

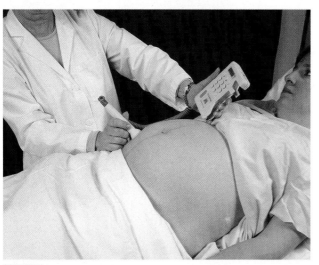

30.12

Normal Range of Findings	Abnormal Findings

Differentiate the FHTs from the slower rate of the maternal pulse and the *uterine souffle* (the soft, swishing sound of the placenta receiving the pulse of maternal arterial blood) by palpating the mother's pulse while you listen. Also, distinguish FHTs from the *funic souffle* (blood rushing through the umbilical arteries at the same rate as the FHTs). The FHTs are a double sound, like the tick-tock of a watch under a pillow, whereas the funic souffle is a sharp, whistling sound heard in only 15% of cases.[6]

Abdominal findings are of interest to the patient. Share them with her. Often she will want to listen to FHTs with her significant other. For a hearing-impaired pregnant patient, place her hand on the fetal monitor to feel the fetal heart vibrating.

Pelvic Examination

Genitalia

Use the procedure for pelvic examination described in Chapter 27. Note the following characteristics. Enlargement of the labia minora is common in multiparous women. Labial varicosities may be present. The perineum may be scarred from a previous episiotomy or lacerations. Note the presence of any rectal hemorrhoids. Note any lesions on the symphysis pubis, labia, or perianal area.

Lesions may indicate an infection, condyloma, or herpes simplex virus.

Speculum Examination

When examining the vagina, you may see Chadwick's sign, the bluish purple discoloration and congested look of the vaginal wall and cervix resulting from increased vascularity and engorgement (Fig. 30.13). Note the vaginal discharge which, in pregnancy, may be heavier in amount but similar to the patient's non-pregnant discharge, and should not be accompanied by itching, burning sensation, or unusual odour (except that, occasionally, chapping of the vaginal area may result from excessive moisture). Perform a wet mount or culture of the discharge when you are uncertain of its normality.

Many cervical infections or STIs are asymptomatic. Any cervical secretions that are purulent or mucopurulent (chlamydia or gonorrhea); yellow or green frothy (trichomoniasis); thin, white, grey, or milky, with a "fishy" odour (bacterial vaginosis); or thick, white, and clumpy (candidiasis) should be treated appropriately during pregnancy. Bacterial vaginosis can lead to preterm labour and rupture of membranes.

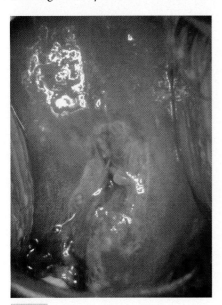

30.13

Normal Range of Findings

Note whether the cervix appears open, smooth, and round with a dotlike external os (in a nulliparous patient) or irregular with an external os that appears more like a crooked line (in a multiparous patient; the result of cervical dilation and possibly lacerations during a previous pregnancy).

Bimanual Examination

As described in Chapter 27, palpate the uterus between the hand that is performing the internal examination and the hand placed on the abdomen. Note the position of the uterus. The pregnant uterus may be rotated toward the right side as it rises out of the pelvis because of the presence of the descending colon on the left. This positioning is called **dextrorotation**. Irregular enlargement of the uterus may be noted at 8 to 10 weeks and occurs when implantation occurs close to a corneal area of the uterus. This appearance is called **Piskacek's sign**. You may also note Hegar's sign, when the enlarged uterus bends forward on its softened isthmus between the fourth and sixth weeks of pregnancy.

Note the size and consistency of the uterus. When the embryo is at 6 weeks of gestation, the uterus may seem only slightly enlarged and softened. At 8 weeks, the uterus is approximately the size of an avocado, approximately 7 to 8 cm across the fundus. At 10 weeks, the uterus is approximately the size of a grapefruit and may reach to the pelvic brim, but is narrow and does not fill the pelvis from side to side. At 12 weeks, the uterus fills the pelvis. After 12 weeks, the uterus is sized from the abdomen. A multigravida uterus may be larger initially, and early sizing of such a uterus may be less reliable for dating.

Softening of the cervix is called Goodell's sign. When examining the cervix, note its position (anterior, midposition, or posterior), degree of effacement (or thinning, expressed in percentages, if the cervix is at least 2 cm long initially), dilation (opening, expressed in centimetres), the consistency (soft or firm), and the station of the presenting part (centimetres above or below the ischial plane; Fig. 30.14, C).

Abnormal Findings

A friable cervix bleeds easily when touched with a cotton swab, Cytobrush, or speculum; friability may be caused by cervicitis. Obtain cultures. Any lesions should be investigated.

CRITICAL FINDINGS

Cervical cancer is the most common cancer in pregnancy. Most women with cervical cancer have a visible cervical lesion. Bleeding on contact is common. Investigate any concerns related to the speculum examination.[39]

Uterine fibroids (leiomyomas) may also be palpated during a bimanual examination.

A shortened cervix is less than 2 cm long.

Cavity of cervix with mucus plug —— Internal os

—— External os

A

— Dilating, effacing cervix

— External os

B

-5 cm
-4
-3
-2
-1
0 cm
+1
+2
+3
+4
+5 cm

— Ischial spine

C

30.14   **A,** Cervix before labour. **B,** Beginning of cervical effacement and dilatation. **C,** Station height of presenting part in relation to maternal ischial spines.

The ovaries rise with the growing uterus. Always examine the adnexa to rule out the presence of a mass, such as an ectopic pregnancy.

To determine tone, ask the patient to squeeze your fingers as they rest in the vagina. Take this opportunity to teach Kegel exercises, with the aim of strengthening the pubococcygeus muscles to prevent, reduce, or improve pelvic floor issues such as urinary incontinence, uterine prolapse, and sexual function. Women can identify the muscle by inserting a finger into the vagina. Alternatively, these muscles can be identified by stopping the flow of urine midstream. The patient should perform this manoeuvre only once to help confirm the function of the muscle group. There are several variations of Kegel exercises, including use of biofeedback. Patients should be encouraged to consider a strategy that will work for them. The patient contracts and relaxes the muscle group in sets of 10 or more, several times a day.

Pelvimetry

Assess the bones of the pelvis for shape and size. The dimensions may indicate the amenability of the bony structure for vaginal birth but are no longer considered a reliable indicator of pelvic capacity. Relaxation of pelvic joints, widening of the pelvis in the squatting position, and capacity of the fetal head to mould to the shape of the pelvis may enable a vaginal birth despite seemingly unfavourable measurements.

To aid in visualizing the pelvis, imagine three planes: (a) the pelvic inlet (from the sacral promontory to the upper edge of the pubis), (b) the midpelvis, and (c) the pelvic outlet (from the coccyx to the lower edge of the pubis; Fig. 30.15). Assessment of each of these pelvic planes, as described in the following techniques, allows you to estimate the adequacy of the pelvis for vaginal delivery.

Adnexal enlargement and pain with palpation occur with ectopic pregnancy or ovarian mass.

Objective Data

| Normal Range of Findings | Abnormal Findings |

■ ■ ■ ■ ■ ■ Sagittal diameter, posterior portion
────── Sagittal diameter, anterior portion
▬ ▬ ▬ ▪ Diagonal conjugate

30.15 Planes of the pelvis.

You may postpone examination of the bony pelvis until the third trimester, when the vagina is more distensible.

There are four general types of pelves: (a) gynecoid, (b) anthropoid, (c) android, and (d) platypelloid (see Table 30.2, p. 879). With your two fingers still in the vagina, note the shape and width of the pubic arch (a 90-degree arch, or 2 fingerbreadths, is desirable). If you are right-handed, move your hand to the right side of the patient's pelvis. If you are left-handed, move it to the left side of the patient's pelvis. Assess the inclination and curve of the side walls and the prominence of the ischial spine (refer to Fig. 30.15 for location of these landmarks).

Move your fingers back and forth between the ischial spines to get an impression of the transverse diameter; 10 cm is desirable. Sweep your fingers down the sacrum, noting its shape and inclination (hollow, J-shaped, or straight). Assess the coccyx for prominence and mobility. From the sacrum, locate the sacrospinous ligament. Assess the length of the ligament; $2\frac{1}{2}$ to 3 fingerbreadths is adequate. Assess the shape and width of the sacrospinous notch. Shift to the other side of the pelvis and assess for similarity to the first side.

The pelvic inlet cannot be palpated, but you can estimate its shape by measuring the **diagonal conjugate**, which indicates the anteroposterior diameter of the pelvic inlet. Having measured the length of the second and third fingers of your examining hand, with your fingers still in the vagina, point these fingers toward the sacral promontory (Fig. 30.16). If you cannot reach the promontory, note the measurement as being greater than the centimetres of length of your examining fingers. A measurement of 11.5 to 12.0 cm is desirable.

Objective Data

Normal Range of Findings	**Abnormal Findings**

TABLE 30.2 The Four Pelvic Types

GYNECOID PELVIS

GYNECOID

Inlet: round or oval
Posterior sagittal diameter of inlet: only slightly less than anterior sagittal diameter
Pubic arch: wide (≥90 degrees)
Ischial spines: not prominent; allowing a transverse diameter of 10 cm or more
Sacrosciatic notch: round and wide
Straight side walls
Posterior pelvis: round and wide

Sacrum: parallel with the symphysis pubis; hollow and concave
Favourable for vaginal delivery
Observed in 50% of all women

ANDROID PELVIS

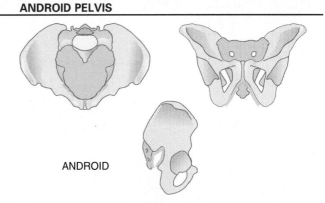

ANDROID

Inlet: heart-shaped
Posterior sagittal diameter of inlet: less than the anterior sagittal diameter
Pubic arch: narrow (<90 degrees)
Ischial spines: prominent; transverse diameter decreases

Sacrosciatic notch: narrow and highly arched
Convergent side walls
Posterior sagittal diameter: decreases from inlet to outlet as sacrum inclines forward
Anterior of pelvis: narrow and triangular; the "male" pelvis
Sacrum: straight and prominent; coccyx may be prominent

Unfavourable for vaginal delivery

ANTHROPOID PELVIS

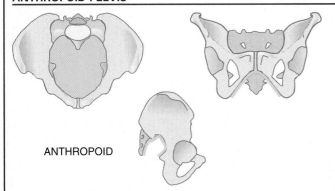

ANTHROPOID

Inlet: oval
Pubic arch: may be somewhat narrow
Ischial spines: usually prominent but not encroaching because of the spaciousness of the posterior segment
Sacrosciatic notch: average height, but wide (approximately 4 fingerbreadths)
Side walls: somewhat convergent
Sacrum: posteriorly inclined, with posterior sagittal diameters long throughout the pelvis

If pelvis is somewhat large, adequate for vaginal birth because posterior pelvis is generous

PLATYPELLOID PELVIS

PLATYPELLOID

Inlet: shaped like a flattened gynecoid pelvis
Pubic arch: wide
Ischial spines: usually prominent but not encroaching because of the already wide interspinous diameter
Sacrosciatic notch: wide and flat

Side walls: slightly convergent
Sacrum: posteriorly inclined and hollow, rendering pelvis short and shallow
Observed in fewer than 3% of all women
Unfavourable for vaginal birth

Data from Varney, H. (1997). *Varney's midwifery* (3rd ed.) Sudbury, MA: Jones & Bartlett.

Objective Data

Normal Range of Findings	Abnormal Findings

= = = Diagonal conjugate

30.16 Diagonal conjugate.

Remove your fingers from the vagina. Having previously measured the width of your own hand across the knuckles, form your hand into a closed fist and place it across the perineum between the ischial tuberosities. Estimate this diameter, which is the **bi-ischial diameter** (also known as the *bituburous* or *intertuberous diameter* and the *transverse diameter of the pelvic outlet*). A measurement greater than 8 cm is generally adequate (Fig. 30.17).

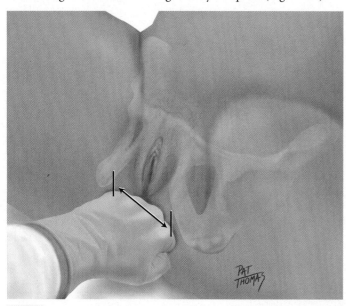

30.17 Bi-ischial diameter.

Normal Range of Findings	Abnormal Findings

Normal Range of Findings

When describing pelvimetry, note all the aforementioned measurements, and state the pelvic type. The pelvis may be described as being "proven" (accommodated) to the weight of the largest vaginally born infant. Alternatively, to describe a small pelvis, you may make the assessment such as "adequate for a 3-kg baby."

Blood Pressure

Measure the BP after the patient has been sitting quietly and before the physical examination, when the patient is most relaxed. With the patient sitting upright and her arm at heart level, check for an elevated BP. Hypertension in pregnancy is defined by a diastolic BP of at least 90 mm Hg as an average of two readings taken in the same arm.[41] "White coat" hypertension is recognized and can be confirmed by a home BP of less than 135/85 mm Hg.

Routine Laboratory and Radiological Imaging Studies

At the first prenatal encounter, discuss options for screening and diagnostic tests. In the first trimester or at booking, all pregnant patients should be offered the following tests: a complete blood cell count; measurement of rubella antibody titre; blood typing; Rh factor determination with antibody screen; syphilis serological study; hepatitis B surface antigen determination; and HIV screen with full counselling and consent. Special populations identified by history and/or work environment can be offered screening for cytomegalovirus, parvovirus, hepatitis C, thyroid-stimulating hormone, ferritin, vitamin B_{12}, and TORCH infection.* Screen for sickle cell anemia, β-thalassemia, α-thalassemia, Tay-Sachs disease, and cystic fibrosis in at-risk populations. Women who work with children benefit from screening for varicella (because immunization is safe), cytomegalovirus, and parvovirus.

A midstream urine culture should be obtained to screen for asymptomatic bacteriuria at 11 to 16 weeks. The value of testing urine for protein at every prenatal visit in women without hypertension is debated.[42,43]

A pelvic examination should be offered to screen for cervical cancer. Consent should be obtained for a cervical culture for chlamydia and gonorrhea. If the patient has a history of preterm birth or symptoms of infection or bacterial vaginosis, add a vaginal screen for culture and sensitivity. Perform a bimanual examination to confirm uterine size for gestational age.

Abnormal Findings

Hypertension is considered chronic if a patient has a documented history of increased BP before pregnancy or a persistent elevation of at least 140/90 mm Hg on two occasions more than 24 hours apart before the twentieth week after conception.[41]

Recommendation is still to test between 11 and 16 weeks for asymptomatic bacteria in pregnancy,[42,43] but dipstick testing for protein and glucose is not reliable.

*TORCH is an acronym for a special group of infections that can be transmitted to the fetus: *t*oxoplasmosis; *o*ther infections, namely, hepatitis B, syphilis, and herpes zoster, the virus that causes chicken pox; *r*ubella; *c*ytomegalovirus; and *h*erpes simplex virus, which causes genital herpes.

Objective Data

Normal Range of Findings	**Abnormal Findings**

Genetic counselling programs vary across Canada. All women should receive timely counselling and be offered appropriate screening and diagnostic procedures per regional availability. It is essential that nurses responsible for preconception and prenatal care be aware of screening options and their optimal timing during pregnancy. The Society of Obstetricians and Gynaecologists of Canada recommends all pregnant women be offered noninvasive screening for Down syndrome, trisomy 18, and open neural tube defects.[44] Invasive diagnostic procedures should be reserved for women whose findings exceed the set screen risk cutoff and for women who will be 40 years old by the EDB; they should also receive counselling about the risks of pregnancy loss with the procedures. Age alone is no longer recommended as an appropriate risk assessment tool.[45] Screening programs offer risk assessment based on biochemical and ultrasound markers. Noninvasive options include (a) first trimester serum markers and ultrasonography for nuchal translucency, plus second trimester serum testing; (b) based on risk factors, a serum test for fetal DNA (Non-Invasive Prenatal Testing [NIPT]) and (c) a two-step integrated approach with first and second trimester serum testing with or without ultrasonography for nuchal translucency. Invasive procedures (amniocentesis and chorionic villi sampling) enable diagnosis of a number of chromosomal abnormalities.

Screening ultrasonography should be offered to all women at 18 to 20 weeks, including a discussion about the risks and benefits, as well as limitations, of ultrasound technology. First trimester ultrasonography for dating is recommended when the history is unclear or complicated by irregular menstrual cycles. Ultrasound studies may also be part of a provincial or regional integrated genetic screening program. Nuchal translucency can be assessed by ultrasonography between 11 and 14 weeks. The single recommended ultrasound study at 18 to 20 weeks provides gestational age assessment that is accurate within 7 to 10 days, describes fetal number, fetal anatomy (including open neural tube defects, soft markers of fetal aneuploidy), amniotic fluid volume, and placental location, in addition to uterine and umbilical arterial blood flow.

Ultrasonography can also help visualize fetal presentation, position, activity, tone, breathing, gender, interval growth, estimated fetal weight, and maternal anatomy, including cervical length and dilation. Additional scans may be indicated at any time for complications such as bleeding, pain, suspected ectopic or molar pregnancy, trauma, fetal concerns, inappropriate fundal height measures, medical complications (including hypertension disorders and diabetes), preterm premature rupture of membranes, and noncephalic presentation.

Additional screening during the second and third trimesters includes an antibody screen for Rh-negative women (at 26 to 28 weeks), hemoglobin (at 28 weeks), gestational diabetes screen (at 24 to 28 weeks), and single vaginal/anal swab for group B streptococcus (at 35 to 37 weeks).

DOCUMENTATION AND CRITICAL THINKING

Focused Assessment: Clinical Case Study 1

Rosa Gallagher (R.G.) is a 27-year-old woman, Grav 2/Para 1, who presents with her husband and daughter for her first prenatal visit.

SUBJECTIVE

R.G. is a full-time homemaker who completed 2 years of postsecondary education. LMP was April 4 of this year (certain of date), with an EDB of January 11 of next year; thus, she is at 10 weeks' gestation today.

Her obstetrical history includes a normal spontaneous vaginal birth 3 years ago of a viable 3.5-kg female infant after an 8-hour labour without anaesthesia, intact perineum. No complications of pregnancy, birth, or postpartum. She breastfed this daughter, Ana, for 1 year. Current pregnancy was planned, and R.G. and her husband are pleased. R.G. is having breast tenderness, and nausea on occasion, which resolves with crackers. No past medical or surgical conditions are present. She denies allergies. Family history is significant only for diet-controlled adult-onset diabetes in two maternal aunts.

OBJECTIVE

General: R.G. appears well nourished and is carefully groomed. English is second language, and she is fluent.
Skin: Light tan in colour, surface smooth with no lesions, small tattoo noted on left forearm.
Mouth: Good dentition and oral hygiene. Oral mucosa pink, no gum hypertrophy. Thyroid gland small and smooth.
Chest: Expansion equal, respirations effortless. Lung sounds clear bilaterally with no adventitious sounds. No CVA [costovertebral angle] tenderness.
Heart: Rate 76 bpm [beats per minute], regular rhythm; S_1 and S_2 are normal, not accentuated or diminished, with soft, blowing systolic murmur grade 2/6 at second left interspace.
Breasts: Tender, without masses, with supple, everted nipples. Breast self-examination reviewed.
Abdomen: No masses; bowel sounds present. No hepatosplenomegaly. Uterus nonpalpable. No inguinal lymphadenopathy noted.
Extremities: No varicosities, redness, or edema. DTRs 2+ and equal bilaterally. BP 110/68 mm Hg, sitting.
Pelvic: Bartholin's glands, urethra, and Skene's glands negative for discharge. Vagina: pink, with white, creamy, nonodorous discharge. Cervix: pink, closed, multiparous, 5 cm long, firm.
Uterus: 10-week size, consistent with dates, nontender, dextrorotated. FHTs heard with Doppler fetoscope, rate 140s.
Pelvis: Pubic arch wide; side walls straight, spines blunt, interspinous diameter >10 cm. Sacrum hollow; coccyx mobile. Sacrospinous ligament 3 fingerbreadths wide. Diagonal conjugate >12 cm, bituberous diameter >8 cm. Spacious gynecoid pelvis proven to 3.5 kg.

ASSESSMENT

Intrauterine pregnancy 10 weeks by good dates, size = dates
R.G. and husband happy with pregnancy; she feels well

PLAN

Prenatal vitamins to begin
Prenatal blood screen and urinalysis
HIV screen offered and accepted
Reviewed comfort measures for nausea
Reviewed warning signs: vaginal bleeding and abdominal pain
Informed of genetic screening options
Return visit in 4 weeks

Focused Assessment: Clinical Case Study 2

Kadija Edris (K.E.) is a 30-year-old Ethiopian woman, Grav 5 TPAL 3204, who presents with an interpreter and her eldest daughter for her first prenatal visit.

SUBJECTIVE

K.E. runs a day care facility within her home. She immigrated to Canada with her family 5 years ago. Her husband is employed. They live in a three-bedroom townhouse in a subsidized housing complex. Her LMP was May 28th of this year, with an EDB of March 5th next year; thus, she is at 11 weeks' gestation today.

K.E. finds it challenging to remember details of her births in Ethiopia, except that one child "died in childbirth." She gave birth to her youngest child after coming to Canada, delivered vaginally, without complications, after 5 hours of labour. She is unsure of the baby's weight at birth. She had FGC [female genital cutting] as a child, so has scarring from her previous births. She is having nausea with occasional vomiting, has breast tenderness, and 1 week ago experienced "pink" vaginal spotting. She is unsure of her family health history. Both parents are deceased, as are all but one of her seven siblings. This pregnancy is unplanned, but she accepts it. She is concerned about transportation to her appointments because her husband works days and she does not drive.

OBJECTIVE

General: K.E. appears well nourished and is carefully groomed. English is her second language, but she understands some. Daughter who is present is well groomed and speaks English.

Skin: Dark tan in colour, smooth surface, small scarring on left arm and both legs. No lesions or tattoos.

Mouth: Poor dentition. Oral mucosa pink, some gum hypertrophy. Thyroid gland small and smooth.

Chest: Expansion equal, respiration effortless. Lung sounds clear bilaterally with no adventitious sounds. No CVA tenderness.

Heart: Rate 84 bpm, regular rhythm; S_1 and S_2 are normal, not accentuated or diminished, with soft, blowing systolic murmur grade 2/6 at second left interspace.

Breasts: Tender, no masses; large everted nipples. No drainage present. Breast self-examination reviewed.

Abdomen: No masses; bowel sounds present in four quadrants. No hepatomegaly or splenomegaly. Uterus nonpalpable. No inguinal lymphadenopathy noted. No healed incisions noted.

Extremities: No lower extremity varicosities, edema, or redness noted. Negative Homan's sign. DTRs 1+. BP 124/76 mm Hg.

Pelvic: Scarring noted where excision of the clitoris occurred (Type I FGM). Bartholin's glands, urethra, and Skene's glands negative for discharge. Vagina pink, with white, creamy, nonodorous discharge. Cervix pink, not friable, closed, and approximately 3 cm long and soft. Vaginal wall muscles lax. No evidence of a cystocele or rectocele. Vaginal examination challenging due to pain related to scarring of perineum.

Uterus: Approximately 11-week size and nontender. Dextrorotated. FHTs not heard with Doppler. Confirmed on ultrasound studies along with dating.

Pelvis: Pubic arch wide; side walls straight, spines blunt, interspinous diameter >12 cm, bituberous diameter >8 cm. Spacious, proven, gynecoid pelvis to ≈3.5 kg.

ASSESSMENT

Intrauterine pregnancy at 11 weeks' gestation by ultrasonography today with positive fetal cardiac activity. Size = dates. Mother aware of potential language and cultural issues. Via interpreter, understands advised prenatal testing, clinic routine, and warning signs and symptoms in pregnancy. Physical examination findings within normal limits.

PLAN

Prenatal vitamins to begin

Routine prenatal blood screening, plus thyroid function tests, vitamin D level, sickle cell screen, and thalassemia screen

HIV, hepatitis B, and rubella screening discussed, offered, and accepted

Reviewed integrated prenatal screening with US [ultrasonography] for NT [nuchal translucency]; understands need to complete within 2 weeks and will discuss with her husband and let us know

Reviewed clinic routines and whom to contact after hours

Reviewed comfort measures for nausea and vomiting; offered medication, declined at this time

Reviewed warning signs: vaginal bleeding, abdominal pain, pain with urination

Will return to clinic within 2 weeks if desires prenatal screening, or 4 weeks if does not

Refer to social worker for financial planning and transportation services

Obtain records from previous pregnancy and birth

Ensure all health care providers are aware of scarring on perineum for future visits in culturally appropriate way[46]

ABNORMAL FINDINGS

TABLE 30.3 Pre-Eclampsia

Pre-eclampsia, a condition specific to pregnancy, rarely occurs before 20 weeks' gestation except in the presence of a molar (gestational trophoblastic) pregnancy. The cause remains unknown, but theories include coagulation abnormalities; vascular endothelial damage; cardiovascular maladaptation; immunological phenomena; dietary deficiencies or excess; and genetic predisposition. Predisposing conditions include familial or personal history of pre-eclampsia; nulliparity; obesity; multifetal gestation; and pre-existing medical genetic conditions such as chronic hypertension, renal disease, type 1 (insulin-dependent) diabetes, factor V Leiden, and thrombophilias such as antiphospholipid antibody syndrome.[a]

Classic symptoms of pre-eclampsia are elevated BP and proteinuria. Edema is common in pregnancy and is no longer considered part of a pre-eclampsia diagnosis.[a] However, when edema of the face (see photo) is of sudden onset and associated with sudden weight gain, diagnosis of pre-eclampsia should be considered. Proteinuria is a late development in pre-eclampsia and an indicator of the severity of the disease. Canadian guidelines for managing hypertension in pregnancy[a] define hypertension as a diastolic BP of >90 mm Hg, by office measurement, with the patient sitting and her arm at the level of the heart according to the fifth Korotkoff sound. Presence of hypertension is necessary for diagnosis of pre-eclampsia, but pre-eclampsia may occur without edema or proteinuria.

Onset and worsening of symptoms may be sudden. Subjective signs may include headaches and vision changes (blurring or seeing spots or flashing lights), caused by cerebral edema, and right upper quadrant or epigastric pain, caused by liver enlargement in which the liver also becomes necrotic and hemorrhagic. Liver enzyme levels become elevated, hematocrit usually increases, and platelet levels drop. Serum creatinine and blood urea nitrogen levels become elevated. Hemolysis occurs, at least partly due to vasospasm. A serious variant of pre-eclampsia, HELLP syndrome (*h*emolysis, *e*levated *l*iver enzymes, and *l*ow *p*latelet count), represents an ominous clinical picture.

Untreated pre-eclampsia may progress to eclampsia, which is manifested by generalized tonic–clonic seizures. Eclampsia may develop as late as 10 days postpartum. Before the syndrome becomes clinically manifested, it affects the placenta through vasospasm and a series of small infarctions. The placenta's capacity to deliver oxygen and nutrients to the fetus may be seriously diminished, and fetal growth may be restricted.

[a]Society of Obstetricians and Gynaecologists of Canada. (2014). Diagnosis, evaluation and management of hypertensive disorders of pregnancy. *Journal of Obstetrics and Gynaecology Canada, 36*(5) 416–438.
BP, Blood pressure.
See Illustration Credits for source information.

TABLE 30.4 Fetal Size Inconsistent With Dates

Disorder/Condition	Description
Size Small for Dates	Fundal height measures smaller than expected for dates.
Inaccuracy of dates	Conception may have occurred later than originally thought. Reconsider the patient's menstrual history, sexual history, contraceptive use, early pregnancy testing, early measurement of the uterus, ultrasonography results, timing of pregnancy symptoms (including the date of quickening), and fundal height measurements. If, after this review, the expected date of birth is correct, then further investigation is required.

Continued

TABLE 30.4	Fetal Size Inconsistent With Dates—cont'd
Disorder/Condition	Description
Preterm labour and birth	Preterm birth occurs before 37 weeks' gestation; it affected 7.8% of pregnancies in Canada in 2013.[a] The cause of preterm labour is unknown: 50% occur in the absence of known risk factors. Pre-existing factors associated with preterm birth include maternal history of previous preterm birth, three or more first trimester pregnancy losses (habitual abortion), second trimester loss, uterine anomalies, and cervical conization. Current pregnancy risk factors include multiple pregnancy, preterm rupture of membranes, polyhydramnios, antepartum hemorrhage, intra-abdominal surgery, urinary tract infection (UTI), tobacco or cocaine use, serious maternal infection, and physical or emotional trauma.[b] Prevention strategies include bed rest, tocolysis, home uterine monitoring, and hydration. Serial ultrasonographic assessments of cervical effacement and use of fetal fibronectin sometimes reassure women who present with threatened preterm labour that they are not likely to give birth immediately; however, it is not yet possible to predict who will proceed to have a preterm birth.
Intrauterine growth restriction (IUGR) or fetal growth restriction	IUGR, a syndrome in which the fetus fails to meet its growth potential, is associated with increased fetal and neonatal mortality and morbidity. Its origin may be fetoplacental, as with chromosomal abnormalities, genetic syndromes, congenital malformations, infectious diseases, and placental disorders; or its origin may be maternal, as with decreased uteroplacental blood flow (as occurs with hypertensive disorders), poor maternal weight gain, poor maternal nutrition, or previous pregnancy with an IUGR infant. Other contributing factors include infectious diseases (rubella, cytomegalovirus); multiple gestation; and environmental toxins such as cigarette smoke and maternal drug and alcohol use.
Fetal position	Fetal position varies until approximately 34 weeks, when the vertex should settle into the pelvis and remain there. The position of the fetus in a transverse lie, or shoulder presentation, results in widening of the maternal abdomen from side to side and decreased fundal height. Fetal malposition may occur with lax maternal abdominal musculature (inability to hold the baby in close), an abnormality in the fetus (e.g., the enlarged head of the hydrocephalic infant), placenta previa (implantation of the placenta over the cervix, blocking fetal descent), or a restricted maternal pelvis.
Size Large for Dates	Fundal height measures larger than expected for dates.
Inaccuracy of dates	Review the same findings as listed for "Size Small for Dates."
Hydatidiform mole	Also termed *gestational trophoblastic neoplasia*, this condition results from abnormal proliferation of trophoblastic tissue associated with pregnancy. In 50% of cases, uterine size is excessive and the gestational age and uterine size do not coincide.
Multiple gestation	The incidence of multiple gestations is rising in Canada (>12 000 in 2011) and other developed countries, mostly because of assisted reproductive technologies and advanced maternal age.[c,d] Up to 12% of twin pregnancies become singletons by the loss of one embryo without symptoms early in the pregnancy.[c] Twin gestations are either monozygotic (division of a single ovum after fertilization) or dizygotic (simultaneous fertilization of two ova). Higher order multiple gestations are rarer; they can be monozygotic, dizygotic, or a combination.[c] The placenta and fetal membranes also differ according to the type of twin pregnancy: (a) monoamniotic or diamniotic and (b) monochorionic or dichorionic. The placentas may be separate or fused.

TABLE 30.4 Fetal Size Inconsistent With Dates—cont'd

Disorder/Condition	Description
	Multifetal pregnancies have many risks: preterm birth and increased risks for congenital anomalies, maternal anemia, or placenta previa. Prenatal care includes more frequent visits to assess fetal growth and development, maternal coping, and amniotic fluid volume. More frequent ultrasounds are used to determine fetal health.[e] Mothers and families need support to cope with greater prenatal care and the increased needs of the infants after birth. Breastfeeding support by a lactation consultant is beneficial, if this is the patient's choice.
Polyhydramnios	An amniotic fluid volume is a maximum volume pocket >8.0 cm or an amniotic fluid index (AFI) >95th percentile or ≥20 cm. The cause is usually idiopathic but may result from fetal anomalies, diabetes in pregnancy, or presence of multiple fetuses.[f]
Oligohydramnios	Oligohydramnios is a reduction in amniotic fluid volume (i.e., an AFI <5 or a single deepest pocket <2 cm).
Leiomyoma (myoma or uterine fibroid)	This is a pre-existing benign tumour of the uterine wall, which is stimulated to enlarge by the estrogen levels of pregnancy. Myomas may be located anywhere in the uterine wall (see Table 27.6, p. 815). When they grow in the outer uterine wall, the myometrium, they may affect the clinician's judgement of where the fundus of the uterus should be measured. A myoma may grow just underneath the endometrial surface into the uterine cavity, displacing the fetus or preventing its descent into the pelvis.
Fetal macrosomia	This is a condition where the infant weighs more than 4 000 g at birth or is >90th percentile for gestational age.[g] Maternal risk factors for fetal overgrowth include a history of a macrosomic infant, maternal obesity (body mass index >30), increased weight gain during pregnancy, multiparity, male fetus, gestational age >40 weeks, ethnicity, maternal age <17 years, and diabetes. Birth risks to the mother include labour complications such as failure to progress, an increased incidence of Caesarean delivery, bladder trauma, and vaginal tissue trauma. Fetal risks include birth trauma such as fractured clavicle and brachial plexus nerve damage from shoulder dystocia, decreased Apgar scores, extended hospitalizations, and possible fetal or neonatal mortality.

[a]Public Health Agency of Canada. (2016). *Health fact sheets: Preterm live births in Canada: 2000 to 2013*. Retrieved from http://www.statcan.gc.ca/pub/82-625-x/2016001/article/14675-eng.htm.

[b]Public Health Agency of Canada. (2012). *Perinatal health indicators for Canada 2011*. Ottawa: Author.

[c]Blackburn, S. T. (2013). *Maternal, fetal, & neonatal physiology: A clinical perspective* (4th ed.). St. Louis: W. B. Saunders.

[d]Vanier Institute of the Family. (2014). *Facts and stats: Multiple births in Canada*. Retrieved from http://vanierinstitute.ca/wp-content/uploads/2015/10/FS_2014-04-16_Multiple-births.pdf.

[e]Lowdermilk, D., Perry, S., Cashion, K., et al. (2012). *Maternity & women's health care* (10th ed.). St. Louis: Elsevier/Mosby.

[f]Creasy, R. K., Resnick, R., Iams, J. D., et al. (2014). *Creasy & Resnick's maternal–fetal medicine: Principles and practice* (7th ed.). Philadelphia: W. B. Saunders.

[g]Gaudet, L., Ferraro, Z. M., Wen, S. W., et al. (2014). Maternal obesity and occurrence of fetal macrosomia: A systematic review and meta-analysis. *Biomed Research International*, 2014:640291. Retrieved from https://www.ncbi.nlm.nih.gov/pmc/articles/PMC4273542/.

See Illustration Credits for source information.

TABLE 30.5	Disorders of Pregnancy
Disorder/Condition	**Description**
Anemia	The most common cause of anemia in pregnancy is iron deficiency. Women should be tested at their first prenatal visit and again between 24 and 28 weeks' gestation.[a] This second testing is done together with gestational diabetes screening. The fetus uses maternal red blood cells for growth and development, and this use increases around week 20. Women at risk for iron deficiency anemia are those with persistent nausea and vomiting who are unable to eat a healthy diet rich in iron, those with multiple gestation, those who have two pregnancies close together, and those with inadequate nutrition before pregnancy. Iron deficiency anemia during pregnancy increases the risk for low birth weight, preterm birth, maternal infections, and perinatal mortality. Severe anemia with maternal hemoglobin (Hgb) less than 120 g/L is associated with abnormal fetal oxygenation.[b,c] Oral iron supplementation is usually sufficient, but some women cannot tolerate this and require intravenous iron administration.
Vaginal bleeding	Some women have bright red, pink, or dark brown spotting at some time during the first trimester. This is not always a sign of pending pregnancy loss, but it may be caused by a blighted ovum, friable cervix, ectopic pregnancy, perigestational hemorrhage, or cervical lesions. In the second and third trimesters, vaginal bleeding may be indicative of placental abruption, placenta previa, uterine rupture, cervical dilation, cervical lesion, or a friable cervix. Risk factors that increase the risk for vaginal bleeding include gestational or chronic hypertension, cocaine use, abdominal trauma, uterine anomalies, prolonged preterm rupture of membranes, prior placental abruption, and cervical cancer.
Spontaneous abortion	An estimated 50% of all pregnancies end in spontaneous abortion (SA) (known as *miscarriage*), with many not recognized clinically.[d] Spontaneous abortion is defined as loss of a fetus weighing less than 500 g before 20 weeks' gestation. Most first trimester losses are attributed to chromosomal abnormalities, while many second trimester losses are attributed to uterine abnormalities. Risk factors for spontaneous abortion include advanced maternal or paternal age, increasing parity, and maternal and paternal exposure to environmental toxicants. Other risk factors are exposure to tobacco, ethanol, and cocaine and other drugs, as well as to therapeutic agents such as chemotherapy, radiation, and anaesthetics.
Incompetent cervix	Cervical incompetence is defined as gradual and painless premature cervical dilation and effacement leading to preterm labour if not detected in time to have a cervical cerclage placed. It may be congenital or acquired after cervical trauma or a cone biopsy.
Hyperemesis	Hyperemesis is excessive vomiting in pregnancy that may last well into the second trimester and beyond. It can interfere with electrolyte levels, acid–base balance, and nutritional status. Dehydration and starvation may ensue and lead to fetal intrauterine growth restriction. Nausea and vomiting are not uncommon in pregnancy, usually resolve between weeks 16 and 20, and may be controlled with dietary and lifestyle changes. Vitamin B_6, ginger, acupuncture, acupressure, or Diclectin can be used with some effectiveness. Diclectin is a delayed-release formulation of doxylamine succinate, 10 mg, with pyridoxine hydrochloride (vitamin B_6), 10 mg. This effective treatment can be offered to alleviate nausea and vomiting. It has a pregnancy risk factor rating of A−. There is no risk to the fetus.[e] Risk factors for hyperemesis include history of previous hyperemesis, molar pregnancy, multiple gestation, emotional stress, history of gastro-intestinal reflux, uncontrolled thyroid disease, primigravida status, and obesity.
Preterm labour	Preterm labour is labour that occurs after 20 weeks' gestation and before completion of 37 weeks' gestation. Preterm labour is a major factor in fetal morbidity and mortality. Some risk factors are chronic urinary tract infections (UTIs), polyhydramnios, multiple gestation, previous preterm labour or preterm birth, smoking, problematic substance use, limited or irregular prenatal care, low weight gain after 20 weeks' gestation, history of cervical conization, low socioeconomic status, being of non-European descent, and uterine infections.
Decreased fetal movement	Fetal movement is one indicator of fetal well-being. Maternal awareness of fetal movement during the third trimester is important; formal counting should be taught to women at risk for adverse perinatal outcomes starting between 26 and 28 weeks' gestation.

TABLE 30.5	Disorders of Pregnancy—cont'd
Disorder/Condition	Description
Psychological illness	Mental illness during pregnancy has significant effects on fetal well-being. According to research reports, 10%–20% of pregnant women experience depression during pregnancy, with most diagnosed in the second and third trimesters. Depression is a risk factor for decreased fetal birth weight and premature birth. Anxiety disorders, eating disorders, and psychotic illness present before and during pregnancy are additional predictors of adverse perinatal outcomes. It is important to understand these disorders and their effect on pregnancy to weigh potential risks from psychiatric medications used to treat these disorders.[f]

[a]March of Dimes Foundation. (2013). *Pregnancy complications: Anemia.* Retrieved from http://www.marchofdimes.com/pregnancy/complications_anemia.html.

[b]Society of Obstetricians and Gynaecologists of Canada. (2007). Fetal health surveillance: Antepartum and intrapartum consensus guideline. *Journal of Obstetrics and Gynaecology Canada, 29*(9 Suppl. 4), S3–S56.

[c]Coad, J., & Conlon, C. (2011). Iron deficiency in women: Assessment, causes, and consequences. *Current Opinion in Clinical Nutrition and Metabolic Care, 14*, 625–634.

[d]McLaughlin Centre for Population Health Risk Assessment. (2013). *Spontaneous abortion.* Ottawa: Institute for Population Health, University of Ottawa.

[e]Society of Obstetricians and Gynaecologists of Canada. (2016). Clinical practice guideline: The management of nausea and vomiting of pregnancy. *Journal of Obstetrics and Gynaecology Canada, 38*(12), 1127–1137.

[f]Pearlstein, T. (2015). Depression during pregnancy. *Best Practice and Research Clinical Obstetrics and Gynecology, 29*, 757–764.

TABLE 30.6	Malpresentations

Vertex (for comparison)

Complete breech

Footling breech

Frank breech

Transverse lie and shoulder presentation

Face presentation

Brow presentation

Compound presentation

Malpresentations may be detected by an experienced examiner, confirmed by the location of fetal heart tones, and further confirmed by ultrasonography. Before 34 weeks' gestation, any position is normal. The vertex presentation is desirable thereafter because spontaneous turning becomes less likely as the fetus grows in proportion to the amount of space and fluid available in the uterus and pelvis.

Summary Checklist: Pregnancy Examination

1. **Collect historical information**
2. **Determine EDB** and current number of weeks of gestation
3. Ask the patient to undress and empty her bladder, **saving her urine for it to be tested** for protein and glucose
4. **Measure weight and height**; calculate prepregnancy BMI, and monitor ongoing weight gain
5. **Perform a physical examination**, starting with general survey
6. **Inspect skin** for pigment changes and scars
7. **Check oral mucous membranes**
8. **Palpate thyroid gland**
9. **Inspect breast changes** and palpate for masses
10. **Auscultate** breath sounds, heart sounds, heart rate, and any murmurs
11. **Check lower extremities** for edema, varicosities, and reflexes
12. **Examine the abdomen:** Measure fundal height; perform Leopold's manoeuvres; auscultate fetal heart tones
13. **Perform the pelvic examination:** Note signs of pregnancy, the condition of the cervix, and the size and position of the uterus
14. **Perform pelvimetry**
15. **Measure the BP**
16. **Obtain** appropriate **laboratory work**
17. **Engage in teaching and health promotion**

REFERENCES

1. Aikawa, H., Tamai, M., Mitamura, K., et al. (2014). Innate immunity in an in vitro murine blastocyst model using embryonic & trophoblast stem cells. *Journal of Bioscience and Bioengineering, 117*(3), 358–365. doi:10.1016/j.jbiosc.2013.09.001.

2. DeCherney, A., Goodwin, T., Nathan, L., et al. (2007). *Current diagnosis and treatment: Obstetrics & gynecology* (10th ed.). New York: McGraw-Hill.

3. Heitmann, K., Nordeng, H., Havnen, G., et al. (2017). The burden of nausea & vomiting during pregnancy: Severe impacts on quality of life, daily life functioning and willingness to become pregnant again—Results from a cross-sectional study. *BMC Pregnancy and Childbirth, 17*, 75.

4. Mindell, J., Cook, R., & Nikolovski, J. (2015). Sleep patterns and sleep disturbances across pregnancy. *Sleep Medicine, 16*, 4.

5. Blackburn, S. T. (2013). *Maternal, fetal, & neonatal physiology: A clinical perspective* (4th ed.). St. Louis: W. B. Saunders.

6. Cunningham, F. G., Leveno, K. J., Bloom, S. L., et al. (2010). *Williams' obstetrics* (23rd ed.). Stamford, CT: Appleton & Lange.

7. Carney, L., Quinlan, J., & West, J. (2014). Thyroid disease in pregnancy. *American Family Physician, 89*(4), 273–278.

8. Geisinger, M., Geurs, N., Bain, J., et al. (2014). Oral health education and therapy reduces gingivitis in pregnancy. *Journal of Clinical Periodontology, 41*(2), 141–148.

9. Soucy-Giguère, L., Tétu, A., Gauthier, S., et al. (2016). Periodontal disease and adverse pregnancy outcomes: A prospective study in a low-risk population. *Journal of Obstetrics and Gynaecology Canada, 38*(4), 346–350.

10. Creasy, R. K., Resnick, R., Iams, J. D., et al. (2014). *Creasy & Resnick's maternal–fetal medicine: Principles and practice* (7th ed.). Philadelphia: W. B. Saunders.

11. Osterman, M., Ilyas, A., & Matson, J. (2012). Carpal tunnel syndrome in pregnancy. *Orthopedic Clinics of North America, 43*, 515–520.

12. Society of Obstetricians and Gynaecologists of Canada. (2011). Genetic considerations for a woman's pre-conception evaluation. *Journal of Obstetrics and Gynaecology Canada, 33*(1), 57–64.

13. Statistics Canada. (2016). *Live births, by age of mother, Canada: Provinces and territories.* Retrieved from http://www5.statcan.gc.ca/cansim/a26?lang=eng&id=1024503&p2=46.

14. Ministry of Health and Long Term Care. (2017). *Teen pregnancy.* Retrieved from http://www.health.gov.on.ca.

15. Society of Obstetricians and Gynaecologists of Canada. (2015). Adolescent pregnancy guidelines. *Journal of Obstetrics and Gynaecology Canada, 37*(8), 740–756.

16. MacSween, K., Whelan, E., & Woolcott, C. (2016). Gestational weight gain and perinatal outcomes in adolescent mothers: A retrospective cohort study. *Journal of Obstetrics and Gynaecology Canada, 38*(4), 338–345.

17. American College of Obstetricians and Gynecologists' Task Force on Hypertension. (2013). *Hypertension: Clinical practice guidelines.* Retrieved from https://www.acog.org/~/media/Task%20Force%20and%20Work%20Group%20Reports/public/HypertensioninPregnancy.pdf.

18. Society of Obstetricians and Gynaecologists of Canada. (2012). Clinical practice guideline: Delayed child-bearing. *Journal of Obstetrics and Gynaecology Canada, 34*(1), 80–93.

19. Statistics Canada. (2017). *Fertility: Fewer children, older moms.* Retrieved from http://www.statcan.gc.ca/pub/11-630-x/11-630-x2014002-eng.htm.

20. March of Dimes. (2016). *Birth defects, Down syndrome.* White Plains, NY: March of Dimes Birth Defects Foundation.

21. Kenny, L., Lavender, T., McNamee, R., et al. (2013). Advanced maternal age and adverse pregnancy outcome: Evidence from a large contemporary cohort. *PLoS ONE, 8*(2), e56583.

22. Registered Nurses' Association of Ontario. (2007). *Embracing cultural diversity in health care: Developing cultural competence.* Retrieved from http://rnao.ca/bpg/guidelines/embracing-cultural-diversity-health-care-developing-cultural-competence.

23. Women and Children First. (2017). *Maternal mortality & safe motherhood.* Retrieved from https://www.womenandchildrenfirst.org.uk/maternal-mortality?gclid=Cj0KEQjw8tbHBRC6rLS024qYjtEBEiQA7wIDeYLv7ew3KTaBN__QD14-L8nZAQHotO_idxyYgWXoMC8aAo2i8P8HAQ.

24. Public Health Agency of Canada. (2013). *Maternal mortality in Canada.* Retrieved from https://sogc.org/wp-content/uploads/2014/05/REVISEDMortality-EN-Final-PDF.pdf.

25. Say, L., Chou, D., Gemmill, A., et al. (2014). Global causes of maternal death: A WHO systemic analysis. *The Lancet. Global Health, 2,* 323–333.

26. Society of Obstetricians and Gynaecologists of Canada. (2013). SOGC clinical practice guideline: Cancer chemotherapy and pregnancy. *Journal of Obstetrics and Gynaecology Canada, 35*(3, 263–278.

27. Keyser, E. A., Staat, B. C., Fausett, M. B., et al. (2012). Pregnancy-related breast cancer. *Reviews in Obstetrics & Gynecology, 5*(2), 94–99.

28. Society of Obstetricians and Gynaecologists of Canada. (2016). Clinical practice guideline: The management of nausea and vomiting of pregnancy. *Journal of Obstetrics and Gynaecology Canada, 38*(12), 1127–1137.

29. Society of Obstetricians and Gynaecologists of Canada. (2007). Fetal health surveillance: Antepartum and intrapartum consensus guideline. *Journal of Obstetrics and Gynaecology Canada, 29*(9, Suppl. 4), S3–S56.

30. Szczypinska, E., & Chadrasekar, P. (2015). *Human T-cell lymphotropic viruses.* Retrieved from http://emedicine. medscape.com/article/219285-overview.

31. Best Start Resource Centre. (2017). *Risks of cannabis on fertility, pregnancy, breastfeeding and parenting.* Toronto: Author.

32. Society of Obstetricians and Gynaecologists of Canada. (2016). Canadian consensus on female nutrition: Adolescence, reproduction, menopause and beyond. *Journal of Obstetrics and Gynaecology Canada, 38*(6), 508–554.

33. Society of Obstetricians and Gynaecologists of Canada. (2016). Clinical practice guideline: In pregnancy. *Journal of Obstetrics and Gynaecology Canada, 38*(7), 667–679.

34. Government of Canada. (2016). *Pregnancy and women's mental health in Canada.* Retrieved from https://www.canada.ca/en/ public-health/services/publications/healthy-living/pregnancy-women-mental-health-canada.html.

35. Canadian Perinatal Surveillance System. (2015). *Effect of maternal weight on pregnancy outcomes.* Retrieved from https://www.canada.ca/en/public-health/services/publications/ healthy-living/effect-maternal-weight-pregnancy-outcomes. html.

36. Society of Obstetricians and Gynaecologists of Canada. (2017). Clinical practice guideline: No. 342—Hepatitis B and pregnancy. *Journal of Obstetrics and Gynaecology Canada, 39*(3), 181–190.

37. Society of Obstetricians and Gynaecologists of Canada. (2016). Clinical practice guideline: Diabetes in pregnancy. *Journal of Obstetrics and Gynaecology Canada, 38*(7), 667–679.

38. Kriebs, J., & Gegor, C. (2005). *Varney's pocket midwife* (2nd ed.). Sudbury, MA: Jones & Bartlett.

39. Hurt, K., Guile, M., Bienstock, J., et al. (2011). *The Johns Hopkins manual of gynecology and obstetrics* (4th ed.). Philadelphia: Wolters Kluwer/Lippincott Williams & Wilkins.

40. VanRooyen, M. J., Scott, J. A., et al. (2011). Emergency delivery. In J. E. Tintinalli, J. S. Stapczynski, & D. M. Cline (Eds.), *Tintinalli's emergency medicine: A comprehensive study guide* (7th ed.; sec. 11, ch. 105). New York: McGraw Hill Medical.

41. Society of Obstetricians and Gynaecologists of Canada. (2014). Clinical practice guideline: Diagnosis, evaluation, and management of hypertensive disorders of pregnancy. *Journal of Obstetrics and Gynaecology Canada, 36*(5), 416–438.

42. British Columbia Perinatal Health Program. (2016). *Prenatal screening for Down syndrome, trisomy 18 and open neural tube defects.* Vancouver: Author. Retrieved from http:// www.perinatalservicesbc.ca/Documents/Guidelines-Standards/ Maternal/PrenatalScreeningGuideline.pdf.

43. Zolotor, A., & Carlough, M. (2014). Update on prenatal care. *American Family Physician, 89*(3), 199–208.

44. Society of Obstetricians and Gynaecologists of Canada. (2007). Clinical practice guideline: Prenatal screening for fetal aneuploidy. *Journal of Obstetrics and Gynaecology Canada, 29*(2), 146–161.

45. Murdoch, B., Ravitsky, V., Ogbogu, U., et al. (2017). Non-invasive prenatal testing and the unveiling of an impaired translation process. *Journal of Obstetrics and Gynaecology Canada, 39*(1), 10–17.

46. Tilley, S. (2015). Nursing care of women who have undergone genital cutting. *Nursing for Women's Health, 19*(5).

31 | CHAPTER

Functional Assessment of the Older Adult

Written by Carla Graf, MS, RN, CNS-BC, and Melissa A. Lee, MS, RN, CNS-BC
Adapted by Dianne Groll, RN, BA, BScH, MScH, PhD

ⓔ http://evolve.elsevier.com/Canada/Jarvis/examination/

Canada has a large and growing population of older adults. In 2015, 16.1% of Canadians were 65 years of age or older.[1] Many older adults lead fulfilling lives without significant physical or cognitive changes. They welcome the opportunity to pursue interests and activities that were previously restricted by the responsibilities of work and family (Fig. 31.1). In the 2015 Canadian Community Health Survey (CCHS), respondents were asked to rate, on a scale from 0 ("very dissatisfied") to 10 ("very satisfied"), how they felt about their life as a whole. More than 89% of people older than age 65 reported being "satisfied" or "very satisfied."[2] Despite the fact that older adults are healthier than ever before, the CCHS revealed that only 45% reported their perceived health as very good or excellent, compared with 56% of individuals aged 45 to 64.[2]

The comprehensive assessment of an older adult requires knowledge not only of normal aging changes but also of the effects of chronic diseases, heredity, and lifestyle. A comprehensive assessment incorporates both the physical examination and assessments of an individuals' mental, functional, social, and economic status; pain; and the physical environment for safety concerns. Professionals from multiple disciplines—including physicians; nurses; physical, occupational, and speech therapists; social workers; case managers; nutritionists; and pharmacists—may participate in the assessment. Early recognition of disabilities and treatable conditions is instrumental in preserving function and quality of life for older adults.

The normal process of aging does not necessarily include disease. However, normal aging changes in addition to chronic and acute illnesses may precipitate transitions from home to settings such as hospitals, skilled nursing facilities, long-term care facilities, and assisted living facilities, in which nursing-focused assessments are performed. The care setting usually determines the types of assessment and instruments used. However, the goal of the functional assessment remains the same—to identify an older adult's strengths and any limitations—so that appropriate interventions will promote independence and prevent functional decline.

FUNCTIONAL ABILITY

Functional ability refers to a person's ability to perform activities necessary to live in modern society, including driving, using the telephone, and performing personal tasks such as bathing and toileting. Functional ability also incorporates the person's physiological and psychological status and the physical and social environments.[3] Functional status is an individual's actual performance of activities and tasks and is dependent on motivation, sensory capacity (i.e., vision and hearing), degree of assistance needed to accomplish the tasks, and cognition. For example, the effect that arthritis might have on a person's ability to exercise may affect physical function. A condition such as Alzheimer's disease may affect problem solving, safety concerns, and motivation, which in turn affect function. The presence or absence of social supports and the safety of the physical setting are environmental issues that affect functional status and possibly the ability to live independently. The interaction of these components provides a "snapshot" of an older adult's functional status at a given point. Functional status is not static; older adults may move continuously through varying stages of independence and disability.

Assessment of function is important for comparison, prognosis, and objective data to determine efficacy of treatments. Medical diagnosis is not sufficient to predict functional abilities. Older adults may not experience the usual symptoms of an acute illness. A decline in functional status may indicate another process, such as an infection.

A functional assessment of an older adult is the basis for care planning, goal setting, and discharge planning. A functional assessment also is needed to determine eligibility for obtaining many services, such as durable medical equipment, home modifications, and inpatient or outpatient rehabilitation services. For an older adult and the family, a functional assessment can identify areas for current and future planning, such as the most appropriate living situation.

A functional assessment includes three overarching domains: **activities of daily living (ADLs)**, **instrumental activities of daily living (IADLs)**, and **mobility**.[3] A

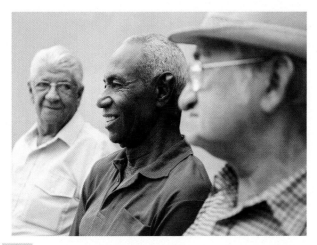

31.1   (© Diego Cervo, 2014/Shutterstock.)

functional evaluation should be systematic, with attention paid to the particular needs of the patient, such as the presence of pain, fatigue, shortness of breath, or memory problems. There are two approaches to use when performing a functional assessment: *asking individuals* about their abilities to perform tasks (using self-reports) or actually *observing* their ability to perform tasks. For patients with memory problems, use of surrogate reporters (proxy reports) such as family members or caregivers may be necessary; the examiner should note that they may either overestimate or underestimate actual abilities.

Activities of Daily Living

ADLs are the tasks necessary for self-care. Typically, ADLs encompass domains of eating/feeding, bathing, grooming (the individual tasks of washing face, combing hair, shaving, cleaning teeth), dressing (lower body and upper body), toileting (bowel and bladder), walking (including propelling a wheelchair), using stairs (ascending and descending), and transferring (such as bed to chair). ADL instruments are designed as self-report, observation of tasks, or proxy/surrogate report.

ADL dependency has been related to the presence of chronic disease such as arthritis and rheumatism; diabetes; urinary incontinence; bronchitis, emphysema, or chronic obstructive pulmonary disease; the effects of stroke; and Alzheimer's disease or other dementia. Therefore, chronic illness must be considered when ADLs and IADLs are assessed.

The Katz Index of ADL

The Katz Index of ADL[4] is based on the concept of physical disability and was intended to measure physical function in older adults and chronically ill patients.[3] It is widely used in both clinical practice and research to measure performance, evaluate treatment outcomes, and predict the need for continuing supervised care.

The Katz Index of ADL was developed as a hierarchical structure. Katz and colleagues believed loss of physical function occurred in the most complex activities first, that these functions were lost in descending order of complexity,

and that they were regained in ascending order.[4] Activities assessed are bathing, dressing, toileting, transferring from bed to chair, continence, and feeding (Fig. 31.2). Only activities that can be performed without help are rated as independent. One point is given for each item rated independent. The tool takes approximately 5 minutes to administer, but its use has limitations. In a hospital setting, a patient cannot demonstrate all the activities and may need to adjust the degree of dependence or independence. The patient's function may be overestimated or underestimated, and small changes in the activities may not be identified.

Because the instrument helps measure current function, it is valuable for planning specific types of assistance. For example, a patient may be unable to bathe independently on hospital discharge but can undertake feeding and transferring to a commode safely and independently. In this case, plan for a home health aide to visit twice weekly to assist with bathing.

Additional Activity of Daily Living Instruments

Additional tools used to assess ADL ability are the Barthel Index,[5] the Functional Independence Measure (FIM),[6] and the Rapid Disability Rating Scale-2.[7] The Barthel Index includes definitions of each task to facilitate ease of scoring and has a more comprehensive assessment of mobility than the Katz Index of ADL. The Barthel Index is often used to follow progress in rehabilitation settings.[3]

The FIM was developed by a consensus panel of physical medicine and rehabilitation staff and has been widely tested on older adults. It can be administered three ways: (a) by telephone, (b) by in-person interview, and (c) by proxy. It is more sensitive to change than other ADL instruments, but formal training in its use is necessary, and it is more time consuming.[3]

The Rapid Disability Rating Scale-2 is completed by a family member or professional caregiver familiar with the abilities of the older adult. It is designed to measure what the patient *actually can do* versus what they might be able to do. You should conduct a session to train the observer in the use of this instrument.

Instrumental Activities of Daily Living

Many IADL instruments have been developed since the 1960s, with the goal of measuring functional abilities necessary for independent community living. IADL tasks typically include shopping, meal preparation, housekeeping, laundry, managing finances, taking medications, and using transportation. These instruments may have cultural and gender biases, especially in older cohorts.[3] IADL instruments focus on tasks historically performed by women (doing laundry, cooking, housework), and most do not address activities traditionally performed primarily by men, such as home repairs, car maintenance, and yard work.

Lawton Instrumental Activities of Daily Living

IADL measures were first developed by Lawton and Brody in 1969 to address higher order components of the Katz Index

---

Katz Activities of Daily Living

Activities

Points (1 or 0)

Independence

(1 Point)

NO supervision, direction, or personal assistance

Dependence

(0 Points)

WITH supervision, direction, personal assistance, or total care

Bathing

Points _____

(1 Point) Bathes self completely or needs help in bathing only a single part of the body such as the back, genital area, or disabled extremity

(0 Point) Needs help with bathing more than one part of the body or with getting in or out of the tub or shower; requires total bathing

Dressing

Points _____

(1 Point) Gets clothes from closet and drawers and puts on clothes and outer garments complete with fasteners; may have help tying shoes

(0 Point) Needs help with dressing self or needs to be completely dressed

Toileting

Points _____

(1 Point) Gets to toilet, gets on and off, arranges clothes, cleans genital area without help

(0 Point) Needs help transferring to the toilet or cleaning self, or uses bedpan or commode

Transferring

Points _____

(1 Point) Moves into and out of bed or chair unassisted; mechanical transferring aids are acceptable

(0 Point) Needs help in moving from bed to chair or requires a complete transfer

Continence

Points _____

(1 Point) Exercises complete self-control over urination and defecation

(0 Point) Is partially or totally incontinent of bowel or bladder

Feeding

Points _____

(1 Point) Gets food from plate into mouth without help; preparation of food may be done by another person

(0 Point) Needs partial or total help with feeding or requires parenteral feeding

Total Points = _____

6 = High (patient independent)

0 = Low (patient very dependent)

Adapted from Gerontological Society of America. Katz S., et al. (1970). Progress in the development of the index of ADL. *Gerontologist, 10* (1, Part 1), 20-30.

31.2

---

of ADL and to measure the more complex ADLs required for a person to adapt to the environment.[3] The Lawton IADL instrument is designed as a self-report measure of performance rather than ability, and was originally developed to determine the most suitable living situation for an older adult. The theory was that competence and maintenance of life skills such as shopping, cooking, and managing finances are a meaningful way to assess function because these abilities are prerequisites for independent living. As with the Katz Index of ADL, the Lawton IADL instrument assumes a hierarchical nature of skill acquisition and loss. The Lawton IADL scale contains eight items (Fig. 31.3); women's functions are scored in all eight domains, whereas men's are scored in five (laundry, housekeeping, and preparing food are omitted). The instrument is useful in acute hospital settings for discharge planning and ongoing assessment in outpatient settings. It would not be useful for residents in institutional settings because many of these tasks are already being managed for the residents. Given that many individuals either live alone or have never subscribed to "traditional" gender roles, it is also extremely likely that most older adults prepare their own food, keep house, and do their own laundry, regardless of the gender they identify with. As such, this assessment may not be the most appropriate for everyone.

Additional IADL Instruments

Other IADL instruments available are the Older Americans Resources and Services Multidimensional Functional Assessment Questionnaire-IADL (OARS-IADL)[8] and the Direct Assessment of Functional Abilities (DAFA).[9] The OARS-IADL assesses five areas of personal function: (a) social, (b) economic, (c) mental health, (d) physical health, and (e) self-care capacity; it is administered as either a self-report or trained observer instrument. The questions are the same for men and women. The DAFA is a 10-item observational instrument for use with adults with dementia.

The Lawton Instrumental Activities of Daily Living Scale

A. Ability to Use Telephone
1. Operates telephone on own initiative; looks up and dials numbers   1
2. Dials a few well-known numbers   1
3. Answers telephone, but does not dial   1
4. Does not use telephone at all   0

B. Shopping
1. Takes care of all shopping needs independently   1
2. Shops independently for small purchases   0
3. Needs to be accompanied on any shopping trip   0
4. Completely unable to shop   0

C. Food Preparation
1. Plans, prepares, and serves adequate meals independently   1
2. Prepares adequate meals if supplied with ingredients   0
3. Heats and serves prepared meals or prepares meals, but does not maintain adequate diet   0
4. Needs to have meals prepared and served   0

D. Housekeeping
1. Maintains house alone with occasional assistance (heavy work)   1
2. Performs light daily tasks such as dishwashing, bed making   1
3. Performs light daily tasks, but cannot maintain acceptable level of cleanliness   1
4. Needs help with all home maintenance tasks   1
5. Does not participate in any housekeeping tasks   0

E. Laundry
1. Does personal laundry completely   1
2. Launders small items, rinses socks, stockings, etc.   1
3. All laundry must be done by others   0

F. Mode of Transportation
1. Travels independently on public transportation or drives own car   1
2. Arranges own travel via taxi, but does not otherwise use public transportation   1
3. Travels on public transportation when assisted or accompanied by another   1
4. Travel limited to taxi or automobile with assistance of another   0
5. Does not travel at all   0

G. Responsibility for Own Medications
1. Is responsible for taking medication in correct dosages at correct time   1
2. Takes responsibility if medication is prepared in advance in separate dosages   0
3. Is not capable of dispensing own medication   0

H. Ability to Handle Finances
1. Manages financial matters independently (budgets, writes checks, pays rent and bills, goes to bank); collects and keeps track of income   1
2. Manages day-to-day purchases, but needs help with banking, major purchases, etc.   1
3. Incapable of handling money   0

Scoring: For each category, circle the item description that most closely resembles the client's highest functional level (either 0 or 1).

From Lawton, M. P., & Brody, E. M. (1969). Assessment of older people: Self-maintaining and instrumental activities of daily living. *Gerontologist, 9* (3, Part 1), 179-186. Copyright © The Gerontological Society of America.

31.3

It requires the patient to demonstrate tasks of money management, shopping, hobbies, meal preparation, awareness, reading, and transportation.[3] The obvious strength of this instrument is the direct observation versus self- or proxy reporting. However, it can take up to an hour and a half to complete, so it would not be feasible to use in an acute-care hospital setting.

Advanced Activities of Daily Living

Advanced activities of daily living (AADLs) are activities that an older adult performs as a family member and a member of society and community; they include occupational and recreational activities. Various AADL instruments commonly include items concerning self-care, mobility, work (either paid or volunteer), recreational activities/hobbies, and socialization.

Measuring Physical Performance

A disadvantage of many ADL and IADL instruments is the self- or proxy report of functional activities. Incorporating an objective standardized measure of performance prevents overestimation or underestimation of abilities. Many physical performance measures also incorporate balance, gait, motor coordination, and endurance, and many are timed.

Although direct observation of the older adult performing the activities has clear advantages, there are some disadvantages. The instruments can be very time consuming; administering them may require training and special equipment; and performing certain activities entails the possibility the individual might fall or sustain an injury during testing. Commonly used physical performance measures include the **Physical Performance Test**,[10] the **performance test activities of daily living**,[11] and the **Timed Up and Go Test**.[12] In a review of 17 functional balance tests, Langley and Mackintosh recommended the Timed Up and Go Test as valid and reliable for the older adult population.[13]

Assessment of Cognition

Assessment of cognitive status in older adults is an important part of the functional assessment. In general, a gradual and mild to moderate decline in short-term memory may be attributable to aging; an older adult may need more time to learn new material or a new task or may need a system for reminders. However, although some decline in memory is a normal part of aging, sudden or severe cognitive decline is not. Altered cognition in older adults is commonly attributed to three disorders: (a) *delirium*, (b) *dementia*, and (c) *depression*. However, other factors, such as certain medications or infection, may also be contributory.

Delirium is a common, life-threatening disordered mental state that, when recognized and treated promptly, is often reversible. Delirium is characterized by an acute decline in attention and cognition that usually develops over a period of hours or days. It is reported to affect as many as 50% of hospitalized older adults, and is common among people receiving palliative care.[14] National guidelines for screening of patients at risk for delirium, and assessment and treatment of delirium, have been developed and can be downloaded free from the Canadian Coalition for Seniors' Mental Health (CCSMH) website (https://ccsmh.ca).[15]

Dementia is a progressive loss of brain function that can occur as a result of diseases such as Parkinson's or Huntington's diseases, stroke (or vascular dementia), or brain injury. The most common form of dementia in Canada is Alzheimer's disease. Individuals with dementia have alterations in short-term and long-term memory, difficulty in finding words and naming objects, problems with judgement and reasoning, and changes in mood, behaviour, and personality. As the Canadian population ages, the proportion of individuals with dementia is expected to increase from 9.2% of adults aged 65 and older in 2014 to 10% in 2033; the resulting economic burden is estimated to be $16.6 billion by 2031.[16]

The Physical, Intellectual, Emotional, Capabilities, Environment and Social (P.I.E.C.E.S.) program was developed for all health care providers to enhance understanding of and care for patients with complex physical and cognitive/mental health needs and behavioural changes. The P.I.E.C.E.S. website (http://pieceslearning.com) offers resources such as videos and learning packages about how to administer and score the Mini-Mental State Examination and how to use the Cornell Scale for Depression in Dementia. The Indigenous Cognition & Aging Awareness Research Exchange (I-CAARE) has developed fact sheets about dementia in Indigenous communities with the help of Indigenous people living with memory loss, their Elders, and caregivers.[17]

For nurses in various settings, cognitive assessments provide continuing comparisons to the individual's baseline to detect any acute changes. The assessments are not diagnostic but are for screening purposes and identify the need for a more comprehensive workup. As with screening for ADLs and IADLs, assessment of cognition helps with determining the best discharge plan. Common assessment instruments are listed in Table 31.1.

As an illness, **depression** (or clinical depression) usually includes persistent feelings of sadness or hopelessness, a loss of interest or pleasure in previously enjoyable activities, or a combination of these. It also includes cognitive and physical changes, such as trouble with concentration (which leads to memory problems), disturbed sleep, decreased energy or excessive tiredness, and decreased appetite. These changes are present for at least 2 weeks and not just ascribable to a "passing mood" or a normal reaction to a sad event. Depression is the most common mental health problem among older adults, and substantial depressive symptoms affect an estimated 15% of those living in the community.[14] Rates of depression are higher in long-term care facilities; up to 44% of residents have an established diagnosis of depression or significant (three or more) depressive symptoms. Always assess for suicidal ideation when depression is present or suspected.

The Registered Nurses' Association of Ontario (RNAO) has developed clinical best practice guidelines related to caregiving for adults aged 65 years and older with delirium,

TABLE 31.1 Common Cognitive Assessment Instruments

NAME OF INSTRUMENT	TYPE OF TEST	DOMAINS COVERED	ADMINISTRATION TIME
Mini-Mental State Examination[a]	Mental status	Orientation, immediate and delayed recall, working memory, language, visuospatial ability	10 minutes
Northern Cultural Assessment of Memory (N-CAM)[b]	Mental status	Mental status examination designed for Indigenous individuals	
Montreal Cognitive Assessment (MoCA)[c]	Mental status	Orientation, general/personal information, working memory	5–10 minutes
Mini-Cog Test[d]	Mental status	Immediate and delayed recall, visuospatial ability	5–10 minutes
Cornell Scale for Depression[e]	Depression with concomitant dementia	Signs and symptoms of major depression in patients with dementia	20 minutes
Geriatric Depression Scale, Short Form[f]	Depression	Depression and changes in level of depression	5–10 minutes
Confusion Assessment Method[g]	Delirium	Acute onset or fluctuating course; inattention, disorganized thinking, altered level of consciousness	Less than 5 minutes
NEECHAM Confusion Scale[h]	Delirium	Processing (attention, command, orientation), behaviour (appearance, motor, verbal), vital function stability	10 minutes
Clock Drawing Test[i]	Mental status	Cognitive and adaptive functioning, memory, ability to process information	2–5 minutes

[a]Folstein, M. F., Folstein, S. E., & McHugh, P. R. (1975). "Mini-Mental State": A practical method for grading the cognitive state of patients for the clinician. *Journal of Psychiatric Research, 12*(3), 189–198.

[b]Crossley, M., Lanting, S., St. Denis-Katz, H., et al. (2012, February). *The Northern Cultural Assessment of Memory (N-CAM): Normative data from an inner-city clinic supports efficacy and validity of a cognitive screen for Aboriginal adults.* In Fortieth Annual Meeting, International Neuropsychological Society, Montreal, Quebec. Retrieved from http://www.the-ins.org/includes/ckfinder/userfiles/files/Linked%20Program_abstracts.pdf.

[c]Nasreddine, Z. S., Phillips, N. A., Bédirian, V., et al. (2005). The Montreal Cognitive Assessment, MoCA: A brief screening tool for mild cognitive impairment. *Journal of the American Geriatrics Society, 53*, 695–699. doi:10.1111/j.1532-5415.2005.53221.x.

[d]Borson, S., Scanlan, J. M., Chen, P., et al. (2003). The Mini Cog as a screen for dementia: Validation in a population-based sample. *Journal of the American Geriatric Society, 51*, 1451.

[e]Alexopoulos, G. A., Abrams, R. C., Young, R. C., et al. (1988). Cornell Scale for Depression in Dementia. *Biological Psychiatry, 23*, 271–284.

[f]Yesavage, J. A., Brink, T. L., Rose, T. L., et al. (1983). Development and validation of a geriatric depression rating scale: A preliminary report. *Journal of Psychiatric Research, 17*, 37–49.

[g]Inouye, S. K., van Dyck, C. H., Alessi, C. A., et al. (1990). Clarifying confusion: The confusion assessment method. *Annals of Internal Medicine, 113*, 941–948.

[h]Neelon, V. J., Champagne, M. T., Carlson, J. R., et al. (1996). The NEECHAM Confusion Scale: Construction, validation, and clinical testing. *Nursing Research, 45*, 324–330.

[i]Shulman, K., Shedletsky, R., & Silver, I. (1986). The challenge of time: Clock drawing and cognitive function in the elderly. *International Journal of Geriatric Psychiatry, 1*, 135–140.

dementia, and depression.[14] The guidelines also include several helpful tools for assessing and screening for delirium, dementia, and depression.

Social Domain

For older adults, quality of life is closely linked to the success of social function. The social domain focuses on relationships within family, social groups, and the community and is composed of multiple dimensions, including sources of formal and informal assistance available from those relationships. A health care provider's knowledge of a patient's day-to-day routines can provide baseline health information and serve as a reference point for detecting functional decline during future encounters.

A comprehensive social assessment (Box 31.1) is typically spread over several evaluation periods. Because more than 80% of all care is provided by family members, the social

BOX 31.1 Components of Social Assessment

- Social network (formal, semiformal, informal)
- Caregiver assessment
- Potential for elder abuse
- Environment
- Spiritual needs

assessment also addresses the assessment of caregivers.[18] Using a multidimensional approach may help to identify potential risks, such as elder abuse.

Social networks consist of informal supports accessible to the older adult. Informal support is based on cultural beliefs regarding who should be providing care, prior relationships, and location and availability of caregivers. Informal support includes family and close long-time friends and is usually provided free of charge. Such caregiving includes domestic work (e.g., cooking, cleaning, shopping) and care of other household members.

Formal supports include programs such as social welfare and other social service and health care delivery agencies, such as those that provide home health care. Semiformal supports such as church societies, neighbourhood groups, and older adult centres also play an important role in social support. The availability of assistance from family or friends frequently determines whether a functionally dependent older adult remains at home or is placed in residential care. It is important to document who would be available to help the older adult if he, she, or they became ill, even for healthy older adults.

Several standardized assessment instruments are available to provide structured assessment. The Duke Social Support and Stress Scale[19,20] is a measure of a patient's perceptions of support and stress in family and nonfamily relationships. It allows the individual to rate perceived support and stress associated with specific social relationships and to further identify the relationships that provide the most support and stress.

A useful way of illustrating an individual's social and personal relationships with the outside world is through an ecomap. Ecomaps are commonly used in nursing, social work, and family counselling. One example of an ecomap, with instructions on how to make one, can be found here: https://www.smartdraw.com/ecomap/.

MAINTAINING INDEPENDENCE

Most older adults reside in the community, in their own homes, and wish to remain in their homes as long as practical (known as "aging in place"). To do so, necessary health and social services need to be present, and other factors need to be considered. Will the home need renovations or modifications such as a chair lift for stairs, or handrails? Are there supports available in the immediate community, such as health care providers, recreational opportunities, and good transportation? According to Statistics Canada, 7.7% of older adults in an economic family arrangement (two or more persons living in the same dwelling and related to each other) and 32.0% of unattached older adults are considered to be living in low-income situations.[21] As such, will the older adult have the income necessary to maintain independence? Is the individual receiving all the benefits older adults are eligible for? The Canada Mortgage and Housing Corporation has excellent resources on its website (https://www.cmhc-schl.gc.ca/en/developing-and-renovating/accessible-adaptable-housing/aging-in-place) for older adults planning on staying in their homes, including a detailed checklist of home modifications to consider.

ENVIRONMENTAL ASSESSMENT

The physical environment of the older adult includes the home environment and community system and is crucial

31.4 (© Monkey Business Images, 2014/Shutterstock.)

for maintaining independence. In the functional assessment, inquire about the safety of the neighbourhood and whether transportation or transportation services are readily available for older adults where they live (Fig. 31.4). The older adult needs access to basic services such as food and clothing stores, pharmacists, financial institutions, health care facilities, and social service agencies. Common environmental hazards increase the risk for falls and fractures. Those hazards include inadequate lighting, loose throw rugs, curled carpet edges, obstructed hallways, cords in walkways, lack of grab bars in the tub and shower, and low and loose toilet seats. Environmental modification can promote mobility and reduce the likelihood of an older adult's falling. Occupational therapists are trained to assess and suggest modification to the environment to improve safety, mobility, and assist with independent living.

Falls

Seniors' Falls in Canada is a comprehensive report on the prevalence of falls, risk factors for falls, and how to conduct a risk assessment for the prevention of falls.[22] Falls are the number one cause of injury-related hospitalizations of older adults in Canada. It is estimated that 20 to 30% of older adults fall every year, with a higher prevalence in those over the age of 85. Females have an increased likelihood of falling compared with males, and this gender difference increases with age. Older adults who fall spend an average of 3 weeks (22 days) in hospital, compared with an average stay of 12 days for nonfall-related hospitalizations. A full 50% of falls occur in the home, and most are due to the interaction of one or more of the following risk factors: environmental (living environment, weather factors [e.g., ice]), biological/intrinsic (acute illness, balance deficits, chronic illness or disabilities, cognitive impairment, poor vision, muscle weakness), behavioural (footwear, excessive alcohol, poor nutrition, risk-taking behaviours), and economic (social isolation, poor socioeconomic status). A comprehensive falls risk assessment should be conducted for all older adults, regardless of their history of falling. Components of an assessment can be found in the *Seniors' Falls in Canada* report. The assessment should include at least a medical history; physical examination; cognitive and functional assessments; environmental hazards assessment; medication review; and an assessment of gait, balance, and strength.

Older adults may have problems not easily detected during an office visit. A home visit can reveal issues, such as household and bathing hazards, social isolation, family/caregiver stress, and nutrition deficits. The Public Health Agency of Canada provides information on home safety for older adults (Box 31.2).

SPIRITUAL ASSESSMENT

Spirituality provides personal answers about the meaning and purpose of one's own life and how to interpret life events and regard them as "bigger than oneself." Spiritual health may improve with age, even as physical and mental health deteriorate. The aging process is part of a person's spiritual journey, with capability for growth.[23] Views on spirituality vary greatly from one adult to another and between people of the same faith or belief system. It is important to acknowledge spirituality as a powerful coping mechanism

during stressful life events, during illness, and at the end of life.[24]

Spiritual assessment is highly individual and may be delayed until a professional–patient relationship has been developed. Open-ended questions provide a foundation for future dialogue. A sample question posed during the initial assessment may be, "Do you consider yourself to be a spiritual person?" If the patient says yes, a follow-up question could be, "How does that spirituality relate to your health or health care decisions?" Involving chaplains or clergy members, when possible and appropriate, can provide the older adult with support and serve as a resource for the clinician.

ASSESSMENT AT THE END OF LIFE

Ideally, all aspects of the social assessment are completed before the approach to end of life. If this is not the case, the depth and completeness of the assessment are dependent on the plan of care. If interviewing is not possible, gather all available data to formulate interventions. Use information from caregivers and other existing sources. Be aware that caregiver stress may be increased during this time.

Medical Assistance in Dying

In June 2016, the Canadian federal government passed legislation allowing medical assistance in dying (Bill C-14). This legislation provides an exemption in the Criminal Code and allows physicians and nurse practitioners to provide medical assistance in dying services. It also allows pharmacists, family members, other people asked by the individual, and other health care providers to provide medical assistance in dying. A physician or nurse practitioner can either directly administer a substance that causes death, or can provide or prescribe a medication the person takes independently.

To be eligible for medical assistance in dying, an individual must be eligible for government health care coverage (not a visitor to Canada), be at least 18 years old, have a grievous and irremediable medical condition, make a voluntary request for medical assistance in dying, and be able to give informed consent.

The Canadian Nurses Association (CNA) has developed a national nursing framework on medical assistance in dying, as well as several other related documents that can be found on its website (https://www.cna-aiic.ca). The Canadian Researchers at the End of Life Network (CARENET) is a group of health care providers from across the country who research care at the end of life (http://www.thecarenet.ca). CARENET has excellent resources for people caring for individuals at the end of life.

HEALTH PROMOTION

Exercise

Staying physically active is key to remaining in good health and remaining independent. *Canadian Physical Activity Guidelines for Older Adults—65 Years & Older* recommends levels of activity that will help reduce the risk of developing chronic illnesses such as diabetes, heart disease, and depression, and help maintain mobility and functional independence.[25] Older adults should aim to accumulate at least 150 minutes of moderate- to vigorous-intensity aerobic physical activity per week. These activities may be performed in bouts of 10 minutes or more. In addition to endurance activities, older adults should try to include muscle and bone-strengthening activities at least 2 days per week as well as physical activities to enhance balance and prevent falls.

Older adults can remain healthy and live independently longer by maintaining and improving their aerobic fitness and endurance. Aerobic fitness is a person's ability to perform a physical activity for 2 minutes or longer. Research has shown that adults who are less active lose 16% of their existing level of aerobic fitness every 10 years.[26] Experts also recommend that older adults perform strength training to maintain their strength, muscle mass, and balance. Loss of muscle mass and inactivity result in an increased risk for disability, falls, and diseases such as diabetes. Health care practitioners should encourage older adults to maintain their physical fitness and mobility by continuing or initiating an exercise program.

Sexual Health

Sexual health assessment in older adults is often overlooked. However, sexual activity is reported by more than 50% of adults aged 65 to 74 and by more than 25% of adults aged 75 to 84.[27] Although the topic can be uncomfortable, it is important to assess older adults for sexual health to ensure they are practising safe behaviours and able to express their sexuality as they desire. Older adults may be at a higher risk for sexually transmitted infections such as human immunodeficiency virus (HIV) infection and acquired immune deficiency syndrome (AIDS). Some older adults are recently divorced or widowed and may enter into new relationships without considering safer sex practices.

Polypharmacy

Polypharmacy is the prescription and use of multiple medications (usually five or more) to deal with concomitant multiple diseases. According to Statistics Canada, 83% of individuals aged 65 to 79 were taking at least one prescription medication, with 30% taking five or more medications.[28] Concurrent use of several prescription medications can lead to adverse drug events such as medication interactions, decreased functional status, cognitive impairment, and falls.

Because many older adult patients require prescription medications, it is very important to assess for inappropriate use of these medications, such as combinations of medications that cancel out each other's effects, or concurrent use of other substances, including alcohol. The Beers Criteria for Potentially Inappropriate Medication Use in Older Adults[29] and the Canadian list of inappropriate practices in prescribing[30] are two commonly used guidelines on inappropriate prescribing and on the potential complications and interactions of specific medications commonly taken by older

adults. The Canadian Geriatrics Society website (http://canadiangeriatrics.ca) provides links to several useful tools. In addition to prescription medications, ask about any other nonprescription or over-the-counter medications, alternative medications or preparations, and alcohol use.

Immunizations and Vaccinations

Immunizations and vaccines are an important part of health promotion for people of all ages, including older adults. Routine immunizations for older adults include annual influenza immunizations; either a varicella (chickenpox) vaccination for those who are seronegative or a herpes zoster (shingles) vaccination for those who are seropositive for, or who have had, chickenpox; and pneumococcal polysaccharide 23-valent for the prevention of pneumococcal disease. Immunizations received in childhood such as pertussis may require a booster shot in adulthood, and diphtheria and tetanus immunizations require boosters every 10 years. Older adults planning on travelling should also be aware of any area-specific recommended immunizations such as hepatitis A.[31] Therefore, it is important to check the immunization history, ensure that it is both complete and up-to-date, and encourage seasonal vaccinations.

 ## SOCIAL DETERMINANTS OF HEALTH CONSIDERATIONS

Be aware that culture influences all parts of each person's life (review Chapter 3). Food habits and dietary beliefs may conflict with dietary recommendations made by health care providers. The response to pain—including how it is perceived, how much is considered tolerable, and the reaction to pain experienced—varies among and within different cultures. How the person interprets the symptoms, meaning, and causes of illness can be defined by the person's culture. It also plays a part in the older adult's choice of when to seek care and may influence how the illness is treated.[32] Individuals may want to try traditional or alternative practices to prevent or treat certain conditions.

Wide differences appear among individuals in every culture. Learn how the older adult's culture aligns with suggested interventions. Culture may influence reliance on family for care, the approach to decision making (e.g., involvement of family and friends), disclosure of medical information (e.g., cancer diagnosis), and end-of-life care (e.g., advance directives, resuscitation preferences, and nutrition).[32]

SPECIAL CONSIDERATIONS

Assessment of the functional status of an older adult can be more time consuming than for younger adults (Table 31.2). It may take longer for an older adult to understand and process the questions and to respond. Presence of physical disabilities, anxiety, depression, pain, or fatigue may necessitate several sessions to complete the assessment. An older adult may need assistance with clothing and may prefer that a family member be present for all or parts of the examination. For older adults who are hospitalized or placed in residential care, consider assessing function during normal activities such as grooming, at mealtime, or during toileting.

An individual with multiple medical problems may tire early and easily, and many medications have adverse effects that contribute to fatigue or affect the attention span. Again, assessments may need to be performed incrementally, such as positioning for comfort and clustering similar tasks to prevent fatigue. Having the person use glasses or hearing aids can mitigate communication difficulties resulting from vision or hearing loss. Provide directions in written format if necessary, and have hearing amplifiers and page magnifiers

---

TABLE 31.2 Comprehensive Older Adult's Evaluation

Name (print): _____
Date of visit: _____
Chief complaint: _____
_____

Today I will ask you about your overall health and function and will be using a questionnaire to help me obtain this information. The first few questions are to check your memory.

Preliminary Cognition Questionnaire:
Record if answer is correct with (+); if answer is incorrect, with (–). Record total number of errors.

	(+, –)
1. What is the date today?	_____
2. What day of the week is it?	_____
3. What is the name of this place?	_____
4. What is your telephone number or room number? *(Record answer: _____)*	_____
If subject does not have phone, ask: What is your street address?	
5. How old are you? *(Record answer: _____)*	_____
6. When were you born? *(Record answer from records if patient cannot answer: _____)*	_____
7. Who is the prime minister of Canada now?	_____
8. Who was the previous prime minister?	_____
9. What was your mother's maiden name?	_____
10. Subtract 3 from 20, and keep subtracting from each new number you get, all the way down.	_____
Total errors	_____

If patient makes more than 4 errors, ask #11. If more than 6 errors, complete questionnaire from informant.

11. Do you think you would benefit from a legal guardian, someone who would be responsible for your legal and financial matters?
    a. No
    b. Has functioning legal guardian for sole purpose of managing money (describe: _____)
    c. Has legal guardian
    d. Yes
    Do you have a living will? Would you like one?
    a. No
    b. Yes

	YES	NO
12. Is your daily life full of things that keep you interested?	_____	_____
13. Have you, at times, very much wanted to leave home?	_____	_____
14. Does it seem that no one understands you?	_____	_____
15. Are you happy most of the time?	_____	_____
16. Do you feel weak all over much of the time?	_____	_____
17. Is your sleep fitful and disturbed?	_____	_____

18. Taking everything into consideration, how would you describe your satisfaction with your life in general at the present time: good, fair, or poor?
    a. Good
    b. Fair
    c. Poor
19. Do you feel you now need help with your mental health: for example, a counsellor or psychiatrist?
    a. No
    b. Has such help *(specify: _____)*
    c. Yes

Continued

TABLE 31.2 **Comprehensive Older Adult's Evaluation—cont'd**

Physical Health Section:

The next few questions are about your health.

20. During the past month (30 days), how many days were you so sick that you couldn't do your usual activities, such as working around the house or visiting with friends?

21. Relative to other people your age, how would you rate your overall health at the present time: excellent, good, fair, poor, or very poor?
    a. Excellent (*Skip to #22*)
    b. Very good (*Skip to #22*)
    c. Good (*Ask #i*)
    d. Fair (*Ask #i*)
    e. Poor (*Ask #i*)
       i. Do you feel you need additional medical services such as a doctor, nurse, visiting nurse, or physiotherapist? *(Circle all that apply)*
          A. Doctor
          B. Nurse
          C. Visiting nurse
          D. Physiotherapist
          E. None

22. Do you use an aid for walking, such as a wheelchair, walker, cane, or anything else? *(Circle aid usually used)*
    a. Wheelchair
    b. Other *(specify: _____)*
    c. Visiting nurse
    d. Walker
    e. None

23. How much do your health troubles stand in the way of your doing things you want to do: not at all, a little, or a great deal?
    a. Not at all (*Skip to #24*)
    b. A little (*Ask #i*)
    c. A great deal (*Ask #i*)
       i. Do you think you need assistance to do your daily activities? For example, do you need a live-in aide or chore worker?
          A. Live-in aide
          B. Chore worker
          C. Has aide, chore worker, or other assistance *(describe: _____)*
          D. None needed

24. Have you had, or do you currently have, any of the following health problems? (If yes, place an "X" in appropriate box and describe; medical record information may be used to help complete this section)

	HISTORY	CURRENT	DESCRIBE
a. Arthritis or rheumatism?			
b. Lung or breathing problem?			
c. Hypertension?			
d. Heart trouble?			
e. Phlebitis or poor circulation problems in arms or legs?			
f. Diabetes or low blood glucose level?			
g. Digestive ulcers?			
h. Other digestive problem?			
i. Cancer?			
j. Anemia?			
k. Effects of stroke?			
l. Other neurological problem? *(Specify: _____)*			
m. Thyroid or other glandular problem? *(Specify: _____)*			
n. Skin disorders such as pressure sores, leg ulcers, burns?			
o. Speech problem?			
p. Hearing problem?			
q. Vision or eye problem?			
r. Kidney or bladder problems or incontinence?			
s. A problem of falls?			
t. Problem with eating or your weight? *(Specify: _____)*			
u. Problem with depression or your nerves? *(Specify: _____)*			
v. Problem with your behaviour? *(Specify: _____)*			
w. Problem with your sexual activity?			

TABLE 31.2   Comprehensive Older Adult's Evaluation—cont'd

   x. Problem with alcohol?
   y. Problem with pain?
   z. Other health problems? *(Specify: _____)*
Immunizations: _____
_____

25. What medications are you currently taking, or have been taking, in the past month? May I see your medication bottles? *(If patient cannot list, ask categories a-r below and note dosage and schedule, or obtain information from medical or pharmacy records and verify accuracy with the patient.)*

ALLERGIES: **PRESCRIPTION (DOSAGE AND SCHEDULE)**

   a. Arthritis medication
   b. Pain medication
   c. Blood pressure medication
   d. Water pills or pills for fluid
   e. Medication for your heart
   f. Medication for your lungs
   g. Blood thinners
   h. Medication for your circulation
   i. Insulin or diabetes medication
   j. Seizure medication
   k. Thyroid pills
   l. Steroids
   m. Hormones
   n. Antibiotics
   o. Medicine for nerves or depression
   p. Prescription sleeping pills
   q. Other prescription medications
   r. Other nonprescription medications

26. Many people have problems remembering to take their medications, especially ones they need to take on a regular basis. How often do you forget to take your medications? Would you say you forget often, sometimes, rarely, or never?
   a. Never
   b. Rarely
   c. Sometimes
   d. Often

Activities of Daily Living:
The next set of questions asks whether you need help with any of the following activities of daily living.
27. I would like to know whether you can do these activities without any help at all, or if you need assistance to do them. *(If yes, describe, including patient's needs.)* Do you need help to:

	YES	NO	DESCRIBE (INCLUDE NEEDS)
a. Use the telephone?			
b. Get to places out of walking distance (using transportation)?			
c. Shop for clothes and food?			
d. Do your housework?			
e. Handle your money?			
f. Feed yourself?			
g. Dress and undress yourself?			
h. Take care of your appearance?			
i. Get in and out of bed?			
j. Take a bath or shower?			
k. Prepare your meals?			
l. Do you have any problem getting to the bathroom on time?			

28. During the past 6 months, have you had any help with such things as shopping, housework, bathing, dressing, and getting around?
   a. Yes *(specify: _____)*
   b. No
Signature of person completing the form: _____

Adapted with permission from Pearlman, R. (1987). Development of a functional assessment questionnaire for geriatric patients: COPE. *Journal of Chronic Diseases, 40*(1), 85S–94S.

available. Face the person as much as possible, speak slowly in a low-pitched voice, and enunciate words clearly. For non–English-speaking patients, be prepared to use the services of interpreters rather than family members.

Older adults are a heterogeneous population. You must be aware of your own attitudes and beliefs about older adults to ensure the functional assessment truly reflects abilities and not the myth that functional decline is a normal outcome of aging. Demonstrating respect and interest and treating the patient as an individual is imperative. Ask how the older adult would like to be addressed. Maximize communication by using terms understandable to the patient, rather than medical jargon. Include the older adult in decision making about how the interview or testing is to be performed; such inclusion establishes rapport and promotes self-esteem. Be aware of body language and behaviours, and be prepared to modify your approach. Touch can also help in establishing rapport and can reduce anxiety, but may not be appropriate for certain cultures.

A functional assessment can be intimidating for older adults. Frustration or embarrassment may arise if some physical manoeuvres cannot be performed or questions cannot be answered during cognitive testing. Older adults may also be fearful about consequences of functional testing, such as losing independence or having a caregiver move into the home. Provide reassurance that not everyone can complete all the tasks or answer all the questions and that, to the extent possible, confidentiality will be honoured.

Ensure adequate space when performing tests of mobility. An older adult may need room to manoeuvre an assistive device. When testing mobility, stand close to the older adult to prevent falls. The environment should be well-lit; avoid high-gloss, shiny, slippery surfaces. Minimize extraneous noises such as those from intercoms, televisions, or high-traffic areas. Warm rooms, access to fluids, proximity to a bathroom, and privacy are important.

Assessing Older Adults With Pain

Pain is not a normal part of aging. If the older adult is feeling pain or discomfort, the knowledge gathered through the assessments will be deficient. Alleviating pain should be a priority over other aspects of the assessment. It may be necessary to administer premedication before portions of the assessment, especially if the assessment requires movement. Another strategy is to use positioning to decrease pain. Ask what position is most comfortable. Providing comfort can help maximize the information gathered. It is paramount to remember that older adults with cognitive impairment do *not* experience less pain. See Chapter 11 for more information about pain in older adults.

Caregivers need to look for verbal and nonverbal signs of pain and consider appropriate pharmacological and non-pharmacological interventions, and assess the effectiveness of these measures. Various pain assessment scales are available for use in cognitively impaired older adults, and can be found in the RNAO's *Delirium, Dementia and Depression in Older Adults: Assessment and Care.*[14]

Assessing Older Adults With Altered Cognition

Cognitive impairment poses unique challenges. The older adult may not be able to actively participate in the evaluation or provide consistent answers. Cognitive impairment may severely restrict the ability for expression. Gathering information from an older adult first-hand is always best but not always feasible. To ensure the information collected is reliable, one strategy is to interview the caregiver or family for subjective assessment data. Another is to arrange opportunities to assess the patient during different times of the day, when the patient may be more clear-headed. If possible, split the assessment into smaller sections at a time. Be flexible.

Adults with cognitive impairment may need questions or directions broken down into single commands, repeated word for word, ongoing verbal cueing, or physical cues. For example, after getting the patient's attention, you might say, "Sit here" and pat the chair. Never assume that the patient cannot respond to questions even when the patient is known to have cognitive impairment. Using yes-or-no questions may prevent frustration. Be relaxed and calm, because an older adult with dementia may mirror your emotions. If a family member or caregiver does need to provide collateral information, avoid collecting it in front of the patient.

CAREGIVER ASSESSMENT

According to Statistics Canada, in 2012, most care for older adults (44%) was provided by people between 45 and 64 years of age, and 20% of caregivers were 65 to 74 years of age.[33] This means that many people providing care to older adults are themselves older adults. A Health Quality Ontario report stated that between 2009–10 and 2013–14, approximately 71% of older Ontarians were cared for by children or spouses of their children; 33% were cared for by spouses; 19% were cared for by other relatives; and 9.2% were cared for by friends and neighbours (because the data recorded up to two caregivers per patient, the percentages do not add up to 100%).[34] As the number of older adults grows (to 27% by 2050), so will the need for families to provide care to them.

According to the Health Quality Ontario report, most caregivers (92%) found the experience rewarding, and 37% found it very rewarding. In contrast, 28% of caregivers found the experience somewhat or very stressful, and one-third reported anger, depression, and distress.[34] Distress was associated with the number of hours of care provided per week, with distress increasing as time providing care increased. Caregiver stress was also greatest when caregiving for a spouse, with almost half (47.2%) reporting distress. In addition to their caregiving responsibilities, 60% of caregivers also had paid work and 28% had children under the age of 18 at home.

Caregivers also face increased financial expenses, such as fees for home care services, transportation costs for medical appointments, medication dispensing, technical aids and equipment, and home modification, which can cause further strain.

Modified Caregiver Strain Index

Directions: Here is a list of things that other caregivers have found to be difficult. Please put a checkmark in the columns that apply to you. We have included some examples that are common caregiver experiences to help you think about each item. Your situation may be slightly different, but the item could still apply.

	Yes, on a regular basis = 2	Yes, sometimes = 1	No = 0
My sleep is disturbed (For example, *the person I care for* is in and out of bed or wanders around at night)			
Caregiving is inconvenient (For example, helping takes so much time or it's a long drive over to help)			
Caregiving is a physical strain (For example, lifting in or out of a chair; effort or concentration is required)			
Caregiving is confining (For example, helping restricts free time or *I* cannot go visiting)			
There have been family adjustments (For example, helping has disrupted *my* routine; there has been no privacy)			
There have been changes in personal plans (For example, *I* had to turn down a job; *I* could not go on vacation)			
There have been other demands on my time (For example, other family members *need me)*			
There have been emotional adjustments (For example, severe arguments *about caregiving)*			
Some behaviour is upsetting (For example, incontinence; *the person cared for* has trouble remembering things; or *the person I care for* accuses people of taking things)			
It is upsetting to find the person I care for has changed so much from his or her former self (For example, he or she is a different person than he or she used to be)			
There have been work adjustments (For example, *I* have to take time off *for caregiving duties)*			
Caregiving is a financial strain			
I feel completely overwhelmed (For example, *I* worry about *the person I care for; I* have concerns about how *I* will manage)			

Total Score =

Words appearing in *italics* represent modifications from the original Caregiver Strain Index from Robinson, B. C. (1983). Validation of a caregiver strain index. *J Gerontol 38*:344-348. Copyright © The Gerontological Society of America.

31.5

Assessment of Caregiver Burden

The health and well-being of the older adult and caregiver are closely linked. For these reasons, part of caring for a frail older adult involves paying attention to the well-being of the caregiver, and all caregivers should be screened for caregiver burden. One formal screening tool is the Modified Caregiver Strain Index (Fig. 31.5), which is used to identify caregivers of any age who need a more comprehensive assessment. It is a brief tool with 13 questions addressing potential strain in employment, financial, physical, social, and time domains.[35]

ELDER ABUSE

Elder abuse is an umbrella term used to describe one or more of the following situations: physical abuse, sexual abuse, emotional or psychological abuse, financial or material exploitation, abandonment, neglect, or a combination of these (Box 31.3). An excellent guide for assessment and prevention of elder abuse and resources available in Canada can be found at the Canadian Network for the Prevention of Elder Abuse website (https://cnpea.ca).

Assessing for Elder Abuse

When interviewing older adults, a general guideline is to ask direct and simple questions (Box 31.4). Structure your assessment questions in a nonjudgemental and nonthreatening manner. Arrange time to interview the patient and caregiver together and separately. This is done not only to detect abusive behaviour but to detect disparities in stories or to assess for caregiver stress. Caregivers may be reluctant to discuss their personal problems in the presence of the person who depends on their care.

BOX 31.3 **Definitions of the Types of Elder Abuse**

- Physical abuse: Hitting and rough handling, as well as purposeful over- or undermedicating, or physical restraints
- Sexual abuse: Any nonconsensual sexual behaviour, either physical or psychological
- Emotional abuse: Somebody threatens, insults, intimidates, or humiliates an older adult, treats the person like a child, or does not allow them to see their family and friends
- Financial or material abuse: Theft or misuse of the older person's money or property
- Violation of rights: Disregard of basic human and legal rights of the individual
- Neglect:
  - Active (intentional withholding of basic necessities of life)
  - Passive (not providing basic necessities because of lack of experience, information, or ability)
- Systemic abuse: Rules, regulations, or policies that harm or discriminate against older adults

Data from Canadian Network for the Prevention of Elder Abuse. (2017). *What is elder abuse?* Retrieved from https://cnpea.ca/en/what-is-elder-abuse/forms-of-abuse.

1. Has anyone ever hurt you?
2. Has anyone ever touched you without your consent?
3. Has anyone ever made you do things you didn't want to do?
4. Has anyone taken anything of yours without asking?
5. Has anyone ever scolded or threatened you?
6. Have you signed any papers that you didn't understand?
7. Is there anyone at home you are fearful of?
8. Has anyone ever refused to help you take care of yourself when you needed help?

From Patterson, C. (1994). Secondary prevention of elder abuse. In Canadian Task Force on the Periodic Health Examination (Ed.), *Canadian guide to clinical preventive health care* (pp. 922–999). Ottawa: Health Canada.

Documentation

Proper and precise documentation is important in recording suspected cases of elder abuse because medical records may become part of the legal record. If possible, document verbatim descriptions of events, and draw or photograph physical findings. Box 31.5 lists a mnemonic (STOP HARM) to help detect, diagnose, and manage elder abuse. For more information on elder abuse, see Chapter 8.

CONCLUSION

This chapter highlights the importance and components of a functional assessment of older adults in a variety of settings. Additional resources for nurses and nursing students can be found at the National Initiative for the Care of the Elderly

Screen for abuse in all older adult patients
Think about risk factors
Ominous danger signs present?
Physical findings
History
Address issue of elder abuse
Report to adult protective services
Manage with prevention and risk factor modification

From Kruger, R. M., & Moon, C. H. (1999). Can you spot the signs of elder mistreatment? *Postgraduate Medicine, 106*(2), 169–183.

(http://www.nicenet.ca) and the Canadian Gerontological Nursing Association (http://www.cgna.net).

REFERENCES

1. Statistics Canada. (2015, July 1). Canada's population estimates: Age and sex. *The Daily.* Retrieved from http://www.statcan.gc.ca/daily-quotidien/150929/dq150929b-eng.htm.
2. Statistics Canada. (2017). *Health fact sheets: Life satisfaction, 2016.* Ottawa: Minister of Industry. Retrieved from http://www.statcan.gc.ca/pub/82-625-x/2017001/article/54862-eng.pdf.
3. Pearson, V. (2000). Assessment of function. In R. Kane & R. Kane (Eds.), *Assessing older persons: Measures, meaning and practical applications* (pp. 17–48). New York: Oxford University Press.
4. Katz, S., Ford, A. B., Moskowitz, R. W., et al. (1963). Studies of illness in the aged. The Index of ADL: A standardized measure of biological and psychosocial functioning. *JAMA: The Journal of the American Medical Association, 185*(12), 914–919.
5. Mahoney, F. I., & Barthel, D. W. (1965). Functional evaluation: The Barthel Index. *Maryland State Medical Journal, 14,* 61–65.
6. Hamilton, B., Granger, C. V., Sherwin, F. S., et al. (1987). A uniform national data system for medical rehabilitation. In M. J. Fuher (Ed.), *Rehabilitation outcomes: Analysis and measurement* (pp. 137–147). Baltimore: Brooks.
7. Linn, M., & Linn, B. (1982). The Rapid Disability Rating Scale–2. *Journal of the American Geriatric Society, 30,* 378–382.
8. Fillenbaum, G. C., & Smyer, M. (1981). The development, validity, and reliability of the ORS, multidimensional functional assessment questionnaire. *Journal of Gerontology, 36,* 428–434.
9. Karagiozis, H., Gray, S., Sacco, J., et al. (1998). The Direct Assessment of Functional Abilities (DAFA): A comparison to an indirect measure of instrumental activities of daily living. *Gerontologist, 38,* 113–121.
10. Reuben, D. B., & Siu, A. L. (1990). An objective measure of physical function of elderly outpatients: The Physical Performance Test. *Journal of the American Geriatrics Society, 38*(10), 1105–1112.
11. Kuriansky, J. B., & Gurland, B. (1976). Performance test of activities of daily living. *International Journal of Aging and Human Development, 7,* 343–352.

12. Mathias, S., Nayak, U. S., & Isaacs, B. (1986). Balance in the elderly patient: The "Get Up and Go" Test. *Archives of Physical Medicine and Rehabilitation, 67*, 387–389.

13. Langley, F. A., & Mackintosh, S. F. H. (2007). Functional balance assessment of older community dwelling adults: A systematic review of the literature. *Internet Journal of Allied Health Sciences and Practice, 5*(4). Retrieved from http://ijahsp.nova.edu/articles/vol5num4/pdf/langley.pdf.

14. Registered Nurses' Association of Ontario (2016). *Delirium, dementia, and depression in older adults: Assessment and care* (2nd ed.). Toronto: Author.

15. Canadian Coalition for Seniors' Mental Health. (2017). *National guidelines for seniors' mental health: The assessment and treatment of delirium.* Retrieved from http://ccsmh.ca/projects/delirium/.

16. Alzheimer Society of Canada. (2018). *Fact sheets.* Retrieved from http://alzheimer.ca/en/Home/News-and-Events/Media-centre/Fact-sheets.

17. Indigenous Cognition & Aging Awareness Research Exchange. (2018). *Dementia factsheets.* Retrieved from https://www.i-caare.ca/factsheets.

18. Hollander, M. J., Liu, G., & Chappell, N. L. (2009). Who cares and how much? The imputed economic contribution to the Canadian healthcare system of middle-aged and older unpaid caregivers providing care to the elderly. *Health Care Quarterly, 12*(2), 42–49.

19. Parkerson, G. R., Jr., Broadhead, W. E., & Tse, C.-K. J. (1991). Validation of the Duke Social Support and Stress Scale. *Family Medicine, 23*(5), 357–360.

20. Department of Community and Family Medicine, Duke University Medical Center. (2017). *Duke Social Support and Stress Scale (DUSOCS).* Retrieved from https://cfm.duke.edu/research/duke-health-measures.

21. Statistics Canada. (2017, May 26). Canadian income survey 2015. *The Daily.* Retrieved from http://www.statcan.gc.ca/daily-quotidien/170526/dq170526a-eng.pdf.

22. Public Health Agency of Canada. (2014). *Seniors' falls in Canada: Second report.* Ottawa: Author. Retrieved from http://www.phac-aspc.gc.ca/seniors-aines/publications/public/injury-blessure/seniors_falls-chutes_aines/assets/pdf/seniors_falls-chutes_aines-eng.pdf.

23. Berggren-Thomas, P., & Griggs, M. J. (1995). Spirituality in aging: Spiritual need or spiritual journey? *Journal of Gerontological Nursing, 21*(3), 5–10.

24. Moore, S. (1998). Spirituality. In A. S. Luggen, S. S. Travis, & S. Meiner (Eds.), *NGNA core curriculum for gerontological advanced practice nurses* (pp. 415–419). Thousand Oaks, CA: Sage.

25. Canadian Society for Exercise Physiology. (2013). *Canada's physical activity guidelines for older adults-65 years & older.* Retrieved from http://www.csep.ca/CMFiles/Guidelines/CSEP_PAGuidelines_older-adults_en.pdf.

26. Public Health Agency of Canada. (2011). *Tips to get active: Physical activity tips for older adults (65 years and older).* Ottawa: Author. Retrieved from http://www.phac-aspc.gc.ca/hp-ps/hl-mvs/pa-ap/assets/pdfs/08paap-eng.pdf.

27. Lindau, S. T., Schumm, L. P., Laumann, E. O., et al. (2007). A study of sexuality and health among older adults in the United States. *New England Journal of Medicine, 357*, 762–774.

28. Rotermann, M., Sanmartin, C., Hennessy, D., et al. (2014). *Prescription medication use by Canadians aged 6 to 79* (Catalogue no. 82-003-X). Ottawa: Statistics Canada.

29. Fick, D. M., Cooper, J. W., Wade, W. E., et al. (2003). Updating the Beers Criteria for Potentially Inappropriate Medication Use in Older Adults. Results of a US consensus panel of experts. *Archives of Internal Medicine, 163*(22), 2716–2724.

30. McLeod, J. P., Huang, A. R., & Tamblyn, R. M. (1997). Defining inappropriate practices in prescribing for elderly people: A national consensus panel. *Canadian Medical Association Journal, 156*(3), 385–391.

31. Alliance for a National Seniors Strategy. (2016). *An evidence-informed national seniors strategy for Canada.* Retrieved from http://www.nationalseniorsstrategy.ca.

32. Jett, K. F. (2011). Cultural influences. In S. E. Meiner (Ed.), *Gerontological nursing* (4th ed., pp. 81–93). St. Louis: Mosby.

33. Sinha, M. (2013). *Portrait of caregivers, 2012* (Catalogue no. 89-652 X). Ottawa: Statistics Canada, Social and Aboriginal Statistics Division. Retrieved from http://www.statcan.gc.ca/pub/89-652-x/89-652-x2013001-eng.htm.

34. Health Quality Ontario. (2016). *The reality of caring.* Toronto: Queen's Printer for Ontario. Retrieved from http://www.hqontario.ca/Portals/0/documents/system-performance/reality-caring-report-en.pdf.

35. Thornton, M., & Travis, S. S. (2003). Analysis of the reliability of the modified Caregiver Strain Index. *The Journals of Gerontology. Series B, Psychological Sciences and Social Sciences, 58*(2), S129.

ILLUSTRATION CREDITS

INSIDE BACK COVER

"Key Laboratory Values" listing: Excerpted from Lewis, S. L., Dirksen, S. R., Heitkemper, M. M., Bucher, L., Camera, I., et al. (2014). *Medical-surgical nursing in Canada* (3rd Canadian ed., pp. 2061–2072). Toronto: Elsevier Canada.

CHAPTER 1

Fig. 1.1: Aleksandra Yakovleva/iStockphoto.

Fig. 1.2: Gregory, D. M., Raymond-Seniuk, C., Patrick, L., & Stephen, T. C. (2014). *Fundamentals: Perspectives on the art and science of canadian nursing*. Philadelphia: Wolters Kluwer Health.

Fig. 1.3: Alfaro-LeFevre, R. (1999). *Critical thinking in nursing: A practical approach* (2nd ed.). Philadelphia: W.B. Saunders.

Fig. 1.4: Rocketclips, Inc./Shutterstock.com.

CHAPTER 2

Unnumbered photo: © Annette J. Browne.

Fig. 2.2: Hamilton, N., & Bhatti, T. (1996). Population health promotion: an integrated model of population health and health promotion. Retrieved from Public Health Agency of Canada website: http://www.phac-aspc.gc.ca/ph-sp/php-psp/index-eng.php.

Fig. 2.3: The Nipissing District Developmental Screen. Reprinted with permission. The Nipissing, Nipissing District Developmental Screen, and NDDS are trademarks of NDDS Intellectual Property Association, used under license. All rights reserved.

CHAPTER 3

Unnum photo: © Annette J. Browne.

Fig. 3.1: © Colleen Varcoe.

Fig. 3.2: © Annette J. Browne.

Fig. 3.3: © Mary Zhang.

Figs. 3.4 and 3.5: © Colleen Varcoe.

Fig. 3.6: © Annette J. Browne.

Fig. 3.7: © Access Alliance Multicultural Health and Community Services, Toronto, Ontario. Reprinted with permission.

Fig. 3.8: © Karol Ghuman.

Fig. 3.9: Kirby, M. J. L. (2002). *The health of Canadians— The federal role. Final report. Volume 6: Recommendations for reform* (Chapter 13). Retrieved from http://www.parl.gc.ca/37/2/parlbus/commbus/senate/Com-e/soci-e/rep-e/repoct02vol6-e.htm#ORDER%20OF%20REFERENCE. Reprinted with permission.

Fig. 3.10: From *The Georgia Straight* (March 6–13, 2008, p. 13). Reprinted with permission.

Fig. 3.11: Adapted from, Macdonald, D., & Wilson, D. (2016). *Shameful neglect: Indigenous child poverty in Canada*. (Fig. 2, p14) Ottawa, ON: Canadian Centre for Policy Alternatives

Fig. 3.12: Courtesy Rachel E. Spector, 2006. From Jarvis, C. (2008). *Physical examination & health assessment* (5th ed., p. 39, Fig. 3.3). St. Louis: W.B. Saunders.

Fig. 3.13: sack/iStockphoto.

Fig. 3.14: © Hospital Employees Union, British Columbia. Reprinted with permission.

Fig. 3.15: © Mark Richards/PhotoEdit.

Fig. 3.16: © Colleen Varcoe.

CHAPTER 4

Fig. 4.1: © Can Stock Photo /monkeybusiness.

Fig. 4.2: Monkey Business Images/Shutterstock.com.

Fig. 4.3: Image Point Fr/Shutterstock.com

Fig. 4.4: © Can Stock Photo / Bialasiewicz.

Fig. 4.5: © Photawa/Dreamstime.com.

Fig. 4.6: © Tony Freeman/PhotoEdit.

CHAPTER 5

Fig. 5.2: Adapted from American Society of Human Genetics. (2004). Retrieved from http://www.ashg.org.

Fig. 5.4: Goldenring J. M., & Rosen, D. S. (2004). Getting into adolescent heads: An essential update. *Contemporary Pediatrics, 21*(1), 64–68, 70, 73–74. Copyright © 2013, Advanstar Communications Inc. 100328:613JM.

CHAPTER 6

Fig. 6.1: Copyright © Dr. Z. Nasreddine. *The Montreal Cognitive Assessment* (MoCA). All rights reserved. Retrieved from http://www.mocatest.org/pdf_files/test/MoCA-Test-English_7_1.pdf. Reprinted with permission.

CHAPTER 8

Fig. 8.2: SpeedKingz/Shutterstock.com.

CHAPTER 9

Fig. 9.14: Courtesy of *The Pantagraph* (August 10, 1998). Bloomington, IL.

CHAPTER 10

Fig. 10.3: Health Canada. (2003). *Canadian guidelines for body weight classifications in adults* (Catalogue No. H49-179/2003E; p. 37). Ottawa: Author. Retrieved from http://

www.hc-sc.gc.ca/fn-an/alt_formats/hpfb-dgpsa/pdf/
nutrition/weight_book-livres_des_poids_e.pdf.

Fig. 10.5: © Pat Thomas, 2006.

Fig. 10.10: Potter, P. A., & Perry, A. G. (2005). *Fundamentals of nursing* (6th ed., p. 650, Fig. 31.10). St. Louis: Mosby.

Fig. 10.22: Canadian Hypertension Education Program (CHEP). (2017). Hypertension Canada's 2017 Guidelines for Diagnosis, Risk Assessment, Prevention, and Treatment of Hypertension in Adults. *Canadian Journal of Cardiology*, 33(5) 557-576.

Art for Table 10.4: (hypopituitary dwarfism; gigantism) from Hall, R., & Evered, D. C. (1990). *Colour atlas of endocrinology* (2nd ed.). London: Mosby; (acromegaly [hyperpituitarism]) Reprinted from the Clinical Slide Collection on the Rheumatic Diseases © 1991, 1995, 1997. Used by permission of the American College of Rheumatology; (anorexia nervosa) Courtesy of George, D. Comerci, M. D.; (Marfan's syndrome) from Manusov, E. G., & Martucci, E. (1994). The Marfan syndrome. *Archives of Family Medicine, 3,* 824. Copyrighted 1994, American Medical Association; (endogenous obesity—Cushing's syndrome) from Wenig, B. M., Heffess, C. S., & Adair, C. F. (1997). *Atlas of endocrine pathology.* Philadelphia: W.B. Saunders; (achondroplastic dwarfism) Jones, A., & Owen, R. (1995). Color atlas of clinical orthopaedics (2nd ed., p. 10, Fig. 3). London, England: Mosby.

CHAPTER 11

Fig. 11.3: Adapted from McCaffery, M., & Pasero, C. (1999). *Pain: Clinical manual* (2nd ed., p. 61, Form 3.2). St. Louis: Mosby.

Fig. 11.4: McCaffery M., & Pasero, C. (1999). *Pain: Clinical manual* (2nd ed., p. 63, Fig. 3.2). St. Louis: Mosby.

Fig. 11.5 [FACES Pain Rating Scale]: Hicks, C.L., von Baeyer, C.L., Spafford, P., van Korlaar, I., Goodenough, B. (2001). The Faces Pain Scale—Revised: Toward a common metric in pediatric pain measurement. *Pain, 93,* 173–183; and Bieri, D., Reeve, R., Champion, G.D., Addicoat, L., Ziegler, J. (1990). The Faces Pain Scale for the self-assessment of the severity of pain experienced by children: Development, initial validation and preliminary investigation for ratio scale properties. *Pain, 41,* 139–150.

Unnumbered figure in Promoting Health box (WHO Pain Ladder): Adapted from World Health Organization. (1996). *Cancer pain relief with a guide to opioid availability.* Geneva, Switzerland: Author. Retrieved from http://whqlibdoc.who.int/publications/9241544821.pdf. Figure also available at http://www.who.int/cancer/palliative/painladder/en/.

CHAPTER 12

Unnumbered photo: © Annette J. Browne.

Fig. 12.1: Excerpts from Health Canada. (2007). *Eating well with Canada's food guide.* © Her Majesty the Queen in Right of Canada, represented by the Minister of Health

Canada. Cat No. H164-38/1-2007E. Retrieved from http://www.hc-sc.gc.ca/fn-an/alt_formats/hpfb-dgpsa/pdf/food-guide-aliment/print_eatwell_bienmang_e.pdf.

Fig. 12.2: From Canadian Malnutrition Task Force. (2017). Canadian nutrition screening tool (CNST). http://nutritioncareincanada.ca/sites/default/uploads/files/CNST.pdf. Ontario, Canada: Canadian Nutrition Society:

Fig. 12.3: Adapted from Canadian Food Inspection Agency. (2009). *Nutrition labelling.* Retrieved from http://www.inspection.gc.ca/english/fssa/labeti/guide/ch5e.shtml#a5_4. Adapted with the permission of the Minister of Public Works and Government Services Canada, 2012.

CHAPTER 13

Fig. 13.1: Lewis, S. L., Dirksen, S. R., Heitkemper, M. M., Bucher, L., & Camera, I. M. (2011). *Medical-surgical nursing: Assessment and management of clinical problems* (8th ed., p. 437, Fig. 23.1). St. Louis: Mosby.

Fig. 13.3, B: Marks, J.G., & Miller, J.J. (2006). *Lookingbill & Marks' principles of dermatology* (4th ed., p. 191, Fig. 13.8) Philadelphia: W.B. Saunders.

Fig. 13.4, A & B: Hurwitz, S. (1993). *Clinical pediatric dermatology: A textbook of skin disorders of childhood and adolescence* (2nd ed., pp. 200, 212). Philadelphia: W.B. Saunders.

Fig. 13.4, C: Lookingbill, D. P., & Marks, J. G. (1993). *Principles of dermatology* (2nd ed., p. 91). Philadelphia: W.B. Saunders.

Fig. 13.5: Images retrieved from the National Cancer Institute database (http://visualsonline.cancer.gov/) and used with permission.

Fig. 13.6: Bloom, A., Watkins, P. H., & Ireland, J. (1992). *Color atlas of diabetes* (2nd ed.). St. Louis: Mosby.

Fig. 13.7: Lookingbill, D. P., & Marks, J. G. (1993). *Principles of dermatology* (2nd ed.). Philadelphia: W.B. Saunders.

Fig. 13.10: Courtesy Lemmi & Lemmi, 2011.

Fig. 13.11: Courtesy Lemmi & Lemmi, 2011.

Fig. 13.13: Courtesy Jane Deacon, RNC, MS, NNP, The Children's Hospital, Denver, CO.

Fig. 13.14: Bowden, V. R., Dickey, S. B., & Greenburg, C. S. (1998). *Children and their families: The continuum of care.* Philadelphia: W.B. Saunders.

Figs. 13.15 and 13.16: Hurwitz, S. (1993). *Clinical pediatric dermatology: A textbook of skin disorders of childhood and adolescence* (2nd ed.). Philadelphia: W.B. Saunders.

Fig. 13.17: Courtesy Lemmi & Lemmi, 2011.

Fig. 13.18: Hurwitz, S. (1993). *Clinical pediatric dermatology: A textbook of skin disorders of childhood and adolescence* (2nd ed.). Philadelphia: W.B. Saunders.

Fig. 13.19: Murray, S. S., & McKinney, E. S. (2010). *Foundations of maternal–newborn nursing and women's health nursing* (5th ed., p. 536, Fig. 20.13). St. Louis: W.B. Saunders.

Fig. 13.20, A & B: Habif, T. P., Campbell, J. L., Jr., Chapman, M. S., Dinulos, J. G. H., & Zug, K. A. (2005). *Skin disease: Diagnosis and treatment* (3rd ed., p. 73). St. Louis: Mosby.

Fig. 13.21: Lookingbill, D. P., & Marks, J. G. (1993). *Principles of dermatology* (2nd ed., p. 89). Philadelphia: W.B. Saunders.

Fig. 13.22: Lookingbill, D. P., & Marks, J. G. (1993). *Principles of dermatology* (2nd ed.). Philadelphia: W.B. Saunders.

Fig. 13.23: Habif, T.P., et al. (2001). Skin disease: Diagnosis and treatment. St Louis: Mosby.

Fig. 13.24: Lookingbill, D. P., & Marks, J. G. (1993). *Principles of dermatology* (2nd ed., p. 75). Philadelphia: W.B. Saunders.

Fig. 13.25: Callen, J. P., & Greer K. E. (1993). *Color atlas of dermatology* (p. 103, Fig. 3.118). Philadelphia: W.B. Saunders.

Art for Table 13.4: Line drawings © Pat Thomas, 2010; (photos of macule, patch, papule, plaque, nodule, tumour, wheal, vesicle, bulla, cyst, and pustule): Courtesy Lemmi & Lemmi, 2011; (photo of urticaria [hives]) from Fireman, P. (1996). *Atlas of allergies* (2nd ed., p. 250, Fig. 16.2). London: Mosby.

Art for Table 13.5: Line drawings © Pat Thomas, 2010; (photos of crust, scale, fissure, erosion, ulcer, excoriation, scar, atrophic scar, lichenification, and keloid): Courtesy Lemmi & Lemmi, 2011.

Art for Table 13.6: (photos of pressure ulcers): Potter, P. A., & Perry, A. G. (2009). *Fundamentals of nursing* (7th ed., p. 1283, Fig. 48.6). St. Louis: Mosby.

Art for Table 13.8: (port-wine stain [nevus flammeus]) from Hurwitz, S. (1993). *Clinical pediatric dermatology: a textbook of skin disorders of childhood and adolescence* (2nd ed.). Philadelphia: W.B. Saunders; (strawberry mark [immature hemangioma]) from Lookingbill, D. P., & Marks, J. G. (1993). *Principles of dermatology* (2nd ed.). Philadelphia: W.B. Saunders; (cavernous hemangioma [mature]) from Habif, T. P., Campbell, J. L., Jr., Chapman, M. S., Dinulos, J. G. H., & Zug, K. A. (2005). *Skin disease: Diagnosis and treatment* (3rd ed., p. 437). St. Louis: Mosby; (telangiectasis spider or star angioma) Courtesy Lemmi & Lemmi, 2011; (venous lake) from Habif, T. P., Campbell, J. L., Jr., Chapman, M. S., Dinulos, J. G. H., & Zug, K. A. (2001). *Skin disease: Diagnosis and treatment* (2nd ed.). St. Louis: Mosby; (petechiae) from Dockery, G. L. (1997). *Cutaneous disorders of the lower extremity* (p. 119, Fig. 9.47). Philadelphia: W.B. Saunders. Reprinted with the permission of the author; (purpura) from Hurwitz, S. (1993). *Clinical pediatric dermatology: a textbook of skin disorders of childhood and adolescence* (2nd ed.). Philadelphia: W.B. Saunders; (ecchymosis) Courtesy Lemmi & Lemmi, 2011.

Art for Table 13.9: (diaper dermatitis) from Hurwitz, S. (1993). *Clinical pediatric dermatology: a textbook of skin disorders of childhood and adolescence* (2nd ed.). Philadelphia: W.B. Saunders; (intertrigo [candidiasis]) and (impetigo) Courtesy Lemmi & Lemmi, 2011; (atopic dermatitis [eczema]) from Hurwitz, S. (1993). *Clinical pediatric dermatology: a textbook of skin disorders of childhood and adolescence* (2nd ed.). Philadelphia: W.B. Saunders; (measles [rubeola] in dark skin) from Feigin, R. D., &

Cherry, J. D. (1998). *Textbook of pediatric infectious diseases* (4th ed.). Philadelphia: Saunders; (measles [rubeola] in light skin) Courtesy Lemmi & Lemmi, 2011; (German measles [rubella]) from Hurwitz, S. (1993). *Clinical pediatric dermatology: a textbook of skin disorders of childhood and adolescence* (2nd ed.). Philadelphia: W.B. Saunders; (chickenpox [varicella]) from Callen, J. P., & Greer K. E. (1993). *Color atlas of dermatology* (p. 170, Fig. 5.34). Philadelphia: W.B. Saunders.

Art for Table 13.10: (primary contact dermatitis) from Lookingbill, D. P., & Marks, J. G. (1993). *Principles of dermatology* (2nd ed., p. 124). Philadelphia: W.B. Saunders; (allergic drug reaction) from Lookingbill, D. P., & Marks, J. G. (1993). *Principles of dermatology* (2nd ed., p. 218). Philadelphia: W.B. Saunders; (tinea corporis [ringworm of the body]) from Hurwitz, S. (1993). *Clinical pediatric dermatology: a textbook of skin disorders of childhood and adolescence* (2nd ed.). Philadelphia: W. B. Saunders; (tinea pedis [ringworm of the foot], labial herpes simplex [cold sores], tinea versicolor, and herpes zoster [shingles]) from Lemmi & Lemmi, 2011; (psoriasis) from Lookingbill, D. P., & Marks, J. G. (1993). *Principles of dermatology* (2nd ed.). Philadelphia: W.B. Saunders; (erythema migrans of Lyme disease) from Swartz, M. H. (2006). *Textbook of physical diagnosis: History and examination* (5th ed.). Philadelphia: W.B. Saunders.

Art for Table 13.11: (basal cell carcinoma; malignant melanoma) from Lookingbill, D. P., & Marks, J. G. (1993). *Principles of dermatology* (2nd ed.). Philadelphia: W.B. Saunders; (squamous cell carcinoma) from Habif, T. P., Campbell, J. L., & Quitadamo, M. J. (2001). *Skin disease: Diagnosis and treatment.* St. Louis: Mosby; (metastatic malignant melanoma) courtesy Lemmi & Lemmi, 2011.

Art for Table 13.12: (AIDS-related Kaposi's sarcoma: patch stage) from Friedman-Kien, A. E. (1989). *Color atlas of AIDS.* Philadelphia: W.B. Saunders.

Art for Table 13.13: (tinea capitis [scalp ringworm]; furuncle and abscess) from Lookingbill, D. P., & Marks, J. G. (1993). *Principles of dermatology* (2nd ed.). Philadelphia: W.B. Saunders; (toxic alopecia) from Hurwitz, S. (1993). *Clinical pediatric dermatology: A textbook of skin disorders of childhood and adolescence* (2nd ed.). Philadelphia: W.B. Saunders; (alopecia areata; traumatic alopecia: traction alopecia; and seborrheic dermatitis [cradle cap]) from Hurwitz, S. (1993). *Clinical pediatric dermatology: A textbook of skin disorders of childhood and adolescence* (2nd ed.). Philadelphia: W.B. Saunders; (pediculosis capitis [head lice]; and trichotillomania) from Callen, J. P., & Greer K. E. (1993). *Color atlas of dermatology.* Philadelphia: W.B. Saunders; (hirsutism) from James, W.D., Berger, T.G., Elston, D.M. (2016). Andrews' diseases of the skin (12th ed.). Philadelphia: Elsevier.

Art for Table 13.14: (scabies; paronychia; onycholysis; pitting; habit-tic dystrophy) courtesy Lemmi & Lemmi, 2011; (Beau's line; splinter hemorrhages) from Callen, J. P., & Greer K. E. (1993). *Color atlas of dermatology.* Philadelphia: W. B. Saunders; (late clubbing) Reprinted from the Clinical Slide Collection on the Rheumatic Diseases. © 1991, 1995, 1997. Used by permission of the American College of Rheumatology.

CHAPTER 14

Unnumbered Figure, Promoting Health: ©David Kawai/ Ottawa Citizen

Fig. 14.8: © Pat Thomas, 2006.

Fig. 14.12, B: Dean, S., Garrett, N., Tyrrell, J. (2008). Management of enlarged cervical lymph nodes. Paediatrics and Child Health, 118(3), 118-122.

Fig. 14.14, B: Courtesy Lemmi & Lemmi, 2011.

Figs. 14.16 and 14.17, A: Murray, S. S., & McKinney, E. S. (2010). *Foundations of maternal–newborn and women's health nursing* (5th ed., pp. 514–15). St. Louis: W.B. Saunders.

Art for Table 14.2: (Hydrocephalus) from Bowden, V.R., Dickey, S.B., & Greenburg, C.S. (1998). Children and their families: the continuum of care. Philadelphia: Saunders; (Down Syndrome) from Hockenberry, M.J. & Wilson, D.: Wong's Essentials of Pediatric Nursing (9th ed.). St. Louis: Mosby; (Fetal alcohol syndrome) from Streissguth, A.P. et al. (1980). Teratogenic effects of alcohol in humans and laboratory animals, Science 209, 353-361; (Fetal alcohol syndrome [line drawing]) Copyright Pat Thomas, 2006. (Atopic [allergic] facies and Allergic salute and crease) from Zitelli, B.J., & Davis, H.W. (2007). Atlas of pediatric physical diagnosis (5th ed.). St Louis: Mosby; (Plagiocephaly) from Pomatto J.K., Calcaterra J., Kelly K.M., et al. (2006). A study of family head shape: environment alters cranial shape. Clinical Pediatrics 45 (1), 55–64, 2006; (Craniosynostosis) from Quiñones-Hinojosa A. (2012). Schmidek and Sweets Operative Neurosurgical Techniques: Indications, Methods and Results (6th ed.). Philadelphia: Saunders.

Art for Table 14.3: (Torticollis [wryneck]) from Zitelli, B.J., & Davis, H.W. (2007). Atlas of pediatric physical diagnosis (5th ed.). St Louis: Mosby; (Thyroid—multiple nodules) from Swartz, M.H. (2005). Textbook of physical diagnosis: history and examination (5th ed.). Philadelphia: Saunders; (Pilar cyst [wen]) from Callen, J.P., et al. (1993). Color atlas of dermatology, Philadelphia: Saunders; (Parotid gland enlargement) from From Meningaud et al. (2007). Kimura's Disease of the Parotid Region. Journal of Oral and Maxillofacial Surgery (65)1, 134-140.

Art for Table 14.4: (Parkinson syndrome) from Glynn M. and Drake W.M. (2012). Hutchison's Clinical Methods: An Integrated Approach to Clinical Practice (23rd ed.). Philadelphia: Saunders/Elsevier Ltd.; (Cushing syndrome) from Kanski, J.J. (2009). Clinical Ophthalmology: a Synopsis (2nd ed.). Elsevier Ltd.; (Bell Palsy [left side]) from Studdiford J.S., Altschuler M. Salzman B., Tully A. (2009). Images from the Wards: Diagnosis and Treatment (1st ed.). Philadelphia: Saunders; (Stroke or "Brain Attack") from Nolte, J., Sundsten, J. (2009). The Human Brain: An

Introduction to Its Functional Anatomy (6th ed.). Philadelphia: Mosby/Elsevier; (Cachectic appearance) courtesy Lemmi and Lemmi, 2011; (Acromegaly) from Liu, G. T., Volpe, N.J., Galetta S.L. (2010). Neuro-Ophthalmology: Diagnosis and Management (2nd ed.). Philadelphia: Saunders.

Art for Table 14.5: (Hypothalamic-pituitary-thyroid axis) © Pat Thomas, 2014; (Hyperthyroidism) from Swartz, M.H. (2005). Textbook of physical diagnosis: history and examination (5th ed.). Philadelphia: Saunders; (Myxedema [hypothyroidism]) from Hall, R., & Evered, D.C. (1990). Color atlas of endocrinology (2nd ed.). St. Louis: Mosby.

CHAPTER 15

Figs. 15.1, 15.2, 15.3, 15.4, 15.18: © Pat Thomas, 2006.

Fig. 15.23: Courtesy Heather Boyd-Monk and Wills Eye Hospital, Philadelphia, PA.

Figs. 15.24 and 15.25: Courtesy Lemmi & Lemmi, 2011.

Fig. 15.30: Zitelli, B. J., McIntire, S.C., & Nowalk, A.J. (2012). *Zitelli & Davis' atlas of pediatric physical diagnosis* (6th ed., p. 739, Fig. 19.18).St. Louis: Mosby.

Fig. 15.31: Albert, D. M., & Jakobiec, F. A. (1994). *Principles and practice of ophthalmology.* Philadelphia: Saunders.

Figs. 15.32 and 15.34: Courtesy Lemmi & Lemmi, 2011.

Fig. 15.33: Swartz, M. H. (2009). *Textbook of physical diagnosis: History and examination* (6th ed., p. 244, Fig. 10.54). Philadelphia: W.B. Saunders.

Fig. 15.35: Friedman, N., & Pineda, R. (1998). *The Massachusetts Eye and Ear Infirmary illustrated manual of ophthalmology.* Philadelphia: W.B. Saunders (p. 535).

Art in Table 15.1: (A, pseudostrabismus; **B,** esotropia; **C,** exotropia) from Zitelli, B. J., McIntire, S.C., & Nowalk, A.J. (2012). *Zitelli & Davis' atlas of pediatric physical diagnosis* (6th ed., pp. 737–40, Figs. 19-12, 19-18, 19-20). St. Louis: Mosby.

Art in Table 15.2: (periorbital edema) from Ibsen, O. A. C., & Phelan, J. A. (1996). *Oral pathology for the dental hygienist* (2nd ed.). Philadelphia: W.B. Saunders; (exophthalmos [protruding eye]) from Scheie, H. G., & Albert, D. M. (1977). *Textbook of ophthalmology* (9th ed.). Philadelphia: W.B. Saunders; (ptosis [drooping upper lid]) Courtesy Lemmi & Lemmi, 2011; (upward palpebral slant) from Zitelli, B. J., McIntire, S.C., & Nowalk, A.J. (2012). *Zitelli & Davis' atlas of pediatric physical diagnosis* (6th ed., p. 101, Fig. 3.37) St. Louis: Mosby; (ectropion; entropion) from Albert, D. M., & Jakobiec, F. A. (1994). *Principles and practice of ophthalmology* (vol. 3, p. 1849). Philadelphia: W.B. Saunders.

Art in Table 15.3: (blepharitis [inflammation of the eyelids]; dacryocystitis [inflammation of the lacrimal sac]) from Friedman, N., & Pineda, R. (1998). *The Massachusetts Eye and Ear Infirmary illustrated manual of ophthalmology.* Philadelphia: W.B. Saunders; (chalazion) Courtesy Heather Boyd-Monk and Wills Eye Hospital, Philadelphia, PA; (hordeolum [stye]) Courtesy Lemmi & Lemmi,

2011; (basal cell carcinoma) from Scheie, H. G., & Albert, D. M. (1977). *Textbook of ophthalmology* (9th ed., p. 449). Philadelphia: W.B. Saunders.

Art in Table 15.6: (conjunctivitis; subconjunctival hemorrhage) courtesy Lemmi & Lemmi, 2011; (iritis [circumcorneal redness]; acute glaucoma) from Scheie, H. G., & Albert, D. M. (1977). *Textbook of ophthalmology* (9th ed., pp. 13, 536). Philadelphia: W. B. Saunders.

Art in Table 15.7: (pterygium) from Albert, D. M., & Jakobiec, F. A. (1994). *Principles and practice of ophthalmology* (vol. 1). Philadelphia: W. B. Saunders; (corneal abrasion) Courtesy Heather Boyd-Monk and Wills Eye Hospital, Philadelphia, PA; (hyphema) from Scheie, H. G., & Albert, D. M. (1977). *Textbook of ophthalmology* (9th ed.). Philadelphia: W. B. Saunders; (hypopyon) from Scheie, H. G., & Albert, D. M. (1977). *Textbook of ophthalmology* (9th ed., p. 391). Philadelphia: W. B. Saunders.

Art in Table 15.8: (central grey opacity: nuclear cataract; star-shaped opacity: cortical cataract) from Friedman, N., & Pineda, R. (1998). *The Massachusetts Eye and Ear Infirmary illustrated manual of ophthalmology*. Philadelphia: W. B. Saunders (pp. 220–21, Figs. 8-4 and 8-6).

Art in Table 15.9: (optic atrophy [disc pallor]; papilledema [choked disc]; excessive cup-disc ratio) from Friedman, N., Kaiser, P.K., & Pineda, R. (2009). *The Massachusetts Eye and Ear Infirmary illustrated manual of ophthalmology*. Philadelphia: W. B. Saunders.

Art in Table 15.10: (arteriovenous crossing [nicking]) from Friedman, N., Kaiser, P. K., & Pineda, R. (2009). *The Massachusetts Eye and Ear Infirmary illustrated manual of ophthalmology* (3rd ed., p. 268, Fig. 10.35). Philadelphia: W. B. Saunders; (narrowed [attenuated] arteries; microaneurysms; exudates) courtesy Lemmi & Lemmi, 2011; (intraretinal hemorrhages) from Friedman, N., Kaiser, P. K., & Pineda, R. (2009). *The Massachusetts Eye and Ear Infirmary illustrated manual of ophthalmology* (3rd ed.). Philadelphia: W. B. Saunders.

CHAPTER 16

Fig. 16.1: © Pat Thomas, 2010.

Fig. 16.3: Courtesy Lemmi & Lemmi, 2011.

Fig. 16.4: © Pat Thomas, 2006.

Fig. 16.9: Adams, G. L., Boies, L. R., & Hilger, P. A. (1989). *Boies fundamentals of otolaryngology: A textbook of ear, nose, and throat diseases* (6th ed.). Philadelphia: W. B. Saunders.

Fig. 16.10: © Pat Thomas, 2006.

Fig. 16.19: Images © Pat Thomas, 2014. Scale from Hickey, J.V. (1986). Neurological and neurosurgical nursing (2nd ed.). Philadelphia: Lippincott.

Art for Table 16.1: (frostbite) Reprinted from the Clinical Slide Collection on the Rheumatic Diseases. © 1991, 1995, 1997. Used by permission of the American College of Rheumatology; (otitis externa: swimmer's ear; cellulitis) Courtesy Lemmi & Lemmi, 2011; (branchial remnant and ear deformity) from Liebert, P. S. (1996). *Color atlas of pediatric surgery* (2nd ed., p. 31, Fig. 2.45). Philadelphia: W. B. Saunders.

Art for Table 16.2: (sebaceous cyst) from Liebert, P. S. (1996). *Color atlas of pediatric surgery* (2nd ed., p. 29, Fig. 2.40). Philadelphia: W. B. Saunders; (tophi) Reprinted from the Clinical Slide Collection on the Rheumatic Diseases © 1991, 1995, 1997. Used by permission of the American College of Rheumatology; (chondrodermatitis nodularis helicis) from Habif, T. P. (2004). *Clinical dermatology: A color guide to diagnosis and therapy* (4th ed., p. 716, Fig. 20.39). St. Louis: Mosby; (keloid) courtesy Lemmi & Lemmi, 2011; (carcinoma) from Callen, J. P., & Greer K. E. (1993). *Color atlas of dermatology*. Philadelphia: W. B. Saunders (p. 111, Fig. 3.140A); (battle sign) from Zitelli, B.J., McIntire, S.C., Nowalk, A.J. (2012). *Atlas of pediatric physical diagnosis* (ed. 6). Philadelphia, Saunders.

Art for Table 16.3: © Pat Thomas, 2014.

Art for Table 16.4: © Pat Thomas, 2010.

Art for Table 16.6: (retracted eardrum) from Adams, G. L., Boies, L. R., & Hilger, P. A. (1989). *Boies fundamentals of otolaryngology: A textbook of ear, nose, and throat diseases* (6th ed., p. 6). Philadelphia: W. B. Saunders; (otitis media with effusion [OME]) from Swartz, M. H. (2009). *Textbook of physical diagnosis: History and examination* (6th ed., p. 320, Fig. 11.34A). Philadelphia: W. B. Saunders; (acute purulent otitis media: early stage; acute purulent otitis media: later stage) from Adams, G. L., Boies, L. R., & Hilger, P. A. (1989). *Boies fundamentals of otolaryngology: A textbook of ear, nose, and throat diseases* (6th ed.). Philadelphia: W. B. Saunders; (perforation) from Swartz, M. H. (2009). *Textbook of physical diagnosis: History and examination* (6th ed., p. 318, Fig. 11.30A). Philadelphia: W. B. Saunders; (insertion of tympanostomy tubes) from Fireman, P. (1996). *Atlas of allergies* (2nd ed., p. 182, Fig. 11.19). London: Mosby; (cholesteatoma; bullous myringitis) from Swartz, M. H. (2009). *Textbook of physical diagnosis: History and examination* (6th ed., pp. 317, 319, Figs. 11.27 and 11.31A). Philadelphia: W. B. Saunders; (illustrations of scarred eardrum, blue eardrum, and fungal infection [otomycosis]) © Pat Thomas, 2010.

CHAPTER 17

Figs. 17.1, 17.2, 17.3, 17.6, 17.19: © Pat Thomas, 2006.

Figs. 17.4, 17.5: © Pat Thomas, 2010.

Fig. 17.7: Martino, R., Silver, F., Teasell, R., Bayley, M., Nicholson G., Streiner, D. L., & Diamant, N. E. (2009). The Toronto Bedside Swallowing Screening Test (TOR-BSST): Development and validation of a dysphagia screening tool for patients with stroke. *Stroke, 40*, 555–561. Retrieved from http://www.neostrokenetwork.com/newportal/LinkClick.aspx?fileticket=rDVxJ5l9NGo%3D&tabid=299.

Fig. 17.10: Fireman, P. (1996). *Atlas of allergies* (2nd ed., p. 151, Fig. 9.27). London: Mosby.

Fig. 17.17: Ibsen, O. A. C., & Phelan, J. A. (1996). *Oral pathology for the dental hygienist* (2nd ed., Slide #106). Philadelphia: W. B. Saunders.

Fig. 17.18: Courtesy Lemmi & Lemmi, 2011.

Fig. 17.24: Zitelli, B. J., McIntire, S.C., & Nowalk, A.J. (2012). *Zitelli & Davis' atlas of pediatric physical diagnosis* (6th ed., p. 780, Fig. 20.13). St. Louis: Mosby.

Figs. 17.25 and 17.26: Courtesy Lemmi & Lemmi, 2011.

Art for Table 17.1: (foreign body; acute rhinitis; allergic rhinitis; nasal polyps) from Fireman, P. (1996). *Atlas of allergies* (2nd ed.). London: Mosby; (perforated septum) from Hawke, M. (1998). *Diagnostic handbook of otorhinolaryngology.* London: Martin Dunitz (p. 122, Fig. 2.60). Reproduced by permission of Taylor & Francis Books UK.

Art for Table 17.2: (cleft lip) from Ibsen, O. A. C., & Phelan, J. A. (1996). *Oral pathology for the dental hygienist* (2nd ed., slide 294). Philadelphia: W. B. Saunders; (herpes simplex 1; angular cheilitis [stomatitis, perlèche]) from Callen, J. P., & Greer K. E. (1993). *Color atlas of dermatology.* Philadelphia: W. B. Saunders; (carcinoma; retention "cyst" [mucocele]) from Hawke, M. (1998). *Diagnostic handbook of otorhinolaryngology.* London: Martin Dunitz (p. 161-62, Fig. 3.6 & 3.7). Reproduced by permission of Taylor & Francis Books UK.

Art for Table 17.3: (baby bottle tooth decay) Courtesy F. Ferguson, Department of Children's Dentistry, School of Dental Medicine, State University of New York at Stony Brook, Stony Brook, NY; (dental caries) Courtesy A. McWhorter, Pediatric Dentistry, Baylor College of Dentistry, Texas A&M University System, Dallas, TX; (epulis; gingival hyperplasia) from Ibsen, O. A. C., & Phelan, J. A. (1996). *Oral pathology for the dental hygienist* (2nd ed.). Philadelphia: W. B. Saunders; (gingivitis) from Callen, J. P., & Greer K. E. (1993). *Color atlas of dermatology* (p. 385). Philadelphia: W. B. Saunders; (meth mouth) from Neville, B. W., Damm, D. D., Allen, C. M., & Bouquot, J. E. (2009). *Oral and maxillofacial pathology* (3rd ed.). St. Louis: W. B. Saunders.

Art for Table 17.4: (aphthous ulcers) from Sleisinger, M. H., & Fordtran, J. S. (1993). *Gastrointestinal diseases: Pathophysiology, diagnosis, and management* (vol. 1, 5th ed.). Philadelphia: W. B. Saunders; (Koplik's spots) from Feigin, R. D., & Cherry, J. D. (1998). *Textbook of pediatric infectious diseases* (4th ed.). Philadelphia: W. B. Saunders; (leukoplakia) from Sleisinger, M. H., & Fordtran, J. S. (1993). *Gastrointestinal diseases: Pathophysiology, diagnosis, and management* (5th ed., vol. 1). Philadelphia: W. B. Saunders; (candidiasis or monilial infection) from Callen, J. P., & Greer K. E. (1993). *Color atlas of dermatology.* Philadelphia: W. B. Saunders; (herpes simplex 1) courtesy Lemmi & Lemmi, 2011.

Art for Table 17.5: (ankyloglossia) from Ibsen, O. A. C., & Phelan, J. A. (1996). *Oral pathology for the dental hygienist* (2nd ed., slide #28). Philadelphia: W. B. Saunders; (geographic tongue [migratory glossitis]; fissured or scrotal tongue) courtesy Lemmi & Lemmi, 2011; (smooth, glossy tongue [atrophic glossitis]) from Adams, G. L., Boies, L. R., & Hilger, P. A. (1989). *Boies fundamentals of otolaryngology: A textbook of ear, nose, and throat diseases* (6th ed., p. 302). Philadelphia: W. B. Saunders; (black hairy

tongue) from Callen, J. P., & Greer K. E. (1993). *Color atlas of dermatology.* Philadelphia: W. B. Saunders (p. 387); (enlarged tongue [macroglossia]) from Zitelli, B. J., & Davis, H. W. (2002). *Atlas of pediatric physical diagnosis* (4th ed.). St. Louis: Mosby. Courtesy Dr. Christine Williams; (carcinoma) from Wenig, B. M., Heffess, C. S., & Adair, C. F. (1997). *Atlas of endocrine pathology.* Philadelphia: W. B. Saunders.

Art for Table 17.6: (cleft palate) from Zitelli, B. J., McIntire, S. C., & Nowalk, A. J. (2012). *Zitelli & Davis' atlas of pediatric physical diagnosis* (6th ed., p. 944, Fig. 23.64,BSt. Louis: Mosby. Courtesy Dr. Michael Sherlock, M. D., Lutherville, MD; (bifid uvula) from Hawke, M. (1998). *Diagnostic handbook of otorhinolaryngology.* London: Martin Dunitz (p. 195, Fig. 3.67); (oral Kaposi's sarcoma) from Friedman-Kien, A. E. (1989), *Color atlas of AIDS.* Philadelphia: W. B. Saunders (p. 38); (acute tonsillitis and pharyngitis) Courtesy Lemmi & Lemmi, 2011.

CHAPTER 18

Fig. 18.2: © Pat Thomas, 2010.

Fig. 18.6: Redrawn from Tanner, J. M. (1962). *Growth at adolescence.* Oxford, UK: Blackwell Scientific.

Fig. 18.8: Callen, J. P., & Greer K. E. (1993). *Color atlas of dermatology.* Philadelphia: W. B. Saunders.

Fig. 18.19: Courtesy Denise Tarlier.

Fig. 18.21: Moore, K. L., Persaud, T.N., & Torchia, M.G. (2013). *Before we are born: Essentials of embryology and birth defects* (8th ed., p. 300, Fig. 19.7). Philadelphia: W.B. Saunders. Courtesy Children's Hospital and University of Manitoba, Winnipeg, Manitoba.

Art for Table 18.3: (dimpling) from Evans, A. J., Wilson, A. R. M., Blamey, R. W., Robertson, J. F. R., Ellis, I. O., & Elston, C. W. (1998). *Atlas of breast disease management: 50 illustrative cases.* Philadelphia: W. B. Saunders; (edema [peau d'orange]; fixation; deviation in nipple pointing) from Mansel, R., & Bundred, N.J. (1995). *Colour atlas of breast diseases.* London: Mosby-Wolfe.

Art for Table 18.6: (mammary duct ectasia; intraductal papilloma; Paget's disease [intraductal carcinoma) from Mansel, R., & Bundred, N.J. (1995). *Colour atlas of breast diseases.* London: Mosby-Wolfe; (carcinoma) from Evans, A. J., Wilson, A. R. M., Blamey, R. W., Robertson, J. F. R., Ellis, I. O., & Elston, C. W. (1998). *Atlas of breast disease management: 50 illustrative cases.* Philadelphia: W. B. Saunders.

Art for Table 18.7: (mastitis; breast abscess) from Mansel, R., & Bundred, N.J. (1995). *Colour atlas of breast diseases.* London: Mosby-Wolfe.

Art for Table 18.8: (gynecomastia) from Lorenzo, G. D., Autorino, R., Perdonà, S., Placido, S.D. (2005). Management of gynaecomastia in patients with prostate cancer: a systematic review. The Lancet 6(12), 972-979; (breast carcinoma in men) from Elshafieya, M.E., Zeeneldinb, A.A., Elsebaia, H.I., Moneerc, M., et al. (2011). Epidemiology and management of breast carcinoma in Egyptian males:

Experience of a single Cancer Institute. Journal of the Egyptian National Cancer Institute 23(3), 115-122.

CHAPTER 19

Figs. 19.1, 19.2, 19.10: © Pat Thomas, 2010.
Fig. 19.11: © Pat Thomas, 2006.
Fig. 19.12: Nichols, F. H., & Zwelling, E. (1997). *Maternal–newborn nursing: Theory and practice*. Philadelphia: W. B. Saunders.

CHAPTER 20

Figs. 20.2, 20.3, 20.4, 20.8, and 20.9: © Pat Thomas, 2006.
Fig. 20.29: © Pat Thomas, 2014.
Art for Art for Promoting Health Box (heart truth logo): The Heart Truth: Awareness and Prevention. Retrieved from http://www.4women.gov/hearttruth.
Art for Table 20.8: Images © Pat Thomas, 2006.
Art for Table 20.9: Images © Pat Thomas, 2006.
Art for Table 20.10: Stenosis images © Pat Thomas, 2006.

CHAPTER 21

Figs. 21.1, 21.2, 21.3, and 20.5: © Pat Thomas, 2010.
Figs. 21.4, 21.6, and 21.22: © Pat Thomas, 2006.
Fig. 21.18, B: Bloom, A., Watkins, P. H., & Ireland, J. (1992). *Color atlas of diabetes* (2nd ed.). St. Louis: Mosby.
Fig. 21.20, B: Courtesy Lemmi & Lemmi, 2011.
Art for Table 21.2: (Raynaud's syndrome; hand cyanosis) courtesy Lemmi & Lemmi, 2011; (lymphedema) Walsh, T. D., Caraceni, A. T., Fainsinger, R., Foley, K. M., Glare, P., Goh, C., …, Rabruch, L. (2009). *Palliative medicine*. Philadelphia: W. B. Saunders (Fig. 87.1).
Art for Table 21.4: (arterial: ischemic ulcer) from Dockery, G. L. (1997). *Cutaneous disorders of the lower extremity*. Philadelphia: W. B. Saunders. Reprinted with the permission of the author; (venous [stasis] ulcer) from Lookingbill, D. P., & Marks, J. G. (1993). *Principles of dermatology* (2nd ed., p. 267). Philadelphia: W. B. Saunders; (diabetes) courtesy Lemmi & Lemmi, 2011.
Art for Table 21.5: (superficial varicose veins; deep vein thrombophlebitis) from Dockery, G. L. (1997). *Cutaneous disorders of the lower extremity*. Philadelphia: W. B. Saunders. Reprinted with the permission of the author.

CHAPTER 22

Figs. 22.1, 22.2, 22.3, 22.4, and 22.5: © Pat Thomas, 2006.
Art for Table 22.2: © Pat Thomas, 2014.
Art for Table 22.3: © Pat Thomas, 2006.
Art for Table 22.4: (umbilical hernia) from Zitelli, B. J., & Davis, H. W. (2007). *Atlas of pediatric physical diagnosis* (5th ed.). St. Louis: Mosby. Courtesy Dr. Thomas P. Foley, Jr.; (epigastric hernmia) from Conroy K., Malata C.M. (2012). Epigastric hernia following DIEP flap breast reconstruction: complication or coincidence? *Journal*

of *Plastic, Reconstructive & Aesthetic Surgery* 65(3), 387-391; (incisional hernia) courtesy Lemmi & Lemmi, 2011; (diastasis recti) from Clark D.A. (2000). *Atlas of neonatology* (ed. 7). Philadelphia: Saunders.

CHAPTER 23

Unn Fig. 23.1: Reproduced by kind permission of Dr K W Heaton, Reader in Medicine at the University of Bristol. 2000 Norgine Ltd.
Fig. 23.1: © Pat Thomas, 2010.

CHAPTER 24

Fig. 24.2: © Pat Thomas, 2006.
Figs. 24.32, C, and 24.33, B: Dieppe, P. A., Cooper, C., & McGill, N. (1991). *Arthritis and rheumatism in practice*. London: Gower Medical Publishing.
Fig. 24.37: Courtesy Lemmi & Lemmi, 2011.
Fig. 24.50: Zitelli, B. J., McIntire, S.C., & Nowalk, A.J. (2012). *Zitelli & Davis' atlas of pediatric physical diagnosis* (6th ed., pp. 853–854, Figs. 21.93B and 21.95). St. Louis: Mosby.
Figs. 24.51, B, and Fig. 24.54: Courtesy Lemmi & Lemmi, 2011.
Art for Table 24.3: (atrophy; dislocated shoulder; joint effusion) from Bunker, T., & Schranz, P. J. (1998). *Clinical challenges in orthopaedics: The shoulder*. London: Martin Dunitz. Reproduced by permission of Taylor & Francis Books UK. (frozen shoulder: adhesive capsulitis) from Peñas C.F., Cleland, J.A., Huijbregts, P.A. (2011). Neck and Arm Pain Syndromes: Evidence-informed screening, diagnosis and management. Philadelphia: Churchill Livingstone; (tear of rotator cuff) from Waldman, S.D. (2010). Physical diagnosis of pain: an atlas of signs and symptoms (ed. 2). Philadelphia: Saunders.
Art for Table 24.4: (olecranon bursitis) from Dieppe, P. A., Cooper, C., & McGill, N. (1991). *Arthritis and rheumatism in practice*. London: Gower Medical Publishing; (gouty arthritis) from Polley, H. F., & Hunder, G. G. (1978). *Rheumatalogic interviewing and physical examination of the joints* (2nd ed.). Philadelphia: W. B. Saunders; (subcutaneous nodules) from Callen, J. P., & Greer K. E. (1993). *Color atlas of dermatology*. Philadelphia: W. B. Saunders; (epicondylitis—tennis elbow) from Skirven, T.M., Osterman, A.L., Fedorczyk, J.M., Amadio, P.C. (2011). Rehabilitation of the Hand and Upper Extremity (ed. 6). St. Louis: Mosby.
Art for Table 24.5: (ganglion cyst) from Callen, J. P., & Greer K. E. (1993). *Color atlas of dermatology*. Philadelphia: W. B. Saunders; (carpal tunnel syndrome with atrophy of thenar eminence; swan-neck and boutonnière deformity) Reprinted from the Clinical Slide Collection on the Rheumatic Diseases. © 1991, 1995, 1997. Used by permission of the American College of Rheumatology; (ankylosis) from Slutsky D.J. (2010). Principles and Practice of Wrist Surgery. Philadelphia: Saunders; (Dupuytren's contracture) from Canale, S.T., Beaty, J.H. (2013). Campbell's

Operative Orthopaedics (ed. 12). St. Louis: Mosby. (ulnar deviation or drift; degenerative joint disease or osteoarthritis) Reprinted from the Clinical Slide Collection, 1991, American College of Rheumatology; (syndactyly; polydactyly) from Liebert, P. S. (1996). *Color atlas of pediatric surgery* (2nd ed.). Philadelphia: W. B. Saunders; gout in the thumb: Courtesy Lemmi & Lemmi 2011.

Art for Table 24.6: (mild synovitis; prepatellar bursitis) from Dieppe, P. A., Cooper, C., & McGill, N. (1991). *Arthritis and rheumatism in practice.* London: Gower Medical Publishing; (swelling of menisci) from Jones, A., & Owen, R. (1995). *Colour atlas of clinical orthopedics* (2nd ed.). London: Mosby-Wolfe; (Osgood-Schlatter disease) from Zitelli, B. J., McIntire, S.C., & Nowalk, A.J. (2012). *Zitelli & Davis' atlas of pediatric physical diagnosis* (6th ed., p. 410, Fig. 21.97, A) St. Louis: Mosby; (postpolio muscle atrophy) courtesy Lemmi & Lemmi, 2011.

Art for Table 24.7: (Achilles tenosynovitis; acute gout) from Dieppe, P. A., Cooper, C., & McGill, N. (1991). *Arthritis and rheumatism in practice.* London: Gower Medical Publishing; (tophi with chronic gout) from Dockery, G. L. (1997). *Cutaneous disorders of the lower extremity.* Philadelphia: W. B. Saunders. Reprinted with the permission of the author; (hallux valgus with bunion and hammertoes) Reprinted from the Clinical Slide Collection, 1991, American College of Rheumatology; (callus; ingrown toenail; plantar wart) Courtesy Lemmi & Lemmi, 2011.

Art for Table 24.8: (scoliosis *[top]*) Courtesy Lemmi & Lemmi, 2011; (scoliosis *[bottom]*) Zitelli, B. J., McIntire, S.C., & Nowalk, A.J. (2012). *Zitelli & Davis' atlas of pediatric physical diagnosis* (6th ed., p. 840, Fig. 21.71, B. St. Louis: Mosby; (herniated nucleus pulposus) from Polley, H. F., & Hunder, G. G. (1978). *Rheumatologic interviewing and physical examination of the joints* (2nd ed.). Philadelphia: W. B. Saunders.

Art for Table 24.9: (congenital dislocated hip) from Zitelli, B. J., McIntire, S.C., & Nowalk, A.J. (2012). *Zitelli & Davis' atlas of pediatric physical diagnosis* (6th ed., p. 850, Fig. 21.89, A–B). St. Louis: Mosby; (talipes equinovarus [clubfoot]) Courtesy A. E. Chudley, M.D.; (spina bifida) from Thompson, D.N.P. (2010). Spinal dysraphic anomalies; classification, presentation and management. Paediatrics and Child Health 20(9), 397-403.

CHAPTER 25

Figs. 25.1, 25.2, 25.3, 25.4, 25.6, and 25.7: © Pat Thomas, 2006.

Fig. 25.5: © Pat Thomas, 2010.

Fig. 25.54, B: Braddom, R.L. (2011). Physical Medicine and Rehabilitation (ed. 4). Philadelphia: Saunders.

Fig. 25.60: Images © Pat Thomas, 2014.

Fig. 25.61 (Canadian Neurological Scale): Côté, R., Hachinski, V. C., Shurvell, B. L., Norris, J. W., & Wolfson, C. (1986). The Canadian Neurological Scale: A preliminary study in acute stroke. *Stroke, 17*(4), 731–737; Côté, R., Battista, R. N., Wolfson, C., Boucher, J., Adam, J., &

Hachinski, V. C. (1989). The Canadian Neurological Scale: Validation and reliability assessment. *Neurology, 39,* 638–643; and Bushnell, C. D., Johnston, D. C. C., & Goldstein, L. B. (2001). Retrospective assessment of initial stroke severity: Comparison of the NIH Stroke Scale and the Canadian Neurological Scale. *Stroke, 32,* 656.

Art for Tables 25.9 and 25.11: © Pat Thomas, 2006.

CHAPTER 26

Figs. 26.1, 26.2 and 26.3: © Pat Thomas, 2006.

Fig. 26.4: Redrawn from Marshall, W. A., & Tanner, J. M. (1970). Variations in the pattern of pubertal changes in boys. *Arch Dis Child, 45,* 22.

Fig. 26.9, B: Courtesy Lemmi & Lemmi, 2011.

Fig. 26.12: Sorrentino, S., Wilk, M., & Newmaster, R. (2013). *Mosby's Canadian textbook for the support worker* (3rd ed., p. 702, Fig. 31.10, B). Toronto: Elsevier Canada.

Art for Table 26.1: Adapted from Tanner, J. M. (1962). *Growth at adolescence.* Oxford, UK: Blackwell Scientific.

Art for Table 26.2: Courtesy Connie Cooper.

Art for Table 26.3: (urethritis [urethral discharge and dysuria]) from Emond, R., Rowland, H.A.K., & Welsby, P. (1995). *Colour atlas of infectious diseases* (3rd ed., p. 161). St. Louis: Mosby-Wolfe; (renal calculi) from Gould, B.E., Dyer, R. (2011). Pathophysiology for the Health Professions (ed. 4). Philadelphia: Saunders.

Art for Table 26.4: (tinea cruris) courtesy Lemmi & Lemmi, 2011; (genital herpes: HSV-2 infection) courtesy Pfizer Laboratories Division, Pfizer Inc., New York. From *A close look at VD: A slide presentation produced as a public service;* (syphilitic chancre) from Emond, R. T., Rowland, H. A. K., & Welsby, P. (1995). *Colour atlas of infectious diseases* (3rd ed., p. 173). London: Mosby-Wolfe; (genital warts) from Habif, T. P., Campbell, J. L., Jr., Chapman, M. S., Dinulos, J. G. H., & Zug, K. A. (2005). *Skin disease: Diagnosis and treatment* (3rd ed.). St. Louis: Mosby; (carcinoma) from Callen, J. P., & Greer K. E. (1993). *Color atlas of dermatology.* Philadelphia: W. B. Saunders.

Art for Table 26.5: (phimosis; hypospadias) from Liebert, P. S. (1996). *Color atlas of pediatric surgery* (2nd ed.). Philadelphia: W. B. Saunders; (paraphimosis) from Keys, C., Lam, J.P.H. (2013). Foreskin and penile problems in childhood. Surgery (Oxford) 31(3), 130-134; (epispadias) from Zitelli, B. J., McIntire, S.C., & Nowalk, A.J. (2012). *Zitelli & Davis' atlas of pediatric physical diagnosis* (6th ed., p. 570, Fig. 14.14, A). St. Louis: Mosby; (Peyronie's disease) courtesy Dr. Hans Stricker, Department of Urology, Henry Ford Hospital, Detroit, MI.

Art for Tables 26.6 and 26.7: © Pat Thomas, 2006.

CHAPTER 27

Fig. 27.13, A: Courtesy Lemmi & Lemmi, 2011.

Fig. 27.15: From Cancer Care Nova Scotia (2014). Screening for Cancer of the Cervix: An Office Manual for Health Professionals. Author: Nova Scotia, Canada.

Art for Table 27.2: (pediculosis pubis [crab lice]; herpes simplex virus-type 2 [herpes genitalis]) from Callen, J. P., & Greer K. E. (1993). *Color atlas of dermatology.* Philadelphia: W. B. Saunders; (red rash-contact dermatitis) Courtesy Pfizer Laboratories Division, Pfizer Inc., New York. From *A close look at VD: A slide presentation produced as a public service;* (syphilitic chancre; abscess of Bartholin's gland) from Emond, R. T., Rowland, H. A. K., & Welsby, P. (1995). *Colour atlas of infectious diseases* (3rd ed.). London: Mosby-Wolfe; (human papillomavirus [HPV] genital warts]) from Habif, T. P., Campbell, J. L., Jr., & Quitadamo, M. J. (2001). *Skin disease: Diagnosis and treatment.* St. Louis: Mosby; (urethral caruncle) from Rimsza, M. E. (1989). An illustrated guide to adolescent gynecology. *Pediatric Clinics of North America, 36*(3), 641.

Art for Table 27.3: (cystocele; uterine prolapse) from Symonds, E. M., & McPherson, M. B. A. (1997). *Diagnosis in colour: Obstetrics and gynecology.* London: Mosby-Wolfe; (rectocele) from Huffman, J. W. (1962). *Gynecology and obstetrics.* Philadelphia: W. B. Saunders.

Art for Table 27.4: (human papillomavirus (HPV, condylomata; polyp; carcinoma) from Symonds, E. M., & McPherson, M. B. A. (1997). *Diagnosis in colour: obstetrics and gynecology.* London: Mosby-Wolfe.

Art for Table 27.5: (candidiasis [moniliasis]) courtesy Lemmi & Lemmi, 2011; (gonorrhea) Courtesy Pfizer Laboratories Division, Pfizer Inc., New York. From *A close look at VD: A slide presentation produced as a public service.*

Art for Table 27.8: (ambiguous genitalia) from Moore, K. L., Persaud, T. N. & Torchia, M. G. (2013). *Before we are born: essentials of embryology and birth defects* (8th ed., p. 184, Fig. 13.25). Philadelphia: W.B. Saunders. Courtesy Dr. Heather Dean, Department of Pediatrics and Child Health, University of Manitoba, Winnipeg, Manitoba.; (vulvovaginitis in child) from Muram, D., Simmons, K.J. (2008). Pattern Recognition in Pediatric and Adolescent Gynecology—A Case for Formal Education. J Pediatr Adolesc Gynecol (21)2, 103-108.

Table 27.1: Adapted from Tanner, J. M. (1962). *Growth at adolescence.* Oxford, UK: Blackwell Scientific.

CHAPTER 29

Art for electronic health recording: from Potter, P.A., Perry, A.G., Stockert, P.,Hall, A. (2015). Essentials for Nursing Practice (ed. 8). St. Louis: Mosby; Minister of Public Works and Government Services Canada (2010): Electronic health records in Canada: An overview of federal and provincial audit reports. Author: Ottawa, Ontario.

CHAPTER 30

Fig. 30.4: from Black, M., Ambros-Rudolph, C.M., Edwards, L., Lynch, P.J. (2008). Obstetric and Gynecologic Dermatology (ed. 3). St. Louis: Mosby.

Fig. 30.13: from Apgar, B.S., Brotzman, G.L., Spitzer, M. (2008). Colposcopy: Principles and Practice (ed. 2). Philadelphia, Saunders.

Art for Table 30.3: (pre-eclampsia) from Symonds, E. M., & McPherson, M. B. A. (1997). *Diagnosis in colour: Obstetrics and gynecology.* London: Mosby-Wolfe.

Art for Table 30.4: (fetal macrosomia) from Meur, S., Mann, N. P. (2007). Infant outcomes following diabetic pregnancies. Paediatrics and Child Health(17) 6, 217-222.

CHAPTER 31

Fig. 31.1: © Diego Cervo, 2014/Shutterstock.

Fig. 31.2: Adapted from Katz, S., Downs, T. D., Cash, H. R., & Grotz, R. C. (1970). Progress in the development of the index of ADL. *Gerontologist, 10*(1, Part 1), 20–30.

Fig. 31.3: Lawton, M. P., & Brody, E. M. (1969). Assessment of older people: Self-maintaining and instrumental activities of daily living. *Gerontologist, 9*(3, Part 1), 179–186. © The Gerontological Society of America.

Fig. 31.5: Thornton, M., & Travis, S. S. (2003). Analysis of the reliability of the Modified Caregiver Strain Index. *The Journal of Gerontology, Series B, Psychological Sciences and Social Sciences, 58*(2), S129. © The Gerontological Society of America.

Page numbers followed by "*f*" indicate figures, "*t*" indicate tables, and "*b*" indicate boxes.

TABLE 1   Serum, Plasma, and Whole Blood Chemistry

TEST	NORMAL VALUES		POSSIBLE CAUSE OF ABNORMALITIES	
	SI UNITS	CONVENTIONAL UNITS	HIGHER VALUE	LOWER VALUE
Bicarbonate (HCO$_3$)	21-28 mmol/L	21-28 mEq/L	Chronic use of loop diuretics, compensated respiratory acidosis, metabolic alkalosis	Acute renal failure, compensated respiratory alkalosis, diarrhea, metabolic acidosis
Bilirubin			Biliary obstruction, hemolytic anemia, impaired liver function, pernicious anemia, prolonged fasting	
• Total	5.1-17 mcmol/L	0.3-1.0 mg/dL		
• Indirect	3.4-12 mcmol/L	0.2-0.8 mg/dL		
• Direct	1.7-5.1 mcmol/L	0.1-0.3 mg/dL		
Blood gases*				
• Arterial pH	7.35-7.45	Same as SI unit	Alkalosis	Acidosis
• Arterial partial pressure of carbon dioxide (PaCO$_2$)	35-45 mm Hg	Same as SI unit	Compensated metabolic alkalosis, respiratory acidosis	Compensated metabolic acidosis, respiratory alkalosis
• Arterial partial pressure of oxygen (PaO$_2$)	80-100 mm Hg	Same as SI unit	Administration of high concentration of oxygen	Chronic lung disease, decreased cardiac output
Carbon dioxide (CO$_2$) content	21-28 mmol/L	21-28 mEq/L	Same as bicarbonate	
Chloride	98-106 mmol/L	98-106 mEq/L	Corticosteroid therapy, dehydration, excessive infusion of normal saline, metabolic acidosis, respiratory alkalosis, uremia	Addison's disease, congestive heart failure, diarrhea, metabolic alkalosis, overhydration, respiratory acidosis, SIADH, vomiting
Cholesterol	<5 mmol/L	<200 mg/dL, age dependent	Biliary obstruction, cirrhosis hypothyroidism, hyperlipidemia, idiopathic hypercholesterolemia, renal disease, uncontrolled diabetes	Corticosteroid therapy, extensive liver disease, hyperthyroidism, malnutrition
• High-density lipoprotein (HDL)				
• Male	>0.75 mmol/L	>45 mg/dL		
• Female	>0.91 mmol/L	>55 mg/dL		
• Low-density protein (LDL)	<3.37 mmol/L	<60-180 mg/dL		
Glucose, fasting	4-6 mmol/L	72-110 mg/dL	Acute stress, cerebral lesions, Cushing's syndrome, diabetes mellitus, hyperthyroidism, pancreatic insufficiency	Addison's disease, hepatic disease, hypothyroidism, insulin overdosage, pancreatic tumour, pituitary hypofunction, postgastrectomy dumping syndrome
Oxygen saturation, arterial (SaO$_2$)	≥95%	Same as SI unit	Increased inspired oxygen, polycythemia vera	Anemia, cardiac decompensation, decreased inspired oxygen, respiratory disorders
Potassium	3.5-5.0 mmol/L	3.5-5.0 mEq/L	Acute or chronic renal failure, Addison's disease, dehydration, diabetic ketosis, excessive dietary or IV intake, massive tissue destruction, metabolic acidosis	Burns, Cushing's syndrome, deficient dietary or IV intake, diarrhea (severe), diuretic therapy, gastrointestinal fistula, insulin administration, pyloric obstruction, starvation, vomiting
Prostate-specific antigen (PSA)	<4 mcg/L	<4 ng/mL	Benign prostatic hypertrophy, prostate cancer, prostatitis	
Proteins			Burns, cirrhosis (globulin fraction), dehydration	Congenital agammaglobulinemia, increased capillary permeability, inflammatory disease, liver disease, malabsorption, malnutrition
• Total	64-83 g/L	6.4-8.3 g/dL		
• Albumin	35-50 g/L	3.5-5 g/dL		
• Globulin	23-34 g/L	2.3-3.4 g/dL		
Sodium	135-145 mmol/L	135-145 mEq/L	Corticosteroid therapy, dehydration, impaired renal function, increased sodium intake in diet or IV, primary aldosteronism	Addison's disease, decreased sodium intake in diet or IV therapy, diabetic ketoacidosis, diuretic therapy, excessive loss from GI tract, excessive perspiration, water intoxication
T$_4$ (thyroxine), total	64-154 nmol/L	5-12 mcg/dL	Hyperthyroidism, thyroiditis	Cretinism, hypothyroidism, myxedema

Continued

TABLE 1 Serum, Plasma, and Whole Blood Chemistry—cont'd

TEST	NORMAL VALUES SI UNITS	NORMAL VALUES CONVENTIONAL UNITS	POSSIBLE CAUSE OF ABNORMALITIES HIGHER VALUE	POSSIBLE CAUSE OF ABNORMALITIES LOWER VALUE
T_4 (thyroxine), free	10-36 pmol/L	0.8-2.8 ng/dL	Hyperthyroidism, metastatic neoplasms	Hypothyroidism
T_3 (triiodothyronine), uptake	24-34 AU	24%-34%		
T_3 (triiodothyronine), total	1.2-3.4 nmol/L	70-205 ng/dL	Hyperthyroidism	Hypothyroidism
Triglycerides	0.45-1.69 mmol/L	40-150 mg/dL	Diabetes mellitus, hyperlipidemia, hypothyroidism, liver disease	Hyperthyroidism, malabsorption syndrome, malnutrition
Urea nitrogen, blood (BUN)	3.6-7.1 mmol/L	10-20 mg/dL	Burns, dehydration, GI bleeding, increase in protein catabolism (fever, stress), renal disease, shock, urinary tract infection	Fluid overload, malnutrition, severe liver damage, SIADH

GI, gastrointestinal; IV, intravenous; SI, Système Internationale; SIADH, syndrome of inappropriate antidiuretic hormone.
*Because arterial blood gases are influenced by altitude, the value for PaO_2 decreases as altitude increases. The lower value is normal for an altitude of 1 mile.

TABLE 2 Hematology

TEST	NORMAL VALUES SI UNITS	NORMAL VALUES CONVENTIONAL UNITS	POSSIBLE CAUSE OF ABNORMALITIES HIGHER VALUES	POSSIBLE CAUSE OF ABNORMALITIES LOWER VALUES
Bleeding time (Ivy method)	1-9 min	Same as SI unit	Aspirin ingestion, clotting factor deficiency, defective platelet function, thrombocytopenia, vascular disease, von Willebrand's disease	
Activated partial thromboplastin time (aPTT)	30-40 sec*	Same as SI unit	Deficiency of factors I, II, V, VIII, IX and X, XI, XII; hemophilia; heparin therapy; liver disease	
Partial thromboplastin time (PPT)	28-35 sec	Same as SI unit	Deficiency of factors I, II, V, VII, and X; liver disease; vitamin K deficiency; warfarin therapy	
Prothrombin time (protime, PT)	11-12.5 sec*	Same as SI unit	Deficiency of factors I, II, V, VII, and X; liver disease; vitamin K deficiency; warfarin therapy	
International normalized ratio (INR)	0.81-1.2	Same as SI unit	Same causes as for higher PT	
Erythrocyte count[†] (altitude dependent)			Dehydration, high altitudes, polycythemia vera, severe diarrhea	Anemia, leukemia, posthemorrhage status
• Male	$4.7\text{-}6.1 \times 10^{12}$/L	$4.7\text{-}6.1 \times 10^6$/mcL		
• Female	$4.2\text{-}5.4 \times 10^{12}$/L	$4.2\text{-}5.4 \times 10^6$/mcL		
Hemoglobin (altitude dependent)[†]			COPD, high altitudes, polycythemia	Anemia, hemorrhage
• Male	140-180 mmol/L	14-18 g/dL		
• Female	120-160 mmol/L	12-16 g/dL		
Platelet count (thrombocytes)[†]	$150\text{-}400 \times 10^9$/L	150,000-400,000/mm³	Acute infections, chronic granulocytic leukemia, chronic pancreatitis, cirrhosis, collagen disorders, polycythemia, postsplenectomy status	Acute leukemia, cancer chemotherapy, DIC, hemorrhage, infection, SLE, thrombocytopenic purpura
White blood cell (WBC) count[†]	$5\text{-}10 \times 10^9$/L	5000-10,000/mm³	Inflammatory and infectious processes, leukemia	Aplastic anemia, autoimmune diseases, overwhelming infection, side effects of chemotherapy and irradiation

COPD, chronic obstructive pulmonary disease; DIC, disseminated intravascular coagulation; SI, Système Internationale; SLE, systemic lupus erythematosus.
*Values depend on reagent and instrumentation used.
[†]Component of complete blood cell count (CBC).